Ophthalmic Surgery

SECTION EDITORS

Bertil Damato, M.D., Ph.D., F.R.C.Ophth.
Honorary Professor
University of Liverpool
Consultant Ophthalmologist
St. Paul's Eye Unit
Royal Liverpool University Hospital
Liverpool, United Kingdom

Robert Alan Goldberg, M.D.
Professor of Ophthalmology
UCLA School of Medicine
Chief, Division of Orbital and Ophthalmic Plastic Surgery
UCLA Medical Center/Jules Stein Eye Institute
Los Angeles, California

Creig S. Hoyt, M.D.
Professor of Ophthalmology
University of California, San Francisco
San Francisco, California

Peter R. Laibson, M.D.
Co-Director, Cornea Service
Wills Eye Hospital/Jefferson Medical College
Philadelphia, Pennsylvania

Stephen A. Obstbaum, M.D.
Professor Clinical Ophthalmology
New York University School of Medicine
Chairman, Department of Ophthalmology
Lenox Hill Hospital
New York, New York

William S. Tasman, M.D.
Chair, Department of Ophthalmology
Jefferson Medical College
Ophthalmologist-in-Chief
Wills Eye Hospital
Philadelphia, Pennsylvania

Giora Treister, M.D.
Professor of Ophthalmology
Director, The MARATIER Institute for the Study of Visual Disorders and Blindness
The Sackler Faculty of Medicine
Director, The Goldschleger Eye Institute
The Sheba Medical Center
The Tel-Aviv University
Tel Hashomer, Israel

George W. Weinstein, M.D.
Ponte Vedra Medical Eye Center
Ponte Vedra, Florida

Third Edition

Ophthalmic Surgery

Principles and Practice

George L. Spaeth, MD
Director, William and Anna Goldberg Glaucoma Service
and Research Laboratories
Louis J. Esposito Research Professor
Wills Eye Hospital/Jefferson Medical College
Philadelphia, Pennsylvania

Illustrations by Birck Cox

Saunders
An Imprint of Elsevier

SAUNDERS
An Imprint of Elsevier

The Curtis Center
Independence Square West
Philadelphia, Pennsylvania 19106

OPHTHALMIC SURGERY ISBN 0-7216-6972-7

Notice

Medicine is an ever-changing field. Standard safety precautions must be followed, but as new research and clinical experience broaden our knowledge, changes in treatment and drug therapy may become necessary or appropriate. Readers are advised to check the product information currently provided by the manufacturer of each drug to be administered to verify the recommended dose, the method and duration of administration, and contraindications. It is the responsibility of the treating physician, relying on experience and knowledge of the patient, to determine dosages and the best treatment for each individual patient. Neither the Publisher nor the editor assume any liability for any injury and/or damage to persons or property arising from this publication.

THE PUBLISHER

First Edition 1982, Second Edition 1990.

Library of Congress Cataloging-in-Publication Data

Ophthalmic surgery : principles & practice / edited by George L. Spaeth ; illustrations by Birck Cox—3rd ed.
p. cm.
Includes bibliographical references.
ISBN 0-7216-6972-7
1. Eye—Surgery. I. Spaeth, George L.
[DNLM: I. Ophthalmologic Surgical Procedures. 2. Eye Diseases—surgery. WW 168 O615 2003]
RE80 .O655 2003
617.7′1—dc21 2002070828

Publishing Director: Richard Lampert
Senior Development Editor: Jennifer Shreiner

TG/MVY

Printed in the United States of America

Last digit is the print number: 9 8 7 6 5 4 3 2

This book is dedicated to my family

Contributors

Juan Carlos Abad, M.D.
Medical Staff, Laser Eye Center of Miami, Miami, Florida
Keratoprosthesis: Beyond Corneal Graft Failure

James J. Augsburger, M.D.
Professor, and Chairman, Department of Ophthalmology, University of Cincinnati Medical Center, Cincinnati, Ohio
Therapeutic Approaches to Ocular Tumors

Kyle C. Balch, M.D.
Formerly Medical Staff, North Florida Regional Medical Center, Gainesville, Florida
Blepharoplasty

William E. Benson, M.D.
Professor of Ophthalmology, Jefferson Medical College; Attending Surgeon, Wills Eye Hospital, Thomas Jefferson University Hospital, and Chestnut Hill Hospital, Philadelphia, Pennsylvania
Retinal Detachment

George W. Blankenship, M.D.
Attending Physician, Holy Spirit Hospital, Camp Hill, Pennsylvania
Proliferative Diabetic Retinopathy; Diabetic Macular Edema

Norbert Bornfeld, M.D.
Professor, Department of Ophthalmology, University of Essen; Chairman, Universitätsklinikum/Augenheilkunde, Essen, Germany
Therapeutic Approaches to Ocular Tumors

Rosario Brancato, M.D.
Professor of Ophthalmology, and Chairman, Department of Ophthalmology and Visual Sciences, University Hospital S. Raffaele, Milano, Italy
Cyclophotocoagulation

Roy D. Brod, M.D.
Associate Clinical Professor of Ophthalmology, Penn State University School of Medicine, Hershey; Chief of Ophthalmology, Lancaster General Hospital, Lancaster, Pennsylvania
Endophthalmitis: Diagnosis, Treatment, Prevention

Reay H. Brown, M.D.
Atlanta Ophthalmology Associates, Northside Hospital, Atlanta, Georgia
Treatment of Excessive or Overfiltering Blebs

Louis B. Cantor, M.D.
Professor, Director of Glaucoma Service, and Residency Program Director, Indiana University School of Medicine, Indianapolis, Indiana
Suprachoroidal Hemorrhage

Roberto G. Carassa, M.D.
Assistant Professor in Ophthalmology, Department of Ophthalmology and Visual Sciences, School of Medicine, University Hospital S. Raffaele, Milano, Italy
Cyclophotocoagulation

Jonathan D. Carr, M.D., M.A.
Medical Director, Laser Eye Consultants, Washington, D.C.
Laser in Situ Keratomileusis: Surgical Technique

Judie F. Charlton, M.D.
Professor of Ophthalmology, West Virginia University, Morgantown, West Virginia
How to Learn New Techniques

George C. Charonis, M.D.
Hellenic Craniofacial Center, Athens, Greece
Eyelid Reconstruction; Orbital and Adnexal Trauma

Thomas A. Ciulla, M.D.
Associate Professor of Ophthalmology, and Co-Director, Retina Service, Indiana University School of Medicine, Indianapolis, Indiana
Vitreoretinal Surgery, Principles: Age-Related Macular Degeneration

Roger A. Dailey, M.D.
Lester T. Jones Chair, Ophthalmic Facial Plastic Surgery, Division Chief, Casey Eye Institute, Oregon Health and Sciences University, Portland, Oregon
Surgery of the Lacrimal System

Bertil Damato, M.D., Ph.D., F.R.C.Ophth.
Honorary Professor, University of Liverpool; Consultant Ophthalmologist, St. Paul's Eye Unit, Royal Liverpool University Hospital, Liverpool, United Kingdom
Therapeutic Approaches to Ocular Tumors

Patrick De Potter, M.D., Ph.D.
Department of Ophthalmology, Cliniques Universitaires St. Luc, Brussels, Belgium
Therapeutic Approaches to Ocular Tumors

Claes H. Dohlman, M.D., Ph.D.
Professor of Ophthalmology, Harvard Medical School; Chief Emeritus, Department of Ophthalmology, Massachusetts Eye and Ear Infirmary, Boston, Massachusetts
Keratoprosthesis: Beyond Corneal Graft Failure

Steven C. Dresner, M.D.
Associate Professor of Ophthalmology, Doheny Eye Institute, University of Southern California Keck School of Medicine, Los Angeles, California
Comprehensive Ptosis Management

Eric J. Dudenhoefer, M.D.
Assistant Chief of Cornea and Refractive Surgery, Department of Ophthalmology, Wilford Hall Medical Center, Lackland Air Force Base, Texas
Keratoprosthesis: Beyond Corneal Graft Failure

Chaim Edelstein, M.D.
Assistant Professor of Ophthalmology, McGill University, Montreal, Quebec, Canada
Blepharoplasty

Jared Emery, M.D.
Retired Professor of Ophthalmology, Baylor College of Medicine, Houston, Texas
Standard Extracapsular Cataract Surgery

Ronald L. Fellman, M.D.
Associate Clinical Professor, Department of Ophthalmology, University of Texas Southwestern Medical Center; Glaucoma Associates of Texas, Dallas, Texas
Trabeculotomy

I. Howard Fine, M.D.
Clinical Associate Professor of Ophthalmology, Casey Eye Institute, Oregon Health and Science University, Portland, Oregon
Clear Corneal Cataract Surgery Incisions

Mitchell S. Fineman, M.D.
Clinical Instructor in Ophthalmology, University of Pittsburgh School of Medicine, Pittsburgh, Pennsylvania
Pars Plana Lensectomy; Open-Globe Injuries

Harry W. Flynn, Jr., M.D.
Professor of Ophthalmology, Department of Ophthalmology, Bascom Palmer Eye Institute, University of Miami School of Medicine, Miami, Florida
Endophthalmitis: Diagnosis, Treatment, Prevention

Wendy A. Franks, M.B., B.Chir, F.R.C.S., F.R.C.Ophth.
Lecturer, Institute of Ophthalmology; Consultant Ophthalmologist and Director of the Glaucoma Service, Moorfields Eye Hospital, London, United Kingdom
Primary Guarded Filtration Procedure Without Antimetabolite

Douglas R. Fredrick, M.D.
Associate Clinical Professor of Ophthalmology, University of California, San Francisco; Director of Pediatric Ophthalmology, San Francisco General Hospital, San Francisco, California
Strabismus Surgery

Neil J. Friedman, M.D.
Clinical Faculty, Stanford University School of Medicine, Stanford, California
Scleral Tunnel Incisions: Principles and Methods

Thomas W. Gardner, M.D.
Professor of Ophthalmology and Cellular and Molecular Physiology, Penn State University College of Medicine, Hershey, Pennsylvania
Proliferative Diabetic Retinopathy; Diabetic Macular Edema

Bruce D. Gaynor, M.D.
Instructor of Ophthalmology, Francs I. Proctor Foundation and Department of Ophthalmology, University of California, San Francisco, San Francisco, California
Nuclear Cracking Techniques

Steven J. Gedde, M.D.
Assistant Professor of Clinical Ophthalmology and Residency Program Director, Bascom Palmer Eye Institute, University of Miami School of Medicine, Miami, Florida
Guarded Filtration Procedure with 5-Fluorouracil

Robert Alan Goldberg, M.D.
Professor of Ophthalmology, UCLA School of Medicine; Chief, Division of Orbital and Ophthalmic Plastic Surgery, UCLA Medical Center/Jules Stein Eye Institute, Los Angeles, California
Orbitotomy: Surgical Approaches; Blepharoplasty; Orbital and Adnexal Trauma

John M. Graney
Owner-Operator, J.G. Machine Company, Woburn, Massachusetts
Keratoprosthesis: Beyond Corneal Graft Failure

Ronald L. Gross, M.D.
Professor of Ophthalmology and The Clifton R. McMichael Chair in Ophthalmology, Baylor College of Medicine and Cullen Eye Institute, Houston, Texas
Argon Laser Peripheral Iridotomy

Michael J. Groth, M.D.
Assistant Clinical Professor, UCLA School of Medicine, Jules Stein Eye Institute, Los Angeles; Clinical Instructor, Wadsworth VA Hospital, Los Angeles; Attending Physician, Jules Stein Eye Institute, UCLA School of Medicine/UCLA Medical Center, Los Angeles; Associate, Saint John's Hospital and Health Care Center; Santa Monica; Active Courtesy, Department of Surgery, Unit of Ophthalmology, Cedar-Sinai Medical Center, Los Angeles; Attending, Surgical, Ophthalmology, Wadsworth VA Hospital, VA Greater Los Angeles Healthcare System, Los Angeles, California
Entropion and Ectropion

Dennis P. Han, M.D.
Professor of Ophthalmology, Medical College of Wisconsin; Director of Vitreoretinal Service Eye Institute, Eye Institute and Medical College of Wisconsin, Milwaukee, Wisconsin
Endophthalmitis: Diagnosis, Treatment, Prevention

Leon W. Herndon, Jr., M.D.
Assistant Professor of Ophthalmology, Duke University Eye Center, Durham, North Carolina
Shallow or Flat Anterior Chamber

Kathy J. Hetzler, B.C.O., F.A.S.O.
Hetzler Ocular Prosthetics, Inc., Indianapolis, Indiana
Enucleation and Evisceration

Dale K. Heuer, M.D.
Professor and Chairman, Department of Ophthalmology, Medical College of Wisconsin; Medical Director, Froedtert and Medical College Eye Institute, Milwaukee, Wisconsin
Aqueous Shunts

Roger A. Hitchings, F.R.C.S., F.R.C.Ophth.
Professor of Glaucoma and Allied Studies, Institute of Ophthalmology, Moorfields Eye Hospital, London, United Kingdom
Primary Guarded Filtration Procedure Without Antimetabolite

Allen C. Ho, M.D.
Associate Professor of Ophthalmology, Thomas Jefferson University; Retina Service, Wills Eye Hospital, Philadelphia, Pennsylvania
Epiretinal Membrane and Macular Pucker; Macular Hole

Richard S. Hoffman, M.D.
Clinical Instructor of Ophthalmology, Casey Eye Institute, Oregon Health and Science University, Portland, Oregon
Clear Corneal Cataract Surgery Incisions

Creig S. Hoyt, M.D.
Professor of Ophthalmology, University of California, San Francisco, San Francisco, California
Strabismus Surgery

John Hungerford, F.R.C.Ophth., D.O.
Consultant Ophthalmologist, St. Bartholomew's Hospital, London, United Kingdom
Therapeutic Approaches to Ocular Tumors

Jeffrey L. Jacobs, M.D.
Attending Physician, Jules Stein Eye Institute, UCLA School of Medicine/UCLA Medical Center, Los Angeles, California
Orbital and Adnexal Trauma

Michael A. Kass, M.D.
Professor and Chairman of Ophthalmology and Visual Sciences, Washington University School of Medicine; Ophthalmologist-in-Chief, Barnes-Jewish Hospital, St. Louis, Missouri
Fornix-Based Conjunctival Flaps for Filtering Surgery

Jonathan W. Kim, M.D.
Clinical Teaching Faculty, Department of Ophthalmology, California Pacific Medical Center; Clinical Research Scientist, Smith-Kettlewell Eye Research Institute, San Francisco, California
Orbitotomy: Surgical Approaches

Yoshiaki Kitazawa, M.D., Ph.D.
Professor Emeritus, Gifu University School of Medicine, Gifu-shi; Head, Akasaka Kitazawa Eye Clinic, Minato-ku, Tokyo, Japan
Guarded Filtration Procedure with Mitomycin C

Douglas D. Koch, M.D.
Professor and The Allen, Mosbacher, and Law Chair in Ophthalmology, Baylor College of Medicine, Houston, Texas
Scleral Tunnel Incisions: Principles and Methods

Günther K. Krieglstein, M.D.
Professor and Chairman, Department of Ophthalmology, Medical School, University of Cologne, Cologne, Germany
Limbus-Based Conjunctival Flap

William R. Lee, M.D., F.R.C.Path.
Emeritus Professor, Tennent Institute of Ophthalmology, University of Glasgow; Senior Research Fellow, Gartnavel General Hospital, Glasgow, United Kingdom
Therapeutic Approaches to Ocular Tumors

Martha Motuz Leen, M.D.
Clinical Assistant Professor, Department of Ophthalmology, University of Washington, Seattle; Surgeon, Harrison Memorial Hospital, Bremerton, Washington
Low Postoperative Intraocular Pressure

Tina G. Li, M.D.
Visiting Assistant Professor of Ophthalmology, UCLA/Jules Stein Eye Institute, Los Angeles, California
Blepharoplasty; Orbital and Adnexal Trauma

Jeffrey M. Liebmann, M.D.
Professor of Clinical Ophthalmology, New York Medical College, Valhalla; Associate Director, Glaucoma Service, and Associate Attending Surgeon, The New York Eye and Ear Infirmary, New York, New York
The Underfiltering Bleb

Mary G. Lynch, M.D.
Professor of Ophthalmology, Emory University School of Medicine; Chief of Ophthalmology, VA Medical Center, Atlanta, Georgia
Treatment of Excessive or Overfiltering Blebs

Samuel Masket, M.D.
Clinical Professor of Ophthalmology, Jules Stein Eye Institute, UCLA, Los Angeles, California
Intraoperative Complications of Phacoemulsification and Small-Incision Cataract Surgery

Travis A. Meredith, M.D.
Sterling A. Barrett Distinguished Professor, and Chairman, Department of Ophthalmology, University of North Carolina, Chapel Hill, North Carolina
Prevention of Infection; Management of Endophthalmitis Associated with Trauma

Darlene Miller, M.P.H., M.T.(A.S.C.P.)
Department of Ophthalmology, University of Miami School of Medicine; Technical Director–Microbiology, Department of Ophthalmology, Bascom Palmer Eye Institute, University of Miami School of Medicine, Miami, Florida
Endophthalmitis: Diagnosis, Treatment, Prevention

Kevin M. Miller, M.D.
Associate Professor of Clinical Ophthalmology, Department of Ophthalmology, UCLA School of Medicine and Jules Stein Eye Institute, Los Angeles, California
Anesthesia for Ophthalmic Surgery

Richard P. Mills, M.D., M.P.H.
Former Chair, and Professor, Department of Ophthalmology, University of Kentucky, Lexington, Kentucky
Low Postoperative Intraocular Pressure

David R. Milstein, M.D.
Assistant Clinical Professor of Ophthalmology, UCLA School of Medicine, Los Angeles, California
Trichiasis

Joseph Moisseiev, M.D.
Clinical Associate Professor of Ophthalmology, The Sackler Faculty of Medicine, The Tel Aviv University, Tel Aviv; Director, The Retina Service, The Goldschlegger Eye Institute, The Sheba Medical Center, Tel Hashomer, Israel
Posterior Segment Trauma: Principles and Practice

Kimberly A. Neely, M.D., Ph.D.
Assistant Professor, Department of Ophthalmology, Hershey Medical Center, The Pennsylvania State University College of Medicine, Hershey, Pennsylvania
Proliferative Diabetic Retinopathy; Diabetic Macular Edema

Thomas Neuhann, M.D.
Professor, Technical University Munich; Head, Eye Department, Red Cross Hospital Munich, Munich, Germany
Capsulorrhexis

John D. Ng, M.D.
Assistant Professor, Department of Ophthalmology, Casey Eye Institute, Portland State, Portland, Oregon
Enucleation and Evisceration

William R. Nunery, M.D.
Clinical Assistant Professor of Ophthalmology, Indiana University School of Medicine; Staff, Methodist Hospital, Indianapolis, Indiana
Enucleation and Evisceration

Stephen A. Obstbaum, M.D.
Professor of Clinical Ophthalmology, New York University School of Medicine; Chairman, Department of Ophthalmology, Lenox Hill Hospital, New York, New York
Nuclear Cracking Techniques

Richard K. Parrish II, M.D.
Professor of Ophthalmology and Associate Dean for Graduate Medical Education, University of Miami School of Medicine, Miami, Florida
Guarded Filtration Procedure with 5-Fluorouracil

David A. Quillen, M.D.
Assistant Professor of Ophthalmology, Penn State University College of Medicine, Hershey, Pennsylvania
Proliferative Diabetic Retinopathy; Diabetic Macular Edema

Christopher J. Rapuano, M.D.
Professor of Ophthalmology, Jefferson Medical College of Thomas Jefferson University; Attending Surgeon, Cornea Service, and Co-Director, Refractive Surgery Department, Wills Eye Hospital, Philadelphia, Pennsylvania
Anterior Segment Trauma; Conjunctival Flap Surgery; Pterygium Surgery; Excimer Laser Phototherapeutic Keratectomy

Carl D. Regillo, M.D., F.A.C.S.
Associate Professor of Ophthalmology, Jefferson Medical College; Director, Clinical Retina Research and Fellowship Testing, Wills Eye Hospital, Philadelphia, Pennsylvania
Retinal Detachment

Robert Ritch, M.D.
Professor of Clinical Ophthalmology, New York Medical College, Valhalla; Chief, Glaucoma Service, and Surgeon Director, New York Eye and Ear Infirmary, New York, New York
The Underfiltering Bleb

J. James Rowsey, M.D.
Director of Corneal Services, Saint Luke's Cataract and Laser Institute, Tarpon Springs, Florida
Radial Keratotomy: Principles and Practice

Thomas W. Samuelson, M.D.
Clinical Associate Professor, University of Minnesota; Attending Surgeon, Minnesota Eye Consultants/Phillips Eye Institute, Minneapolis, Minnesota
Coincident Cataract and Glaucoma Surgery

Stanley M. Saulny, M.D.
Ophthalmic Facial Plastic Surgery Fellow, Casey Eye Institute, Oregon Health and Sciences University, Portland, Oregon
Surgery of the Lacrimal System

Carol L. Shields, M.D.
Associate Professor of Ophthalmology, Jefferson Medical College; Attending Surgeon, Ocular Oncology Service, Wills Eye Hospital, Philadelphia, Pennsylvania
Therapeutic Approaches to Ocular Tumors

Jerry A. Shields, M.D.
Professor, Jefferson Medical College; Director, Ocular Oncology Service, Wills Eye Hospital, Philadelphia, Pennsylvania
Therapeutic Approaches to Ocular Tumors

Norman Shorr, M.D.
Clinical Professor of Ophthalmology, UCLA School of Medicine, Los Angeles; Director, Beverly Hills Ambulatory Surgery Center, Beverly Hills, California
Orbitotomy: Surgical Approaches; Blepharoplasty

Scott C. Sigler, M.D.
Associate Professor and Residency Director, Department of Ophthalmology, University of Oklahoma College of Medicine, Oklahoma City, Oklahoma
Surgery of the Lacrimal System

H. Kaz Soong, M.D.
Associate Professor, Cornea and External Disease and Refractive Surgery, University of Michigan Medical School, University of Michigan, W.K. Kellogg Eye Center, Ann Arbor, Michigan
Corneal Transplantation

George L. Spaeth, M.D.
Director, William and Anna Goldberg Glaucoma Service and Research Laboratories, Louis J. Esposito Research Professor, Wills Eye Hospital/Jefferson Medical College, Philadelphia, Pennsylvania
Introduction; Indications for Surgery; Laser Suture Lysis; Laser Peripheral Iridoplasty; Neodymium: YAG Laser Iridotomy; Incisional Iridectomy; Cyclocryotherapy

Stanley W. Stead, M.D.
Professor, Department of Anesthesiology, University of California, Davis, School of Medicine; Associate Director, Perioperative Services, University of California, Davis, Medical Center, Sacramento, California
Anesthesia for Ophthalmic Surgery

Raymond Stein, M.D., F.R.C.S.(C)
Assistant Professor, University of Toronto; Chief of Ophthalmology, Scarborough Hospital; Co-Director, Bochner Eye Institute, Toronto, Ontario, Canada
Photorefractive Keratectomy

Roger F. Steinert, M.D.
Associate Clinical Professor, Harvard Medical School; Surgeon, Massachusetts Eye and Ear Infirmary; Private Practice, Ophthalmic Consultants of Boston, Boston, Massachusetts
Phaco Chop

R. Doyle Stulting, M.D., Ph.D.
Professor of Ophthalmology and Director of Cornea Services, Emory University School of Medicine, Atlanta, Georgia; Editor, *Cornea*
Laser in Situ Keratomileusis: Surgical Technique

Bridget Sundell, M.D.
Northern Refractive Surgery, Duluth, Minnesota
Temporal Artery Biopsy

Jennifer U. Sung, M.D.
Assistant Professor, Wilmer Ophthalmological Institute, Johns Hopkins University School of Medicine, Baltimore, Maryland
Epiretinal Membrane and Macular Pucker

Troy M. Tanji, M.D.
Assistant Clinical Professor of Surgery, Division of Ophthalmology, University of Hawaii John A. Burns School of Medicine, Honolulu, Hawaii
Aqueous Shunts

Keith P. Thompson, M.D.
Associate Professor of Ophthalmology, Emory University School of Medicine; Medical Director, Emory Vision, Atlanta, Georgia
Laser in Situ Keratomileusis: Surgical Technique

Carlo E. Traverso, M.D.
Professor and Chair, University Eye Clinic, Genoa, Italy
Argon Laser Trabeculoplasty: What it is and How it Works

Giora Treister, M.D.
Professor of Ophthalmology, and Director, The MARATIER Institute for the Study of Visual Disorders and Blindness, The Sackler Faculty of Medicine, The Tel-Aviv University, Tel-Aviv; Director, The Goldschleger Eye Institute, The Sheba Medical Center, The Tel-Aviv University, Tel Hashomer, Israel; Founder and Past President, The International Society of Ocular Trauma
Posterior Segment Trauma: Principles and Practice

Nicolas Uzcategui, M.D.
Clinical Instructor of Ophthalmology, Doheny Eye Institute, University of Southern California Keck School of Medicine; Clinical Instructor of Ophthalmology, Division of Pediatric Ophthalmology, Childrens Hospital of Los Angeles, Los Angeles, California
Comprehensive Ptosis Management

Rebecca Heaps Ward, M.D.
Active Staff, Chester County Hospital, West Chester, Pennsylvania
Fornix-Based Conjunctival Flaps for Filtering Surgery

George O. Waring, M.D.
Professor of Ophthalmology and Director of Refractive Surgery, Emory University School of Medicine, Atlanta, Georgia
Laser in Situ Keratomileusis: Surgical Technique

David A. Weinberg, M.D.
Assistant Professor of Surgery (Ophthalmology), University of Vermont College of Medicine; Director, Orbital and Ophthalmic Plastic Surgery and Neuro-Ophthalmology, Fletcher Allen Health Care, Burlington, Vermont
Temporal Artery Biopsy

M. Edward Wilson, M.D.
Pierre G. Jenkins Professor of Ophthalmology and Pediatrics, and Chairman, Department of Ophthalmology, and Director, Albert Florens Storm Eye Institute, Medical University of South Carolina, Charleston, South Carolina
Surgery for Pediatric Cataracts

Tamara Wygnanski-Jaffe, M.D.
Instructor, The Sackler Faculty of Medicine, The Tel-Aviv University, Tel Aviv; Faculty, Pediatric Ophthalmology Service, The Goldschleger Eye Institute, The Sheba Medical Center, Tel Hashomer, Israel
Posterior Segment Trauma: Principles and Practice

Tetsuya Yamamoto, M.D.
Professor and Chairman, Department of Ophthalmology, Gifu University School of Medicine, Gifu-shi, Japan
Guarded Filtration Procedure with Mitomycin C

Preface

There is a central body of knowledge regarding ophthalmic surgery. This core of knowledge incorporates the overwhelming bulk of everything that ophthalmic surgeons need to know. It is advantageous that no collection of knowledge about ophthalmic surgery can be fully comprehensive and completely current. It is advantageous because the defining characteristic of great surgeons is that they know the essentials, have magnificent technique, and have the personal characteristics that typify champions: meticulous preparation, courage, intense concentration on the essential issues, ability to visualize, a realistic understanding of their own strengths and weaknesses, a passion for excellence, adaptability, marvelous physical skills, and, finally (the most difficult characteristic to describe), an appropriate sense of timing—when to do something and when not to do it. Great innovators are occasionally but infrequently great surgeons. Knowing everything about everything does not make a surgeon great. Knowing that which needs to be known, however, is essential.

Ophthalmic Surgery is a textbook about knowing what needs to be known. The material has been prepared by a group of surgeons who are among the best in the world—the most knowledgeable, the most skillful, and the most appropriate.

It is intended to provide the comprehensive ophthalmologist and the subspecialist with the core of information that is one of the components of being a great surgeon. We have specifically not included every procedure, because it is not necessary to perform every procedure in order to give patients the best care available.

I thank the co-authors, all of them busy people, who have taken the time to share their knowledge so that their colleagues may be successful in helping patients lead healthy lives.

George L. Spaeth, M.D.

Contents

SECTION V Oculoplastic Surgery

SECTION IX Trauma

Giora Treister, M.D.

SECTION I

George W. Weinstein, M.D.

Principles of Ophthalmic Surgery

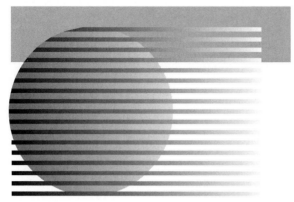

CHAPTER 1

Introduction

GEORGE L. SPAETH, M.D.

The techniques of ophthalmic surgery have proliferated so rapidly that a single surgeon cannot possibly be fully competent in all aspects. Nevertheless, most surgical eye diseases can be properly managed with relatively few procedures. The average ophthalmic surgeon need not be competent in every aspect of surgery in order to give good care. For example, a surgeon who is fully proficient in peripheral iridectomy, trabeculectomy, cataract extraction through a clear corneal incision, and cyclophotocoagulation can provide most glaucoma patients fine care.

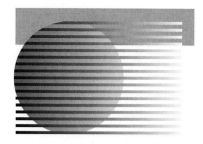

In this text we emphasize *selectivity.* For example, a guarded filtration procedure (trabeculectomy) is the only filtration procedure described as standard treatment for glaucoma. The choice is not meant to imply that other, similar procedures are of lesser worth. It is, rather, a statement that a guarded filtration procedure is probably *as satisfactory* as any other operative procedure in its class, and that experience with other operations of a similar nature is unnecessary for the average surgeon.

Inclusion of a procedure in the text should not be taken as a tacit comment that all surgeons ought to be performing that procedure. All surgeons vary in the range and comprehensiveness of their competency: some are better craftspersons, some are better technicians, and some have better judgment.

A selection of classic, comprehensive, and specialized texts is included (see References).

THE ARTISAN, THE TECHNICIAN, AND THE COMPLETE SURGEON

That both art and science are essential parts of medical practice is a well-established concept. It is also clear that the development of technology is a characteristic feature of the past hundred years. This period stressed the scientific method as a fundamental aspect of medical care. During the latter half of the 19th century the image of the surgeon changed from prognosticator to effective medical scientist. Before that time the surgeon was revered and rewarded primarily because of his ability to support his patient during difficult times; this required mastery of the art, or craft, of medicine. Many individuals benefited as well from the mechanical skills of surgeons, but all too often the limitations of the technology of the time predetermined that the result would be of limited help. Thus the great surgeon of the past was fundamentally a great artisan or craftsman.

Craftsmanship requires knowledge of the tools and materials used in performing one's craft. In the craft of surgery these include surgical instruments, anesthesia, knowledge of the treatment of injury and disease, and the indications for and techniques used in many types of operative procedures. The surgeon must also understand the patient—his or her nature, needs, and wishes—and the unique qualities of each patient and each interaction.

The artisan is personally involved with his or her work, which therefore carries with it a subjective component. Artisans recognize that each work created is unique. Technologists, on the other hand, attempt to remove themselves as much as possible from their work. Technology implies objectivity, standardization, and uniformity of results. The results of the technologist are relatively easy to measure, and hence performance is relatively easy to evaluate. On the other hand, the quality of the artist's or craftsperson's product is difficult to measure. Is, for example, Cellini's rococo salt cellar a "better job" than Cro-Magnon man's flint arrowhead or Calder's starkly simple mobiles? Furthermore, the *process* of creating is as important to the craftsperson as the product itself. The artisan surgeon learned by apprenticeship. He taught by example. His major activity was demonstrating care. His product was not so much "cure" as it was "care."

Great surgeons today are still great artisans, but the technological revolution has dramatically changed the surgeons' role. It provided the means for them to be more effective. No longer did they study the arts, but rather physics, chemistry, and statistics. Truly astounding improvements in the surgical product resulted from this technology revolution. Unfortunately the art of medicine has been neglected. Even the science (e.g., the methodology of the scientifically designed clinical trial) is still not adequately used. As a result, surgeons do not have as much scientifically valid information to answer their basic questions as could be hoped for: How much does intraocular pressure need to be lowered to prevent further glaucoma damage? When should a hyphema be drained? These are among the hundreds of unanswered questions. They are unanswered because surgeons have not brought to their craft the lessons of the technological and scientific revolution as completely as possible. Clinical impression, apprenticeship, and example continue to be the primary sources of information for surgeons. Thus, in response to the question "Why do you do X?" the surgeon's answer is almost invariably either "Because X is the way I was trained" or "Because X seems to work for me."

Even though fundamental questions remain unanswered, the ability of the surgeon to be effective has increased dramatically. The benefit to the patient of cataract extraction in association with an intraocular lens implantation can be literally miraculous.

Technology by itself is inadequate and incomplete. What is needed, especially in the coming years, is the conjunction of the art of the craftsperson with the science of the technician. Fortunately the two methodologies are not mutually exclusive; in fact, they are complementary. *First and foremost, the humanity and grace of the surgeon as master craftsperson must not be lost.* Both attributes are necessary.

Learned surgeons realize all too well that even now the ability to cure completely is only seldom within their grasp, and recognize that the patient is often more disabled by the emotional reaction to the disease than by the disease itself. Surgeons understand the uniqueness of each patient and each patient's response to disease. They recognize the critical importance of the relationship between patient and surgeon. The responsibility of the surgeon is still to support the patient during difficult times, to comfort, and to care. Superimposed on this responsibility is an obligation for the surgeon to assess his or her craft in a scientifically valid way, to know the *science* of surgery as well as the craft. Surgeons must add the skills of the technician to those of the craftsperson. They must learn more about the tools. And they must learn more about the material, that is, the patients. The medical student needs to learn about human nature and the human condition, while at the same time becoming a superb technician. Both attributes are necessary.

Students who consider medicine as a career should be encouraged to spend their time learning who they are, why they are, and how they relate to the spiritual and material world in and around them, and especially to other people. Technical skills grow best when grafted on a whole, healthy, vital tree; considered by themselves, technical skills become lifeless tools, appropriated primarily for the profit of those who possess them. Such is the antithesis of caring.

Surgeons should not be timid. They must act decisively and authoritatively—this is an integral part of the craft. They must consider and balance the available information, making sure that they use appropriate means to obtain as much information as necessary to make a prudent decision, and then they must act. If the surgeon is unsure whether the visual field has really deteriorated in a glaucomatous patient who appears to be under marginal control, the field should be repeated; if the surgeon is unsure regarding the quality of the visual field examination, the test should be evaluated by someone able to assure a valid examination. We are accountable for what we do not do as well as for what we do. All too frequently physicians and surgeons hide unjustifiably under the cloak of "First, do no harm." The truly caring surgeon must be willing to risk harm to achieve an anticipated improvement. To let, for example, a glaucoma patient's vision slip away because the surgeon is afraid of the risks of surgery is as damaging to the patient as it is to perform a procedure that is unnecessary.

To sum up, we hope that this text will help all surgeons bring to their craft adequate knowledge of surgical technique. The provision of that information is a primary purpose of this volume. We have attempted to make the material as accurate and objective as possible. Earlier editions of this text dealt in great detail with issues such as the use of the operating microscope, and how to hold and use specific instruments. These subjects have changed little and do not warrant repeating. They are *not* unimportant, and readers are encouraged to consult other readily available sources in this regard. Here, we have concentrated on presenting what the ophthalmic surgeon needs to know in order to perform competently in the first decade of the 21st century.

We hope every surgeon will recognize his or her obligation to develop new knowledge, and to use, whenever feasible, the methodology of the valid clinical trial. Had we all done so, we would already have become far more effective than we are. We further hope that there will be sufficient agreement with the content of this text that it can serve as a set of guidelines to be used appropriately by surgeons to judge the quality of their own performance and the performance of others. We are not only obligated to perform well ourselves, but, as members of a privileged profession, we must also assure that we do everything within our power to protect patients from those who are unknowledgeable or unscrupulous, or both. When we fail to act corporately in such a manner we fail society just as seriously as we fail our patient individually when we act incompetently or in a manner that is not in the patient's best interest.

THE PROVISION OF SERVICES: INPATIENT VERSUS OUTPATIENT SURGERY AND SPECIALIZED CARE

What services are advised, including whether surgery is best performed in an outpatient or an inpatient setting, is determined by considering what is deemed best for the patient.

"Best" includes convenience, competence, the assurance that complications will be correctly handled, and considerations of cost. But *value* is a more appropriate consideration than cost itself. It is not in the best interest of the patient or society to provide care that is unnecessarily costly, unnecessarily risky, or incompetent. The true cost cannot be measured by the expense of the procedure. Surgery that is performed more competently in the broadest sense of the word "competence" results in a better outcome, avoids subsequent procedures, hospitalizations, loss of function, and loss of wages. A procedure that is less costly but less likely to result in a good outcome for the long term may actually be vastly more expensive both for the patient and society.

Considerations of cost, then, are far more complex than mere considerations of how much a particular procedure is reimbursed.

Decisions regarding the need for particular services, including specialized care, referrals, and hospitalization, have traditionally been made primarily by the patient, with substantial advice and guidance from the physician. Today, that principle has been challenged. Third-party payers make decisions regarding what services are appropriate. Insurance companies and other agencies often will not pay for care that they have not approved before being given. These considerations are a response to concerns about the cost of medical care in comparison to available funds in an increasingly capitalistic world economy. The belief is that doctors, hospitals, and other caregivers and care facilities have demonstrated that they will not keep costs down, at least partially because they have an interest in not doing so. Efforts to keep care affordable, then, have been transferred elsewhere, either to government or to private payers, the thinking being that such agencies will have a greater interest and skill in making care affordable. Theoretically, at least, government is intended to be an advocate for its citizens, while private payers are advocates primarily for the owners of the corporation. The consequence of this shift has been a need for caregivers to justify the cost of their services. This justification methodology has introduced a "third estate" into the practice of medicine, so there are now patients, caregivers, and intermediaries, the usual function of the intermediary being related to the economics of the care. From the physician's and the patient's point of view, the intermediaries often seem to be impediments rather than facilitators of care. Regardless of the merits or demerits of these changes, they exist. The critical point is that their existence does not change surgeons' responsibility, which is to the patients for whom they are caring. The patient and the surgeon must first decide how they wish to proceed, that is, what they jointly consider best for that particular patient in a particular situation. After that decision has been made, then the patient, the surgeon, and the surgeon's staff must work to make their decision a reality. If the payer says "no," then the payer needs to be persuaded to say "yes." If the payer refuses to say "yes" despite major efforts by the surgeon and the patient, then it should be documented in writing that the payer said "no," and that the payer has thus assumed a legal responsibility for the health of the patient. Ideally, the services should be provided even when the cost will not be covered by the payer. For example, when the patient and the physician believe that inpatient surgery is essential, then the surgery should be done in an inpatient setting. However, "should" represents the ideal, and that ideal is not always achievable. In some situations, patients, caregivers, and care facilities simply do not have the funds to give appropriate care. First and foremost, surgeons must act as their patients' advocates, they must struggle to do what they believe is best for the patients, "best," as already mentioned, being a comprehensive definition that includes all those factors that are related to achieving the outcome desired by the patient (Table 1–1). These include clear articulation of the patient's wants, clear understanding of the options and probable outcomes, considerations of cost, convenience, complications of

TABLE 1–1. Requirements for the Best Patient Care

1. Clear definition of the patient's needs and wants
   Patient's major concerns
   Patient's major expectations and wants
   Patient's major hopes
2. Clear consideration of options
   Proper diagnosis
   Understanding the likely course if untreated
   Understanding the various likely courses if treated
   Appropriate options explained
   Desired and possible outcomes explained
3. A competent surgeon or surgical team
   Knowledgeable
   Procedurally skillful
   Ethical
4. Adequate facilities
   Accessible
   Technologically satisfactory
   Safe
5. Consideration of effects (short- and long-term) on the patient
   Patient's family and dependents
6. Appropriate postoperative care, including provisions for emergencies, complications, and follow-up
7. That it be affordable
8. That it be convenient
9. Continuing patient care and education
10. Continuing attention to monitoring and improving competence of the surgeon and the adequacy of facilities
    Learning new knowledge
    Learning new skills
    Pondering what is appropriate

surgery, ease and need of postoperative care, including complications, and the effect of the surgical episode, not just on the patient but also on the patient's family, friends, and dependents.

SYSTEMS OF CARE

Systems intended to streamline and lower the cost of surgery are being developed. For example, preoperative and postoperative care is delegated by some surgeons to associates, employees, or nonmedical practitioners. Whether such systems are proper is determined by how well they work. That is, do they provide the "best" care, the definition of "best" including economic considerations (Table 1–1). Not all patients want the same type of care; some prefer the most complex and most expensive, and others would choose simpler, less expensive care. The surgeon must not misrepresent the services offered. The patient must understand fully just what the surgeon will and will not do. A clearly articulated contract must be established. If the patient gets what he or she wants, the physician–patient relationship may be proper.

In actuality the matter is far more complex. The fears and anxieties of the patient, and the larger fund of knowledge of the physician in comparison to the patient, put the patient in a vulnerable position, one that can all too easily be exploited by the health care providers or the "third estate" (payors). An ancient tradition has evolved in which groups of healers put self-imposed regulations on the behavior of the members in their group. Present-day professional codes of ethics reflect these behavioral guides, all of which have one aspect in common: protection of the patient. However, a problem implicit in this system is that enforcement is difficult because of a reluctance of physicians to be "whistle-blowers"—with all the risks involved—and a legal system that makes litigation easy.

A major change in the past 10 or so years has been the development of "alternative" or "complementary" forms of care. Some physicians have even suggested that these alternative forms be primary, with resort to medical means only where "simpler" methods fail. There is much logic in much of what is written in this regard. Surgeons must be willing to acknowledge that self-care is essential and that one aspect of self-care is the use of nonmedical approaches. Patients should be encouraged to seek help from other reputable practitioners—medical or nonmedical—so long as there is a rational basis for the methodology. Acupuncture, chiropractic, therapeutic touch, dietary therapy—these and many other systems can help a person become healthy.

We are currently witnessing the working out of the tensions involved in changing health care systems. The goal is to incorporate the patient's wishes, maintain physicians' high standards of performance and integrity, and provide care that is appropriate, accessible, and affordable. To date this goal has seen successes and failures. But it is against this shifting backdrop that decisions need to be judged for appropriateness. As long as the ultimate standard is a sincere effort to put the interest of the patient first, the behavior is likely to be appropriate.

WHO SHOULD DO THE SURGERY?

Many factors enter the decision of where and by whom a particular surgical procedure is best performed. A most important consideration is that the patient have confidence in his or her surgeon. Admittedly, some patients will not have confidence in anybody, but such situations are rare.

Whenever feasible, surgery should be performed at a facility close to the patient's home. The surgical experience itself can be upsetting, and the support that comes from familiar surroundings is nourishing, especially for the very young and the very old. When surgery is performed at a distance from the patient's home, postsurgical complications can make the situation difficult, the patient asking himself whether it is worth continuing the difficult and tiring trips to the operating surgeon or concluding that it is wiser—or at any rate overwhelmingly more convenient—to return to the local physician. Surgery also tends to be more expensive when performed at a distance.

On the other hand, some factors favor referral, *even* in cases in which the patient has confidence in the local surgeon. If the patient or the local surgeon believes that another surgeon is more competent in performing the procedure required, the consideration of a referral should definitely arise. It has been demonstrated that substantially fewer postoperative complications occur in referral centers than in peripheral institutions. Furthermore, and this is a factor not to be underestimated, although most patients are aware that complete success is not an invariable part of surgical treatment and are, therefore, prepared to accept results less desirable than hoped for, the entire foundation for such acceptance on the part of the patient is unwavering faith that the quality of care received was satisfactory. Many people are unable to cope with a poor result unless they profoundly believe that they have had "the best care." Surgeons who find themselves caring for a patient who is frankly, or even peripherally, skeptical about the competence of his or her surgeon are courting catastrophe for themselves and for their patients when they decide to proceed themselves with the surgery. No surgeon is obligated to perform surgery when referral services are reasonably available.

When the facilities or the personnel for competent surgery are not available, it is often better to avoid surgery. A patient with useful vision but uncontrolled glaucoma will not be helped by a botched filtering procedure; nor will the person with 20/200 vision caused by keratoconus or vitreous hemorrhage be benefited by a poorly performed corneal graft or vitrectomy.

EVALUATING OUTCOMES: CLINICAL TRIALS

Was the surgery a success? How good are the outcomes of a new procedure? These are questions that need to be answered. They are not, however, answered easily. There is a science to evaluating outcomes. Let us start by discussing the clinical trial.

The basic principles of the valid clinical trial are as follows:

1. To limit variables
2. To eliminate bias
3. To make specific and sensitive measurements
4. To study comparable groups by valid statistical methods

First, let us consider, for example, the surgeon who is trying to decide whether to use proline or nylon to repair corneal lacerations. Available information does not answer his question. He must design a study that will measure *only* the effect of the suture material itself; that is, he must first limit the variables. Thus he cannot use proline in one manner and nylon in another; for example, he cannot use interrupted proline sutures and running nylon sutures, for were he to do so, he would be studying the technique of placing suture material and not the type of suture material itself. He cannot use steroids postoperatively in the eyes of patients sutured with proline and not in those in whom nylon was used. With the one exception of the type of suture material used, *every aspect* of the surgical technique must ideally be the same in the two groups studied.

Second, the surgeon must eliminate bias. Bias can be of several types. It may occur in the design, the operation, or the interpretation phases of the study. The surgeon who wants to prove that nylon is preferable to proline would consciously or unconsciously evaluate patients differently, being more critical regarding the use of proline. When a reaction was between "mild" and "moderate," the case with the nylon suture would be considered "mild," whereas the proline suture would be graded as "moderate." This type of bias is generally understood, and masking techniques can help to eliminate it. Nevertheless, masked surgical studies are seldom done.

Bias can invalidate a study in many other ways. For example, if the surgeon decided to use proline for the first hundred cases and nylon for the second hundred cases, the results would be unfairly biased in favor of the nylon because the surgeon would be likely to improve the surgical technique during the period of the study. On the other hand, if the surgeon had never used nylon but was very familiar with proline, it would not be fair to compare the surgical result in patients in whom nylon was used by the surgeon for the first time with those in whom he had used the suture with which he was far more comfortable. Or consider the surgeon who decides to use proline on all Monday cases and nylon on all Friday cases, believing that to be a convenient way of "randomizing" the study. But it is quite possible that knowingly or unknowingly this surgeon has traditionally scheduled more difficult cases on Monday, so that complications will not occur over the weekend. Therefore, the patients are not truly randomized, and the groups are not validly comparable.

To eliminate bias one must use a system that assures true randomness of selection and objectivity of evaluation.

Third, the surgeon must make measurements that are sensitive and specific enough to reflect accurately what is actually happening. For example, the surgeon may decide that the criterion of the "success" of a cataract extraction is postoperative visual acuity. Assume that the results show the mean visual acuity postoperatively in the patients in whom proline was used (Group P) and in those in whom nylon was used (Group N) to be the same. The surgeon, therefore, concludes that there is no difference between the groups, and thus that the proline and nylon sutures are equally "good." However, measurement of visual acuity may, in fact, be too crude a standard by which to determine subtle differences in the two results. For example, the mean astigmatic correction in Group N could be larger than that in Group *P*, perhaps even twice as large, with statistical significance of $P < .001$. If this were the case, it would be clear that a real difference did exist in the surgical result obtained when using proline sutures versus that obtained when using nylon. Thus, for this experiment, determining the degree of acuity was not an adequately sensitive measurement for finding the real difference that occurred.

Fourth, for the results of a clinical trial to be valid the surgeon must study comparable groups. The surgeon cannot validly conclude, because no endophthalmitis developed in the 50 cases in which he used proline sutures and Dr. X reported 3 cases of endophthalmitis in his 50 cases using nylon, that proline is a better suture material. It is highly unlikely that two groups that have as their only common denominator the need for repair of a corneal laceration will be sufficiently similar that they can be validly compared. Although this seems so obvious that it is almost embarrassing to mention, it is surprising how many articles appear in ophthalmic journals each month in which one author states that his procedure is "better" because his results were superior to those of Dr. X. Even assuming that both surgeons limited the variables, eliminated bias, and measured accurately enough to detect actual differences, comparisons between the two groups are little more than "interesting" unless the two populations studied are truly comparable. Furthermore, comparison must be made using valid statistical methods. Only by using such techniques can the investigator accurately assess the likelihood that the observed finding was a consequence of the variable tested and not a chance occurrence.

Of equal importance is the lack of significance of a negative result. Assume, for the sake of argument, that proline causes severe hypersensitivity reactions in 2% of cases, whereas nylon causes no hypersensitivity reactions. At the end of a study comparing proline and nylon sutures the surgeon identifies in Group P two cases that have had troublesome allergic reactions, but no such cases in Group N. When he analyzes the data by standard statistical methods, he finds that Group P and Group N are not statistically different; therefore, he concludes that the tendency of the two sutures to cause allergic reactions is the same. But in fact his study did not prove *that;* his study showed only that he did not have enough cases to observe differences of a small, but perhaps real magnitude. The statement "This study did not reveal any difference between Group N and Group

P" *must not* be interpreted as saying that Group N and Group P are the same. One cannot generalize negative findings any more than one can say that because all dogs are animals, all animals are dogs.

An important point regarding the interpretation of statistical results is that one must keep in mind the difference between *mathematical* significance and *clinical* significance. For example, Group P may have had a final astigmatic correction of 0.87 ± 0.1 diopters, while Group N showed 1.00 ± 0.1 diopters of postoperative astigmatism. The difference is highly significant statistically, but clinically it makes virtually no difference whether a patient has a cylinder of 0.87 D or one of 1.00 D. Therefore, to conclude that proline is a better suture than nylon because it was shown statistically that it produced less astigmatism *is mathematically correct, but clinically incorrect.*

It is important to provide *absolute numbers* when presenting data. Percentages are not adequate. A paper stating that "67% of patients treated with operation Q improved" may sound convincing until the reader learns that only three patients were treated.

The reader must also beware of imprecise statements. For example, the period of follow-up will influence the nature and validity of the results. A statement such as "cases were reexamined up to 18 months after surgery" is of little value. Perhaps only one case was examined 18 months postoperatively, all the others having been reevaluated 1 month after surgery. This could be entirely possible within the framework of the sentence given, so the reader must be careful not to assume that reevaluation of all cases was made 18 months after surgery.

This discussion of outcomes and clinical trials is brief, but it should indicate to the reader that the bulk of published and oral communication regarding surgical results represents only "clinical impression." This is even more of a problem when considering the outcomes of one's own surgery. "Clinical impression" is a weak foundation, because it is so frequently wrong.

We surgeons are so eager to have results that we forget that the method of study determines the validity. If we were to restrict ourselves to correctly studying one thing at a time, the fund of useful information would increase far more rapidly than it has. Taking the nylon sutures versus proline sutures question as an example, if we wanted to determine which was better we would first master the techniques of using both proline and nylon sutures. Next, we would use one or the other in the same way in strictly comparable groups, varying nothing else and introducing cases randomly. Finally, using measurements that were sufficiently *specific* and *sensitive* to indicate the changes that had occurred, we would analyze the data by statistically valid techniques. Even after we had carried out such an elegant clinical trial, however, we would still not be justified in generalizing our conclusions too broadly. All that we could state with authority would be that either proline or nylon *appeared* to be better when used in a particular way in a particular population by a particular surgeon. However, because the conclusion would probably be valid as a result of our having fulfilled the four basic requirements of the clinical trial, it would serve as a block on which further studies could be built. Such investigations can be done by any surgeons who design and manage their studies well.

PRINCIPLES OF TRAINING

The ophthalmic surgeon is first a member of an amazing and magnificent universe, second a person, third a physician, and fourth an ophthalmic surgeon. It is all too easy, as our time becomes preoccupied by the daily excitement and real rewards of practicing ophthalmology, to pervert this order and distort our perspectives. Our first responsibility is to be conscious of the universal interconnectedness of everything, or to a universal God, and the second, to our species and the fundamental unit of that species, the family in the most comprehensive sense—our loved ones and all those who need us. Third, as physicians we have a special obligation toward those who need help with their emotional and physical health. Fourth, we are ophthalmic surgeons. Proper training thus begins in the home and progresses to a comprehensive education that assures the development of social skills and stresses the humanities and their interrelations with the sciences, and finally to the specifics of health and disease.

Ophthalmic patients are afflicted with a full range of conditions that require medical, surgical, and emotional care. Although ophthalmic surgery demands special training and skills, without which surgeons cannot practice their craft properly, the ophthalmic surgeon must first possess the general knowledge regarding health and disease that is needed by all physicians. This is usually acquired by satisfactory completion of an accredited medical school program, with an additional year of general medical and surgical experience before starting a full-time residency in ophthalmology.

Specific training in ophthalmic surgery begins with the residency period. Learning new procedures, during residency or later in one's career, is discussed in detail in Chapter 4. Ideally, the resident's surgical experience should span the entire 3 years of this training, during which considerable time is spent in the role of assistant to senior instructors. Later the trainee should perform as the primary surgeon in a wide variety of ophthalmic operative procedures. One satisfactory mode of progression is that shown in Table 1–2.

No matter how carefully planned and supervised the program, complications will inevitably occur; the intelligent ophthalmic surgeon should learn from these unfortunate events. In fact, the surgeon who has not had broad exposure to the complications of surgery will not be adequately prepared to cope with them when they occur. It should be remembered that the skillful teacher can lead the neophyte surgeon through difficult experiences; the confidence that grows out of the knowledge of the correct way to handle such situations is an essential component of the fully developed surgeon. Furthermore, learning surgeons must develop first-hand familiarity with the humbling truth that the surgical result may be less beneficial than hoped for by the patient

TABLE 1–2. Optimal Mode of Training Ophthalmic Surgeons

1. Practical experience in a supervised clinic (helping to diagnose and select patients for surgery)
2. Observation of surgery
3. Practice with eye bank and animal eyes
4. Further observation as first assistant to surgeons teaching full range of preoperative, operative, and postoperative care
5. Highly supervised surgical experience incorporating diagnosis, examination techniques, indications for surgery, details of surgical techniques, and continuing postoperative care
6. Broad surgical experience with gradually increasing autonomy
7. Experience teaching surgical procedures, including preoperative and postoperative care

or the surgeon, or both. Training programs that avoid cases of great complexity or cases in which a poor result could seriously hamper the patient's life-style cannot claim to be doing more than a superficial job of introducing the physician to the field of surgery.

A resident's first really difficult procedure should, if at all possible, be performed in a setting in which the necessary supervision and support are present. Considerable experience with such surgery is preferable before the resident surgeon is allowed to function independently. Both the surgeon who completes a residency training program and the patient who expects to benefit from this encounter with the surgeon are justified in believing that the ophthalmologist who finishes an accredited ophthalmic residency program should be able to manage the great majority of surgical problems encountered.

Many or most of the details, and even some of the principles, learned by the student will change with time. The ophthalmic surgeon must maintain a highly flexible approach to the learning situation. Modifications and improvements develop at such a remarkable rate that every surgeon must realize that a technique widely used today will probably be outdated in the near future. A large number and variety of postgraduate courses are now available; these should be used by the mature surgeon. Constant self-criticism (not self-doubt) and reevaluation of principles and practice are required for continuing growth.

A profound understanding of himself or herself and his or her world is the final element that leads to the development of the surgeon as a great contributor to the world (Table 1–3).

THE SURGICAL EVENT

The surgical event encompasses far more than just the time spent in the operating room.[1] *The surgical event starts with the decision to do surgery and does not end until the changes initiated by the surgery are stable.* The operating surgeon is responsible for the entire surgical event. He or she may delegate care during that period but must continue to supervise all care. The surgeon is the manager and is responsible for the management of the patient during the surgical event. To repeat, the surgical event is not limited to what takes place in the operating room. It is entirely appropriate for the surgeon to share and to delegate; it is not appropriate to "comanage." The surgeon is in charge and is responsible until the patient is discharged to the care of somebody else. For example, it may be appropriate for a technician, a junior physician, or an optometrist to participate in the care of a patient following a cataract extraction. Those participants are under the supervision of the operating surgeon and are responsible to the operating surgeon; they may be authorized to perform much of the postoperative care, but the operating surgeon remains accountable. In some cases it is not feasible for the patient to remain under the care of the operating surgeon, in which case it is appropriate for the patient's care to be transferred to another physician. That physician, then, is the new manager and becomes fully responsible for the patient's care. Any new manager will probably wish to maintain close contact with the operating surgeon, and when such a transfer occurs it must be clear to the operating surgeon, the new caregiver, and the patient. Such a transfer should not occur without prior planning and approval of all the participants. In such situations the patient must know prior to the time of the surgery that a transfer will occur, and the new caregiver must have been contacted and have agreed to become the new manager.

The duration of a surgical event varies from patient to patient and procedure to procedure. For example, with the standard phacoemulsification the duration is approximately 6 weeks, whereas with a Neodymium:YAG laser iridotomy the duration is approximately 1 week.

TABLE 1–3. Aspects of the Accomplished Craftsperson

Understands the *purposes* of the craft.
Knows the *technical* aspects of the craft.
Is familiar with the *materials* used.
Recognizes the *limitations* of the craft.

DIAGNOSIS

The first step in the proper performance of surgery is correct diagnosis. Correct diagnosis demands adequate evaluation of the patient. Unless this evaluation provides the surgeon with the information needed to make an appropriate decision, optimal results will not be achieved.

Because facilities vary widely from place to place, there may be circumstances in which it may not be feasible to obtain the most sensitive diagnostic examinations possible for a particular patient. When this is the case, the surgeon must remember the shortcomings of the examination and must not credit the data with false validity. Consider, for example, the patient on appropriate medical therapy who has an intraocular pressure of 40 mm Hg, and moderately advanced glaucomatous cupping of the optic nerve head; equipment for a visual field examination is not available, but confrontation fields fail to document field loss. Under such circumstances the surgeon would be ill-advised to rely on the confrontation field as evidence of normal function. Although clearly other factors also must be considered in the patient just described, surgery would appear to be the most reasonable option, despite the *apparently* normal visual fields.

In the overwhelming majority of cases it is, however, possible to gather enough valid information to arrive at a reasonably sure diagnosis. All appropriate efforts should be made; it is my impression that the most common cause of an unsatisfactory surgical result is inadequate evaluation of the patient and the patient's expectations.

PREPARATION OF THE PATIENT

The surgeon must adequately prepare the patient, and in some instances the patient's family, for any proposed surgery. The idea of surgery on the eyes is, for most people, frightening. Blindness is generally disabling to the spirit as well as to the body. It is the ophthalmologist's duty, therefore, to explain tactfully to the patient the nature of the problem and to present the available options for managing it. Such a discussion should include the possibility of treatment by nonsurgical means, the nature of surgical options with attention toward reasonable prognosis, the effect the surgery would probably have on the patient's life-style, associated risks, and the anticipated costs.

The surgeon should remember that a surgical procedure can be considered a violation of the patient's "privacy" in the strictest sense of the word. The patient should make the ultimate decision as to whether or not surgery is to be performed and by whom. It is the physician's responsibility to advise the patient of a condition that necessitates surgery, to offer the possibility of a surgical correction, and to provide enough information to permit the patient to make an appropriate decision. The information should be presented in a clear-cut, reassuring manner, so that the patient will not automatically shy away from the idea of necessary surgery. The risks of performing surgery should be explained, but always in a format in which they are weighed against the risks of *not* performing surgery. It is a mistake to tell a patient that he has an X percent chance of losing sight in surgery without also telling him that he has about a Y percent chance of losing sight if the surgery is *not* performed. When such comparative risks are explained, the patient will, in most instances, make a decision in line with the surgeon's own opinion.

In some cases a patient is reluctant to make the surgical decision himself. The physician must then take on this burden. In my experience this is a rare event. It usually indicates incomplete discussion between the surgeon and the patient. When a surgeon believes that a patient is unable to decide what is in his or her own best interest, the surgeon usually underestimates the patient and overestimates his own rights and abilities. Patients must be encouraged to participate in deciding which option is most appropriate. When the patient chooses not to do so, it is not only the physician's right, but an *obligation* to make what he or she judges to be the most reasonable decision.

When a patient's conclusion differs from that of the surgeon, it is quite possible that it is because of lack of confidence in the surgeon. In such instances the surgeon is probably best advised to ask the patient if a consultation is desired. Surgeons should not wait for their patients to request such a consultation, for patients are frequently reluctant to do so.

A variety of forms can be used to help provide patients with the necessary information regarding diagnosis, hospitalization, and recovery. Although brochures prepared by professional firms and various agencies are available, it is a relatively simple thing for surgeons to prepare such forms themselves. The forms are then more likely to be fully pertinent. Such information, however, should never be considered a substitute for direct communication between patient and surgeon.

INFORMED CONSENT

Informed consent involves important medical and ethical considerations as well as strictly legal ones. The following discussion deals primarily with the ethical aspects of informed consent, with the meaning of the phrase, and with its importance for the patients, the physicians, and the medical profession.[1]

Informed consent is, in many ways, at the heart of the American system of medical and surgical practice. It essentially means that the patient understands the risks and the benefits involved in a proposed procedure. Such understanding demands knowledge and discussion. It also requires a contract between the patient and the surgeon. The patient and the physician become partners, both of whom are primarily interested in the patient's health. The enhancement of this partnership as a meaningful relationship may be the best way to ensure high-quality medical care.

In the Commonwealth of Pennsylvania informed consent is defined as

> The consent of a patient to the performance of health care services by a physician or podiatrist: Provided: That prior to the consent having been given, the physician or podiatrist has informed the patient of the nature of the proposed procedure or treatment and of those risks and alternatives to treatment or diagnosis that a reasonable patient would consider material to the decision whether or not to undergo treatment or diagnosis.

Exceptions to the rule exist, and the law states that physicians will not be held liable for failing to obtain informed consent in the following circumstances:

a. In the case of an emergency that prevents consulting the patient.

b. When furnishing the information to the patient would have resulted in a seriously adverse effect on the patient or on the therapeutic process, to the material detriment of the patient's health.

c. In the case of a minor, when in the physician's judgment an attempt to secure the consent of the parent or legal guardian would result in delay of treatment that would increase the risk to the minor's life or health.

Consent for the treatment of minors should be obtained from the patient's parent or guardian, although exceptions may be made if the minor is (a) 18 years of age or older, (b) one who has graduated from high school, (c) one who has married, or (d) one who has been pregnant.*

Informed consent is not merely the obtaining of a signature on a piece of paper.[2–4] In fact, the act of having a patient sign a written consent for surgery unfortunately sometimes serves as means to avoid obtaining truly informed consent.

The form can improperly substitute for the actual consent. This is rather like the practice of going to church in order to avoid the more difficult responsibilities of being a participating member of a religious faith.

Some physicians appear to believe that the major purpose of obtaining a signed "informed consent" is to prevent malpractice suits. The extreme mental and emotional stress that often accompanies such lawsuits makes prevention of them a deservedly important goal. However, simply because a patient signs a consent form does not eliminate the possibility of litigation. The patient may state at a later date that he did not really understand the form. In fact, it has been shown that patients forget more than they recall the information given to them preoperatively.[5] An informed consent form in itself will not effectively prevent malpractice suits from being filed.

On the other hand, the process of obtaining true informed consent from a patient—that is, the meaningful interchange of information, anticipations, hopes, and fears that should precede a request to sign any form—does help to limit the likelihood that suit will be brought at a later date. It must be remembered that the form is only documentation of the discussion; the form is not the consent.

Some patients, of course, will bring suit even when the physician has been expert, thorough, and caring in obtaining informed consent; a properly executed consent form may provide protection for the surgeon or his institution at a later date.

Failure to obtain adequate informed consent is not the basis for many malpractice claims—only 2.5% according to one study.[6] Most plaintiffs' lawyers plead lack of informed consent as a last-resort allegation in weak cases, and do not, as a rule, use it as a primary charge against a negligent doctor.

Paradoxically, there are risks to the patient in obtaining informed consent. The individual who stands to be helped by cataract extraction, for example, may decline surgery when he hears his surgeon say, "You may lose your eye." Information itself changes people's moods and feelings. The suggestible patient who is fully informed of the difficulties that occasionally plague people with unilateral aphakia may convince himself that he cannot be rehabilitated. Were such patients less completely apprised of the risks, they would probably manage quite satisfactorily. Furthermore, some patients who are functioning well become incapacitated when burdened with greater knowledge of their illness. We must remember that both the manner of obtaining informed consent and the information itself can be damaging to the patient.

The effects on the physician, and consequently on the patient, of a litigative climate should also be recalled. The anxieties produced in the physician by this situation are not conducive to good medical practice.

Surgical care should *never* be based solely on medicolegal considerations. Surgeons must, in each case, exercise their reasonable judgment based on understanding of the case. This is not to say that surgeons should be unaware of what is considered to be "standard practice." Surgeons are, in fact, unlikely to be found negligent when practicing according to the accepted standard. When surgeons choose to deviate from this standard, they should be aware of that deviation and be able to justify it. When standard care is not chosen, the proper concern is not whether litigation will ensue, but rather why such a deviation is in the patient's best interest. The history of medicine makes it clear that *standard* levels of care are not always *optimal* levels of care. Conscientious physicians must constantly be evaluating the benefits and risks of the care they are offering. It is often the case that improvement in care will result only when deviations from that standard are made. Such alterations must be reasonable and in the best interests of the patient.

One of the prerequisites to obtaining informed consent is sufficient knowledge on the part of both doctor and patient (Table 1–4). The physician must adequately understand the medical and surgical aspects of the case

TABLE 1–4. Requirements for Obtaining Appropriate Informed Consent

1. Sufficient knowledge by the surgeon
   a. Adequate understanding of the medical and surgical aspects of the case under consideration
   b. Adequate understanding of the patient's needs and wishes
   c. Adequate understanding of the surgeon's own motivations
2. Willingness of the surgeon to discuss matters with the patient
3. Willingness of the patient to discuss matters with the surgeon
4. Ability of the surgeon to communicate information to the patient and of the patient to comprehend it
5. Sufficient time for discussion of the patient's and surgeon's concerns, and for the information to be assimilated

*Pennsylvania Health Insurance Corporation Bulletin #2B, November 1978.

under consideration and a reasonable comprehension of the patient's needs and wishes. Both the patient and the surgeon should compare the anticipated risks and benefits of not performing surgery.

Not only must surgeons have adequate knowledge of the medical aspects of each case, they must also be aware of their personal motivations influencing the choice of whether to perform or not perform surgery. The major intent of the surgeon should be to help the patient. However, the surgeon is subjected to the full range of influences that affect human decisions; occasionally some may be of almost overwhelming weight. Included among these are pressures from the patient or the patient's family and friends, economic considerations, hope of acquiring new knowledge, curiosity regarding a new instrument or procedure, prestige associated with performing particularly difficult surgery, and the pleasure of conquering a difficult challenge. None of these is a justifiable reason for surgery, since none passes the criteria that are the standard for ethical care, specifically, *is the action thought to be in the best interest of the patient and is the action agreeable to the patient.* On the other hand, there are considerations that may put pressure on the surgeon to avoid operating; these include concern that surgery will damage the patient, timidity based on previous unfortunate experiences with similar surgery, worry that an unfavorable result will bring damaging litigation, and reluctance to refer the patient elsewhere for economic or psychological reasons. Thus the pressures are not solely economic. To perform surgery is stressful and fatiguing. When compensation for the performance of surgery is present, whether in the form of academic promotion, public acclaim, or economic reward, the surgeon will be driven toward electing to do surgery; when compensation is inadequate, or when the physician may be penalized for operating unsuccessfully, then the desire to perform surgery is greatly diminished. The latter case is by no means necessarily preferable to the former. To deny a patient the possibility for improvement by means of surgery is just as unfortunate as to perform surgery when it is not likely to help. The patient has the best chance of receiving proper treatment in a system in which (a) surgeons are knowledgeable regarding both medical care and themselves, (b) rewards and punishments are acceptable to both patients and physicians alike, and (c) the patient is knowledgeable enough to assess the quality of care.[3]

Some patients do not want to be informed. Occasional patients will be articulate about this, saying something like, "Doctor, don't tell me anything; just do what you need to do." In such a situation it is usually best for the physician to try to determine why the patient does not want to know. There may be a significant underlying emotional difficulty that, in some cases, may be more important than the patient's ophthalmic problem. When patients remain adamant about not knowing, surgeons may understandably be reluctant to proceed with recommended treatment, recognizing that although they may have patient consent, it is not truly informed consent. Nevertheless, under such circumstances surgeons should not delay in proceeding with what, in their opinion, appears to be the appropriate therapy. It is advisable in such circumstances to put a note on the patient's chart to the effect that the patient specifically asked not to be informed of the details. In most cases, such a patient request should be honored; patients may well know themselves better than the physician does, and may anticipate that a recitation of the risks of the surgery, even if done compassionately, might induce such fear that they would decide against doing what in fact would be in their own best interest. Such patients may well prefer to trust completely the physician's recommendation. Clearly such trust should never be exploited, but it should be honored. In such cases physicians should feel free to follow recommendations.

Physicians are not always cognizant of the absolutely central role they play in patient care. Physicians and surgeons have not been replaced by computers, or computed tomography scanners, or surgical microscopes. These technological masterpieces occasionally get in the way of the physician-patient relationship, and may even substitute for particular aspects of it, but they can never meaningfully replace it.

In summary, informed consent is an essential part of medical practice, for four rather different reasons. First, it is the physician's ethical responsibility to be honest with the patient.[4] Second, it is the patient's right to make decisions regarding his or her destiny, and the patient is not in a position to do this without appropriate knowledge. Third, the process of obtaining informed consent is one of the most important practical ways of assuring high standards and ongoing improvement of quality of medical care. Finally, the physician is legally obligated to obtain such consent.

PREOPERATIVE STUDIES

Adequate knowledge of a patient's state of health before performance of surgery is clearly essential to achieving a successful result. For example, the presence of an enlarged prostate could lead to serious urinary retention in patients who require the use of agents that induce marked diuresis. A history should be taken preoperatively that includes questions about systemic medications being taken by the patient, known or suspected allergies and drug reactions, bleeding abnormalities, and previous surgical experiences. For example, because the use of aspirin is widespread, very specific questions should be asked regarding the use of aspirin-containing compounds. It is important to question in detail in this regard, because the patient may be unaware of the aspirin content of his or her medication, and most patients are unaware that aspirin can predispose to serious bleeding complications at the time of surgery and postoperatively. A list of aspirin-containing compounds is given in Table 1–5.

Pertinent questions should also be asked regarding the patient's general health and family and social life. A brief but skillful physical examination is usually appropriate. Laboratory studies should be limited to those that bear directly on the patient's state of health. The

TABLE 1–5. Aspirin-Containing Medications

Aspirin	Warfarin
Alka-Seltzer	Naprosyn
Ascriptin	Indocin
Bayer compounds	Diflunisal
Encaprin	Midol
Measurin	Fiorinal
Aleve	Empirin
Zorprin	Ecotrin
Salsalate	Easprin
Doan's Pills	Feldene
Ibuprofen	Tolectin
Anacin	Advil
Excedrin	

need for these will clearly vary with the patient, the anticipated surgical procedure, and the facilities available.

For cases in which general anesthesia is thought advisable, the anesthesiologist should evaluate the patient preoperatively. Even when only local anesthesia is to be used, a visit from the anesthesiologist or nurse is helpful.

ANESTHESIA

Adequate anesthesia is important to the successful outcome of a surgical procedure. Previous practice has generally been to administer medication (e.g., a sedative, an antiemetic, and an analgesic) before the surgery, to reduce anxiety and produce a general feeling of well-being. However, it is not at all certain that such medication is necessary. Experiences with outpatient surgery suggest that many patients need little or no premedication. The general tendency now is to use general anesthesia or to use minimal sedation in association with local anesthesia. The surgeon who uses potent medications that are effectively the equivalent of general anesthesia must take appropriate preoperative, postoperative, and intraoperative precautions. Procedures performed under local anesthesia are probably best accomplished when there is careful psychological preparation of the patient, an appropriately soothing and confidence-inspiring atmosphere during the preoperative and operative periods, excellent technique of administration of the anesthetic agent, and administration of the minimal amount of short-acting medication. The goal is to have the patient relaxed and cooperative during surgery, and completely alert and ready for ambulation (should that be appropriate) immediately after surgery.

Principles regarding the use of anesthesia and anesthetic techniques are discussed in detail in Chapter 5.

OPERATIVE TECHNIQUES

General principles that apply to virtually all operative techniques are discussed in Chapter 3. Specific principles and techniques are covered in each of the chapters dealing with the individual suspecialties.

POSTOPERATIVE CARE

The final phase of the surgical procedure begins at the conclusion of the operation and extends through the postoperative recovery phase until healing is complete.

ACTIVITY AND PATCHING

The level of activity in the early postoperative period varies markedly depending on the procedure. With most ophthalmic surgery, there is little need for limitation of activity in the postoperative period, though there are marked exceptions, such as patients who need highly specific positioning following surgery for macular degeneration. Early ambulation should be encouraged to prevent the host of problems that arise with prolonged bedrest, a special concern in the elderly. Most patients should be up and about the same day as surgery.

Modern wound closure also reduces the need for eye patches. Although a firm patch may make a patient more comfortable by preventing movement of the lids and excess tearing, it has the negative effect of increasing the temperature around the eye, thus providing a better environment for bacterial growth. Where a facial nerve block has not been employed there is usually no need for any patch. The general rule is that eye patches should be used only as long as they are essential to protect the eye. The use of protective glasses to prevent inadvertent bumps to the eye is often appropriate. But by and large the older "shield" should be limited to bedtime use where necessary and is best not used during the day.

POSTOPERATIVE MEDICATION

There is no "routine" postoperative medication to fit the needs of all patients. Each case must be considered separately. The surgeon must be familiar with the advantages and disadvantages of various therapeutic agents. The tremendous importance of proper postoperative medication cannot be over-emphasized. A successful operative procedure can be ruined by incorrect postoperative therapy; on the other hand, a marginally successful operation can often be salvaged by proper medication. (This emphasis on postoperative care was a teaching of E. B. Spaeth.) Sedation and analgesia should be kept to a minimum. Aspirin in any form is often contraindicated because of its tendency to encourage bleeding. Medications should not be used as a substitute for the psychological support and reassurance that can come from all those who participate in the patient's postoperative care, but most essentially from the surgeon.

DISCHARGE AND REHABILITATION

Time of discharge varies with the surgery and the patient. The surgeon's task is not complete until the patient has been fully rehabilitated. This aspect of the surgical procedure may be the most challenging; it may persist for the remainder of the patient's life.

One of the weakest aspects of many training programs is the lack of exposure of the learning surgeon to the patient in the postoperative period. The neophyte simply does not have the chance to see the unfortunate and long-lasting distress often caused by so-called successful, but ill-chosen surgery. *The art of proper selection of surgery demands exposure to patients in the postoperative period.* An additional problem in this regard is that the inexperienced surgeon may fail to fully realize the great need for immediate recognition of complications, together with institution of remedial steps, and the tremendous importance of reassuring and comforting the patient.

The recognition and management of specific complications are dealt with later in this text. As we conclude this brief introduction to the general aspects of ophthalmic surgery, it is pertinent, however, to review some of the general causes for the unfortunate events that may reduce the benefits of a surgical experience. These are listed in Table 1–6.

Probably the single most important factor that affects the surgical outcome is the character of the surgeon, which largely determines the nature of the other characteristics listed. There is a deep fundamental validity in the inscription on the monument in the Sanctuary of Aesculapius:

> These are the duties of a physician; first [to repeat] the Paeonian chants and to heal his mind and give assistance to himself before giving it to anyone [else], and not to look upon [his patient] or make approaches in a manner contrary to divine laws and to the oath. He would cure with moral courage and with the proper moral attitude. He would not [be spiritually] unequipped when as helper he handles lovely matrons and maidens, burn in his breast with desire [in a manner unworthy of a true] physician. . . . Having become such a one in his judgment, he would be like God saviour equally of slaves, of paupers, of rich men, of princes, and to all a brother, such help he would give. For we are all brothers. Therefore he would not hate anyone, nor would he harbor envy in his mind, nor increase his pretensions.*

TABLE 1–6. Causes for a Surgical Result That is Less than Optimal

The Surgeon (partially controllable by the medical profession)
- Poor surgeon–patient relationship
- Poor diagnostic skill
- Lack of technical knowledge or skill
- Insufficient medical care
- Inadequate facilities
- Lack of surgical judgment

The Medical Setting (partially controllable by the medical profession and the hospital administration)
- Poor facilities
- Inadequate nursing care

The Patient (partially controllable by public education)
- Ignorance of the disease
- Unwillingness to understand the disease
- Refusal to cooperate in a program of appropriate treatment

The Nature of the Disease Itself (partially controllable by increased knowledge)

External Forces
- Societal conditions that could be controlled (e.g., malnutrition)
- Conditions that appear to be uncontrollable (e.g., accidents)

REFERENCES

Classic Texts

1. American Academy of Ophthalmology Code of Ethics, San Francisco, 1989.
2. Stanley B, Guido J, Stanley M, et al.: The elderly patient and informed consent. JAMA 1984;252:1302.
3. Ost DE: The "right" not to know. J Med Philos 1984;9:301.
4. Bockelmann P: Zur rechtlichen situation bei prophylaktischen Massnahmen in der Ophthalmologie. Klin Mbl Augenheilk 1978; 173:129.
5. Curran WJ: Law-Medicine Notes: Malpractice claims: New data and new trends. N Engl J Med 1979;300:26.
6. Fasanella RM (ed.): Eye Surgery: Innovations and Trends, Pitfalls, Complications. Springfield, Ill: Charles C Thomas; 1977.
7. Fifth Symposium of the Ophthalmic Microsurgery Study Group. London, June 1974: Microsurgery of Cataract Vitreous and Astigmatism. In Kersley J, Pierse D (eds.), Advances in Ophthalmology, vol 33. Basel: S Karger; 1976.
8. Fox SA: Ophthalmic Plastic Surgery, 5th Edition. New York: Grune & Stratton; 1976.
9. Heilmann K, Paton D: Atlas of Ophthalmic Surgery. Stuttgart: Thieme; 1985.
10. Helveston EM: Atlas of Strabismus Surgery. St. Louis: CV Mosby; 1977.
11. Iliff CE, Iliff WJ, Iliff NT: Oculoplastic Surgery. Philadelphia: WB Saunders; 1979.
12. Jaffe NS: Cataract Surgery and Its Complications, 4th Edition. St. Louis: CV Mosby; 1984.
13. Jones LT, Wobig JL: Surgery of the Eyelids and Lacrimal System. Birmingham: Aesculapius Publishing Co; 1976.
14. Klein R, Katzin H: Microsurgery of the Vitreous: Comparisons of Instrumentation, Techniques and Philosophies. Baltimore: Williams & Wilkins; 1978.
15. Krasnov MM: Mikrochirurgie der Glaukome. Leipzig: Thieme; 1977.
16. L'Esperance FA: Ocular Photocoagulation: A Stereoscopic Atlas. St. Louis: CV Mosby; 1975.
17. Machemer R, Asbert TM: Vitrectomy, 2nd Edition. Current Ophthalmology Monographs. New York: Grune & Stratton; 1979.
18. Spaeth GL: Ophthalmic Surgery: Principles and Practice. Philadelphia: WB Saunders, 1982.
19. Stallard HH: Eye Surgery. Bristol: John Wright & Sons; 1946. (Fifth Edition, published 1973).
20. Stanley B, Guido J, Stanley M, et al.: The elderly patient and informed consent. JAMA 1984;252:1302.
21. Troutman RC: Microsurgery of the Anterior Segment of the Eye: The Cornea, vol 2. St. Louis: CV Mosby; 1977.
22. Troutman RC: Microsurgery of the Anterior Segment of the Eye. St. Louis: CV Mosby; 1974.
23. Weinstein GW, Drews RC: The Surgery of Intraocular Lenses. Thorofare, N.J.: Slack Inc.; 1977.

*Translated by James H. Oliver. Bull. History of Medicine, 7:315, 1939.

CHAPTER 2

Anesthesia for Ophthalmic Surgery

STANLEY W. STEAD, M.D. and KEVIN M. MILLER, M.D.

As important to most eye surgery patients as the outcome of their surgery are their concerns about pain or the consequences of moving inadvertently during the procedure. Patients are generally more apprehensive about procedures performed on their eyes than procedures performed on other parts of their bodies. Therefore, ocular anesthesia presents challenges to the ophthalmologist and anesthesiologist not seen in other surgical specialties (Table 2–1). In this chapter, we will review the preparation of eye surgery patients, local and general anesthetic techniques including selection criteria for the appropriate anesthetic, and management of pediatric patients and those undergoing special surgical procedures.

TABLE 2–1. Special Concerns in Ocular Anesthesia

Patient anxiety related to decreased vision
Elderly patients with multiple systemic diseases
Pediatric patients, often premature with congenital syndromes
Limited access to the patient and the need for immobility during surgery
Intraocular pressure and anesthetic agent interactions
Oculocardiac reflexes

PREOPERATIVE EVALUATION

Whether performing a minor surgical procedure under topical anesthesia (such as radial keratotomy, chalazion excision, etc.), a cataract procedure under local anesthesia with sedation, or a procedure requiring general anesthesia (such as in children), effective communication between the patient and the ophthalmologist is crucial. Minor surgical treatment of a young, healthy patient may be performed in an unmonitored procedure room without anesthesia and should not require extensive preoperative evaluation. Most ophthalmic surgery patients are at the extremes of age and represent a high-risk population. Although the procedures themselves are of relatively low systemic risk, the importance of a thorough preoperative evaluation cannot be overemphasized. In review of malpractice litigation in cataract surgery, failure of the anesthesiologist, ophthalmologist, and internist to coordinate perioperative patient care resulted in 16% of the successful claims against physicians.[1]

We recommend the following principles:

1. To ensure that the patient is not acutely ill and to optimize all reversible medical conditions, every preoperative patient should have an appropriate and thorough medical history and physical examination preferably performed by the patient's personal physician.
2. The individual performing the anesthesia should interview the patient (a) to review medical history and laboratory data, (b) to determine whether further testing or consultation is needed, (c) to

formulate a perioperative anesthetic plan, and (d) to discuss the plan with the patient.

3. Avoid ordering a routine battery of laboratory studies, which can be wasteful and may lead to unnecessary further evaluation on the basis of false-positive results.
4. In some instances, patients with severe, chronic, life-threatening disease will demand ophthalmic surgery, even if there is an increased risk of a major complication or death. In these circumstances, explain the risks, be certain that informed consent is obtained, and perform the procedure under local or monitored anesthesia care if at all possible.

OPHTHALMIC EMERGENCIES

Most ophthalmic procedures need not be done on an emergent basis. This is important to understand because the anesthetic plan depends on the NPO status (i.e., nothing by mouth in the preoperative hours) and general condition of the patient. In the patient with a full stomach or one with a situation that can be reversed or improved by nonsurgical means, it is better to delay surgery. This does not apply to true emergencies where therapy should be instituted within a matter of minutes (e.g., central retinal artery occlusion caused by orbital hemorrhage). Many ophthalmic conditions are considered urgent, and therapy should be instituted within a matter of one to several hours. Ophthalmic conditions where therapy can be instituted within days or sometimes within weeks are considered semiurgent situations.

LOCAL ANESTHESIA

Local anesthetic agents can be administered topically, intraocularly, or by injection. It is important to understand the relative potencies and recommended maximum dosages of the various agents. Maximum dosages may be modified depending upon the method of administration or the concomitant use of vasoconstrictors (Table 2–2).

TOPICAL ANESTHESIA

With the evolution of less invasive, relatively atraumatic, and short duration procedures, topical anesthesia may be used satisfactorily in patients who are able to understand sensations that may be experienced during surgery.[2,3] Patients should be able to tolerate the lid speculum and operating microscope light and be able to follow instructions during surgery. The surgeon must be well trained and able to communicate the anticipated sensations at each step, a process termed "vocal local." The surgeon must be aware that, while topical medications achieve anesthesia of the conjunctiva, cornea, and anterior sclera, they do not anesthetize the eyelids, posterior sclera, intraocular tissues, or extraocular muscles. It is therefore important to avoid excessive manipulation of the globe, placement of bridle sutures, cautery, and manipulation of the iris and lens. How well patients respond during tonometry and A-scan ultrasonography appears to be a good predictor of how they will tolerate phacoemulsification and lens implantation under topical anesthesia.[4]

Monocular patients are particularly suited for topical anesthesia surgery because of their unique need for quick recovery of vision from the operated eye. Most patients in the age range typical for cataract development are good candidates for topical surgery. Inappropriate candidates include the very young, the mentally retarded, those with a strong blink reflex, those with whom the surgeon has difficulty communicating, and those for whom surgery will be long (greater than 30 to 40 minutes) or difficult (small pupils, hard lenses, weak zonules).

Topical anesthesia is administered by placing several drops of a single anesthetic agent into the superior and inferior conjunctival fornices just prior to sterilizing the eye chemically. Earlier application of drops is disad-

TABLE 2–2. Local Anesthetic Agents

Generic	Trade Name*	Equieffective Concentration (%)	Duration after Injection (min)	Recommended Maximum Dose in 70 kg Adult (mg)
Amino Esters				
Cocaine		4	30 ± 10	200
Procaine	Novocaine	2	45 ± 15	1000
2-Chloroprocaine	Nesacaine	2	30 ± 10	1000
Tetracaine	Proparacaine	0.25	30 ± 15	200
Amino Amides				
Lidocaine	Xylocaine	1	100 ± 20	350
Prilocaine		1	120 ± 40	900
Mepivacaine	Carbocaine	1	120 ± 30	500
Bupivacaine	Marcaine	0.25	200 ± 30	150
Etidocaine		0.25	170 ± 60	300

*Representative proprietary names.

vantageous as it may lead to drying, superficial punctate keratopathy, and a difficult view during surgery. It is helpful to massage the eye through closed eyelids while the sting of the anesthetic is subsiding and inform or remind the patient of the pressure sensation that will be experienced during surgery. Just before the eyelids are draped, additional drops can be applied to suppress the sting of the antiseptic agent, to stop reflex tearing, and to improve adhesion of the drape to the eyelids. During surgery the patient is instructed to fixate a light within the operating microscope to keep the eye still. Additional drops of anesthetic agent can be applied as needed during surgery.

Topical anesthesia of the eye can be achieved with any of the available topical agents including tetracaine (0.5%) and proparacaine (0.5%). Injection agents such as bupivacaine (0.75%), carbocaine (4%), and lidocaine (1.0-4.0%) can also be applied topically. Lidocaine that is pH adjusted with sodium bicarbonate to 7.2 achieves a higher anterior chamber concentration than standard lidocaine (pH = 5.2).[5] The duration of effect of most agents is 20 to 40 minutes. The amount of superficial punctate keratopathy probably differs from agent to agent. Rosenthal has described a technique that involves placement of a small saturated piece of Weckcel or instrument-wipe sponge in the superior and inferior fornices to preserve corneal clarity.[6] Alternately, Bloomberg has placed a ring saturated with local anesthetic on the parilimbal area.[7]

Advantages of topical anesthesia include avoidance of orbital or intraocular injection, elimination of the need for a patch on the eye after surgery, avoidance of temporary vision loss from the eye undergoing surgery, and lack of a need to interrupt anticoagulant or antiplatelet therapy. As relative disadvantages, patients are distinctly aware of the surgical procedure, conscious of the eyelid speculum and microscope light, subject to discomfort or pain with intraocular manipulation or intraocular pressure fluctuation, and capable of extraocular movements.

TOPICAL PLUS INTRAOCULAR ANESTHESIA

Intraocular anesthesia can be administered as a routine adjunct to topical anesthesia, or it can be reserved for patients who experience discomfort under topical anesthesia. The reported benefit of intraocular anesthetic injection is a reduction of the visceral pain associated with pressure fluctuations in the anterior chamber and with surgical manipulations of the iris, ciliary body, and lens, particularly phacoemulsification and lens insertion. In a prospective, randomized, placebo-controlled clinical trial, Gills reported that preservative-free lidocaine (1%, 0.1 cc) was statistically superior to balanced salt solution in controlling intraoperative discomfort.[5] Injection of 0.5 cc was more effective than injection of 0.1 cc. Neither was associated with endothelial cell loss.

As a cautionary note, anterior chamber injection of bupivacaine (0.75%), preservative-free lidocaine (4%), and proparacaine (0.5%) produced corneal thickening and opacification in a rabbit model that was clinically and statistically significant when compared to injection of balanced salt solution.[8] Tetracaine (0.5%) was minimally toxic to the endothelium in this study. The anesthetic agents in this experimental study were not irrigated from the rabbit eyes after injection, thereby providing worst-case toxicity scenario. Benzalkonium chloride is known to be toxic to the corneal endothelium, so agents injected intraocularly should be free of this preservative.[9]

Intraocular anesthesia is administered through a 1-mm paracentesis or side-port incision. The drug may be directed posterior to the iris to achieve a maximal effect on the iris and ciliary body proprioceptors. After 15 to 30 seconds the agent is washed out by injection of viscoelastic material. Non-preserved lidocaine (1%) has been studied the most, but use of preservative-free tetracaine has been reported.[2] Patient selection criteria and surgical considerations are the same as for surgery performed under topical anesthesia alone, but some consideration should be given to avoidance of intraocular anesthesia in patients with a low endothelial cell count.

Topical plus intraocular anesthesia produces anesthesia of the conjunctiva, cornea, anterior sclera, iris, and ciliary body. There is decreased sensitivity to the light of the surgical microscope and decreased sensitivity to intraocular pressure fluctuation. Not anesthetized are the posterior intraocular structures (unless the lens–zonule barrier is disrupted) and the extraocular muscles. Transient blindness may occur if anesthetic reaches the retina.

ORBITAL INJECTION ANESTHESIA

Principal variations of orbital anesthesia are parabulbar injection, peribulbar injection, and retrobulbar injection. Orbital injection anesthesia attains anesthesia of the conjunctiva, cornea, sclera, intraocular structures, and extraocular muscles. There is little or no sensitivity to the light of the surgical microscope and no sensitivity to intraocular pressure fluctuation. Extraocular muscles are anesthetized and extraocular movements are greatly decreased or fully eliminated. As a result, orbital injection anesthesia is suitable for patients who prefer to have no sensation in the area undergoing surgery and patients who are not qualified for either topical anesthesia or topical plus intraocular anesthesia.

Usually, the patient is unaware or only minimally conscious of the eyelid speculum and microscope light. The surgeon has less requirement for communication with the patient, and there is less need for patient cooperation and control of extraocular movement. Therefore, this technique is appropriate for patients who are anxious, young, or patients with a mental or psychological deficit. It is suitable for complicated surgical procedures with extensive intraocular manipulation, and for lengthy procedures (greater than 30 to 40 minutes in duration).

Orbital injection anesthesia permits use of a superior rectus suture or cautery and does not restrict the extent of anterior intraocular or posterior intraocular manipulation.

Advantages of orbital injection anesthesia are full anesthesia of the eye and extraocular structures of the orbit, as well as the suitability for surgical procedures of relatively great complexity and duration. Disadvantages of orbital injection anesthesia are the need for a patch on the eye during the postoperative period of recovery from anesthesia, advisability of decreasing or interrupting anticoagulant or platelet-modifying therapy, and specific complications of the orbital injection.

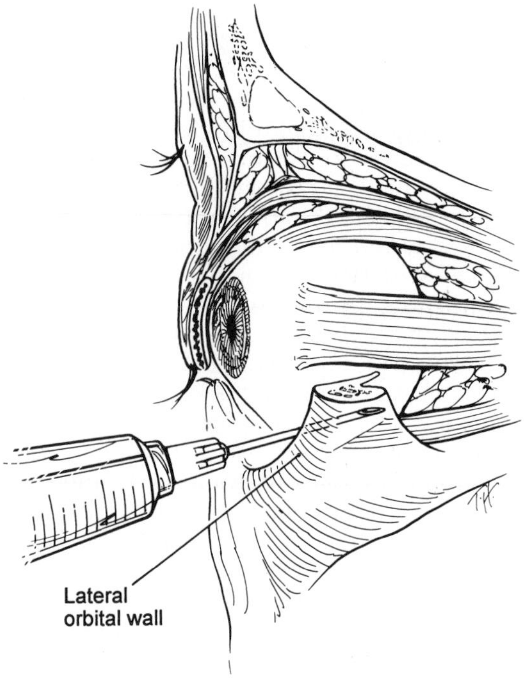

Figure 2–1. Peribulbar anesthesia. Peribulbar anesthesia described by Davis and Mandel uses a 24-mm, 23 to 26-gauge needle. Injection is made with the eye in the primary position, needle insertion in the inferotemporal eyelid and orbit, and penetration 3 to 4 mm posterior to the equator of the globe.

PARABULBAR ANESTHESIA

Parabulbar anesthesia was described by Bergman in 1993.[10] This entails initial topical anesthesia, a limbal sub-tenon dissection, and use of a blunt metal cannula in the sub-tenon space to produce retrobulbar flush anesthesia. The technique uses bupivacaine (0.75%, 2.5 ml) and lidocaine (2.0%, 2.5 ml).

Topical plus parabulbar anesthesia was modified by Greenbaum and Aleman.[11] Topical anesthesia is followed by a postlimbal sub-tenon incision (1 mm in length) in the inferotemporal or inferonasal quadrant. The Greenbaum flexible polyethylene cannula is passed posteriorly in the sub-tenon space, and retrobulbar flush anesthesia is administered. The retrobulbar flush anesthesia uses bupivacaine (0.75%, 1.25 ml) and lidocaine (2.0 or 4.0%, 1.25 ml).[11]

PERIBULBAR ANESTHESIA

Peribulbar anesthesia, described by Davis and Mandel, consists of a preperibulbar injection of lidocaine (0.2%, 2 ml) warmed to body temperature and injection with a 12-mm 27-gauge needle into the inferotemporal orbicularis area and anterior orbit.[12] A subsequent peribulbar injection is composed of bupivacaine (0.75%, 6 ml), lidocaine (1.0%, 3 ml) and hyaluronidase (1 ml). Using a 24-mm, 23 to 26 gauge needle, injection is made with the eye in the primary position, needle insertion in the inferotemporal eyelid and orbit, and penetration 3 to 4 mm posterior to the equator of the globe (Fig. 2–1). An average of 8 ml (range 4 to 10 ml) is injected and followed by a period of orbital compression. Waiting 10 to 25 minutes after the injection before commencing surgery is recommended.

In a prospective multicenter study of 16,224 consecutive peribulbar blocks, supplemental blocks were used in 661 (5.0%) cases, and complications were rare.[12]

RETROBULBAR ANESTHESIA

For retrobulbar anesthesia, Beatie and Stead recommended sedation and analgesia with intravenous propofol by bolus (0.24 to 0.4 mg/kg) and infusion (60 to 80 µg/kg/min) and intravenous alfentanil bolus (3.0 to 5.0 µg/kg) and infusion (0.75 to 1.0 µg/kg/min) (Table 2–3).[13] Straatsma described retrobulbar anesthesia with bupivacaine (0.75%, 1.5 ml) and lidocaine (2.0%, 1.5 ml) with hyaluronidase (5 units/ml). Injection with a 31-mm, 26-gauge needle is carried out with the eye in the primary position (Fig. 2–2). Injection begins at the inferotemporal orbital margin and the needle is aimed at the lower edge of the superior orbital fissure. Typically the needle is directed 45 degrees from the sagittal plane and 10 degrees superiorly (Fig. 2–3). After insertion 3 mm beyond the posterior surface of the globe and aspiration, 3.0 ml of anesthetic solution is injected slowly (1 ml/10 seconds).[14] On withdrawal, orbicularis akinesia may be achieved with injection of 1.5 ml of the same anesthetic solution slowly (1 ml/20 seconds) anterior to the septum orbitale. After injection, orbital compression is maintained for several minutes and the effect of injection is evaluated in 5 to 7 minutes. Supplemental injection may be advisable in about 5% of cases.

Some physicians apply manual compression to assist the spread of local anesthesia after ophthalmic nerve blocks. Manual compression, or a mechanical compression device (such as Honen's) may also be used to produce a "soft eye" (i.e., an eye with decreased intraocular pressure) before surgery. Compression has been used with great safety over a number of years however, persistent case reports can be found implicating orbital compression as the cause of postoperative ptosis and, more importantly, impaired retinal circulation.[15,16] When compression on the globe is used, the pressure exerted should be substantially below dia-

TABLE 2-3. Recommended Sedation for Injection Anesthesia

Age	Alfentanil Dose	Propofol Dose
***Alfentanil/Propofol Bolus*[11]**		
< 50 yrs	5 μg/kg	0.40 mg/kg
50–70 yrs	4 μg/kg	0.32 mg/kg
> 70 yrs	3 μg/kg	0.24 mg/kg
Type of Local Injection	**Alfentanil Dose**	**Propofol Dose**
***Alfentanil/Propofol Infusion Rate*[11]**		
Discrete nerve block(s)	0.75 μg/kg/min	60 μg/kg/min
Large field blocks	1.00 μg/kg/min	80 μg/kg/min

stolic blood pressure to ensure that vascular impairment does not occur.

SAFETY OF PERIBULBAR AND RETROBULBAR ANESTHESIA

Safety and efficacy of orbital anesthesia, particularly peribulbar and retrobulbar injection, has been enhanced by studies of orbital anatomy, computed tomography (CT) imaging of orbital injection needles in situ, and CT imaging of orbital anesthetic solution spread. In such studies, CT images of orbital injection needles in situ demonstrated the advantages of fixation in the primary position of gaze, which increased the distance between injection pathway and both the optic nerve and the ophthalmic artery.[17] Furthermore, anesthetic solutions in the retrobulbar and peribulbar space spread radially into all parts of the retrobulbar space and anteriorly into the preseptal tissue of the eyelids.[18]

Outcome of retrobulbar anesthesia has been reported in a number of large case series. Among these are a report of 12,000 orbital anesthetic injections,[19] a description of 12,500 consecutive retrobulbar injections,[20] and a report of over 50,000 orbital injections.[21] Serial sections of orbital specimens reveal no fascial "cone" or intramuscular septum (Fig. 2–4). Peribulbar and retrobulbar injection are, in fact, the same.

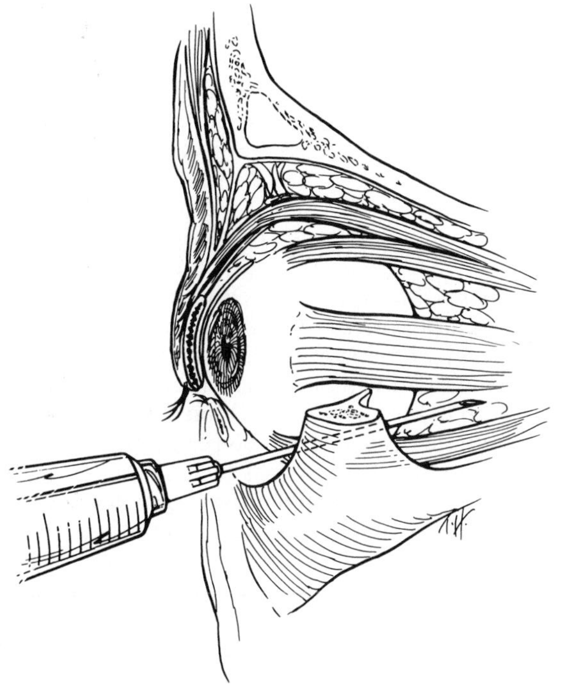

Figure 2–2. Retrobulbar anesthesia. Straatsma described retrobulbar anesthesia as injection with a 31-mm, 26-gauge needle carried out with the eye in the primary position. Injection begins at the inferotemporal orbital margin, and the needle is aimed at the lower edge of the superior orbital fissure.

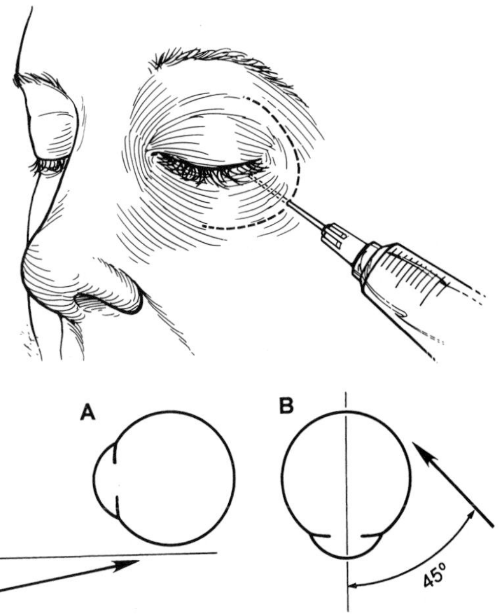

Figure 2–3. Retrobulbar anesthesia. In retrobulbar anesthesia, the needle is inserted in at the inferotemporal orbital margin. The needle is directed approximately 45 degrees from the sagittal plane and 10 degrees superiorly. The needle is advanced 3 mm beyond the posterior surface of the globe and after aspiration, the anesthetic solution is injected slowly.

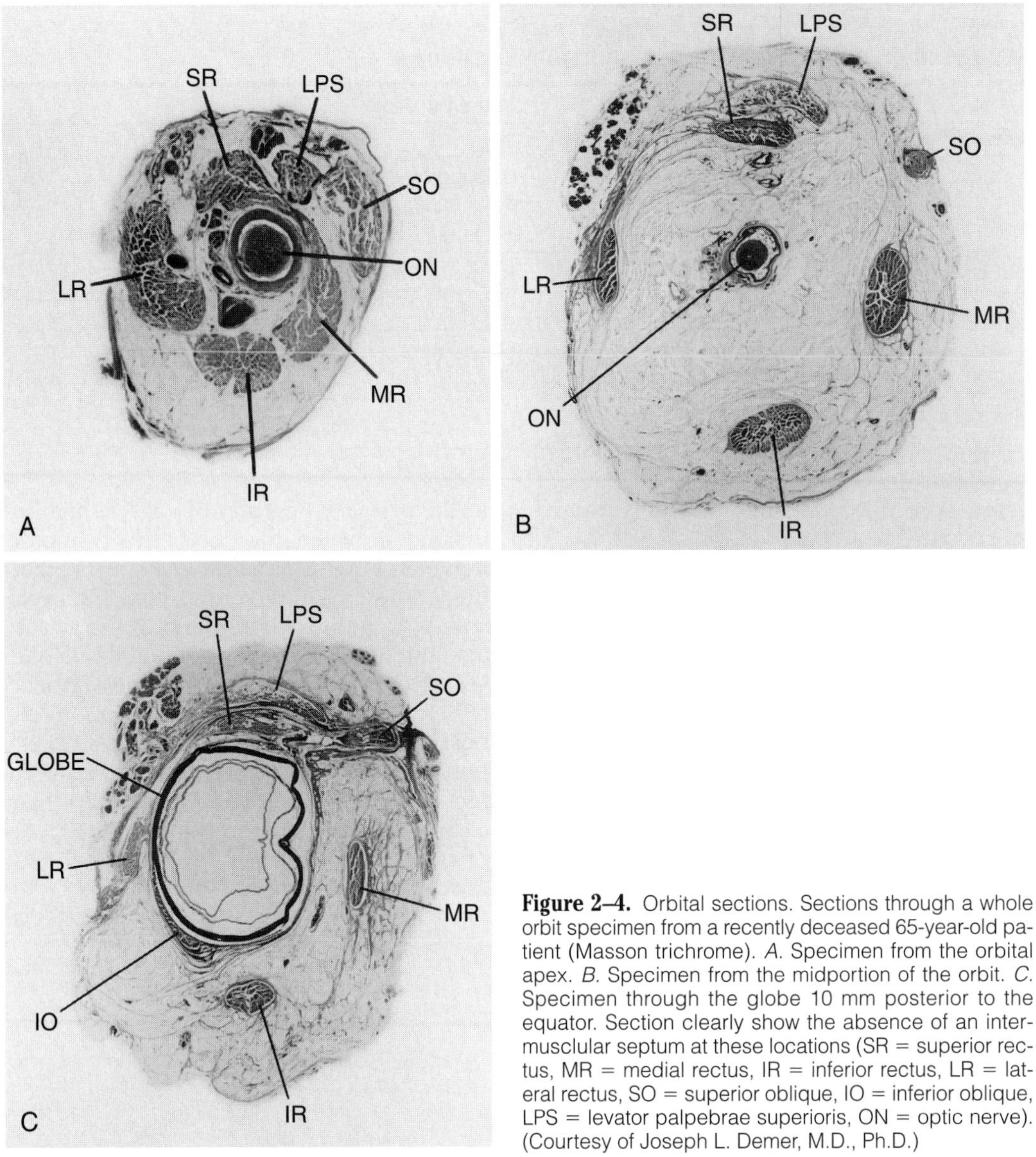

Figure 2–4. Orbital sections. Sections through a whole orbit specimen from a recently deceased 65-year-old patient (Masson trichrome). *A.* Specimen from the orbital apex. *B.* Specimen from the midportion of the orbit. *C.* Specimen through the globe 10 mm posterior to the equator. Section clearly show the absence of an intermuscular septum at these locations (SR = superior rectus, MR = medial rectus, IR = inferior rectus, LR = lateral rectus, SO = superior oblique, IO = inferior oblique, LPS = levator palpebrae superioris, ON = optic nerve). (Courtesy of Joseph L. Demer, M.D., Ph.D.)

Complications of a significant nature are rare. Reported complications include venous and arterial hemorrhage, scleral perforation, vascular occlusion, optic nerve lesion, brain stem anesthesia, and extraocular muscle abnormality.[22,23] Special care must be taken in the presence of certain anatomic factors, particularly the presence of a large myopic globe with an axial length greater than 26 or 27 mm, and in patients with severe or inadequately controlled systemic vascular disease.[22]

FACIAL NERVE BLOCKS

Because small incision surgical techniques for both cataract and vitreoretinal procedures are common place, facial nerve blocks are used less and less frequently. Even with the use of an eyelid retractor, patients may squeeze their eyelids shut during ophthalmic surgery. The orbicularis occuli is the muscle that mediates the squeeze. It is innervated by branches of the facial nerve. Various facial nerve blocks have been developed to insure akinesia of the eyelids.

In the modified van Lint block, the needle is inserted 1 cm lateral to the lateral orbital rim (Fig. 2–5), and 2 to 4 ml of anesthetic is injected deeply on the periosteum just lateral to the superolateral and inferolateral orbital rim.[24] For the O'Brien facial nerve block, the mandibular condyle is palpated inferior to the posterior zygomatic process and anterior to the tragus of the ear as the patient opens and closes the jaw.[25] The needle is inserted perpendicular to the skin about 1 cm to the periosteum. As the needle is withdrawn, 3 ml of anesthetic is injected.

A facial nerve block that provides the most complete akinesia is that described by Spaeth.[26] This is preferable to the Nadbath-Rehman block, because it provides equally complete akinesia, but with less risk. In the Spaeth block the facial nerve is anesthetized where it

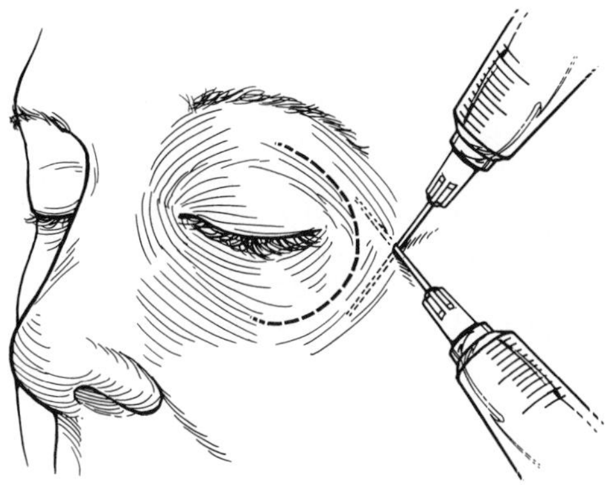

Figure 2–5. Modified Van Lint technique of facial nerve block. In the modified Van Lint block, the needle is inserted 1 cm lateral orbital rim, and 2 to 4 ml of anesthetic is injected deeply on the periosteum just lateral to the superolateral and inferolateral orbital rim.

crosses the posterior edge of the mandible, thus catching the nerve before it divides (Fig. 2–6). To perform the Spaeth block, the fingers are placed along the posterior border of the mandible as superiorly as possible. The needle is placed just anterior to the most superior finger; the bone should be felt quickly as the needle penetrates. If not, the needle is withdrawn and landmarks rechecked before a second attempt is made. After the bone is reached, traction on the plunger assures the vessel has not been punctured. Then 5 mL of anesthetic is injected. Although not necessary, the needle can be pulled back until it rests under the skin and then directed slightly superior towards the outer canthus for a distance of 1½ inches, where an additional 5 mL is injected. An almost complete unilateral facial palsy should be evidenced by 30 seconds.

The local anesthetic solution used most at our institution is a combination of bupivacaine 0.75% and lidocaine 2% in a 1:1 ratio with epinephrine. Hyaluronidase is added to speed tissue penetration. Alternately, mepivicaine 2% with epinephrine may be used. In all cases injection should be slow (1 ml per 10 sec) so as to minimize discomfort to the patient.

GENERAL ANESTHESIA

General anesthesia is used in approximately 35% of the ophthalmic surgery cases at our institution. The most common indications for general anesthesia are lengthy vitreoretinal surgery and pediatric strabismus surgery. Indications for general anesthesia include the following:

- Inability of the patient to cooperate with Monitored Anesthesia Care (MAC; e.g., children, adults with mental or psychological deficits, tremor, inability to lie supine, etc.)
- Complete ocular akinesia desired by surgeon
- Lengthy procedure (longer than 3 to 4 hours)
- Surgical field not amenable to regional, local, or topical anesthesia
- Regional block technically difficult or contraindicated (e.g., large myopic globe, coagulopathy, etc.)
- Following inadvertent intrathecal or intravascular injection of local anesthetic
- Surgeon or patient preference

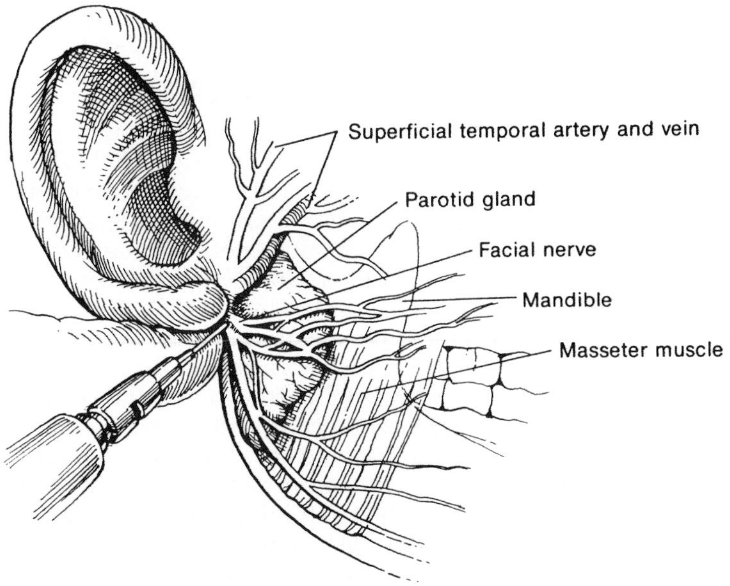

Figure 2–6. In the Spaeth modification of the O'Brien technique, the facial nerve is blocked where it crosses the posterior edge of the mandible, thus catching the nerve before it divides. This provides more complete paralysis of the inferior orbicular muscle.

Controversy exists as to the relative safety of general and regional anesthesia in ophthalmic surgery. The two techniques have shown no postoperative differences with regard to patient memory,[27] cognitive function,[28] or oxygen saturation.[29] The incidences of death and major complications are also similar.[30] However, regional anesthesia has been reported to be associated with fewer episodes of intraoperative oxygen desaturation, hemodynamic fluctuation,[28] postoperative nausea and vomiting (PONV),[30] and initial postoperative pain.[31] Regional anesthesia for ophthalmic surgery has also been shown to be free of the hormonal stress responses associated with general anesthesia.[32,33] With these considerations in mind, it is prudent to avoid general anesthesia, if possible, in patients with severe cardiovascular or pulmonary disease and in those who are prone to PONV.

The goals of general anesthesia for ophthalmic surgery include a smooth induction with stable intraocular pressure, avoidance or treatment of severe oculocardiac reflexes, maintenance of a motionless field, a smooth emergence, and avoidance of PONV. These goals can be accomplished in a variety of ways, using inhalation anesthesia, intravenous agents or a combined technique. Muscle relaxants are indicated during intraocular microsurgery when the slightest patient movement can be disastrous.

"Deep extubation" is a term used to describe the extubation of a patient before complete awakening has occurred. It is indicated whenever there is a compromised globe, intravitreal gas or whenever it is essential to avoid an increase in intraocular pressure from tracheal stimulation. Deep extubation is accomplished just after the patient has passed through anesthesia "stage 2," which is classically described as "delirium," into "stage 1," "analgesia." This stage of anesthesia is characterized by slow regular breathing with diaphragm and intercostal muscles, and the presence of a lid reflex. A patient extubated at this time experiences amnesia, analgesia, and sedation. Extubations at this point have a minimum of tracheal stimulation, but there is a small possibility of aspiration because airway reflexes have not completely returned. Therefore, a patient with a full stomach (having recently ingested food or drink prior to surgery), or a patient with a compromised airway is not a good candidate for deep extubation.

COMPLICATIONS OF OCULAR ANESTHESIA

OCULOCARDIAC REFLEX

The oculocardiac reflex (OCR) is caused by traction on the extraocular muscles, manipulation of the globe, or an increase in intraocular pressure. It is most commonly described as occurring during eye muscle surgery, but it is common during retinal detachment repair and enucleation as well. The oculocardiac reflex has also been observed after retrobulbar block and retrobulbar hemorrhage. The oculocardiac reflex may be manifested as bradycardia, and also by bigeminy, ectopic beats, nodal rhythms, atrioventricular block, and asystole. These dysrhythmias may persist as long as the stimuli are present. Repeated stimuli cause fatigue with diminished vagal effects.

Diagnosis of the OCR relies upon continuous monitoring of the electrocardiogram. Treatment varies based upon the severity of the reflex. If the reflex manifests itself as bradycardia or infrequent ectopic beats, and the blood pressure remains stable, no treatment may be justified. If the dysrhythmias become significant, cessation of the surgical stimuli is indicated. Commonly, the procedure may resume after a brief pause. The OCR fatigues easily and usually there is little or no activity after a brief pause in surgical stimuli. When OCR is severe, treatment with anticholinergics (glycopyrrolate or atropine) is indicated. Caution must be exercised with large doses of atropine, because more severe, prolonged tachydysrhythmias may result.[34]

INTRAOCULAR PRESSURE

Intraocular pressure may be increased significantly during induction or emergence from general anesthesia. Coughing, straining, bucking, breath-holding, obstructed airway, or Valsalva maneuvers can elevate the intraocular pressure as much as 30 to 40 mm Hg. Similarly, external pressure from the face mask will increase intraocular pressure.

Many anesthetic agents, both inhalational and intravenous, alter the production or drainage of the aqueous humor and consequently can affect the intraocular pressure (Table 2–4).

Succinylcholine causes a 6 to 12 mm Hg increase in intraocular pressure, which can be sustained for 5 to 10 minutes.[35-38] This pressure increase, ascribed to the contraction of the extraocular muscles leading to compression of the globe, could lead to extrusion of intraocular contents in a patient with an open globe injury. Therefore, although recent studies suggest that this agent does not stimulate extraocular muscle contraction, the use of succinylcholine is not advised for induction in cases of open globe injury.

ANESTHESIA FOR PEDIATRIC PROCEDURES

Anesthesia for pediatric ophthalmology encompasses a diverse group of patients and procedures. It has been said that pediatric ophthalmic anesthesiology can be considered a subspecialty in and of itself.[39] Many ophthalmic procedures that are done in adults with MAC require general anesthesia in the pediatric population.

For a variety of conditions, examination under anesthesia (EUA) is required for the young child. Because anesthetic agents, laryngoscopy, and intubation can affect the intraocular pressure, most ophthalmologists prefer to measure pressure before a deep level of anesthesia has been reached and intubation has been performed. This is accomplished by positioning the mask so that there is unobstructed access to the eye. If neces-

TABLE 2-4. Common Anesthetic Drugs and Their Effect on Intraocular Pressure

Agent	Dose	Route	Effect on Intraocular Pressure
Unknown or No effect			
Alfentanil	5 mcg/kg	Intravenous	No effect
Atracurium	0.4–0.5 mg/kg	Intravenous	No effect
Atropine	0.4–1.0 mg	Intramuscular	No effect
Flumazenil	0.0025 mg/kg	Intravenous	No effect
Glycopyrrolate	0.2–0.4 mg	Intravenous	No effect
Merperidine	50–100 mg	Intramuscular	May increase, normally no effect
Nitrous Oxide	70%	Inhalation	No effect
Remifentanil	0.5 mcg/kg	Intravenous	No effect
Scopolamine	0.4 mg	Intramuscular	No effect
Vecuronium	0.08–0.1 mg/kg	Intravenous	No effect
Drugs that Increase Intraocular Pressure			
Ketamine	1–2 mg/kg	Intravenous	Increased
Ketamine	5 mg/kg	Intramuscular	Slight increase
Succinylcholine	1–2 mg/kg	Intravenous	18% increase
Drugs that Decrease Intraocular Pressure			
Chlorpromazine	10–25 mg	Intramuscular	20%–30% decrease
Curare	0.5–0.6 mg/kg	Intravenous	Slight decrease
Dexmedetomidine	1 mcg/kg	Intravenous	40% decreased
Diazepam	10 mg	Intravenous	Decrease
Dilaudid	1–2 mg	Intravenous	Decrease
Desflurane	6–12%	Inhalation	30% decrease
Droperidol	5–10 mg	Intravenous	12% decrease
Enflurane	1% with N_2O	Inhalation	35%–40% decrease
Etomidate	0.3 mg/kg	Intravenous	30% decrease
Fentanyl	50–100 mcg	Intramuscular	20% decrease
Haloperidol	0.5 mg	Intravenous	15% decrease
Halothane	1 MAC	Inhalation	14%–33% decrease
Isoflurane	1%–3%	Inhalation	40% decrease
Lidocaine	1.5 mg/kg	Intravenous	Decrease
Metocurine	0.3–0.4 mg/kg	Intravenous	Slight decrease
Metocurine + Pancuronium	0.4–0.5 mg/kg	Intravenous	Slight decrease
Midazolam	0.15 mg/kg	Intravenous	25% decrease
Morphine	8–15 mg	Intramuscular	Decrease
Pancuronium	0.05 mg/kg	Intravenous	Slight decrease
Propofol	1–2 mg/kg	Intravenous	Decrease
Pentothal	3–5 mg/kg	Intravenous	30% decrease
Methohexital	6 mg/kg	Intravenous	Decrease
Sevoflurane	1%–3% with N_2O	Inhalation	40% decrease
Sufentanil	1–2 mcg/kg	Intravenous	Decrease
Thiamylal	4–5 mg/kg	Intravenous	Decrease
Thiopentone	2.5 mg/kg	Intravenous	30% decrease

sary, the mask can be removed to allow measurement of the pressure and then replaced.

Strabismus surgery frequently stimulates the oculocardiac reflex (OCR). This reflex is elicited by traction on the extraocular muscles and is manifested primarily as bradycardia, but also by bigeminy, ectopic beats, nodal rhythms, atrioventricular block, and asystole. In many cases, no treatment is necessary. However, if the dysrhythmias become significant, cessation of the surgical stimuli is indicated. When OCR is severe, treatment with anticholinergics (glycopyrrolate or atropine) is necessary.

Postoperative nausea and vomiting have been reported to occur in more than 50% of pediatric strabismus patients. Many different anesthetic techniques and anti-emetic regimens have been used in an attempt to decrease this high incidence. Propofol infusion has been shown to be effective in many cases, and has become widely used in outpatient surgical settings, with halothane discontinued following induction of anesthesia.

Postoperative emesis is multifactorial; which patients should get prophylactic antiemetics is controversial. We recommend prophylaxis for those patients with a history of motion sickness, previous history of postoperative nausea, obesity, and anxiety. We recommend 0.1 mg/kg ondansetron, a selective 5HT3 receptor antagonist.

ANESTHESIA FOR VITREORETINAL PROCEDURES

Vitreoretinal surgery offers challenges to the anesthesiologist because the surgery is often lengthy and many of the patients are diabetic and/or hypertensive.[40] Although general anesthesia has been used traditionally, local anesthesia with MAC has increased in popularity. If necessary, the retrobulbar block can be supplemented intraoperatively with a parabulbar sub-tenon's injection using a blunt 19-gauge cannula.[41] When general anesthesia is used, there are advantages to supplementation with long-acting parabulbar anesthesia administered by the same technique. This eliminates the risk of scleral perforation and reduces the amount of pain and nausea in the postoperative period.[42]

Frequently, intravitreal gas (SF6 or C3F8) is administered after retinal reattachment. If nitrous oxide is being used as an anesthetic, and is administered after injection of the gas bubble, the N_2O will enter the intraocular gas bubble, expanding the size of the bubble. This can cause transient elevation of the intraocular pressure. However, when the nitrous oxide is discontinued, the pressure will normalize; however, the gas bubble will also shrink and this could lead to inadequate tamponade. Therefore, N_2O should be discontinued at least 20 minutes before intravitreal gas injection.

KEY POINTS

1. Although the ophthalmic surgical procedure is considered "low-risk" in terms of blood loss, third-spacing of fluids, and postoperative pain, the patient population as a whole tends to be a "high-risk" group, which necessitates appropriate preoperative medical consultation.
2. Whereas true emergencies such as central retinal artery occlusion caused by orbital hemorrhage require immediate therapy, urgent situations such as penetrating injuries to the globe can be delayed in many cases for several hours, to allow time to carry out an appropriate anesthetic plan regarding NPO status and the general condition of the patient.
3. Neither regional nor general anesthesia has been demonstrated to be safer in ophthalmic surgery; however, regional anesthesia offers some advantages, such as less postoperative nausea and vomiting, greater cardiopulmonary stability, quicker return to ambulation, and prolonged postoperative analgesia.
4. Pressure on the globe or traction on the extraocular muscles can stimulate the oculocardiac reflex and cause bradycardia, AV block, ventricular ectopy, or asystole.
5. Deep inhalational or thiopental anesthesia can decrease the intraocular pressure, whereas ketamine or succinylcholine can increase the pressure, which in an open globe injury may result in extravasation of intraocular contents.
6. Complications of the peribulbar/retrobulbar orbital anesthesia for akinesia and anesthesia of the eye include retrobulbar hemorrhage, globe perforation, increased intraocular pressure, accidental intravascular injection with CNS excitation and convulsions, and subarachnoid extension with resultant obtundation and respiratory arrest.
7. Nitrous oxide should not be used for 20 minutes before the use of intravitreal gas in vitreoretinal surgery, and should be avoided for 3-4 weeks thereafter to prevent expansion and a significant increase in intraocular pressure.

BIBLIOGRAPHY

1. Bruce RA Jr: Ocular anatomy. In Bruce RA Jr, McGoldrick KE, Oppenheimer P (eds.), Anesthesia for Ophthalmology, Birmingham, Alabama, Aesculapius Publishing; 1982.
2. Campbell DNC, Lim M, Kerr Muir M, et al.: A prospective randomized study of local versus general anaesthesia for cataract surgery. Anaesthesia 1993;48:422–8.
3. Donlon JV: Local anesthesia for ophthalmic surgery: patient preparation and management, Ann Ophthalmol 1980,12:1183.
4. Duncalf D: Anesthesia and intraocular pressure, Bull NY Acad Med 1975;51:374,.
5. Stead SW: Complications in ophthalmic anesthesiology, Semin Anesth 1996;15:171–82.

REFERENCES

1. Kraushar MF, Turner MF: Medical malpractice litigation in cataract surgery. Arch Ophthalmol 1987;105:1339.
2. Fine IH, Fichman RA, Grabow HB: Clear-Corneal Cataract Surgery and Topical Anesthesia. Thorofare, N.J.: Slack, Inc;1993.
3. Patel BCK, Burns TA, Crandall A, et al.: A comparison of topical and retrobulbar anesthesia for cataract surgery. Ophthalmology 1996;103:1196–203.
4. Fraser SG, Siriwadena D, Jamieson H, Girault J, et al.: Indicators of patient suitability for topical anesthesia. J Cataract Refract Surg 1997;23:781–3.
5. Zehetmayer M, Rainer G, Turnheim K, et al.: Topical anesthesia with pH-adjusted versus standard lidocaine 4% for clear corneal cataract surgery. J Cataract Refract Surg 1997;23:1390–3.
6. Rosenthal KJ: Deep, topical, nerve-block anesthesia. Cataract Refract Surg 1995;21:499–503.
7. Bloomberg LB, Pellican KJ: Topical anesthesia using the Bloomberg SuperNumb Anesthetic Ring. Cataract Refract Surg 1995;21:16–20.
8. Judge AJ, Najafi K, Lee DA, Miller KM: Corneal endothelial toxicity of topical anesthesia. Ophthalmology 1997;104:1373–9.
9. Britton B, Hervey R, Casten K, et al.: Intraocular irritation evaluation of benzalkonium chloride in rabbits. Ophthalmic Surg 1976;7:46–55.
10. Bergman L: Significant developments in local anesthesia. In Highlights of Ophthalmology, Boyd BF (ed.) 1995;23(6):56.
11. Aleman CE: Significant developments in local anesthesia, Boyd BF (ed.), Highlights of Ophthalmology, 1995;23:65.
12. Davis DB, Mandel MR: Efficacy and complication rate of 16,224 consecutive peribulbar blocks. J Cataract Refract Surg 1994; 20:327–37.
13. Beatie CD, Stead SW: Cardiorespiratory stability and amnesia with propofol and alfentanil sedation. Anesthesiology 1992;77.
14. Straatsma BR: Current concepts of cataract surgery and lens implantation—inferotemporal retrobulbar anesthesia: minimizing patient discomfort. In Koo CY, Ang BC, Cheah WM, et al. (eds.), New frontiers in ophthalmology. Proceedings of the XXVI International Congress of Ophthalmology, Singapore, March 1990. Exerpta Medica 1991;103–6.
15. Kaplan LJ, Jaffee NS, Clayman HM: Ptosis and cataract surgery. Ophthalmology 1985;92:237–42.
16. Atkinson WS: Akinesia of the orbicularis. Am J Ophthalmol 1953;26:1255–8.
17. Unsöld R, Stanley J, DeGroot J: The CT topography of retrobulbar anesthesia. Anatomic-clinical correlation of complications and suggestion of a modifed technique. Graefes Arch Klin Ophthalmol 1981;217:125–36.

18. Ropo A, Nikki P, Ruusuvaara P, Kivisaari L: Comparison of retrobulbar and periocular injections of lignocaine by computerised tomography, Br J Ophthalmol 1991;75:417–20.
19. Hamilton RC, Gimbel HV, Strunin L: Regional anesthesia for 12,000 cataract extraction and intraocular lens implantation procedures, Can J Anaesth 1988;35:615–23.
20. Edge KR, Nicoll JMV: Retrobulbar hemorrhage after 12,500 retrobulbar blocks. Anesth Analg 1993;76:1019–22.
21. Gills JP, Loyd T: Anesthesia for ophthalmic surgery. In Gills JP, Hustead RF, Sanders DR (eds.), Thorofore, N.J.: Slack, Inc.; 1993: 128–31.
22. Duker JS, Belmont JB, Benson WE, et al.: Inadvertent globe perforation during retrobulbar and peribulbar anesthesia: patient characteristics, surgical management, and visual outcome. Ophthalmology 1991;98:519–26.
23. Hunter DG, Lam GC, Guyton DL: Inferior oblique muscle injury from local anesthesia for cataract surgery. Ophthalmology 1995;102:501–9.
24. Van Lint: Paralysis palperbrale temporaire provoquée dans l'operation de la cataracte. Ann Occul 1914;151:420.
25. O'Brien CS: Local anesthesia in ophthalmic surgery. Trans Sect Ophthalmol AMA 1927;237:253.
26. Spaeth GL: A new method to achieve complete akinesia of the facial muscles of the eyelids. Ophthalmic Surg 1976;7:105–9.
26a. Nadbath RP, Rehman I: Facial nerve block. Am J Ophthalmol 1963;55:143.
27. Karhunen U, Jonn G: A comparison of memory function following local and general anesthesia for extraction of senile cataract. Acta Anaesthesiol Scand 1982;26:291.
28. Campbell DNC, Lim M, Kerr Muir M: A prospective randomised study of local versus general anaesthesia for cataract surgery. Anaesthesia 1993;48:422–8.
29. McCarthy GJ, Mirakhur RK, Elliott P: Postoperative oxygenation in the elderly following general or local anaesthesia for ophthalmic surgery. Anaesthesia 1992;47:1090–2.
30. Lynch S, Wolf GL, Berlin I: General anesthesia for cataract surgery: a comparative review of 2217 consecutive cases. Anesth Analg 1974;53:909.
31. Koay P, Laing A, Adams K, et al.: Ophthalmic pain following cataract surgery: a comparison between local and general anesthesia. BJ Ophthalmol 1992;76:225–7.
32. Barker JP, Robinson GC, Vafidis GC, et al.: Local analgesia prevents the cortisol and glycaemic response to cataract surgery. Br J Anaesth 1990;64:442.
33. Barker JP, Vafdis GC, Robinson PN, Hall GM: Plasma catecholamine response to cataract surgery: a comparison between general and local anaesthesia. Anaesthesia 1991;46:642.
34. Katz RL, Bigger JT: Cardiac arrhythmias during anesthesia and operation. Anesthesiology 1970;33:193–213.
35. Cook JH: The effect of suxamethonium on intraocular pressure. Anaesthesia 1981;36:359.
36. Petruscak J, Smith RB, Breslin P: Mortality related to ophthalmical surgery. Arch Ophthalmol 1973;89:106.
37. Wynands JE, Crowell DE: Intraocular tension in association with succinylcholine and endotracheal intubation, Can Anaesth Soc J 1960;7:39.
38. Arthur DS, Dewar KMS: Anaesthesia for eye surgery in children, Br J Anaesthesiol 1980;52:681.
39. Brucker AJ, Saran BR, Maguire AM: Perilimbal anesthesia for pars plana vitrectomy. Am J Ophthalmol 1994;117:599–602.
40. Murat J, Chauvaud D: Evaluation of a simplified protocol of local regional anesthesia for the surgery of the posterior segment. Ophthalmol 1993;16:254.

CHAPTER 3

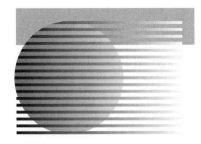

Prevention of Infection

TRAVIS A. MEREDITH, M.D.

Postoperative infection remains a feared complication of intraocular surgery, and strategies to prevent its occurrence remain important in surgical management. The incidence of postoperative endophthalmitis has remained about the same in series spanning more than 20 years from major eye institutes.[1,2] Intraocular surgery is complicated by infection in approximately 0.08% of elective cases, relatively rare as compared with rates of 2% to 3% in abdominal surgery. Infection rates vary by procedure: cataract extraction, 0.072%; secondary lens implantation, 0.03%; penetrating keratoplasty, 0.11%; glaucoma procedures, 0.061%; pars plana vitrectomy, 0.051%.[2] The rate of infection is nearly 100 times greater after repair of penetrating trauma, ranging from 1% to as high as 30%, depending on the circumstances of the injury.[3,4]

The source of pathogens in elective surgery is usually the patient's own conjunctival flora[5]; in ocular trauma, organisms from the site of the injury may also be introduced into the eye. In studies of the normal conjunctival flora most subjects harbor potential pathogens[6]; the most common isolates are staphylococci. Coagulase-negative staphylococci are by far the predominating cause of culture-positive endophthalmitis.[7] Chronic infections of the conjunctiva, lids, canaliculus, and lacrimal sac[8] increase the likelihood of introducing pathogenic bacteria into the eye during surgery. Cultures of anterior chamber aspirates after cataract extraction have found positive cultures in 5% to 43% of cases.[9–11] That endophthalmitis is a relatively rare event by comparison suggests that the eye clears these bacteria well[12] and has other mechanisms that prevent infection.

Contamination from materials used in surgery causing subsequent infection is a less common event. Epidemics resulting from contaminated solutions have been reported,[13–15] however, and instruments or intraocular lenses can occasionally transmit pathogens. Donor corneas may also be a source of infection.[16]

In addition to preoperative factors, higher rates of postoperative infection have been linked to features of the surgical procedure itself. Eyes with a capsular tear, those requiring vitrectomy at cataract extraction, and eyes implanted with lenses with polypropylene haptics have each been demonstrated to have greater risk of postoperative infection.[17]

Certain patients have a higher risk of endophthalmitis. Diabetic patients[2] and those who are immunosuppressed by either medications or HIV infection have an increased risk.

STRATEGIC RATIONALE

Because introduction of bacteria into the eye at the time of surgery is the cause of most cases of endophthalmitis, the strategic goals are these: (1) reduce the number of bacteria in the operating field and on materials introduced into the eye; (2) provide subsequent antibiotic treatment to reduce the likelihood of frank infection either from bacteria that entered the eye or those that could gain access in the immediate postoperative period. Treatment of preexisting infection of the external eye and adnexae is of obvious importance. The prophylactic use of antiseptics and antibiotics, usually in tandem, is designed to reduce bacteria on the skin and conjunctiva (Table 3–1). Antiseptics kill on contact, while a longer exposure of the bacteria to antibiotics is necessary for killing. The operating field should be isolated from the surrounding area by draping, and meticulous intraoperative sterile technique is essential.

TABLE 3–1. Prophylaxis of Elective Intraocular Surgery

Treatment of preexisting lid and lacrimal disease
Use of plastic-backed adhesive drapes
Topical povidone-iodine applied to the periorbital skin, lashes, and conjunctival sac
Preoperative and postoperative topical antibiotics; possible use of subconjunctival antibiotics

PREPARATION OF THE PATIENT

When elective surgery is scheduled the examination should specially address potential sources of postoperative infection. Chronic blepharitis, styes, or dacryocystitis are findings that should delay surgery until they are effectively treated. In years past preoperative face scrubs the night before surgery were routine in some institutions. Though probably not frequently employed in the era of same-day surgery, they may have a role in preparation of the patient with poor personal hygiene.

The technique for the preoperative preparation of the patient in the operating room may vary from institution to institution, but certain features are common. Some surgeons prefer to cut the eyelashes, because long lashes may rub on instruments as they are introduced into the eye. Antisepsis with povidone-iodine has been demonstrated to decrease the bacterial population of the conjunctival sac and eyelids.[18,19] Placement of two drops of povidone-iodine 5% into the conjunctival sac for 1 to 2 minutes during preparation has been demonstrated to reduce the incidence of endophthalmitis significantly when compared to conjunctival antisepsis with silver protein solution.[19] The lids and lashes are prepared separately with cotton-tipped swabs soaked in povidone-iodine 5% or 10%, and the skin is then scrubbed with gauze pads in a broad area extending to the upper lip, the hairline, and across the nose to the opposite canthus. The povidone-iodine is then washed out of the conjunctival sac, and the lids and skin are dried with sterile gauze and cotton-tipped swabs.

A variety of drapes are available to isolate the periorbital skin from the rest of the face. The most important step is careful application of an adhesive-backed plastic drape to seal off the operative area. If possible the lashes should be turned under the drape to keep them out of the operative field.[20]

ANTIBIOTIC PROPHYLAXIS

ROUTINE INTRAOCULAR SURGERY

In ophthalmology the preponderance of evidence favors prophylactic use of perioperative antibiotics to reduce the incidence of postoperative infection,[21] but the choice of antibiotic, route of administration, dosing frequency, and timing of administration are not well defined by any clinical studies. The benefits of prophylaxis must be weighed against the risks of toxic and allergic reactions, the emergence of resistant bacteria, and the cost–benefit ratio of the antibiotic administered. In routine cataract surgery the incidence of endophthalmitis is approximately one in 1200 cases, and one half of the affected eyes recover 20/50 vision.[22] Thus the potential risks and costs of aggressive prophylaxis must be balanced against the fact that serious visual loss from postoperative infection will occur in only about one in 2400 cataract operations. In traumatic cases the incidence of infection is much higher and the outcome significantly worse, thus altering the equation. The number of cataract extractions in the United States on a yearly basis is approaching 1.5 million, and when other intraocular procedures are added both the cost and the potential impact of widespread antibiotic prophylaxis on bacterial populations is significant.

Evidence from general surgery demonstrates that prophylactic systemic antibiotics given within the two hours before incision significantly reduce the incidence of postoperative infection, and such treatment is therefore recommended for many cases.[23,24] Preoperative topical antibiotics have been demonstrated to reduce conjunctival bacterial counts,[25,26] which in turn might be expected to reduce bacterial introduction into the eye and subsequent development of endophthalmitis. Consistently sterilizing the ocular surface preoperatively is extremely difficult,[26] and the best to be hoped for is a reduction in the total number of organisms. One study performed in the era of intracapsular cataract extraction demonstrated a tenfold increase in endophthalmitis in patients not given topical antibiotics prior to surgery compared to a treated group.[1]

Because there are multiple species of bacteria in the conjunctival sac, broad-spectrum antibiotic prophylaxis is necessary. Fluoroquinolones, aminoglycosides, or combinations of antibiotics are preferred for preoperative administration. The routine use of vancomycin has been strongly discouraged by the Centers for Disease Control and Prevention (CDC) because the emergence of vancomycin-resistant staphylococci will pose a serious and difficult problem for infectious disease management in general.[20,27]

Antibiotics are frequently given at the end of the surgical procedure by topical drops, subconjunctival injection, or collagen shield. The logical goal of this strategy is to kill organisms already in the eye, or to kill those on the ocular surface, which might subsequently migrate through the surgical wound. Although aqueous humor antibiotic concentrations are higher after subconjunctival injection than after topical administration, there is still marginal penetration of most anti-biotics into postsurgical eyes.[28–33] In animal studies ceftazidime,[34] gentamicin,[35] or ciprofloxacin[36] given subconjunctivally have been demonstrated, however, to reduce the incidence of infection compared with controls. One study from a university eye service demonstrated a lower incidence of endophthalmitis in patients treated at the end of surgery with subconjunctivalinjections of penicillin G.[37] In two large series from cataract camps in India and

Pakistan, all patients were given preoperative topical antibiotics. In one study of 54,000 patients there was no decrease in endophthalmitis in those patients also given postoperative subconjunctival antibiotic injections.[38] In a second series of 23,900 patients, patients given both preoperative topical antibiotics and subconjunctival injections had lower rates of infection than those given only topical antibiotics.[39] Great care must be taken, however, because inadvertent penetration of the eye with the needle, when administering a subconjunctival injection can deliver potentially devastating concentrations of drug into the eye.[40]

Collagen shields offer another alternative for delivering antibiotic to the surface of the eye after surgery. The actual efficiency of delivering antibiotic to the anterior chamber and the efficacy in reducing the incidence of endophthalmitis has not been reported. Both collagen shields and subconjunctival administration have some risk of delivering unacceptably high concentrations of antibiotic into the eye when adequate closure of the cataract wound has not been achieved.

Adding antibiotic to the infusion fluid for cataract surgery has been advocated (Table 3–2).[41] One study demonstrated a slight but statistically insignificant reduction of bacterial counts in the eyes treated with this regimen,[42] and endophthalmitis has been reported despite use of antibiotics in the infusion fluid.[43] There are few data on safe dosages for this route, and the possibility of a dosage error is a major problem.[44] In some surgical centers many cases are performed using a single bag of infusion fluid mixed at the beginning of the day; a dosage error in mixing the antibiotic into the solution will thus affect multiple patients. Furthermore, the choice of an appropriate antibiotic is difficult. The target organisms are predominately gram-positive, particularly coagulase-negative staphylococci. A significant number of these organisms are resistant to beta-lactam antibiotics. Vancomycin has the broadest gram-positive coverage for potential pathogens, but it should be avoided for prophylaxis in line with CDC recommendations. Intraocular gentamicin is known to produce macular infarction.[40] Given the low incidence of severe visual loss from postoperative endophthalmitis, this route of administration should be used judiciously until studies prove it to be safe and effective.[20]

TABLE 3–2. Considerations for Intraocular Antibiotic Prophylaxis

Pro	Con
Attempt to reduce incidence of intraocular infection	Failure to be 100% effective
	Potential for iatrogenic harm (dilutional errors, allergic reactions)
	Cost
	Promotion of emergence of resistant microorganisms

ROUTINE EXTRAOCULAR SURGERY

Surgery of the lids, orbit, and lacrimal system is rarely complicated by postoperative infection. Standard preoperative antisepsis and draping are employed, and perioperative antimicrobial therapy is used less frequently than in intraocular surgery. The decision to administer either preoperative or postoperative antimicrobials is usually made on a case-by-case basis.

Some surgeons will often give oral antibiotics after lacrimal surgery. In orbital surgery, if the procedure becomes prolonged, intraoperative antibiotics and postoperative antibiotics are sometimes administered intravenously. Other criteria for administration of postoperative antibiotics would depend on the surgeon and could include the presence of a large amount of devitalized tissue, inadvertent contamination of the operative field, an excessively long operating time, heavy use of intraoperative cautery, or extensive flap preparation with poor vascular supply.

CONTAMINATED WOUNDS

Antimicrobial treatment is commonly recommended after penetrating trauma. Clinical series in which this issue has been examined have demonstrated that patients with posttraumatic endophthalmitis have usually received systemic antibiotics that failed to prevent the infection.[45,46] Should patients with penetrating trauma routinely be given antibiotics and, if so, which medications and by which routes? In the absence of data from controlled trials a definitive answer is not possible, but the weight of evidence seems to suggest a beneficial although limited effect.

An ideal antibiotic regimen for treatment in this setting would have the following characteristics: (1) activity against commonly encountered gram-positive organisms, especially *Bacillus*, streptococci, and staphylococci; (2) activity against gram-negative bacteria; (3) good intraocular penetration after intravenous administration; (4) low toxicity after intraocular injection; (5) demonstrated prophylactic efficacy in animal and human trials. Unfortunately no single antimicrobial or combination of antibiotics meets all these criteria.

The best choice of antimicrobial agents depends in part on the route of administration.

Topical Antibiotics

Topical administration of antimicrobials before surgery may be considered in some cases. When the cornea is lacerated so that the full-strength antibiotic may gain access to the anterior chamber, topical administration should probably be avoided. When the globe is ruptured and the penetration site is beneath the conjunctiva, antibiotic administration may help to reduce the bacterial load in the operative field during the surgical repair. A broad-spectrum choice such as an aminoglycoside or combination antibiotic is commonly used.

Subconjunctival Antibiotics

Antibiotics are commonly given subconjunctivally at the close of surgery. Their penetration into the eye from this location is limited[28–30,34] and the beneficial effects are probably limited to the anterior chamber and the external eye.

Intravenous Antibiotics

Most texts on trauma and many authors[45–47] recommend intravenous antibiotic treatment in penetrating trauma, despite lack of any trials to demonstrate efficacy. Treatment is clearly not uniformly effective because most patients who develop infection have received antibiotics. A major difficulty is the poor penetration of antibiotics into the vitreous cavity after intravenous administration. Although inflammation increases intraocular penetration, not all antibiotics enter the eye equally well. In experimental studies of traumatized eyes, aminoglycosides have particularly poor penetration.[48,49] One study demonstrated no effect in preventing experimental *Pseudomonas* endophthalmitis.[50] Administration of intravenous amikacin for the treatment of endophthalmitis in the endophthalmitis vitrectomy study (EVS) was not associated with improved visual outcomes.[51] Therefore aminoglycosides for intravenous administration should probably be abandoned.

Cefazolin has been studied in pig and swine models[48,52–54] of ocular trauma. Trauma leads to a breakdown of the blood–retina barrier and was shown to significantly increase the penetration of cefazolin into the anterior chamber and vitreous cavity after repeated doses. Intravenous cefazolin was begun 1 hour after inoculation of *Staphylococcus epidermidis* into an eye with a standardized penetrating injury.[53] Repeated dosing over two to three days prevented development of infection as compared to controls. Many staphylococci, *E. coli, Klebsiella,* and *Proteus* organisms are susceptible to cefazolin. However, *Bacillus* organisms are not sensitive and over half of the staphylococcal organisms from hospital microbiology laboratories, and many coagulase-negative staphylococci are not sensitive. Thus the utility of cefazolin against the most important pathogens causing traumatic endophthalmitis is limited.

Ciprofloxacin penetration into the vitreous cavity was enhanced by trauma in a swine model to levels that exceeded the minimal inhibitory concentrations for *Staph. epidermidis, Bacillus,* and *Proteus,* but not for *Staph. aureus, Pseudomonas,* or *Streptococcus pneumoniae.*[55] Unfortunately, staphylococci are rapidly developing resistance to ciprofloxacin; more than 40% of recent coagulase-negative isolates and up to 60% of *Staph. aureus* isolates have not been sensitive.

Vancomycin has been demonstrated to penetrate into the vitreous cavity of inflamed eyes[56] but has not been studied in traumatized eyes. Vancomycin has good coverage for streptococci, staphylococcal organisms, and for *Bacillus,* and is therefore probably the best choice for systemic administration.

Ceftazidime also penetrates into inflamed eyes and has good gram-negative coverage, particularly against *Pseudomonas,* but it has poor gram-positive action.[57,58] Ceftazidime was demonstrated to prophylactically modulate an experimental *Pseudomonas* infection when administered within 4 hours of bacterial inoculation, but not when given 8 hours after bacteria were introduced into the vitreous cavity.[50]

Intraocular Antibiotics

Intraocular injections for potentially contaminated wounds have been advocated by some authors,[45] but because of potential complications this route of administration has not gained widespread acceptance. The main concerns are toxicity from the injected antibiotics (especially the aminoglycosides), and injury to the eye if a needle inserted for injection cannot be visualized because of the effects of the trauma. Nevertheless, very high concentrations of antibiotics can be attained by this route, and intraocular antibiotics are effective for treating established infections. In a study of infection in a swine model, intraocular injection of ciprofloxacin 100 μg prevented or modulated experimental *Bacillus* infections when the drug was given 1 or 6 hours after bacterial inoculation.[55]

High-risk cases such as foreign bodies in farm environments, penetrating injuries in rural settings, injuries contaminated with vegetable matter, and injuries from dental prostheses should probably be considered for intraocular treatment. Intraocular injections may be made at the close of a procedure when the needle tip can be visualized so that the risk of iatrogenic mechanical damage is reduced. At the close of vitrectomy surgery, injections may be made into the fluid-filled cavity. In our current state of knowledge, vancomycin 1 mg and either amikacin 200–400 mcg or ceftazidime 2.25 mg are likely to provide a significant intraocular concentration, which should cover most of the likely pathogens.

Surgical Intervention

Timing of surgical intervention for primary repair of injury may play a role in reducing the risk of traumatic endophthalmitis. One study demonstrated a significant number of positive cultures from eyes undergoing vitrectomy for intraocular foreign body even though subsequent infection did not develop.[59] In a study of microbial contamination at the time of open globe repair, anterior chamber fluid was positive in one third of cases, although no cases of endophthalmitis developed.[60] Although it cannot be known how many of these eyes would have developed infection without surgery and antibiotics, the findings suggest that earlier surgery may reduce the risk of infection. A review of a large number of cases of intraocular foreign bodies demonstrated that surgery carried out more than 24 hours after the trauma had a risk of infection four times higher than surgery performed within the first 24 hours.[61]

REFERENCES

1. Allen HF, Mangiaracine AB: Bacterial endophthalmitis after cataract extraction. II. Incidence in 36,000 consecutive operations with special reference to preoperative topical antibiotics. Trans Am Acad Ophthalmol Otolaryngol 1973;77:581–8.

2. Kattan HM, Flynn HW, Pflugfelder SC, et al.: Nosocomial endophthalmitis survey: Current incidence of infection following intraocular surgery. Ophthalmology 1991;98:227–38.
3. Boldt HC, Pulido JS, Blodi CS, et al.: Rural endophthalmitis. Ophthalmology 1989;96:1722–6.
4. Brinton GS, Topping TM, Hyndiuk RA, et al.: Posttraumatic endophthalmitis. Arch Ophthalmol 1984;102:547–50.
5. Speaker MG, Milch FA, Shah MK: Role of external bacterial flora in the pathogenesis of acute postoperative endophthalmitis. Ophthalmology 1991;98:639–50.
6. Taomy JA, Moller S, Weiss-Bentzon M: Bacterial flora in relation to cataract extraction. Acta Ophthalmol 1975;53:458–75.
7. Han DP, Wisniewski SR, Wilson LA, et al.: Spectrum and susceptibilities of microbiologic isolates in the Endophthalmitis Vitrectomy Study. Am J Ophthalmol 1996;122:1–17.
8. Lopez PF, Beldavs RA, Al-Ghamdi S, et al.: Pneumococcal endophthalmitis associated with nasolacrimal obstruction. Am J Ophthalmol 1993;116:56–62.
9. Dickey JB, Thompson KD, Jay WM: Anterior chamber aspirate cultures after uncomplicated cataract surgery. Am J Ophthalmol 1991;112:278–82.
10. Sherwood DR, Rich WJ, Jacob SJ, et al.: Bacterial contamination of intraocular and extraocular fluids during cataract extraction. Eye 1989;3:308–12.
11. Samad A, Solomon LD, Miller MA, Mendelson J: Anterior chamber contamination after uncomplicated phacoemulsification and intraocular lens implantation. Am J Ophthalmol 1995;120:143–50.
12. Maylath FR, Leopold IH: Study of experimental intraocular infection. I. The recoverability of organisms inoculated into ocular tissues and fluids. II. The influence of antibiotics and cortisone, alone and combined, on intraocular growth of these organisms. Am J Ophthalmol 1955;40:86–101.
13. O'Day DM: Value of a centralized surveillance system during a national epidemic of endophthalmitis. Ophthalmology 1985;92:309–14.
14. Pettit TH, Olson RJ, Foos RY, Martin WJ: Fungal endophthalmitis following intraocular lens implantation: A surgical epidemic. Arch Ophthalmol 1980;98:1025–39.
15. Stern WH, Tamura E, Jacobs RA, et al.: Epidemic postsurgical *Candida parapsilosis* endophthalmitis: Clinical findings and management of 15 consecutive cases. Ophthalmology 1985;92:1701–9.
16. Cameron JA, Antonios SR, Cotter JB, et al.: Endophthalmitis from contaminated donor corneas following penetrating keratoplasty. Arch Ophthalmol 1991;109:54–9.
17. Menikoff JA, Speaker MG, Marmor M, Raskin EM: A case-control study of risk factors for post-operative endophthalmitis. Ophthalmology 1991;98:1761–8.
18. Apt L, Isenberg SJ, Yoshimori R: Outpatient topical use of povidone-iodine in preparing the eye for surgery. Ophthalmology 1989;96:289–92.
19. Speaker MG, Menikoff JA: Prophylaxis of endophthalmitis with topical povidone-iodine. Ophthalmology 1991;98:1769–75.
20. Alfonso EC, Flynn HW Jr: Controversies in endophthalmitis prevention: The risk for emerging resistance to vancomycin. Arch Ophthalmol 1995;113:1369–70.
21. Starr MB, Lally JM: Antimicrobial prophylaxis for ophthalmic surgery. Surv Ophthalmol 1995;39:485–501.
22. Endophthalmitis Vitrectomy Study Group: Results of the Endophthalmitis Vitrectomy Study: A randomized trial of immediate vitrectomy and of intravenous antibiotics for the treatment of postoperative bacterial endophthalmitis. Arch Ophthalmol 1995;113:1479–96.
23. Wenzel RP: Preoperative antibiotic prophylaxis. N Engl J Med 1992;326:337–9.
24. Classen DC, Evans RS, Pestontnik SL, et al.: The timing of prophylactic administration of antibiotics and the risk of surgical wound infection. N Engl J Med 1992;326:281–6.
25. Whitney CR, Anderson RD, Allansmith MR: Preoperatively administered antibiotics: Their effects on bacterial counts of the eyelids. Arch Ophthalmol 1972;87:155–60.
26. Fahmy JA: Bacterial flora in relation to cataract extraction. V: Effects of topical antibiotics on the preoperative conjunctival flora. Acta Ophthalmol (Copenh) 1980;58:567–75.
27. CDC [Centers for Disease Control and Prevention]: Recommendations for preventing the spread of vancomycin resistance. MMWR Morb Mortal Wkly Rep 1995;44:1–13.
28. Barza M, Kane A, Baum J: Intraocular penetration of gentamicin after subconjunctival retrobulbar injection. Am J Ophthalmol 1978;85:541–7.
29. Barza M, Kane A, Baum JL: Intraocular levels of cefamandole compared with cefazolin after subconjunctival injection in rabbits. Invest Ophthalmol Vis Sci 1979;18:250–5.
30. Barza M, Lynch E, Baum JL: Pharmacokinetics of newer cephalosporins after subconjunctival and intravitreal injection in rabbits. Arch Ophthalmol 1993;111:121–5.
31. Barza M, Kane A, Baum J: Ocular penetration of subconjunctival oxacillin, methicillin, and cefazolin in rabbits with staphylococcal endophthalmitis. J Infect Dis 1982;145:899–903.
32. Donnenfeld ED, Perry HD, Snyder RW, et al.: Intracorneal, aqueous humor and vitreous humor penetration of topical and oral ofloxacin. Arch Ophthalmol 1997;115:173–6.
33. Donnenfeld ED, Schrier A, Perry HD, et al.: Penetration of topically applied ciprofloxacin, norfloxacin, and ofloxacin into the aqueous humor. Ophthalmology 1994;101:902–5.
34. Shockley RK, Fishman P, Aziz M, et al.: Subconjunctival administration of ceftazidime in pigmented rabbit eyes. Arch Ophthalmol 1986;104:266–8.
35. Elliott RD, Katz HR: Inhibition of pseudophakic endophthalmitis in a rabbit model. Ophthalmic Surg 1987;1987:538–41.
36. Parks DJ, Cyryin AS, Sarfarazi FA, Katz HR: Subconjunctival ciprofloxacin inhibits pseudophakic endophthalmitis in a rabbit model. Invest Ophthalmol Vis Sci 1991;34(Suppl 4):706.
37. Kolker AE, Freeman MI, Pettit TH: Prophylactic antibiotics and post-operative endophthalmitis. Am J Ophthalmol 1967;63:434–9.
38. Christy NE, Lall P: A randomized, controlled comparison of anterior and posterior periocular injection of antibiotic in the prevention of postoperative endophthalmitis. Ophthalmic Surg 1986;17:715–8.
39. Christy NE, Sommer A: Antibiotic prophylaxis of postoperative endophthalmitis. Ann Ophthalmol 1979;1261–5.
40. Campochiaro PA, Conway BP: Aminoglycoside toxicity: A survey of retinal specialists. Arch Ophthalmol 1991;109:946–50.
41. Gills JP: Filter and antibiotics in irrigating solution for cataract surgery. J Cataract Refract Surg 1991;17:385
42. Ferro JF, de-Pablos M, Logrono MJ, et al.: Postoperative contamination after using vancomycin and gentamicin during phacoemulsification. Arch Ophthalmol 1997;115:165–70.
43. Townsend-Pico WA, Meyers SM, Langston RHS, Costin JA: Coagulase-negative staphylococcus endophthalmitis after cataract surgery with intraocular vancomycin. Am J Ophthalmol 1996;121:318–9.
44. Jeglum EL, Rosenberg SB, Benson WE: Preparation of intravitreal drug doses. Ophthalmic Surg 1981;12:345–9.
45. Affeldt JC, Flynn HW Jr, Forster RK, et al.: Microbial endophthalmitis resulting from ocular trauma. Ophthalmology 1987;94:407–13.
46. Brinton GS, Topping TM, Hyndiuk RA, et al.: Posttraumatic endophthalmitis. Arch Ophthalmol 1984;102:547–50.
47. Parrish CM, O'Day DM: Traumatic endophthalmitis. Int Ophthalmol Clin 1987;112–19.
48. Alfaro DV, Pince K, Park J, et al.: Systemic antibiotic prophylaxis in penetrating ocular injuries. Retina 1992;2:S3–S6.
49. Yoshizumi MO, Leinwand MJ, Kim J: Topical and intravenous gentamicin in traumatically lacerated eyes. Graefe's Arch Clin Exp Ophthalmol 1992;230:175–7.
50. Liang C, Meredith TA, Aguilar HE: Prophylaxis of experimental *Pseudomonas* endophthalmitis with intravenous ceftazidime. Invest Ophthalmol Vis Sci 1994;35:156.
51. Endophthalmitis Vitrectomy Study Group: Results of the Endophthalmitis Vitrectomy Study: A randomized trial of immediate vitrectomy and of intravenous antibiotics for the treatment of postoperative bacterial endophthalmitis. Arch Ophthalmol 1995;113:1479–96.
52. Alfaro DV, Liggett PE: Intravenous cefazolin in penetrating eye injuries I. Effects of trauma and multiple doses on intraocular delivery. Graefe's Arch Clin Exp Ophthalmol 1994;232:238–41.
53. Alfaro DV, Runyan T, Kirkman E, et al.: Intravenous cefazolin in penetrating eye injuries II. Treatment of experimental posttraumatic endophthalmitis. Retina 1993;13:331–4.
54. Nossov PC, Alfaro DV, Michaud ME, et al.: Intravenous cefazolin in penetrating eye injuries. Retina 1996;16:246–9.

55. Alfaro DV, Davis J, Kim S, et al.: Experimental *Bacillus cereus* posttraumatic endophthalmitis and treatment with ciprofloxacin. Br J Ophthalmol 1996;80:755–8.
56. Meredith TA, Aguilar HE, Shaarawy A, et al.: Vancomycin levels in the vitreous cavity after intravenous administration. Am J Ophthalmol 1995;119:774–8.
57. Meredith TA: Antimicrobial pharmacokinetics in endophthalmitis treatment; studies of ceftazidime. Trans Am Ophthalmol Soc 1993;91:653–99.
58. Aguilar HE, Meredith TA, Shaarawy A, et al.: Vitreous cavity penetration of ceftazidime after intravenous administration. Retina 1995;15:154–9.
59. Mieler WF, Ellis MK, Williams DF, Han DP: Retained intraocular foreign bodies and endophthalmitis. Ophthalmology 1990;97:1532–8.
60. Ariyasu RG, Kumar S, La Bree LD, et al.: Microorganisms cultured from the anterior chamber of ruptured globes at the time of repair. Am J Ophthalmol 1995;119:181–8.
61. Thompson JT, Parver LM, Enger CL, Mieler WF, et al.: Infectious endophthalmitis after penetrating injuries with retained intraocular foreign bodies. Ophthalmology 1993;100:1468–74.

CHAPTER 4

How to Learn New Techniques

JUDIE F. CHARLTON, M.D.

There are two primary reasons for an ophthalmic surgeon to acquire new skills in diagnostic and therapeutic procedures. The most obvious is to provide enhanced patient care. Another less obvious reason is to advance the practice of medicine. The more people offering their time, energy, and ideas to a procedure, the more the procedure will improve. There are multiple secondary reasons for acquiring new skills, such as retention of licensure and board certification. Most states require a minimum number of continuing medical education (CME) credits. While continuing education can be achieved through refresher courses, the acquisition of new skills may better serve patients. The American Board of Ophthalmology now requires recertification every 10 years. Although there is no section on skills testing as part of recertification, knowledge on new widely accepted treatment modalities will be expected.

More emphasis is being placed on the quality of training received by surgeons. For example, laser refractive surgery certification is required by the federal Food Drug Administration, and the laser refractive industry has limited those who may offer such certification. Hospitals are becoming more stringent about those to whom they grant privileges, and about criteria for expanding the privileges of their current staff to new procedures. Stronger emphasis is given to helping physicians become better teachers.[1] The American College of Surgeons (Chicago, Illinois) sponsors yearly workshops on "Surgeons as Educators." Accredited CME courses try to link submitting completed evaluation forms to receiving CME credit. This is done in an effort to provide feedback to the instructor on how to improve the course.

There are many reasons to learn new surgical skills. However, the problems associated with such learning may be formidable, even awesome, with major risks to both the patient and the surgeon.[2] Residency programs are specifically designed to facilitate such learning in a manner that protects patients. Fellowship learning programs are also good ways to learn special skills effectively, and they are relatively safe for both patient and surgeon. In a surgicenter environment with little or no apparent monitoring of results, it may be tempting to try to learn procedures without appropriate safeguards. Not only is this unethical, it is also unwise, putting the surgeon at risk for devastating problems.

With the explosion of technology, practitioners need to assess which new procedures deserve their resources of time, money, and energy. For example, the use of therapeutic ultrasound to treat patients with glaucoma was preceded with a large marketing push before the research and incidence of risks were well known. The procedure has now been abandoned, and physicians who used it may have learned to proceed more wisely.

When investigating a new technique, peer review literature should be weighted more heavily than the information supplied by the industry. Also the American Academy of Ophthalmology (655 Beach Street, San Francisco, CA 94109-1336) provides excellent "Procedure Assessments."

Individual surgeons need to weigh the success of new treatments against risks and expense. Surgeons should also consider how many of their patients are likely to benefit from the new procedure. If patient volume is small, it is likely a better resource of time, money, and office space to refer patients to a physician experienced and equipped in the new technique.

Once you decide to acquire a new skill, the question arises of what is the most effective strategy for acquiring that skill. Two basic elements must be considered: didactic knowledge and skills transfer.

DIDACTIC KNOWLEDGE

Didactic knowledge should be aimed toward understanding the basic science fundamentals of why the procedure works. Historical information should also be given to help the physician gain a perspective on how the procedure evolved, and especially what has been tried without success. The goals are to advance knowledge and to avoid repeating failures. Didactic knowledge should also include patient-selection criteria, risks and their rates of occurrence, preoperative and postoperative treatment, recuperation, success rates, and expense to the physician, to the hospital, and to the patient. Practitioners should become familiar with alternative therapies and be able to defend their choice of recommended treatment (Table 4–1).

WHERE TO ACQUIRE DIDACTIC KNOWLEDGE (Table 4–2)

Courses

The American Academy of Ophthalmology, subspecialty societies, and provide industry lectures. These are especially helpful when associated with panel discussions and question/answer periods.

Journals

With medical literature computer searches now available on the Internet, individuals in private practice can easily acquire references (Medline, Grateful Med, CD-ROM, OphthaLine). It is also possible to get help with locating the references and getting copies of the articles (PMIC, Practice Management Information Corporation, Los Angeles, CA, www.medicalbook store.com). Peer reviewed journals are an excellent source of information. For journals that are not peer reviewed, look for evidence of statistical analysis, and an indication of whether the study was done prospectively or retrospectively. Avoid articles that report procedures "in my hands" and patient series with small numbers. Also take into consideration whether the author has proprietary interest. Such an author virtually always has a conflict of interest, specifically making himself or herself appear more competent than others. Bias is inevitable.

TABLE 4–1. Didactic Knowledge

Basic science
Historical perspective
Patient selection
Risks
Preoperative and postoperative management
Recuperation
Success rates
Costs
Alternative treatments

TABLE 4–2. Sources of Didactic Information

Courses
Journals
Textbooks
American Academy of Ophthalmology materials
Computer interactive video programs
Computer Internet exchange

Textbooks

Because of the delay in publishing, textbooks may not be as good a source of information on "cutting edge" procedures as journals. They are, however, a better resource for tried-and-true procedures, and offer more permanence.

American Academy of Ophthalmology Materials

The AAO provides monographs and procedure assessments that are written and critically reviewed by leaders in the field. The series LEO: Lifelong Education of the Ophthalmologist is also valuable.

Computer Interactive Video Programs

Interactive programs turn learning into an active process rather than a passive one. There are a few companies developing interactive video programs for the education of ophthalmologists (Lifelearn Eyecare, Waterloo, Ontario, Canada). The effectiveness of interactive video programs is not established in the area of ophthalmology; however, one study comparing the knowledge of physiology graduate students after completing an interactive video program versus participating in a laboratory experience showed that the knowledge acquired was equal and that the video program allowed the students to complete the exercise in 30% less time.[3]

Computer Internet Exchange

Posting questions on the Internet on a common web site may generate many opinions at once and offer review by multiple other practitioners. The responses, however, are usually incomplete and the information unsubstantiated. Even well-known resources are biased.

Computer Internet Web Pages

Multiple Web pages provide information on eye diseases, many written for the lay public. Because these usually are not peer reviewed, the reputation of the source of information is of paramount importance. Web sites sponsored by national organizations such as the American Academy of Ophthalmology and subspecialty organizations such as the American Glaucoma Society provide reliable information that is appropriate for either patients or practioners. Internet Ophthalmology (www.ophthal.org) is a nonprofit organization devoted to the education of international eye care providers. In contrast to those reputable web sites, there are also multiple sites presenting patient testimonials. Some Web sites are sponsored by proprietary centers and are flavored with information to attract business.

SKILLS TRANSFER

Certain new techniques may be variations of an already mastered procedure. Simply seeing diagrams or watching a video may be adequate preparation for performing such amended procedures. Procedures with which a surgeon has no similar experience will require hands-on practice, preferably with a skilled individual who can interact with the learner.

Surgery requires three-dimensional visualization, movement, and tactile feedback. It is difficult to gain skills from one-dimensional media forms (Table 4–3).

TEXTBOOKS WITH THREE-DIMENSIONAL ATLASES

The authors of some texts realize the importance of three-dimensional views in mastering new techniques. For example, the textbook by Richard MacKool[4] comes with stereo discs and a view finder to use while reading the text.

VIDEO TAPES

Video tapes are not only convenient, they also can be played multiple times. Especially helpful are video tapes that include inserts showing hand position in the corner of the screen. Be wary of heavily edited tapes; it is beneficial if the demonstrating surgeon shows not only a complication-free case, but also one with complications. Good sources of video tapes are the Video Journal of Ophthalmology (St. Louis, MO) and the Video Journal of Cataract and Refractive Surgery (Robert Osher, M.D., Cincinnati Eye Institute, Cincinnati, OH).

TABLE 4–3. Skills Transfer

Textbooks
Video tapes
Observation of a skilled surgeon
Wet lab
Practice eyes

OBSERVING IN THE OPERATING ROOM

Most hospitals have no legal or liability problems with observers in the operating room. Such observation allows good interchange between surgeons. There may be privilege problems, however, for scrubbing in on a case. A variation of this concept is that used by ORBIS. An airplane maintained by this nonprofit organization is equipped with an operating room. It travels around the world and has local surgeons sit in a video classroom while the faculty and local surgeons operate. The surgery is transmitted live via video to the video classroom, where the observing surgeons can watch. An intercom allows for two-way conversation.

WET LABS

The American Academy of Ophthalmology, subspecialty societies, teaching hospitals and the ophthalmic industry often offer wet labs with their courses. Some equipment manufacturing sites have continuous wet labs up and running which practitioners may visit. Recently there have been firms developed that specialize in skills transfer and certification. For example, CRS Education (14988 N 78th Way, #108, Scottsdale, AZ 85260) provides training and certification in the area of refractive surgery. When participating in wet labs, physicians should take care to note the instruments and supplies used. Because the wet lab cannot be replayed or reread, it is helpful to make a list of the steps and procedures for reference at a later time. To learn procedures involving extraocular muscles or conjunctiva as a critical part of their procedure, the use of live animals is necessary. Since these skills must be learned on live animals, it is best done at wet lab courses or at academic centers where individuals skilled in the humane handling of animals under institutional review board guidelines are involved.

PRACTICE EYES

Plastic practice eyes are commercially available. These can be set up rapidly, need few supplies, and have no risk of infection. Unfortunately, they don't resemble natural eye tissue very well. Eye banks will supply practitioners with donor eyes that are not suitable for transplantation. Fees for these eyes vary from state to state, and the eyes may not have been tested for possible communicable infection such as HIV and hepatitis. Usually only a few donors eyes are available at any time, and they should be used within four days. The great advantage of donor human eyes is that the tissue most resembles that of living human tissue. Animal

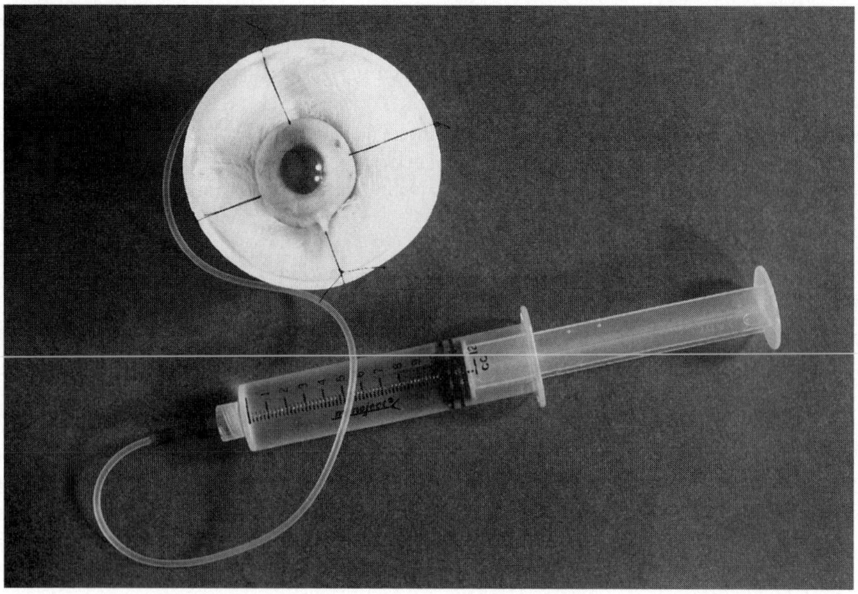

Figure 4–1. Practice eye fixated to Styrofoam cup.

eyes are available from commercial suppliers who are supplied by butchers. The butchers usually only slaughter certain animals on certain days of the week. Customarily there is a minimum number of eyes that must be ordered at one time, usually 25 eyes or more. Species to choose from usually consist of rabbit, sheep, cow, and pig. Eyes can be supplied either fresh or frozen. The fresh animal eyes better simulate living human tissue than do plastic model eyes, but they must be used within four days for the best results. Post mortem changes that occur in both human donor and animal eyes include hypotony, corneal edema, opacified corneal epithelium, myopic iris, and floppy lens support. These problems can be improved upon by a variety of techniques (some simple and some complex) depending on how good a model is needed.[5,6]

Stabilization of the Eye and Maintenance of Intraocular Pressure

The eye may be stabilized in a paper cup, Styrofoam block, or a practice head. It works best if the muscle insertion stumps are pinned or anchored with bridle sutures to the support structure (Fig. 4–1). The intraocular pressure can be best adjusted by inserting a butterfly needle (23-gauge or 25-gauge) through the optic nerve into the vitreous cavity (Fig. 4–2). The butterfly needle is then connected to a syringe filled with a saline solution (preferably a balanced salt solution such as BSS, Alcon Laboratories, Fort Worth, TX). Distilled water is not suitable because it will cause further opacification of the cornea. This system works best if there is a hole in the bottom of the support structure through which the butterfly needle can transverse.

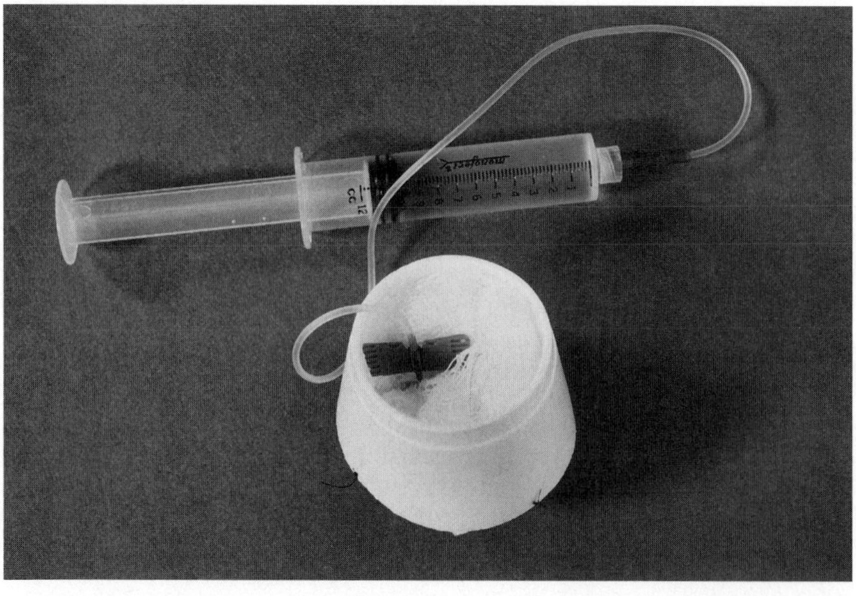

Figure 4–2. Intraocular pressure of practice eye is maintained with balanced salt solution delivered through the optic nerve by a butterfly needle. A hole in the bottom of the container allows for easy access.

Simple Technique for Short Anterior Segment Procedures

To alleviate the opacification from edema, the cornea can be dehydrated with glycerin. The corneal epithelium may also be removed if the cornea remains cloudy. Irrigating the cornea with water will further opacify the cornea, but glycerin (Ophthalgan, Wyeth-Ayerst, Philadelphia, PA) may be applied repeatedly if necessary. If the procedure involves irrigation into the anterior chamber, a saline solution such as BSS should be used, because distilled water would further cloud the cornea. If a rabbit eye in a living rabbit is being used, a small amount of heparin may be added to the anterior chamber at entry. Rabbits often have a virulent fibrinous response in the aqueous, and this can be tempered by the heparin. With any animal model, there may be problems with iris prolapse at the incision site if the intraocular pressure is too high in the vitreous cavity. A peripheral iridectomy can help should this occur. If a viscoelastic material is used in the procedure, an economical substitute can be methylcellulose 2.5% (Goniosol, Ciba Vision, Duluth, GA).

Complex Fixation Technique Necessary for Posterior Segment Work

The following technique described by Gerd, Auffran, and associates[5] at the Center for Research on Ocular Therapeutics and Biodevices is complex, but it offers superior results. Hyperosmotic dextran is used as a dehydrating agent. It is injected into the anterior chamber, the corneal epithelium is removed, and the eye is immersed in the dextran solution for at least 30 minutes. The injected dextran mechanically opens the pupil. The intraocular pressure is maintained with balanced salt solution via injection by the optic nerve as described above. The eye is fixated in a training head, and the dextran in the anterior chamber is removed and substituted with viscoelastic material. Formalin 10% is instilled into the anterior chamber with the viscoelastic substance for 5 to 10 seconds to fixate the iris. Both the viscoelastic material and the formalin are removed. After removal of the lens by an extracapsular cataract extraction technique, the anterior chamber and lens bag are filled with the viscoelastic substance. The iris is fixated yet again with a stronger agent, Karnovsky fixative. This too is removed after 5 to 10 seconds. Further procedures such as IOL insertion or posterior segment procedures can then be performed.

Keratoprosthesis

Posterior segment procedures can also be performed on cadaveric eyes using the keratoprosthesis to bypass the post mortem cloudy cornea and, possibly, the lens.[6]

THE FUTURE

VIRTUAL REALITY

The Georgia Institute of Technology and the Massachusetts Institute of Technology[7] are both developing an eye surgery simulation system that provides both visual and force feedback while a surgeon operates on a computer model of the eye in a virtual environment. Virtual surgical instruments are controlled by a handheld tracking stylus with options to change instruments. A cataract extraction procedure is simulated in which a knife makes the initial incision, and a phacoemulsifier breaks up and removes the lens. The system also permits the simulated grasping of tissue with forceps and cutting tissue with scissors. In the virtual environment, the eye and the surgical instruments exist only as computer models. Interaction between the instruments and the eye model depend upon the tool selected and the location of the instrument in the anatomy. Depth of incisions are quantified, and the user is alerted when the instruments violate predefined limits.

The force feedback system produces a compliment resistance matched to eye bank eyes in an attempt to characterize some of the forces experienced by the surgeon. This technique allows the surgeon to acquire skills more quickly in a harm-free environment. Although such a system will initially be an expensive setup, it allows the surgeon freedom to use the system multiple times at his or her convenience. It also allows an inexperienced surgeon to compare his virtual performance to that of more highly skilled surgeons.

TELEMEDICINE

High-resolution images can be transmitted via telephone lines to remote monitors. A novice surgeon can observe an experienced surgeon and interact with the surgeon during the course of the procedure. Such interaction can also work in reverse; the experienced surgeon can watch the trainee perform his or her first live case and offer verbal assistance.

ETHICAL CONSIDERATIONS

When a new skill has been studied and practiced in an experimental setting, ethical considerations must be taken into account before the first human clinical application. The American Academy of Ophthalmology issued an excellent "Advisory Opinion of the Code of Ethics" on the subject Learning New Techniques Following Residency (September 1997). The advisory addresses both the "learning curve" and responsibilities to the patient.

> Appropriate patient selection is a particularly important factor in assuring success with early cases, in building confidence in performing the technique, and in avoiding complications. Patient selection should initially be made on the basis of anticipated technical difficulty. Additionally, patient personality should also be considered; those who exert additional pressures through their anxiety, impatience, or a demanding style are not suitable candidates.
>
> Of special consideration is the process of providing appropriate informed consent. The ophthalmologist should disclose his/her level of experience as a surgeon and

level of experience with a new technique. An experienced surgeon can appropriately inform the patient that he/she is modifying or improving a portion of an otherwise familiar procedure. When discussing success rates for a given procedure, it may be appropriate to provide data from more experienced surgeons as long as the less experienced surgeon does not imply these success rates are his/her own. The patient should be made aware of a mentor's role, if any, as part of the surgical team.

Medicine is a life-long learning opportunity. While many procedures have "learning curves," these curves can be shortened if education is thorough and appropriate. Complications should be anticipated, and the surgeon must master techniques for dealing with them. With proper planning, education, and practice, unexpected events need not end with negative results. It is encouraging that a review of residents learning phacoemulsification concluded that, with proper training and supervision, the rate of surgical complications is acceptably low when compared to manual lens extraction.[8] To learn a new technique, the ophthalmologist should strive for a quality educational experience, adequate preparation, and practice to deliver quality care.

REFERENCES

1. Whitman N, Schwenk TL: The Physician as a Teacher, 2nd Edition. Salt Lake City, Whitman Associates; 1997.
2. Organ CH, Porter JM: General Surgery. JAMA 1998;280:496.
3. Fawver AL, Branch CE, Trentham L, et al.: A comparison of interactive videodisc instruction with live animal laboratories. Am J Physiol 1990;259:S11.
4. MacKool RJ: The Stereoatlas of Phacoemulsification and IOL Implantation. Woodbury, NY: Stereo Arts Press; 1990.
5. Auffarth GU, Wesendahl TA, Solomon KD, et al.: A modified preparation technique for closed-system ocular surgery of human eyes obtained postmortem. Ophthalmology 1996;103:977.
6. Eckardt U, Eckardt C: Keratoprosthesis as an aid to learning surgical techniques on cadaver eyes. Ophthalmic Surg 1995;26:358.
7. Hunter IW, Jones LA, Sagar MA, et al.: Ophthalmic microsurgical robot and associated virtual environment. Comput Biol Med 1995;25:173.
8. Tarbet KJ, Mamalis N, Theurer J, et al.: Complications and results of phacoemulsification performed by residents. J Cataract Refract Surg 1995;21:661.

SECTION II

Stephen A. Obstbaum, M.D.

Cataract

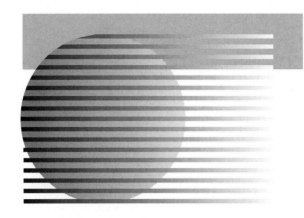

CHAPTER 5

Clear Corneal Cataract Surgery Incisions

I. HOWARD FINE, M.D. and RICHARD S. HOFFMAN, M.D.

The availability of foldable intraocular lenses (IOLs) that can be inserted through small unsutured phacoemulsification incisions[1] has created an increasing trend away from scleral tunnel incisions in favor of clear corneal incisions for cataract removal and lens insertion.[2] Scleral tunnel incisions have several technical disadvantages, among them (1) the need to perform conjunctival incisions and scleral dissections; (2) the need for cautery to provide a bloodless operative field, especially in patients who are receiving anticoagulants or who have bleeding dyscrasias; (3) increased difficulty with oarlocking of the phaco tip and distortion of the cornea because of the length of scleral tunnel incisions. Any of these features may complicate the phacoemulsification procedure.

HISTORY

A historical review of sutureless clear corneal cataract surgery would not be complete without understanding the evolution of small cataract incisions. Richard Kratz is generally credited with being the first surgeon to move from the limbus to the sclera in order to increase the appositional surfaces and thereby enhance wound healing and reduce surgically induced astigmatism.[3,4] L. J. Girard and R. F. Hoffman were the first surgeons to name the posterior incision a "scleral tunnel incision" and, together with Kratz, were the first to make a point of entering the anterior chamber through the cornea, creating a "corneal shelf."[5] The corneal shelf was designed to prevent iris prolapse. In 1989 M. S. McFarland used this incision architecture and recognized that scleral tunnel incisions sized to accommodate foldable IOLs allowed for phacoemulsification and the implantation of lenses without the need for suturing.[6] W. F. Maloney, who was a fellow under Kratz, advocated the addition of a corneal shelf to his incisions, which he described as strong and waterproof (Fig. 5–1).[7] Paul Ernest recognized that McFarland's long scleral tunnel incision terminated in a well-defined corneal entrance. He hypothesized that the posterior lip or "corneal lip" of the incision acted as a one-way valve, which explained the mechanism of self-sealability (Ernest PH. Presentation at the Department of Ophthalmology, Wayne State University School of Medicine, Detroit, Mich., February 28, 1990). In April 1992, I. Howard Fine presented his self-sealing temporal clear corneal incision at the annual meeting of the American Society of Cataract and Refractive Surgery.[8] Finally, in May 1992, at the Island Ophthalmology Seminar, Robert Kellan demonstrated on videotape a technique that he referred to as the "scleral-less incision." It was essentially a corneal limbal stab incision through the conjunctiva and the limbus, entering the anterior chamber through clear cornea, leaving a corneal shelf or lip (Fig. 5-2*A* and *B*).

Through the years, many surgeons have favored corneal incisions for cataract surgery. In 1967, Charles Kelman stated that the best approach for performing

This chapter is an updated and revised version of a previous publication in Ophthalmic Surgery and Lasers. Permission for publication has been given by Slack, Inc.

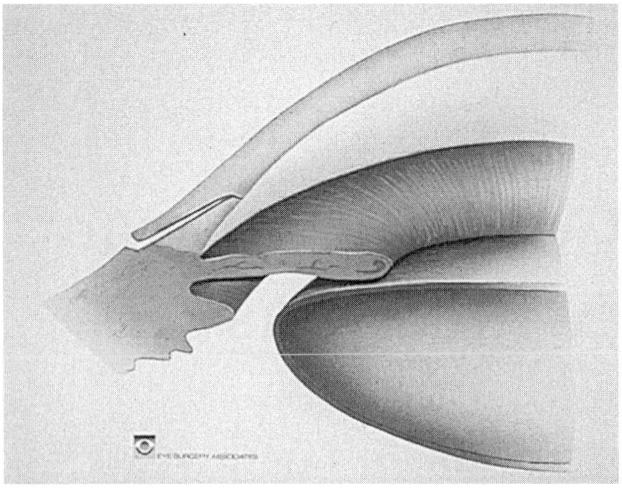

Figure 5–1. Cross-sectional view of the "corneal shelf" incision. Incision begins in sclera, is beveled into clear cornea, and enters the anterior chamber, producing a corneal shelf, which is watertight and prevents iris prolapse.

cataract surgery was with phacoemulsification through a clear corneal incision utilizing a triangular-tear capsulotomy and a grooving and cracking technique in the posterior chamber.[9] At the same time, H. Harms and G. Mackenson in Germany published an intracapsular technique that used a corneal incision in an atlas of Ocular Surgery Under the Microscope.[10] R. Troutman was an early advocate of controlling surgically induced astigmatism at the time of cataract surgery by means of the corneal-incision approach.[11] In England, E. J. Arnott used clear corneal incisions and a diamond keratome for phacoemulsification, although he had to enlarge the incision for introducing an IOL.[12] A. Galand in Belgium used clear corneal incisions for extracapsular cataract extraction in his "envelope" technique,[13] and R. Stegman of South Africa has a long history of using the cornea as the site for incisions for extracapsular cataract extraction (Stegmann R: Personal communication, December 3, 1992). Finally, perhaps the leading proponent of clear corneal incisions for modern era phacoemulsification was Kimiya Shimizu of Japan.[14]

Fine's personal experience with corneal incisions began in 1979 when he used the temporal clear cornea as the site for secondary anterior chamber intraocular lens implantation. The temporal approach was preferred because of the vagaries and disturbed anatomy present at the superior limbus in eyes that had previous intracapsular cataract extraction. When foldable lenses became available in 1986, he employed sutured clear corneal incisions for phacoemulsification and foldable IOL implantation in patients who had preexisting filtering blebs. After these procedures, a marked reduction in surgically induced astigmatism was noted, even though these incisions were corneal rather than scleral. In 1992, Fine began routinely using clear corneal cataract incisions for phacoemulsification and foldable IOL implantation, with incision closure using a tangential suture modeled after John Shepherd's technique.[15] Within a very short time, the tangential suture was abandoned in favor of self-sealing corneal incisions.[16]

INDICATIONS

In the beginning, the use of clear corneal incisions was limited to patients with preexisting filtering blebs, patients on anti-coagulants or with blood dyscrasias, or patients with cicatrizing diseases such as ocular pemphigoid or Stevens-Johnson syndrome. Later, because of the natural fit of clear corneal cataract incisions with topical anesthesia, the indications for clear corneal cataract surgery expanded. With the ability to avoid injection into the orbit and the use of intravenous medications, patients who had cardiovascular, pulmonary, and other systemic diseases that might have contraindicated cataract surgery became surgical candidates. Subsequently, through the safety and increasing use of clear corneal incisions by pioneers in the United States, including C.H. Williamson, J.R. Shepherd, R.G. Martin, and H.B. Grabow,[17] these incisions became more and more popular and began to be used around the world.

Studies using topographical analyses of these incisions by E. Rosen demonstrated that clear corneal incisions 3 mm in width or less were topographically astigmatism-neutral.[18] This led to greater interest in these incisions because of increasing use of surgical tech-

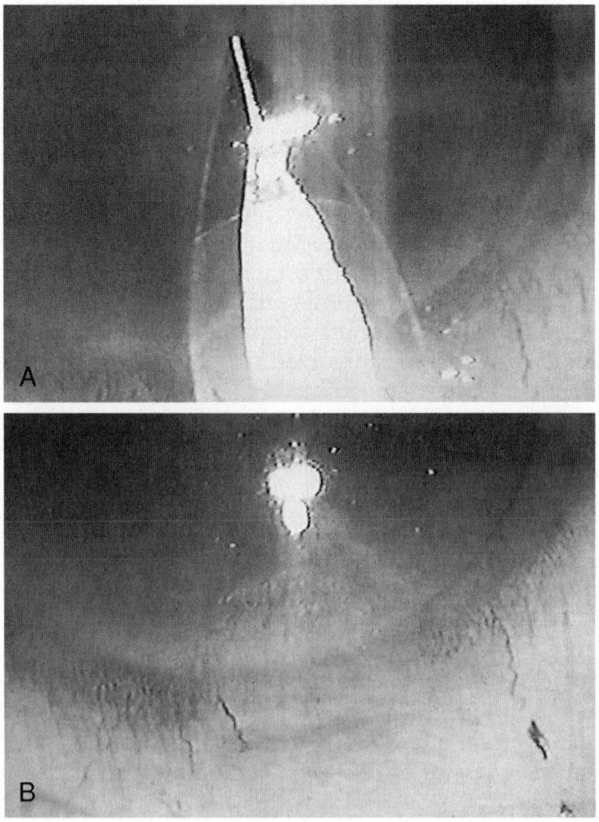

Figure 5–2. *A.* Kellan's corneal limbal stab incision through conjunctiva and the limbus *(B)*. Corneal limbal incision following removal of the steel keratome.

niques, including T-cuts, arcuate cuts, and limbal relaxing incisions, for managing preexisting astigmatism at the time of cataract surgery. Without astigmatism neutrality in the cataract incision, the predictability of adjunctive astigmatism-reducing procedures would be decreased, making it more difficult to achieve the desired result. In the initial studies and with the ultimate use of multifocal IOLs, the need for astigmatism neutrality was again a factor in stimulating interest in clear corneal incisions. Finally, the availability of phakic IOLs and the need for control of astigmatism at the time of implantation of these lenses has led many surgeons to consider clear corneal incisions as the route for phakic IOL implantation.

Other advantages of the temporal clear corneal incision include better preservation of preexisting filtering blebs,[19] preservation of options for future filtering surgery, increased stability in the refractive results because of the neutralization of the forces from lid blink and gravity, the ease of approach to the incision site, the lack of need for bridle sutures and resultant iatrogenic ptosis, and, finally, the location of the lateral canthal angle under the incision, which facilitates drainage.

CLASSIFICATIONS

Early on there was criticism surrounding the use of self-sealing clear corneal incisions because of the fear of a possible increase in the incidence of endophthalmitis secondary to poor wound healing and sealability. This potential controversy stimulated many studies into the strength and safety of clear corneal incisions compared to limbal and scleral tunnel incisions. Unfortunately, because of a lack of standardization in the definition of what constitutes a limbal incision versus clear corneal incision, considerable confusion has been generated in this area, making it difficult for surgeons to communicate and compare the relative claims of their individual techniques. Based on Hogan's Histology of the Human Eye ["The conjunctival vessels are seen with the slit lamp as fine arcades that extend into clear cornea for about 0.5 mm beyond the limbal edge"][20] and topographical studies of incisions done by Menapace[21] in Vienna, Fine has categorized these incisions using the parameters of location and architecture.[22] An incision is termed *clear corneal* when the external edge is anterior to the conjunctival insertion, *limbal corneal* when the external edge is through conjunctiva and limbus, and *scleral corneal* when it is posterior to the limbus (Fig. 5–3). In addition to the anatomic designation of the external incision, these incisions are also classified by their architecture as being *single plane* when there is no groove at the external edge of the incision, *shallow grooved* when the initial groove is less than 400 microns, and *deeply grooved* when it is deeper than 400 microns (Figs. 5–4 and 5–8). To reduce the confusion and to facilitate communication regarding these incisions; we believe they should be classified as *clear corneal, limbal corneal,* or *scleral corneal* incisions and either *single planed, shallow grooved,* or *deep grooved.*

Location

- **Clear Corneal Incision-**
  Entry anterior to conjunctival insertion
- **Limbal Corneal Incision-**
  Entry through conjunctiva & limbus
- **Scleral Corneal Incision-**
  Entry posterior to the limbus

Figure 5–3. Classification of corneal tunnel incisions by external incision location.

Architecture

- **Single Plane (No groove)**
- **Shallow Groove (< 400 μ)**
- **Deep Groove (> 400 μ)**

Figure 5–4. Classification of corneal tunnel incisions by wound architecture.

CONTROVERSIES

One of the most controversial criticisms of clear corneal incisions has been their relative strength compared to limbal or scleral incisions. Ernest demonstrated that rectangular clear corneal incisions in cadaver eye models were less resistant to external deformation utilizing pinpoint pressure than square limbal or scleral tunnel incisions.[23,24] Subsequently, Mackool demonstrated that once the incision width was 3.5 mm or less and the length 2 mm or greater, there was equal resistance to external deformation in clear corneal incisions and scleral tunnel incisions.[25] In Ernest's work as well, as incision sizes became smaller, the force required to cause failure of the incision became very similar for limbal and clear corneal incisions, a finding that could be used to further document the safety of incisions of 3 mm or less.

A major criticism of these cadaver studies is that there is a lack of functioning endothelium contributing to wound sealing. Other investigators have also indicated that cadaver eye incision strength cannot be compared to incisions in vivo.[18] In comparisons of in vivo posterior limbal incisions and clear corneal incisions Ernest found that deep grooved incisions performed better than shallow grooved or single-plane incisions and that posterior limbal incisions performed better than clear corneal incisions when challenged by pinpoint pressure.[26]

Many surgeons have called into question the validity of pinpoint pressure as a clinically relevant test for cataract wound strength because it is not likely that patients would challenge their own incisions by pressing on them with something as fine as the instruments used to apply pinpoint pressure in these studies. Regardless of whether more posteriorly placed incisions demonstrate increased strength compared to clear corneal incisions, the real question is whether that added strength is clinically significant or relevant. Fine

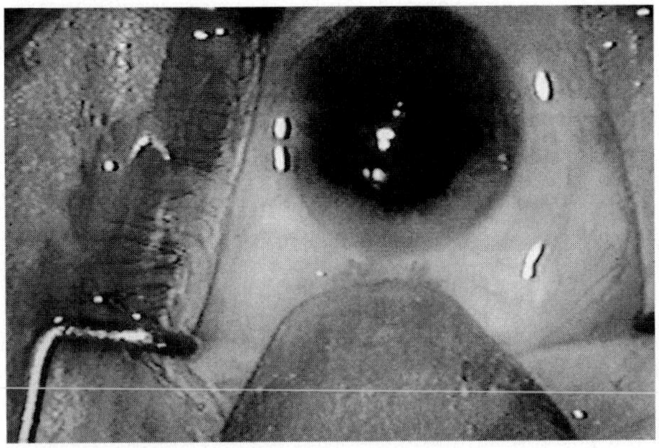

Figure 5–5. Demonstration of self-sealability of clear corneal incision to the challenge of a blunt "knuckle."

and others have demonstrated the stability of clear corneal incisions when pressure from a knuckle or a fingertip, the most likely means by which patients would challenge these incisions, was applied (Fine IH: New thoughts on self-sealing clear corneal cataract incisions. Presented at Hawaii '96; Maui, Hawaii, January 22, 1996) (Fig. 5–5). In addition, it is well known that a 1-mm "hypersquare" paracentesis will leak the day after surgery if pinpoint pressure is applied to its posterior lip; however, the likelihood of any paracentesis incision leaking spontaneously or with blunt pressure the day after surgery is highly unlikely.

One final point of controversy regards the studies in cat eyes performed by Ernest and Tipperman.[27] These studies revealed a fibrovascular response in incisions placed in the limbus, with extensive wound healing in 7 days, compared to a lack of fibrovascular healing in clear corneal incisions. This study has been used to propose greater safety for limbal incisions than for clear corneal incisions. Unfortunately, the real issue is not healing but sealing. We feel that as long as an incision is sealed at the conclusion of surgery and remains sealed, the time before complete healing of the incision is accomplished is practically irrelevant. This conclusion is reinforced by the documented 7-day period in which limbal incisions are not truly "healed." An analogy can be drawn between sealing of the clear corneal incision and the sealing that takes place during laser-assisted in-situ keratomileusis. With the latter procedure, there is no fibrovascular healing of the clear corneal interface, which has little effect on the strength, effectiveness, or safety of the wound; this, in fact, presents an advantage by limiting scarring and an inflammatory healing response. Ultimately, the safety of one incision over another in the clinical setting will only be determined with the findings of a difference in the rate of incision-related complications, which to date have not been demonstrated.

One distinct disadvantage of limbal corneal incisions is the greater likelihood of ballooning of conjunctiva, which can make visualization of anterior chamber structures during the surgical procedure more difficult. In addition, studies by Park[19] demonstrated that violation of the conjunctiva threatens the integrity not only of preexisting filtering blebs but of the conjunctiva that would participate in filtering surgery at some future date. Finally, the presence of subconjunctival hemorrhage, although not important with respect to the ultimate function of the eye, may be of cosmetic importance to the patient and may affect the survival of filtering blebs.

Contraindications for clear corneal incisions include the presence of radial keratotomy incisions that extend to the limbus and that might be challenged by clear corneal incisions,[28] marginal degenerations associated with thinning of the peripheral cornea, and perhaps advanced corneal endothelial dystrophy.

PREOPERATIVE EVALUATION

Certain studies that may be of value as part of a preoperative work-up include endothelial cell counts in patients with endothelial dystrophies, and perhaps computerized corneal topography when refractive surgical procedures are to be combined with cataract surgery in the management of preexisting astigmatism, especially when refractive and keratometric measurements do not coincide.

TECHNIQUES

Single plane incisions, as first described by Fine,[29] were made with a 3.0-mm diamond knife. After pressurization of the eye with placement of viscoelastic material through a paracentesis, the blade was placed on the eye in such a way that it completely applanated the eye with the point placed at the leading edge of the anterior vascular arcade. The knife was moved in the plane of the cornea until its shoulders, which are 2 mm posterior to the point of the knife, touch the external edge of the incision. At this point, a dimple-down technique was employed to initiate the cut through Descemet's membrane. After the tip enters the anterior chamber, the initial plane of the knife was reestablished to cut through Descemet's membrane in a straight-line configuration (Fig. 5–6).

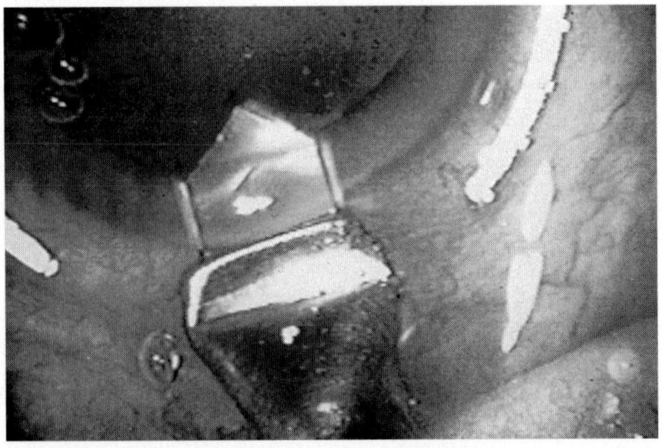

Figure 5–6. Diamond keratome enters the anterior chamber after "dimpling down" to incise Descemet's membrane. After the tip enters the anterior chamber, the initial plane of the knife is reestablished to cut through Descemet's membrane in a straight-line configuration.

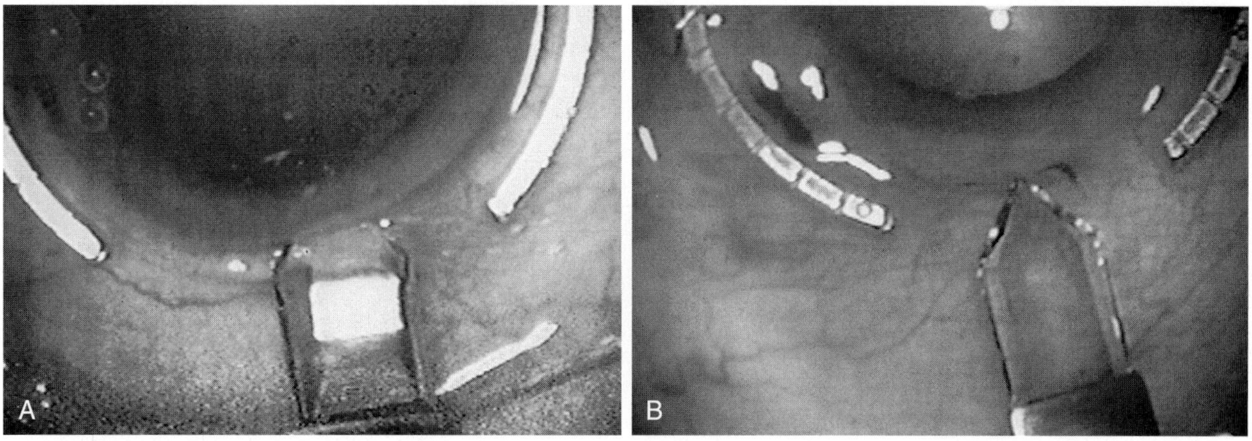

Figure 5–7. *A.* Guarded diamond knife produces grooved incision in temporal clear cornea. *B.* Tip of diamond keratome is placed in grooved incision as the posterior lip of the incision is depressed to produce shallow and deep grooved incisions.

Williamson was the first to use a shallow 300- to 400-micron grooved clear corneal incision (Fig. 5–7*A* and *B*).[30] The rationale for the Williamson incision was that it led to a thicker external edge to the roof of the tunnel and less likelihood of tearing. Langerman later described the single-hinge incision, in which requirements for the initial groove were 90% of the depth of the cornea anterior to the edge of the conjunctiva.[31] Initially he used a depth of 600 microns and subsequently made the tunnel itself superficially in that groove, believing that this led to enhanced resistance of the incision to external deformation (Fig. 5–8). Minimal differences in surgically induced astigmatism have been demonstrated between beveled and hinged clear corneal incisions.[32]

Adjunctive techniques were employed to combine refractive surgery incisions with clear corneal cataract incisions. Fine continued to use the temporal location for the cataract incisions and added one or two T-cuts made by a Feaster knife with a 7-mm optical zone for the management of preexisting astigmatism. Other investigators, including Lindstrom and Rosen, rotated the location of the incision to the steep axis to achieve some flattening at the steepest axis to address preexisting astigmatism. Kershner used the corneal incision in the temporal half of the eye by starting with a nearly full-thickness T-cut, through which he then made his corneal tunnel incision. For a large degree of astigmatism, he used a paired T-cut in the opposite side of the same meridian.[33] Finally, the popularization of limbal relaxing incisions by Gills[34] and Nichamin[35] added another means of reducing preexisting astigmatism by using the groove for the limbal relaxing incision as the site of entry for the clear corneal cataract incision. This has been found to be a simple and practical approach for reducing preexisting astigmatism at the time of cataract surgery.[36]

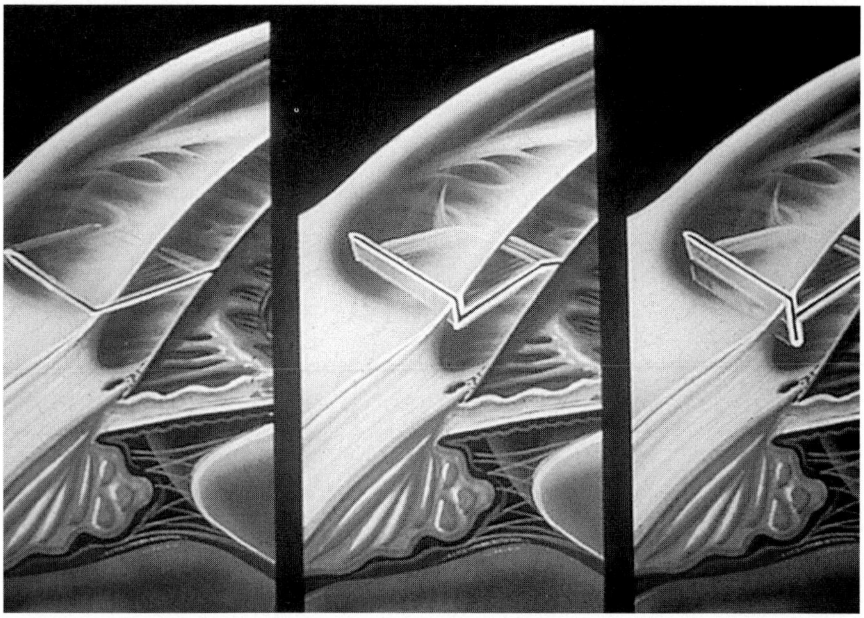

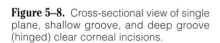

Figure 5–8. Cross-sectional view of single plane, shallow groove, and deep groove (hinged) clear corneal incisions.

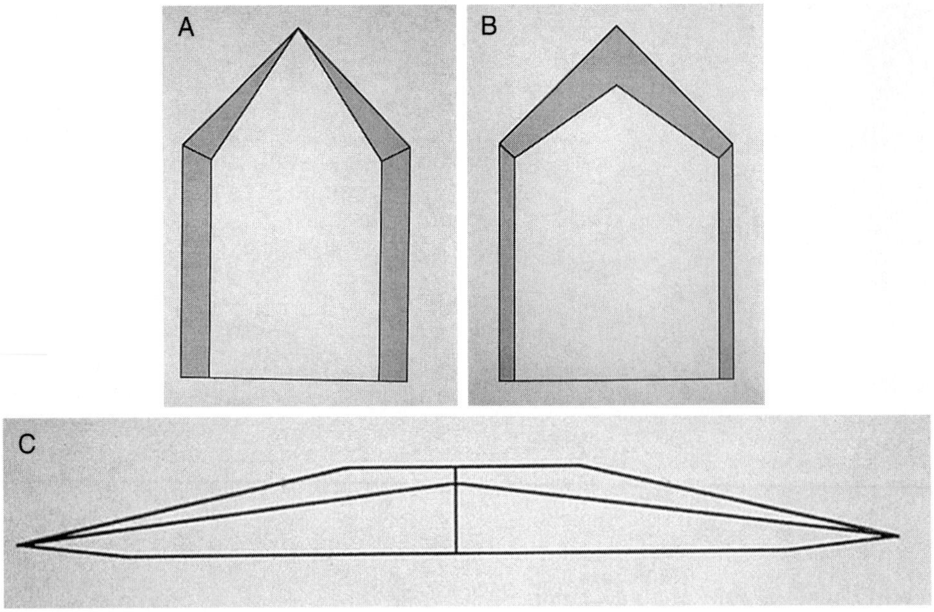

Figure 5–9. Schematic representation of top view *(A)* and bottom view *(B)* of the 3.0-mm Rhein 3-D diamond keratome. The front profile of the keratome *(C)* demonstrates the differential slopes on the anterior and the posterior aspects of the blade, which allow the forces of tissue resistance to create the proper incision architecture.

New technology blades that have been developed have helped perfect incision architecture. The Fine Triamond knife was developed in conjunction with Mastel Instruments so that the incision could be made with an extremely sharp, thin, and narrow knife without a necessity for dimpling down, which sometimes led to tearing of tissue or scrolling of Descemet's membrane. Subsequently, in conjunction with Rhein Medical, the 3-D blade was developed. This knife had differential slope angles to the bevels on the anterior versus the posterior surface (Fig. 5–9*A, B,* C), resulting in an ability to just touch the eye at the site of the external incision location and advance the blade in the plane of the cornea. The differential slopes on the anterior and posterior aspects of the blade allowed the forces of tissue resistance to create an incision characterized by a linear external incision, a 2-mm tunnel, and a linear internal incision. All of this could be accomplished without the need to dimple down or distort tissues to create the proper incision architecture.[37] The trapezoidal 3-D blade also allows enlargement of the incision to 3.5 mm for IOL insertion without altering incision architecture (Fig. 5–10). Histologic studies of clear corneal incisions performed with steel keratomes and diamond keratomes have shown greater disruption of corneal stromal tissue with steel keratomes and greater likelihood of severe stromal damage after insertion of foldable IOLs, suggesting that diamond keratomes may have a beneficial effect on incision healing.[38,39]

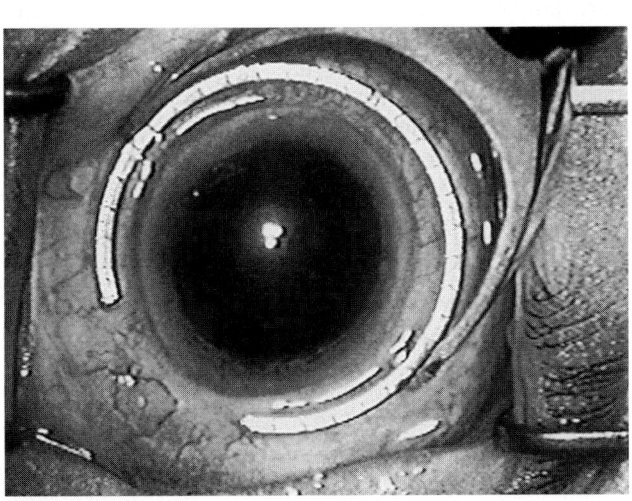

Figure 5–11. The Fine-Thornton fixation ring is ideal for globe fixation during paracentesis placement, clear corneal incision creation, and lens insertion.

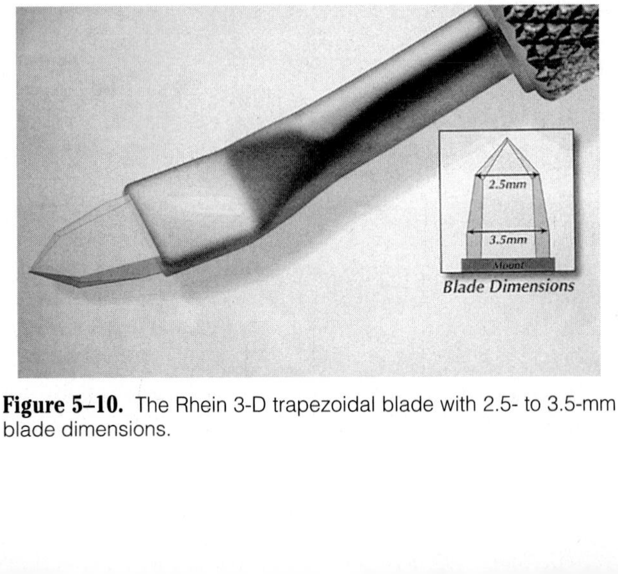

Figure 5–10. The Rhein 3-D trapezoidal blade with 2.5- to 3.5-mm blade dimensions.

Although we prefer the Fine/Thornton fixation device, which was developed by taking 8 mm of arc length out of the Thornton refractive surgery fixation ring (Fig. 5–11), other surgeons have used the side port incision for fixation to stabilize the eye during incision

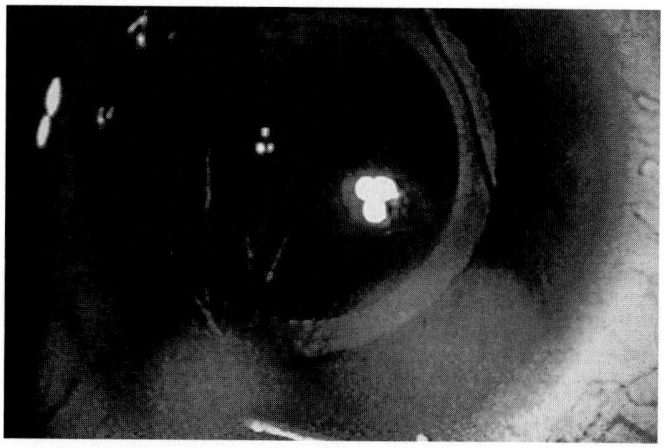

Figure 5–12. Stromal hydration of the incision is created by placing the tip of a 26-gauge cannula in the side walls of the incision and gently irrigating balanced salt solution into the stroma. This is performed at both edges of the incision to help appose the roof and the floor of the incision.

construction. Recently, Maloney and Wallace have collaborated on the design of a paracentesis knife, which provides for fixation and stabilization of the globe for cataract incision construction through clear cornea. The disadvantage of this knife resides in the fact that the paracentesis must be at least one quadrant away from the clear corneal incision in order to maximize stabilization of the globe.

Following phacoemulsification, lens implantation, and removal of residual viscoelastic material, stromal hydration of the clear corneal incision can be performed to help seal the incision.[16] Stromal hydration is accomplished by placing the tip of a 26- or 27-gauge cannula in the side walls of the incision and gently irrigating balanced salt solution into the stroma (Fig. 5–12). This maneuver is performed at both edges of the incision to help appose the roof and the floor of the incision. Once apposition takes place, the hydrostatic forces of the endothelial pump will help seal the incision. In those rare instances of questionable wound integrity, a single 10-0 nylon suture is placed to ensure a tight seal.

INTRAOPERATIVE AND POSTOPERATIVE COMPLICATIONS

Although clear corneal and scleral incision cataract surgery share many of the same intraoperative and postoperative complications, clear corneal incisions by nature of their architecture and location have some unique associated complications. If the surgeon incidentally incises the conjunctiva at the time of the clear corneal incision, ballooning of the conjunctiva can develop, which may compromise visualization of anterior structures. When this occurs, a suction catheter is usually required by the assistant in order to aid in visualization. Early entry into the cornea might result in an incision of insufficient length to be self-sealing, and thus placement of a single suture may be required to assure a secure wound at the conclusion of the procedure. Late entry may result in a corneal tunnel incision sufficiently long that the phacoemulsification tip would create striae in the cornea and compromise visualization of the anterior chamber. In addition, incisions that are too short or improperly constructed can result in an increased tendency for iris prolapse.

Manipulation of the phacoemulsification handpiece intraoperatively may result in tearing of the roof of the tunnel, especially at the edges, resulting in potential compromise of the ability for the incision to self-seal. Tearing of the internal lip can also result in compromised self-sealability or in rare instances, small detachments or scrolling of Descemet's membrane at the anterior edge of the incision. Of greater concern has been the potential for incisional burns.[40,41] When incisional burns develop in clear corneal incisions, there may be a loss of self-sealability, and closure of the wound may induce an excessive degree of astigmatism. In addition, manipulation of the incision can result in epithelial abrasion, which can compromise self-sealability because of the lack of a fluid barrier by an intact epithelium. Without an intact epithelial layer, the corneal endothelium does not have the ability to help appose the roof and floor of the incision through hydrostatic forces.

Postoperatively, hypotony might result in some compromising of the ability for these incisions to seal. Wound leaks and iris prolapse have been very infrequent postoperative complications[42] and are usually present in incisions greater than 3.5 mm in width. In a large survey performed for the American Society of Cataract and Refractive Surgery by Masket,[43] there was a slightly increased incidence of endophthalmitis in clear corneal cataract surgery compared to scleral tunnel surgery. However, the survey failed to note the incision sizes in those cases where endophthalmitis in clear corneal incisions had occurred; thus it is possible that any increase in the incidence of endophthalmitis is associated with unsutured clear corneal incisions greater than 4.0 mm in width.

POSTOPERATIVE CLINICAL COURSE AND OUTCOMES

The usual postoperative regime involves examination on the first postoperative day and a second examination at 10 to 14 days, at which time spectacle correction is prescribed. Administration of drops postoperatively include instillation two to three times a day of a fluoroquinolone, prednisolone acetate and Voltaren ophthalmic solution. The antibiotic and steroid are discontinued at 10 to 14 days. The Voltaren is continued for an additional 10 weeks for its theoretical benefit in suppressing lens epithelial cell division and biosynthesis of collagen precursors.[44]

Numerous studies have been performed documenting the safety and low magnitudes of astigmatism induced by these incisions depending on their size. Masket has documented by vector analysis 0.50 diopter of induced cylinder and less than 0.25 diopter of cylinder change in the surgical meridian using 3.0×2.5 mm self-sealing temporal clear corneal incisions. He was also able to demonstrate the refractive stability of these incisions 2 weeks after surgery.[45] Kohnen compared the surgically induced astigmatism of 3.5-mm, 4.0-mm, and 5.0-mm grooved temporal clear corneal incisions and found a mean induced astigmatism of 0.37 D, 0.56 D, and 0.70 D, respectively, after 6 months.[46] A similar study by Pfleger revealed even smaller degrees of induced astigmatism from 3.2-mm, 4.0-mm, and 5.2-mm temporal clear corneal incisions with the 3.2-mm incision demonstrating astigmatic neutrality with only 0.09 D of induced cylinder.[47]

In addition to comparing the effects of different sized temporal clear corneal incisions on induced astigmatism, numerous studies have evaluated the relative astigmatic effects of incision location in regards to clear corneal incisions versus corneoscleral incisions, and the temporal versus superior meridian. Nielsen evaluated surgically induced astigmatism from 3.5-mm and 5.2-mm temporal and superior clear corneal incisions and compared them with 3.5-mm and 5.2-mm corneoscleral incisions at the superior location.[48] The 3.5-mm clear corneal incisions induced roughly 0.5 D of with-the-rule or against-the-rule drift, depending on temporal or superior location. Larger degrees of astigmatism were induced with the larger clear corneal incisions. He found that the refractive effect of clear corneal incisions was stable between postoperative day 1 and postoperative week 6, making their astigmatic keratotomy effect more useful and predictable if one wished to consider preoperative cylinder when selecting incision type or location.

Cillino compared the astigmatic effects of unsutured 5.2-mm temporal clear corneal incisions with 5.2-mm superior corneoscleral incisions and found comparable degrees of induced astigmatism.[49] Rainer, however, has found a small but significant degree of surgically induced astigmatism continuing up to 5 years postoperatively with 5.0-mm superior scleral incisions.[50] Although the use of unsutured 5.2-mm clear corneal incisions is considered controversial because of a possible increase in rates of wound complications and endophthalmitis, Holweger has demonstrated that absorbable sutured 5.0-mm clear corneal incisions were topographically comparable to 3.5-mm sutureless clear corneal incisions 6 to 8 months postoperatively, making this incision and closure technique a viable option for surgeons.[51]

When temporal clear corneal incisions of 3.2 mm or less have been compared with superiorly placed scleral tunnel incisions of the same size, similar degrees of low induced astigmatism have been documented for the two incision locations.[52,53] In contrast, similarly sized incisions when compared with regard to temporal versus superior clear corneal location have demonstrated more meridional flattening in the superior axis than in the temporal axis.[54–56] This has also been demonstrated in the oblique superolateral clear corneal incision compared with a temporal incision, confirming the bias for the temporal location for clear cornea incisions when astigmatic neutrality is desired.[57]

Although small clear corneal incisions appear to have similar astigmatic effects as superior corneoscleral incisions, recent concern has surrounded the possibility of increased endothelial cell loss with these incisions. Grabow reported an increased incidence of endothelial cell loss for superior clear corneal incisions, which increased linearly with increasing ultrasound times.[58] Amon discovered a significant increase in endothelial cell loss in 3.5-mm temporal clear corneal incisions when compared to 3.5-mm superior scleral tunnel incisions.[59] However, a recent study by Dick and coauthors found that the total endothelial cell loss at1 year with clear corneal incisions compared favorably with endothelial cell loss rates of other cataract extraction techniques.[60] As ultrasound times decrease in the future with advancing technologies and techniques such as lens chopping and the use of power modulations,[61] endothelial cell loss rates should become insignificant.

CONCLUSION

Clear corneal cataract incisions are becoming a more popular option for cataract extraction and intraocular lens implantation throughout the world. Through the use of clear corneal incisions and topical and intracameral anesthesia, we have achieved a technique that is the least invasive of any in the history of cataract surgery and visual rehabilitation that is almost immediate. Clear corneal incisions have had a proven safety record and relative astigmatic neutrality with the smaller incision sizes. In addition, corneal incisions result in an excellent cosmetic outcome and should increase in popularity, especially as newer modalities such as phakic IOLs increase in popularity.

REFERENCES

1. Fine IH: Architecture and construction of a self-sealing incision for cataract surgery. J Cataract Refract Surg 1991;17:672–6.
2. Leaming DV: Practice styles and preferences of ASCRS members-1997 survey. J Cataract Refract Surgery 1998;24:552–61.
3. Colvard DM, Kratz RP, Mazzocco TR, Davidson B: Clinical evaluation of the Terry surgical keratometer. Am Intraocular Implant Soc J 1980;6:249–51.
4. Masket S: Origin of scleral tunnel methods. [Letter to the Editor] J Cataract Refract Surg 1993;19:812–3.
5. Girard LJ, Hoffman RF: Scleral tunnel to prevent induced astigmatism. Am J Ophthalmol 1984;97:450–6.
6. McFarland MS: Surgeon undertakes phaco, foldable IOL series sans sutures. Ocular Surg News 1990;8.
7. Maloney WF, Grindle L: Textbook of Phacoemulsification. Fallbrook, Ca.: Lasenda Publishers; 1988:31–39.
8. Brown DC, Fine IH, Gills JP, et al.: The future of foldables. Ocular Surg News 1992; August 15 (Suppl); Panel discussion held at the 1992 annual meeting of the American Society of Cataract and Refractive Surgery.
9. Kelman CD: Phacoemulsification and aspiration: A new technique of cataract removal: A preliminary report. Am J Ophthalmol 1967;64:23.
10. Harms H, Mackensen G: Intracapsular extraction with a corneal incision using the Graefe knife. In Ocular Surgery Under the Microscope. Stuttgart: Thieme; 1967:144–53.
11. Paton D, Troutman R, Ryan S: Present trends in incision and closure of the cataract wound. Highlights Ophthalmol 1973;14:3, 176.

12. Arnott EJ: Intraocular implants. Trans Ophthalmol Soc UK 1981; 101:58–60.
13. Galand A: La technique de l'enveloppe. Liege, Belgium: Pierre Mardaga; 1988.
14. Shimizu K: Pure corneal incision. Phaco & Foldables 1992;5;6–8.
15. Shepherd JR: Induced astigmatism in small incision cataract surgery. J Cataract Refract Surg 1989;15:85–8.
16. Fine IH: Corneal tunnel incision with a temporal approach. In Fine IH, Fichman RA, Grabow HB (eds.), Clear-Corneal Cataract Surgery & Topical Anesthesia. Thorofare, N.J.: Slack, Inc.; 1993:5–26.
17. Fine IH, Fichman RA, Grabow HB: Clear-Corneal Cataract Surgery & Topical Anesthesia. Thorofare, N.J.: Slack, Inc.; 1993.
18. Rosen ES: Clear corneal incisions: A good option for cataract patients. A Roundtable Discussion. Ocular Surg News February 1, 1998.
19. Park HJ, Kwon YH, Weitzman M, Caprioli J: Temporal corneal phacoemulsification in patients with filtered glaucoma. Arch Ophthalmol 1997;115:1375–80.
20. Hogan MJ, Alvarado JA, Weddell JE (eds.): Histology of the Human Eye: An Atlas and Textbook. Philadelphia: WB Saunders; 1971:118–119.
21. Menapace RM: Preferred incisions for current foldable lenses and their impact on corneal topography. Abstract. Cataract Workshop on the Nile, Luxor-Aswan, Egypt; November 20, 1996.
22. Fine IH: Descriptions can improve communication. Ophthalmology Times 21:30,4; December 15, 1996.
23. Ernest PH, Lavery KT, Kiessling LA: Relative strength of scleral corneal and clear corneal incisions constructed in cadaver eyes. J Cataract Refract Surg 1994;20:626–9.
24. Ernest PH, Fenzl R, Lavery KT, Sensoli A: Relative stability of clear corneal incisions in a cadaver eye model. J Cataract Refract Surg 1995;21:39–42.
25. Mackool RJ, Russell RS: Strength of clear corneal incisions in cadaver eyes. J Cataract Refract Surg 1996;22:721–5.
26. Ernest PH, Neuhann T: Posterior limbal incision. J Cataract Refract Surg 1996;22:78–84.
27. Ernest P, Tipperman R, Eagle R, et al.: Is there a difference in incision healing based on location? J Cataract Refract Surg 1998; 24:482–6.
28. Budak K, Friedman NJ, Koch DD: Dehiscence of a radial keratotomy incision during clear corneal cataract surgery. J Cataract Refract Surg 1998;24:278–80.
29. Fine IH: Self-sealing corneal tunnel incision for small-incision cataract surgery. Ocular Surgery News May 1, 1992.
30. Williamson CH: Cataract keratotomy surgery. In Fine IH, Fichman RA, Grabow HB (eds.), Clear-Corneal Cataract Surgery & Topical Anesthesia. Thorofare, N.J: Slack, Inc.; 1993:87–93.
31. Langerman DW: Architectural design of a self-sealing corneal tunnel, single-hinge incision. J Cataract Refract Surg 1994;20:84–8.
32. Vass C, Menapace R, Rainer G, et al.: Comparative study of corneal topographic changes after 3.0 mm beveled and hinged clear corneal incisions. J Cataract Refract Surg 1998;24:1498–504.
33. Kershner RM: Clear corneal cataract surgery and the correction of myopia, hyperopia, and astigmatism. Ophthalmology 1997;104: 381–9.
34. Gills JP, Gayton JL: Reducing pre-existing astigmatism. In Gills JP (ed.), Cataract Surgery: The State of the Art. Thorofare, N.J.: Slack, Inc.; 1998:53–66.
35. Nichamin L: Refining astigmatic keratotomy during cataract surgery. Ocular Surgery News April 15, 1993.
36. Budak K, Friedman NJ, Koch DD: Limbal relaxing incisions with cataract surgery. J Cataract Refract Surg 1998;24:503–8.
37. Fine IH: New blade enhances cataract surgery. Techniques Spotlight. Ophthalmology Times September 1, 1996.
38. Jacobi FK, Dick B, Bohle R: Histological and ultrastructural study of corneal tunnel incisions using diamond and steel keratomes. J Cataract Refract Surg 1998;24:498–502.
39. Radner W, Menapace R, Zehetmayer M, Mallinger R: Ultrastructure of clear corneal incisions. Part I: Effect of keratomes and incision width on corneal trauma after lens implantation. J Cataract Refract Surg 1998;24:487–92.
40. Fine IH: Special Report to ASCRS Members: Phacoemulsification incision burns. Letter to American Society of Cataract and Refractive Surgery members, 1997.
41. Majid MA, Sharma MK, Harding SP: Corneoscleral burn during phacoemulsification surgery. J Cataract Refract Surg 1998;24: 1413–15.
42. Menapace R: Delayed iris prolapse with unsutured 5.1 mm clear corneal incisions. J Cataract Refract Surg 1995;21:353–7.
43. Endophthalmitis: State of the prophylactic art. Eyeworld News, August 1997, pp 42–3.
44. Nishi O, Nishi K, Fujiwara T, Shirasawa E: Effects of diclofenac sodium and indomethacin on proliferation and collagen synthesis of lens epithelial cells in vitro. J Cataract Refract Surg 1995;21:461–5.
45. Masket S, Tennen DG: Astigmatic stabilization of 3.0 mm temporal clear corneal cataract incisions. J Cataract Refract Surg 1996; 22:1451–5.
46. Kohnen T, Dick B, Jacobi KW: Comparison of the induced astigmatism after temporal clear corneal tunnel incisions of different sizes. J Cataract Refract Surg 1995;21:417–24.
47. Pfleger T, Skorpik C, Menapace R, et al.: Long-term course of induced astigmatism after clear corneal incision cataract surgery. J Cataract Refract Surg 1996;22:72–7.
48. Nielsen PJ: Prospective evaluation of surgically induced astigmatism and astigmatic keratotomy effects of various self-sealing small incisions. J Cataract Refract Surg 1995;21:43–8.
49. Cillino S, Morreale D, Maurceri A, et al.: Temporal versus superior approach phacoemulsification: Short-term postoperative astigmatism. J Cataract Refract Surg 1997;23:267–71.
50. Rainer G, Vass C, Menapace R, et al.: Long-term course of surgically induced astigmatism after 5.0 mm sclerocorneal valve incision. J Cataract Refract Surg 1998;24:1642–6.
51. Holweger R, Marefat B: Corneal changes after cataract surgery with 5.0 mm sutured and 3.5 mm sutureless clear corneal incisions. J Cataract Refract Surg 1997;23:342–6.
52. Oshima Y, Tsujikawa K, Oh A, Harino S: Comparative study of intraocular lens implantation through 3.0 mm temporal clear corneal and superior scleral tunnel self-sealing incisions. J Cataract Refract Surg 1997;23:347–53.
53. Poort-van Nouhuijs HM, Hendrickx KHM, van Marle WF, et al.: Corneal astigmatism after clear corneal and corneoscleral incisions for cataract surgery. J Cataract Refract Surg 1997;23:758–60.
54. Long DA, Monica ML: A prospective evaluation of corneal curvature changes with 3.0 to 3.5 mm corneal tunnel phacoemulsification. Ophthalmology 1996;103:226–32.
55. Simsek S, Yasar T, Demirok A, et al.: Effect of superior and temporal clear corneal incisions on astigmatism after sutureless phacoemulsification. J Cataract Refract Surg 1998;24:515–8.
56. Roman SJ, Auclin F, Chong-Sit DA, Ullern M: Surgically induced astigmatism with superior and temporal incisions in cases of with-the-rule preoperative astigmatism. J Cataract Refract Surg 1998;24:1636–41.
57. Rainer G, Menapace R, Vass C, et al.: Corneal shape changes after temporal and superolateral 3.0 mm clear corneal incisions. J Cataract Refract Surg 1999;25:1121–6.
58. Grabow HB: The clear-corneal incision. In Fine IH, Fichman RA, Grabow HB (eds.), Clear-Corneal Cataract Surgery & Topical Anesthesia. Thorofare, N.J.: Slack, Inc.; 1993;29–62.
59. Amon M, Menapace R, Vass C, Radax U: Endothelial cell loss after 3.5 mm temporal clear corneal incision and 3.5 mm superior scleral tunnel incision. Eur J Implant Refract Surg 1995;7:229–32.
60. Dick HB, Kohnen T, Jacobi FK, Jacobi KW: Long-term endothelial cell loss following phacoemulsification through a temporal clear corneal incision. J Cataract Refract Surg 1996;22:63–71.
61. Fine IH, Packer M, Hoffman RS: The use of power modulations in phacoemulsification: Choo choo chop and flip. J Cataract Refract Surg 2001;27:188–97.

CHAPTER 6

Scleral Tunnel Incisions: Principles and Methods

NEIL J. FRIEDMAN, M.D. and DOUGLAS D. KOCH, M.D.

Cataract surgery has progressed rapidly over the past two decades as technology and techniques have evolved. With the advent of phacoemulsification and foldable intraocular lenses, there has been a trend toward smaller incision and sutureless surgery.[1] One of the developments that has allowed this to occur successfully is the change in wound architecture. Each step of a cataract procedure builds on the previous step; therefore, to construct a successful operation, a stable foundation is required: this is the wound. The focus of this chapter is the scleral tunnel incision, with specific attention to the design and technique of wound construction.

WOUND CONSTRUCTION

The surgeon's choice among the many techniques for making the cataract wound depends in large part on the type of procedure to be performed, whether intracapsular, extracapsular, or phacoemulsification. Although most cataract extractions are performed using phacoemulsification, there are situations in which extracapsular or intracapsular cataract extraction (ECCE or ICCE) is necessary. Therefore, it is important that the surgeon be familiar with a variety of techniques to meet any situation. One of the advantages of the scleral tunnel incision is its versatility. It is used for cataract removal as well as for secondary intraocular lens (IOL) implantation or IOL exchanges, and it can be placed superiorly, obliquely, or temporally. The components of the cataract incision include location, size, shape, and architecture; each will be examined in turn.

LOCATION

Location of the wound refers to both the position relative to the limbus and the quadrant in which the incision is placed. The anterior–posterior location with respect to the limbus is important, but first it is useful to review the limbal anatomy because these landmarks are commonly used for proper wound placement and construction.

The width of the surgical limbus, like that of the cornea, is different in different meridians, being wider vertically and narrower horizontally. Superiorly, it is approximately 2 mm in width and comprises two 1-mm regions: an anterior blue zone, which overlies clear cornea, and a posterior white zone, which overlies the trabecular meshwork. The midlimbal dividing line between these two zones corresponds to Schwalbe's line, which is the termination of Descemet's membrane. The limbal boundaries are the anterior limbal border (ALB), which corresponds to the conjunctival insertion and overlies Bowman's membrane, and approximately 2 mm posteriorly, the posterior limbal border, which overlies the scleral spur/iris root (Fig. 6–1).

Incisions for ICCE and ECCE are traditionally limbal and placed 1 to 2 mm posterior to the ALB, whereas scleral incisions are longer and located 2 to 3.5 mm posterior to the ALB. This scleral location for the incision was introduced by Kratz,[2] and Girard and Hoffman[3] later coined the term "scleral tunnel." The advantages of a longer scleral dissection are increased wound healing and decreased induced astigmatism.

Incisions produce tissue gape, which causes corneal flattening in the meridian of the incision and steepen-

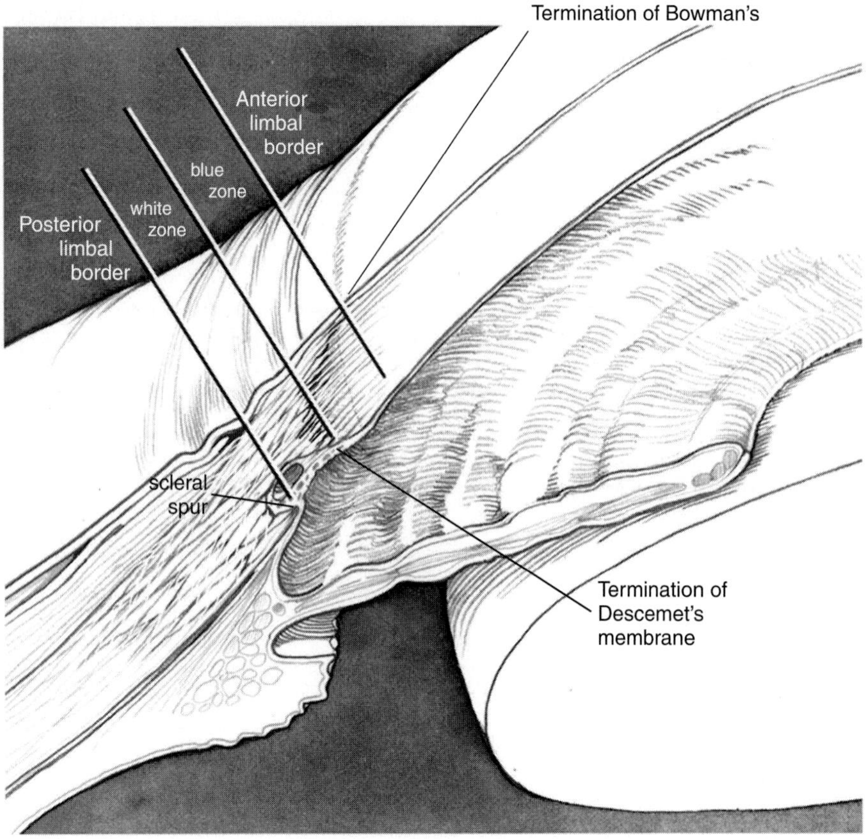

Figure 6–1. Anatomy of the surgical limbus.

ing in the meridian 90 degrees away.[4] The amount of induced change depends on the distance of the incision from the center of the cornea, the size[5] of the incision, and its shape.[6] Specifically, astigmatism is inversely proportional to the incision distance from the limbus and directly proportional to the cube of the incision length.[7,8] These interrelationships are demonstrated by Paul Koch's concept of the incisional funnel for creating astigmatically neutral wounds (Fig. 6–2).[9]

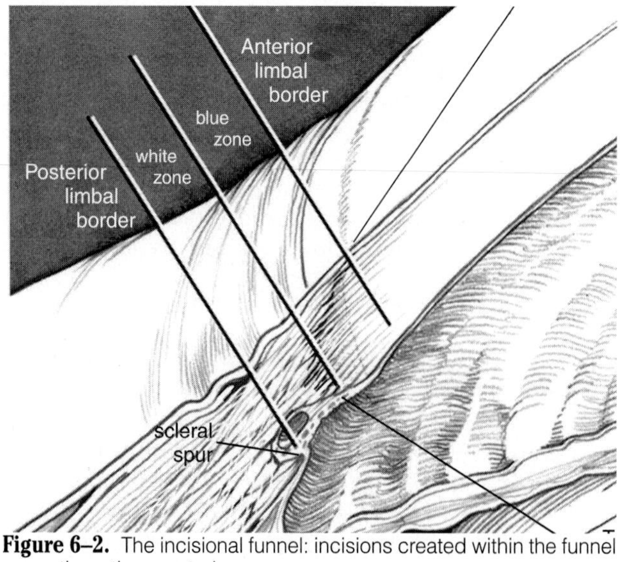

Figure 6–2. The incisional funnel: incisions created within the funnel are astigmatism neutral.

The other component of incision location is the clock hour position at which the wound is centered. Traditionally, the scleral tunnel is placed superiorly; however, with surgeons paying increasing attention to the patient's preexisting astigmatism, wound placement on the steep corneal meridian is becoming more common. In fact, temporal scleral incisions have been shown to be more stable than identical superior incisions.[10] Other factors, such as the presence of a prominent brow, deep-set orbit, corneal opacity, or filtering bleb, also need to be considered when choosing the appropriate position for the incision.

SIZE

The size of the incision is determined by the procedure (largest for ICCE and smallest for phacoemulsification), sometimes by the location, and in the case of phacoemulsification, by the IOL design. For curvilinear/circumlimbal incisions, which are used for ICCE and ECCE, the size of the wound depends on the location because the length (arc > chord) increases as the incision is moved posteriorly. As a result, it is often helpful to designate ICCE and ECCE wound size by extent in clock hours rather than length in millimeters. For phacoemulsification using a scleral tunnel, the incision width is 3 to 7 mm in chord length. The advantage of a smaller incision is reduced astigmatic effect, and, in fact, incisions that are smaller than 3.5 mm are astigmatically neutral (i.e., they induce less than 0.5 D of astigmatic change).[11]

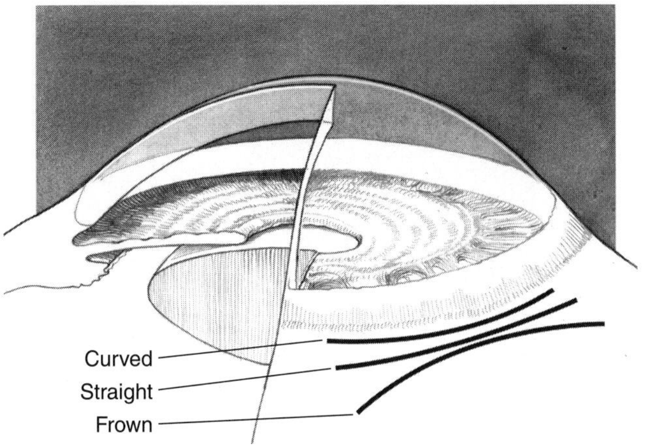

Figure 6–3. Incision shape demonstrating curved, straight, and frown incisions.

SHAPE

The shape of the external incision can take one of many forms and, like location and size, shape can affect astigmatism. As mentioned above, ICCE and ECCE wounds are typically curved and follow the limbus. The groove of the smaller scleral tunnel incision can be curved, straight (most common), frown,[6] keyhole,[12] or chevron[13] in shape (Fig. 6–3). Those that curve away from the limbus are more stable with respect to late postop against-the-wound astigmatic drift.

ARCHITECTURE

The wound architecture is described by the different incision planes. Incisions may be perpendicular or bevelled with one, two, three, or four planes (Fig. 6–4*A* and *B*). Biplanar wounds have a greater surface area than uniplanar ones, and therefore are presumably more stable. The initial groove is a partial-thickness usually perpendicular incision followed by a bevelled entry into the anterior chamber. The three-plane incision (perpendicular-bevelled-perpendicular), introduced by Gormaz[14] for corneal surgery, consists of an internal corneal lip. The four-plane incision, introduced by Dobree[15] and Swan,[16] is similar to the three plane incision but is made in the sclera (the conjunctival incision is included in the plane count). McFarland[17] later created a self-sealing scleral tunnel incision by emphasizing the corneal lip, which functions as a one-way valve.

TECHNIQUE

Although a modified scleral tunnel incision can be used to create a more stable ECCE wound, the scleral tunnel incision is used primarily for phacoemulsification. This section will describe in detail the technique for creating a self-sealing scleral tunnel (four-plane) incision.

A fornix-based conjunctival flap (plane 1) is created by performing a peritomy to expose a scleral bed of a size appropriate to accommodate the desired incision size. This is begun at one margin of the wound by tenting the conjunctiva and Tenon's fascia with 0.3-mm forceps, making a radial snip with Westcott scissors through both tissue layers, bluntly dissecting Tenon's fascia from the underlying sclera, and then cutting the limbal attachments. The initial radial cut usually provides enough relaxation of the tissues for proper exposure; however, it may be necessary to either lengthen this incision or create a second identical relaxing incision at the other end. Hemostasis is then achieved with light Wetfield cautery to blanch the exposed episcleral and scleral vessels. Care should be taken to avoid heavy cautery, as this can cause astigmatism from excessive collagen shrinkage.

The sclera is securely grasped with 0.12-mm toothed forceps or a scleral twist. To fixate the globe for the scleral incision, it is necessary to grasp the sclera securely with 0.12-mm toothed forceps. Gentle upward

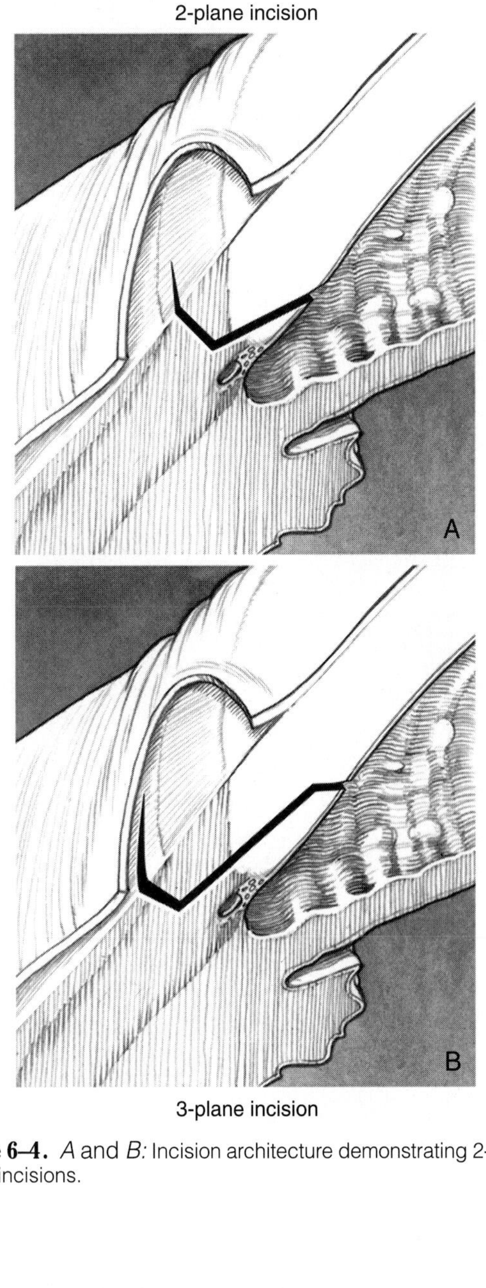

Figure 6–4. *A* and *B:* Incision architecture demonstrating 2- and 3-plane incisions.

traction prevents indenting the globe and raising the intraocular pressure during the procedure. The field is dried with a Weck cell sponge to enhance visualization of the scleral fibers during dissection, and calipers are used to measure the exact size of the desired wound at 2- to 3.5-mm posterior to the ALB. A sharp metal or gem blade, typically an angled blade or a Crescent blade, or a guarded diamond knife, is then positioned perpendicular to the sclera and used to create a ½ to ¾ depth scleral groove (plane 2). This should be done in one continuous stroke at equal depth.

Another blade, typically a bevel-up rounded Crescent blade, is then placed at the correct depth in the groove and gently "wiggled" side-to-side with forward pressure to achieve a scleral pocket dissection into clear cornea just anterior to the vascular arcade (plane 3) (Fig. 6–5). Careful attention must be paid to the orientation of the blade to assure that the dissection remains at the desired depth along its entire extent. It is necessary to follow the curve of the sclera forward and readjust when the cornea, with its steeper curvature, is approached. This is accomplished by keeping the heel of the blade down, or the tip up, because bevel-up knives tend to dive downward.

The final portion of the scleral tunnel incision is the entry into the anterior chamber, or the internal incision (plane 4). Prior to this step, many surgeons prefer to create a paracentesis and replace the aqueous humor with a viscoelastic agent. This maneuver pressurizes the eye and prevents sudden collapse of the anterior chamber when the eye is entered with the keratome, thus avoiding potential damage to the iris, lens capsule, or corneal endothelium from contact with the blade. The internal incision is performed so that a corneal lip is formed, and this functions as a one-way valve, imparting a self-sealing character to the wound. To achieve this, a 2.5- to 3.2-mm metal or diamond keratome is advanced under the scleral flap to the anterior border of the tunnel in clear cornea. The tip is then angled downward by elevating the heel of the instrument. This creates a dimpling in the cornea, visible as striae (in deep stroma and Descemet's membrane) radiating from the tip of the keratome, and is termed the "dimple down" maneuver (Fig. 6–6). When this effect is visible the blade is advanced, and as soon as the tip enters the anterior chamber, the keratome must be reoriented parallel to the iris so that a straight incision is created in Descemet's membrane. The blade is advanced to its shoulders and then removed. If the keratome is angled downward, upward, or tilted sideways while incising Descemet's membrane, the resulting internal incision will be in the shape of an arrowhead, a V, or an S, and the internal valve function may be compromised.

After the lens and residual cortex have been removed, the internal incision may need to be enlarged to accommodate the IOL. This is usually accomplished with a keratome, a Crescent knife, or a superblade, cutting on the inward stroke and keeping the tip in the anterior chamber to avoid catching and stripping Descemet's membrane. The internal incision is opened in this manner to the full extent of the external incision (Fig. 6–7).

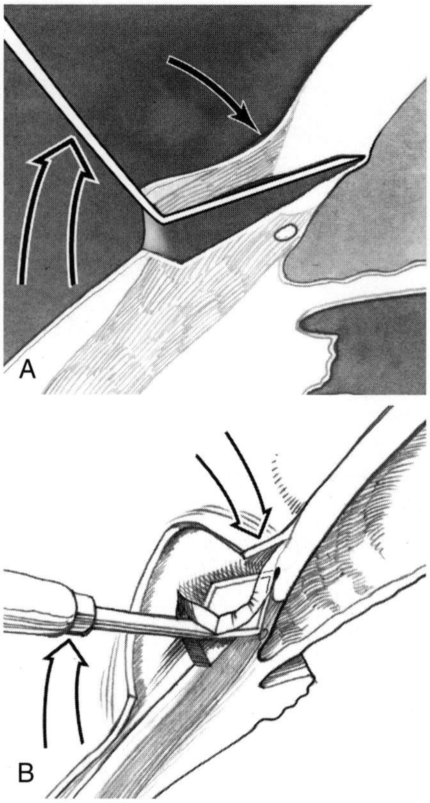

Figure 6–6. The "dimple down" maneuver created with the keratome prior to entry into the anterior chamber.

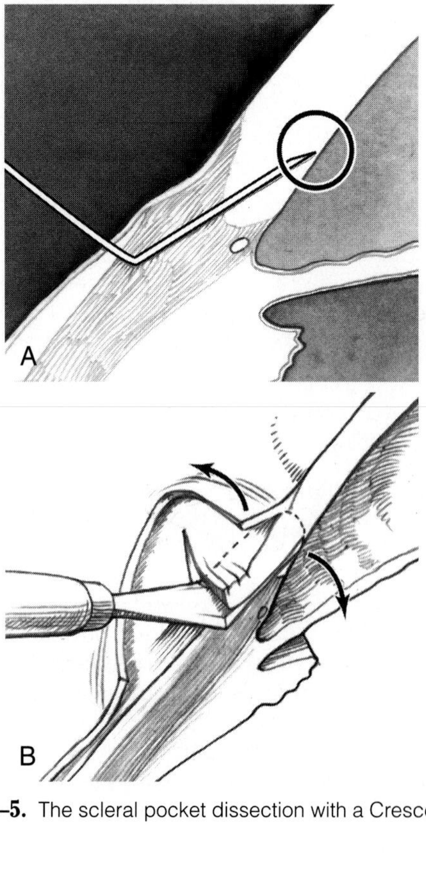

Figure 6–5. The scleral pocket dissection with a Crescent knife.

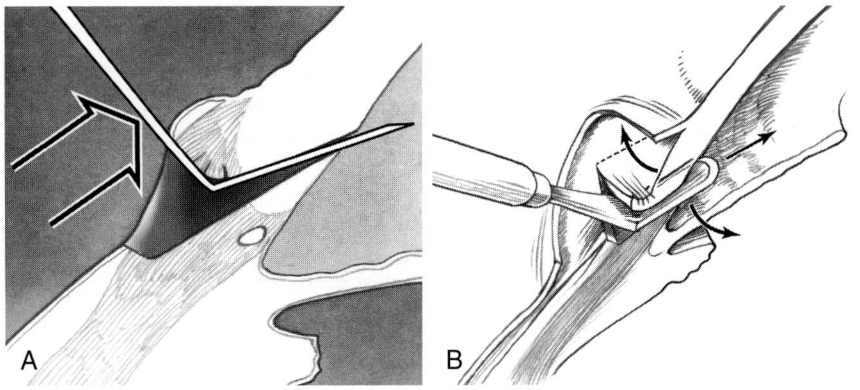

Figure 6–7. Enlarging the internal incision with a Crescent knife.

At the conclusion of the operation, the wound is tested for watertightness and self-sealability by applying pressure with a microsurgical sponge. Depending on the result and the size of the wound, any one of a variety of suturing techniques may be employed to secure the incision.

WOUND CLOSURE

Scleral tunnel incisions may be sutured or left sutureless. Small self-sealing wounds are commonly not sutured, whereas larger incisions typically are (even if found to be watertight). Various suturing techniques can be used, including running, interrupted, and continuous horizontal (Fig. 6–8). Like wound location, size, and shape, the closure can also influence astigmatism. Furthermore, all wounds to different degrees result in against-the-wound drift with time,[4] and it may therefore be beneficial to secure all incisions to limit or prevent such an effect.

Shepherd[18] first described the single horizontal suture for 4-mm incisions. This vertical mattress stitch merely apposes the scleral flap to the underlying bed, and because it is oriented tangential to the cornea, it is astigmatism neutral. Several similar wound closure techniques have since been reported for larger incisions

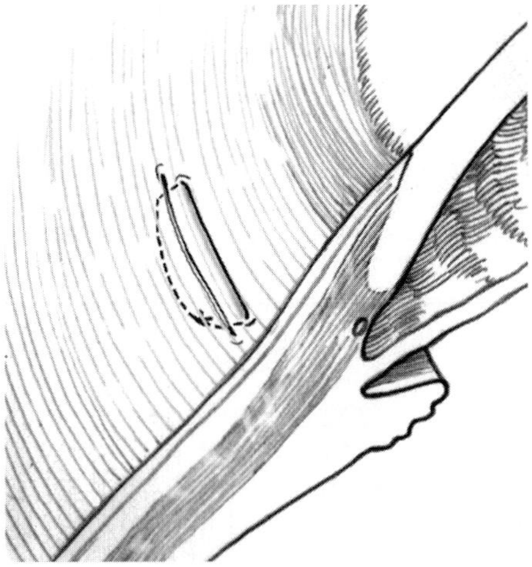

Figure 6–8. Wound closure with a horizontal suture.

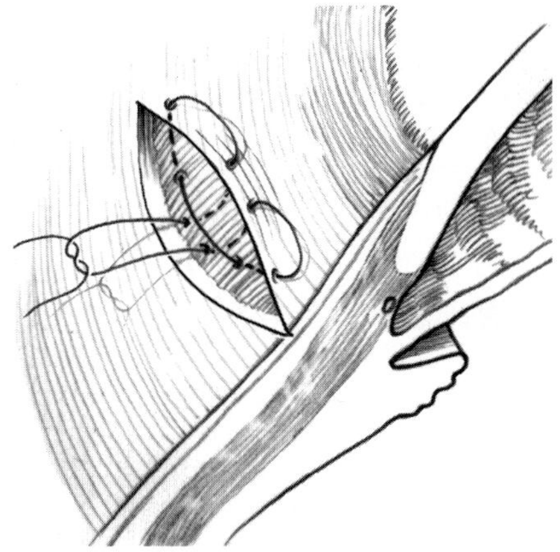

Figure 6–9. Wound closure with the horizontal anchor suture.

(5 to 7 mm), including the infinity suture,[19] the horizontal anchor suture (Fig. 6–9),[20] and the horizontal overlap suture.[21] Alternatively, larger wounds can be closed with a running shoelace stitch or interrupted sutures; the latter permit selective suture cutting postoperatively to adjust any induced astigmatism. Small incisions that require a suture to ensure watertightness in the immediate postoperative period can be closed with an absorbable material (e.g., polyglycolic acid [Vicryl, Biosorb]). Degradation of the suture material over time eliminates any prolonged suture-induced astigmatism and the risk of a late suture breakage and erosion.

COMPLICATIONS

A number of problems may occur during construction of a scleral tunnel. An initial scleral groove that is too deep (full-thickness) will cause scleral disinsertion with exposure of the ciliary body. This situation can lead to problems with hemostasis as well as poor wound stability, and suture repair is required. Similarly, the subsequent pocket may be too deep, predisposing to early or posterior entry into the anterior chamber, resulting in difficulties with iris prolapse. In contrast, a scleral pocket that is too thin or shallow may result in buttonholing the roof of the tunnel, causing problems with watertight wound closure. In either case (too deep or too shallow a scleral tunnel), if the problem is recognized early, it will be possible to redissect a more suitable plane to achieve the desired tunnel thickness and entry site into the anterior chamber. Alternatively, the initial wound may be closed with suture and the process attempted in an adjacent location.

The length of the scleral tunnel is also important. A dissection that extends too far into the cornea results in an excessively anterior entry into the eye, causing problems with decreased instrument maneuverability and the production of corneal striae, which interfere with visibility during subsequent steps. A dissection that enters too posteriorly may compromise the self-sealability of the wound and can also predispose to iris prolapse during the surgery.

Other complications related to wound construction include filtration, bleeding (with resultant hyphema), Descemet's detachment, and induced astigmatism. Thus, it is essential to be careful and precise in each aspect of wound preparation so that a properly positioned, well-designed scleral tunnel is produced and potential problems are avoided.

CONCLUSION

The importance of mastering the scleral tunnel incision cannot be overemphasized, for a well-constructed wound provides the stable foundation on which to build the rest of the operation. Once the components (location, size, shape, and architecture) are understood, a variety of wound designs can be created. A particular design should be chosen and tailored to the individual situation, taking into account the patient's orbital anatomy, ocular pathology, and preexisting astigmatism. If these principles and techniques are followed, the surgery will be successful for the surgeon and patient alike.

REFERENCES

1. Leaming D: Practice styles and preferences of ASCRS members—1995 survey. J Cataract Refract Surg 1996;22:931–9.
2. Colvard D, Kratz R, Mazzocco T, Davidson B: Clinical evaluation of the Terry surgical keratometer. Am Intraocular Implant Soc J 1980;6:249–51.
3. Girard L, Hoffman R: Scleral tunnel to prevent induced astigmatism. Am J Ophthalmol 1984;97:450–6.
4. Koch DD, Lindstrom RL: Controlling astigmatism in cataract surgery. Semin Ophthalmol 1992;7:224–33.
5. Steinert RF, Brint SF, White SM, Fine IH: Astigmatism after small incision cataract surgery. A prospective, randomized, multicenter comparison of 4- and 6.5-mm incisions. Ophthalmology 1991; 98:417–23.
6. Singer JA: Frown incision for minimizing induced astigmatism after small incision cataract surgery with rigid optic intraocular lens implantation. J Cataract Refract Surg 1991;17:677–88.
7. Armeniades C, Boriek A, Knolle GE Jr: Effect of incision length, location, and shape on local corneoscleral deformation during cataract surgery. J Cataract Refract Surg 1990;16:83–7.
8. Gills J, Sanders D (eds.): Small-Incision Cataract Surgery: Foldable Lenses, One-Stitch Surgery, Sutureless Surgery, Astigmatic Keratotomy. Thorofare, N.J.: Slack, Inc; 1990:147–50.
9. Koch PS: Structural analysis of cataract incision construction. J Cataract Refract Surg 1991;17:661–7.
10. Kohnen T, Mann PM, Husain SE, et al.: Corneal topographic changes and induced astigmatism resulting from superior and temporal scleral pocket incisions. Ophthalmic Surg Lasers 1996;27:263–9.
11. Samuelson SW, Koch DD, Kuglen CC: Determination of maximal incision length for true small-incision surgery. Ophthalmic Surg 1991;22:204–7.
12. Kershner R: Sutureless one-handed intercapsular phacoemulsification: The keyhole technique. J Cataract Refract Surg 1991;17: 719–25.
13. Pallin S: Chevron sutureless closure: A preliminary report. J Cataract Refract Surg 1991;17:706–9.
14. Gormaz B: Corneal "flap" incision for cataract operation. Br J Ophthalmol 1958;42:486–93.
15. Dobree J: Scalpel and scissors: A flanged incision for cataract extraction. Br J Ophthalmol 1959;43:513–20.
16. Swan K: Surgical anatomy in relation to glaucoma. In Clark W (ed.), Symposium on Glaucoma: Transactions of the New Orleans Academy of Ophthalmology, 1957; St. Louis: Mosby; 1959.
17. McFarland M: Surgeon undertakes phaco, foldable IOL series sans sutures. Ocular Surgery News 1990.
18. Shepherd JR: Induced astigmatism in small incision cataract surgery. J Cataract Refract Surg 1989;15:85–8.
19. Fine IH: Infinity suture: Modified horizontal suture for 6.5 mm incisions. In Gills J, Sanders D (eds.), Small-Incision Cataract Surgery: Foldable Lenses, One-Stitch Surgery, Sutureless Surgery, Astigmatic Keratotomy. Thorofare, N.J.: Slack, Inc.; 1990:191–6.
20. Masket S: Horizontal anchor suture closure method for small incison cataract surgery. J Cataract Refract Surg 1991;17:689–95.
21. Fishkind W: Horizontal overlap suture: A new astigmatism-free closure, focus on phaco. Ocular Surgery News 1990:8.

CHAPTER 7

Capsulorrhexis

THOMAS NEUHANN, M.D.

With the advent of modern extracapsular cataract surgery techniques through Binkhorst and Charles Kelman, better and more controlled anterior capsulectomy techniques were needed to make controlled manipulation of the nucleus and aspiration of cortex possible. The "can-opener" technique and the "letter box" technique became the most widely used approaches. The need for yet better controlled techniques arose when surgeons realized that positioning and stability of the lens was not optimal when the lens was not placed in the capsular bag. With the aforementioned techniques they could well be placed in the capsular bag, but it soon became apparent that in a sizeable number of cases they did not stay there because one or more peripheral tears in the anterior capsular margin frequently occurred, which eventually allowed the lens haptic to slip out of the bag. Capsulorrhexis was primarily developed to solve that problem.[1,2]

TERMINOLOGY

The term "kapsulorrhexis" was proposed by Neuhann to make clear that he was describing a truly new surgical technique and a new surgical principle (namely tearing instead of cutting), not just another modification of existing techniques. It is derived from the Greek word καψυλη = membrane and ρηγνυναι = to tear. Howard Gimbel originally called his technique "continuous tear capsulotomy." Bringing the two terms together yields "CCC" for continuous curvilinear (more general than circular) capsulorrhexis."

PRINCIPLE AND ADVANTAGE OF CAPSULORRHEXIS

The basis of capsulorrhexis is the property of the lens capsule to mechanically behave like cellophane: Tearing it perpendicular to a smooth margin is difficult, but it tears readily from a sharply pointed edge; also, such a tear can be directed as desired. If a hole in the lens capsule has a smooth continuous edge, the remaining part will stay under the same tension, as if no hole were present.

The obvious advantages of this are:

1. No tags or flaps of anterior capsule interfere with surgery, especially the aspiration of cortical remnants.
2. The forces exerted onto the capsule, and thereby onto the zonules, are lessened.
3. The capsular bag is deeply open during surgery with a closed-system approach: The posterior capsule is ballooned posteriorly and thus held on stretch, reducing the danger of its getting snagged and broken; the anterior capsule remains on stretch horizontally, maintaining intracapsular space for surgical maneuvers.

4. Radial tears are less likely to occur with an intact capsulorrhexis.
5. It is the prerequisite for a secure, verifiable, reproducible, and permanent intracapsular implantation and fixation of artificial lenses.
6. Even in the event of a posterior capsular rupture, an intact or at least mainly intact capsulorrhexis margin may allow for secure intraocular lens implantation into the ciliary sulcus, yet still benefiting from most of the advantages of capsular fixation.
7. It can be learned "by doing" without exposing the patient—nor the physician—to any risk.

REGULAR TECHNIQUE

There are three basic choices a surgeon must make for establishing a standard technique:

1. The instrument: a cystotome of some sort or a forceps
2. The access: via the main incision or via a side-port paracentesis
3. The medium: irrigation with fluid or viscoelastic material

Although all three options may theoretically be freely combined, there are two primary choices:

1. With a bent needle or cystotome, through a side paracentesis, under fluid (or viscoelastic) irrigation
2. With a forceps, through the main incision (or a side port/paracentesis), under viscoelastic irrigation

For the first option, I bend a 23-gauge needle to about a one-quarter circle and bend the tip 45 degrees away from the bevel. With the needle mounted on an infusion handpiece, I connect it to the gravity-fed infusion at its maximum height. With the infusion continuously running, the anterior chamber can be entered through the side port, the size of which should just about permit passage of the needle. The chamber can thus be perfectly formed and made as deep as possible. I then use the needle tip to perforate the anterior capsule near the center, and slit it in a curvilinear manner with the cutting edge of the needle so that the desired radius of the capsulorrhexis is reached in a blend-in manner. When about to reach the desired circumference, I lift the capsule from underneath close to the leading tear edge, pushing upward and forward to propagate the tear. This creates enough of a flap to permit flipping it over, engaging it from the back side—its epithelial side—which now faces upwards, toward the cornea. I then allow the needle to engage the flap by exerting enough pressure to create the necessary friction for engagement, but not enough pressure to cause the needle tip to perforate. With the capsular flap thus engaged, it is possible to tear it in a circular fashion by appropriately influencing the tear vectors. The more distant the point of engagement lies from the leading edge of the tear, the more centripetally one must tear; the closer the point of engagement is to the leading edge, the more directly the tear will follow the direction of traction. It is therefore most advisable, to regrasp the tear frequently close to the leading edge, a basic principle that governs the entire technique and its variations. After I bring the tear around full circle, I blend it into itself, automatically coming from the outside edge inward, a basic prerequisite to avoid a discontinuity.

The same technique can be employed with the anterior chamber filled with a viscoelastic substance. One would follow the same guidelines—except that the infusion of viscoelastic is not continuously running. When using viscoelastic material to maintain the chamber, it is important to keep the capsular flap of increasing size spread flat over its undersurface so that the edge of the tear is always clearly visible. Disregarding this detail may lead to a crimped flap, frozen in the viscoelastic, and possibly mixed with dug-up cortex. These procedural errors may make identification of the tear edge difficult if not impossible, leading to loss of control over the flap.

For the **forceps technique** use of a viscoelastic substance is essential to maintain the anterior chamber. With a forceps of the Utrata type, access must be through the main incision, which for that purpose must be fully widened to at least 3 mm. With a forceps of a vitrectomy-type construction, such as the Koch forceps, a paracentesis opening of appropriate size is sufficient. Otherwise, the forceps technique follow the same principles and guidelines as outlined above for the needle technique.

A capsulorrhexis forceps has the advantage of permitting direct grasping of the capsule, which makes the technique easier for many surgeons. The disadvantage is the possible loss of good visualization for the reasons described above for the needle technique under viscoelastic infusion. Furthermore, the forceps technique makes loss of viscoelastic inevitable. This leads to some flattening of the anterior chamber and consequently a forward movement of the lens. This, in turn, leads to an increase of the outward-pulling vector forces inherent in the lens capsule, which makes it more and more difficult to keep the tear from running outwards. Knowing the danger means preventing it: Refilling the chamber with viscoelastic as losses occur can prevent this source of loss of control over the capsular tear. Additionally, using instruments that open only at the tip (vitrectomy-type, Koch capsulorrhexis forceps) will help to prevent such mishaps.

Two additional aspects of capsulorrhexis technique merit discussion.

THE QUESTION OF THE IDEAL SIZE

Most surgeons prefer a size that will just cover the margin of the optical part of the IOL, completely sealing it to the capsular bag.
Ideally, the size should

- be as large as possible: The larger the opening, the less the danger of posterior synechiae between the capsulorrhexis margin and the iris pigment layer, which may lead to chronic low-grade iritis with recurring precipitates on the intraocular lens surface.

- allow the anterior capsular margin to just cover the optical part of the intraocular lens, completely sealing it into the capsular bag.

Limitations to obtain the ideal size include

- the size of the pupil.
- the central insertion of the zonular fibers.

An asymmetrical opening that partly covers the optic margin is to be avoided because it may cause decentration.

LEARNING CAPSULORRHEXIS

One of its major advantages is that capsulorrhexis can be learned "by doing" without exposing the patient to any additional risk. No matter which technique of anterior capsulotomy the surgeon employs, the procedure proceeds along the given guidelines. If the tear starts moving in an unwanted direction, the surgeon can revert to his or her standard (previous) technique.

DIFFICULT SITUATIONS

Capsulorrhexis is best learned under ideal conditions—i.e., good to adequate pupillary dilatation, clear red reflex, adequate chamber depth, and no active back pressure.

There are four physical types of difficulties for capsulorrhexis:

- Small pupil
- No red reflex
- Positive back pressure
- Extreme elasticity: the infantile/juvenile capsule

Although these features frequently occur in various combinations, let us look at each one of these situations separately in order to make the basic principles of management clear.

SMALL PUPIL

In addition to precluding visualization of the capsular area and where the surgeon wishes to place the tear, the small pupil in most instances also causes reduction of the red reflex.

Measures to increase the pupillary diameter may include injection of atropine or epinephrine into the anterior chamber; filling the chamber with viscoelastic material; peeling off the fibrous lining of the posterior aspect of the pupil, which often limits its dilatation; dilatation of the pupil with self-retaining hooks; or local dilatation of the pupil by placing a second instrument through a second paracentesis and manipulating the capsule, sliding along the pupillary edge with the progression of the tear. Pulling the tear around behind the iris without actually seeing the tear edge is possible, but it requires considerable experience. In any case, the diameter of the capsulorrhexis should be the same in all cases—i.e., considerably larger than the "small" pupil, in order to avoid the development of synechiae between the iris and the rhexis margin.

NO RED REFLEX

When there is no adequate reflex from the fundus to retroilluminate the surgical site for visualization, other clues must be used to "detect" the capsular margin and so control the tear at every moment. First, inclining the eye slightly with regard to the observation and illumination paths can sometimes produce enough of a red reflex to safely proceed. Also, side illumination—in addition to or instead of coaxial illumination—can be helpful. Often, there is some benefit from the "orange-skin"-like specular reflex of the coaxial light source on the capsule: Constant manipulation of the eye in such a way that the progressing tear edge remains in that reflex zone outlines the tear very clearly. Also, the surgeon should always choose the highest magnification that does not interfere with the necessary overview. Finally, proceeding slowly, in small steps and with frequent regrasping will help the surgeon maintain control of the flap.

Recently, dyeing of the capsule has been proposed (with indocyanine green, fluorescein, methylene blue, gentian violet, and trypan blue). Of all the dyes tested, trypan blue is clearly the first choice. It is instilled under an air bubble onto the anterior capsule, and any excess is flushed after a few seconds. This dyes the capsule well enough to improve visibility.

POSITIVE FORWARD PRESSURE

The problem with positive back pressure is that it has a very pronounced tendency to force the tear outward. Therefore, the procedure should involve an intentionally small diameter to begin with—which can be widened as soon as the pressure is relieved—and continuous pronounced centripetal traction in small steps, with frequent regrasping close to the tear edge. Exerting counterpressure by pushing the lens back with viscoelastic material is helpful.

The *intumescent lens* combines the difficulties of forward pressure with those of a lack of red reflex. Filling of the anterior chamber with a thick viscoelastic substance is advisable to block opaque liquefied cortex from leaking into the aqueous humor and compromising visibility. Usually, the forceps technique is preferable, because the cortex is more or less liquefied and therefore presents no resistance to the needle tip. Capsular dyeing has become the method of choice in visualizing these "white cataracts." Sometimes it is possible to decompress the lens by making a small puncture in the anterior lens vertex and aspirating some of the liquid content to take the distensive forces off the anterior capsule; this maneuver, however, carries a significant risk of causing an uncontrollable tear to the periphery. Gimbel has shown that sometimes one can initially perform a can-opener capsulotomy, the margin of which is torn out with a secondary rhexis—if it then is still without radial tears.[6]

THE INFANTILE/JUVENILE CAPSULE

The infantile/juvenile lens capsule is characterized by extreme elasticity. As the surgeon tears on a flap, the capsule will first distend considerably, before propagating the tear; once the tear starts, therefore, it can easily get lost outwardly, as a result of the traction "preload" and the elastic tension, which create a pronounced outward pulling vector force. It is therefore advisable to plan a tear smaller than one really wishes it to be, because it will become wider by itself. The surgeon should progress slowly and in small steps, with frequent regrasping of the margin and pronounced centripetal tearing.

Should a discontinuity in the rhexis margin occur, because of the increased elasticity, it is less likely to progress peripherally when due caution is maintained during surgery.

The only situation in which capsulorrhexis is indeed principally impossible is the case of the totally fibrosed capsule. Heavy fibrosis or fibrous plaques extending so far peripherally that it is not possible to tear around them without hitting zonules mandate the use of scissors to cut through the fibrosis. The scissor-cut should end just at the margin of the fibrosis, from which point the opening should be continued as a tear.

SPECIAL SURGICAL TECHNIQUES

Following the principles described above has led to the development of "tricks" that may prove helpful in certain situations.

"BIMANUAL FORCEPS"

Sometimes it is difficult to grasp and manipulate the capsular flap with just the needle tip. In such situations, the surgeon may prefer to change to a forceps technique, perhaps only intermittently. However, when removing the irrigating cystotome, the lens diaphragm can come forward, causing the tear to divert outwardly. To avoid this problem, a bifurcated spatula of the Bechert type can be introduced into the chamber through an opposite paracentesis, the capsular flap pinched between needle tip and fork-notch, and, thus grasped, the flap can be manipulated as with a forceps.

BIMANUAL/BI-INSTRUMENTAL CAPSULORRHEXIS

When the zonules are very weak, pulling centripetally on the flap may risk disinsertion of the capsule. Holding the flap with capsular forceps with one hand and gently pushing the peripheral margin outward, centrifugally, makes it possible to propagate the tear with less stress on the zonules.

POSTERIOR CAPSULORRHEXIS

Leaving the posterior capsule intact is one of the major advantages of extracapsular surgery. Nevertheless, this is a goal that cannot always be attained. The posterior capsule must be opened in the case of a dense, nonremovable posterior capsular opacification that will doubtlessly interfere significantly with vision (very rare, but occurring) or infantile cataract. The most frequent cause, however, is accidental posterior capsular rupture/defect. In all of these cases, the necessary/inevitable opening in the posterior capsule should have the same quality, if possible, as that of the anterior capsule. That is, it should not be further extendable, which requires the surgeon to maintain a continuous smooth margin, and that can be accomplished by applying the exact same technique of capsulorrhexis to the posterior capsule. In intended cases, the posterior capsule should be nicked (without perforating) with a needle tip, so that viscoelastic material can be injected through the first tiny triangular defect in order to separate and posteriorly displace the anterior vitreous face. At that point the posterior capsular triangle can be grasped by capsular forceps and torn out circularly/curvilinearly.

When an unintended capsular defect occurs, it can be blunted—and thus prevented from extending—by the same technique, as long as it is limited enough to permit this. This technique will then preserve a tire-shaped capsular bag into which an intraocular lens can be implanted securely, maintaining all the advantages of intracapsular implantation.

"RHEXIS-FIXATION"

In the case of a posterior capsular rupture that cannot be saved, another "trick" may maintain most of the advantages of capsular implant fixation: If the anterior capsulorrhexis margin is intact, the intraocular lens can be implanted into the ciliary sulcus, the optic part being captured, "buttoned-in" backwards through the capsulorrhexis. This provides secure mechanical fixation of the lens by the capsule and centration in relation to the capsular opening, the lens haptics only acting supportively. The lens is also in the same position as though intracapsularly implanted, which maintains the correct refractive effect.

COMPLICATIONS AND PITFALLS

Three classical intraoperative complications can occur with capsulorrhexis:

- Discontinuity of the anterior capsular margin
- Tear into the zonules
- Diameter too small

Two classical postoperative complications can also occur:

- Purse-string contraction
- Incarceration of viscoelastic

DISCONTINUITY OF THE ANTERIOR CAPSULAR MARGIN

The major factors in discontinuity of the anterior capsular margin are completing the capsulorrhexis "from inside outwards," nicking an originally intact margin with a second instrument during lens extraction, or braking the rim with the activated phaco tip.

A discontinuity in an otherwise intact CCC-margin will in most cases extend into a radial tear into the capsular fornix; it will do so very readily, because the distensive forces concentrate on this single point of weakness. The risk of this radial tear extending around the capsular fornix into the posterior capsule increases with rarification and friability of the zonules and with all maneuvers that distend the anterior capsular opening (such as hydrodissection and hydroexpression of the nucleus), nuclear fracturing techniques that rely on pushing the nuclear parts widely apart, and all implantation-associated maneuvers. The most important rule is to ***always close the circle from outside inwards.*** This will automatically occur, when the surgeon starts the tear somewhere in the center of the capsule, as described above. If the flap breaks off during the course of tearing, it becomes crucial to grasp the remaining flap and continue the outward-pointing tear edge.

When a discontinuity occurs, timely recognition is of key importance! Its edge must then instantly be grasped with forceps and blunted by blending the margin into the main contour. When a tear has occurred into the capsular fornix, utmost caution is warranted not to distend the tear further. Placing a relaxing counterincision opposite the first tear may be considered.

A radial tear does not preclude capsular bag implantation, if manipulations are appropriately gentle. The lens haptics should be placed at an angle 90 degrees from the radial tear. For plate haptic lenses such a tear is a relative contraindication.

TEAR INTO THE ZONULES

If the tear hits zonular fibers, either because it is too close to the periphery of the capsule or because zonules are inserting abnormally centrally, then it cannot readily be continued. Further tearing will have the effect of tearing paper against a ruler and will risk deviation of the tear to the periphery.

With the help of high microscope magnification, an optimized red reflex, or a specular reflex and optimal focusing, the causative zonule(s) can be identified and their insertions removed from the capsule with the needle or forceps tip. Then it becomes possible to bring the tear more centrally and to continue it. Sometimes this situation can also be managed by grasping the flap close to its edge and briskly pulling it centrally; this maneuver, however, carries a higher risk and is advised only when the more controlled approach does not seem possible.

CAPSULORRHEXIS WITH TOO SMALL A DIAMETER

If the surgeon realizes that the diameter of the CCC is smaller than desired, it is possible simply to continue the tear in a spiral manner until the desired diameter is reached.

PURSE-STRING CONTRACTION

The remaining lens epithelial cells on the back surface of the anterior capsule postoperatively undergo fibrous metaplasia. The contraction of this fibrous layer is normally counteracted by the centrifugal forces of the zonular apparatus. However, when either the zonules are weak (as in pseudoexfoliation, trauma, or retinitis pigmentosa, for example) or when the fibrosis is excessive (e.g., after increased postoperative inflammation, with some silicone lenses and other factors), or in combinations of both, the anterior capsular opening may contract ("capsular phimosis"). In cases identified at risk for excessive contraction the surgeon should aim for a relatively large opening, implant lenses with stiff haptics and an overall diameter of about 13 mm, consider implantation of a capsular expansion ring (or even two), and perhaps even avoid using silicone as a lens material. Postoperatively, the patient should be monitored closely and at the first sign of contraction the anterior capsular margin should be incised with a Nd:YAG laser at three or four equidistant locations. Extension of these discontinuities need not be feared at this stage, due to the fibrous lining itself and the already secure sealing of the intraocular lens.

INCARCERATION OF VISCOELASTIC MATERIAL

Residual viscoelastic material may become trapped behind an implant, when its margin is completely covered by the capsulorrhexis. The implant will act as a valve, permitting the influx of aqueous behind the lens, but not the efflux of the thick viscoelastic–aqueous mixture. This finding is more pronounced with plate haptic lenses, but it can happen with all types of implants.

The consequence may be gross inflation of the capsular bag, with posterior ballooning of the posterior capsule and anterior displacement of the intraocular lens. This complication can best be avoided by complete removal of the viscoelastic material, actively aspirating it from behind the lens. When it has occurred, the material can be released into the anterior chamber by puncturing the anterior capsule beyond the optical margin. If this cannot be achieved, the posterior capsule must be punctured, releasing the material into the vitreous. Timely recognition of this complication helps avoid difficulties in rectifying it because of too distended a capsular bag.

The technique of capsulorrhexis has established itself as the standard technique for the opening of the anterior capsule in phacoemulsification, if not all techniques of extracapsular cataract extraction. It is not so much definitive technique, as a general principle, which can be made to work for every surgeon's personal technical preferences as well as for every clinically occurring situation with very few exceptions. It is not only a prerequisite of predictable and permanent capsular fixation of intraocular lenses, it also greatly facilitates surgery itself.

REFERENCES

1. Assia EI, Apple DJ, Barden A, et al.: An experimental study comparing various anterior capsulectomy techniques. Arch Ophthalmol 1991;109:642–7.
2. Assia EI, Apple DJ, Tsai JC, Lim ES: The elastic properties of the lens capsule in capsulorrhexis. Am J Ophthalmol 1991;111:628–32.
3. Colvard DM, Dunn SA: Intraocular lens centration with continuous tear capsulotomy. J Cataract Refract Surg 1990;16:312–4.
4. Davison JA: Capsular bag distension after endophacoemulsification and posterior chamber intraocular lens implantation. J Cataract Refract Surg 1990;16:99–108.
5. Fritsch E, Bopp S, Lucke K, Laqua H: Pars-plana-Kapselresektion zur Therapie des okulären Hypotoniesyndroms durch Kapselschrumpfung mit Ziliarkörpertraktion. Fortschr Ophthalmol 1991;88:802–5.
6. Gimbel HV, Neuhann T: Continuous curvilinear capsulorrhexis. J Cataract Refract Surg 1991;17:110–1.
7. Harris DJ, Specht CS: Intracapsular lens delivery during attempted extracapsular cataract extraction: Association with capsulorrhexis. Ophthalmology 1991;98:623–7.
8. Hausmann N, Richard G: Investigations on diathermy for anterior capsulotomy. Invest Ophthalmol Vis Sci 1991;32:2155–9.
9. Krag S, Thim K, Corydon L: Stretching capacity of capsulorrhexis: An experimental study on animal cadaver eyes. Eur J Implant Refract Surg 1990;2:43–5.
10. Neuhann T: Theorie und Operationstechnik der Kapsulorrhexis. Klin Mbl Augenheilk 1987;190:542–5.
11. Thim K, Krag S, Corydon L: Stretching capacity of capsulorrhexis and nucleus delivery. J Cataract Refract Surg 1991;17:27–31.
12. Waltz KL, Rubin ML: Capsulorrhexis and corneal magnification (letter). Arch Ophthalmol 1992;110:170.

CHAPTER 8

Standard Extracapsular Cataract Surgery

JARED EMERY, M.D.

Indications

Techniques
Preparation
Conjunctival Incision
Scleral Incision

Anterior Capsulectomy
Removal of the Nucleus
Removal of the Cortex
Implantation of Intraocular Lens
Wound Closure

Extracapsular cataract surgery, strictly speaking, includes both phacoemulsification and standard or planned extracapsular extraction. By convention the terms *standard extracapsular* or *planned extracapsular* refer to an operation in which the lens nucleus is delivered intact through a limbal incision of about 10 mm, in contrast to *phacoemulsification,* in which the nucleus is ultrasonically fragmented and aspirated through a 3-mm incision.

During the past two decades phacoemulsification and standard extracapsular cataract surgery have replaced intracapsular extraction, except for rare instances, such as subluxated lenses or the possibility of patient sensitivity to lens material. Phacoemulsification was preferred by 12% of U.S. cataract surgeons in 1985, 52% of surgeons in 1990, and 86% of surgeons in 1995.[1] Preference by U.S. surgeons for the standard extracapsular cataract operation stabilized at 14% in 1994 and 1995 (see Fig. 8–1). In some cases it can be the safest operation. For 2 years I have used temporal clear corneal phacoemulsification in more than 99% of cases, but I believe that every cataract surgeon should be skilled in extracapsular cataract surgery. The techniques presented in this chapter were developed and honed over several recent years during which I used planned extracapsular surgery in most cases.

INDICATIONS

The extracapsular operation can be used successfully for almost any cataract. The method is not appropriate for luxated or subluxated lenses. Its main disadvantages, compared with phacoemulsification, include greater induced astigmatism and less stability of postoperative refraction.[2–4] Its main advantage is that it can, in some cases, provide a greater margin of safety. In cases where operative exposure is difficult, corneal clarity is compromised, the pupil dilates poorly, there are posterior synechiae, or zonular integrity is in question (as after pars plana vitrectomy), many surgeons will have a greater margin of safety with the extracapsular procedure.

As a rule, the procedure of choice is the one that is likely to give the most successful result. For example, proceeding with a phacoemulsification made difficult by poor exposure might involve a higher likelihood of capsular rupture with vitreous loss than might have been the case had the patient been treated by large-incision extracapsular extraction. The careful surgeon will judge each case in advance, and will choose phacoemulsification or planned extracapsular surgery based upon the expectation that it will produce the best result for the patient. In most cases this decision can be made before surgery; for some cases, however, the choice might become necessary during the operation. The extracapsular technique of Emery, to follow, allows the surgeon to switch from phacoemulsification to large-incision planned extracapsular surgery at any stage of the operation.

TECHNIQUES

The best cataract surgical techniques give consistent reproducible results. The surgeon remains in control. The

This chapter originally appeared in Steinert RF (ed). Cataract Surgery: Technique, Complications & Management. Copyright © 1995, W.B. Saunders Company.

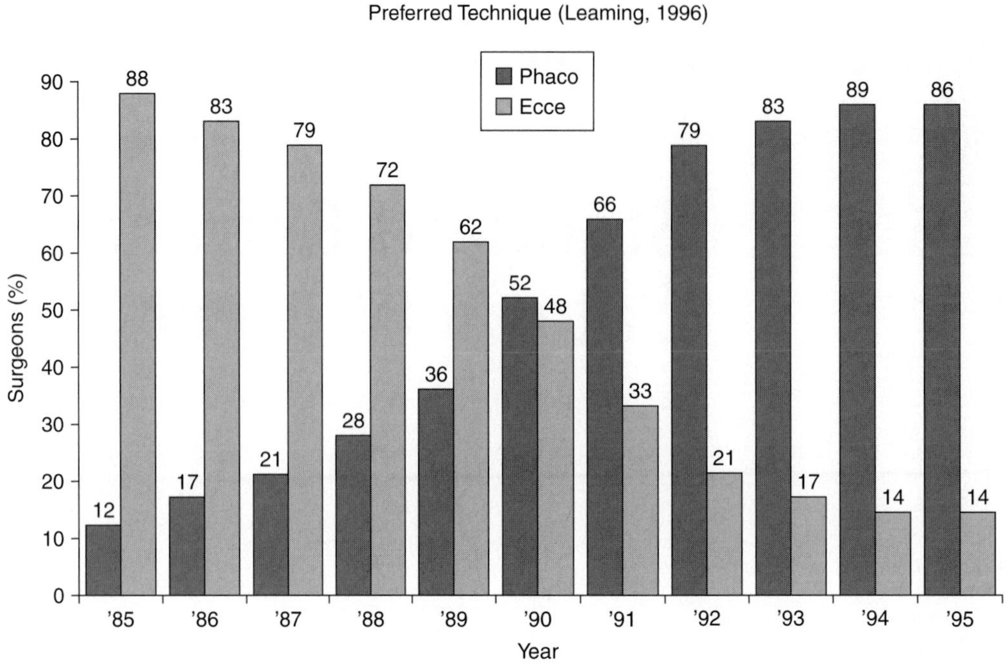

Figure 8–1. U.S. surgeons' preferred cataract extraction technique. Phaco = phacoemulsification; ECCE = standard or planned extracapsular extraction. (From Emery, A: *In* Steinert RF [ed], Cataract Surgery: Technique, Complications, & Management. Philadelphia, WB Saunders, 1995, with permission.)

operation accomplishes removal of the nucleus with minimal stress on the zonules, secure placement of an intraocular lens within an intact capsular bag, and closure with a watertight incision that gives minimal astigmatism. The procedure should be as simple as possible to promote success, and should apply, with minimal variations, to all types of cases.

PREPARATION

After aseptic preparation of the operative site, dry the lid margins with cellulose sponges. Apply a large unperforated plastic drape (3M) to the open lids, and incise (Fig. 8–2).

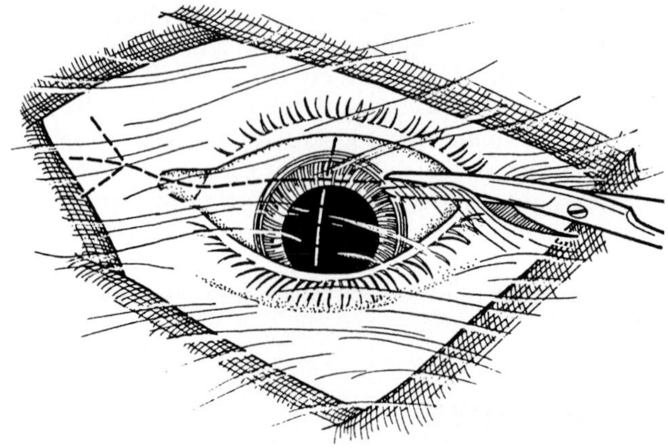

Figure 8–2. Technique for incision of plastic drape. (From Emery, A: *In* Steinert RF [ed], Cataract Surgery: Technique, Complications, & Management. Philadelphia, WB Saunders, 1995, with permission.)

Retract the upper and lower lids, using Jaffe wire lid specula. Attach a rubber band to each speculum and use a hemostat to clip the rubber band to the drapes, applying the least amount of tension needed to give adequate exposure of the globe. Place 4-0 black silk sutures beneath the insertions of the superior and inferior rectus muscles. Tuck in the flaps of the drape and attach the sutures to the rubber bands (Fig. 8–3). Use only the necessary tension to produce adequate exposure above the superior limbus, and to maintain visibility of the inferior limbus.

CONJUNCTIVAL INCISION

Make a fornix-based flap to expose the limbus using a 7-mm peritomy with oblique relaxing incisions extending from the limbus about 3 mm posteriorly as illustrated in Figure 8–4.

Apply light wet-field cautery to obliterate all visible surface vessels *posterior* to the intended incision site, which will be approximately 3 mm posterior to the anterior limbus (Fig. 8–5). Clean the limbus with a Tooke knife to "squeeze" residual blood from vessels near the limbus. Avoid fraying the scleral surface with excessive scraping.

SCLERAL INCISION

Using calipers, measure a 10-mm chord length on the sclera with the points positioned 3 mm posterior to the limbus (Fig. 8–6). Make a 10-mm partially penetrating incision using a 30 degree disposable steel microsurgical blade. The incision groove will run parallel with the

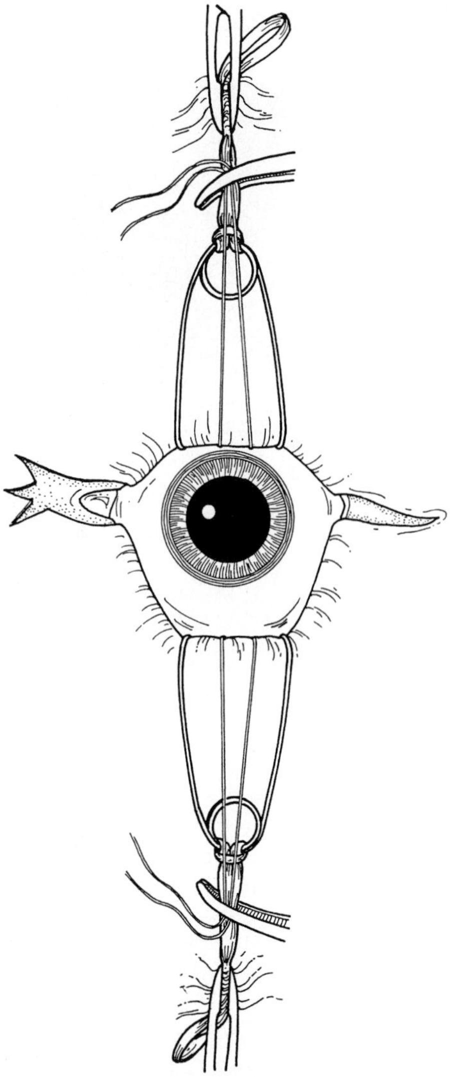

Figure 8–3. Surgeon's view of placement of Jaffe wire lid specula and rectus sutures. Note that good exposure of the operative site is achieved while still allowing visibility of the inferior limbus. (From Emery, A: *In* Steinert RF [ed], Cataract Surgery: Technique, Complications, & Management. Philadelphia, WB Saunders, 1995, with permission.)

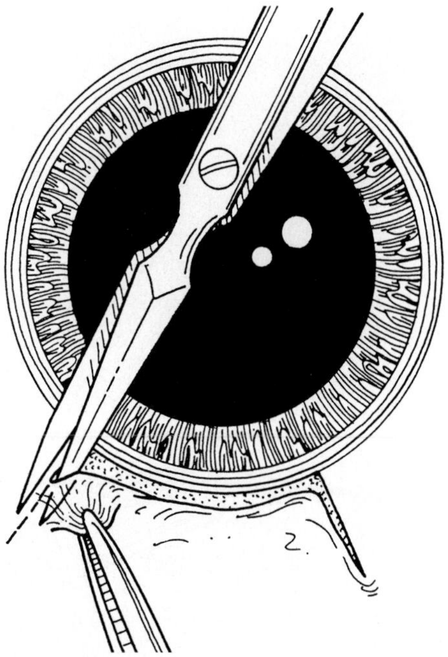

Figure 8–4. Expose the superior limbus with a 7-mm peritomy and oblique relaxing incisions. (From Emery, A: *In* Steinert RF [ed], Cataract Surgery: Technique, Complications, & Management. Philadelphia, WB Saunders, 1995, with permission.)

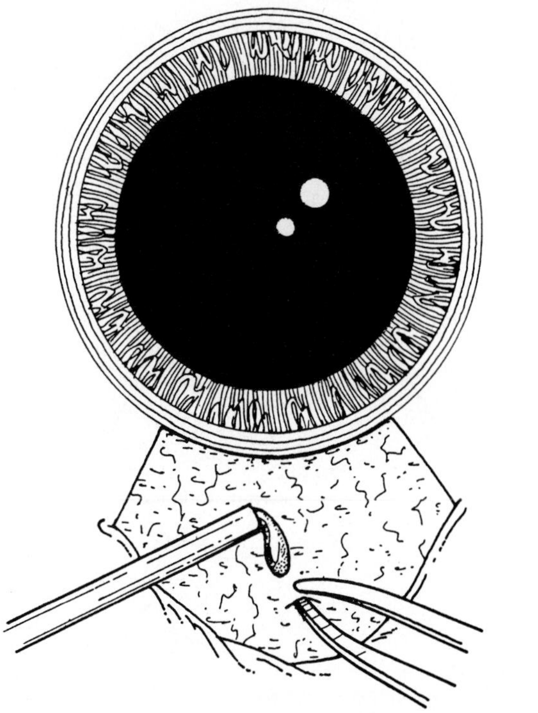

Figure 8–5. Cauterize surface vessels posterior to the incision site. (From Emery, A: *In* Steinert RF [ed], Cataract Surgery: Technique, Complications, & Management. Philadelphia, WB Saunders, 1995, with permission.)

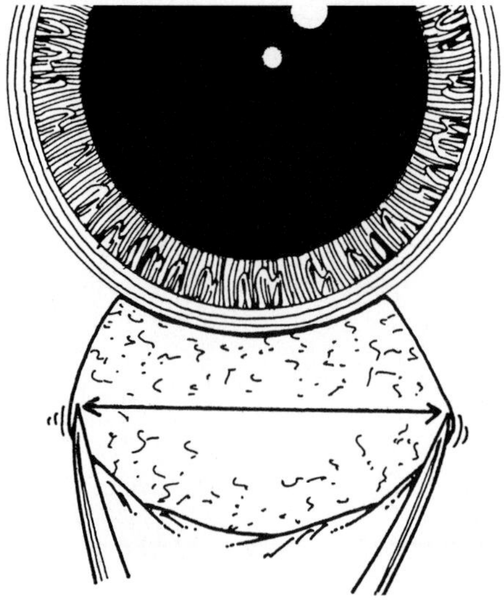

Figure 8–6. Incision site: a 10-mm chord length 3 mm posterior to the limbus. (From Emery, A: *In* Steinert RF [ed], Cataract Surgery: Technique, Complications, & Management. Philadelphia, WB Saunders, 1995, with permission.)

limbus and 3 mm posterior to the anterior limbal margin (Fig. 8–7). The groove should be perpendicular to the globe and of approximately 75% depth.

Make a lamellar scleral dissection using a disposable Crescent blade (Alcon 8065-940002). Begin this dissection at the base of the pre-placed groove. Dissect the flap anteriorly, beginning at the apex of the groove. Continue on a tangent to the globe for approximately 1 mm along the entire length of the groove. Then extend the tunnel in one location, wherever access is easiest (Fig. 8–8). Gradually proceed with the dissection anteriorly, being careful to depress the heel of the Crescent blade to avoid premature penetration at the point where the corneoscleral curvature steepens. Continue the incision anteriorly into clear cornea just beyond (central to) the limbal arcade (Figs. 8–8 and 8–9). There should be about 4 mm of scleral/corneal dissection to the point of anterior chamber entry. Keeping the blade fully inserted as in Figure 8–8, gently extend the plane of dissection right and left to the full 10-mm width; stabilize the globe by grasping the sclera posterior to the groove. Avoid grasping the scleral flap, as it might tear. Judge the depth of the scleral/corneal dissection by viewing the blade through the translucent sclera. Keep the sclera moist to give greater visibility of the blade (Figs. 8–8 and 8–9).

Use a disposable phaco blade to penetrate the anterior chamber, making an incision parallel with the iris plane. It helps to aim the point of the blade somewhat posteriorly until initial penetration is achieved; this will avoid sliding the blade up along corneal lamellae and entering the anterior chamber more centrally than desired. After penetration, level out the blade so that it remains parallel with the plane of the iris and then push in to make a 1.5-mm opening. You will extend this incision later, after the anterior capsulectomy (Fig. 8–10).

ANTERIOR CAPSULECTOMY

Fully inflate the anterior chamber with a viscoelastic substance such as sodium hyaluronate. Use a 27-gauge

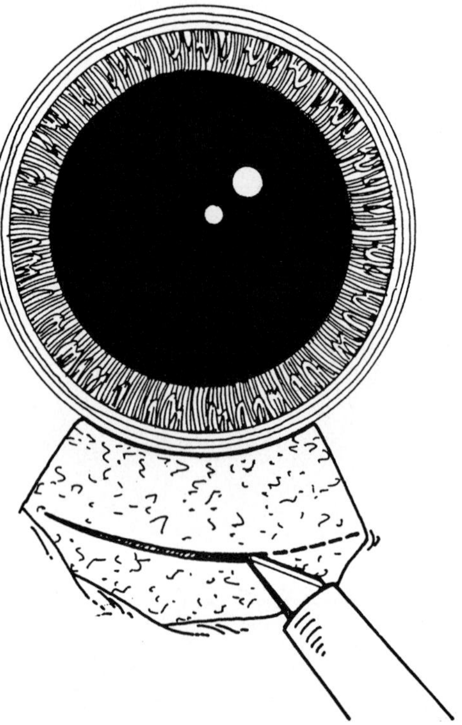

Figure 8–7. Place incision groove parallel with the limbus 3 mm posterior to the anterior limbal margin. (From Emery, A: *In* Steinert RF [ed], Cataract Surgery: Technique, Complications, & Management. Philadelphia, WB Saunders, 1995, with permission.)

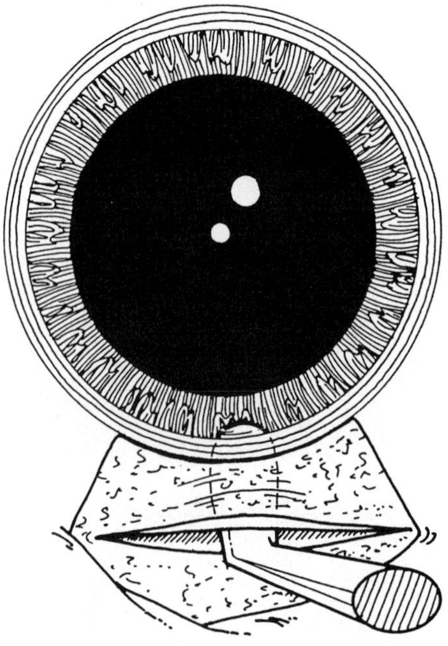

Figure 8–8. Dissection of scleral tunnel using a Crescent blade. (From Emery, A: *In* Steinert RF [ed], Cataract Surgery: Technique, Complications, & Management. Philadelphia, WB Saunders, 1995, with permission.)

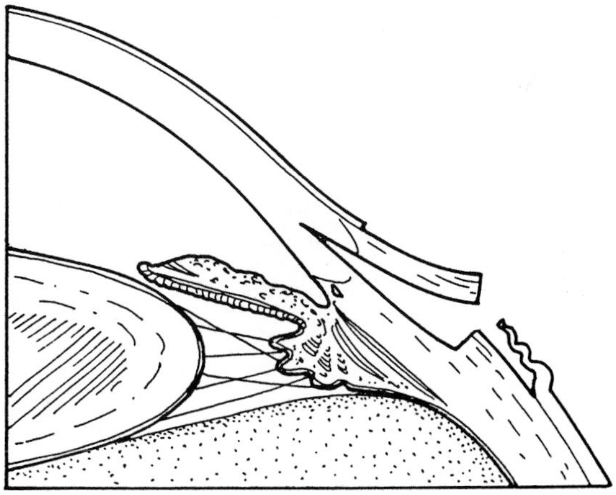

Figure 8–9. Cross-sectional view showing depth and extent of scleral tunnel. (From Emery, A: *In* Steinert RF [ed], Cataract Surgery: Technique, Complications, & Management. Philadelphia, WB Saunders, 1995, with permission.)

disposable needle with a small micro-hook at its tip to create a circular 6- or 7-mm circular anterior capsulectomy. Make very small "bites" directed in parallel with the pupillary margin. Each bite after the first should begin on top of the anterior capsule about 1 mm from the adjacent capsular incision (Fig. 8–11). A fluid movement of the micro-hook should first puncture the capsule with slight posterior pressure and then sweep parallel with the pupillary margin until the tear joins the adjacent incision.

The capsulectomy should be about 6 mm in diameter. Smaller diameter openings lead to rather large tears of the peripheral capsule that tend to destabilize the lens implant. An opening of 6 mm gives a reasonable margin of peripheral anterior capsule while allowing the nucleus to prolapse with less pronounced radial tearing.

After completion of the circular anterior capsulectomy, re-insert the blade used to make the original entry into the anterior chamber and extend the entry site to about 3 mm. Inject additional viscoelastic material before this step as needed. To skip this step, make the initial entry 3-mm wide. The 1.5-mm initial entry was suggested to help retain the viscoelastic material and maintain the depth of the anterior chamber throughout the capsulectomy. Remove the fragment of anterior capsule using toothless forceps. Insert the Crescent blade and extend the third plane of the incision parallel with the iris plane to the full 10-mm width of the previous flap dissection (Fig. 8–12). Use pushing strokes of the Crescent blade to cut the third plane; this helps make a watertight valve incision.

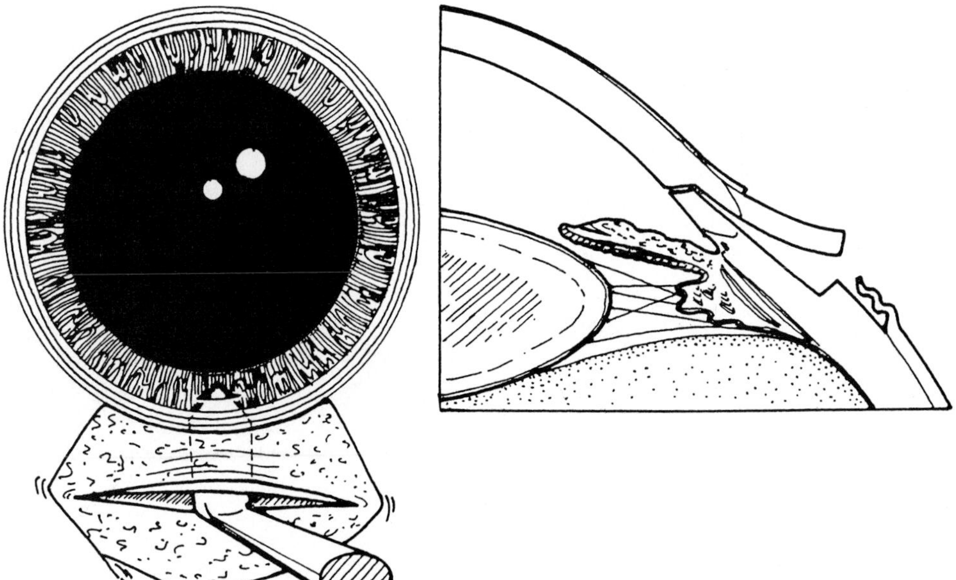

Figure 8–10. Plane three of the incision: penetration into the anterior chamber using a disposable "phaco" blade. Inset shows cross-sectional view of incisional planes. (From Emery, A: *In* Steinert RF [ed], Cataract Surgery: Technique, Complications, & Management. Philadelphia, WB Saunders, 1995, with permission.)

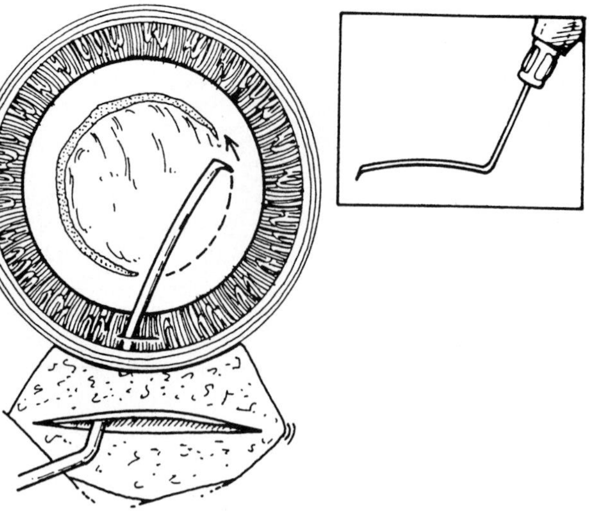

Figure 8–11. Anterior capsulectomy. For this, bend a 27-gauge disposable needle into the configuration shown in the inset. Attach the needle to a small syringe which serves as a handle. (From Emery, A: *In* Steinert RF [ed], Cataract Surgery: Technique, Complications, & Management. Philadelphia, WB Saunders, 1995, with permission.)

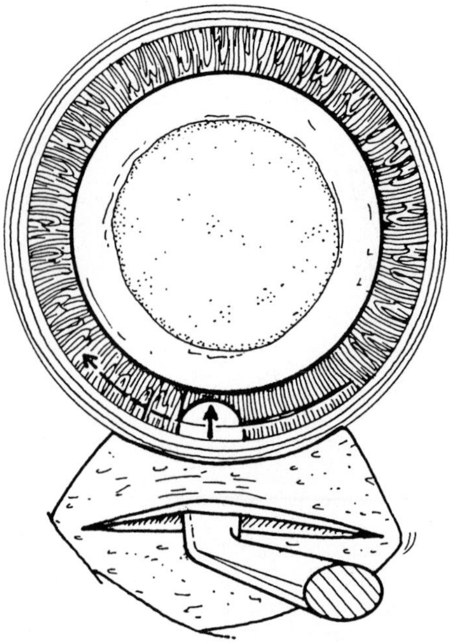

Figure 8–12. Extend plane three of the incision with the Crescent blade. (From Emery, A: *In* Steinert RF [ed], Cataract Surgery: Technique, Complications, & Management. Philadelphia, WB Saunders, 1995, with permission.)

REMOVAL OF THE NUCLEUS

Put three interrupted 9-0 black silk sutures across the lips of the scleral groove, taking about a 1-mm bite on each side. Place the sutures so that, when tied, they will be equally spaced across the wound, giving four 2.5-mm openings for passage of the irrigation/aspiration instrument (Fig. 8–13). Loop the sutures around the margins of the groove as shown in Figure 8–13.

Using a McIntyre 26-gauge cannula attached to an irrigating cystotome handpiece, prolapse the superior lens nucleus into the anterior chamber: Pass the McIntyre 26-gauge cannula into the anterior chamber at the 12 o'clock position. Move the tip to the 2 o'clock position

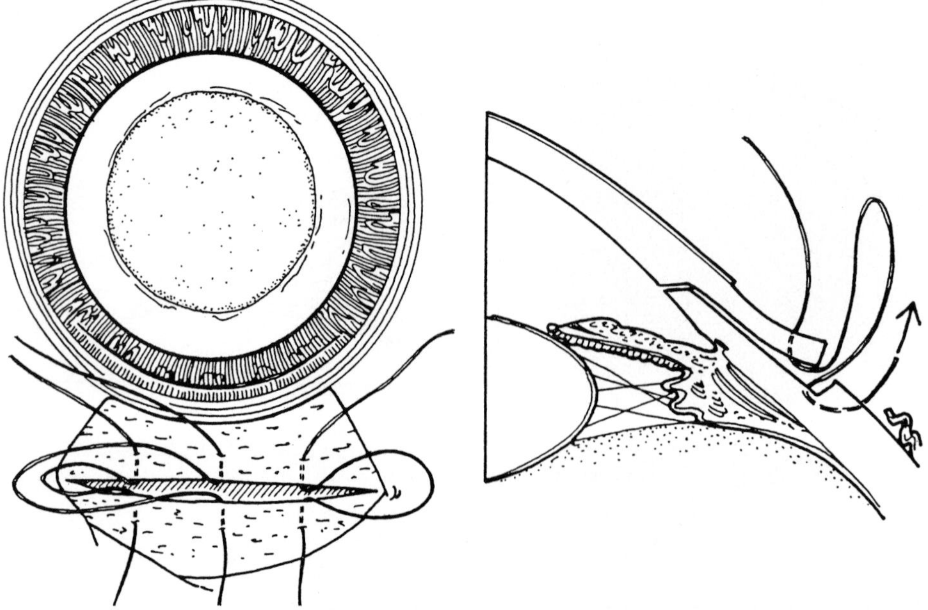

Figure 8–13. Technique for placement of three interrupted 9-0 black silk sutures. (From Emery, A: *In* Steinert RF [ed], Cataract Surgery: Technique, Complications, & Management. Philadelphia, WB Saunders, 1995, with permission.)

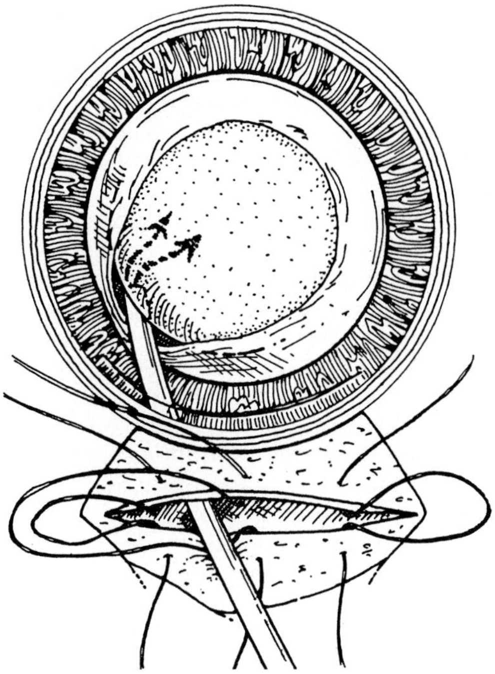

Figure 8–14. Technique for prolapse of superior nucleus into the anterior chamber using the McIntyre 26-gauge cannula with irrigation. (From Emery, A: *In* Steinert RF [ed], Cataract Surgery: Technique, Complications, & Management. Philadelphia, WB Saunders, 1995, with permission.)

and slide it beneath the margin of the anterior capsular leaflet. Retract the leaflet toward the lens equator rather firmly, so that the cannula will pass beyond the equator. Then, press slightly posterior with the whole shaft of the cannula (not just the tip) while gently irrigating with gravity flow through the handpiece. Maintain posterior pressure against the scleral wound while holding the shaft of the instrument parallel with the plane of the iris to help bring the nucleus forward. The lens nucleus will begin to cleave from the posterior capsule, allowing the tip of the cannula to pass beneath the equator of the nucleus. After cleavage begins and irrigation forms a space between the edge of the nucleus and the posterior capsule, lift slightly on the edge of the nucleus to enhance the cleavage; then slide the cannula slightly to the right in the cleavage, lift on the edge of the nucleus again, depress slightly and slide into the cleavage to the right again, lift again on the nucleus and so on, repeating this movement slowly, allowing the nucleus to cleave and be lifted away from the posterior capsule. The movement should be slow and deliberate to give the nucleus time to separate gently from the posterior capsule. Continue this movement until the superior one quarter to one half of the nucleus emerges through the pupil into the anterior chamber (Figs. 8–14 and 8–15).

Attach a Knolle-Pearce irrigating lens loop (Storz E0631) to the irrigating handpiece, and adjust the bottle height to get a rapid drip of fluid. Pass the lens loop through the incision, and then gently beneath the nucleus, allowing time for the fluid to dissect ample space between the nucleus and the posterior capsule. Lift slightly on the nucleus, slide into the cleavage plane, lift slightly again, slide into the cleavage plane, and so on. Repeat this sequence until the nucleus floats up away from the posterior capsule and toward the wound. The lens loop should now be positioned beneath the central nucleus. Hesitate until fluid builds up and pushes the nucleus against the internal lip of the wound. Then withdraw the loop while applying slight posterior pressure; at the same time lift slightly on the anterior scleral lip with forceps held in the free hand. Most nuclei come readily through a 10-mm incision, but an occasional large, hard, compact nucleus comes

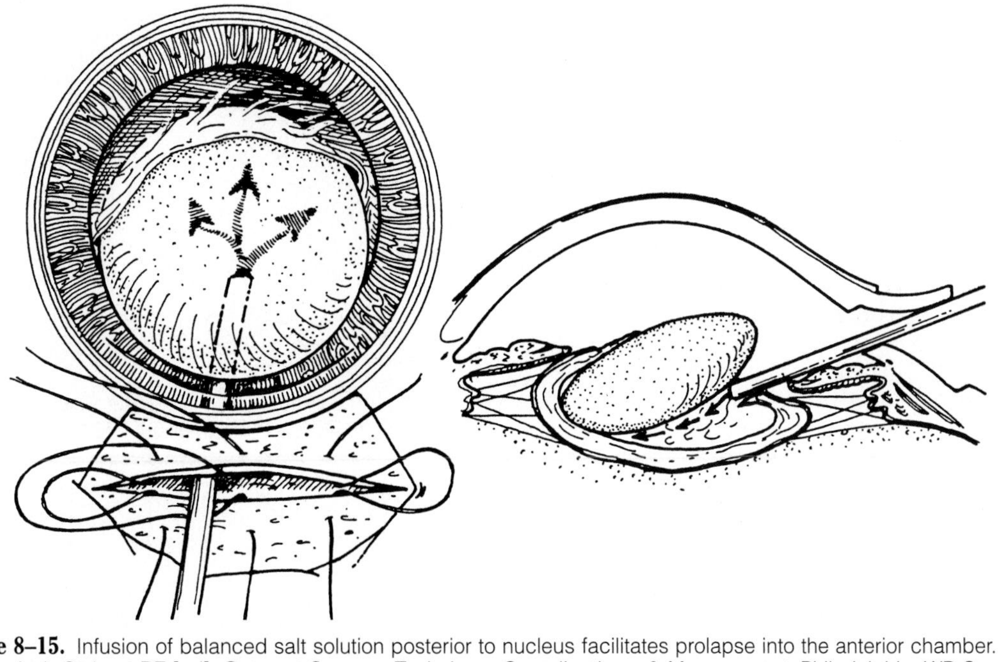

Figure 8–15. Infusion of balanced salt solution posterior to nucleus facilitates prolapse into the anterior chamber. (From Emery, A: *In* Steinert RF [ed], Cataract Surgery: Technique, Complications, & Management. Philadelphia, WB Saunders, 1995, with permission.)

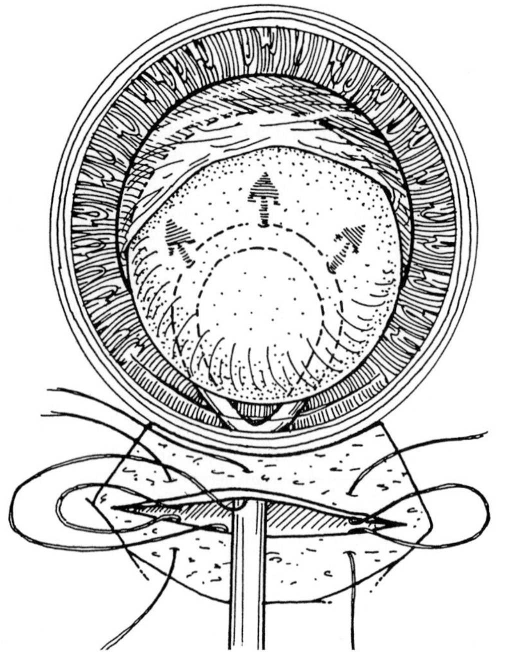

Figure 8–16. Pass lens loop gently beneath nucleus. Pause while fluid separates nucleus from posterior capsule; nucleus floats up toward wound. (From Emery, A: *In* Steinert RF [ed], Cataract Surgery: Technique, Complications, & Management. Philadelphia, WB Saunders, 1995, with permission.)

out more readily after the scleral incision is extended to a width of 11 mm (Figs. 8–16 and 8–17).

Commonly, a rumpled shell of epinuclear cortex strips away from the nucleus as it passes out of the eye and remains adjacent to the internal lip of the wound. Irrigate this loose cortex from the anterior chamber using a Randolph cannula attached to a squeeze bottle of balanced salt solution.

REMOVAL OF THE CORTEX

Tie the three pre-placed 8-0 silk sutures. Use an automated irrigation/aspiration device such as that found with equipment supplied for phacoemulsification or extracapsular surgery. Insert the tip of the irrigation/aspiration device through any of the 2.5-mm wound segments between the 9-0 sutures as needed for easy access. Insert the instrument with the aspiration hole aimed anteriorly.

Place the tip of the instrument gently beneath the iris and into the capsular fornix while keeping close to the posterior capsule to avoid aspirating the free anterior capsular flap. This allows the cortex in the capsular fornix to occlude the opening as aspiration begins, helping prevent aspiration of the anterior capsular leaflet. About a second after initiating gentle aspiration, withdraw the tip of the aspiration device into the pupillary space to verify that cortex is attached to it. Once the irrigation port is aspirating cortex and is free of other unwanted attachments, the aspiration vacuum can be increased to complete aspiration of the attached cortical fragment. Remove the cortex sequentially from adjacent sites until all has been removed. As each fragment is aspirated, slowly bring the tip of the instrument into the center of the pupil to strip cortex away from the posterior capsule and simultaneously aspirate it.

Begin aspirating cortex at the 6 o'clock position and then remove it gradually as illustrated (Figs. 8–18 through 8–21) until the only remaining cortex is adjacent to the wound. Usually cortex adjacent to the wound can be removed by inserting the aspiration tip at the far right-hand side of the incision to remove cortex next to the left-hand part of the incision, and vice versa. If cortex near the wound is adherent, irrigate it using a curved Binkhorst aspiration cannula attached to a syringe. This usually loosens it so that it can be more easily removed by the aspiration tip (Figs. 8–18 through 8–21). If these maneuvers do not remove the cortex, aspirate it carefully using a curved Binkhorst cannula attached to a syringe containing balanced salt solution after inflating the capsular bag with Healon.

Polish the posterior capsule with a Kratz scratcher (Fig. 8–22). Any cortex that can be readily removed will be rubbed off the capsule. If residual fibrotic material does not readily come away, this may be left for later YAG laser capsulotomy. With an appropriate aspiration device that includes a "capsule vacuuming" mode, residual cortical material can be vacuumed away from the posterior capsule with reasonable safety (Fig. 8–23).

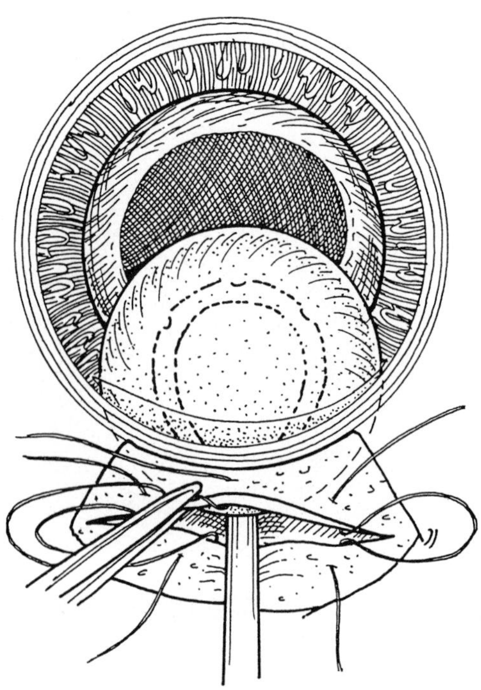

Figure 8–17. Irrigation fluid pushes nucleus against internal lip of wound, then lens loop draws nucleus through wound. (From Emery, A: *In* Steinert RF [ed], Cataract Surgery: Technique, Complications, & Management. Philadelphia, WB Saunders, 1995, with permission.)

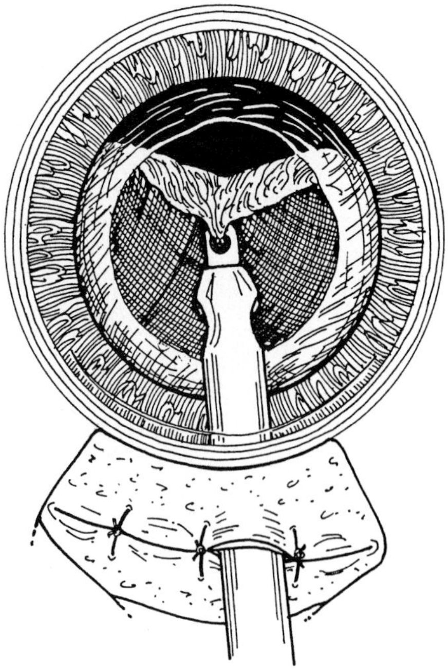

Figure 8–18. Remove residual cortex from posterior capsule using irrigation/aspiration instrument beginning at the 6 o'clock position (surgeon's view). (From Emery, A: *In* Steinert RF [ed], Cataract Surgery: Technique, Complications, & Management. Philadelphia, WB Saunders, 1995, with permission.)

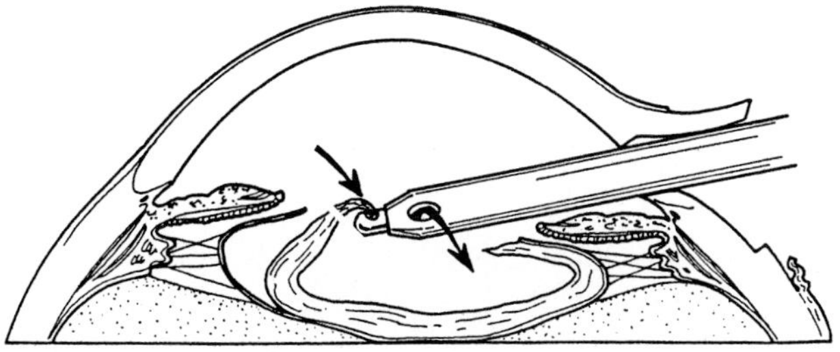

Figure 8–19. Cross-sectional view of cortical aspiration. (From Emery, A: *In* Steinert RF [ed], Cataract Surgery: Technique, Complications, & Management. Philadelphia, WB Saunders, 1995, with permission.)

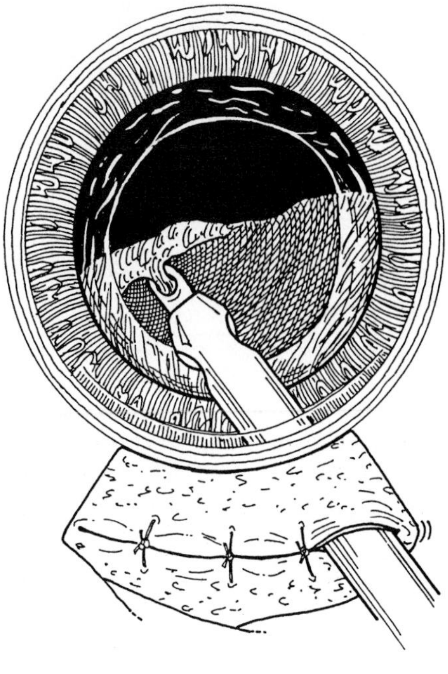

Figure 8–20. Cortex at 3 o'clock and 9 o'clock is removed after the inferior cortex. (From Emery, A: *In* Steinert RF [ed], Cataract Surgery: Technique, Complications, & Management. Philadelphia, WB Saunders, 1995, with permission.)

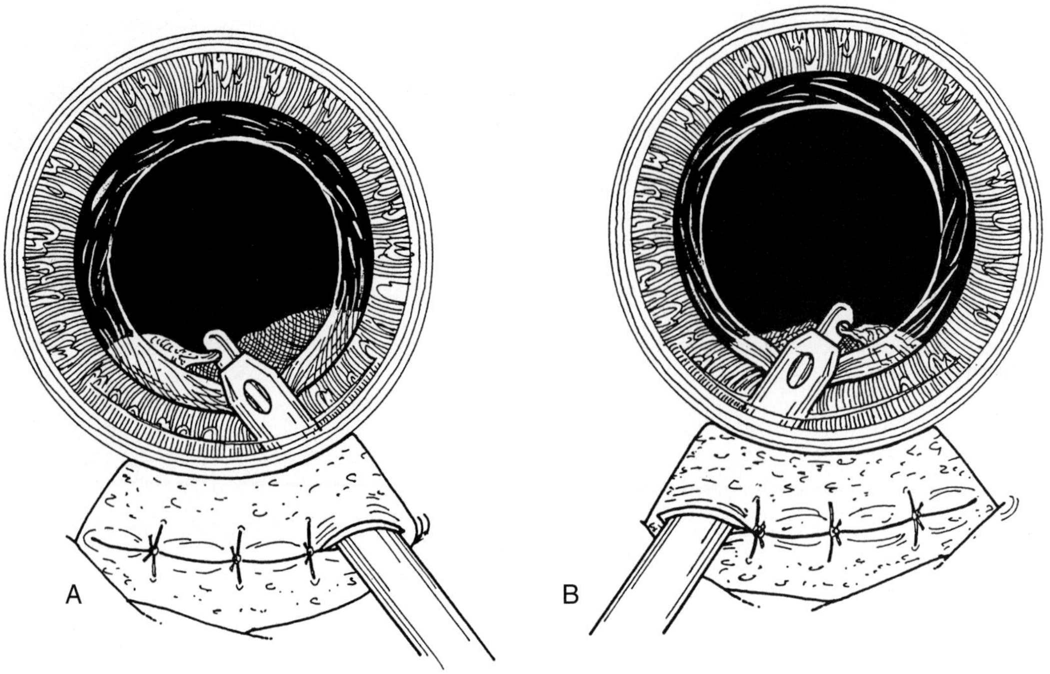

Figure 8–21 Aspiration of 12 o'clock cortex is made easier by inserting the irrigation/aspiration instrument through the far right-hand site of the incision to remove cortex at the 12–1 o'clock position *(A)* and through the far left of the incision to remove cortex at the 11–12 o'clock position *(B)*. (From Emery, A: *In* Steinert RF [ed], Cataract Surgery: Technique, Complications, & Management. Philadelphia, WB Saunders, 1995, with permission.)

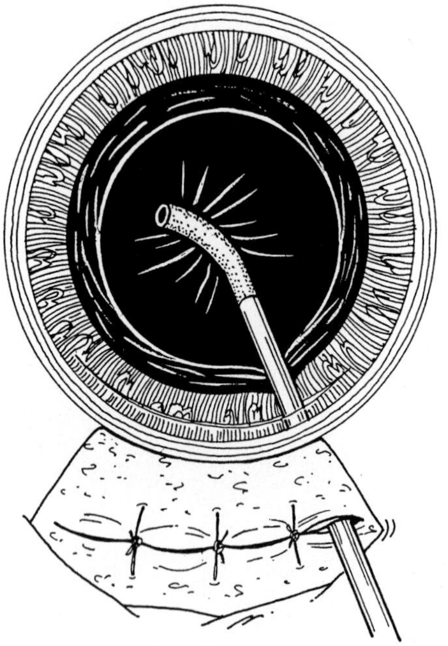

Figure 8–22. Polish the posterior capsule with a Kratz scratcher. (From Emery, A: *In* Steinert RF [ed], Cataract Surgery: Technique, Complications, & Management. Philadelphia, WB Saunders, 1995, with permission.)

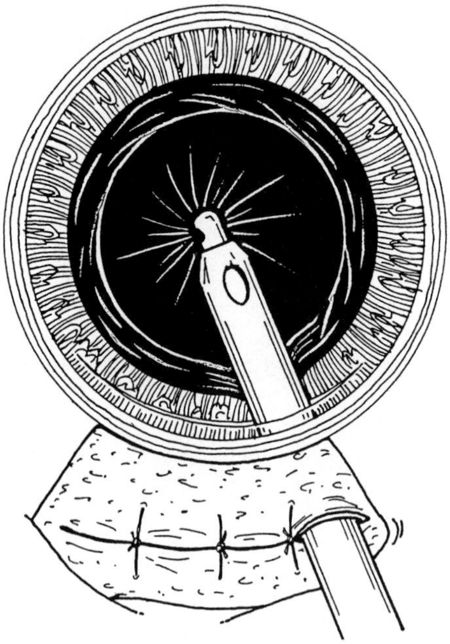

Figure 8–23. Aspiration of residual cortical material using irrigation/aspiration instrument and "capsule vacuuming" mode. (From Emery, A: *In* Steinert RF [ed], Cataract Surgery: Technique, Complications, & Management. Philadelphia, WB Saunders, 1995, with permission.)

IMPLANTATION OF INTRAOCULAR LENS

Inflate the anterior chamber with a viscoelastic material like sodium hyaluronate: Fill the central anterior chamber; then, add additional viscoelastic beneath the anterior capsular flap to inflate the capsule for "in-the-bag" insertion. If the lens implant is to be placed into the ciliary sulcus, as when there is a rupture of the posterior lens capsule, viscoelastic material should be used to flatten the residual anterior capsular flap against the posterior capsule to permit inflation of the space of the ciliary sulcus, rather than inflating the lens capsule as described above.

In preparation for lens insertion, remove the 11 o'clock and 12 o'clock temporary 9-0 silk sutures. Holding the lens with lens-insertion forceps such as Bechert forceps, slide the lens into the anterior chamber. As the optic passes through the wound, tilt it to position the haptic to pass into the capsular bag (or sulcus, if desired). The inferior haptic should slide close to the posterior capsule and into the bag (or sulcus) as the optic passes through the wound incision (Fig. 8–24). As the right hand releases the optic, the left hand, holding the superior haptic, pushes it in and to the left, thereby rotating the inferior haptic of the lens somewhat toward the 7 o'clock or 8 o'clock position.

After releasing the optic, grasp the superior haptic of the lens at its midpoint. In the left hand use a blunt iris hook (Katena K3-5422) (Fig. 8–25). Grasp the residual margin of the anterior capsule along with the margin of the iris and retract slightly toward the wound, using the blunt iris hook in the left hand while passing the superior haptic into the anterior chamber using the right hand with a vector of movement toward the position of the iris hook (Fig. 8–26). This causes the lens to rotate into a horizontal position. The superior haptic is flexed sufficiently to clear the margin of the iris and the anterior capsule and to pass beneath the edge of the iris hook, which can in effect "shoe-horn" the superior

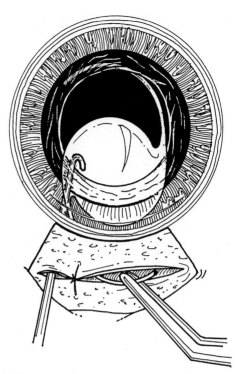

Figure 8–25. A blunt iris hook guides the superior haptic into the capsular bag. (From Emery, A: *In* Steinert RF [ed], Cataract Surgery: Technique, Complications, & Management. Philadelphia, WB Saunders, 1995, with permission.)

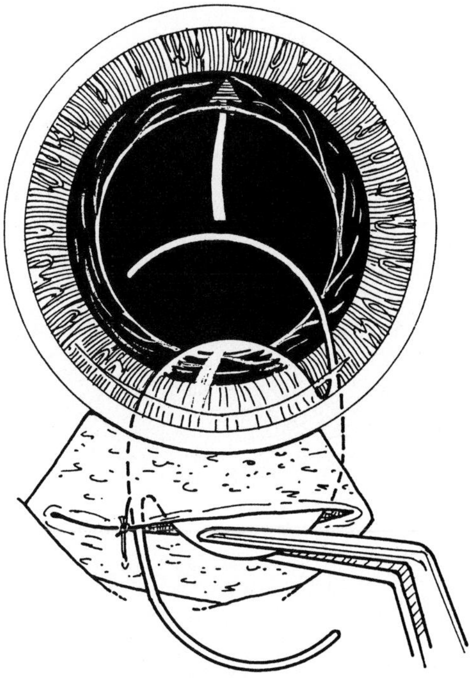

Figure 8–24. Technique for implantation for intraocular lens using viscoelastic material. (From Emery, A: *In* Steinert RF [ed], Cataract Surgery: Technique, Complications, & Management. Philadelphia, WB Saunders, 1995, with permission.)

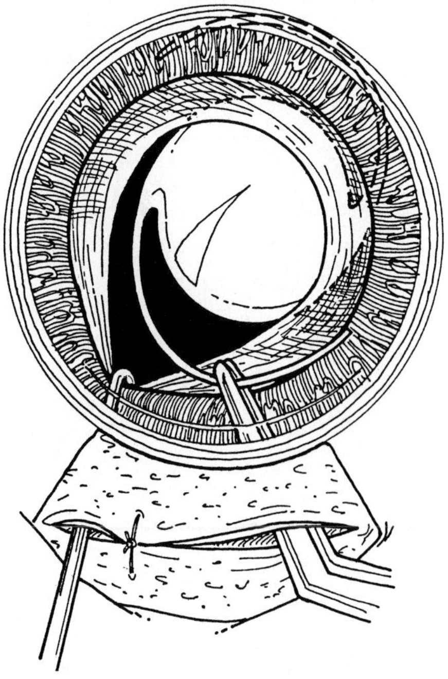

Figure 8–26. The iris hook can retract the anterior capsule and iris if necessary to allow accurate placement of the superior haptic into the capsular bag. (From Emery, A: *In* Steinert RF [ed], Cataract Surgery: Technique, Complications, & management. Philadelphia, WB Saunders, 1995, with permission.)

haptic into the capsular bag by gliding the haptic beneath the hook. Once the superior haptic has been released into the capsule bag, a Sinskey hook can be used to rotate the lens slightly clockwise to settle it into a central position. Minimize manipulation of the lens to avoid dislocating a haptic from the bag into the ciliary sulcus.

WOUND CLOSURE

Place a corneal cover over the central cornea to block light from the microscope. Leave the temporary 9-0 suture in place at the 1 o'clock position; close the incision to the right of that suture with a running 10-0 nylon suture placed in a shoelace fashion as illustrated in Figure 8–27. In that figure, the initial penetration point of each bite of the suture is labeled sequentially to demonstrate how the suture is placed. The first bite starts within the lips of the wound and passes through only the posterior lip; the final bite passes only through the anterior lip, thereby allowing the two suture ends to come together and be tied within the wound. Begin each suture bite after the first about 1 mm from the anterior lip of the incision. Pass the needle through the flap, then intralamellarly along the bed of the sceral dissection, and finally through intact sclera. Exit 1 mm posterior to the scleral grove. Bury the knot within the lips of the wound next to the 9-0 suture.

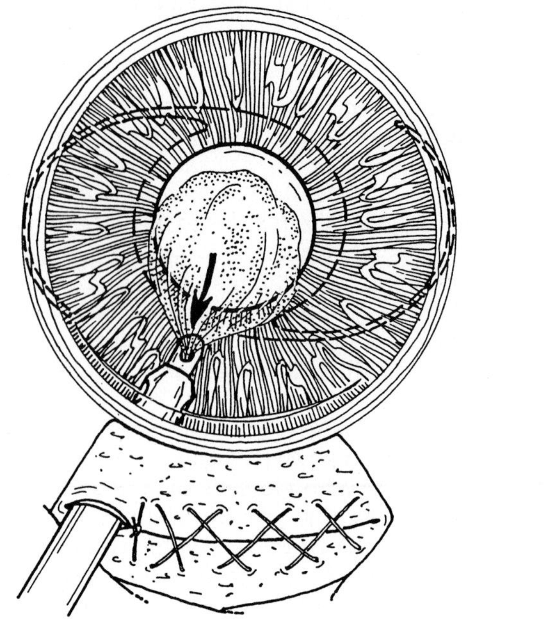

Figure 8–28. Removal of viscoelastic material through remaining unsutured part of wound. Inject intraocular carbachol 0.01% to constrict pupil after removal of the viscoelastic substance. (From Emery, A: *In* Steinert RF [ed], Cataract Surgery: Technique, Complications, & Management. Philadelphia, WB Saunders, 1995, with permission.)

Aspirate residual viscoelastic material by passing the irrigation/aspiration instrument through the incision remaining open to the left of the temporary suture (Fig. 8–28). Inject intraocular carbachol 0.01% (Miostat) to constrict the pupil. Close the remainder of the wound with a 10-0 nylon suture using a modified shoelace configuration as indicated in Figure 8–29. Close the conjunctival flap by applying Wetfield coaptation forceps in the usual fashion along the oblique cuts nasally and temporally (Fig. 8–30).

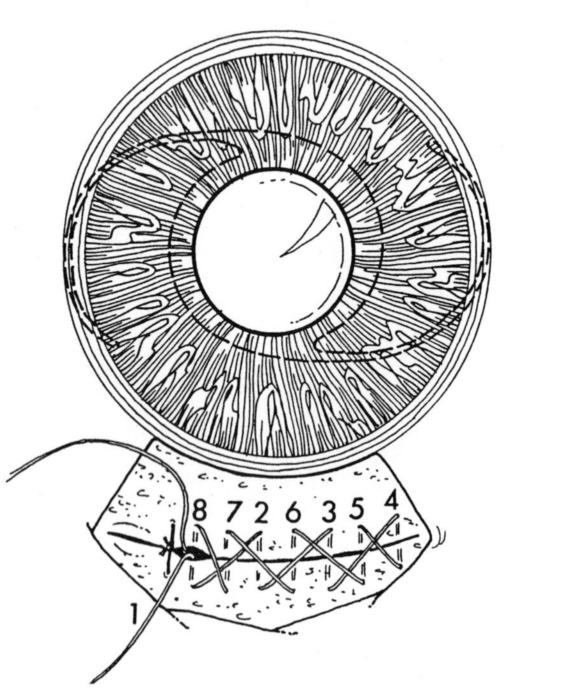

Figure 8–27. Technique for placement for shoelace suture—each bite is numbered in order. Suture is tied with knot in wound. (From Emery, A: *In* Steinert RF [ed], Cataract Surgery: Technique, Complications, & Management. Philadelphia, WB Saunders, 1995, with permission.)

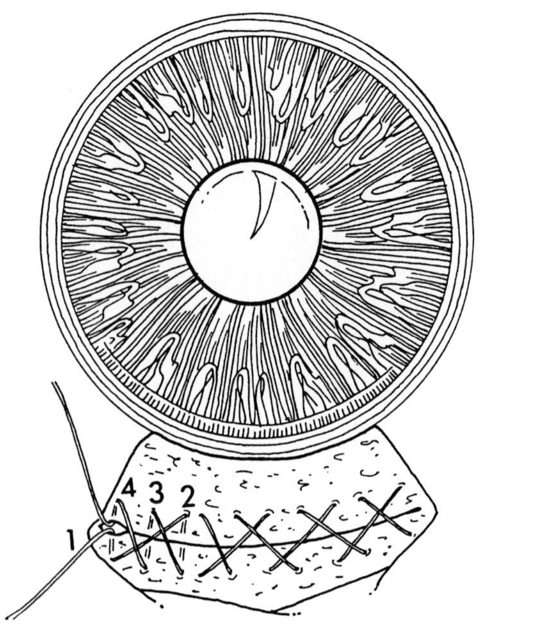

Figure 8–29. Remove remaining 9-0 silk suture, and place 10-0 nylon shoelace suture as indicated, with each bite numbered in order of placement. (From Emery, A: *In* Steinert RF [ed], Cataract Surgery: Technique, Complications, & Management. Philadelphia, WB Saunders, 1995, with permission.)

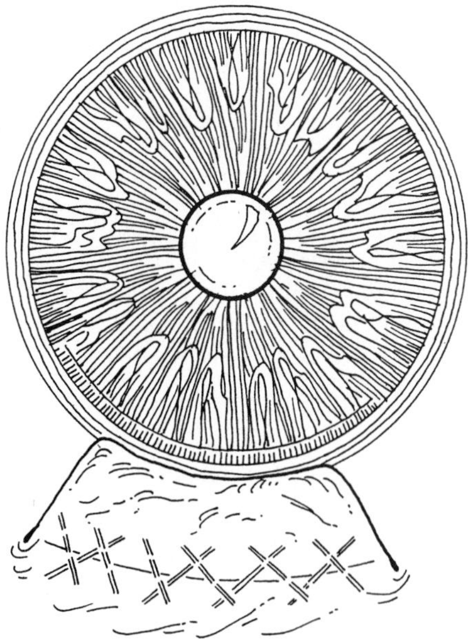

Figure 8–30. Appearance showing constricted pupil (carbachol) and conjunctival flap in place. (From Emery, A: *In* Steinert RF [ed], Cataract Surgery: Technique, Complications, & Management. Philadelphia, WB Saunders, 1995, with permission.)

REFERENCES

1. Leaming DV: Practive styles and preferences of ASCRS members—1995 survey. J Cataract Refract Surg 1996;22:931.
2. Werblin TP: Astigmatism after cataract extraction: 6-year follow up of 6.5- and 12-millimeter incisions. Refract Corneal Surg 1992;8:448.
3. Watson A, Sunderraj P: Comparison of small-incision phacoemulsification with standard extracapsular cataract surgery: Postoperative astigmatism and visual recovery. Eye 1992;6(Pt 6):626.
4. Steinert RF, Brint SF, White SM, et al.: Astigmatism after small incision cataract surgery. A prospective, randomized, multicenter comparison of 4- and 6.5-mm incisions. Ophthalmology 1991;98:417.

CHAPTER 9

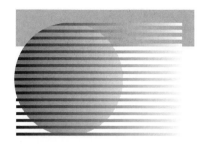

Nuclear Cracking Techniques

BRUCE D. GAYNOR, M.D. and STEPHEN A. OBSTBAUM, M.D.

EVOLUTION OF PHACOEMULSIFICATION

In 1967, Kelman introduced a surgical technique to remove a cataract using ultrasonic vibration.[1] A single instrument was inserted through a 3-mm incision and the anteriorly luxated nucleus was emulsifed in the anterior chamber in order to avoid damaging the posterior capsule.[2,3] Although phacoemulsification was adopted by some surgeons, most ophthalmologists used extracapsular cataract extraction to remove the intact nucleus. The nucleus was either expressed by applying pressure to the globe or removed using a lens loop or irrigating vectis and then evacuated from the anterior chamber through a 10-mm incision. During the 1970s and 1980s, ophthalmologists recognized the benefits of an intact posterior capsule but wanted to avoid the difficulty of emulsifying dense nuclei and damaging the cornea during anterior chamber lens fragmentation. Also, the potential advantages of small-incision surgery were lost because of the unavailability of an intraocular lens (IOL) that could be passed through a 3-mm incision.

Undaunted by these problems, skilled, innovative surgeons continued to modify and master the techniques of phacoemulsification. The site of emulsification moved from the anterior chamber to the iris plane and then to the capsular bag. Subsequently, a supracapsular technique was introduced. Another important advance was introduction of viscoelastic agents that coated tissues, moved tissues, and maintained space,[4-8] and these agents remain as essential adjuncts in modern cataract surgery. More efficient instruments and microcomputer programs to increase the safety of phacoemulsification have increased the popularity of this technique. Finally, the adoption of small-incision surgery provided major advantages, including greater intraoperative ocular stability, less surgically induced astigmatism, rapid visual rehabilitation, and rapid resumption of normal functional activities.[9,10]

NUCLEUS REMOVAL

From the inception of phacoemulsification, various techniques have been advocated to facilitate nucleus removal. This discussion is limited to a description of nucleofracture using sculpting techniques; chopping techniques are covered in Chapter 10. Often, various approaches are combined by phacosurgeons to individualize their approach.

Kelman initially advocated anterior chamber phacoemulsification to protect the posterior capsule.[1] With this approach, the nucleus is elevated from the capsular bag into the anterior chamber through the anterior capsulotomy and emulsified. Specular microscopy studies have shown that anterior chamber phacoemulsification, prior to the introduction of viscoelastic agents, was associated with a significant reduction in endothelial cell counts.[5,11,12] These observations and others prompted development of phacoemulsification techniques that are performed in the iris plane or capsular bag.

Iris plane phacoemulsification is a two-handed technique that is performed deeper in the anterior chamber than Kelman's procedure and is at a greater distance from the endothelium. After a wide anterior capsulotomy, the nucleus is tilted to allow access to the superior nucleus edge. The nucleus is then emulsified from the periphery toward the center of the lens. This method of phacoemulsification promoted the concept of bimanual lens nucleus removal.

Nucleus cracking was first described by Shepherd in 1990 and was called "in situ fracture."[13] With this technique, cruciate grooves are created in the nucleus, creating quadrants. These quadrants are then separated by placing instruments deep into the grooves to crack the deeper nuclear plates. These smaller, more manageable nuclear segments are then drawn to the deeper central portion of the chamber and emulsified through the capsulorrhexis opening. The term *in situ* refers to fracturing and emulsification of the nucleus within the capsular bag. Central to this technique is the adoption of the continuous-tear capsulotomy to avoid the peripheral tears that are often seen with a "can-opener" capsulotomy. Although this technique is widely used today, temporal clear corneal incisions with topical anesthesia are often used instead of the scleral pocket incision originally described by Shepherd.

Gimbel introduced the "divide-and-conquer" technique that begins with the creation of a large central crater that is sculpted deep enough to allow for bimanual fracturing using a second instrument such as a cyclodialysis spatula.[14] Once fracturing of the nucleus is ensured, the nucleus is rotated 90 degrees and another crack is created. Emulsification is then performed on the small pieces of the nucleus that were previously disassembled. These techniques are particularly helpful for managing moderate to hard nuclei. The softer nucleus does not crack as readily because instruments cut through, rather than crack, these less resistant nuclei.

Fine's less resistant "chip and flip" technique is applicable to softer nuclei.[15] A central bowl is developed in the nucleus that extends only to the delineation of the central nucleus or to the "golden halo." A second instrument, introduced through the paracentesis, engages the superior portion of the nuclear bowl to expose the internal portion of the nuclear rim inferiorly. Emulsification of the nuclear rim one clock hour at a time as the nucleus is rotated results in the creation of a nuclear plate or chip that is then elevated and emulsified.

In each of these techniques the epinucleus is removed by aspiration alone or with manual phacoemulsification and aspiration. The goal is to evacuate the capsular bag, maintain the intact capsulorrhexis opening, and encourage predictable placement of an IOL.

BASIC PRINCIPLES OF NUCLEUS CRACKING

The defining characteristic of phacoemulsification techniques performed through an intact capsulorrhexis is that the lens elements are removed in a meaningful sequential fashion. Whether a divide-and-conquer or a chopping technique is used, the idea is to create small nuclear segments that can easily be removed, to evacuate the epinucleus from the capsular bag, and finally, to perform cortical clean-up to prepare the bag for IOL implantation.

Divide-and-conquer techniques require deep sculpting into the nuclear substance. As the nucleus is sculpted, changes in the red-reflex occur that help determine the optimum depth for easy cracking of lens material. The groove is generally made slightly wider than the width of the phacoprobe. The advantage of fashioning the groove in this manner is that it removes sufficient nuclear substance while leaving resistant chasm walls to allow an easy two-handed, two-instrument cracking maneuver or use of a nucleus cracker. Central sculpting using a shaving technique is accomplished with relatively low vacuum and power, but with adequate flow to remove emulsified tissue. Once an appropriately thinned plate is created, the crack is readily performed. Secondary grooves or troughs can then be made to generate several smaller pie-shaped nuclear segments that are easily removed.

Segmental evacuation is a controlled way to remove the disassembled nucleus. With this approach, the vacuum is increased and the flow is increased while the phacopower may remain stable. Because flow helps to bring the nuclear elements to the phaco-tip, and vacuum promotes effective aspiration, the segmental nuclear fragments are brought centrally, in the deepest portion of the anterior chamber, for removal. With harder nuclei, greater phaco-power may be required than with soft nuclei, but in either case, mobilization of a manageable nuclear mass facilitates the phaco process.

Cracking the nucleus into wedge-shaped pieces allows most of the phaco to be performed in the central part of the chamber at some distance from the lens equator. With newer phaco instruments, excellent purchase of the nuclear segments is obtained by controlling the flow and vacuum levels. In many instances, much of the segment can be removed by phacoaspiration with application of relatively little phacoenergy. The amount of phacoenergy used will depend on the density of the nucleus, but generating small nuclear fragments can help minimize the amount required. This principle is also applicable to the phaco-chop techniques discussed in Chapter 10.

In summary, nucleus cracking techniques facilitate nucleus removal through an intact capsulorrhexis. Mobilization of nuclear fragments after creating deep troughs permits their removal using phacoaspiration while minimizing the use of phacoenergy. This is a safe, controlled technique that can be mastered by most ophthalmic surgeons.

REFERENCES

1. Kelman CD: Phacoemulsification and aspiration. A new technique of cataract removal. A preliminary report. Am J Ophthalmol 1967;64:23–35.
2. Kelman CD: Phacoemulsification in the anterior chamber. Ophthalmology 1979;86:1980–1982.
3. Kelman CD: Phaco-emulsification and aspiration. A progress report. Am J Ophthalmol 1969;67:464–477.
4. Holmberg AS, Philipson BT: Sodium hyaluronate in cataract surgery. II: Report on the use of Healon in extracapsular cataract surgery using phacoemulsification. Ophthalmology 1984;91:53–57.
5. Glasser DB, Katz HR, Boyd JE: Protective effects of viscous solutions in phacoemulsification and traumatic lens implantation. Arch Ophthalmol 1989;107:1047–1051.
6. Craig MT, Olson RJ, Mamalis N, et al.: Air bubble endothelial damage during phacoemulsification in human eye bank eyes: The protective effects of Healon and Viscoat. J Cataract Refract Surg 1990;16:597–601.
7. Glasser DB, Osborn DC, Nordeen JF, et al.: Endothelial protection and viscoelastic retention during phacoemulsification and intraocular lens implantation. Arch Ophthalmol 1991;109:1438–1440.
8. Lane SS, Naylor DW, Kullerstarnd LJ, et al.: Prospective comparison of the effects of Occucoat, Viscoat and Healon on intraocular pressure and endothelial cell loss. J Cataract Refract Surg 1991;17:21–26.
9. Heslin KB, Guerriero PN: Clinical retrospective study comparing planned extracapsular cataract extraction and phakoemulsification with and without lens implantation. Ann Ophthalmol 1984;16:956–962.

10. Steinert RF, Brint SF, White SM, Fine IH: Astigmatism after small incision cataract surgery. A prospective, randomized multicenter comparison of 4 and 6.5 mm incisions. Ophthalmology 1991;98: 417–424.
11. Kraff MC, Sanders DR, Lieberman HL: Specular microscopy in cataract and intraocular lens patients. A report of 564 cases. Arch Ophthalmol 1980;98:1782–1784.
12. Kraff MC, Sanders DR, Lieberman HL: Monitoring for continuing endothelial cell loss with cataract extraction and intraocular lens implantation. Ophthalmology 1982;89:30–34.
13. Shepherd JR: In situ fracture. J Cataract Refract Surg 1990;16: 436–440.
14. Gimbel HV: Divide and conquer nucleofractis phacoemulsification: Development and variations. J Cataract Refract Surg 1991;17:281–291.
15. Fine IH: The chip and flip phacoemulsification technique. J Cataract Refract Surg 1991;17:366–371.

CHAPTER 10

Phaco Chop

ROGER F. STEINERT, M.D.

Over the past decade, phacoemulsification has evolved from a "one-handed" technique to a number of a variants, most of which involve use of instruments in both hands.

In 1993, Kunihiro Nagahara introduced the concept of a new technique for nuclear disassembly during phacoemulsification. His insight was that natural cleavage planes within the nucleus had not been used previously (Fig. 10–1*A*). By impaling the nucleus on the *phacoemulsification tip,* and thereby stabilizing it, a second "chopping" instrument could be passed from the *equatorial edge* of the outer *nucleus* toward the center. The nucleus was split readily by the second instrument. Nagahara made an analogy to the technique of chopping or, more accurately, splitting, a log with a wedge, taking advantage of the wood's natural cleavage plane (Fig. 10–1*B*).

EVOLUTION OF PHACO CHOP

STOP AND CHOP

Several surgeons were stimulated by Nagahara's method and evolved techniques intended to improve the reliability and repeatability of the "phaco chop." Paul Koch found that the initial chop, intended to bisect the nucleus, was the most difficult to perform. He reverted to creating an initial deep trough with the phaco tip and then cracking the trough with two instruments, identical to the beginning of the *quadrant cracking* technique. At this point, however, Koch *stopped* the quadrant cracking approach and then began *chopping* the remaining pieces of nucleus; he called this technique "stop and chop" (Fig. 10–2).[1] It remains popular with many surgeons, and it is an important transition for almost anyone learning the phaco chop technique, because it eliminates the most difficult step: the initial chop.

CHOP AND DEBULK

To maximize protection of the corneal endothelium, and continue to perform phacoemulsification in the posterior chamber an iris plane, the surgeon should create some central space in order to use the chopping technique to disassemble the nucleus posterior to the iris. Similar to disassembly of a jigsaw puzzle, taking the pieces apart becomes easier once the first piece is removed. In addition, most of the ultrasound power is used to phacoemulsify the central hard nucleus, not the periphery. Steinert described a technique that began identically to Nagahara's with an initial phaco chop to bisect the nucleus.[2] This is a more efficient maneuver than creating the trough and splitting it, as in the "stop and chop" technique. After the initial chop, however, the central hard nucleus is emulsified along the fault line of the initial crack. In softer nuclei, very little central material is removed at this step. In harder, larger nuclei, more central nucleus can be removed at this step; in very advanced cataracts, the center is bowled out toward the periphery before the surgeon begins to chop further (Fig. 10–3).

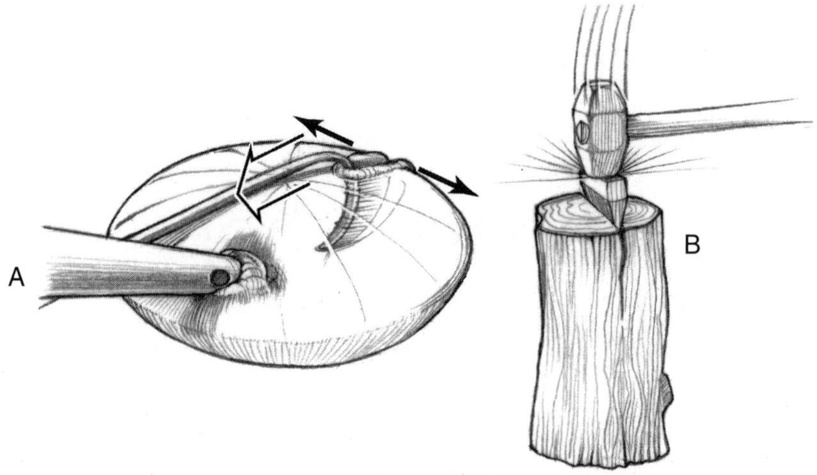

Figure 10–1. *A.* Nagahara's insight was to split the nucleus along its natural cleavage planes. *B.* The principle of chopping is the same as using a wedge to split a log along its natural planes.

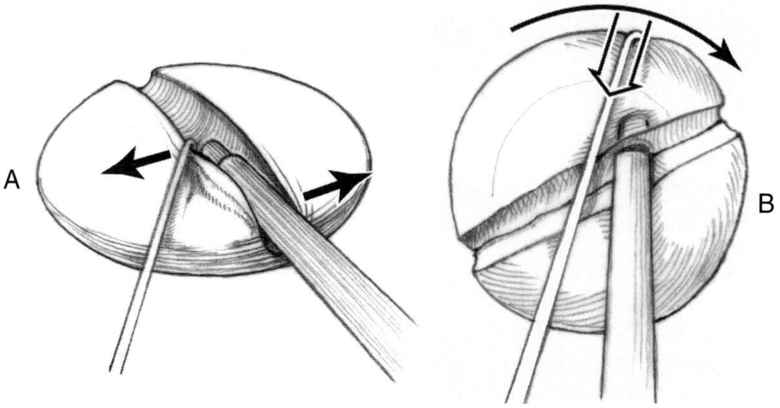

Figure 10–2. *A.* Paul Koch's "stop and chop" technique begins with a groove and cracking of the nucleus in half, identical to the start of "divide-and-conquer" nuclear fracture. *B.* The nucleus is rotated 1 to 2 clock hours, and the surgeon *stops* the "divide-and-conquer" technique and begins to "chop."

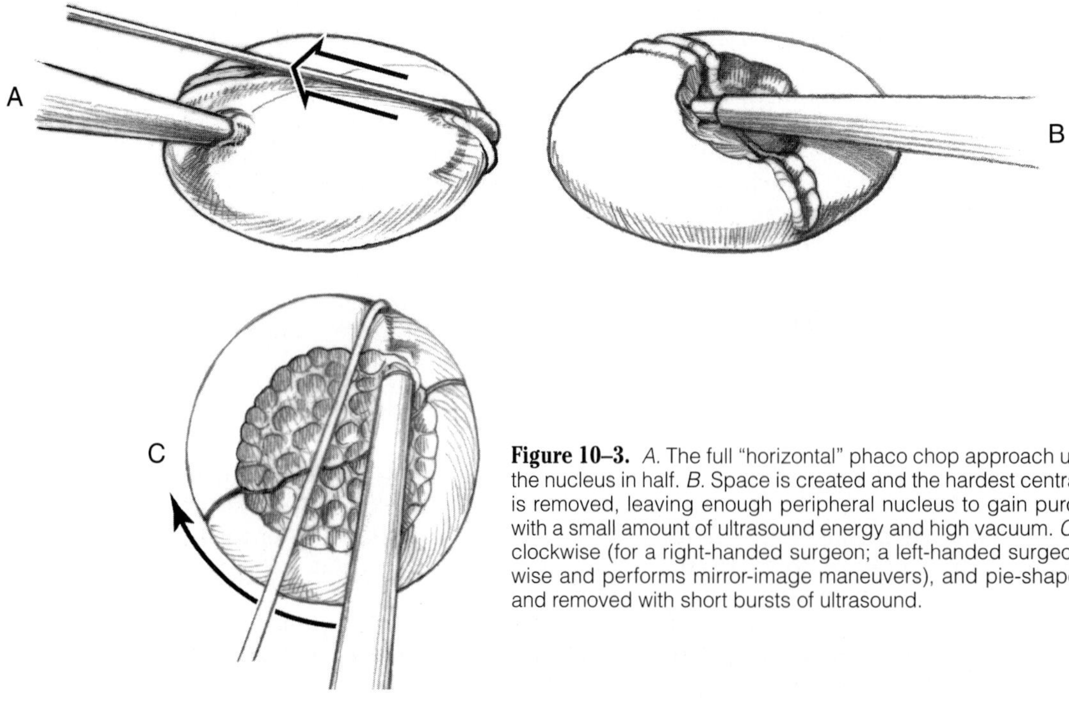

Figure 10–3. *A.* The full "horizontal" phaco chop approach uses the chopper to split the nucleus in half. *B.* Space is created and the hardest central portion of the nucleus is removed, leaving enough peripheral nucleus to gain purchase by the phaco tip with a small amount of ultrasound energy and high vacuum. *C.* The nucleus is rotated clockwise (for a right-handed surgeon; a left-handed surgeon rotates counterclockwise and performs mirror-image maneuvers), and pie-shaped wedges are split off and removed with short bursts of ultrasound.

CIRCUMFERENTIAL SEQUENTIAL DISASSEMBLY

Both Koch and Steinert found that the chop technique was better applied as a progressive chopping of small wedges in a circumferential direction, rather than chopping four full quadrants as originally described by Nagahara. Because of the bulk, the large nuclear pieces remain stable within the posterior capsular sac. Therefore, control of the phacoemulsification process is enhanced.

Howard Gimbel earlier described several techniques of nuclear fracture the principles of which have been incorporated in phaco chop as it has evolved.[3] Gimbel pointed out the importance of debulking the central nucleus, forming a narrow trough for soft nuclei and a larger crater for hard nuclei. In addition, he demonstrated the ability to break off pieces of the peripheral nucleus with lateral separation movements after engaging them with the phacoemulsification tip, proceeding in a circumferential direction. Gimbel called this technique "nucleofractis." In essence, a phaco chop is the nucleofractis technique, greatly facilitated by the second "chopping" instrument instead of relying on forceful lateral movements of the phacoemulsification tip.

HIGH VACUUM PHACO CHOP

In addition to incorporating central debulking and using progressive circumferential chopping steps, Steinert recognized that using high vacuum during chopping further improves nuclear control and reduces the total ultrasound energy required. High vacuum allows the surgeon to grasp and hold the nuclear wedges and draw them toward the central zone of safety before completing the emulsification. Moreover, the manual energy input from the phaco chop combined with the energy input from the high vacuum, reduces the total amount of ultrasonic energy required. Overall, the technique appears to be safer and more controlled. Because of its efficiency, the nuclear disassembly step of phacoemulsification cataract surgery is generally substantially faster than alternative techniques such as quadrant cracking.[4–6]

PHACO QUICK CHOP ("VERTICAL PHACO CHOP")

Vladimir Pfeifer of Slovenia is generally credited with originating the fundamental concept of creating vertical forces that fragment the nucleus. This technique has been developed and taught by Davis Dillman as "phaco quick chop." Nagahara's concept is to stabilize the nucleus with the phaco tip and then pull the chopping instrument in the *horizontal* plane from the equator toward the center. *Vertical* chop differs by embedding the phaco tip as deeply as possible into the nucleus, and then impaling the anterior nucleus on a sharp-tipped chopping instrument at a point in front of and adjacent to the phaco tip. The chopping tool pushes downward sharply while the phaco tip lifts upward (Fig. 10–4*A*). Each instrument moves about one half of the total amount of vertical separation needed to generate a fissure. As soon as the vertical (anteroposterior) split begins to develop, the two instruments also spread horizontally slightly to complete cleavage of the two sections (Fig. 10–4*B*). The surgeon then continues the vertical chop to break off smaller sections of nucleus for

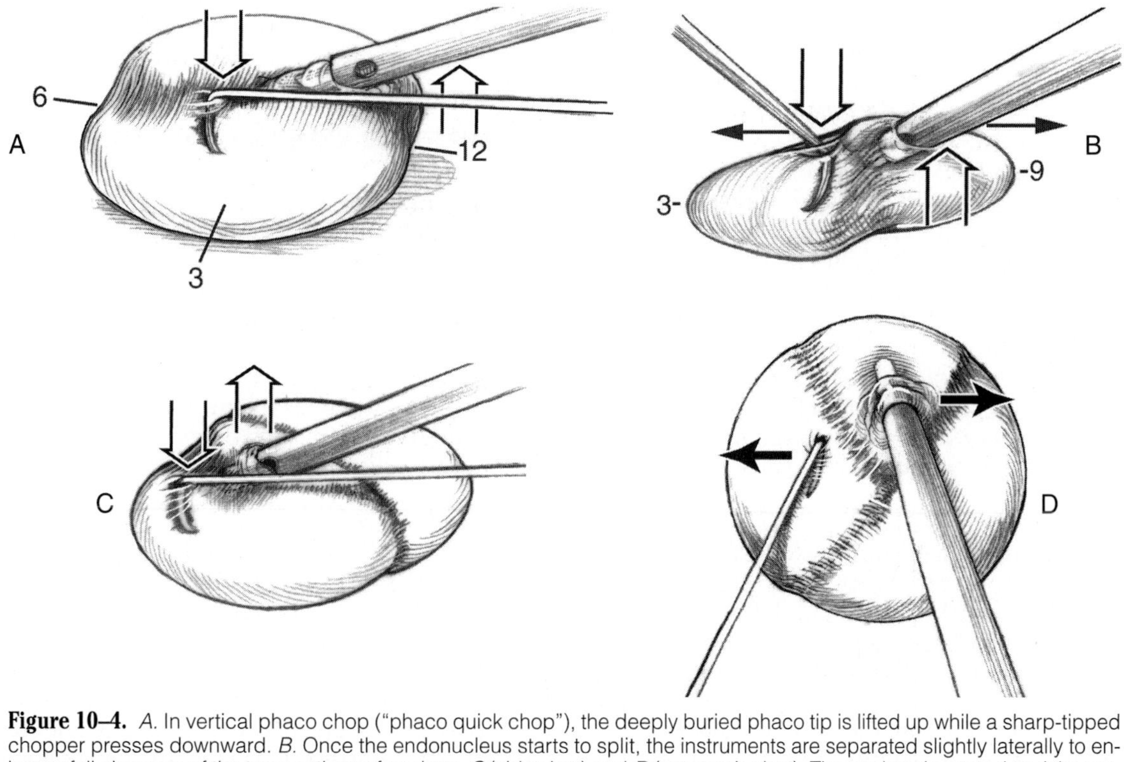

Figure 10–4. *A*. In vertical phaco chop ("phaco quick chop"), the deeply buried phaco tip is lifted up while a sharp-tipped chopper presses downward. *B*. Once the endonucleus starts to split, the instruments are separated slightly laterally to enhance full cleavage of the two sections of nucleus. *C* (side view) and *D* (surgeon's view). The nucleus is rotated and the vertical chop maneuver is repeated to create smaller nuclear fragments that can be removed with ultrasound and aspiration.

emulsification, progressing circumferentially as in the technique described earlier (Fig. 10–4C).

The principal advantage of vertical chopping is elimination of the need to pass the chopper under the anterior capsule out to the equator of the nucleus. Because neither the anterior capsular edge nor the equator can always be seen, some surgeons dislike having to rely on tactile feedback and judgment of distances under the iris. On the other hand, vertical chopping works best in moderate-density nuclei; it often fails in softer nuclei, where the phaco tip and chopper pull through the nucleus, or in hard nuclei, where so much force is required that, when cleavage does occur, the abrupt movement threatens the integrity of the posterior capsule and/or zonules.

The "complete phaco surgeon" should be comfortable with both horizontal and vertical chopping maneuvers, as each has its place.

TECHNIQUE OF PHACO CHOP

The basic concept of Nagahara's phaco chop, as it is usually practiced, is illustrated in Figure 10–5. The nucleus is stabilized with the phacoemulsification tip, on which it is then impaled under moderate vacuum (typically 50 to 80 mm Hg) at low ultrasonic power, at a point just off-center, about 1 mm toward the incision. The irrigation sleeve should be retracted more than is customary for the traditional "divide and conquer" nuclear fracture to permit the phaco top to advance to the depth of the mid-nucleus (1.5 to 2 mm). As the nucleus is being impaled on the phaco tip, the phaco handpiece is markedly tipped in the vertical direction, as if the surgeon is aiming for the optic nerve head. The chopping instrument is passed through a paracentesis that is about 1½ clock hours from the incision. The chopper can be used to assist the proper location for impaling the nucleus by pressing it lightly against the nuclear surface, thus gently shifting the nucleus about 1 mm away from the incision.

The chopper is advanced under the anterior capsule until it can pass around the equator of the nucleus at the nucleus/epinucleus border, about 180 degrees opposite the paracentesis. If the border can be visualized as either a "golden ring" (small nucleus) or a dark ring (large nucleus) as a result of effective hydrodelineation in combination with a large pupil, the copper can be placed into this ring, which indicates the equator of the nucleus, under direct visualization (Fig. 10–5*A* and *B*). If the nucleus is very large or the pupil does not adequately dilate, the surgeon will nevertheless be able to *feel* an abrupt change as the chopper tip passes from the hard nucleus to the relatively soft epinucleus. The chopping instrument will shift posteriorly by at least 1 mm when this border is encountered (Fig. 10–5C).

The chopping instrument is then drawn across the center of the nucleus, beginning at a point opposite the paracentesis and moving toward the paracentesis (Fig. 10–5*D*). Once the center of the nucleus is fully transected, the nucleus fractures readily. The chopper tip should be at least at half depth in the nucleus anteroposteriorly as well as chopping across half of the nucleus radially. The impaled phaco tip will also have weakened the central nucleus which contributes to a successful chopping hemisection of the nucleus. This basic chop maneuver works well in nuclei ranging from low to high density.

The next step is to debulk the center of the nucleus. If the lens is of mild to moderate density, debulking is restricted to a zone no larger than a conventional trough. In that manner, the peripheral nuclear pieces retain enough integrity for the circumferential peripheral chopping maneuvers. If the lens is firmer, however a crater or bowl must be phacoemulsified to further debulk the center (Fig. 10–5*E*). In all cases, it is important to leave sufficient firm peripheral nuclear material to allow the nucleus to be safely engaged during the progressive circumferential chopping.

Circumferential peripheral nuclear chopping then proceeds. For a right-handed surgeon, the heminucleus being chopped should be located to the surgeon's left, and the nucleus rotated in a clockwise direction. The phacoemulsification tip engages the leading edge of the heminucleus, and then the chopper transects the peripheral wedge, leaving the wedge engaged in the phacoemulsification tip (Fig. 10–5*F*). For a left-handed surgeon, the maneuvers are performed in a mirror-image fashion, with the direction of the nuclear rotation counterclockwise.

The size of the pie-shaped wedges of nucleus to be chopped depends on the density of the nucleus. The pie-shaped pieces can be created in virtually any size, but the harder the nucleus, the smaller the fragments should be. For 2+ nuclear density, create only three wedges in each heminucleus; for a very dense 4+ nucleus, create 6 to 8 wedges. If a piece is chopped and then appears to be too large, it can be chopped again. The goal is to create "bite-sized" pieces that are appropriate for the phacoemulsification tip.

CHOPPING INSTRUMENTS

A large number of chopping instruments have been developed. Although this variety can confuse a novice, it also gives the surgeon many options for solving technical problems. Once a surgeon becomes comfortable with a chopping instrument, however, there is little value in further change.

Original chopping instruments were fashioned out of Sinskey hooks, with the tip rebent to a length of approximately 1.5 mm. This type of instrument is generally not recommended because the very fine gauge wire of a Sinskey hook can cut through a nucleus, whereas the absence of any bulk in the wire prevents the full realization of the potential of phaco chop. Recall that Nagahara's fundamental principle was that the chopping instrument should act like a wedge. Most models of chopping instruments have a thicker gauge than the Sinskey hook, often with a sharp internal cutting surface, thus obtaining the desired splitting effect.

Chopping instruments may have only one sharpened surface, generally directed along the shaft of the chopper,

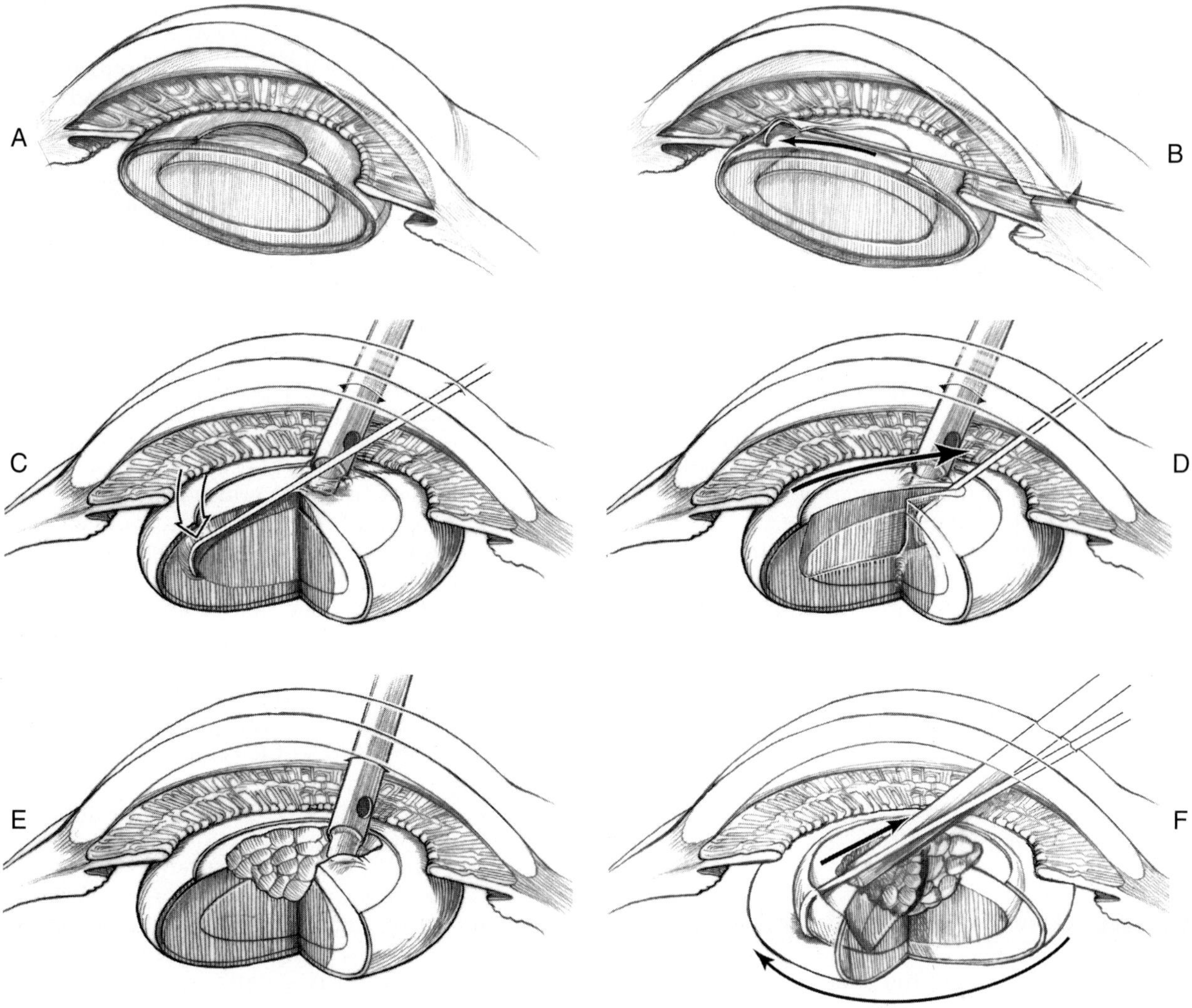

Figure 10–5. *A* (cross-section view). With a widely dilated pupil and small to moderate sized endonucleus, hydrodelineation will create a separation of the endonucleus from the epinucleus, seen as a golden ring or a black ring, depending on the illumination and red reflex. *B* (cross-section view). The surgeon directs the chopper under the anterior capsule and down into the ring. *C* (a quarter-section view to reveal inner nucleus). If the pupillary dilation is smaller than the size of the endonucleus, then the surgeon must advance the tip of the chopper without being able to see the equator. With experience, the surgeon will develop a good sense of how much the chopper needs to be advanced to reach the zone of the ring and will be able to feel when the chopper tip reaches this point and is able to drop. *D*. The phaco tip is used to impale the nucleus and is advanced to the depth of the mid-nucleus. The chopper is pulled toward the phaco tip, splitting the nucleus in half. *E*. The central, hardest portion of the nucleus is removed. The harder the nucleus, the larger the area sculpted. Enough nuclear material must remain that the phaco tip can engage and become occluded on the periphery, while the chopper breaks off pie-shaped wedges for removal *(F)*.

or two or three surfaces may be sharpened, allowing more successful "lateral chopping" maneuvers. The shaft may also be angled for right- or left-handed approaches.

Steinert designed a curved chopping instrument (Fig. 10–6; Rhein Medical, Tampa, FL) that incorporates all of the principles of the phaco chop and also facilitates keeping the chopper engaged in the center of the nucleus. The curved distal element acts in the same manner as a cat's claw or a farmer's hoe. The chopper naturally engages the curved equator of the nucleus, which can be felt by the surgeon. The claw configuration then keeps the chopper engaged deeply within the nucleus, unlike the straight choppers which tend to rise up and out of the nucleus as they pass toward the center.

THE PHACOEMULSIFICATION NEEDLE

For many years, phacoemulsification instrument manufacturers progressively increased the angle of the phacoemulsification tip in order to gain increased "cutting power." The phaco chop technique has reversed that trend. The greater the angle of the phacoemulsification tip, the more the tip must be buried into the nuclear fragment to obtain occlusion, which is necessary for stabilizing the nucleus before the initial phaco chop and for engaging and controlling the peripheral circumferential wedges. In fact, Nagahara worked with one company to return to a true zero degree phacoemulsification tip

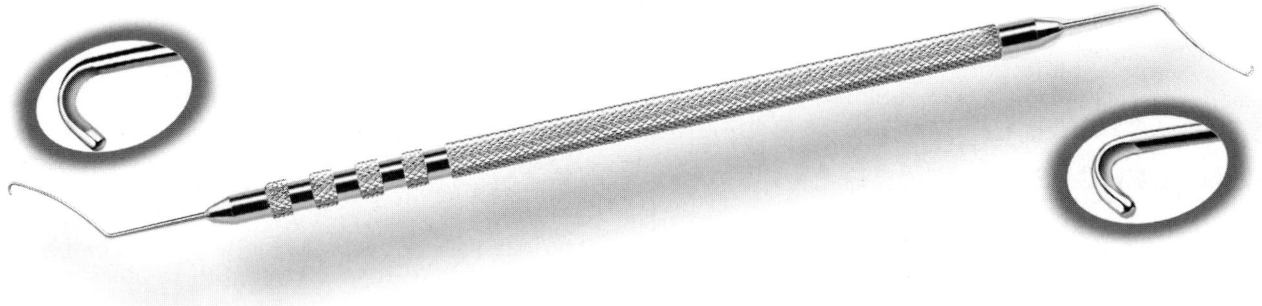

Figure 10–6. The Steinert double-ended claw chopper. One end is 1.5 mm in length, for chopping most nuclei; the other end is 1.75 mm long for chopping large, hard nuclei. (Courtesy of Rhein Medical, Inc., Tampa, FL.)

(Allergan, Inc., Irvine, CA). That tip greatly facilitates obtaining occlusion of the circumferential nuclear fragments and aiding their manipulation.

Why does this not reduce ultrasound unacceptably? Phacoemulsification handpieces have greatly increased in power over recent years. More importantly, however, better understanding of ultrasonics had led to manipulations in the configuration of the phacoemulsification tip to improve the efficiency of ultrasonification of the nucleus by means of cavitation. For example, Nagahara's zero degree tip has an internal bevel that vastly improves ultrasound power through internal cavitation as well as by reducing the cross-sectional area of the phacoemulsification needle tip.

TRANSITION TO PHACO CHOP

Before endeavoring to use the phaco chop technique, the surgeon should first become proficient in anterior *capsulorrhexis, hydrodissection,* and *hydrodelineation.* The nucleus must be freely mobile to allow free rotation once chopping begins. An intact and well-defined circular tear anterior capsulotomy provides a clear landmark for the surgeon, and it also provides strength for extra manipulation.[7] Hydrodelineation frees the nucleus from the epinucleus, which is necessary for chopped fragments to be removed, as well as disclosing the location of the nuclear equator, as noted earlier.

The surgeon who wishes to learn phaco chop should begin by chopping the second half of the nucleus in a case where the first half has been removed with a conventional divide-and-conquer quadrant technique (Fig. 10–7*A*). The second half of the nucleus is usually quite mobile at that point, and the basic technique and tactile feel of phaco chop can be appreciated within several cases by chopping the second half of the heminucleus (Fig. 10–7*B*).

Once the surgeon feels comfortable with chopping the second heminucleus, the next step is to perform the "stop and chop" technique for both halves of the heminucleus, but retaining the initial trough and split hemisection of the divide-and-conquer approaches (Fig. 10–2).

The last step in the progress to full phaco chop is to bisect the nucleus with the phaco chopper (Figs. 10–3*A* and 10–5*D*). Although some surgeons have found this to be the most challenging aspect of mastering the technique, it also is the most rewarding. Full phaco chop

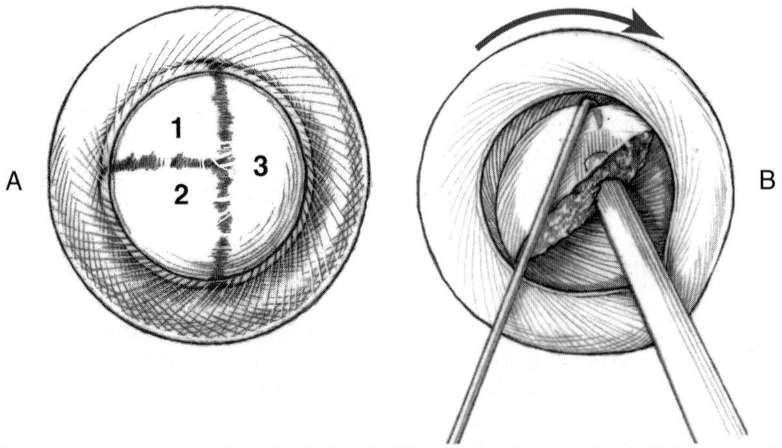

Figure 10–7. *A.* To begin learning phaco chop, the first half of the nucleus (pieces 1 and 2) is removed using the standard divide-and-conquer technique; the second heminucleus (3) remains undivided. *B.* The second half of the nucleus can be chopped with good direct visualization.

markedly improves the efficiency of the disassembly of the nucleus, chiefly because it eliminates the multiple steps of rotation and trough creation required by the standard quadrant cracking techniques.

CHALLENGES IN PHACO CHOP

SMALL PUPILS

When the patient has small pupils, the novice surgeon will be insecure about the inability to visualize the periphery during chopping maneuvers. Small pupil cases should only be undertaken with phaco chop after the surgeon has gained reasonable experience on more straightforward cases with large pupils and moderate density nuclei. Once this skill is achieved, however, chopping is preferred over the quadrant cracking divide and conquer technique because chopping does not require peripheral passes with the ultrasound tip, and it is not dependent on a good red reflex.[8,9]

THE 4+ NUCLEUS

Chopping a 4+ hard nucleus can be particularly difficult, both because a hard nucleus is also a thick nucleus and because of the physical properties of a hard *brunescent* nucleus.[10] Nevertheless, chopping offers distinct advantages in phacoemulsification of very advanced cataracts.[11] Because the nucleus is thick, a standard 1.5-mm length phaco chopper will not have adequate length to pass through its center (Fig. 10–8*A*). As a result, a superficial vertical split will occur, but the deeper layer of the nucleus may split in a more lateral fashion, creating a posterior plate (Fig. 10–8*B*). If this occurs, the surgeon needs to identify which half of the nucleus is above the plate and which half is attached to the plate. The heminucleus that is above the plate should be removed first, which then allows the larger fragment to be mobilized and chopped. Several chopping instruments are now available with longer tips on the order of 1.75 to 2 mm, which greatly facilitates successful chopping of thicker nuclei. These choppers, although longer, are still well short of endangering the posterior capsule, considering that a brunescent nucleus is at least 3.5 mm thick (Fig. 10–8*C*).

A very hard nucleus tends to have a posterior "leathery" quality. Chopped fragments contain bridging strands that keep nuclear fragments attached to each other. These posterior strands represent epinucleus that has partially hardened, with strong adhesion to the posterior nucleus which has a tough, strand-like quality. When these strands occur, they are readily seen against the red reflex as they bridge two chopped nuclear fragments (Fig. 10–8*D*). The surgeon can rotate the phaco chopper 90 degrees in his or her fingers, carefully pass the chopper posterior to the nuclear fragment, and transect the bridging fibers (Fig. 10–8*E*). It is this maneuver that has led to variations of phaco chop generally known as "posterior cracking."

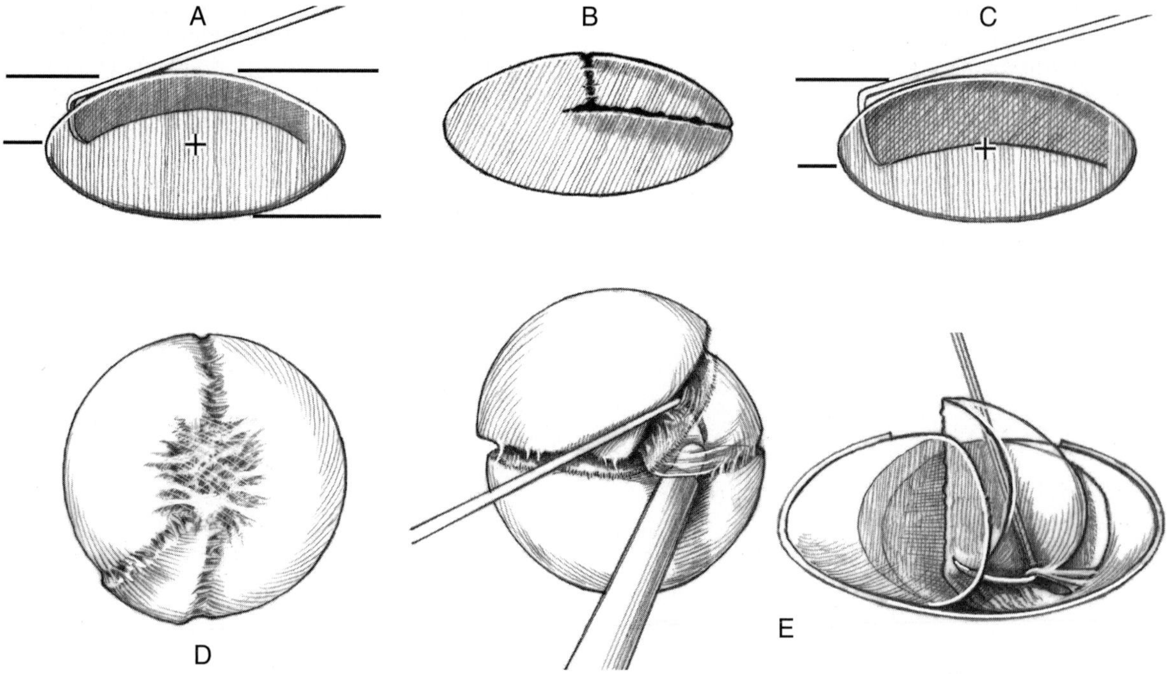

Figure 10–8. *A.* A thick, advanced nuclear cataract cannot be broken up effectively with a standard chopping instrument because the length of the tip is inadequate to split the center of the nucleus. *B.* If the thick nucleus splits at all, a short-tipped chopper will tend to split the upper portion of the nucleus, but the fracture line below that point will lateralize, leaving a posterior nuclear plate attached to one portion of the two halves of the nucleus. *C.* A longer chopper will have a better likelihood of cleanly splitting the nucleus. The extra length of the chopper tip is far removed from the posterior capsule and will not penetrate to that level. *D* (posterior view). In advanced nuclear sclerosis, "leathery" posterior nuclear strands will bridge across a chopped wedge and interfere with its removal, particularly at the posterior apex. *E 1.* (surgeon's view) and *2.* (side view). The chopper can be rotated 90 degrees, parallel to the posterior capsule, and used to snap across these strands and free the nuclear wedge.

ZONULAR ABNORMALITIES

Once experience is gained with phaco chop, it is the preferred technique in cases of *pseudoexfoliation* syndrome or after trauma, when zonules are weak or absent.[12–15] Because horizontal chopping creates opposing forces between the two instruments, it minimizes forces on the zonules.[16]

COMPLICATIONS OF PHACO CHOP

MULTIPLE INCOMPLETE CHOPS

A surgeon inexperienced at phaco chop often tends to "scratch" the nucleus without accomplishing front-to-back cleavage. This can occur for two reasons: The first is failure to pass the chopper far enough into the periphery to allow the chopper to "hook" and engage the equator. The surgeon can test for this position by gently pulling on the chopper and verifying that the nucleus moves with it. The second common problem is allowing the chopper to ride up and out of the nucleus. The claw-shaped chopper was designed by Steinert to help overcome this tendency. For all chopper styles, the surgeon needs to learn to maintain appropriate posterior pressure on the chopping instrument.

When incomplete chops do occur, leaving incompletely cleaved fragments, the surgeon must remain patient. Concentrating on proper technique, it is important to continue rotating, attempting to chop a new area. In addition, the chopper can be used to hook a fragment and help bring it toward the phaco tip in the central zone. This maneuver is particularly helpful when the vacuum is inadequate, or when complete occlusion cannot be achieved, and the nuclear fragment keeps "falling back," away from the phaco tip.

POSTERIOR CAPSULE RUPTURE

The most feared complication of phaco chop is rupture of the posterior capsule with the chopper. In fact, this is rare, and should not occur at all with adherence to the principles of phaco chop. The phaco chop instrument is typically only 1.5 mm along and, even in phaco chop instruments that have been elongated for dealing with a 4+ nucleus, the length never exceeds 2.0 mm (see Fig. 10–8*A* and *C*). The conventional lens is thicker than this in the periphery, and increases to between 3 and 4 mm centrally (and sometimes even thicker). As a result, the phaco chopping instrument is well away from the posterior capsule. Many of the phaco chop instruments have a blunted tip, which is also less likely to engage the poserior capsule.

ANTERIOR CAPSULE/ZONULAR RUPTURE

A more common complication is misjudging the location of the anterior capsule, such that the phaco chopper is anterior to the peripheral anterior capsule rather than within the capsular bag (Fig. 10–9*A*). This mistake can be avoided by placing the phaco chopping instrument against the nucleus centrally, within the capsulorrhexis, and then keeping a small amount of posterior pressure against the nucleus as the chopper is passed peripherally. In a very hard nucleus with almost no anterior cortex, little space is present between the

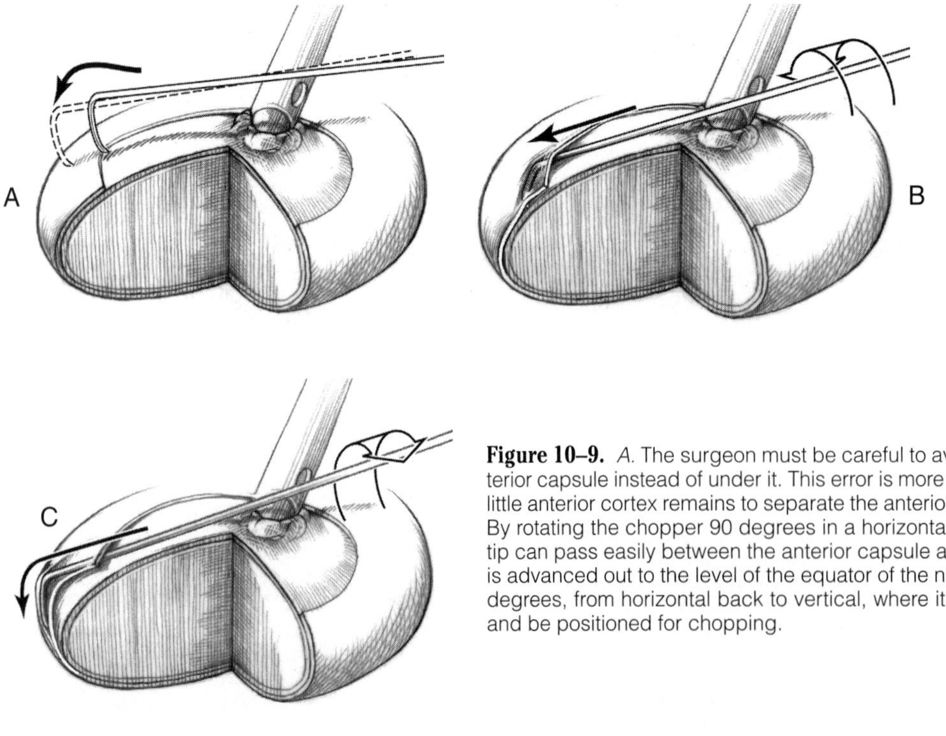

Figure 10–9. *A*. The surgeon must be careful to avoid passing the chopper over the anterior capsule instead of under it. This error is more likely in a large, dense cataract where little anterior cortex remains to separate the anterior capsule from the anterior nucleus. *B*. By rotating the chopper 90 degrees in a horizontal position parallel to the iris plane, the tip can pass easily between the anterior capsule and the nucleus. *C*. As the chopper tip is advanced out to the level of the equator of the nucleus, the tip is then rotated back 90 degrees, from horizontal back to vertical, where it will pass around the nuclear equator and be positioned for chopping.

anterior capsule and the nucleus. In this case, the surgeon should rotate the phaco chopping instrument 90 degrees within the surgeon's fingers so that it can slip under the anterior capsule in a "flat" position (Fig. 10–9*B*). As the chopper passes to the edge of the endonucleus, it is then rotated back 90 degrees to the vertical chopping position (Fig. 10–9*C*).

CONCLUSIONS

With careful attention to detail in following the progressive learning technique suggested above, any two-handed phaco surgeon should be able to master the maneuvers of phaco chop. Phaco chop is faster and, as a result, ultrasound time is reduced, with the reduction in corneal endothelial damage and the potential for rupture of the posterior capsule.

Moreover, because phaco chop is a technique that involves stabilizing the nucleus with a phaco instrument centrally and then applying centripetal forces with the phaco chopper against the ultrasound tip, there is much less zonular stress than in standard cracking techniques. After phaco chop is mastered, it becomes a central element in the phacoemulsification surgeon's technique.

REFERENCES

1. Koch PS, Katzen LE: Stop and chop phacoemulsification. J Cataract Refract Surg 1994;20:566–570.
2. Steinert RF: "Phaco chop." *In* Steinert RF et al. (eds): Cataract Surgery: Technique, Complications, and Management, Philadelphia, WB Saunders, 1995, p 166.
3. Gimbel HV: Divide and conquer nucleofractis phacoemulsification: development and variations. J Cataract Refract Surg 1991;17: 281–291.
4. Pirazzoli G, D'Eliseo D, Ziosi M, Acciarri R: Effects of phacoemulsification time on the corneal endothelium using phacofracture and phaco chop techniques. J Cataract Refract Surg 1996;22: 967–969.
5. DeBry P, Olson RJ, Crandall AS: Comparison of energy required for phaco-chop and divide and conquer phacoemulsification. J Cataract Refract Surg 1998;24:689–692.
6. Ram J, Wesendahl TA, Auffarth GU, Apple DJ: Evaluation of in situ fracture versus phaco chop techniques. J Cataract Refract Surg 1998;24:1464–1468.
7. Gimbel HV, Neuhann T: Development, advantages, and methods of the continuous circular capsulotomy technique. J Cataract Refract Surg 1990;16:31–37.
8. Lumme P, Laatikainen LT: Risk factors for intraoperative and early postoperative complications in extracapsular surgery. Eur J Ophthalmol 1994;4:151–158.
9. Joseph J, Wang HS: Phacoemulsification with poorly dilated pupils. J Cataract Refract Surg 1993;19:551–556.
10. Hayashi K, Nakao F, Hayashi F: Corneal endothelial cell loss after phacoemulsification using nuclear cracking procedures. J Cataract Refract Surg 1994;20:44–47.
11. Vasavada A, Singh R: Step-by-step chop in situ and separation of very dense cataracts. J Cataract Refract Surg 1998;24:156–159.
12. Lunne P, Laatikainen L: Exfoliation syndrome and cataract extraction. Am J Ophthalmol 1993;116:51–55.
13. Osher RH, Cionni RJ, Gimbel HV, et al.: Cataract surgery in patients with pseudoexfoliation syndrome. Eur J Implant Refract Surg 1993;5:46–50.
14. Fine IH, Hoffman RS: Phacoemulsification in the presence of pseudoexfoliation: Challenges and options. J Cataract Refract Surg 1997;23:160–165.
15. Moreno J, Duch S, Lajara J: Pseudoexfoliation syndrome: Clinical factors related to capsular rupture in cataract surgery. Acta Ophthalmol 1993;71:181–184.
16. Masket S (ed.): Consultation Section. J Cataract Refract Surg 1998;24:1289–1298.

CHAPTER 11

Intraoperative Complications of Phacoemulsification and Small-Incision Cataract Surgery

SAMUEL MASKET, M.D.

This chapter is devoted to intraoperative complications specific to phacoemulsification and small-incision cataract surgery. Uncomplicated cataract surgery generally assures rapidly achieved and stable results, but such success may not hold true in cases with severe or improperly managed surgical complications. Surgeons in training or those in transition to phacoemulsification should recognize that "acceptable" rates of complications may be achieved at all levels of experience. The key factors are appropriate instruction, adequate practice in the laboratory, careful attention to surgical detail, and an awareness of potential complications.

PREOPERATIVE ASSESSMENT

Favorable complication management should begin with prevention. Careful preoperative evaluation of the cataract patient may reveal conditions that are likely to lead to complications. With appropriate surgical planning and execution, intraoperative calamities can be avoided.

The patient's medical history may, as an example, reveal chronic obstructive pulmonary disease (COPD) with attendant frequent coughing; the risk of intraoperative coughing and an associated elevation of orbital pressure can be prevented by pretreating the patient with inhalants or parenteral medications. Likewise, a patient known to be significantly claustrophobic may require general anesthesia or special draping for comfortable, safe, and successful surgery. Thus prior knowledge and planning may anticipate problems and prevent surgical complications, including the need to convert the patient to general anesthesia intraoperatively, potentially with the eye already incised. As another example, patients treated with anticoagulants may be better served by a clear corneal entrance under topical anesthesia than with an orbital injection and sclerocorneal incision. In essence, knowledge of the patient's medical history may be a significant aid in the prevention of operative complications.

Ocular history taking may also reveal added risk factors for undesired surgical events. A case in point is that significant blunt trauma earlier in life may be associated with zonular weakness and potential disinsertion during capsulotomy, nuclear rotation, cortical clean-up, etc. Although the presurgical examination is likely to uncover obvious signs of prior trauma (Table 11–1), many cataract patients after trauma may have only subtle findings. Awareness of the history, however, arms the surgeon with preparedness for zonular weakness, and appropriate steps during surgery may allow the outcome to be routine. Ophthalmologists must not lose sight of the fact that assessment of the patient's history is a most salient aspect of proper treatment for all conditions, including cataract.

TABLE 11-1. Traumatic Zonulysis

Phacodonesis
Iridoplegia
Pupillary sphincter tears
Iridodialysis
Recession of angle
Secondary glaucoma
Retinal dialysis

ANESTHETIC COMPLICATIONS

Anesthesia for phacoemulsification may be accomplished by general, regional, subconjunctival, topical, or intracameral methods. Systemic complications of ocular anesthesia are not specific for phacoemulsification, but their potential should not be overlooked when employing small-incision surgery. Appropriate patient support systems must be in place if intravenous agents are contemplated or if regional anesthetics are injected, because both may be associated with central nervous system consequences including apnea and death. Qualified personnel must be available to manage anesthetic complications, although the ultimate responsibility for the patient remains with the surgeon.

Given that topical and intracameral anesthetic methods are increasingly popular, patient cooperation is a consequential variable in the progress of surgery. The necessary interaction between patient and surgeon may be hindered when oversedated or very anxious patients move excessively or fail to control ocular movements. Surgery may be interrupted and an alternative method of anesthesia initiated. Deep sub-Tenon's ("parabulbar") infiltration may be performed at any time during small-incision surgery because the self-sealing wound generally employed during phacoemulsification can allow for globe manipulation yet maintain the anterior chamber. In that context it is wise to pressurize the chamber before anesthetic infiltration. With sub-Tenon's instillation, small amounts of anesthetic will suffice since the parabulbar method affords direct access to the retrobulbar space.[1] Moreover, excessive subconjunctival anesthetic may induce chemosis with subsequent pooling of fluid on the cornea, which produces horrific reflections that interfere with the surgeon's view, potentially complicating surgery.

INCISIONAL COMPLICATIONS

Incisions for phacoemulsification cataract surgery may vary from slightly above 2.0 mm to 7.0 mm, depending on the ultrasonic tip and machinery, implant style and material, and implant insertion instruments. Likewise, the meridional location for the incision may vary with surgeon preference and be placed fully in clear cornea, at the limbus, or originate in the sclera with anterior dissection into the cornea (sclerocorneal tunnel). While each style may be associated with specific operative problems, complications common to all methods include incisions that are too small, too large, too deep, too superficial, too anterior, too posterior, or inadequately sealed.

Given the rapidly expanding interest in small incisions, particularly in clear cornea, many surgeons have downsized the chamber entry to eliminate iatrogenic astigmatism and to assure hermetic sealing of corneal incisions. Specialized reduced-diameter phacoemulsification tips (0.9 mm) are required to work through incisions smaller than 2.8 mm. Standard, larger tips (1.1 mm) may be "forced" into the eye, but incisions that are too small and too tight may not allow adequate inflow and result in corneal burns, with potentially disastrous astigmatism and wound leaks (Fig. 11–1). Corneal burns may also be induced by inadequate fluid exchange through the phaco tip. Most often this occurs with advanced nuclear brunescent cataracts, which require prolonged ultrasound time and high energy. It will also occur when the surgeon fully occludes the tip by impaling or "lollipopping" an ultrafirm cataract, because the hard consistency of the lens clogging the tip precludes the egress of lens emulsate. Furthermore, blockage prevents the flow of balanced salt solution (BSS) through the tip, and so the cooling function of BSS ceases with occlusion. This phenomenon may occur more frequently when surgeons employ "chopping" maneuvers in favor of grooves for nuclear dissection; nuclear "chopping" requires tip occlusion, which may potentiate clogging, whereas groove dissection does not, as a rule, involve tip occlusion.

Corneal or corneoscleral incisional burns are apparently more common, perhaps in part because surgeons are adapting new surgical methods while employing older styles of equipment or using techniques inappropriate for the specific case. For the former, standard phaco tips with silicone sleeves require a keratome incision of at least 2.8 mm; a 3.2-mm incision assures adequate inflow and is generally recommended by manufacturers. For the latter, surgeons should consider the density of the cataract before deciding on the method for nuclear division and removal. Since groove dissection surgical methods do not require occlusion of the

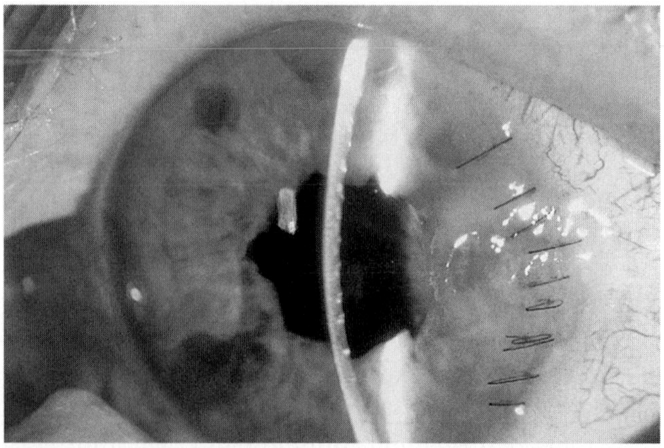

Figure 11–1. Postoperative consequences of an incisional burn. Clinical slit-lamp photograph demonstrates corneal edema, corneal striae, and probable high corneal astigmatism after incisional burn with the need for multiple suture closure (photograph courtesy of Douglas D. Koch, M.D.).

tip, very advanced brunescent cataracts are perhaps better managed by a traditional quadratic "divide-and-conquer" method. Finally, wound burns may develop if the gravity-fed infusion bottle is too low, resulting in adequate inflow. This may occur when surgeons inappropriately opt for a "low-flow" system in the face of a dense cataract and/or when using a very highly retentive viscoelastic agent, which may also contribute to clogging of the tip.[2] In essence, adequate ingress and egress of infusate must be a surgical priority; the amount necessary varies with nuclear density, viscoelastic substance, surgical method, and phaco tip style. By and large, corneal wound burns are iatrogenic and most likely occur because surgeons inappropriately "mix and match" techniques and equipment. This dreaded complication should be avoidable by employing the appropriate surgical method and devices for the given situation.

Management of incisional burns varies with the extent of the damage. The most significant concern is to assure a watertight seal at the close of surgery. Generally, this can be accomplished by using sutures to approximate the roof and floor of the incision. Sutures may be placed radially or circumferentially as needed. In severe burns, however, the amount of tissue shrinkage may require the use of scleral patch grafts or relaxing incisions, or both. Graft material may be obtained from banked sclera or from other areas of the operative eye, taking partial-thickness lamellae. Conjunctival closure should be performed diligently after securing the corneoscleral incision. Surgeons should encourage the patient to tolerate the induced astigmatism, since it tends to wane over time; only after stabilization of corneal curvature should corrective keratorefractive procedures be considered.

Incisions that are too large create excess fluid egress during emulsification or aspiration maneuvers. As a result, the chamber may shallow and the incision lack self-sealing ability. An oversized incision generally results when the surgeon uses a free-hand knife rather than a specifically measured keratome, or, when a sharp-sided diamond keratome is employed and the blade extends the incision laterally if the surgeon fails to maintain the blade position during both entry and exit. Here, too, the cause is iatrogenic and may be avoided with the use of proper technique and an appropriate keratome.

Incisions that begin with a vertical groove that is too deep, particularly in the case of sclerocorneal tunnels, risk entering the ciliary body, risk inducing chamber hemorrhage resulting from an entrance that is too posterior, and risk physical instability after surgery with significant and evolving iatrogenic astigmatism. Shallow incisions, on the other hand, primarily risk external "buttonholes," which may cause wound leakage. In the case of scleral tunnels, a buttonhole may be sewn closed and covered with the conjunctiva. However, clear corneal tunnels, which are less forgiving, may be difficult to manage when buttonholes are induced by a tunnel that is too thin externally.

Incisions that are placed too far centrally have their chamber entrance closer to the corneal apex than is necessary or wise. As a result striae will form on the corneal surface during chamber maneuvers. Striae make visualization extraordinarily difficult for the surgeon. In this situation, prevention is the best answer to the problem. Generally, eyes that are underfilled with viscoelastic material prior to chamber entrance have low intraocular pressure and are prone to long incisional tracts and anterior entries. In addition to striae, the surgeon may be burdened with "oarlocking" from a very long tunnel. The restrictions imposed by a very long tunnel may make it difficult to perform capsulorrhexis and other intracameral maneuvers; furthermore, long, tight, and restricting tunnels promote incisional burns.

Sclerocorneal incisions that are too posterior in their entrance may pierce the chamber in vascular tissue, possibly inducing hyphema. Moreover, with an entrance that is too far posterior, surgery may be complicated by the annoyance of intraoperative iris prolapse. A surgeon needs to experience iris prolapse only once to recognize that the protruding iris will hinder the progress of surgery. Furthermore, any mechanical stimulus to the iris may result in a release of prostaglandins with ensuing miosis. In addition, the posterior iris pigment layer may separate and eventually wash away, the iris will be cosmetically deformed, and the process will evolve in a "snowballing" manner unless the incision is sutured and another entrance is selected. Iris prolapse is generally preventable by carrying the incision adequately anterior into the clear cornea. Should prolapse occur, early recognition and management (suture closure, alternative incision site, iridotomy for the pupillary block, or mechanical protection of the iris with a modified Sheet's glide) can reduce the surgeon's stress and preserve the patient's cosmesis. Another potential problem develops when incisions, whether corneal or sclerocorneal, are too far posterior at their internal entrance to the chamber. Such incisions are unlikely to self-seal because they lack a sufficient internal corneal valve (Fig. 11–2). A large concern about inadequately sealed incisions with clear corneal entries is that they have no external (conjunctival) barrier against the ingress of microbes after surgery. Truly self-sealing incisions, however, are generally hermetic.

An additional consideration with respect to incision complications is the development of a detachment of Descemet's membrane. This potentially serious threat to corneal clarity is induced by incisions that are too central or too narrow, causing the surgeon to "stuff" instruments through the incision into the chamber. Also, incisions that are made with dulled knives may cause detachment of Descemet's membrane. Alternatively, the surgeon may "catch" an edge of Descemet's with the phaco tip or its sleeve on chamber entrance, an event than can be avoided by deepening the entrance space with viscoelastic material. Care must be taken, however, because improper viscoagent injection may induce a Descemet's detachment if the cannula does not completely enter the chamber.[3] Early recognition of a small "scroll" of Descemet's membrane may allow the surgeon to prevent further central extension with postoperative corneal decompensation. If the problem occurs early in the surgery, another site may opened. Often, however, working carefully, or enlarging the incision slightly, will prevent significant progression of

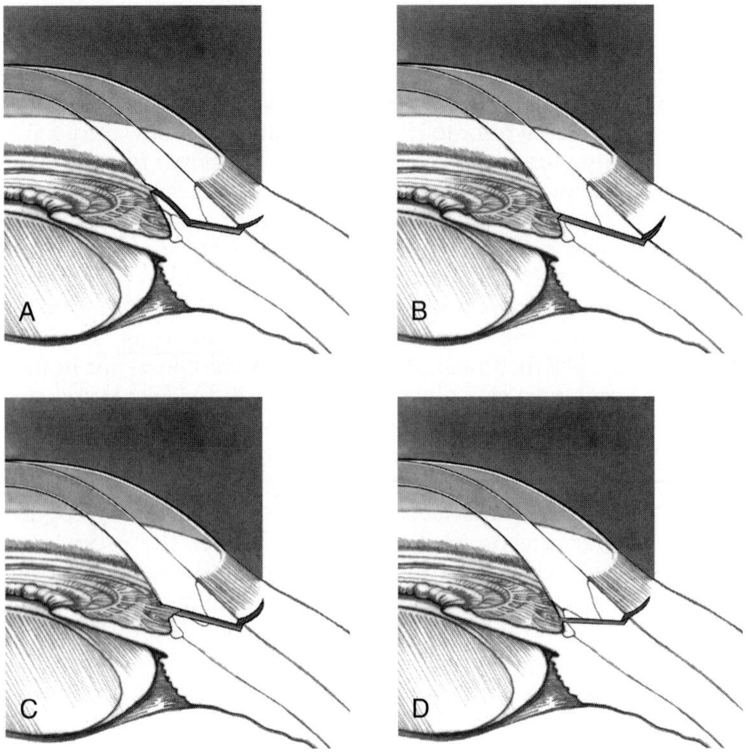

Figure 11–2. Schematic cross-sectional representation of incision profiles. *A*. *A* competent internal corneal valve incision that will self-seal after surgery and prevent iris prolapse intraoperatively. *B*. A schematic corneal valve that can prevent iris prolapse during surgery but is unlikely to self-seal. *C*. An incision without any internal valve; it is incompetent with respect to both prevention of iris prolapse and self-sealing, *D*.

the detachment. Management of a large Descemet's detachment requires repositioning with air, long-acting gases (SF_6, for example), or viscoelastic material administered through sideport incisions with or without through-and-through corneal sutures.[4]

Iatrogenic astigmatism is a long-term complication of cataract surgery that is induced by the style, location, and size of the cataract incision. Its causes, prevention, and management are discussed in Chapter 6.

COMPLICATIONS RELATED TO ANTERIOR CAPSULORRHEXIS

An anterior capsulotomy that is too small (generally, less than 3.5 mm in diameter) may cause difficulty with nuclear manipulation during phacoemulsification and with lens implantation, both situations leading to zonular stress with potential disinsertion of the capsular bag, anterior displacement of vitreous, nuclear loss, and late implant decentration. Furthermore, should the capsulotomy be too small, the edge may be caught and torn during emulsification, during attempted removal of subincisional cortex, or with lens implantation; resultant radial tears in the capsule will compromise the integrity of the capsular bag and, if unrecognized may extend around the lens equator to the posterior capsule during surgical manipulations. Management of radial tears in the capsulorrhexis (see below) requires an alteration of surgical strategy and, as in the case of most complications, will be more successfully managed with early recognition. While an adequately sized capsular opening will obviate complications, the undersized capsulorrhexis is readily enlarged with the use of long, sharp-pointed scissors (Gills-Welch) to initiate a new capsular edge, which can then be torn with capsule forceps (Fig. 11–3). This step may be performed before or after nuclear management, or even after lens

Figure 11–3. Schematic drawing of technique to enlarge anterior capsulorrhexis if anterior capsular opening is insufficient.

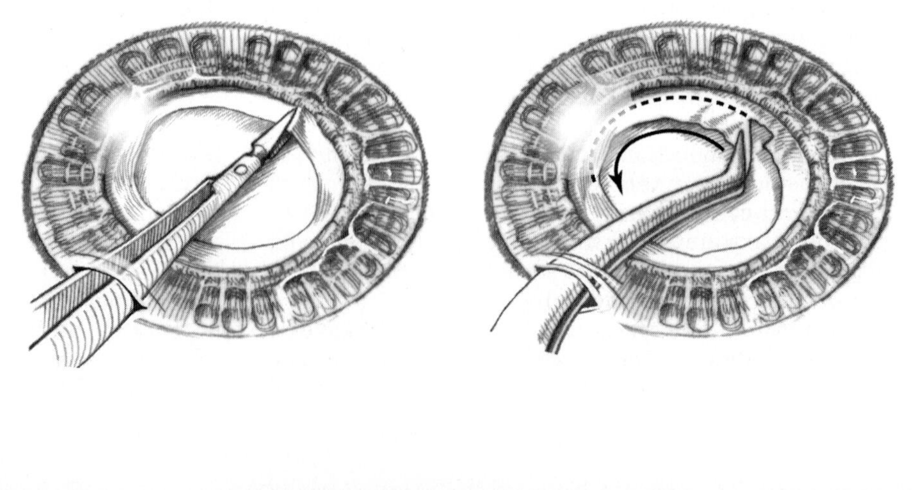

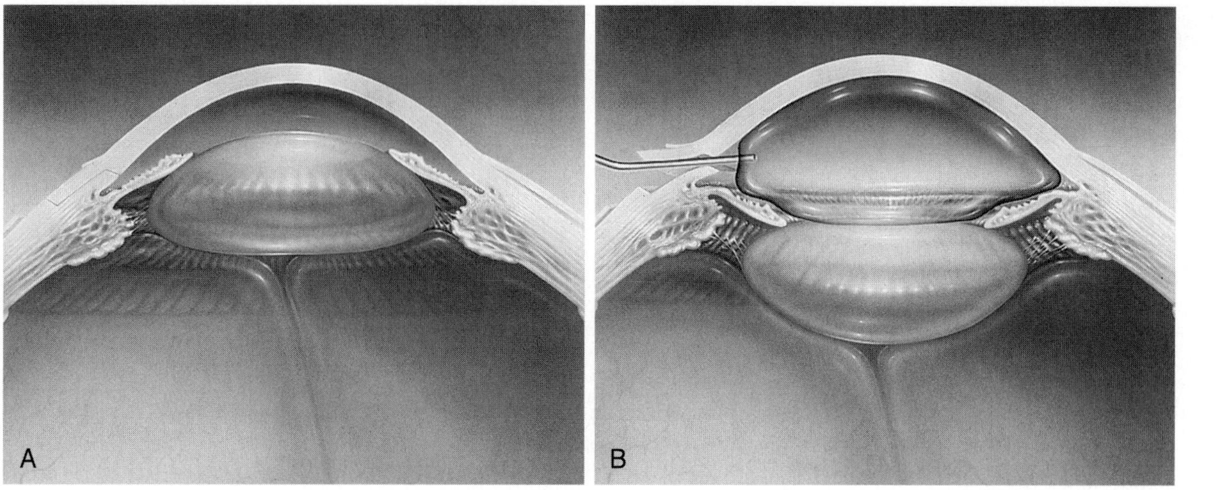

Figure 11–4. *A*. The anterior capsule has assumed a convex configuration; capsular tears can often extend peripherally as they tend to "run downhill." *B*. The anterior capsule has flattened to a scaphoid shape in response to the addition of a highly retentive viscoelastic agent (courtesy Upjohn Pharmacia).

implantation, because a small capsulotomy is more likely associated with postoperative complications of capsulorrhexis.[5]

Loss of control of the capsular tear with subsequent radialization during capsulorrhexis is arguably the most common complication of smooth-edged anterior capsulotomy. This is more likely to occur with surgeon inexperience, "positive" posterior pressure, pediatric or young adult eyes, intumescent and white cataracts, intraoperative shallowing of the anterior chamber, poor visualization, small pupils, long scleral tunnel incisions, or attempting to generate too large a capsulorrhexis. The common pathway to difficulty in controlling the fate of the capsular tear occurs when the anterior lens capsule assumes a convex shape (Fig. 11–4*A*). Subsequently, the capsular tear is likely to extend peripherally as there is a tendency for the capsulotomy to "run downhill." While this may be unavoidable in certain situations, rendering the anterior capsule scaphoid or flat (Fig. 11–4*B*) in the routine case affords the surgeon far greater control of the fate and direction of the tear. This may be attained with a highly retentive and cohesive viscoagent, use of capsule forceps that conform to the shape of the anterior segment, avoiding external pressure on the eye, and employing an incision that avoids oarlocking. If too large a capsulorrhexis is attempted, the tear may extend peripherally when unusually tough zonules are encountered, forcing the tear along the zonular axis. Because anatomic studies have demonstrated that the zonules insert anteriorly to approximately a 6.0 mm central clear zone, this represents a safe upper limit for capsulorrhexis in most situations.

While many surgeons find that the use of a cystitome provides adequate control for routine capsulorrhexis, and allows the capsulotomy to be performed through a very small chamber entrance, making viscoelastic insertion optional, an errant capsular tear may be redirected and the capsulorrhexis salvaged with the use of capsule forceps. When the capsular tear cannot be redirected, the capsulotomy is best completed with scissors or with a cystitome in a "canopener" fashion. Should radialization of the anterior capsulotomy occur, or the canopener method become necessary, the surgical plan of attack must be modified, because the chief concern is posterior extension of an anterior capsular tear with loss of lens material into the posterior segment. Generally, hydrodissection, which increases the hydrostatic forces in the capsular bag, is best avoided to prevent extension of the tear. In this situation, an iris plane or anterior chamber emulsification method might be the safest approach, because endolenticular phaco methods require hydrodissection. Alternatively, the experienced surgeon may be comfortable with very gentle and slow hydrodissection despite a radial tear in the anterior capsulotomy. In such a case, the specific meridian of the radial tear dictates the strategy. As an example, a radial tear in the 6-o'clock position, mandates that lens cracking maneuvers be performed from 3 o'clock to 9 o'clock to avoid further stress on the radial rent. Periodic observation of the condition of the anterior and posterior capsules will allow the surgeon to "bail out" and bring the lens nucleus into the anterior chamber should conditions so mandate. Once control of the nucleus is established, a decision to perform anterior chamber emulsification or manual lens removal can be made; the presurgical condition of the corneal endothelium should be one factor in the decision-making process.

In addition to the capsular difficulties that may be encountered with certain patient types or surgical conditions, special consideration should be given to cases in which postoperative anterior capsular contraction is likely. Typically, risk factors include pseudoexfoliation, uveitis, diabetes, retinitis pigmentosa, and any condition associated with weakened zonules. In such cases it is also possible that during the capsulorrhexis the surgeon will gain insight into the strength of the natural lens support system. If the lens is particularly

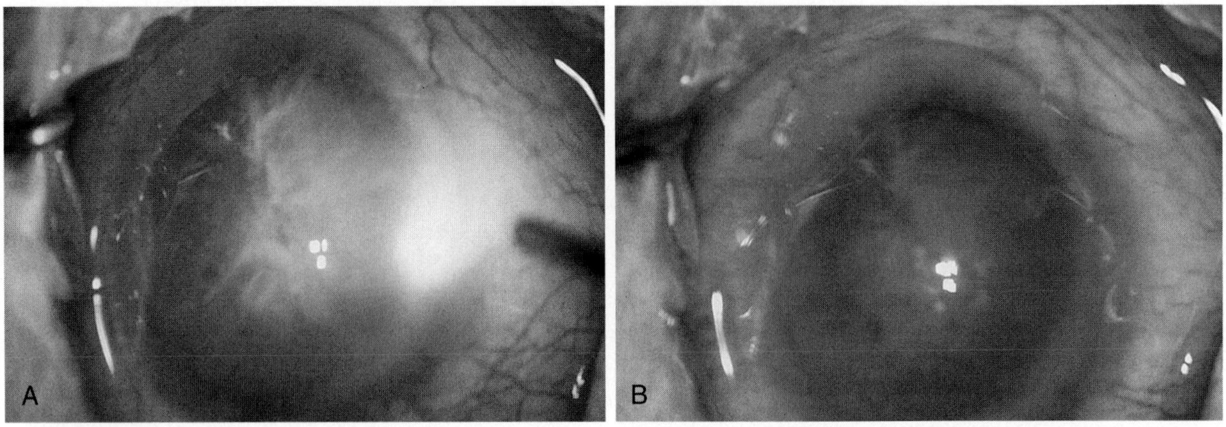

Figure 11–5. *A.* Intraoperative view of the anterior capsule of a mature cataract. The retinal endoilluminator, placed to the right, enhances details of the capsule. *B.* Same view as in A, without endoilluminator. Details of the anterior capsule are not visible.

loose, alternative surgical plans for cataract removal and lens implantation must be considered.

Ultradense nuclear cataracts or those that are white mature, hinder the surgeon's view during capsulorrhexis because they preclude a red reflex. While a number of methods to aid the view of the capsule have been proposed, a simple system is the use of tangential illumination of the anterior segment during capsular maneuvers. A retinal endoilluminator is generally available in ophthalmic operating theaters; held adjacent the limbus, the light source greatly facilitates the view of the capsular tear (Fig. 11–5*A* and 5*B*). Even better is the visible contrast between the white cortex and the capsule afforded by the use of capsule-staining materials like indocyanine green (ICG) and trypan blue.[6]

A final condition of note with regard to the anterior capsulotomy is myotonic dystrophy. In this disorder, the anterior capsule is particularly difficult to incise because it has a rubbery consistency and high tensile strength. On occasion, even a very sharp cystotome will fail to incise the capsule. Myotonic dystrophy may be considered as an indication for the use of the Nd:YAG laser, or diathermy capsulotomy to initiate the anterior capsulotomy.

COMPLICATIONS ASSOCIATED WITH HYDRODISSECTION

Hydrodissection is employed to free the lens material from its attachments to the lens capsule. Adequate hydrodissection allows the lens to be rotated freely within the confines of the capsular sac with relative impunity. Most nuclear disassembly methods of phacoemulsification depend on hydrodissection to bring the lens nucleus into position for sculpting, fracturing, chopping, etc., although some surgeons recommend so-called nonrotational nuclear cracking in certain cases. Hydrodissection is generally performed within the lens cortex, freeing the nucleus for rotation while leaving the cortical layer behind with the lens capsule. An alternative method, described by Fine, and referred to as "cortical cleaving hydrodissection" uses the injected fluid to free the cortex from the capsule so that it adheres to the epinucleus and will exit during (epi)nuclear removal.[7] In this manner, it is not necessary to perform cortical "clean-up" as a distinct step in the surgery. Nevertheless, many surgeons find it difficult to fully cleave the cortex from the capsule and are satisfied when hydrodissection allows full rotation of the lens nucleus. Finally, incomplete hydrodissection, may lead to zonular rupture or loss during attempted spinning of the lens. Many surgeons rotate the nucleus with two hooks or similar instruments after hydrodissection to assure its completion.

Laceration of the anterior capsular rim can occur during hydrodissection if the capsule is unusually fragile, as in cases of pseudoexfoliation, if the cannula has sharp edges or burrs at its orifice, or if the surgeon is too aggressive in lifting the capsular flap in performing cortical cleaving hydrodissection. This iatrogenic complication is avoidable with the use of specially designed blunt cannulas, particularly those that are flattened to reduce their diameter in one dimension. Certainly, care must be taken to avoid excessive lift on the capsule.

While some surgeons advocate hydroexpression of the lens nucleus for manual extracapsular cataract extraction or even for some styles of phacoemulsification (phaco flip), most popular surgical techniques leave the lens nucleus in situ and use hydrodissection only to free it from its capsular attachments. Excessive and/or too rapid hydrodissection can force the lens nucleus out of the capsular bag and into the anterior chamber. Emulsification under those circumstances runs a greater risk of damage to the corneal endothelium and the iris. Additionally, if a large and firm nucleus is prolapsed through a relatively small anterior capsular opening, the capsulotomy may inadvertently develop a radial tear. Complications associated with hydrodissection are uncommon but include prolapse of the lens out of the capsular bag, radial tears of the anterior capsule, and "blowing out" the posterior capsule. Slow injection of fluid while allowing the cannula to gently depress the posterior lip of the incision will generally prevent complications of hydrodissection. After delivering fluid judiciously, the surgeon may observe the nucleus rise toward the corneal dome. At that juncture, the hydrodissection cannula can be used to push the nucleus posteriorly, forcing the trapped fluid to further dissect the cleavage plane. Generally, it is also useful to hydrodissect the subincisional region either with a U-shaped cannula or the use of the standard cannula placed through the paracentesis.

Posterior capsule "blow out" is a rare but serious iatrogenic complication of hydrodissection. It may occur when fluid is injected too aggressively into an eye with a fully mature nuclear cataract. In these cases, there is little to no cortex and no epinuclear shell. As a result, none of the injected fluid will be absorbed by the lens material and the capsular bag will bear the mechanical burden of the expanding fluid wave. Rapid injection of a high volume of fluid, particularly with highly retentive viscoelastic agents in the anterior chamber, allows the weakest point, the posterior capsule, to rupture once intralenticular hydrostatic pressure reaches a certain, but unknown threshold. Posterior capsular rupture may be evidenced by dislocation of the lens immediately or after attempted rotation and phacoemulsification of the lens nucleus. Another clinical sign, the "pupil snap" may be noted with rupture of the posterior capsule after hydrodissection.[8] In this situation the pupil is seen to constrict rapidly by as much as 30% of its original size.

Rupture of the posterior capsule may also occur during hydrodissection in cases of posterior polar cataract.[9] This anomaly, which may be associated with posterior lenticonus, has a congenital defect in the posterior capsule in approximately 25% of cases. During aggressive hydrodissection, the herniated or weakened portion of the posterior lens capsule may "blow out" easily. Presurgical evaluation of cases with posterior polar cataract should include examination for the "Dalgit-Singh sign," which may portend a capsular defect.[10] This clinical sign is marked by the presence of small satellite cataracts surrounding the central posterior polar lesion. Singh's theory suggests that an already present capsular defect allows the permeation of aqueous into the lens with the subsequent formation of duplicated cataracts. To prevent loss of nuclear material into the posterior segment in cases with posterior polar cataract, most surgeons agree that the use of hydrodelineation (see below) to separate the nucleus from the epinuclear and cortical shells will protect the posterior capsule. Following endonuclear removal, gentle viscodissection can cleave the cortex and epinucleus from the capsule while providing for viscoelastic plug over the potential capsular defect. Irrespective of the technique used, this case type represents a surgical challenge with a high likelihood for posterior capsular rupture.

Hydrodelineation separates the lens nucleus into epinuclear and endonuclear portions for purposes of dividing the lens circumferentially into softer peripheral and firmer central parts. There are no common complications associated with hydrodelineation.

COMPLICATIONS RELATED TO THE IRIS

Given good pupil dilation, damage to the iris during phacoemulsification is a rare event. However, poor wound construction can lead to iris prolapse (see above) with potential iris damage. Additionally, however, damage to the iris during phacoemulsification may occur from thermal or mechanical injury. "Phaco burns" of the iris (Fig. 11–6) may typically occur with shallow chambers or in cases of prolonged phacoemulsification of very hard nuclei. Generally, the damage is more of an aesthetic than a functional concern. This is particularly true if the emulsification has been performed through a superior entrance and the iris injury is covered by the upper eyelid. With temporally oriented surgery, however, phacothermal injury to the iris may take on functional as well as aesthetic significance if iatrogenic iris defects create multiple pupils or otherwise reduce the function of the pupil or iris. Anticipation of potential heat injury to the iris may allow a defensive strategy on the part of the surgeon. Maintaining a deep chamber, employing an incision that affords adequate fluid exchange, creating a chamber entrance slightly more central than usual, adding viscoelastic material frequently during emulsification, and using a modified Sheet's glide may all add to the protection of the iris.

Mechanical damage to the iris typically occurs in patients with small pupils. The iris may be aspirated into the port and very quickly emulsified. Generally, the iris tissue is not cut cleanly by the phaco needle but will take on a stringy appearance and unravel much like a spool of yarn. The fine wisps of iris tissue seem to have an almost magnetic attraction to the aspiration port. Often it is difficult to avoid further aspiration of the iris unless these "strings" are cut with scissors to prevent further unspooling of the iris stroma. The resultant iris damage tends to be more an aesthetic problem than a functional one; however, large defects in the pupillary sphincter may result in postoperative glare.[11] Care must be taken to avoid aspiration and emulsification of the iris during

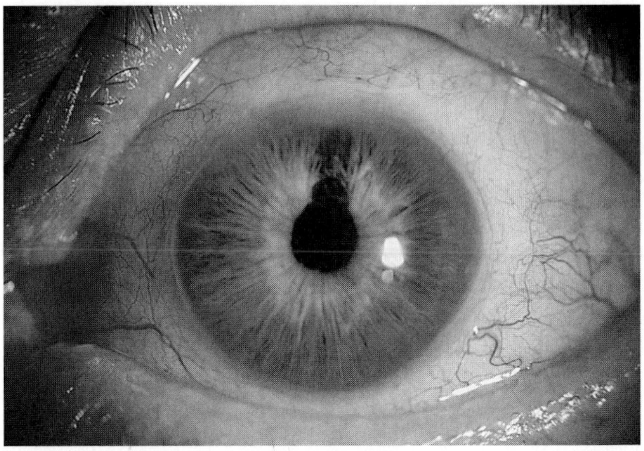

Figure 11–6. Clinical photograph of patient after phacoemulsification of ultrafirm nucleus, shallow anterior chamber, and small pupil resulting in superior iris thermal damage.

nuclear removal. There are a host of methods for managing the small pupil. Four-quadrant divide-and-conquer phacoemulsification can be performed within the central 3 mm of the chamber and the method avoids the need to reach into the more peripheral aspects of the capsular bag. A good motto is, "never phaco where you can't see." Lastly, with respect to the small pupil, surgical methods employing pupil stretching, pupil expanders, and highly retentive viscoagents can allow the surgeon to safely enlarge the pupil for emulsification while maintaining a functionally adequate sphincter to prevent postoperative disabling glare.

COMPLICATIONS RELATED TO THE ZONULAR APPARATUS

Weakened or absent zonules may exist prior to surgery or develop intraoperatively as an iatrogenic complication. There are a variety of causes for presurgical zonular weakness as may be noted in Table 11–2. Given an appropriate history, the surgeon can prepare a surgical plan. However, if the surgeon does not suspect a zonular dehiscence or if the condition occurs intraoperatively, surgery may change from routine to complex. Patients with a history of ocular trauma or those with pseudoexfoliation represent the greatest likelihood for intraoperative stripping of zonules. The patient's history and ocular examination should prepare the surgeon for possible zonular problems. Routine gonioscopy in cases of prior trauma might uncover unsuspected angle recession or subclinical luxation of the lens. Likewise, the characteristic peripupillary fluff of material (Fig. 11–7) characteristic of the pseudoexfoliation syndrome should alert the surgeon to potential weakness of the zonule and its attachment to the lens capsule. Moreover, early in the course of surgery, during the capsulorrhexis for example, it is often possible to sense zonular weakness during capsular manipulations. A tell-tale sign is the presence of radial striations of the anterior capsule during the initial puncture. Under circumstances of weak zonules, copious but slow hydrodissection must be performed to completely free the nucleus within the capsular bag. Otherwise, nuclear rotation might serve to further weaken zonular attachments. It is probably wise to reduce the height of the infusion bottle and slow the aspiration flow to avoid sudden deepening and shallowing of the chamber, which can add to zonular stress. Increased phacoemulsification power and use of a sharp-angle cutting tip, perhaps 45 degrees, can prevent additional zonular stress during emulsification. Care must be taken during "cortical clean-up" to avoid aspiration of the loosely attached capsule. It must be remembered that lens cortex irrigation-aspiration involves high levels of vacuum, up to 500 mm Hg. It is therefore wise to consider using a "dry technique" with single-bore cannulas after filling the capsular bag with a highly retentive viscoagent. Generally, it is best to avoid silicone lenses in cases with compromised zonules because the silicone, in contact with the subcapsular lens epithelial cells, may stimulate capsular fibrosis and phimosis of the anterior capsulotomy, resulting in centripetal traction on the zonules. Alternative choices would include foldable acrylic lenses, which generate less fibrotic reaction, or a rigid one-piece polymethylmethacrylate (PMMA) lens that further expands the capsular bag and retards postoperative contraction. The long axis of the lens should be placed in the meridian of the zonular disinsertion so that the lens can act as a stent against late capsular contraction and implant decentration.

TABLE 11-2. Causes of Presurgical Zonule Weakness

Loose/missing zonules
Pseudoexfoliation
Trauma
Marfan's syndrome
Homocystinuria
Familial
Postsurgical
Post-inflammatory
Idiopathic

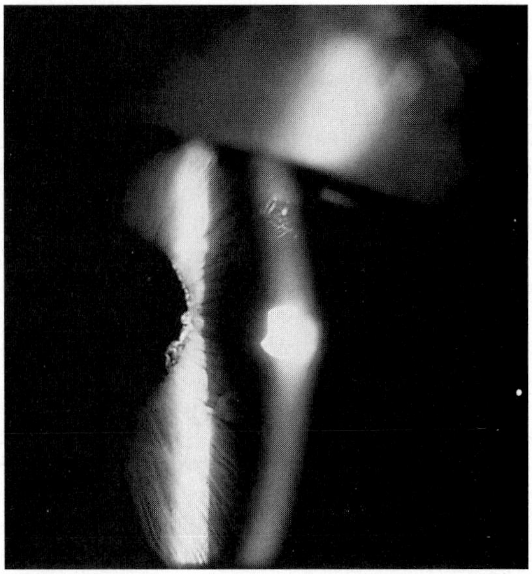

Figure 11–7. Clinical photograph of a patient with pseudoexfoliation syndrome. The pupil is small, and "fluffy" material near the pupil margin indicates the presence of pseudoexfoliation.

Recently, PMMA expansile rings for the capsular bag have gained popularity for the management of weak zonules.[12] These devices, manufactured and widely used in Europe, may be placed within the confines of the capsular bag after capsulorrhexis or at any stage of surgery after a successful capsulorrhexis. Capsular tension rings, in concept, equalize the stress on the zonules over 360 degrees. This device is not manufactured or distributed in the United States because it does not have the approval of the U.S. Food and Drug Administration, a fact that U.S. eye surgeons planning its use must consider. Potentially, endocapsular rings allow phacoemulsification and small-incision surgery to be performed when there are as many as 6 clock hours of zonular dehiscence. Without use of an endocapsular ring, it is probably wisest not to attempt that form of surgery in cases beyond 3 clock hours of zonular loss.

An important surgical concept in cases with zonular dehiscence is that if vitreous prolapses into the anterior chamber, at any time during surgery, then phacoemulsification must be halted in favor of management of the vitreous. Phacoemulsification in the presence of vitreous can have major consequences with respect to posterior segment structures. Continued aspiration of vitreous with the phaco handpiece can lead to giant retinal tears, retinal avulsion, and even phacoemulsification of retinal tissue.

COMPLICATIONS ASSOCIATED WITH NUCLEAR EMULSIFICATION

During nuclear emulsification, as discussed above, thermal and mechanical injuries may occur to the incisional tissue and to the iris; however, the primary concern during emulsification is damage to the capsular and zonular structures.

The cornea may be subjected to damage if the emulsification tip contacts the endothelium or if the nucleus or its remnants abrade the endothelial surface during surgery. For that reason, most surgeons attempt to avoid damage to the cornea with the use viscoelastic agents and by performing emulsification within the confines of the capsular bag. Capsular damage may take the form of a radial tear in the anterior capsule or a rent in the peripheral or posterior capsule. Radial extension of the anterior capsulotomy, if recognized early, may not interfere with the surgical plan, except to influence the choice of implant type (see below). However, if a radial tear of the anterior capsulorrhexis is not recognized, and if significant force is applied in the axis of the radial tear during surgery, the tear may extend around the equator to the posterior capsule; potential vitreous prolapse into the anterior segment and loss of nuclear material posteriorly are possible consequences. Damage to the anterior capsule during nuclear emulsification may occur in the subincisional region if emulsification proceeds too close to the incision. This maloccurrence may be prevented by performing phacomaneuvers distally from the midplane. Additionally, the anterior capsule may be damaged at its distal aspect of the chamber should the emulsification process be too superficial rather than within the lens substance. Novice surgeons often sweep the tip toward the underside of the cornea during distal nuclear sculpting, a habit that should be discouraged in order to protect the anterior capsule, iris, and cornea.

Management of radial tears in the anterior capsule during phacoemulsification should vary with the density of the nucleus and the axis of the tear. If the nucleus is firm and likely to require considerable manipulation for its removal, the lens should be debulked before attempting disassembly. Alternatively, it may be wise to bring the nucleus into the anterior chamber by careful viscodissection and lens rotation in order to perform anterior chamber emulsification, putting the least possible stress on the capsular bag. The preoperative status of the corneal endothelium must be considered. Additionally, a highly retentive dispersive viscoelastic agent can help guard against iris and corneal damage during anterior chamber or iris plane nuclear emulsification.

Damage to the posterior capsule may occur at virtually any phase of surgery, but, in the absence of presurgical capsular pathology, should be avoidable, occurring in approximately 3% of cases.[13] The management of posterior capsular tear during phacoemulsification is dependent in large part on the volume of nucleus remaining, the size of the posterior capsular rent, and the presence or absence of vitreous anterior to the capsular tear. Therefore, early recognition of the capsular defect is the most important aspect of management of posterior capsular rents. A few clinical signs that may, on occasion, be noted include sudden deepening of the chamber concomitant with pupil expansion, difficulty in nuclear rotation after previously easy rotation, tilting of the nucleus, and visibility of the equator of the nucleus.

Small capsular tears that are recognized with little residual nuclear material and no vitreous present in the chamber are best managed with a calm approach and an appropriate plan. The phacoemulsification tip should remain in the chamber and the infusion bottle greatly lowered. Sudden withdrawal of the tip may allow ocular hypotony, chamber shallowing, anterior migration of vitreous, and enlargement of the posterior capsular rent. Alternatively, the tip can be maintained in the chamber (with a lowered infusion bottle) while the surgeon simultaneously places a bolus of viscoelastic material into the chamber through the side port to maintain chamber depth and ocular pressure before removal of the phaco tip. Once the tip is removed, the surgeon can inspect the degree of damage and carry out an alternative plan. The essential factor is to tamponade and protect the anterior hyaloid. A highly retentive viscoagent or Sheet's glide may be placed over the small capsule rent and the remaining lens material removed either manually, with the I/A handpiece, or with the phaco tip, exercising great care. It may be necessary to use the viscoagent through the side port as a second instrument during continued emulsification. The nature of the retained nuclear material should dictate the best course of action.

On the other hand, should vitreous be present in the anterior chamber, phacoemulsification is contraindicated. In that situation, the vitreous should be removed in a bimanual fashion[14] prior to managing the remaining nuclear fragments. Although many surgeons prefer an anterior approach for vitrectomy, a pars plana entry for the vitrectomy port is useful because it allows removal of only that vitreous prolapsed into the anterior segment. Generally, the chamber is infused through the side port during vitreous removal. Although it may be possible, in theory, to continue nuclear emulsification after vitrectomy, a wiser approach is to place a modified Sheet's glide over the capsular rent and use mechanical means, such as a lens spoon, to withdraw the nuclear remnants through an enlarged incision. The surgeon must never express lens material in the presence of an open capsule or zonular dehiscence. Such maneuvers invite further loss of vitreous through the incision with concomitant loss of nuclear material into the posterior segment.

If the capsule is ruptured very early in the emulsification process, heralded by the presence of vitreous in the chamber or other clinical signs (see above) management must be aimed at preventing loss of the nucleus into the vitreous. Given a large dense nuclear remnant, it is best to enlarge the incision, radialize the anterior capsulotomy, and place a lens loop or spoon underneath the nucleus and remove it manually. Another maneuver to prevent posterior nuclear loss is to place a blunt spatula through a pars plana sclerotomy behind the lens and elevate the nucleus into the anterior chamber, as has been suggested by Kelman.[15] Alternatively, should the lens material be soft enough to allow its eventual removal through the pars plana, the cataract surgeon may opt to toilet the anterior segment of vitreous, place an implant in the sulcus above the anterior circular capsulotomy, and close the eye for later pars plana nuclear removal by a posterior segment surgeon.

The most significant concern of a capsular rent remains "the dropped nucleus." In this situation, all or a portion of the lens nucleus falls into the vitreous cavity. Management of this complication is somewhat controversial, in that some anterior segment surgeons prefer to attempt nuclear removal at the time of original surgery by "floating" the nucleus into the anterior chamber with fluid or by scooping it with a lens loop or spoon, eventually completing the complicated surgery in one operation. Others strongly urge that it is safer to leave the nucleus in the posterior segment, toilet the anterior segment of vitreous and lens remnants, and refer the patient for future vitreoretinal surgery. A lens implant may be placed at the time of the initial surgery unless the retained nuclear material is unusually large and firm, requiring removal through the anterior segment en masse, rather than by fragmentation through the pars plana. Given the technical advances in pars plana vitrectomy, and the wide availability of posterior segment specialists, it appears wiser to involve a vitreoretinal consultant in management of these rare but potentially vision-threatening cases.[16] In reality, the prognosis is generally favorable with appropriate handling and varies largely with the presence or absence of subsequent retinal detachment. The cataract surgeon, in the interests of continuity of care and patient rapport, might find it beneficial to attend the secondary surgery, particularly if lens implantation is needed. More likely than not, the vitreoretinal specialist would prefer that the cataract surgeon place the intraocular lens.

It serves well for the cataract surgeon to adopt a presurgical contingency plan in the event of a dropped nucleus. Because vitreoretinal referral is almost always wise, it is good policy to establish an ongoing relationship with a qualified posterior segment surgeon. Generally, there is no urgency for referral, but in some cases it may be convenient if the vitrectomy is performed as a continuation of the cataract surgery. Otherwise, it is safe to allow several days to pass before the patient is seen by the retinal specialist; secondary surgery, if necessary, should be scheduled after corneal clearing, control of intraocular pressure, and control of inflammation. It has been established that the timing for secondary surgery does not significantly affect the outcome.

Methods and devices for lens implantation after posterior capsule rupture vary with the condition of the remaining capsule and the other anterior segment structures. Ideally, a localized posterior capsular tear may be converted into a continuous circular posterior capsulorrhexis. Given the tensile strength of a continuous circular tear, the lens implant may be placed within the capsular bag in the same fashion as in an uncomplicated case (Fig. 11–8). If, however, the rent in the posterior capsule extends to the periphery or cannot be converted to a capsulorrhexis, it is unwise to place the lens in the capsule because posterior dislocation may occur. With an intact anterior capsulorrhexis, a lens implant may be positioned in the ciliary sulcus, irrespective of the condition of the posterior capsule. Some surgeons prefer to leave the implant loops anterior to the capsule and capture the optic behind the anterior capsulorrhexis. In this manner, the optic is held firmly in place and has little tendency to contact the posterior iris surface. Implant selection for the ciliary sulcus must take into account a change in effective lens power when the lens is placed closer to the posterior corneal surface. Additionally, sulcus-placed lenses, particularly those with polypropylene loops demonstrate a tendency for posterior iris chafing.[17] Should the anterior and posterior capsules be damaged to the extent that they cannot hold a posterior chamber lens, the surgeon must choose between an anterior chamber lens, an iris-supported lens, or a posterior chamber lens sewn to the iris or sclera.

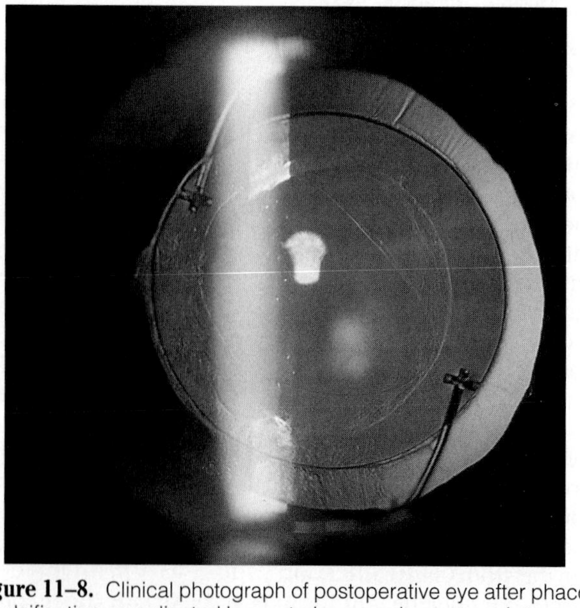

Figure 11–8. Clinical photograph of postoperative eye after phacoemulsification complicated by posterior capsular rupture. Intraoperative posterior capsulorrhexis allowed for "in the bag" implantation of a foldable intraocular lens. The posterior capsulorrhexis is noted to be smaller than the anterior capsulotomy.

COMPLICATIONS ASSOCIATED WITH CORTEX REMOVAL

Lens cortex removal is generally a simple and uncomplicated step of modern cataract surgery. However, the surgeon must recognize that the vacuum and flow rate levels typically used during cortical clean-up are considerably higher than those employed for nuclear removal. As a result, accidental aspiration of the capsule may induce a capsular tear or zonular dehiscence. Some surgeons experience capsule rupture more often during cortical removal than during nuclear emulsification. Capsular tears may be avoided if the surgeon is vigilant and avoids a "let-down" after nuclear emulsification. Alternative means to prevent capsule damage include the use of cortical cleaving hydrodissection which, when successful, precludes cortical removal as a separate surgical step. Another plan is to implant the lens prior to cortex aspiration. Generally, the greatest chance for difficulty occurs during attempted removal of the subincisional cortex. However, in addition to the above methods to facilitate cortical clean-up, the surgeon may use specialized bimanual cannulas through side ports to obviate the difficulty of working beneath the main incision.[18]

Finally, in cases with pseudoexfoliation or other causes for weakened zonules, inadvertent aspiration of the anterior capsular rim may cause disinsertion of the capsular sac. In cases with very weak zonules a capsular expansile ring may be placed prior to cortex removal. Alternatively, viscodissection of the cortex may be performed and the cortex removed through single-bore cannulas without the need for mechanized irrigation and aspiration. The latter technique is considered a "dry method" of cortex removal, which is also useful for removal of cortex in cases with posterior capsule tears.

COMPLICATIONS ASSOCIATED WITH LENS IMPLANTATION

Given that rigid one-piece PMMA intraocular lenses are used in conjunction with all forms of extracapsular cataract surgery, this section is limited to intraoperative complications associated with foldable lenses because they are the type employed with phacoemulsification. Intraoperative complications associated with foldable lenses may result from damage to the implant optic or haptics or from damage to anterior segment structures.

A unique facet of foldable lens implants is that they generally require special handling with folding and inserting devices, sometimes specific for a given implant. In fact, discussion of foldable lenses must include consideration of the tools needed to place them inside the eye. Two basic types of devices are available. The first consists of a pair of forceps, one to fold the implant and the second to grasp the folded lens and pass it through the incision. Generally, these instruments have been designed for specific lens materials, sizes, and styles. Lens implants may be fractured, if the folding or inserting devices are inappropriate for the lens used. For example, there have been reports of acrylic lenses fracturing with the use of Fine Type II universal forceps (Rhein Medical, Tampa, FL).[19] Given the fact that this device was designed for second-generation foldable silicone lenses, its performance with acrylic lenses could be suspect. Warming acrylic lenses to 37 degrees facilitates their folding and implantation.

Cartridge injector systems are also in common use for foldable lenses. Typically, they are associated with the use of one-piece plate haptic silicone lens implants, but they have been adapted to looped lenses as well. Plate haptic lenses owe a considerable amount of their popularity to the ease of implantation afforded by a injector system. The lenses may be loaded by a surgical assistant and handed to the surgeon ready for implantation. This is in distinction to the use of forceps for folding and implanting of lenses which often require the surgeon's personal manipulation. Although plate haptic lenses may be associated with late postoperative complications (decentration and posterior dislocation), the seductive simplicity of their implantation is sufficient to retain common use. Intraoperative complications associated with injected plate haptic lenses include partial or complete fracture of the plate supports, rupture of the anterior capsulotomy, and renting of the posterior capsule. Lacerations of the optic or plates may reduce optical performance or lead to implant decentration; removal of the lens at the time of surgery may be necessary, varying with the extent of the damage. It has been observed that incomplete fractures will not progress after surgery. With respect to tears in the anterior capsular rim induced during implantation or manipulation of the intraocular lens, plate haptic lenses will show a strong tendency to decenter, in many cases with discontinuity of the capsulorrhexis. It is best to remove the lens and consider an alternative style should this rare occurrence be observed. Additionally, the posterior or peripheral capsule may be damaged if the implant exits abruptly from the cartridge. Likewise, in this situation the intraocular lens must be removed and an alternative style placed. Any capsular defect *contraindicates* the use of a plate haptic lens implant.

COMPLICATIONS ASSOCIATED WITH "POSITIVE PRESSURE"

The devastating complication of expulsive suprachoroidal hemorrhage, known to occur in up to 1% of cases during large incision cataract extraction, is essentially a nonoccurrence with small-incision cataract surgery, given reduced ocular hypotony, reduced operating time, and a self-sealing incision that will allow intraocular pressure to tamponade an effusion-hemorrhage. However, phacoemulsification surgeons will, on rare occasions, encounter "positive posterior pressure," from external forces on the globe (tight drapes, lid speculum, traction sutures), suprachoroidal effusion, or posteriorly misdirected balanced salt solution. Whatever the cause, the surgeon should cease working and evaluate the situation. In the case of external pressure or misdirected infusion, the eye will be noted to soften after removal of the phaco handpiece from the eye. Continued elevation of intraocular pressure suggests an effusion. The self-sealed incision will allow the intraocular pressure to elevate and will generally tamponade and terminate the effusion. After some period of time the surgeon may wish to continue or postpone the completion of surgery, depending on the condition of the eye.[20] During the waiting period, examination of the posterior segment (if possible) should be performed to distinguish between suprachoroidal effusion and misdirection of the infusate. In the former situation, indirect ophthalmoscopy will reveal a subretinal elevation. In case of the latter, it may be possible to continue surgery after a short interval or by removing fluid from the posterior segment by way of a pars plana tap, if that technique is within the expertise of the surgeon. In either case, it may be prudent to postpone surgery even for a short period of time while observing the patient's intraocular pressure and retinal vasculature.

REFERENCES

1. Greenbaum S: Anesthesia for cataract surgery: parabulbar and (sub-Tenon's) anesthesia. In Greenbaum S (ed.), Ocular Anesthesia. Philadelphia, WB Saunders; 1997:30–6.
2. Osher R: Slow motion phacoemulsification approach. J Cataract Refract Surg 1993;19:667.
3. Masket S, Tennen DG: ND:Yag laser optical membrane opening for retained Descemet's membrane after penetrating keratoplasty. J Cataract Refract Surg 1996;22:139–41.
4. Kremer I, Stiebel H, Yassur Y, Weinberger D: Sulfur hexafluoride injection for Descemet's membrane detachment in cataract surgery. J Cataract Refract Surg 1997;23:1449–53.
5. Masket S: Postoperative complications of capsulorrhexis. J Cataract Refract Surg 1993;9:721–4.
6. Horiguchi M, Miyake K, Ohta I, Ito Y: Staining of the lens capsule for circular continuous capsulorrhexis in eyes with white cataract. Arch Ophthalmol 1998;116:535–7.
7. Fine IH: Cortical cleaving hydrodissection. J Cataract Refract Surg 1992;18:508–12.
8. Yeoh R: The "pupil snap" sign of posterior capsule rupture with hydrodissection in phacoemulsification. Case report. Br J Ophthalmol 1996;80:486.
9. Osher R, Yu B, Koch DD: Posterior polar cataracts: a predisposition to intraoperative capsular rupture. J Cataract Refract Surg 1990;16:157–62.
10. Singh D: Posterior capsular abnormalities co-existing with cataract: the quiz show. In Singh D, Worst J, Singh R, Sing IR (eds.), Cataract and IOL. New Delhi: Jaypee Brothers, 1993:160–7.
11. Masket S: Relationship between postoperative pupil size and disability glare. J Cataract Refract Surg 1992;18:506–7.
12. Cionni RJ, Osher RH: Endocapsular ring approach to the subluxed cataractous lens. J Cataract Refract Surg 1995;21:245–9.
13. Powe NR, Schein OD, Gieser SC, et al.: Synthesis of the literature on visual acuity and complications following cataract extraction with intraocular lens implantation. Arch Ophthalmol 1994;112:239–52.
14. Koch PS: Managing the torn posterior capsule and vitreous loss. Int Ophthalmol Clin 1994;34:113–30.
15. Kelman C: Posterior capsule rupture: PAL technique. Video J Cataract Refract Surg 1996;12.
16. Smiddy WE, Flynn Jr HW: Managing retained lens fragments and dislocated posterior chamber IOLs after cataract surgery. In Focal Points, Clinical Module for Ophthalmologists. San Francisco, American Academy of Ophthalmology 1996;XIV:7.
17. Masket S: Pseudophakic posterior iris chafing syndrome. J Cataract Refract Surg 1986;12:252–6.
18. Brauweiler HP, Kessler AS, Duhr R: "No stitch" surgery for conventional intraocular lenses. Ophthalmochirurgie 1991;3:75–82.
19. Carlson KH, Johnson DW: Cracking of acrylic intraocular lens during capsular bag insertion. Ophthalmic Surg Lasers 1995;26:572–3.
20. Davison JA: Acute intraoperative suprachoroidal hemorrhage in capsular bag phacoemulsification. J Cataract Refract Surg 1993;19:534–7.

CHAPTER 12

Surgery for Pediatric Cataracts

M. EDWARD WILSON, M.D.

The surgical treatment of pediatric cataracts has undergone dramatic changes in the last two decades. New technology and advanced microsurgical techniques have reduced the morbidity of childhood cataracts. However, cataract surgery in children remains complex and challenging. In addition, the visual system in these small patients is often immature and the eyes are actively growing and developing. Achieving a consistently good visual outcome from the treatment of childhood cataracts remains difficult for even the most talented and diligent ophthalmologist. A major reason for inconsistent visual outcomes is that, unlike the treatment of adult cataracts, the timing of cataract surgery in children is of paramount importance. Timing of surgical intervention affects the visual result to a much greater extent than the surgical technique or method of postoperative optical correction employed by the surgeon. In a young child, a cataract does not merely blur the image received by the retina, it also disrupts the development of the visual pathways in the central nervous system.[1] In addition to causing amblyopia, visual deprivation can disrupt the delicate feedback loop relationship that the growing eye has with the visual environment. This mechanism, known as *emmetropization,* is controlled in part by genetics and in part by a powerful environmental component. Visual images that guide the axial length of the eye to its focal plane can be disrupted by cataract formation. Abnormal axial growth has been documented even in the absence of amblyopia as a result of the effects of unequal visual inputs to the two eyes.[2,3] Complexities of timing aside, when surgical removal of a pediatric cataract is planned, unique features of a child's eye must be considered. These include changing axial length, corneal curvature, and lenticular refracting power[4] (Figs. 12–1 to 12–3); increased tissue reactivity; lower scleral rigidity; smaller size (microphthalmia in many); and a long life span after cataract removal. In addition, the pre- and postoperative examinations are often much more challenging than in adults. Surgery usually requires general anesthesia, and postoperative trauma to the eye will be difficult to control.

Despite these differences and difficulties, advances in surgical technique and in methods used for postoperative optical rehabilitation have drastically improved the prognosis for children with visually significant cataracts, especially if they are detected and treated promptly. However, the surgeon and the patient's family must be aware that associated ocular or systemic anomalies can often also affect the visual outcome. Procedurally, cataract surgery in children is evolving and often requires the use of a combination of techniques

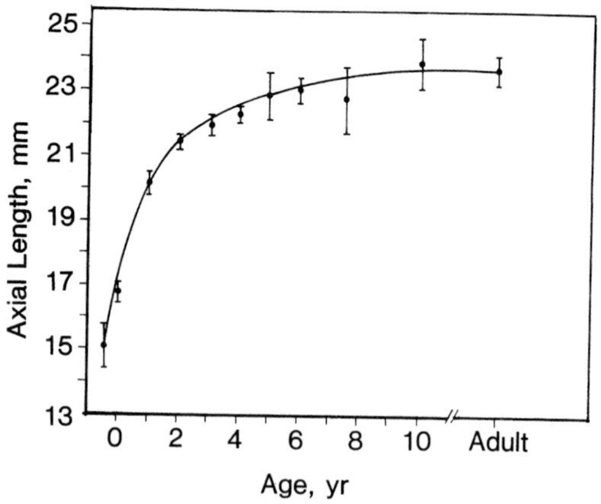

Figure 12–1. Axial length plotted with respect to age. Dots represent mean values for age group indicated; bars, standard deviations. (From Gordon RA, Donzis PB: Refractive development of the human eye. Arch Ophthalmol 1985;103:785–9.)

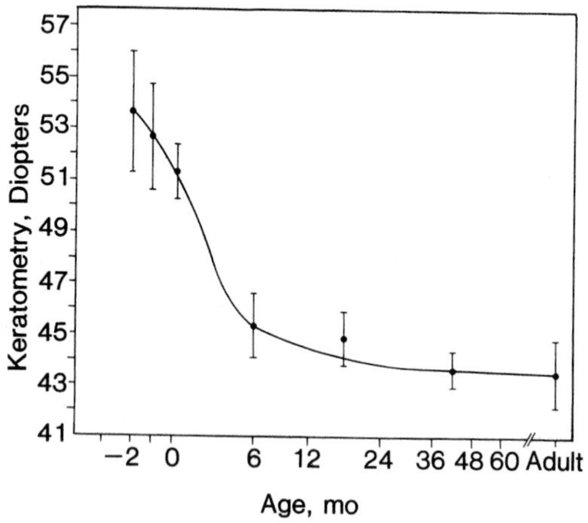

Figure 12–2. Keratometry values plotted with respect to age on logarithmic scale. Negative number represents months of prematurity; dots, mean value for age group indicated; bars, standard deviations. (From Gordon RA, Donzis PB: Refractive development of the human eye. Arch Ophthalmol 1985;103:785–9.)

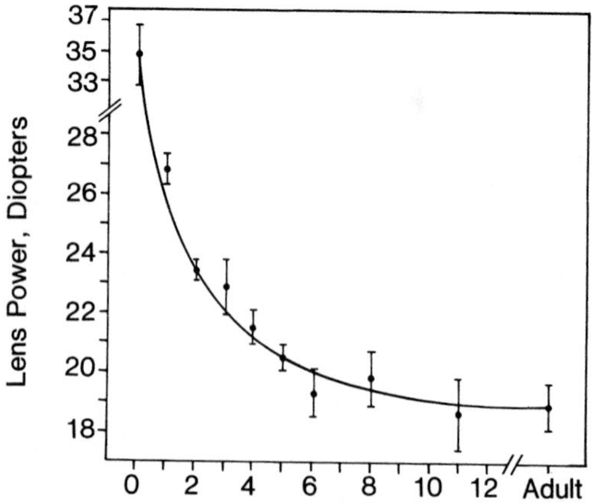

Figure 12–3. Mean values (dots) and standard deviations (bars) for lens power as determined by modified SRK (Sanders-Retzlaff-Kraff) formula, plotted with respect to age. (From Gordon RA, Donzis PB: Refractive development of the human eye. Arch Ophthalmol 1985; 103:785–9.)

designed for children and techniques designed for adults which have been modified for the unique features of the growing eye.[5] Although this chapter will concentrate on the surgical procedure for the removal of childhood cataracts, the surgeon must always remember the importance of amblyopia management to assure the best possible visual outcome for the child.

CHARACTERIZING CHILDHOOD CATARACTS BY TYPE

Not all pediatric cataracts are alike. Consistency of classification is needed in order to compare clinical reports in the literature and properly communicate with other pediatric surgeons.[6] It is the contention of many pediatric ophthalmologists that cataract type underlies critical determinates of outcome, such as age of onset, severity of preoperative visual impairment, amblyogenic potential, and risk of complications[7] (Table 12–1).

Fetal nuclear cataracts are congenital, usually presenting as a dense, white central opacity of 3 to 3.5 mm (Fig. 12–4). Birch and Stager[8] have shown that there is a 6-week period, beginning at birth, during which treatment of dense, congenital, unilateral cataracts is maximally effective. Bilateral congenital fetal nuclear cataracts often result in permanent nystagmus if they are not removed prior to the age of fixation development (approximately 3 months of age). In addition, fetal nuclear cataracts are often associated with microphthalmia, a condition thought to predispose these children to childhood glaucoma.[7,9]

In contradistinction, lamellar cataracts are usually acquired after the fixation reflex has developed and usually occur in normal sized eyes. They present as larger (5-5.5 mm) opacities representing a variably opaque layer of cortex surrounding a usually clear fetal nucleus. When bilateral, they are most often familial and follow an autosomal dominant inheritance pattern. When not familial, a metabolic work-up is indicated to rule out galactosemia, galactokinase deficiency, or more rarely, hypocalcemia or hypoglycemia[10] (Table 12–2). Other important pediatric cataract types (see Table 12–1) include posterior lentiglobus (Fig. 12–5), the most common unilateral childhood cataract presenting in a normal-sized eye, and PHPV (persistent hyperplastic primary vitreous) (Fig. 12–6), which usually presents unilaterally in a microphthalmic eye.

INDICATIONS FOR SURGERY

In a neonate, infant, or toddler, a dense axial opacity 3 mm or larger will most certainly lead to deprivation amblyopia if left untreated. Such opacities usually blacken the central retinoscopic reflex and appear white when viewed at the slit lamp. If medically feasible, surgical removal within 2 to 4 weeks of detection is indicated. Preoperative strabismus in such patients has been associated (in my practice) with a poor prognosis for recovery of normal or near-normal visual acuity.

TABLE 12-1. Classification of Childhood Cataracts

Cataract Type	Usual Laterality	Microphthalmos or Microcornea	Hereditary	Visual Prognosis
Total/diffuse	Bilateral	Occasional	Frequently	Variable
Anterior Polar	Uni- or bilateral	Occasional	Rarely	Good
Lamellar	Bilateral	Rare	Frequently	Good
Nuclear	Bilateral	Occasional	Frequently	Moderate
Posterior Lentiglobus	Unilateral	Rare	Rarely	Good
Persistent Hyperplastic Primary Vitreous	Unilateral	Frequent	Rarely	Poor
Traumatic	Unilateral	N.A.	N.A.	Variable

Reprinted with permission from Ruttum MS: Childhood Cataracts. American Academy of Ophthalmology, Focal Points, Clinical Modules for Ophthalmologists, March 1996; Volume 14/1.

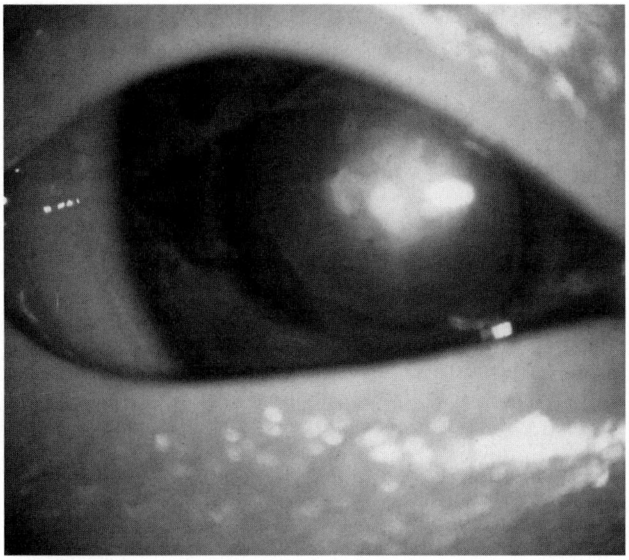

Figure 12–4. Congenital fetal nuclear cataract in a neonate.

TABLE 12-2. Routine Screening in Children with Bilateral Cataracts

Test	Disorder
Chromosome analysis	Down syndrome and other disorders
Examination of parents, siblings	Hereditary cataracts
Serum calcium	Hypoparathyroidism
TORCHS titers	Toxoplasmosis, rubella, cytomegalovirus, herpes
Urine amino acids	Lowe syndrome
Urine reducing substances	Galactosemia

Reprinted with permission from Ruttum MS: Childhood Cataracts. American Academy of Ophthalmology, Focal Points, Clinical Modules for Ophthalmologists, March 1996; Volume 14/1.

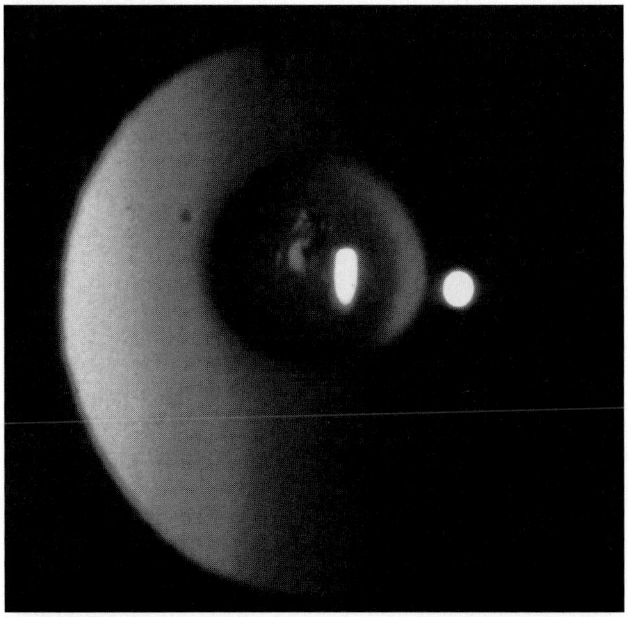

Figure 12–5. Early posterior lentiglobus. A progressive bulging of the posterior capsule precedes a progressive opacification of the posterior cortex of the lens.

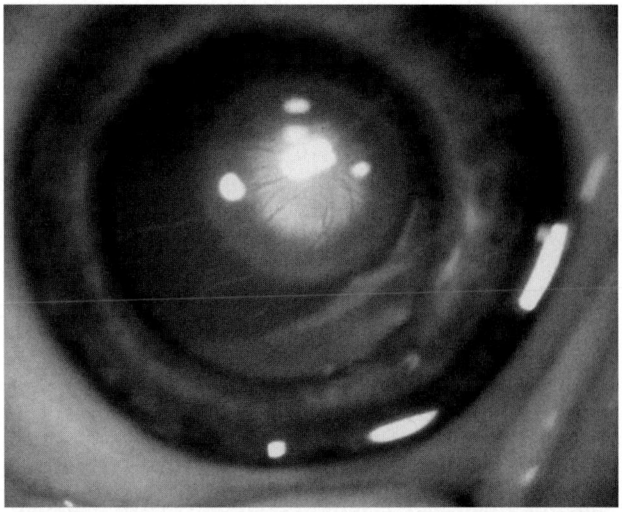

Figure 12–6. Persistent hyperplastic primary vitreous (PHPV) is seen here with associated lenticular changes and vascularity. The eye was also markedly microphthalmic.

When children beyond infancy present with dense, central opacities of uncertain duration and Snellen visual acuity can not be accurately measured, surgery is indicated within a few weeks of detection. Partial cataracts are sometimes managed initially with nonsurgical methods. A trial of patching may be indicated if the level of visual loss seems disproportionate to the density and size of the cataract. Pharmacologic pupillary dilatation can occasionally be helpful as an adjunctive or temporizing treatment.

The threshold for surgical removal of a partial cataract in a child capable of Snellen visual acuity has often been stated to be 20/70 or 20/80. However, individual judgments need to be made (especially in children too young for Snellen visual acuity testing) based on documented progression of the partial cataract and on the child's visual functioning, visual needs, and expected best visual outcome. In addition, emmetropization can be disrupted by cataracts of even moderate density resulting in abnormal axial elongation. Therefore, prolonged observation of a visually significant childhood cataract can lead to amblyopia, secondary strabismus, and axial growth abnormalities induced by visual deprivation. On the other hand, because surgical removal of a childhood cataract eliminates accommodation and may create large amounts of anisometropia, the overly aggressive surgeon also risks amblyopia, secondary strabismus, and axial growth abnormalities. This dilemma underscores the importance of the timing of surgical intervention for childhood cataracts. In my opinion, however, childhood cataracts are seldom removed too early but are frequently removed too late.

CORRECTING POSTOPERATIVE APHAKIA

APHAKIC SPECTACLES

Eyeglasses have been used for many years to correct *bilateral* aphakia in infants and young children. Many patients have achieved excellent visual acuity and satisfactory visual functioning over many years with this form of aphakic correction. Glasses are generally not an acceptable long-term treatment for *unilateral* aphakia but may be used temporarily in conjunction with patching therapy in aphakic children not tolerating a contact lens. Even for the bilaterally aphakic patient, optical distortion and a ring scotoma make aphakic spectacles less than ideal for optimal performance of activities of daily living. In addition, the glasses are costly, difficult to fit, and cosmetically unsatisfactory for many families (Fig. 12–7). Nonetheless, spectacles clearly provide the highest degree of safety.

CONTACT LENSES

Contact lenses are an important and useful modality for correcting pediatric aphakia. They remain the mainstay of aphakic correction in infancy.[1,10] However, contact lenses require the most parental involvement. An emotional, physical, and financial commitment is required for the insertion, removal, and care of the lenses. A major advantage is that their power can be easily adjusted as the child's growing eyes elongate. Because most axial change occurs in the first 2 or 3 years of life, this adjustability is of a greater advantage early in life. In addition, contact lenses provide the monocular aphakic patient an optical correction with minimal image size disparity between the two eyes.

Silicone (Silsoft) contact lenses are the easiest to fit. Most children under age 1 year can be fit with a lens of 7.50 base curve. Older children are most often fit with a base curve of 7.70. A fluorescein pattern may be used during the fitting sequence as needed. Lens movement with blinking is the most critical and important factor to evaluate during fitting. If too much movement is seen, a steeper lens can be tried. If little or no movement is seen, a flatter lens is indicated. Lenses with too steep a fit have been reported to cause the "suck on syndrome." This complication may have been due to problems with the early silicone lens manufacturing process[11] and has been virtually eliminated with the use of Silsoft lenses. Suitability for extended wear is another advantage of silicone lenses. Although continuous wear of a month or more between removal and cleaning is safe, parents are usually instructed to remove the lens once per week.

Silicone lenses also have major disadvantages. Silicone is hydrophobic, and the poor wettability of the first-generation silicone lenses produced an irregular surface where mucus collected and built up. Modern Silsoft lenses have an improved hydrophillic surface coating. However, this surface may still break down with time, the length varying from lens to lens and from patient to patient. When breakdown occurs, mucus builds up, clarity is reduced, and a new lens is required. Silicone lenses are also expensive and are man-

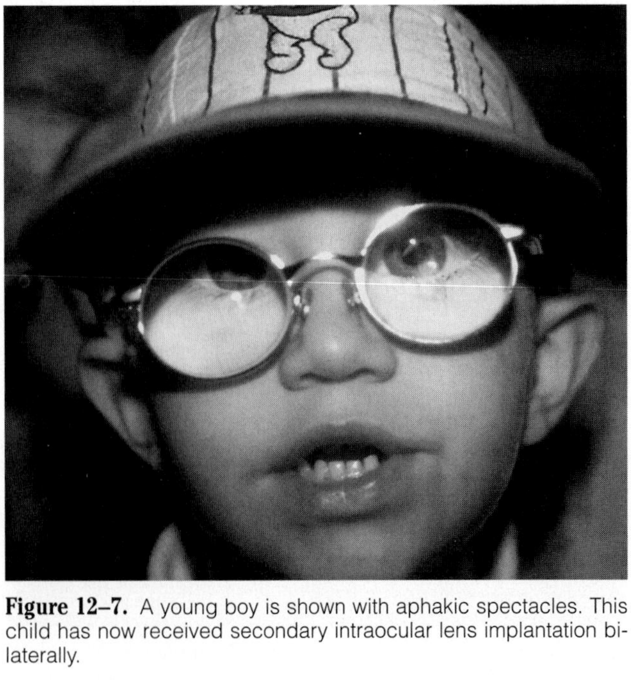

Figure 12–7. A young boy is shown with aphakic spectacles. This child has now received secondary intraocular lens implantation bilaterally.

ufactured in a limited number of powers. The Silsoft silicone lens is 11.3 mm in diameter and is available in lens powers from +20 to +32 in three diopter steps and from +12 to +20 in 1 diopter steps.

Rigid gas-permeable contact lenses have the advantage of low cost and can be customized with regard to power and base curve. The disadvantage of rigid gas-permeable contact lenses is that they must be removed daily and are more difficult for the parents to insert. Both silicone and rigid gas-permeable contact lens have impressive track records of safety. However, the risk of ulcerative keratitis is greater whenever any contact lens is worn overnight.[1]

The major disadvantages of contact lenses for the correction of aphakia are poor compliance and lens loss. Baker[11] reported an average silicone lens loss of only 0.75 lenses per year with a range of 0 to 4. However, Neumann et al.[12] reported a daily wear lens loss rate of 4.2 lenses per year during the first year of lens use and then 2 lenses per year during the second year of lens use. While it is generally agreed that lens loss is less frequent with the silicone contact lenses,[11] the surface coating breaks down quickly with some patients and may add to the frequency of lens replacement. In addition to lens loss, noncompliance is a particular problem for children with monocular aphakia. Assif and co-workers[13] reported that only 44% of children with unilateral aphakia were wearing their contact lens when they returned for follow-up appointments. Loss of the lens, conjunctival erythema, and a poor fit were among the reasons cited for this noncompliance. With noncompliance comes increased amblyopia and sensory strabismus.

EPIKERATOPLASTY

Epikeratoplasty was introduced in the early 1980s as an alternative means of optically correcting aphakic eyes. Epikeratophakia is a simplification of two keratorefractive techniques, keratophakia and keratomileusis, which were originally described by Barraquer.[14,15] In this procedure, donor cornea is frozen and carved to form the epikeratophakic tissue lens. This tissue lens is then sutured directly onto the anterior stromal surface of the host cornea. The central epithelium of the host cornea is removed and a peripheral pocket is dissected to receive the tissue lens. Because Bowman's layer of the host cornea is left intact in this procedure, the tissue can be removed and replaced if the need arrives. The disadvantage of epikeratoplasty is that the tissue lens remains hazy for an extended time after surgery, placing these eyes at increased risk for amblyopia. This procedure has fallen into disuse for correcting pediatric aphakia because of the difficulty in achieving the target refracting power and the prolonged haziness of the host–donor interface.

INTRAOCULAR LENS IMPLANTATION

Early attempts at intraocular lens (IOL) implantation in children resulted in frequent complications secondary to poor lens design and poor quality control.[16] As a result, surgeons have been slow to implant IOLs in these growing eyes. As late as 1991, IOL implantation in childhood was not well accepted, especially by the pediatric ophthalmic community.[17] In 1994, however, 46% of 234 pediatric ophthalmologists responding to a survey indicated that they were implanting IOLs in children.[18] In addition, 27% of 1,039 adult cataract specialists were implanting IOLs in pediatric patients.[18] The numbers are undoubtedly greater today. Many surgeons who remained skeptical in the recent past, have now become advocates of selective IOL use in children. A growing number of case series have now been published supporting the safety and effectiveness of intraocular lenses for children beyond infancy.[19–26]

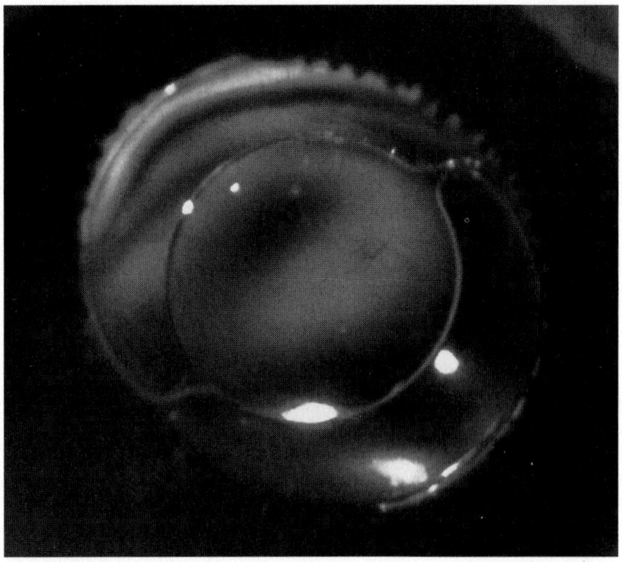

Figure 12–8. A modern flexible all polymethyl methacrylate (PMMA) capsular C design intraocular lens 12 mm overall length is shown after being inserted into the capsular bag of a fresh pediatric autopsy eye.

Among the many reasons for the increased use of IOLs in children, three have been recently cited.[27] First, appropriately sized (11.5–12.0 mm), more flexible polymethyl methacrylate (PMMA) implants are now available and can be inserted much more easily into the capsular bag of the child[28] (Fig. 12–8). Despite their increased flexibility, newer lens designs retain enough "memory" to resist the intense equatorial capsular fibrosis seen in children after implantation.[29] In addition, PMMA as an implant material now has a track record of biocompatibility that extends to 30 or more years. Heparin surface-modified (HSM) PMMA lenses are now available in the United States. These lenses have been shown to be more biocompatible than unmodified lenses in a randomized trial of pediatric cataract patients.[30] The HSM PMMA IOLs are my lenses of choice for sulcus fixation or complicated cases with more anticipated postoperative inflammation.

Recently, the Acrysof IOL (ALCON, Fort Worth, Texas), a PMMA-like foldable acrylic lens, has become my lens of choice for routine cases when "in-the-bag" fixation is employed. The biocompatibility of the acrylic lenses may equal or exceed the tried-and-true

PMMA lenses. The acrylic lenses are easier to insert in a small eye and can be implanted through a much smaller corneal or scleral wound.

The second reason for the increased use of IOLs in children is the perceived safety of capsular fixation of an IOL even over the extended life span of a child. Capsular fixation provides sequestration of the implant away from vascularized tissues. While ciliary sulcus fixation of the IOL may also be safe, uveal contact for a lifetime is not ideal. The preference for capsular fixation over ciliary sulcus placement has resulted in more IOLs being implanted in children at the time of cataract extraction, even at very young ages. Finally, better management of the anterior and posterior capsules at the time of implantation has improved outcomes and decreased complications when an IOL is placed in the eye of a child. These advances will be discussed later in this chapter.

Within certain arguable parameters, IOL implantation is now within the standard of care for children of all ages. In fact, primary IOL implantation is rapidly becoming the most common means of optical correction for children after cataract surgery.[27] However, there remains concern about the unknown risks of an IOL over the long lifespan of a child. The younger the child, the more this concern arises. In addition, predicting the refractive change over time in children is difficult because individual variation is common. While IOL implantation is becoming commonplace, especially in children older than age 2 years, a very conservative surgeon should not be unduly criticized for choosing not to implant an IOL.

In contrast to older children, IOL implantation in infancy continues to be hotly debated. Increased tissue reactivity and marked axial length and refractive changes have been cited as contraindications to IOL use in the first 2 years of life.[31] However, Dahan and Salmenson[32] reported 13 patients who had posterior chamber IOLs implanted at age 18 months or younger. With follow-up ranging from 1.2 years to 4.5 years, the IOLs were well tolerated with no additional surgical intervention needed. Primary posterior capsulectomy and anterior vitrectomy were performed in these patients at the time of IOL placement. Oliver and co-workers[33] included patients as young as 10 months of age in their posterior chamber lens implantation series. Other than a greater propensity for posterior capsule opacification, the IOLs were as well tolerated in the infants and toddlers as they were in the older children. Metge and co-workers[34] reported placing posterior chamber IOLs bilaterally in six patients aged 4 to 6 months. With a mean follow-up of 2.5 years, no complications related to the surgery were seen. More recently, Knight-Nanan and co-authors[35] reported that six eyes with congenital cataracts implanted with IOLs between 4 weeks and 28 weeks of age had central, steady and maintained fixation postoperatively with a mean follow-up of 66.4 weeks. My initial experience with IOL implantation in the first 2 years of life was published in 1998.[36] Twenty-two eyes of 17 patients were reported, with implant ages from 12 days to 22 months. Follow-up ranges from 2 to 36 months (average 14 months). No difference in complications or reoperation rates were noted when the pseudophakic patients were compared to an age-matched aphakic group operated at our institution over a similar time frame. Also, no significant difference in axial growth rate was noted when pseudophakic eyes were compared with the fellow phakic eye in patients having unilateral IOL implantation (Fig. 12–9).

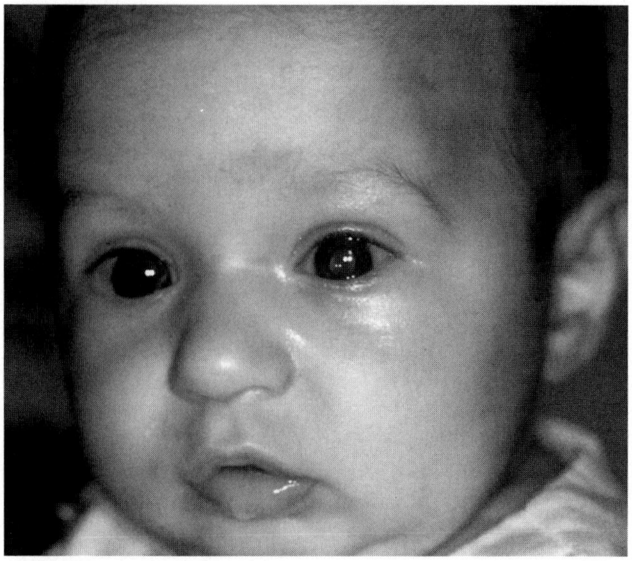

Figure 12–9. A young infant is shown 1 day after cataract extraction and intraocular lens implantation in the left eye.

Although these reports indicate that IOL implantation is technically feasible even in early infancy, problems remain. Because the axial growth of the eye is dramatic in early infancy, IOL power selection is difficult. Keratometry, usually very stable after 12 months of age, is still undergoing rapid change in early infancy.[4] When implanting an IOL in the first few months of life, 10 or more diopters of residual hyperopia may be necessary to avoid high myopia later. To reach emmetropia early in life and avoid hyperopia, I have begun placing an IOL of moderate power (26 D on average) into the capsular bag and a second IOL of lower power (10 D on average) into the ciliary sulcus. The sulcus lens is to be removed after sufficient eye growth has occurred. I have applied this "piggyback" strategy to 13 of the 40 early infant eyes I have implanted. A preliminary report describes these patients with 5 to 48 months of follow-up (20 months on average).[37] Nine of the sulcus IOLs have undergone planned removal. It is still not clear what effect this polypseudophakia will have on visual outcome. A multi-center randomized clinical trial is being planned in hopes of answering the question of whether primary IOL implantation or the use of contact lenses with secondary IOL implantation at an older age produces better outcomes in unilateral congenital cataracts.

Knight-Nanan et al.[35] recommend the use of an IOL that is lower by 6.00 D than one needed for emmetropia to compensate for the expected myopic shift when implanting infants younger than 1 year of age. The residual refractive errors are managed with spectacles. This parallels our own experience. However, when an IOL is implanted in the first months of life, we are often faced with residual hyperopia as high as 10 D. A contact lens may be needed for a few months until the residual hyperopia decreases to the 4 D to 6 D range. Spectacles can then be more easily used. Because contact lens wear is easy in early infancy and much more difficult as the toddler age is approached, this treatment scheme has been successful.

For children beyond age 2, data are available to help the surgeon predict the growth of the eye on average.[4,26,38] When operating on children between the ages of 2 and 8 years, many surgeons have advised selecting an IOL power that will leave mild to moderate hyperopia, milder with increasing age.[21,25,39–41] Enyedi and associates[42] have suggested aiming for a postoperative refraction of +6.00 at age 1 year, +5.00 at age 2, +4.00 at age 3, +3.00 at age 4, +2.00 at age 5, +1.00 at age 6, and plano at age 7. Others have advocated aiming for emmetropia regardless of age when operating beyond age 2.[19,20,22,43] This approach avoids potentially amblyogenic residual hyperopia, but it is likely to lead to the development of significant myopia later.

Modern theoretical IOL formulas are usually used in adults to calculate the IOL power most likely to achieve the desired postoperative refraction. In a recent study we applied the SRK II, SRK-T, Holladay, and Hoffer Q formulas to measurements from 47 consecutive IOL implantations in children.[44] The eyes were divided into short (less than 22 mm axial length), medium (axial length ≥ 22 mm but less than 24 mm) and long (≥ 24 mm) groups. While the average error (1.2 D to 1.4 D for all formulas) was larger than usually expected in adults, no formula outperformed any other. The errors were as often below the target refraction as above it. All axial length and keratometry measurements were made under anesthesia to avoid error from poor patient cooperation.

SURGICAL TECHNIQUES

HISTORICAL OVERVIEW

Manual aspiration of congenital and juvenile cataracts was popularized by Scheie[45] in 1960, and it remained the procedure of choice until the mid 1980s. In 1983, Parks[46] advocated the use of a vitreous suction cutter to perform a posterior capsulectomy and anterior vitrectomy when removing a congenital or juvenile cataract. This procedure revolutionized cataract surgery in infants. Where recurrent membrane formation had been very common, second surgeries became rare. Removal of all but 2 mm of the peripheral posterior lens capsule with a vitreous suction cutter was recommended, as well as a generous anterior vitrectomy. Although this procedure reduced the risk of amblyopia by virtually eliminating secondary membranes, it was incompatible with primary capsular fixation of an IOL or secondary sulcus fixation of an IOL. In anticipation of secondary sulcus fixated posterior chamber intraocular lens at an older age, most pediatric ophthalmic surgeons today modify the Parks procedure to leave enough residual capsule to support the IOL when it is later placed in the ciliary sulcus.

The initial reluctance of the pediatric ophthalmic community to endorse primary implantation of posterior chamber IOLs in children was related in part to the perceived need for an intact posterior capsule. Surgeons experienced in removing neonatal and infantile cataracts feared returning to the days of dense secondary membranes and frequent repeat surgeries. Technical advances have now resulted in several options for opening the posterior capsule without eliminating the possibility of IOL placement within the capsular bag. In addition, even when the posterior capsule is left intact, the combination of more complete cortical removal and the presence of an intraocular lens in the capsular bag has resulted in a lower incidence of, or at least a delay in posterior capsule opacification as compared to data utilizing Scheie's procedure. Controversy still exists concerning when the modified Parks style surgery (with or without an IOL placement) should yield to a more adult-like procedure leaving the posterior capsule intact. This is discussed in further detail later in this chapter when surgical options for the posterior capsule are presented.

ANESTHESIA

Most pediatric cataract surgery is done under general endotracheal anesthesia. As such, the possibility exists for Valsalva or even vomiting in the early postoperative period. This, along with inevitable rubbing of eyes, helps to justify the use of sutures to close the surgical wound even if it appears to be self-sealing (see below under Wound Considerations). Children also have a very active Bell's phenomenon if they become somewhat light under anesthesia. For this reason, many pediatric surgeons still use a superior rectus traction suture during cataract surgery.

WOUND CONSIDERATIONS

Children have thin sclera and markedly decreased scleral rigidity when compared with adults. Scleral collapse results in increased vitreous upthrust. Collapse of the anterior chamber and prolapse of iris tissue are also much more common when operating on pediatric eyes. Therefore, wounds should be constructed to provide a snug fit for the instruments that pass into the anterior chamber. When an IOL is not being implanted, two stab incisions are usually made at or near the limbus. These incisions should not be larger than necessary for the instruments being used. For instance, a micro-vitreoretinal (MVR) blade creates a 20-gauge opening that is ideal for a 20-gauge vitrector/aspirator to enter the anterior chamber. A 20-gauge blunt-tipped irrigating cannula (I use a Nichamin cannula) can also be used through a separate MVR blade stab incision. If the instrument positions need to be reversed, the snug fit is

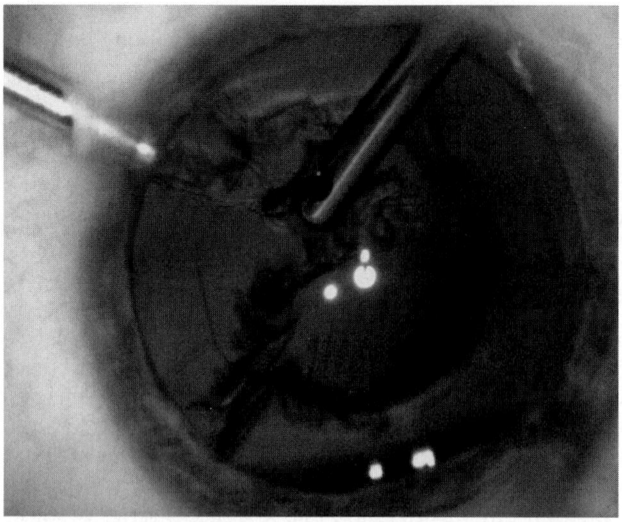

Figure 12–10. A 20-gauge blunt-tipped irrigating cannula and a side port vitrector are placed into the anterior chamber through incisions made with an MVR blade to achieve a snug fit. The instrument positions can be reversed if necessary to facilitate cortex removal. A vitrector cut anterior capsulotomy can be seen.

maintained (Fig. 12–10). An anterior chamber entry of 2.6 mm or less can facilitate manual anterior capsulotomy and cortical aspiration with a phacoemulsification or irrigation/aspiration handpiece. When an intraocular lens is being implanted, a corneal or scleral tunnel wound can be employed.

For scleral wounds, a half-thickness scleral incision is made initially approximately 2 or 2.5 mm from the limbus and dissected into clear cornea. It is enlarged to the size necessary for IOL insertion. As compared to older, curvilinear limbal wounds, scleral tunnel wounds decrease the incidence of iris prolapse into the wound during surgery and assist the surgeon in preventing collapse of the anterior chamber, which occurs with greater frequency in the soft eyes of children. Unlike adults, scleral tunnel incisions do not self-seal. Closure is recommended using a synthetic absorbable suture such as 10-0 Biosorb or Vicryl (Fig. 12–11). Gimbel[47] recommends that the surgeon assess the internal incision with a gonioprism to look for "fish-mouthing" of the internal aspect of the corneal lip secondary to low scleral rigidity in children. According to Gimbel, when fish-mouthing is seen a special suturing technique is required that insures closure of the internal corneal lip. Scleral tunnel incisions are also thought to heal with more strength and stability over time than large curvilinear limbal incisions.

For corneal wounds, a linear groove is made at the tip of the conjunctival vessels where they enter the clear cornea. A tunnel is dissected into the corneal stroma as described above. Even if these corneal wounds appear to be self-sealing, 10.0 synthetic absorbable sutures are recommended because children commonly rub their eyes during the postoperative period. I have found the "near clear" corneal tunnel incision to be an ideal wound for implantation of foldable acrylic lenses in children of all ages. If a rigid lens is to be implanted, requiring a wound larger than 4 mm, I prefer to use a scleral tunnel.

The temporal wound presents the same advantages in children as it does in adults, but the location is more easily traumatized by children. The superior approach allows the wound to be protected by the brow and the Bell's phenomenon in the trauma-prone childhood years. For these reasons, I place corneal or scleral tunnel wounds superiorly in children.

VISCOELASTIC SUBSTANCES

A high molecular weight viscoelastic substance such as sodium hyaluronate 14 mg/per ml (Healon GV, Pharmacia Ophthalmics) is most commonly used in pediatric cataract surgery to effectively resist the increased tendency for anterior chamber collapse due to decreased scleral rigidity and an increased vitreous upthrust. This viscoelastic material helps to maintain a deep anterior chamber and a lax anterior capsule, facilitating attempts at manual anterior capsulorrhexis. Also, the initially convex posterior capsule is effectively held back during IOL insertion. Without a high molecular viscoelastic substance, an IOL inserted in a manner acceptable for an adult eye will result in inadvertent sulcus placement secondary to the posterior vitreous pressure and posterior capsule convexity. The trabecular meshwork in children clears viscoelastic substances more easily, on average, than in adults. However, efforts should still be made to remove all of the viscoelastic material because postoperative intraocular pressure spikes have been documented by us and others when Healon GV is inadequately removed.[48]

Healon V (Pharmacia Ophthalmics) is now becoming available to surgeons in the United States. Anterior chamber stability in the child's eye will be markedly

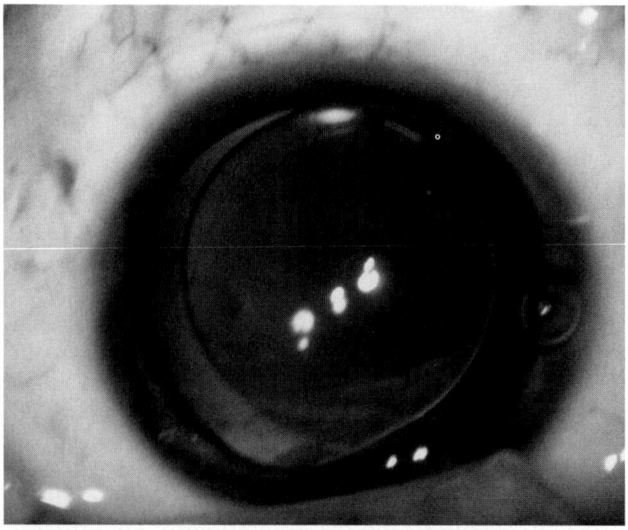

Figure 12–11. A 6.2-mm scleral tunnel has been used to insert an all PMMA intraocular lens of 12-mm overall length with a 6-mm optic. Two X-shaped sutures of 10-0 synthetic absorbable suture were used for closure. This child was 6 years old at the time of implantation.

improved with this new viscoelastic material. Extra care must be taken, however, to remove it completely. Its increased viscosity will lead to intraocular pressure elevation if any of the substance remains in the anterior chamber.

ANTERIOR CAPSULOTOMY TECHNIQUES

The anterior capsule in children is very different from that in adults. A recent review of anterior capsulotomy techniques for use in pediatric eyes has been published.[49] The ideal anterior capsulectomy technique in pediatric patients would be one that is easy to perform and that results in a low incidence of radial tears. While a manual continuous curvilinear capsulorrhexis (CCC) is ideal for adults, it is more difficult to perform in young eyes. The pediatric capsule is very elastic and requires the application of more force before tearing begins. When performing a CCC, control of the capsulectomy and prevention of extensions out toward the lens equator are inversely related to the force needed to generate the tear. Despite these difficulties, manual CCC, when it can be controlled and completed, remains the "gold standard" because it creates an edge that results in the lowest incidence of radial tears. As in adults, radial tears extending outward from the anterior capsulectomy margin can promote decentration of the IOL by allowing one of the haptics to exit the capsular bag. This is known as the "pea pod" effect.[50] Because children have a greater tissue reactivity and more intense capsular fibrosis, asymmetric loop fixation may result in an even higher rate of decentration in children than in adults.

Because manual CCC is more difficult to control in young children, some surgeons have reverted back to a "can-opener" style anterior capsulectomy. However, as stated above, the need for a continuous circular edge to the anterior capsulectomy may be even greater in children than it is in adults. Wasserman et al.[51] have shown that between one and five radial tears occur in virtually 100% of adult cases in which a "can-opener" capsulectomy is performed. Histopathologic studies have confirmed that asymmetric IOL fixation with one haptic outside the capsular bag occurs in up to 50% of cases where a "can-opener" anterior capsulectomy was performed and often is associated with IOL decentration.[52] Therefore, it is likely that the use of a can-opener style capsulotomy in children will result in an unacceptable rate of IOL decentration.

A mechanized circular anterior capsulectomy tested in both laboratory and clinical settings has proved to be a good alternative to CCC for young children, where the CCC may be difficult to control (Fig. 12–12).[53,54] This technique, known as vitrectorrhexis, is best performed using a vitrector tip attached to a Venturi pump irrigation and aspiration system. The capsulectomy is not started with a bent-needle cystotome; rather, the vitrector tip is placed through a tight-fit stab incision at the limbus or through a scleral tunnel. Irrigation is provided with a sleeve surrounding the vitrector or through a separate stab incision. A cut rate of 150 cycles per minute is recommended. With the cutting port oriented posteriorly, the center of the anterior capsule is aspirated into the cutting port to create an initial opening. Any nuclear or cortical material that spontaneously exits the capsular bag anteriorly is easily aspirated without interrupting the capsulectomy technique.[55] The capsular opening is enlarged using the cutter in a gentle circular fashion. The cutter is kept just anterior to the capsular edge, aspirating the capsule up into the cutting port rather than engaging the capsular edge directly. Visualization of the capsular edge during enlargement of the capsulectomy is excellent because the aspirating capability of the vitrector continuously removes lens cortex as it enters the anterior chamber. A smooth round capsulectomy can be produced that resists radial tearing. I have used this technique to perform more than 150 successful anterior capsulectomies in children (Fig. 12–13).

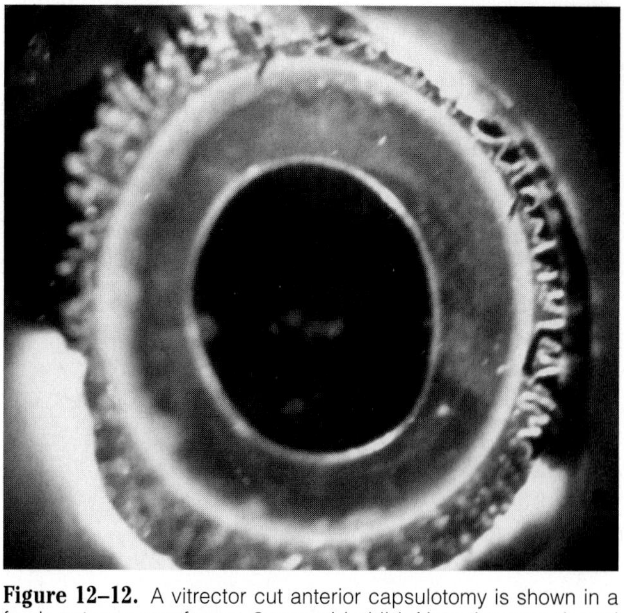

Figure 12–12. A vitrector cut anterior capsulotomy is shown in a fresh autopsy eye from a 2-year-old child. Note the smooth and somewhat rolled edge.

The vitrectorrhexis may produce a slightly scalloped edge initially. However, after the lens is removed and viscoelastic material is placed in the capsular bag, the scalloped edge rolls outward, creating a smooth edge (Fig. 12–14*A* and *B*). Right-angled edges should be avoided because they will frequently lead to radial tears. Capsular tags oriented toward the center of the circle, however, will merely roll outward when the viscoelastic substance reinflates the capsular bag and will not predispose to radial tears.[56,57]

A continuous curvilinear capsulotomy can also be created by a high-frequency endodiathermy. Although designed to produce an anterior capsulotomy in adults, this technique is well suited for the elastic pediatric anterior capsule. The instrument was invented by Kloti,[58–60] is manufactured by Oertli (Berneck, Switzerland). The handpiece is 0.6 mm in diameter. The platinum tip is insulated. A high-frequency modulation (500 kHz) signal is delivered with amperage and voltage preselected and

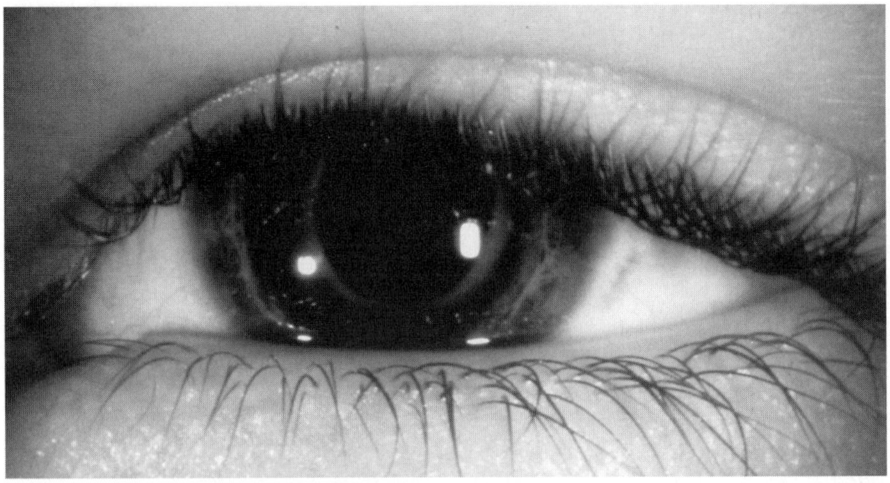

Figure 12–13. A vitrector cut anterior capsulotomy is seen 1 year after intraocular lens implantation. The same eye is pictured here as in Figure 12–11. Note the smooth, round edge of the vitrectorhexis.

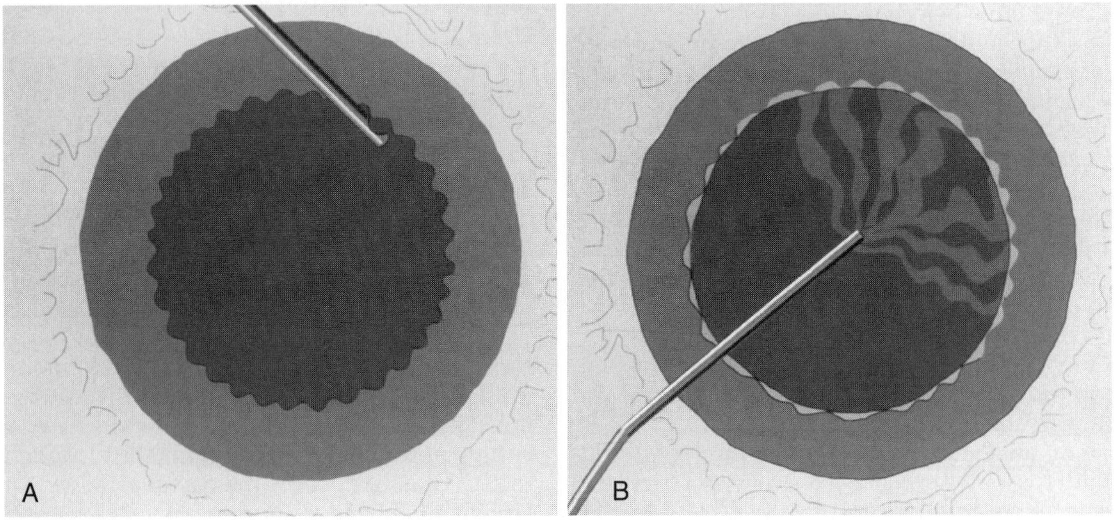

Figure 12–14. Artist drawing of a vitrector cut capsulotomy showing a scalloped edge *(A)* which rolls back when the capsular bag is filled with viscoelastic material *(B)* creating a smooth and somewhat rolled edge. (From Wilson ME, Bluestein EC, Wang XH, et al.: Comparison of mechanized anterior capsulectomy and manual continuous capsulorrhexis in pediatric eyes. J Cataract Refract Surg 1994;20:602–6.)

fixed within the unit by the manufacturer. A low mean energy is delivered, which minimizes the cutting energy and decreases heat generation. The base of the needle tip is placed in contact with the anterior capsule as the tip is activated by pressing the foot pedal. The capsulotomy size and shape are controlled by the surgeon as the tip is moved along a circular path (Fig. 12–15*A–D*). Gas bubbles form as the capsule is cut, but they do not usually interfere with visualization of the capsulotomy edge. The procedure is performed under a layer of viscoelastic agent. The capsular edge tends to roll up slightly, which creates a slightly larger capsulotomy than that initially cut with the instrument tip.[61] Initial studies have found no damage to corneal endothelial cells.[62] Recent studies using adult cadaver eyes and pig eyes have found the radio frequency diathermy capsulotomy edge to be less extensible than a manual CCC edge.[63,64] While neither of these studies were performed on pediatric lens capsules, the studies using pig eyes may correlate closely with results obtained clinically in pediatric patients. The pig anterior capsule is thicker and more elastic than the human adult anterior capsule and therefore is a useful model for pediatric eyes. It is noteworthy that the extensibility and strength of the diathermy anterior capsulotomy edge in the pig eye is markedly greater than in the adult human eye.[63] Our studies have shown a close correlation between the anterior capsule extensilibility of pig eyes and human infant eyes obtained post mortem.[65] As suggested by Taylor,[61] I have found the Kloti diathermy unit to be a useful alternative to manual CCC in selected children.

LENS REMOVAL

Pediatric cataracts are soft. Phacoemulsification is rarely if ever needed. Lens cortex and nucleus usually aspirate easily with an irrigation/aspiration or vitrectomy hand-

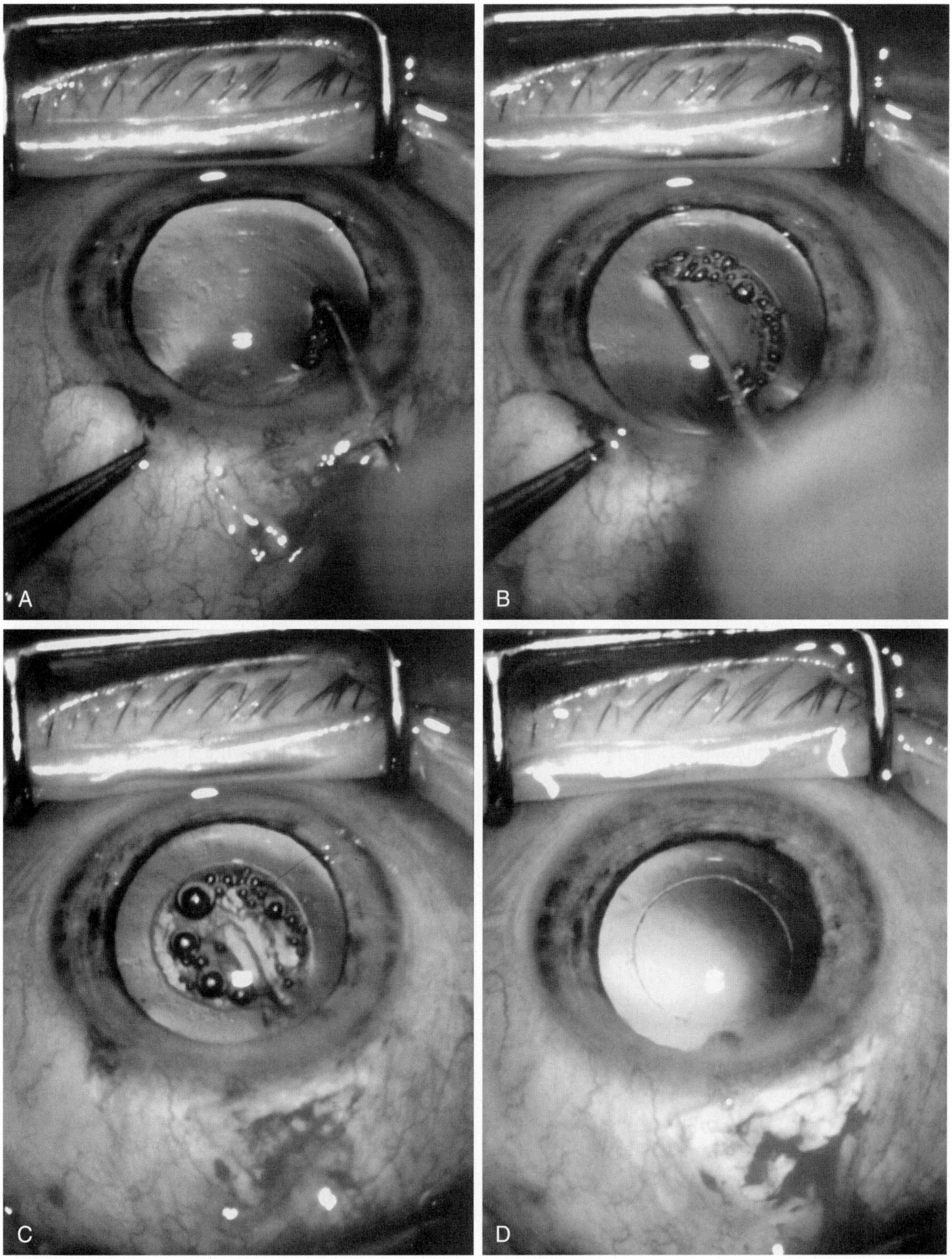

Figure 12–15. A continuous curvilinear capsulotomy can be created by a high-frequency endodiathermy. The base of the needle tip is placed in contact with the anterior capsule as the tip is activated by pressing the foot pedal *(A)*. The tip is moved along a circular path *(B)*. Gas bubbles form as the capsule is cut in a continuous circle *(C)*. The intact capsulotomy edge tends to roll up slightly, creating a larger capsulotomy than initially cut with the instrument tip *(D)*. (Photos courtesy of Garth Taylor, M.D.)

piece. With the vitrector, bursts of cutting can be used intermittently to facilitate the aspiration of the more "gummy" cortex of young children. The phacoemulsification handpiece can also be very useful when aspirating pediatric lens material. Hydrodissection is less useful in children than in adults. A fluid wave can sometimes be generated in older children but not reliably in infants and toddlers. Cortical material strips easily from the pediatric capsule even in the absence of hydrodissection. Attempts at hydrodelineation should be discouraged in children because it does not aid in lens removal and may lead to capsular rupture.

PRIMARY INTRAOCULAR LENS IMPLANTATION

Capsular fixation of the intraocular lens is strongly recommended for children. Care should be taken to avoid asymmetric fixation with one haptic in the capsular bag and the other in the ciliary sulcus. In contrast to adults, dialing of an IOL into the capsular bag can be difficult in children. Vitreous upthrust from scleral collapse often results in an IOL that dials out of, rather than into, the capsular bag.

Sulcus fixation of an intraocular lens in a child appears to be safe, but the long-term consequences of contact with vascularized uveal tissue is not ideal. To help assure lens centration and reduce the possibility of erosion into the ciliary body, prolapse of the optic through an intact anterior capsulotomy is recommended when sulcus fixation of an IOL in a child is necessary.

SECONDARY INTRAOCULAR LENS IMPLANTATION

Most children undergoing secondary intraocular lens implantation have had a primary posterior capsulectomy and anterior vitrectomy. If adequate peripheral capsular support is present, the implant is placed into the ciliary sulcus. Because the sulcus is only 0.5 to 1.0 mm larger than the evacuated capsular bag, most IOLs designed for capsular fixation can also be placed in the ciliary sulcus. However, I prefer a larger IOL for sulcus fixation (such as the Pharmacia 722C with a 6.5 mm optic and 13 mm overall length) than for capsular fixation in children.

Viscodissection may be all that is needed to break synechiae between the iris and the residual capsule. However, extensive synechiae can be present in children requiring much more manipulation of the iris than in primary IOL implantation. Iris pigment dispersion and iris bleeding can complicate the dissection. I have found the phaco-chop instruments useful when extensive anterior synechiae need to be broken. Although both the Acrysof acrylic lens and the all-PMMA lenses can be safely implanted in the sulcus of children, I prefer HSM all-PMMA lenses for the pediatric sulcus. Prolapsing the IOL optic through the fused anterior and posterior capsule remnants is useful in preventing pupillary capture and assuring lens centration. In some cases, the anterior and posterior capsular remnants can be dissected apart, allowing the IOL to be placed in the capsular bag.[66] An exuberant Soemmering's ring formation will often separate the anterior and posterior capsule leaflets and maintain the peripheral capsular bag. This material can be aspirated cleanly after the anterior capsule edge is lifted off of the posterior capsular edge to which it is usually fused.

When inadequate capsular support is present for sulcus fixation in a child, implantation of an IOL is not recommended unless every contact lens and spectacle option has been explored fully. Although the long-term safety is unknown, modern flexible open loop anterior chamber lenses are tolerated well in children when their anterior segment is developmentally normal. Sewing an IOL into the ciliary sulcus in a child has been tolerated well in some patients, but an increased risk of pupillary capture was noted in a recent pediatric series.[66a]

MANAGEMENT OF THE POSTERIOR CAPSULE

Management of the pediatric posterior capsule, especially when implanting an IOL at the time of the primary surgery, remains controversial. Primary posterior capsulectomy and anterior vitrectomy during pediatric lensectomy were popularized by Parks[46] in the early 1980s. This led to a dramatic decrease in the need for secondary surgery for congenital cataracts. Pediatric ophthalmologists are accustomed to removing a portion of the posterior capsule and the anterior vitreous at the time of lensectomy. An increase in late complications from primary capsulectomy and vitrectomy have not been reported. Adult cataract surgeons are often more reluctant to perform a primary capsulectomy and vitrectomy for fear that the risk of retinal detachment or cystoid macular edema will be increased. In point of fact, these complications are exceedingly rare after pediatric cataract surgery with or without a primary capsulectomy and vitrectomy. Neodymium:YAG laser posterior capsulotomy is usually necessary in children when the posterior capsule is left intact. This procedure also carries a risk of retinal detachment and cystoid macular edema. In addition, larger amounts of laser energy are often needed for children than for adults, and the posterior capsule opening may close requiring repeated laser treatments or a secondary pars plana membranectomy.

Dahan and Salmenson[32] have recommended posterior capsulotomy and anterior vitrectomy in every pediatric cataract patient younger than eight years old. Metge and co-workers[34] showed that a posterior capsulectomy without a central vitrectomy did not prevent the development of a secondary membrane. The opacification rate was not significantly decreased by a posterior capsulectomy alone. Only when an anterior vitrectomy was added did the opacification rate fall. Gimbel and DeBrof[67,68] recommend performing a posterior capsulorrhexis with IOL optic capture. This technique is designed to help prevent secondary membrane formation without necessitating a vitrectomy. It also ensures centration of the posterior chamber IOL because the haptics remain in the capsular bag and the optic is captured in the posterior capsular opening.

In contrast, Atkinson and Hiles[69] recommended leaving the posterior capsule intact even in very young children and performing Nd:YAG capsulotomy under a second general anesthesia in the early postoperative period. Later, however, the same group reported a 41% need for a repeat laser capsulotomy when this protocol was followed.[20] Interestingly, Plager and co-workers[26] reported that in their patients, the incidence of posterior capsule opacification began to increase markedly at approximately 18 months after surgery independent of the age at the time of cataract extraction. They recommended a primary posterior capsulectomy and anterior vitrectomy at the time of primary lens implantation in children who are not expected to be suitable candidates for awake Nd:YAG laser capsulotomy within 18 months of surgery.

When a decision is made to perform a primary posterior capsulectomy, several options are available.[39,70] The posterior capsular opening can be made using a manual PCCC technique or using an automated vitrector or the Kloti radiofrequency bipolar unit. The manual technique and the mechanized vitrector technique can each be performed either before or after the IOL has been placed in the eye. The radiofrequency bipolar unit is not easily manipulated beneath an IOL and is therefore usually used on the posterior capsule prior to IOL insertion. In most instances, an anterior vitrectomy is performed simultaneously with the posterior capsulectomy. The exception to this rule is the posterior optic capture technique, which at least theoretically, makes the anterior vitrectomy more elective than required.[67,68]

I prefer to leave the posterior capsule intact at the time of primary IOL placement for children older than age 6. For younger children, I prefer to place the IOL in the capsular bag with the posterior capsule still intact. The corneal or scleral tunnel is then closed securely using synthetic absorbable suture. With the irrigating cannula placed back into the anterior chamber, the central posterior capsule and anterior vitreous are removed through the pars plana as reported by Buckley and coworkers (Fig. 12–16).[25] An MVR blade is used to make a stab incision between 2 and 3 mm posterior to the limbus. The vitrector is then placed in the vitreous cavity through this pars plana incision. With irrigating fluid in the anterior chamber, the posterior capsule bows posteriorly and is easily engaged with the vitrector handpiece. I use a cutting speed of 350-500 cuts per minute. The pars plana technique gives me maximum control and allows me to create a larger posterior capsular opening than I would have felt safe making from the anterior approach. In addition, there is no risk of leaving vitreous in the anterior chamber or having an inadvertent wick of vitreous to the anterior wound. Therefore, the long-term risk of retinal detachment and cystoid macular edema may actually be less when vitreous is cut from this posterior approach than with an anterior approach. The pars plana entry site is closed with an 8-0 synthetic absorbable suture. As with the anterior vitrectorrhexis, a Venturi pump system is recommended when employing this pars plana technique.

When operating through the pars plana, the anatomy of the child's eye must be considered. At term, the newborn pars plana is only 1.5 mm to 2.0 mm wide, and it enlarges to 3 mm by 6 months of age. Surgery in infants can safely be performed through the iris root (0.5 mm posterior to the limbus), pars plicata, or pars plana. I prefer to enter 2 mm posterior to the limbus in children 1 year of age or younger, 2.5 mm in children up to age 4 years, and 3 mm thereafter. The entry angle is toward the center of the vitreous when entering at 3 mm, but it must be adjusted toward the optic disc when a more anterior entry site is used.[71–73]

POSTOPERATIVE ROUTINE

Postoperatively, pediatric eyes are characterized by increased tissue reactivity, especially when iris manipulation has been necessary during surgery. However, with modern surgical techniques, fulminant anterior uveitis after pediatric cataract surgery is not common. Intensive topical steroid use is standard, as is cycloplegia for the early postoperative period. Although some surgeons add systemic steroids postoperatively, no study has documented their superiority over topical therapy alone.

My perioperative routine includes a drop of 5% povidone-iodine at the beginning and at the end of the surgical procedure. I use a miotic at the completion of surgery only when I am concerned about pupillary capture (sulcus fixation) or vitreous in the anterior segment. Miotics can theoretically create increased anterior segment inflammation. Atropine ointment and topical steroid ointment are usually placed on the eye, and a light patch and Fox shield are placed over the eye. I delete the atropine if I have placed the lens in the sulcus, because I have seen pupillary capture after atropine use postoperatively in these patients. Beginning the next morning, I prescribe topical steroid drops six times a day and atropine once per day for 4 weeks. A topical antibiotic is added for the first several days. The atropine is stopped at 2 to 4 weeks, and the topical steroid is tapered and discontinued after 4 weeks. I have not used systemic steroids for postoperative inflammation

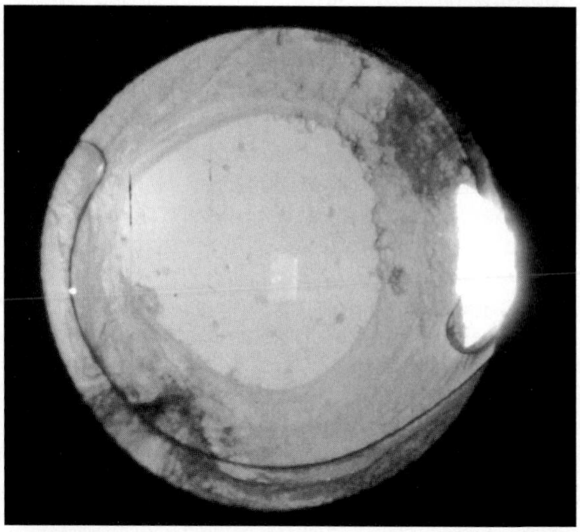

Figure 12–16. A primary vitrector cut posterior capsulectomy is shown in a young child 3 years after surgery.

control. Glasses or a Fox shield are worn over the eye continuously for the first week. I then recommend protective glasses during high-risk activity for life.

COMPLICATIONS OF CATARACT SURGERY IN CHILDREN

ENDOPHTHALMITIS

Endophthalmitis has been reported after cataract surgery in children, but it is exceedingly rare. The over-all risk is probably similar to that in the adult population. The risk of endophthalmitis may be lower than the risk associated with anesthesia in some neonates. Therefore, some ophthalmologists have opted to perform bilateral cataract surgery under one anesthesia in medically unstable infants. This point remains controversial.

RETINAL DETACHMENT

Rhegmatogenous retinal detachments are a rare late complication of cataract surgery in children. The interval from infantile cataract surgery to retinal detachment in one series ranged from 23 to 34 years.[74–77] The incidence appears to be decreasing as surgical techniques advance and evolve. Retinal detachments following infantile cataract surgery are usually secondary to oval or round holes along the posterior vitreous base.[1] Most reported cases have a history of multiple reoperations performed in the years prior to the introduction of automated lensectomy and vitrectomy.

GLAUCOMA

Chronic aphakic glaucoma is detected an average of 5 to 6 years after infantile cataract surgery with an incidence as high as 24%.[70] Microphthalmic eyes appear to be at the highest risk. Recently, Walton[79] has documented the development of a characteristic acquired filtration angle deformity in children with glaucoma following early lensectomy. Significant residual lens tissue and the need for reoperation were both correlated with a higher incidence of glaucoma. Because the relationship between the drainage angle and the iris lens diaphragm appear to be altered in Walton's cases, the question has been raised about whether an intraocular lens would somehow help preserve the proper relationship between the iris and the drainage angle, resulting in a lower incidence of aphakic glaucoma.

Much more rarely, angle closure glaucoma can occur as a result of pupillary block caused by a fibrin membrane extending across the pupil or vitreous prolapsing into the anterior chamber. Patients with microphthalmic eyes are more at risk for this complication as are patients who have been noncompliant with the application of topical corticosteroids postoperatively. A deep anterior vitrectomy in microphthalmic infants also affords some protection. Synechiae between the iris and the intraocular lens have also been reported to cause a pupillary block glaucoma.[80]

POSTERIOR CAPSULE OPACIFICATION

Posterior capsule opacification occurs much more commonly in children than in adults, as discussed earlier. A recent report has indicated an age-independent dramatic rise in the incidence of posterior capsule opacification beginning at 18 months after surgery and reaching nearly 100% over time.[26]

SECONDARY MEMBRANE

Pupillary membranes can occur postoperatively in children whether an IOL has been implanted or not. Microphthalmic eyes with microcoria operated in early infancy are at greatest risk, especially when mydriatic/cycloplegic agents have not been used postoperatively. Secondary membranes in children are usually thicker than simple posterior capsule opacification and are not usually opened successfully with an Nd:YAG laser. When an IOL is in place, secondary membranes may form over the anterior and/or posterior surface of the implant. Intraocular surgery is usually necessary to remove these membranes. The incidence of secondary membranes after neonatal or infantile cataract surgery has been reduced dramatically by minimizing the manipulation of the iris intraoperatively, by applying topical corticosteroids and cycloplegic agents at frequent intervals postoperatively, and by performing an adequate anterior vitrectomy and posterior capsulectomy.

POSTOPERATIVE INFLAMMATION

A mild to moderate anterior uveitis invariably occurs after cataract surgery in children. With modern surgical techniques and limited iris manipulation, however, most children have only mild postoperative inflammation. Because children have increased tissue reactivity, extensive manipulation of the iris and lens during surgery can result in a fulminant inflammatory response. Frequent topical steroids and even systemic steroids may be needed in selected cases.

PUPILLARY ABNORMALITIES

An irregular shape of the pupil is a relatively common complication of childhood cataract surgery. Synechiae may form from the pupillary edge to the remaining anterior capsule or to an intraocular lens. Postoperative mydriasis and the frequent administration of topical corticosteroids helped to prevent these synechiae. Because some surgeons use a vitreous cutting instrument during lensectomy, the iris sphincter can be damaged by the cutter, resulting in an irregular pupil. Some microphthalmic eyes have microcoria with a fibrotic iris sphincter. Intraoperative pupilloplasty may be necessary in these cases.

Pupillary capture of an IOL optic is much more common in children than in adults. It occurs most often with small IOL optic sizes and with ciliary sulcus placement. Placing the IOL in the capsular bag helps prevent pupillary capture. Prolapsing the optic of a secondary sulcus fixated IOL through the anterior capsule can also protect against pupillary capture. When pupillary capture of an IOL optic is associated with dense adhesions between the iris border and the residual capsule, optic prolapse is also useful to prevent recurrence of the capture.

INTRAOCULAR LENS DEPOSITS

Multiple small deposits are seen occasionally on the surface of an IOL optic implanted in a child. The deposits can be pigmented or nonpigmented but usually are not visually significant. They occur much more commonly in children with dark irises, and when compliance with postoperative medications has been poor.

INTRAOCULAR LENS DECENTRATION

Decentration of an intraocular lens can occur because of traumatic zonular loss or inadequate capsular support. Asymmetric fixation of an IOL with one haptic in the capsular bag and the other in the ciliary sulcus can also lead to decentration. Complete IOL dislocation can occur after trauma.

CYSTOID MACULAR EDEMA

Cystoid macular edema (CME) appears to be rare after cataract surgery in children. Hoyt and Nickel[81] in 1982 described CME developing commonly in infantile eyes after lensectomy and anterior vitrectomy, but the appearance was atypical and the CME was not documented photographically. The following year, Gilbard and associates[82] reported no CME in 25 eyes after pars plicata removal of congenital cataracts. No subsequent paper has documented clinically significant CME after pediatric cataract surgery even when an anterior vitrectomy is performed.

SIGNIFICANT RESIDUAL REFRACTIVE ERROR

Uncorrected aphakia after pediatric cataract surgery can cause or worsen amblyopia. When a child is left aphakic, an effort should be made to document time intervals when the prescribed aphakic spectacles or aphakic contact lenses are not worn. Even short intervals of uncorrected aphakia are potentially very damaging to the prognosis for amblyopia treatment. When an IOL is implanted, a smaller quantity of residual hyperopia may be present. Correction of residual hyperopia and any significant astigmatic error is necessary to optimize visual development and recovery from amblyopia. Because young children's eyes continue to grow axially after cataract surgery and IOL implantation, significant late myopia will be more and more common as the years pass. Glasses or contact lenses will be used for more correction of the secondary myopia in most cases. However, the development of new corneal and intraocular refractive procedures will provide new options for correcting significant late myopia.

CONCLUSION

Some aspects of pediatric cataract surgery differ very little from adult surgery; other aspects differ markedly. Combining surgical techniques designed for children with techniques designed for adults (modified for the soft, growing eyes of children) helps to promote optimal surgical results. Visual outcome is affected more by the timing of surgical intervention and the success of amblyopia therapy, however, than by the techniques chosen to remove the lens and rehabilitate the eye optically. Children have a very long life span after cataract surgery and are, therefore, unique clinical responsibilities of the ophthalmologist. While we aggressively search for better and more effective ways to habilitate or rehabilitate small cataractous eyes, we must also be cautious. When operating on children, surgeons must avoid the temptation to apply new untested techniques, therapies, or devices before an adequate assessment of the benefit to risk ratio has been carefully considered.

REFERENCES

1. Lambert SR, Drack AV: Infantile cataracts. Survey of Ophthalmology 1996;40:427–58.
2. Sinskey RM, Stoppel JO, Ammin PA: Ocular axial length changes in a pediatric patient with aphakia and pseudophakia. J Cataract Refract Surg 1993;19:787–8.
3. Huber C: Increasing myopia in children with intraocular lenses (IOL): An experiment in form deprivation myopia? Eur J Implant Refract Surg 1993;5:154–8.
4. Gordon RA, Donzis PB: Refractive development of the human eye. Arch Ophthalmol 1985;103:785–9.
5. Wilson ME: Management of aphakia in childhood. American Academy of Ophthalmology, Focal Points, Clinical Modules for Ophthalmologists, March 1999; Volume 17/1.
6. Parks MM: Visual results in aphakic children. Am J Ophthalmol 1982;94:441–9.
7. Parks MM, Johnson DA, Reed GW: Long term visual results and complications in children with aphakia: A function of cataract type. Ophthalmology 1993;100:826–41.
8. Birch EE, Stager DR: The critical period for surgical treatment of dense, congenital, unilateral cataracts. Invest Ophthalmol Vis Sci 1996;37:1532–8.
9. Wallace DK, Plager DA: Corneal diameter in childhood aphakic glaucoma. J Pediatr Ophthalmol Strabismus 1996;33:230–4.
10. Ruttum MS: Childhood cataracts. American Academy of Ophthalmology, Focal Points, Clinical Modules for Ophthalmologists, March 1996; Volume 14/1.
11. Baker JD: Visual rehabilitation of aphakic children. II. Contact lenses. In Dutton J, Flamovits T (eds.), Viewpoints. Surv Ophthalmol 1990;34:366–71.
12. Neumann D, Weissman BA, Isenberg SJ, et al.: The effectiveness of daily wear contact lenses for the correction of infantile aphakia. Arch of Ophthalmol 1993;111:927–30.

13. Assaf AA, Wiggins R, Engle K, et al.: Compliance with prescribed optical correction in cases of monocular aphakia in children. Saudi J Ophthalmol 1994;8:15–22.
14. Morgan KS: Visual rehabilitation of aphakic children: IV. Epikeratophakia. In Dutton J, Flamovits T (eds.), Viewpoints. Surv Ophthalmol 1990;34:379–84.
15. Barraquer JI. Keratomileusis and keratophakia. In Corneoplastic Surgery: Proceedings of the Second International Corneo-Plastic Conference, Rycroft PV (ed.), New York:Pergamon Press;1969: 409–43.
16. Apple DJ, Kincaid MC, Mamalis N, et al.: Intraocular lenses: evolution, designs, complications, and pathology. Baltimore: Williams & Wilkins; 1989:370–7.
17. Rosenbaum AL: Consultation Section. J Cataract Refract Surg 1991;17:515.
18. Wilson ME, Bluestein EC, Wang XH: Current trends in the use of intraocular lenses in children. J Cataract Refract Surg 1994;20: 579–83.
19. Gimbel HV, Ferensowicz M, Raanan M, et al.: Implantation in children. J Pediatr Ophthalmol Strabismus 1993;30:69–79.
20. Brady KM, Atkinson CS, Kilty LA, et al.: Cataract surgery and intraocular lens implantation in children. Am J Ophthalmol 1995; 120:1–9.
21. Crouch ER Jr, Pressman SH, Crouch ER: Posterior chamber intraocular lenses: Long-term results in pediatric cataract patients. J Pediatr Ophthalmol Strabismus 1995;32:210–8.
22. Koenig SB, Ruttum MS, Lewandowski MF, et al.: Pseudophakia for traumatic cataracts in children. Ophthalmology 1993;100: 1218–24.
23. Sinskey RM, Stoppel JO, Amin P: Long-term results of intraocular lens implantation in pediatric patients. J Cataract Refract Surg 1993;19:405–8.
24. Kora Y, Inatomi M, Fukado Y, et al.: Long-term study of children with implanted intraocular lenses. J Cataract Refract Surg 1992; 18:485–8.
25. Buckley EG, Klombers LA, Seaber JH, et al.: Management of the posterior capsule during pediatric intraocular lens implantation. Am J Ophthalmol 1993;115:722–8.
26. Plager DA, Lipsky SN, Snyder SK, et al.: Capsular management and refractive error in pediatric intraocular lenses. Ophthalmology 1997;104:600–7.
27. Wilson ME: Intraocular lens implantation: Has it become the standard of care for children? Ophthalmology 1996;103:1719–20.
28. Wilson ME, Apple DJ, Bluestein EC, et al.: Intraocular lenses for pediatric implantation: Biomaterials, designs and sizing. J Cataract Refract Surg 1994;20:584–91.
29. Apple DJ, Solomon KD, Tetz MR, et al.: Posterior capsule opacification. Surv Ophthalmol 1992;37:73–116.
30. Basti S, Aasuri MK, Reedy MK, et al.: Heparin surface-modified intraocular lenses in pediatric cataract surgery: Prospective randomized study. J Cataract Refract Surg 1999;25:782–7.
31. Rush DP, Bazarian RA: Intraocular lenses in children. Adv Clin Ophthalmol 1994;1:263–74.
32. Dahan E, Salmenson BD: Pseudophakia in children: Precautions, techniques, and feasibility. J Cataract Refract Surg 1990;16:75–82.
33. Oliver M, Milstein A, Pollack A: Posterior chamber lens implantation in infants and juveniles. Eur J Implant Refract Surg 1990; 2:309–14.
34. Metge P, Cohen H, Chemila JF: Intercapsular implantation in children. Eur J Cataract Refract Surg 1990;2:319–23.
35. Knight-Nanan D, O'Keefe M, Bowell R: Outcome and complications of intraocular lenses in children with cataract. J Cataract Refract Surg 1996;2:730–6.
36. Hutchinson AK, Wilson ME, Saunders RA: Outcomes and ocular growth rates after intraocular lens implantation in the first 2 years of life. J Cataract Refract Surg 1998;24:846–52.
37. Wilson ME, Lall-Trail JK, Peterseim MM, Englert JA: Pseudophakia and polypseudophakia in the first year of life. J AAPOS 2001;5:238–45.
38. McClatchey SK, Parks MM: Myopic shift after cataract removal in childhood. J Pediatr Ophthalmol Strabismus 1997;34:88–95.
39. Basti S, Ravishankar V, Gupta S: Results of a prospective evaluation of three methods of management of pediatric cataracts. Ophthalmology 1993;103:713–20.
40. Vasavada A, Chauhan H: Intraocular lens implantation in infants with congenital cataracts. J Cataract Refract Surg 1994;20:592–7.
41. Wilson ME: Clinician's Corner. In Ruttum MS, Childhood cataracts. American Academy of Ophthalmology, Focal Points, Clinical Modules for Ophthalmologists, March 1996; Volume 14/1:10.
42. Enyedi LB, Peterseim MW, Freedman SF, Buckley EG: Refractive changes after pediatric intraocular lens implantation. Am J Ophthalmol 1998;126:772–81.
43. Greenwald MJ: Clinician's Corner. In Ruttum MS, Childhood cataracts. American Academy of Ophthalmology, Focal Points, Clinical Modules for Ophthalmologists, March 1996; Volume 14/1:10.
44. Andreo LK, Wilson ME, Saunders RA: Predictive value of regression and theoretical IOL formulas in pediatric intraocular lens implantation. J Pediatr Ophthalmol Strabismus 1997;34: 240–3.
45. Scheie HG: Aspiration of congenital or soft cataracts: A new technique. Am J Ophthalmol 1960;50:1048–56.
46. Parks MM: Posterior lens capsulectomy during primary cataract surgery in children. Ophthalmology 1983;90:344–5.
47. Gimbel HV, Sun R, DeBrouff BM: Recognition and management of internal wound gape. J Cataract Refract Surg 1995;21:121–4.
48. Englert JA, Wilson ME: Postoperative intraocular pressure elevation after the use of Healon GV in pediatric cataract surgery. J AAPOS 2000;4:60–1.
49. Wilson ME: Anterior capsule management for pediatric intraocular lens implantation. J Pediatr Ophthalmol Strabismus 1999;36: 1–6.
50. Apple DJ, Assia EI, Wasserman D, et al.: Evidence in support of the continuous tear anterior capsulectomy (capsulorrhexis technique). In Cangelosi GC (ed.), Advances in Cataract Surgery. New Orleans Academy of Ophthalmology. Thorofare, N.J.: Slack, Inc; 1991;21–47.
51. Wasserman D, Apple DJ, Castaneda VE, et al.: Anterior capsular tears and loop fixation of posterior chamber intraocular lenses. Ophthalmology 1991;98:425–31.
52. Assia EI, Legler UFC, Merrill C, et al.: Clinicopathologic study of the effect of radial tears and loop fixation on intraocular lens decentration. Ophthalmology 1993;100:153–8.
53. Wilson ME, Bluestein EC, Wang XH, et al.: Comparison of mechanized anterior capsulectomy and manual continuous capsulorrhexis in pediatric eyes. J Cataract Refract Surg 1994;20:602–6.
54. Wilson ME, Saunders RA, Roberts EL, et al.: Mechanized anterior capsulectomy as an alternative to manual capsulorhexis in children undergoing intraocular lens implantation. J Pediatr Ophthalmol Strabismus 1996;33:237–40.
55. Wilson ME: Mechanized anterior capsulotomy vs manual capsulorrhexis. Letter to the Editor (reply). J Cataract Refract Surg 1996;22:3–4.
56. Assia EI, Apple DJ, Tsai JC, et al.: Mechanism of radial tear formation and extension after anterior capsulectomy. Ophthalmology 1991;98:432–7.
57. Krag S, Thim K, Corybon L, et al.: Biomechanical aspects of the anterior capsulotomy. J Cataract Refract Surg 1994;20:410–16.
58. Kloti R: Bipolar wet field diathermy and microsurgery. Klin Monatsbl Augenheilkd 1984;184:442–4.
59. Kloti R: Anterior high frequency (HF) capsulotomy. Part I: Experimental study. Klin Monatsbl Augenheilkd 1992;200:507–10.
60. Coester C, Kloti R, Speiser P: Anterior high frequency (HF) capsulotomy. Part II: Clinical surgical experience. Klin Monatsbl Augenheilkd 1992;200:511–4; 344–5.
61. Taylor GA: Continuous curvilinear capsulotomy by high frequency endodiathermy. Ophthalmic Pract 1993;11/6:113–4.
62. Gassman F, Fchinmelpfennig B, Kloti R: Anterior capsulotomy by means of bipolar radio frequency endodiathermy. J Cataract Refract Surg 1988;14.
63. Krag S, Thim K, Corydon L: Diathermic capsulotomy versus capsulorrhexis: A biomechanical study. J Cataract Refract Surg 1997; 23:86–90.
64. Morgan JE, Ellingham RB, Young RD, et al.: The mechanical properties of the human lens capsule following capsulorrhexis or radio frequency diathermy capsulotomy. Arch Ophthalmol 1996;114:1110–5.
65. Andreo LK, Wilson ME, Basti S, et al.: Elastic properties and electron microscopic appearance of manual and vitrector-cut anterior capsulotomy in an animal model of pediatric cataract. J Cataract Refract Surg 1999;25:534–9.

66. Wilson ME, Englert JA, Greenwald MJ: In-the-bag secondary intraocular lens implantation in children. J AAPOS 1999;3:350–5.
66a. Lam DSC, Ng JSK, Fan DSP, et al.: Short term results of scleral intraocular lens fixaton in children. J Cataract Refract Surg 1998;24:1474–9.
67. Gimbel HV, DeBroff DM: Posterior capsulorrhexis with optic capture: Maintaining a clear visual axis after pediatric cataract surgery. J Cataract Refract Surg 1994;20:658–64.
68. Gimbel HV: Posterior capsulorhexis with optic capture in pediatric cataract and intraocular lens surgery. Ophthalmology 1996;103:1871–5.
69. Atkinson CS, Hiles DA: Treatment of secondary posterior capsular membrane Nd:YAG laser in a pediatric population. Am Journal Ophthalmol 1994;118:496–501.
70. Wang XH, Wilson ME, Bluestein EC, et al.: Pediatric cataract surgery and IOL implantation techniques: a laboratory study. J Cataract Refract Surg 1994;20:607–9.
71. Maguire AM, Trese MT: Lens-sparing vitreoretinal surgery in infants. Arch Ophthalmol 1992;110:284–6.
72. Ferrone PJ, De Juan E: Vitreous hemorrhage in infants. Arch Ophthalmol 1994;112:1185–9.
73. Peyman GA, Raichand M, Oesterle C, Goldberg MF: Pars plicata lensectomy and vitrectomy in the management of congenital cataracts. Ophthalmology 1981;88:437–9.
74. Jagger JD, Cooling RJ, Fison LG, et al.: Management of retinal detachment following congenital cataract surgery. Trans Ophthalmol Soc UK 1983;103:103–7.
75. Kanski JJ, Elkington AR, Daniel R: Retinal detachment after congenital cataract surgery. Br J Ophthalmol 1974;58:92–5.
76. McLeod D: Congenital cataract surgery: A retinal surgeon's viewpoint. Aust NZJ Ophthalmol 1986;14:79–84.
77. Toyofuku H, Hirose T, Schepens CL: Retinal detachment following congenital cataract surgery. Arch Ophthalmol 1980;98:669–75.
78. Simon JW, Metge P, Simmons ST, et al.: Glaucoma after pediatric lensectomy/vitrectomy. Ophthalmology 1991;98:670–4.
79. Walton DS: Pediatric aphakic glaucoma: A study of 65 patients. Trans Am Ophthalmol Soc 1995;93:403–20.
80. Vajapyee RB, Angra SK, Titiyal JS, et al.: Pseudophakic pupillary block glaucoma in children. Am J Ophthalmol 1991;11:715–8.
81. Hoyt CS, Nickel B: Aphakic cystoid macular edema: Occurrence in infants and children after transpupillary lensectomy and anterior vitrectomy. Arch Ophthalmol 1982;100:746–9.
82. Gilbard SM, Peyman GA, Goldberg MF: Evaluation for cystoid maculopathy after pars plicata lensectomy-vitrectomy for congenital cataracts. Ophthalmology 1983;90:1201–6.

SECTION III

Peter R. Laibson, M.D.

Cornea

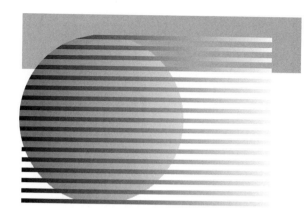

CHAPTER 13

Anterior Segment Trauma

CHRISTOPHER J. RAPUANO, M.D.

The conjunctiva and cornea, the external ocular structures, are the first layers of the eye to be involved in ocular trauma. They may be only superficially involved, or more extensive damage may occur. The degree of damage, which depends on the exact force and type of injury, varies from superficial corneal or conjunctival abrasions to full-thickness corneal lacerations, which may involve the iris, lens, sclera, vitreous and retina. In addition, intraocular foreign bodies may be involved. The particular approach to each patient suffering from anterior segment trauma depends on the history and physical examination.

An accurate history is very important to aid the physician in determining the severity of the injury and the necessary work-up and treatment. Eyes involved in chemical injuries should be copiously irrigated with a neutral solution, such as normal saline, after quickly obtaining a pH reading from the cul-de-sac. In addition, every attempt should be made to learn the exact composition of the chemical, to aid in determining the severity of the injury and subsequent treatment. Irrigation proceeds until the pH normalizes. Eyes involved with trauma from a foreign body, a piece of which may still be in the eye, need to have an intraocular foreign body (IOFB) ruled out by examination or imaging studies. In general, if the presence of an IOFB cannot be ruled out by examination, an ocular and orbital computed tomography (CT) scan should be obtained. When a metal foreign body may be present, a magnetic resonance imaging (MRI) scan is contraindicated.

A slit-lamp examination is necessary to determine the type and extent of any ocular injury, but a penlight examination may be all that is feasible if the patient cannot get to a slit lamp because of other injuries. If it is determined that surgical repair is required, the remainder of the ocular examination can be deferred to the operating room. Slit-lamp examination should differentiate between a conjunctival/corneal abrasion, conjunctival laceration, partial-thickness corneal laceration, full-thickness corneal laceration, scleral laceration, iris damage or prolapse, lens damage, vitreal or retinal involvement, and the presence of an IOFB. Care must be taken when evaluating conjunctival lacerations, to make certain there is no underlying full-thickness scleral laceration, which is not always easy as there is often significant subconjunctival hemorrhage. Partial-thickness corneal lacerations are Seidel negative and demonstrate normal anterior chamber depth. Full-thickness corneal lacerations are typically Seidel positive with a shallower anterior chamber than the fellow eye. Full-thickness corneal lacerations can, however, be deceiving. They may be self-sealing, and consequently Seidel negative, with a normal anterior chamber depth. In general, to determine the risk of intraocular infection, it is important to differentiate partial-thickness from full-thickness corneal trauma. Slight pressure at the limbus may demonstrate leaking and confirm a full-thickness laceration, although it is best not to manipulate the globe excessively if the laceration is not leaking.

Corneal and conjunctival abrasions are treated medically with topical antibiotics, and occasionally pressure patching, and require close follow-up. Most conjunctival lacerations are also treated medically in a similar manner, but large conjunctival lacerations (>10 mm) can be sutured with absorbable suture (e.g., 8-0 Vicryl). Most partial-thickness corneal lacerations can also be treated with topical antibiotics and close follow-up. Large, deep, or gaping partial-thickness lacerations are best treated by surgical closure, to minimize corneal scarring and irregularity.

Injuries that do not perforate the cornea or sclera generally do not require systemic antibiotics to prevent endophthalmitis. In contrast, full-thickness corneal and scleral lacerations are treated with systemic antibiotics (in addition to topical antibiotics) to minimize the chance of endophthalmitis. The route of the systemic antibiotics is presently under debate; in general, intravenous antibiotics covering gram-positive and gram-negative organisms as well as anaerobes are administered preoperatively and for 3 to 5 days postoperatively, followed by oral antibiotics for an additional 4 to 7 days. More recently, oral fluoroquinolones, which have excellent intraocular penetration, have been used in place of intravenous antibiotics at certain institutions. The answer to the question of which regimen is best is not yet known. Tetanus prophylaxis is not controversial and may be required, depending on the patient's immunization history.

SURGICAL REPAIR

Not all full-thickness corneal lacerations require surgical repair, although they do require systemic antibiotic prophylaxis. Small, self-sealing, or minimally leaking corneal lacerations with deep chambers can be followed closely without surgical repair. If the laceration has not stopped leaking in 1 or 2 days, however, surgical repair should be seriously considered.

Several general rules need to be followed in the repair of ruptured globes. Minimal pressure should be placed on the eye during examination, surgical preparation of the patient, placement of the eyelid speculum, and surgical repair itself. Retrobulbar anesthesia is generally contraindicated as bleeding, or the bolus of anesthetic itself, could cause extrusion of intraocular contents through the wound; general anesthesia is therefore preferred. Depolarizing muscle relaxants should be avoided because they can increase intraocular pressure and cause expulsion of the intraocular contents. If general anesthesia is not possible, a combination of facial and subconjunctival blocks is safest. Topical anesthesia can be used for certain lacerations in cooperative patients. Cultures of purulent material should be obtained prior to surgical repair.

When a surgeon is faced with an open globe, sterile cellulose sponges and fine forceps must be used in evaluating the extent of the damage and determining whether intraocular contents, such as iris or vitreous, are extruding from the wound. The surgeon should always keep in mind that a small, unsuspected foreign body may be present. A game plan can then be formulated to approach the repair. A prime goal of surgery is to reposition the ocular structures to their proper anatomic location, if at all possible.

IRIS PROLAPSE

When the iris has prolapsed, every effort should be made to reposit it. Occasionally, the iris can be replaced through the wound from the external surface. Introduction of a small amount of viscoelastic material may be useful, but too much will force more iris out than in. If the anterior chamber is not flat, or if an anterior chamber can be created with a small amount of viscoelastic material, a small limbal paracentesis can be fashioned with a blade, using extreme care not to damage the iris or lens. Through the paracentesis, a cyclodialysis spatula can be inserted and used to gently tug the externalized iris into the eye. This procedure is usually most effectively performed with a sweeping motion from the iris root toward the pupil. Care should be taken not to create an iridodialysis. Iris that is completely macerated or appears infected should be amputated, and not reposited. In eyes with long-standing iris prolapse, the iris may be covered with epithelium. This epithelium needs to be completely removed prior to repositing the iris back into the eye.

CORNEAL SUTURING

Once any iris prolapse is reposited, and the paracentesis is performed, the corneal laceration is repaired with interrupted sutures. It is typically sutured with deeply placed 10-0 nylon. The first suture is placed at an anatomic landmark, such as at the limbus, or at an angle in the laceration, to assure proper surgical alignment. Otherwise, the first suture should be placed in the middle of the laceration. Ensuing sutures should bisect the remaining wound until it is secure and watertight. Attempts should be made to place sutures outside the center of the visual axis. Stellate lacerations are difficult to repair and may require triangular, "X," or purse-string sutures to obtain a watertight seal. The knots are buried just beneath the epithelium in the superficial stroma. The anterior chamber is re-formed with physiological saline and any anterior synechiae are lysed with a cyclodialysis spatula either through the wound or via the paracentesis tract. A Seidel test is performed at the end of surgery to insure a watertight closure. In severely traumatized corneas there may be extensive loss of tissue, requiring a donor patch graft or even a penetrating keratoplasty.

LENS INVOLVEMENT

The lens may be involved in anterior segment trauma, and often it is difficult to determine the exact extent of lens damage at the time of the initial evaluation and surgical repair. If there is doubt regarding whether a traumatic cataract is present, the lens should be left alone at the time of primary wound repair. If, on the other hand, fluffy cortical lens material is present in the anterior chamber, lens removal at the time of surgical repair should be seriously considered. Cataract removal at the time of initial repair may be difficult if visualization is limited by the corneal trauma. In addition, the extent of the anterior capsular opening is unknown and the lens zonule and posterior capsule may be compromised, often making the surgery complex.

The laceration should be repaired first, and then a separate limbal incision created to remove the cataract. Occasionally, the anterior capsular opening can be converted into an intact capsulorrhexis. More often, a "can-opener" type capsulotomy is required. Usually, most of the lens nucleus can be aspirated with the phacoemulsification tip, with minimal ultrasound power. The cortical lens material can then be removed with manual or automated irrigation/aspiration. During the lens removal there should be a high index of suspicion for zonular dehiscence, capsular breaks, and vitreous prolapse.

If a cataractous lens is removed primarily, it is more problematic to place an intraocular lens implant because accurate keratometric and axial eye length measurements may be unavailable. In addition, there is a small theoretical increase in the risk of intraocular infection when a foreign lens implant is present. However, when accurate keratometric and axial eye length readings are available for the involved or the fellow eye, many surgeons insert intraocular lens implantsat the time of corneal laceration repair and cataractremoval.

VITREOUS PROLAPSE

When vitreous prolapse is present, an anterior vitrectomy is required, a procedure that is best performed with an automated vitrectomy instrument. The goal of the vitrectomy is to clear the wound and anterior chamber of vitreous, if possible.

Depending on the extent of the injury and vitreous involvement, vitrectomy can be performed through the corneal wound, or a separate limbal incision can be made. The wound needs to be closed before a limbal vitrectomy can be performed. When a vitrectomy is performed, or in any severely inflamed eyes, a peripheral iridectomy is helpful to prevent pupillary block glaucoma.

CORNEOSCLERAL LACERATIONS

When the sclera is involved, a conjunctival peritomy is required, and the full extent of the scleral laceration must be explored and repaired. When a corneal laceration extends to the limbus, the adjacent sclera needs to be explored for possible involvement. As mentioned earlier, the limbal sutures are placed first, because that anatomical landmark is readily apparent. While corneal sutures are 10-0 nylon, limbal sutures are usually 9-0 nylon and scleral sutures are 8-0 or 9-0 nylon. Any ciliary body and retinal tissue present in the wound is reposited, unless it is infected or necrotic.

INTRAOCULAR FOREIGN BODIES

Foreign bodies embedded in the superficial cornea can be removed at the slit lamp or in the operating room, depending on the severity of other injuries. Deeply embedded corneal foreign bodies are generally removed in the operating room. Not all foreign bodies require removal. Small, inert (e.g., glass) foreign bodies that are outside the visual axis and difficult to remove may be left in place and followed closely. Foreign bodies that extend into or are completely within the anterior chamber should be removed. Foreign bodies that enter the eye and fall into the inferior anterior chamber are often hidden in the inferior angle and iris folds, and may only be apparent on examination with gonioscopy. The injection of a viscoelastic substance into the anterior chamber is extremely helpful in stabilizing the anterior chamber and limiting the movement of a foreign body. Occasionally, a deeply imbedded corneal foreign body or a foreign body in the anterior chamber can be lifted out anteriorly through the corneal wound, but more often removal requires a separate limbal incision. The limbal incision tends to be much larger than the surgeon might predict for most foreign body removals. Care must be taken not to lose the foreign body behind the iris or to damage the lens during surgical removal. Removal of magnetic metallic foreign bodies may be helped with the use of a heavy duty, electric foreign body magnet.

Injections of subconjunctival antibiotics covering gram-positive and gram-negative organisms should be accomplished at the end of surgery. The use of subconjunctival steroids is controversial, because they may increase the risk of endophthalmitis.

POSTOPERATIVE CARE

Topical and systemic antibiotics are used for 7 to 10 days postoperatively. Cycloplegic agents may be helpful. Topical steroids can be added on postoperative day 1 if the wound is not leaking, if there is significant inflammation, and if there is no sign of infection. If a small wound leak is present in the first days after surgery, aqueous suppressants and occasionally pressure patching or a bandage soft contact lens is applied and the patient is followed closely. If a large wound leak is present, or a small wound leak is not improving for several days, re-repair in the operating room may be required. Occasionally a surgical grade tissue adhesive, such as isobutylcyanoacrylate can be applied to seal such a leak and allow for fibrosis to occur. Close follow-up for the first several days is mandatory to monitor the healing process and rule out infection. It is important to evaluate the posterior segment, either by examination or B-scan ultrasonography, within 1 to 2 weeks of the trauma.

CHAPTER 14

Conjunctival Flap Surgery

CHRISTOPHER J. RAPUANO, M.D.

Even though great advances have been made in topical antibiotic and antiviral therapy, artifical tear preparations, and soft contact lenses over the recent years, chronic corneal surface disease remains a formidable clinical problem. Conjunctival flap surgery, as a way to improve chronically compromised corneal surfaces, is a procedure that is often underutilized by the anterior segment surgeon. It is an effective method to replace damaged or nonexistent epithelium with more resilient conjunctiva. Used for appropriate indications with meticulous attention to surgical technique, this family of procedures is extremely useful for the surgeon to master.

Eyes with chronic, noninfected corneal epithelial defects that are not responding to medical management are excellent candidates for conjunctival flap surgery. The eye may or may not have significant corneal ulceration, but active corneal perforation should not be present. In some cases of chronic active stromal ulceration, for example in herpes simplex necrotizing keratitis, conjunctival flaps have been invaluable. Some surgeons have advocated the use of conjunctival flaps in the presence of indolent fungal infections not responding to aggressive anti-fungal therapy. Such surgery has often worked to quiet the eye, but viable fungal organisms have been recovered under conjunctival flaps. In eyes with chronic painful bullous keratopathy with poor visual potential, or that are not otherwise candidates for penetrating keratoplasty, a conjunctival flap is often an excellent long-term solution. The goal is to stabilize the eye, not to improve vision, at least not immediately.

The disadvantages of conjunctival flap surgery include its somewhat tedious surgical procedure, its less than ideal cosmetic appearance at first, and the diminished ability of the physician to view the intraocular contents. Significant postoperative ptosis may also develop. In addition, topical medications may not penetrate the eye as effectively. With experience, the surgeon will fine-tune the technique and be able to create relatively thin flaps, which allow better cosmetic results as well as improved visualization of the interior of the eye. Recently, amniotic membrane grafts have been used with moderate success to cover corneas with bullous keratopathy.[1]

There are numerous techniques to cover the cornea with conjunctiva. The purse-string method, in which the limbal conjunctiva is undermined for 360 degrees and sutured with a purse-string suture over the central cornea, tends to develop healing difficulties in the area of the suture and to retract more readily. Two more effective methods are the thin total conjunctival flap popularized by Gunderson[2] and the partial conjunctival flap. A general principle of these conjunctival flaps is total epithelial removal under the areas to be flapped. Dissection of a thin layer of conjunctiva with an appropriate peritomy and achieving minimal tension on the flap are important. Finally the flap is sutured securely into position.

SURGICAL TECHNIQUE

TOTAL CONJUNCTIVAL FLAP

Typically local anesthesia is used, including a facial block and peribulbar or retrobulbar blocks, but general anesthesia can also be employed. An eyelid speculum creating good exposure of the superior bulbar conjunctiva is required. The entire corneal epithelium needs to be removed. This debridement is usually easily accomplished with a sharp rounded blade (e.g., Beaver No. 57).

Any necrotic stroma also needs to be excised without creating a descemetocele or perforation. The debridement is best performed at the beginning of the surgery so as not to neglect to perform it after the flap is created. In addition, any bleeding near the limbus will have time to undergo hemostasis while the flap is being fashioned.

A traction suture (e.g., 6-0 Mersilene or Vicryl on a spatulated needle) is placed in clear cornea just inside the superior limbus, allowing downward rotation of the globe during flap dissection. The superior bulbar conjunctiva is ballooned away from Tenon's capsule with 1 to 2 cc of local anesthesia (e.g., 1% to 2% lidocaine). It should be injected through a fine needle from a location lateral to the edge of the flap so as not to create a "buttonhole" in the flap. Using the traction suture, the eye is rotated downward. A 3- to 4-mm horizontal incision is made with Wescott scissors 12 to 14 mm superior to the limbus through conjunctiva, but not into Tenon's fascia. Then blunt and sharp dissection is performed with the Wescott scissors separating conjunctiva from Tenon's, ideally in the plane created by the local anesthesia (Fig. 14–1*A*). The dissection is carried out in a meticulous fashion to the limbus. Care is required to not shred the superior edge of the flap. Buttonhole formation should also be avoided, although this may be difficult in areas of conjunctival scarring from previous surgery or trauma. Once most or all of the conjunctiva is dissected down to the superior limbus, the horizontal superior conjunctival incision can be extended several millimeters toward the canthi nasally and temporally (Fig. 14–1*B*). The nasal and temporal portions of the flap then need to be undermined. Once the entire flap has been created, the conjunctival dissection is continued forward to poke through the conjunctiva at the superior limbus. A conjunctival peritomy is then performed for 360 degrees. A small amount of undermining of the inferior limbal conjunctiva often makes the peritomy and subsequent suturing of the inferior half of the conjunctiva easier. The limbus is then debrided of any remaining epithelium.

Once the entire corneal epithelium has been removed, the whole flap has been undermined, and the peritomy carried out for 360 degrees, the flap is gently brought down to cover the cornea. It is first sutured inferiorly to episclera and the inferior conjunctiva in two to four locations, depending on the amount of traction. Interrupted or horizonal mattress sutures (e.g., 8-0 or 9-0 Vicryl) can be used. Once the episcleral sutures have secured the flap inferiorly, any gapes in the con-

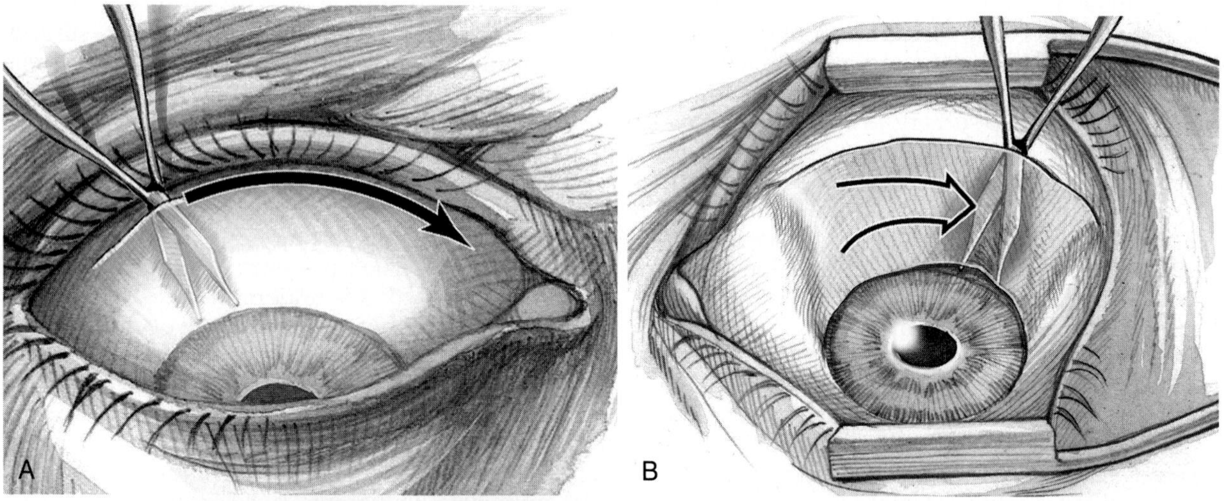

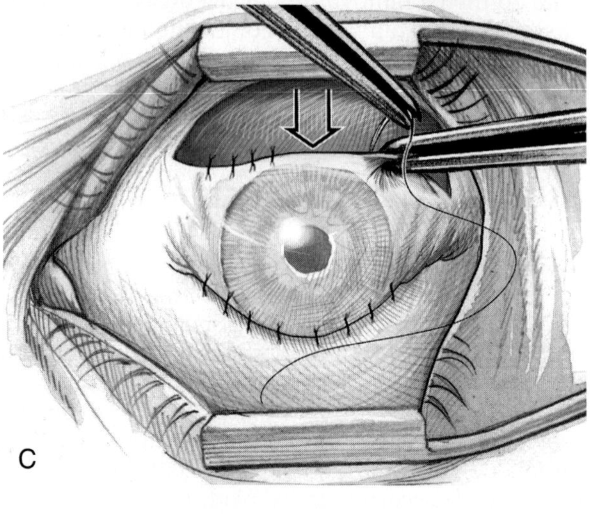

Figure 14–1. *A.* The epithelium has been debrided and the superior conjunctiva ballooned with local anesthesia. While the limbal traction suture is used to pull the eye downward, a small conjunctival incision is made 12 to 14 mm superior to the limbus, and blunt and sharp dissection are used to create a thin flap. *B.* Once the dissection has reached the limbus, the superior incision is extended nasally and temporally. *C.* After the entire flap is fashioned, a 360 degree conjunctival peritomy is performed. The flap is brought down over the cornea and sutured to episclera and conjunctiva inferiorly, and episclera superiorly. Care should be taken to avoid buttonholes and excessive traction on the flap.

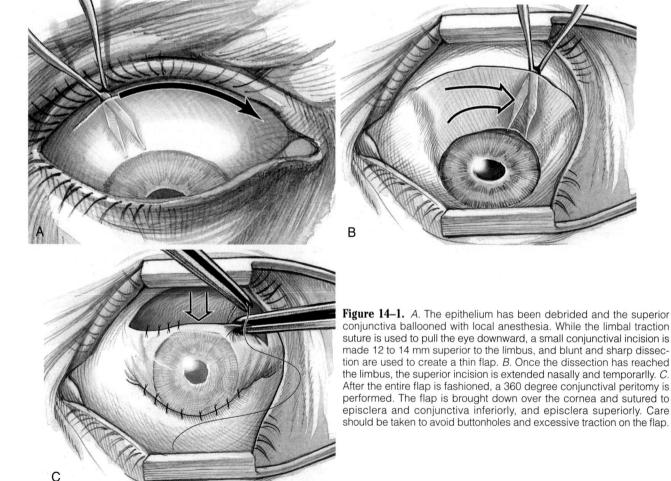

junctival closure can be sutured with simple interrupted sutures. Superiorly, multiple interrupted or horizontal mattress sutures are used to secure the flap to Tenon's and the episclera (Fig. 14–1C). Subconjunctival antibiotics and steriods are injected inferiorly at the conclusion of surgery.

Buttonholes of the flap are the most common intraoperative complication. Great care should be taken to avoid them by careful flap dissection, always paying attention to both the inferior and superior surfaces of the flap. Buttonholes can lead to flap retraction. When buttonholes occur, they should be closed with fine nonabsorbable interrupted or purse-string sutures (e.g., 10-0 or 11-0 nylon).

PARTIAL CONJUNCTIVAL FLAP

A partial conjunctival flap is occasionally all that is necessary to solve the corneal epithelial problem. A localized chronic epithelial defect, bullous keratopathy, or ulceration may be amenable to partial conjunctival flap therapy.

A similar technique is required, including debriding the epithelium from the area to be flapped and undermining enough conjunctival tissue to cover the involved area without significant traction. A peripheral conjunctival relaxing incision is often necessary to release enough traction. The main difference between a partial and a total conjunctival flap is that in a partial flap an edge of conjunctiva is being sutured into the cornea. Therefore it is helpful to create a ledge of cornea into which to suture the conjunctiva. A groove is made into healthy cornea at the edge of the intended extension of the flap with a diamond or metal blade and a small triangle of cornea is removed to create the ledge. Once the flap is created, the edge is sutured into the corneal ledge (e.g., using 9-0 Vicryl). The peripheral edge is sutured to episclera as with a full conjunctival flap (Fig. 14–2). If a bridge flap is being created, a ledge can be created at each edge of the conjunctiva being sutured to cornea.

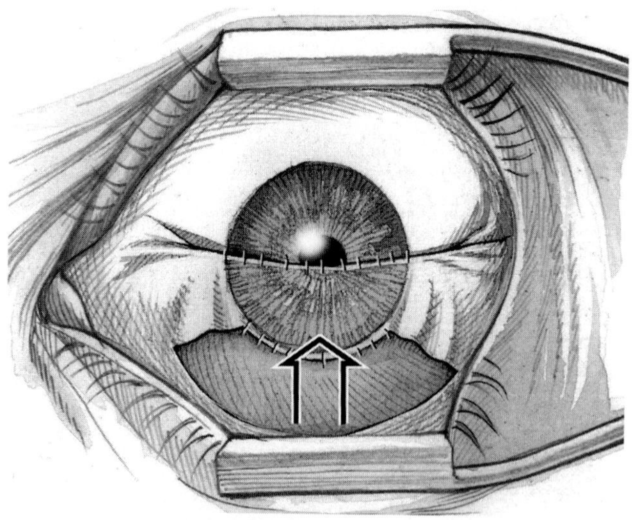

Figure 14–2. An inferior partial conjunctival flap has been fashioned. The superior aspect of the flap was sutured to a ledge of cornea. A conjunctival relaxing incision was created inferiorly, and the inferior aspect of the flap was sutured to the episclera inferiorly.

POSTOPERATIVE CARE

Postoperative treatment includes topical antibiotic and corticosteriod ointment at first, and then drops. Postoperative complications include retraction of the flap, commonly from unrecognized buttonholes or inadequate suturing. Fluid accumulation under the flap can occur when a perforation or leaking descemetocele was not detected preoperatively. Epithelial cyst formation can occur if epithelial cells remain and proliferate under the flap.

Conjunctival flaps are generally permanent solutions to chronic problems. However, they may be removed once the underlying condition has resolved. Some corneal scarring typically remains, and a penetrating keratoplasty may be required to significantly improve vision. Occasionally, penetrating keratoplasties have been performed with success through very thin flaps.

REFERENCES

1. Pires RT, Tseng SGC, Prabhasawat P, et al.: Amniotic membrane transplantation for symptomatic bullous keratopathy. Arch Ophthalmol 1999;117:1291–7.
2. Gunderson T: Conjunctival flaps in the treatment of corneal disease with reference to a new technique of application. Arch Ophthalmol 1958:60:880–7.

CHAPTER 15

Pterygium Surgery

CHRISTOPHER J. RAPUANO, M.D.

A pterygium is a degenerative wing-like fibrovascular growth of tissue encroaching onto the surface of the cornea. It is generally thought to originate from a pinguecula, a degenerative mass at the limbus that does not invade the cornea. Pterygia, like pingueculae, occur in the palpebral fissure, generally nasally, but occasionally temporally or, less often, simultaneously nasally and temporally. A pterygium may be stable or may grow progressively across the cornea to cover the visual axis. Histopathologically, pingueculae and pterygia are characterized by elastotic degeneration; that is, they stain with elastin but are not sensitive to elastase.

Pterygia are likely a result of actinic degeneration of the conjunctiva and cornea related to ultraviolet light exposure, possibly exacerbated by other environmental factors such as wind and dust. Pterygia are much more common in people who live close to the equator than those in more temperate climates. There is also a higher incidence of pterygia in people chronically exposed to sunlight and wind, such as farmers and fishermen.

The management of the pterygium depends on the patient's symptoms and the pterygium's rate of progression. Inflamed pterygia often respond to ocular lubrication; a short course of topical corticosteroids can be useful.

Indications for surgical excision of pterygia include chronic inflammation not responding to medical therapy and enlargement causing visual loss or an intolerable cosmetic appearance. Occasionally small pterygia can cause cosmetically significant redness and inflammation and require surgical removal. In addition, some pterygia can cause symptomatic contact lens intolerance. The primary indication for surgical removal of pterygia is threat of or actual visual loss. Pterygia can impair vision by causing significant corneal astigmatism or by actually invading the visual axis. When a pterygium is noted to be progressing toward the visual axis, even if no significant loss of vision has occurred, surgical removal is often performed before the pterygium extends so close to the center of the cornea that surgical removal involves the visual axis. Pterygium surgery should not be taken lightly, however, as significant potential complications exist, not the least of which is recurrence of the pterygium, occasionally worse than the original disease.

SURGICAL TECHNIQUE

PRIMARY PTERYGIUM

The goals of pterygium surgery are to remove the pterygium, restore the conjunctival anatomy, leave the cornea as smooth and clear as possible, and prevent recurrences. Historically there have been, and there continue to be, numerous techniques to achieve these goals. The lack of consensus on the preferred surgical approach is due to recognition that no one surgical method is far superior to the rest. The following will describe the widely used technique of pterygium excision and conjunctival transplant.

Anesthesia is usually achieved with a peribulbar or retrobulbar block, but occasionally topical anesthesia can be used. A facial block is helpful to achieve the best exposure to harvest the conjunctival transplant. After an eyelid speculum is inserted, a traction suture (e.g., 6-0 Mersilene or Vicryl on a spatulated needle) is placed in clear cornea at the "12-o'clock" limbus. Hand-held or other cautery or a surgical marking pen is used

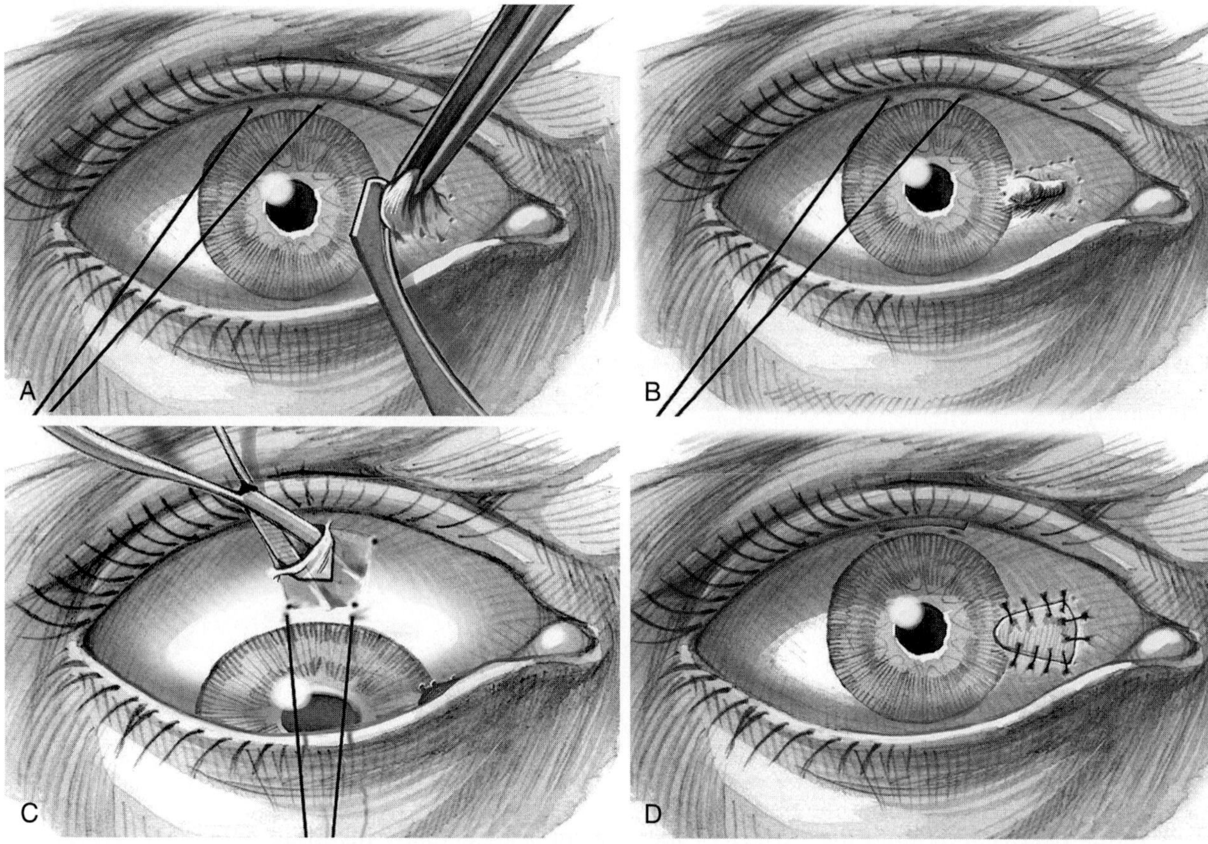

Figure 15–1. *A.* A superior limbal traction suture is in place. Light conjunctival cautery marks have been placed to outline the pterygium prior to undermining it with local anesthesia. *B.* A rounded end blade is used to create a plane between the pterygium and the cornea. A forward-to-backward pushing motion is generally most successful in producing a smooth surface. *C.* After marking the four corners of the conjunctival graft and injecting local anesthesic to separate the conjunctiva from Tenon's layer, the surgeon uses Wescott scissors to create the conjunctival graft. *D.* Multiple sutures are used to secure the conjunctival graft.

to outline the edge of the pterygium to be excised (Fig. 15–1*A*). Care is required to cauterize just conjunctiva, and not sclera. Attempts should be made not to excise the plica semilunaris and caruncle. Local anesthesia (e.g., lidocaine 1% to 2%) is then used to balloon the pterygium, separating it from the sclera. The landmarks of the pterygium are lost, but the cautery or pen marks will still be visible. Following the cautery or pen marks, Wescott scissors are used to incise the conjunctival portion of pterygium, down to bare sclera. This portion of the pterygium is then dissected off bare sclera to the limbus, where it is still attached to the globe. Typically, there is a small amount of bleeding, which clots on its own, but judicious cautery may be used when necessary. Care needs to be taken not to cut the rectus muscle. This warning is especially important in excision of recurrent pterygia.

The corneal portion of the pterygium is then excised. The goal is to find or create a smooth plane between the pterygium and the cornea. A rounded blade (e.g., Beaver No. 57) is used to push (not cut) the most central aspect of the pterygium toward the limbus in attempt to find this plane (Fig. 15–1*B*). This forward-to-backward pushing motion is continued until the entire corneal aspect of the pterygium reaches the limbus and connects to the conjunctival pterygium dissection. Occasionally, a plane is not easily found and some side-to-side cutting with the blade is necessary, although all attempts should be made to achieve a smooth corneal surface. The entire pterygium is then removed from the eye and placed flat on a firm platform, such as a piece of cardboard from the suture package, and fixed in formalin and sent for pathologic examination. A large diamond burr (e.g., 4- to 5-mm diameter) on a handheld drill can be applied in a circular motion to smooth the corneal surface.

The rolled edges of the remaining conjunctiva are unraveled with forceps, and the conjunctival defect is then measured with calipers. The globe is rotated downward with the limbal traction suture and the superior bulbar conjunctiva away from the pterygium excision is exposed. Cautery or a surgical marking pen is used to mark four corners of the conjunctival graft to be created just slightly larger than the conjunctival defect to be filled. Here, too, care must be taken to mark just the conjunctiva, and not the sclera. From a site outside the graft area, local anesthesia (e.g., lidocaine 1% to 2%) is injected to balloon the conjunctiva, separating it from Tenon's capsule. Ideally, one plane is created in the area from which the graft will be harvested. Wescott scissors are used to enter the plane created by the local anesthesic at one of the superior corners, just outside a cautery or pen mark. A small (e.g., 2- to 3-mm) opening is created, and careful blunt dissection is performed with the Wescott scissors, always attempting to stay in the same plane (Fig. 15–1*C*). Some sharp dissection is usually required. The graft should be relatively thin without buttonholes. The dissection should continue until the entire graft area is undermined and free from Tenon's. Then the edges of the conjunctival graft can be cut, but the graft should not be moved from its location yet. Once the graft is totally free, the area to be grafted is reexamined to make sure it is clear of significant clot or active bleeding. Fine forceps are then used to gently slide the conjunctival graft to its new location, making certain to keep the epithelial side up. Once in place, the conjunctival transplant is stretched into position. The cautery or pen marks at the corners of the graft should be visible if it is right side up.

The conjunctival transplant is then sutured into position using nonabsorbable (e.g., 9-0 nylon) or absorbable (e.g., 8-0 or 9-0 Vicryl) sutures. The first sutures are positioned through the two limbal corners of the graft, into episclera, and then into conjunctiva to place the limbal edge of the graft on gentle stretch. The next two sutures secure the posterior corners of the graft to the bulbar conjunctiva. Additional sutures are placed to close the wound edges. A typical conjunctival graft measures approximately 6 × 8 mm and may require 8-15 sutures (Fig. 15–1*D*). If the limbal edge is on good stretch, no additional sutures are required on that edge. Occasionally, a horizontal mattress suture is helpful to tack down the limbal graft edge. Suture knots are generally not buried, as that makes removal, if necessary, much more difficult. It is important to suture the graft to conjunctival edges, and not just Tenon's, as these two tissues may appear similar. Any large buttonholes should be sutured with fine nonabsorable suture (e.g., 10-0 or 11-0 nylon). Routine postoperative subconjunctival corticosteroids and antibiotics are used.

RECURRENT PTERYGIUM

Recurrent pterygia are difficult to treat for a variety of reasons. The most important is that the pterygium in that eye is now known to have a tendency to recur. Second, there tends to be more scarring of both the cornea and the sclera underlying the pterygium. This additional scarring makes surgical removal on the corneal side more involved, as a smooth surgical plane is often impossible to find, potentially resulting in more corneal irregularity and scarring. In addition, surgical excision on the scleral side is more difficult, resulting in more bleeding and a greater danger that the surgeon will unintentionally cut underlying tissue. Great care needs to be taken to lift up on the pterygium when excising it, so as not to incise the underlying rectus muscle, which is often adherent to a recurrent pterygium. Severe recurrences can be so extensive that they limit rotation of the globe and require extensive dissection. If a conjunctival graft was performed during the previous operation, the superior bulbar conjunctiva will also be more difficult to dissect to fashion another conjunctival graft. If there is severe enough conjunctival scarring to make the conjunctival graft impossible to fashion, then it may be taken from the fellow (uninvolved) eye. This possibility needs to be discussed with the patient prior to surgery. Alternatively, an amniotic membrane graft may be used to cover the bare sclera.

If the corneal scarring is still severe once the recurrent pterygium (or rarely the primary pterygium) is removed from the cornea, then a lamellar keratoplasty may be required. The following is a brief description; details can be found elsewhere in this chapter. Once the pterygium has been excised from both the cornea and the sclera, and it is determined that the central cornea is too scarred or irregular to function properly (and too severe to be a good candidate for subsequent excimer laser phototherapeutic keratectomy), the area of pathology is measured. A circular graft is most commonly performed. A partial-thickness trephination is then performed, encompassing the area of pathology, ideally ending outside the visual axis. The scarred anterior cornea is removed with a Martinez dissector, leaving as smooth a lamellar bed as possible. The lamellar graft is then sutured into position using interrupted nonabsorbable sutures (e.g., 10-0 nylon) burying the knots on the recipient side. If there is a large area of bare sclera remaining, a conjunctival graft is also performed.

POSTOPERATIVE CARE

Postoperative care includes topical antibiotics and corticosteroids. Initially, ointments are preferred over drops (e.g., combination tobramycin/dexamethasone 4 to 6 times a day) as they tend to be more comfortable and aid in reepithelialization. Once both corneal and conjunctival reepithelialization has occurred, the medication can be changed to corticosteroid drops, which are tapered slowly over several months. Absorbable sutures tend to fall out over several weeks. Nonabsorbable sutures should be removed between 3 and 6 weeks postoperatively.

Postoperative complications include corneal infiltrate and/or ulceration in the area of the pterygium excision. The larger the corneal epithelial defect and the more irregular the remaining corneal surface, the higher the risk for healing problems. Routine antibiotic use is usually successful in preventing this complication, but should it occur, the infiltrate should be scraped for smears and cultures and treated with intensive topical antibiotics. Delayed healing of the superior bulbar conjunctival defect is rare, but that area must be evaluated on each early postoperative visit. Occasionally, additional lubrication or even temporary punctal occlusion may be required to enhance conjunctival healing. Infrequently, poor healing of the conjunctival graft can also occur. Large buttonholes, poor wound apposition, and excessive tension on the graft causing cheese-wiring of sutures all increase the chances of early graft healing problems. During the first two postoperative weeks there is often significant edema of the conjunctival graft. Continued frequent use of topical corticosteroids leads to resolution of the edema, which does not affect graft survival as long as the sutures holding the conjunctival transplant do not loosen prematurely. Significant graft swelling can cause dellen formation, which needs to be treated with aggressive lubrication.

The most common, and feared, complication of pterygium surgery is recurrence. Occasionally, a recurrent pterygium can be as bad as, or worse than, the original. The fear of recurrence is the reason most surgeons perform a conjunctival graft as a primary procedure with a pterygium excision, as this additional surgery reduces the recurrence rate from upwards of 70% to 80% to 5% to 15%. In an elderly person, where the recurrence rate is lower, with a small conjunctival portion of the pterygium, the conjunctival graft may be omitted, as it increases the difficulty and duration of surgery. Other adjunctive therapies have been used in the past, including thiotepa and beta irradiation, but these have largely been abandoned because of poor results or significant complications. Topical mitomycin C has been used postoperatively for days to weeks after bare scleral pterygium excision with very good results. This adjunctive therapy, however, has been associated with rare but devastating ocular complications. More recently, topical mitomycin C has been used both on bare sclera and under conjunctival flaps applied just during surgery (similar to the way it is used during glaucoma procedures). The jury is still out on the results of these techniques, but improvements on the current imperfect pterygium procedures are always welcome.

CHAPTER 16

Excimer Laser Phototherapeutic Keratectomy

CHRISTOPHER J. RAPUANO, M.D.

Anterior corneal pathology has been treated successfully by lamellar keratectomy for many years. Traditionally, lamellar keratectomy has been performed using a blade to remove the offending corneal tissue. When an anatomic surgical plane can easily be found, these blade keratectomies can be extremely successful. Two common problems are the difficulty treating small areas of pathology with a relatively large blade and the irregular base that often remains, especially if a smooth surgical plane cannot be found. Recently, the excimer laser has been used to treat superficial corneal opacities with good success.[1] When the excimer laser is used to treat anterior corneal pathology it is termed phototherapeutic keratectomy (PTK).

INDICATIONS AND CONTRAINDICATIONS

Indications for PTK include anterior corneal conditions affecting visual function. "Anterior" is typically defined as the superficial one third of the cornea, but the best results are obtained in patients whose pathology involves less than 15% to 20% corneal thickness. For safety, the cornea should be at least 250 microns thick at the end of the surgery, but again, the best results are in patients whose bulk of pathology does not extend to near the 250 micron level. More specifically, indications for PTK include epithelial basement membrane and Bowman's membrane dystrophies such as anterior basement membrane dystrophy and Reis-Bucklers dystrophy. Additionally, stromal dystrophies, such as lattice and granular dystrophies, the bulk of which involves the anterior ⅕ of the cornea, are also good candidates for PTK. Anterior stromal scars, which appear after corneal ulcers, ethylene diamine tetraacetic acid (EDTA) chelation of band keratopathy, trauma or surgery (e.g., pterygium surgery), are also fairly good candidates for PTK as long as the cornea is not too thin to start with. While the excimer laser can remove calcium from the corneal surface, it often leaves an extremely irregular base because the density of band keratopathy is not uniform. In addition, sodium EDTA chelation does an excellent job of removing superficial calcium without damaging underlying tissue. Consequently, PTK is generally not used primarily for band keratopathy, but it can be successful in treating residual anterior corneal scarring after EDTA chelation.

Elevated corneal lesions, such as Salzmann's nodular degeneration and keratoconus nodules can respond remarkably well to PTK. Remember, these lesions may also respond nicely to simple lamellar keratectomy with a blade, as a surgical plane is often easily found. Extremely irregular corneal surfaces can also be treated with PTK, but they tend to be associated with areas of significant thinning, so often are not good candidates for such surgery. In addition, it is difficult, although not impossible, to effectively smooth very irregular corneas. Recurrent erosions also respond well to PTK, although simpler, easier, and less expensive options such as epithelial debridement, anterior stromal puncture, and diamond burr polishing of the involved area should also be considered.

As with any corneal surgery, caution should be taken in patients with potential corneal healing abnormalities, such as neurotrophic corneas (e.g., after herpes simplex or herpes zoster keratitis), exposure keratitis, severe keratoconjunctivitis sicca or blepharitis, collagen vascular conditions (e.g., rheumatoid arthritis) and diabetes mellitus. Additionally, patients with herpes simplex keratitis are at risk for recurrence of the herpes after PTK.

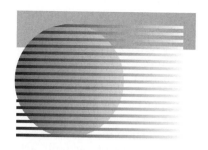

SURGICAL TECHNIQUE

The specific surgical approach for PTK differs depending on the particular corneal pathology. In general, understanding and mastering the treatment techniques for three types of corneal conditions allow the surgeon to expertly treat most, if not all, appropriate corneal pathology. The three different categories of corneal conditions are (1) relatively smooth central anterior stromal opacity (e.g., lattice dystrophy), (2) elevated corneal opacity (e.g., Salzmann's nodular degeneration), and (3) central recurrent erosions. Treatment of many corneas may require a combination of these three techniques.

Relatively smooth central anterior corneal opacities, such as the anterior stromal corneal dystrophies, are excellent candidates for PTK. Often these corneas have a few opacities in the mid-stroma or even the deep stroma, but the bulk of the pathology, causing most of the visual loss or painful symptoms, is quite anterior. Typically the deep opacities are separated by areas of clear cornea, while the superficial opacities are more confluent. Corneas with a significant amount of confluent opacity in the deep stroma, such as often occurs in patients with macular and Schnyder's crystalline dystrophies, are not ideal candidates for PTK.

The goal of PTK is to clear the confluent superficial opacities centrally, with a minimal amount of tissue removal. Therefore, deep opacities are typically left in place. In most of these eyes the epithelial surface is rather smooth, so the epithelium is not removed manually, but rather with the excimer laser. The anterior stromal opacities often protrude into the posterior surface of the epithelium, so the epithelium actually acts as a smoothing or masking agent. A large-diameter ablation zone (e.g., 6-7 mm) is centered over the entrance pupil, and the epithelium and anterior stroma are ablated (Fig. 16–1*A*). Preoperatively, an estimation of the depth of the pathology needs to be determined at the slit lamp, and a certain percentage of this estimated depth, such as 50% to 75%, is ablated (Fig. 16–1*B*). The patient is then brought to a slit lamp, where the effect of the laser treatment is assessed. Typically, more ablation needs to be done and the patient is repositioned under the laser and another treatment is performed (Fig. 16–1C). This "ablate and check" technique, which often requires several trips to the slit lamp during the procedure, is continued until the superficial opacity is re-

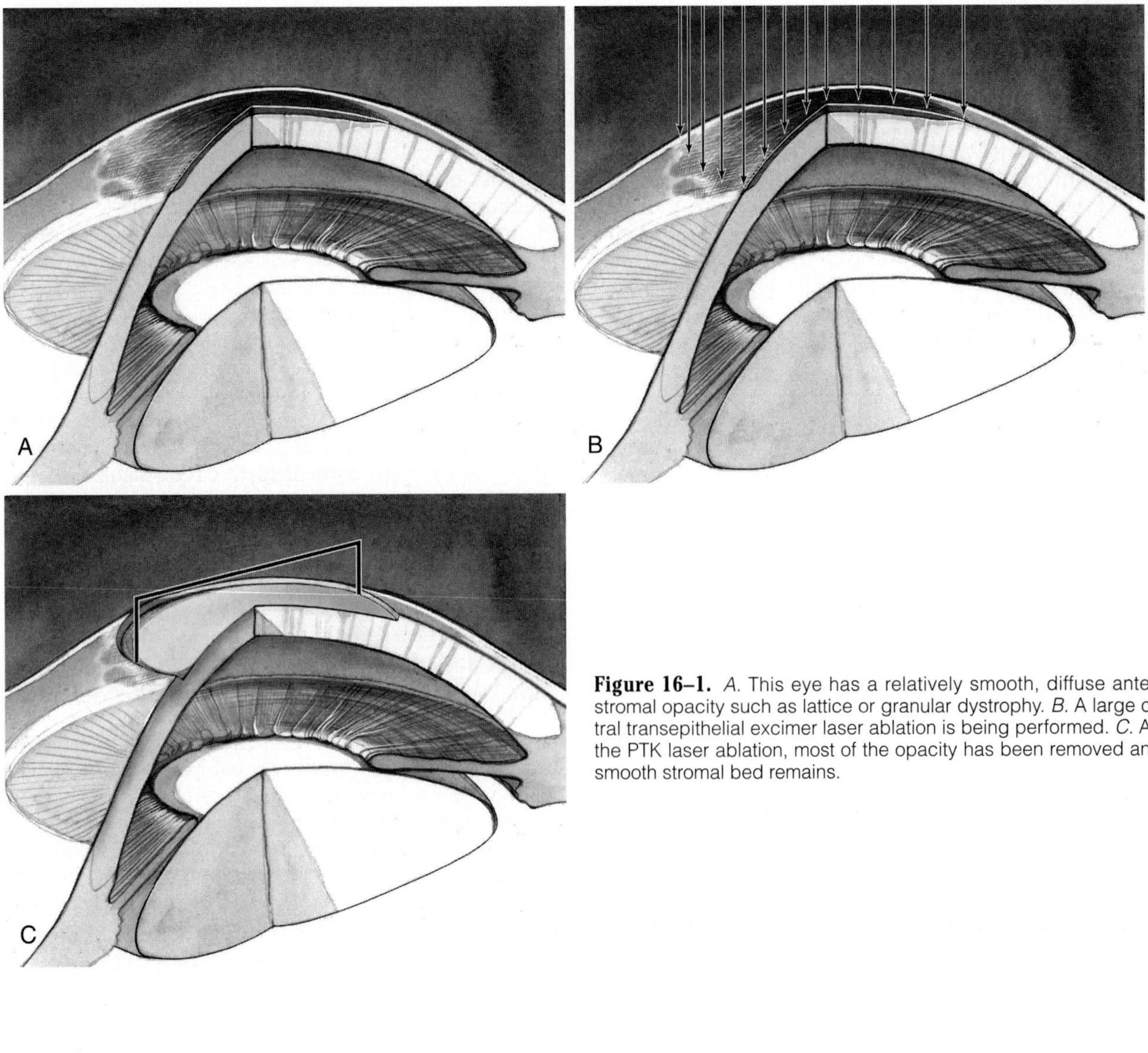

Figure 16–1. *A.* This eye has a relatively smooth, diffuse anterior stromal opacity such as lattice or granular dystrophy. *B.* A large central transepithelial excimer laser ablation is being performed. *C.* After the PTK laser ablation, most of the opacity has been removed and a smooth stromal bed remains.

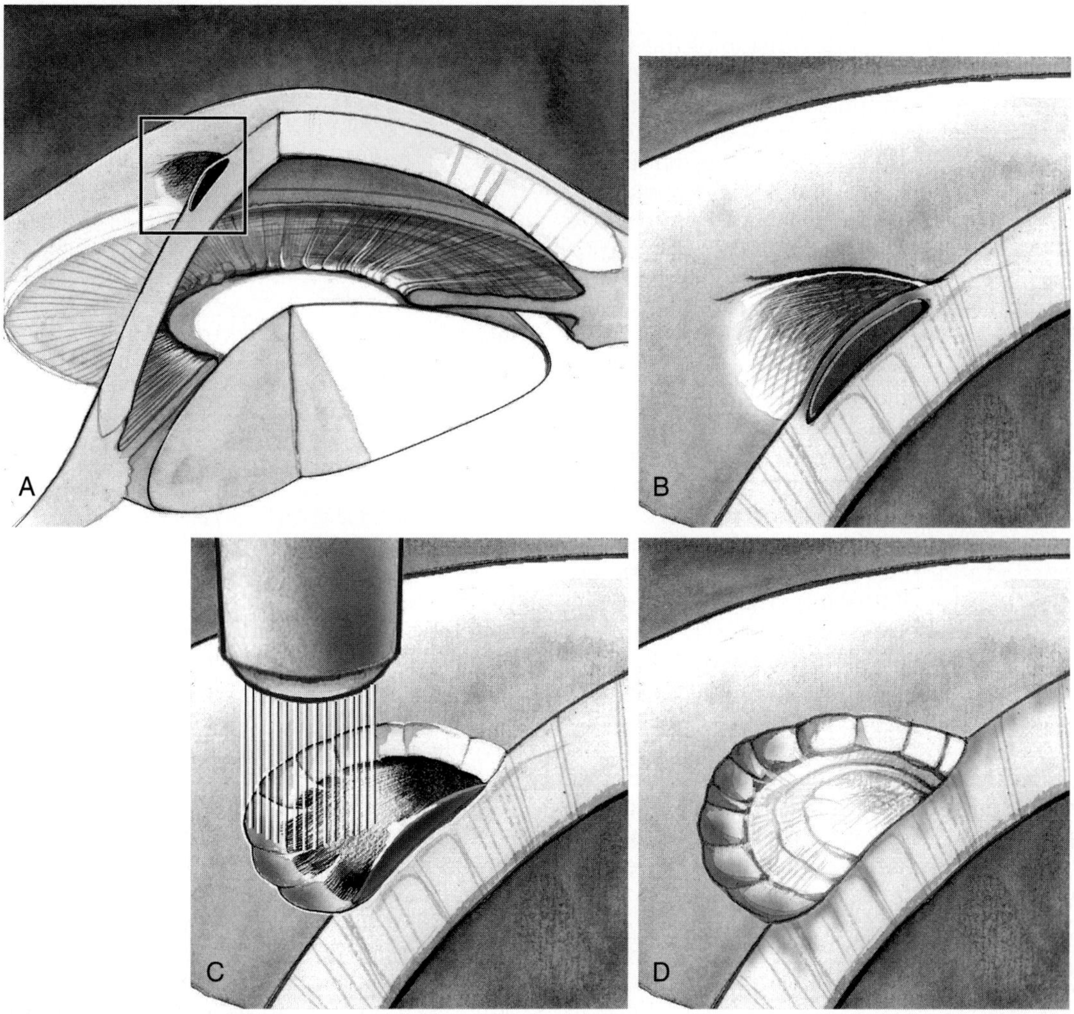

Figure 16–2. *A.* This eye has a localized elevated lesion, such as a Salzmann's nodule. *B.* A high-magnification view of an anterior stromal lesion. *C.* After removal of the epithelium from the surface of the nodule, excimer laser ablation is applied to "shave" down the lesion. *D.* After the PTK laser ablation a smooth stromal bed results.

moved. The surgeon must understand that deep opacities will still be present and must resist the temptation to ablate every single opacity (thereby creating severe flattening and induced hyperopia) if that was not the intention preoperatively.

Elevated corneal opacities, such as keratoconus nodules or Salzmann's nodular degeneration, are often treatable with mechanical superficial keratectomy with a blade (Fig. 16–2*A* and *B*). The advantage in using a blade is that when an anatomic plane can be found, the lesion can be removed relatively simply, leaving an extremely smooth underlying surface. The disadvantage is that when a plane cannot be found, the remaining corneal tissue is often very irregular, predisposing to scarring and impaired vision. Mechanical superficial keratectomy can be attempted, and if a smooth plane cannot be created, a PTK can be performed. For PTK, the epithelium is removed from the top of the elevated lesion, but left in place adjacent to the elevation (Fig. 16–2*C*). A small-diameter ablation zone (e.g., 0.6 to 2.0 mm diameter), depending on the size of the elevation, is then centered on the top of the elevation, and the laser is used to "chip away" at the pathology (Fig. 16–2*D*). The laser beam is aimed at the lesion and slowly moved in a circular fashion around the pathology to fire more at the most elevated areas and less at the lower areas, smoothing the pathology down. The surrounding epithelium is used as a masking agent, preventing the laser from thinning the normal tissue next to the elevation. Masking fluid, in the form of mild to moderately viscous artificial tear solutions, can be placed where additional thinning is not desired. Here, too, an "ablate and check" technique is used to make certain the surgical result is optimal. Once the elevated area is flattened, a larger-diameter (e.g., 4 to 6 mm) ablation zone can be used to smooth the entire area if necessary, taking care not to create significant thinning and flattening.

The third technique is to treat recurrent erosions. In general, PTK is a treatment of last resort for this condition. Here, the epithelium is aggressively debrided over the region of the erosion, extending slightly into "normal" tissue. An ablation zone large enough to encompass the entire debrided area is chosen. A 5-6 micron depth ablation is performed in the debrided area to partially remove Bowman's membrane. One caveat is that when the visual axis is involved, it is probably best if the edge of the ablation ends outside of the visual axis. It would be better to enlarge the ablation zone to keep the edge out of the pupillary area. Although it is uncommon that a required treatment is larger than the largest ablation zone of the laser, it does occur. In this case, care must be taken not to significantly overlap the 5-6 micron ablations to assure as smooth a surface as possible, with the least amount of induced irregularity.

Because one of the common side effects of excimer laser PTK is induced hyperopia, some surgeons have attempted treatments to minimize it. This complication typically occurs in deep, central ablations. In these cases Stark et al.[2] suggested that deepening the periphery of the ablation might eliminate some of the corneal flattening and secondary hyperopia. They described a technique with which a 2-mm diameter circular ablation was used to straddle the large (usually 6-mm diameter) central ablation and deepen the periphery of the large ablation zone (Fig. 16–3). In this manner there might be less induced flattening. The success of the technique is difficult to evaluate because (1) treatment of each cornea's pathology is different and (2) the anti-hyperopia treatment is not currently standardized. Exactly how much peripheral deepening occurs is directly dependent on the individual surgeon's technique. However, many surgeons believe that this anti-hyperopia treatment tends to reduce the amount of induced hyperopia, and most surgeons agree that the best way to reduce the chance and degree of induced hyperopia is by removing less tissue.

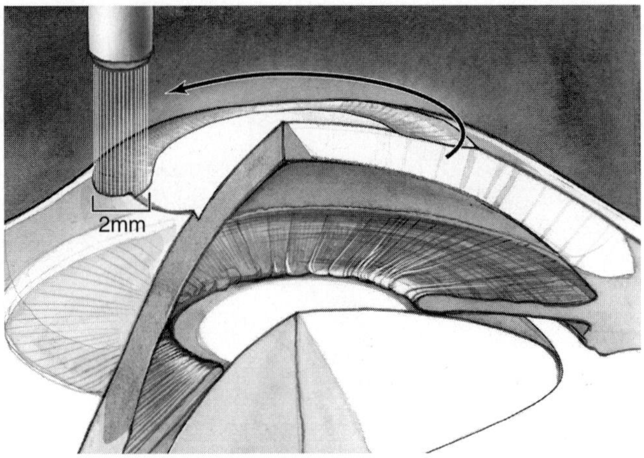

Figure 16–3. An anti-hyperopia treatment can be successful in decreasing induced hyperopia. A 2-mm circular ablation is placed straddling the edge of the large central ablation.

POSTOPERATIVE CARE

Phototherapeutic keratectomy patients need to be followed closely in the postoperative period to make certain the epithelium heals as expected, without a corneal infiltrate or ulcer. These eyes are not "normal" (like most refractive excimer laser patients eyes) and often have healing difficulties. The postoperative regimen generally includes topical antibiotic drops or ointment. Topical corticosteriods and nonsteroidal antiinflammatory medications can be used, but they may impede reepithelialization. Bandage soft contact lenses are often helpful in decreasing postoperative pain, but they have been associated with increased risk of infectious keratitis. Consequently, pressure patching or intensive antibiotic ointment for several days is commonly used. Most surgeons are treating patients with a history of herpes simplex keratitis with prophylactic oral antiviral medications postoperatively to prevent recurrent herpes.

Postoperative complications include the possibility of increased corneal opacity if there is an overly aggressive healing response. Another potential complication is induced refractive error—typically, induced hyperopia, but not infrequently irregular astigmatism, and rarely myopia. Patients with significant irregular astigmatism or induced hyperopia or myopia may require a soft or rigid gas-permeable contact lens postoperatively to achieve their best vision. Patients should understand that dystrophies will recur after PTK, just as they do after traditional lamellar keratectomies and lamellar and penetrating keratoplasties.[3] Superficial recurrences can, however, often be treated with repeat PTK.

Overall, the best candidates for PTK are patients with superficial (top 10% to 20%) stromal opacities, without significant corneal irregularity and thinning, and patients with small elevated central lesions not amenable to treatment with a blade. It is explained to patients that PTK is relatively minimally invasive attempt at correcting their corneal abnormality that is typically, but not always, successful. Additional, more invasive, surgery, such as lamellar or penetrating keratoplasty, may be required to achieve improved visual function.

REFERENCES

1. Rapuano CJ: Excimer laser phototherapeutic keratectomy: long-term results and practical considerations. Cornea 1997;16:151–7.
2. Stark WJ, Chamon W, Kamp MT, et al.: Clinical follow-up of 193-nm ArF excimer laser photokeratectomy. Ophthalmology 1992;99:805–12.
3. Dinh R, Rapuano CJ, Cohen EJ, Laibson PR: Recurrence of corneal dystrophy after excimer laser phototherapeutic keratectomy. Ophthalmology 1999;106:1490–7.

CHAPTER 17

Corneal Transplantation

H. KAZ SOONG, M.D.

Corneal transplantation involves replacement of host corneal tissue with either full-thickness (penetrating keratoplasty; PKP) or partial-thickness (lamellar keratoplasty; LKP) donor corneal tissue. Although the first successful penetrating keratoplasty in humans was performed as recently as the beginning of the 20th century, the notion of transplanting corneal tissue and attempts at such existed at least as early as the beginning of the 19th century. It was not until the second half of the 20th century that substantial advances were made in this field. Up to the mid-1950s, penetrating keratoplasty was considered a medical novelty that was justified only for relatively desperate clinical situations. With the recent advances in microsurgery and suture materials, as well as the advent of topical corticosteroids, the number of keratoplasties performed each year has increased dramatically.

HISTORY

There is considerable contention and debate over who first came forth with the concept of replacing diseased or scarred corneas with living tissue. Guillaume Pellier de Quengsy first suggested replacing the diseased cornea with a thin glass disc (in essence, a keratoprosthesis) in 1789 and Erasmus Darwin, grandfather of the famed Charles Darwin, first suggested replacing a scarred cornea with a small piece of living donor corneal tissue; Franz Reisinger published the results of his experiments on corneal transplantation in rabbits and chickens in Germany in 1824.[1–3] S. L. Bigger successfully replaced the scarred cornea of his pet gazelle with a healthy donor cornea from another gazelle in 1837.[2] Richard Kissam, a New York ophthalmologist and general practitioner, was the first to operate on a human using a pig donor cornea; however, the graft became opaque shortly thereafter.[2] Some of the major advances in the field of general surgery in this early period, coinciding with the early development of corneal transplantation, included the advent of ether and chloroform inhalation anesthesia, topical cocaine anesthesia, local infiltrative anesthesia, and antiseptic surgery. These important companion discoveries were undoubtedly instrumental in accelerating the progress of corneal transplantation.

Considerable amounts of experimental work using living corneal grafts ensued. Von Hippel was the first to improve vision with LKP, consisting of a full-thickness rabbit donor cornea placed into a human recipient lamellar bed.[2] He was also the first to use a circular trephine. A successful penetrating corneal graft in a human was performed by Zirm in a laborer with bilateral lye burns to the cornea.[4] Ironically, alkali burns like this are now known to have one of the worst transplantation prognoses. Professor Anton Elschnig of Prague, with his extensive experimental and clinical work in the 1920s through the 1930s, is credited with refining the crude technique into an elegant, reliable procedure. Filatov, Tudor Thomas, Paton, Franceschetti, Paufique, Sourdille, Castroviejo, Arruga, and the Barraquer brothers, all eminent surgeons, based much of their

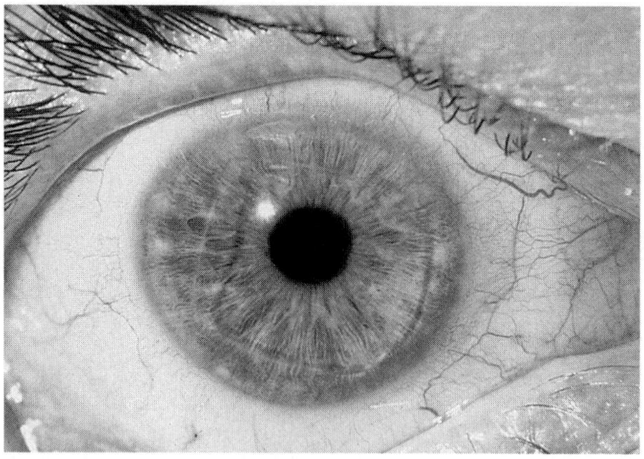

Figure 17–1. Square penetrating graft, performed by Dr. Ramon Castroviejo in 1962 for keratoconus, remains clear 33 years later (photograph taken in 1995).

knowledge and methodologies on the foundation laid by Elschnig.[2] Ramon Castroviejo, a Spanish ophthalmologist practicing in New York City, initiated detailed grafting methodologies, expounding the use of the square graft (Fig. 17–1), and developing and refining keratoplasty instrumentation. A. Edward Maumenee extensively studied the immunology and physiology of corneal graft rejection. Claes H. Dohlman came from Sweden to the United States and established the first cornea fellowship program in 1961, emphasizing the importance of both clinical and research training.

With more recent ophthalmological advances consisting of microscopic surgery, non-absorbable sutures, corticosteroids, tissue-preservation/eyebanking strategies, and progress in immunology, the success of corneal transplantation has grown rapidly over the last 30 years. Paralleling these advances, clinical indications for corneal transplantation surgery have also expanded considerably.

At present, the Eye Bank Association of America records show somewhere in the order of 40,000 PKPs being performed in the United States and Canada each year. This number has been relatively stable in the past 6 years, with corneal edema associated with problematic intraocular lenses (IOLs), i.e., pseudophakic bullous keratopathy (PBK), being the most common indication. The preponderance of PBK in the late 1980s until present as an indication for PKP appears to correlate closely with the dramatic increase in the number of cataract extractions performed in the late 1970s and early 1980s, some of which were complicated initially by the widespread use of prototypical IOLs. As the problematic IOLs, in particular the closed-loop anterior chamber lenses, were discontinued in the mid-1980s, the incidence of PBK has been on the wane.[5] However, with the increasing life expectancies of the present IOL recipient population, even patients with state-of-the-art posterior chamber IOLs may eventually, in theory, manifest PBK as a result of merely living longer.

In the 1950s, when only a small number of PKPs were being performed, keratoconus, corneal scarring, and regrafts were the most common indications for PKP. Comparatively fewer grafts for Fuchs' dystrophy, herpetic scarring, and aphakic bullous keratopathy (ABK) were performed in this era because of the relatively poor prognosis for graft survival. At the same time, the number of regrafts appeared to be on the rise, paralleling the increasing overall numbers of PKPs being performed. With corneal transplantation methodology in its relative infancy, and with the poor availability of donor tissue during this era, the indications for PKPs were biased toward corneal pathologies which had relatively favorable prognoses. With additional advances in corneal transplantation techniques, the introduction of corticosteroids and antiviral agents, and the establishment of increasingly sophisticated eyebanking techniques and networks, the following trends were noted: (1) the expected unmitigated increase in regrafts has not occurred, (2) the need for grafts in herpetic scarring has decreased (owing to decreased incidence of herpetic corneal scarring), while the prognosis for PKP in herpetic eyes has improved, (3) the prevalence of grafts for keratoconus has not changed, and (4) the number of grafts for ABK and PBK has recently reached a peak, and may well be decreasing.[6–8] Table 17–1 shows the relative frequencies of clinical indications for PKP in the United States in 2000.

TABLE 17–1. Corneal Transplant Recipient Diagnoses (77 U.S. Eye Banks Reporting–2000)

Indications for Penetrating Keratoplasty	
Pseudophakic Corneal Edema	19.6%
Endothelial Corneal Dystrophies	14.9%
Ectasias/Thinnings	14.5%
Regraft unrelated to Allograft Rejection	7.3%
Regraft related to Allograft Rejection	4.8%
Noninfectious Ulcerative Keratitis	3.4%
Corneal Degenerations	3.1%
Aphakic Corneal Edema	2.7%
Stromal Corneal Dystrophies	2.1%
Mechanical Trauma	1.7%
Viral/Post-Viral Keratitis	1.4%
Congenital Opacities	1.0%
Microbial/Post-Microbial Keratitis	0.8%
Syphilitic/Post-Syphilitic Keratitis	0.3%
Chemical Injuries	0.3%
Other	21.9%
Indications for Lamellar Keratoplasty	
Unspecified Anterior Stromal Scarring	30.1%
Ulcerative Keratitis or Perforation	27.5%
Keratoconus	13.2%
Corneal Degenerations	12.4%
Trauma	12.4%
Pterygium	2.6%
Post-Keratectomy	1.3%
Reis-Buckler's Dystrophy	0.5%

Source: Eye Bank Association of America, Year 2000 Statistical Report (EBAA, 1015 18th Street, NW, Suite 1010, Washington, DC, 20036).

CLINICAL INDICATIONS FOR KERATOPLASTY

A major objective of penetrating keratoplasty is to remove corneal opacities from the visual axis. Other objectives include correction of abnormal contour or corneal thinning, relief of corneal pain, and removal of infectious or neoplastic foci.

At present, a prevalent cause of corneal opacification is corneal edema associated with cataract surgery (mostly PBK, and less often, ABK). Corneal edema resulting from endothelial decompensation in Fuchs' corneal dystrophy is a relatively common indication for PKP in predominantly Caucasian countries, whereas it is uncommon in Asian and African nations, reflecting a definite racial propensity in this disease. Other causes of corneal opacification that may need keratoplasty include non-Fuchs' corneal dystrophies (e.g., Bowman's layer, stromal, and non-Fuchs' endothelial dystrophies), post-infectious corneal scarring (e.g., following herpetic, bacterial, fungal, or parasitic disease), congenital opacities, traumatic scars, interstitial keratitis, corneal graft failure due to immune rejection and non-immunologic causes, and postoperative complications of noncataract surgeries (e.g., glaucoma, refractive, and retina surgeries). Some examples of keratoplasty indications not involving corneal opacification, include keratoconus, high postoperative astigmatism not correctable with contact lenses or with refractive surgery, ectasia, corneal infections not responding to medical therapy, relief of corneal pain in eyes with intact visual potential, and irregular corneal astigmatism or distortion after surgery, trauma, infection, or inflammation.

In general, corneal disorders having little or no associated inflammation and vascularization have the best prognostic outcomes after keratoplasty; therefore, avascular scars, edema, and ectasia tend to do very well after surgery. Examples include keratoconus, inactive scars, Fuchs' dystrophy, certain stromal dystrophies, and early postcataract extraction corneal decompensation. Better than 90% corneal transplant success rates may be expected with these indications. Although inactive herpetic keratopathy, advanced corneal edema, and interstitial keratitis carry slightly less favorable prognoses, the overall prognoses are nevertheless still quite good. Acute corneal melting with or without perforation and active keratitis of any etiology, in contrast, tend to have poor prognoses. Operating on actively inflamed eyes carries an increased risk of immune rejection, corneal melting, persistent epithelial defects, cystoid macular edema (CME), intractable glaucoma, phthisis, and cyclitic membrane formation. Similarly, problems associated with operating on infected corneas include the retention of microbial organisms in the host cornea and the risk of converting a keratitis into an endophthalmitis. Corneas with significant stromal vascularization have an increased risk of developing suture problems (early loosening, "cheesewiring," and vascularization along the suture tracks) and immune-mediated graft rejection after PKP. Eyes with multiple additional ocular disorders (e.g., glaucoma, phthisis, iridocorneal adhesions, rubeosis irides, retrocorneal fibrous membrane formation, conjunctival scarring, ocular surface diseases, and epithelial downgrowth) tend to have poor prognoses with PKP. These factors must be taken into consideration before deciding to proceed with keratoplasty. Examples of keratoplasty candidates with relatively dismal success rates are those with chemical burns (particularly alkali burns), Stevens-Johnson syndrome, and ocular cicatricial pemphigoid. Less than half of these patients maintain clear, functional grafts after PKP or LKP. Good intraocular pressure control, correction of any ocular surface disorders, and elimination or reduction of corneal inflammation may improve the prognosis in many of the high-risk cases. Avoiding keratoplasty during the acute phase of the corneal disease and allowing the eye ample time to quiet down before performing keratoplasty will also improve the surgical outcome.

On the other hand, if there is concurrent intraocular disease producing progressive irreversible damage to the eye with time, PKP (combined with the proper intraocular surgical intervention) may need to be performed even while the corneal pathology is still in its mild stages and even while the vision is still good. An example of such a case is an eye with early PBK which has a problematic IOL causing progressive CME. Even if the visual acuity were better than 20/50, it may be advisable to perform a combined PKP and IOL explantation or exchange before the CME becomes irreversible. Whether or not to operate this early is understandably a dilemma and a difficult judgment call for the surgeon. As another example, if a patient is functionally disabled by anisometropia in the presence of corneal disease, keratoplasty may be performed early to allow restoration of binocular vision, provided that other options (such as contact lenses) are not viable.

Purely cosmetic keratoplasty in a blind eye is contraindicated in almost all instances. Oftentimes, better cosmesis may be achieved with a cosmetic prosthesis placed over the diseased cornea (contact lens or scleral shell) or over a ball or hydroxyapatite implant following enucleation or evisceration. Painful bullous keratopathy in a blind eye may be relieved with an extended-wear bandage contact lens (although long-term use may be complicated by the risk of infectious keratitis), with retrobulbar absolute alcohol injection (although ptosis, akinesia, and extraorbital extension of alcohol are possible complications), or with a Gundersen conjunctival flap, cauterization of the corneal bullae, or enucleation. Keratoplasty is a relative contraindication in individuals who are at high risk for anesthesia. Additionally, considering the risks of self-inflicted trauma, poor compliance with postoperative care regimens, and loss to follow-up, patients with severe mental retardation, psychosis, senility, alcoholism, and drug addiction are considered relatively poor candidates for PKP. Patients who engage in contact sports or work in high-risk environments for eye trauma may have to curtail such activities or even drastically alter their life-styles after PKP. If adequate visual improvement may be achieved with LKP in an individual who is at a high risk for eye trauma (e.g., a severely retarded Down's syndrome patient with keratoconus), the nonpenetrating procedure is definitely a safer alternative to PKP.

EYE BANKING AND DONOR SELECTION

The first successful human corneal transplant by Zirm in 1905 involved the use of fresh corneal tissue from a boy whose eye was enucleated for penetrating scleral injury. For approximately the next 30 years, all human keratoplasties were done with fresh corneal tissue from living donors whose eyes were enucleated because of trauma or disease not involving the anterior segment.

In 1937, Filatov from the Ukraine introduced the use of whole globes from cadavers stored at 4°C in a moist chamber. This led to a vast increase in the number of donor eyes available for keratoplasty and resulted in the establishment of eye banks to procure, store, and distribute tissue. The duration of storage was still limited to 24 to 48 hours, forcing PKPs to be done on a relatively exigent basis.

The advent of McCarey-Kaufman (M-K) medium in the mid-1970s allowed extension of storage time to up to 4 days at 4°C. Instead of the whole globe being preserved, only the corneo-scleral button was immersed in M-K tissue-culture medium. Dextran was added as a deturgescing osmotic agent, and an antibiotic was added to reduce bacterial growth. Subsequent advances in corneal storage media consisted of the addition of chondroitin sulfate to improve cell survival and stabilization, and the addition of antioxidants. More recent storage media (e.g., Optisol) contain vitamins, amino acids, antioxidants, and ATP precursors, which putatively improve cell survival, reduce autolysis, and maintain ultrastructural integrity. Although storage in Optisol is said to be safe up to 2 weeks, most surgeons prefer to use the stored corneas within 7 days.

Cryopreservation and organ culture preservation are seldom used these days in the United States. Cryopreservation is expensive and technically complicated. Both the freezing and thawing procedures in this technique demand fastidious timing and special precautions to avoid damage to endothelial cells. However, this method allows the tissue to stay viable at −70°C for more than 1 year. Organ cultured corneal tissue is maintained at 34°C incubation, allowing active cellular metabolism to take place during the preservation period. Drawbacks include the complexity of both the equipment and the procedure, possibly a higher microbial contamination rate, and the greater degree of opacity and edema of the stroma at the time of PKP (although the corneas eventually deturgesce and clear after transplantation). The organ culture method is used in several European eye banks and has shown successful preservation in excess of 1 month.

The donor cornea preserved in storage medium is examined by slit-lamp biomicroscopy. An excellent overall morphological assessment of the endothelium, stroma, and epithelium is possible with this method. Storage containers for excised corneoscleral buttons may consist of either glass bottles or plastic viewing chambers. The latter provide superior viewing optics, allowing better appreciation of the anatomical details for either slit-lamp examination or specular microscopy. The tissue is evaluated according to the Eye Bank Association of America (EBAA) guidelines for noting and rating epithelial integrity, epithelial and stromal opacities, presence of foreign bodies and infectious infiltrates, evidence of previous anterior segment surgery, degree of stromal clarity and thickness, presence of Descemet's membrane folds, and extent of endothelial guttae, snail tracks, and precipitates. Specular microscopy of the endothelial cells provides a detailed, microscopic analysis of individual cell morphology and an estimate of cellular density (normally between 2000 and 3500 cells/mm^2; Fig. 17–2). Viewing the specular reflection of the endothelium with the ordinary clinical slit lamp is possible, but it requires practice and experience. Whole globes may also be studied in this fashion, but the quality, optics, and ease of a whole-globe examination are significantly inferior to a corneoscleral button examination. A specular microscopic examination may sometimes be useful in determining whether tissue with dubious parameters (e.g., long death-to-preservation time or advanced age of the donor) is acceptable for transplantation. A major disadvantage of specular microscopic examination is the somewhat restricted field of view offering only a small sampling area. Although specular microscopy is used at many eye banks in the United States, it is perhaps too impractical and expensive for use in developing countries where a dire donor tissue scarcity and a restricted budget often go hand in hand.

In the United States, the EBAA has established donor screening standards which are periodically reviewed by a committee of eye bank medical directors.

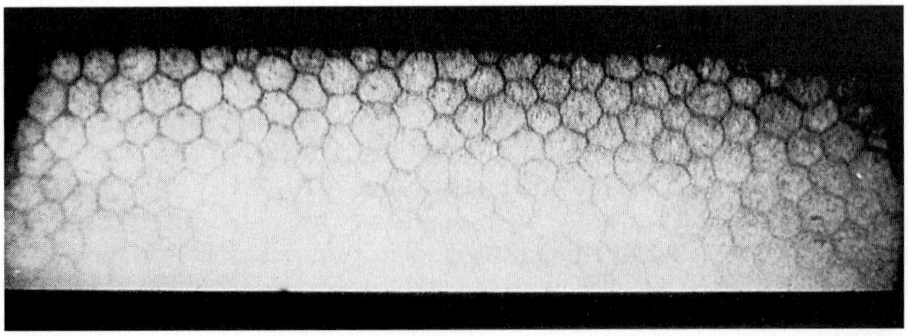

Figure 17–2. In vitro specular micrograph of healthy donor corneal endothelial cells from a 2-year-old donor, showing compact cellular mosaic pattern with uniformly sized, hexagonally shaped individual cells (cellular density = 3015 cells per mm^2).

Other nations have their own eye bank donor acceptance guidelines. Although rarely disease is transmitted from donor to recipient by corneal transplantation (perhaps because of the relative isolation of the cornea from the blood circulation), the transfer of infectious disease and malignancies have nevertheless been reported in the literature. Viral infections, such as rabies and Creutzfeldt-Jakob disease, have been transmitted to the recipient, but the incidence is infinitesimally low. Human immunodeficiency virus (HIV) is, to date, not known to have been transmitted to a corneal transplant recipient. Even in cases in which corneas from donors in the early phases of HIV infection prior to seroconversion were unwittingly transplanted, the recipients remained disease-free.[9] Several corneas from HIV-positive donors have already been inadvertently transplanted[10]; as of the present time, none of these corneal transplant recipients have seroconverted. Recipients of visceral organ transplants from HIV-positive donors, on the other hand, have not been as fortunate; some have seroconverted after transplantation. It is possible that the inoculum level of virus in the donor cornea may be below the threshold needed for infection, perhaps owing in part to the corneal avascularity. Routine hepatitis B and C serological screening has effectively prevented the transmission of hepatitis during corneal transplantation in the United States. In two reported cases, malignancies have been transferred to the recipient via corneal transplantation. Retinoblastoma was transmitted in one case[11] and adenocarcinoma in another.[12] Many individuals who have died of metastatic malignancies have been cornea donors, yet the incidence of transmission of neoplastic disease remains negligible.

Other parameters influencing the acceptance of corneal tissue for transplantation include donor age and death-to-preservation time. Also, the cadaver should be placed in a cold morgue or have ice packs placed over the closed eyelids as soon as possible after death. Although tissue from donors younger than 2 years of age has extremely high endothelial cell densities, it should not be used for adult recipients because of the excessive mechanical compliance and thinness, which may complicate trephination and cause suturing difficulties at the graft–host junction that may lead to poor wound apposition. Infant corneas, in particular, are floppier in consistency, smaller in diameter, and steeper in curvature than adult corneas; thus they are associated with induction of high myopia when used in adult recipients. Infant tissue, however, is ideal for use in pediatric PKP recipients. In general, most eye banks and surgeons prefer to age-match donor and recipients, but this is not a rigid guideline. Some surgeons like to use older donor corneas (e.g., >50 years of age) in keratoconus patients, exploiting the inherent donor corneal rigidity to reduce postoperative myopia and astigmatism. Because keratoconus recipients usually are younger than 35 years of age and have abundant, healthy endothelial cells, the endothelial counts of the older donor become less crucial; however, tissue over 60 years of age is generally not used for younger keratoconus patients.

SURGERY

PREOPERATIVE EVALUATION OF THE KERATOPLASTY PATIENT

Taking a careful and detailed clinical history is of paramount importance during the preoperative evaluation. Information about the pre-morbid visual acuity may elucidate the chronology of the visual deficit, and may provide information on amblyopia, retinal and macular disease, glaucoma, and optic neuropathy. A history of iritis, glaucoma, trauma, dry eyes, herpetic infection, and previous operations may require special alterations of surgical technique and postoperative care.

A history of the patient's general health and demeanor would be very helpful in planning the type of anesthesia. Cardiac, pulmonary, and endocrinological disease may require that specific anesthesia precautions be taken, whereas the presence of uncontrolled, severe systemic disease may contraindicate surgery altogether. The patient's systemic medications may influence blood coagulation, wound healing, and tear production. A history of allergies to some medications may preclude the use of certain intraoperative and postoperative drugs.

The patient's present and anticipated future activities of daily living (e.g., employment, hobbies, and environment) from a visual and physical standpoint should be assessed. The individual's visual needs, as well as visual difficulties, are important factors to consider in making the final plans for surgery, especially vis-à-vis the type of operation to be done and when to do it.

The clinical examination begins with a comprehensive visual assessment consisting of Snellen acuity measurement and refraction for both distance and near vision. Additional testing for glare, contrast sensitivity, and potential acuity may sometimes be helpful. Potential retinal acuity assessment techniques, such as Maddox rod imaging, directional light projection, two-point light discrimination, color perception, entoptic phenomenon studies, laser interferometry, the Guyton-Minkowski potential acuity meter studies, and electrophysiologic tests may aid in the overall investigation of visual function. A swinging flashlight test may uncover defects in the optic nerve pathways. If the corneal pathology is primarily refractive in nature (e.g., keratoconus and scar-related corneal astigmatism), additional useful testing may include keratometry or computed corneal topography.

The external examination may reveal eyelid and/or lacrimal problems, such as blepharitis, rosacea, scarring, lagophthalmos, ectropion, entropion, floppiness, trichiasis, and epiphora. A detailed slit-lamp biomicroscopic examination should search for tear film abnormalities, conjunctival scarring (seen in Stevens-Johnson syndrome, ocular cicatricial pemphigoid, chemical injury, radiation and thermal burns, severe atopic disease, and previous conjunctival surgery), corneal staining or vascularity, and anterior chamber abnormalities (e.g., synechiae and iritis). The presence of these findings may connote, depending on the severity and chronicity, a relatively poor prognosis for PKP. Corrective surgery or medical therapy prior to PKP may be necessary to improve the outcome of surgery. In limbal stem cell–deficient patients, such as those with congenital aniridia or chemical burns, human amniotic membrane or limbal stem cell transplantation may be employed prior to PKP. The peripheral cornea, which will constitute the host side of the graft–host junction, should be checked for extreme thinning. If the thinning is severe, the graft may need to be placed eccentrically to avoid having to place sutures in the ectatic region. In some cases, a lamellar reinforcing graft done before PKP restores the corneal thickness in the host cornea to allow easier and more secure suturing during PKP.

The status of the crystalline lens or the IOL should be assessed for possible cataract extraction or IOL repositioning, explantation, or exchange concurrent with PKP. Intraocular lens types that should be removed are closed-loop anterior chamber lenses, pupillary-plane iris-supported lenses (e.g., Worst-Medallion), and, occasionally, problematic posterior chamber lenses (e.g., dislocated IOLs or those causing uveitis, glaucoma, bleeding, or extremely high refractive errors). Intraocular lens strength measurements may not be as predictive of the final refractive status when IOL implantation is combined with PKP. A combination of good clinical judgment, reasonable choice of cataract/IOL formulas, and personalization of Binkhorst or SRK equations (using regression analysis to estimate the PKP surgeon's refractive tendencies) may enhance the predictability, but high refractive errors are still a major problem in combined PKP/IOL cases.[13] The decison to render the eye myopic, emmetropic, or hyperopic should be influenced by the patient's need and the refractive status of the contralateral eye. The condition of the iris and iridocorneal angle may be a determinant of whether to implant an open-loop, single-piece anterior chamber IOL (Kelman-style), an iris-sutured posterior chamber IOL, a transclerally sutured posterior chamber IOL, or to not implant an IOL at all.

The intraocular pressure may be measured by applanation, pneumo, and MacKay-Marg tonometry, or estimated by finger palpation. When the corneal surface is excessively distorted and precludes accurate applanation, the latter three methods are preferable. Palpational estimates may provide a general appraisal of intraocular pressure, but unless extenuating circumstances are present, these should not be the primary measuring method. The prevalence of glaucoma is high in eyes needing PKP. This is related in part to the older age group of the recipients and in part to the frequent history of prior inflammation and/or ophthalmic surgery. An intraocular pressure higher than 20 mm Hg necessitates better glaucoma control before PKP, by either medical or surgical means. In most eyes, the intraocular pressure tends to rise either immediately or gradually after PKP, making it necessary to keep the preoperative pressure control much below 20 mm Hg to buffer the eye against possible postoperative pressure increases. Reducing the amount of viscoelastic material used during surgery or using a less viscous brand may help avert a major pressure spike after surgery. A visual field examination and an assessment of the optic nerve (if visible) should be attempted prior to surgery in patients with glaucoma.

The retina is examined by direct and indirect ophthalmoscopy for the presence of CME, macular degeneration, retinopathies, and detachments. If the media are clear, fluorescein angiography may provide crucial information on macular disease. If the media are excessively cloudy, B-scan ultrasonography may provide some anatomic clues to the status of the posterior pole. Detection of significant macular, retinal, and optic nerve pathology before grafting may avoid major visual disappointments after PKP.

The patient must be warned before surgery that vision immediately after removal of the bandage on the day after surgery may be blurry, sometimes more so than before the surgery. This avoids unnecessary panic and frustration. The PKP patient should be told that, unlike cataract surgery, the vision may take several months to improve and that new spectacle lenses may not be prescribed for several months until the refraction stabilizes. Patients are also informed that a small percentage of patients may eventually need contact lens correction or astigmatic keratotomy. A well-informed patient is a happier one.

PREPARATION OF THE RECIPIENT EYE

In phakic patients where the lens is to be left intact, it is common practice to instill miotics (e.g., pilocarpine 1% to 2% every 15 minutes for a total of three doses) within two hours prior to PKP. Constriction of the pupil reduces the risk of injury to the crystalline lens and may in some instances facilitate centration of the trephine. In phakic patients undergoing concomitant cataract extraction with or without implantation of an IOL, the pupil needs to be dilated fully with topical mydriatics/cycloplegics (e.g., phenylephrine 2.5% and a second agent such as tropicamide 1% or cyclopentolate 1% every 15 minutes for a total of three doses; CAUTION: 10% phenylephrine should be avoided because of the increased risk of cardiac arrhythmias and infarctions) within 2 hours of surgery. For those patients requiring open-sky vitrectomy, IOL explantation, or IOL exchange the pupils may be dilated. I prefer to leave them undilated if I am to implant an anterior chamber IOL or an iris-sutured posterior chamber IOL. Under open-sky conditions, the pupil can easily be manipulated with instruments or absorbent cellulose spears without prior pharmacologic dilation. Topical antibiotics may be used before PKP, although there is no conclusive scientific evidence that preoperative prophylactic antibiotics are beneficial. Several studies have shown that topical application of povidone-iodine at the time of surgical preparation may be more effective than prophylactic antibiotics in reducing conjunctival bacterial flora.[14,15] Good akinesia and anesthesia of the globe and eyelids are essential for PKP surgery. The surgery is longer than cataract surgery and the open-sky conditions render the eye more susceptible to developing major, unprotected expulsive hemorrhage. For these reasons, I often give a retrobulbar anesthetic injection even when performing the surgery under general anesthesia. This serves three purposes: (1) to reduce the intraoperative vagal stimulation during manipulation of the globe, (2) to eliminate the chance of rectus or eyelid muscle contraction and secondary expulsion of intraocular contents during the vulnerable open-sky period should the patient cough or buck as a result of inadvertent lightening of general anesthesia, and (3) to enhance the degree and duration of postoperative analgesia. The PKP should be aborted if any amount of retrobulbar hemorrhage or a pronounced amount of preseptal hemorrhage is present after local anesthetic injection, as the eye under open-sky conditions is more susceptible to expulsion of intraocular contents than under small-wound surgery such as phacoemulsification. Unlike small-incision cataract surgery with a self-sealing tunnel wound, an intraoperative arterial hemorrhage under open-sky conditions can devastate the eye with frightening rapidity. Anticoagulants, including aspirin and other oral nonsteroidal anti-inflammatory drugs (NSAIDs) should be stopped at a sufficient time before surgery to reduce the chances of intraoperative hemorrhaging. Adequate softening of the globe, especially before open-sky cataract surgery (triple procedure), not only facilitates the operation but also enhances the safety of the procedure. For the same reason, sterile drapes should be applied loosely and the surgeon should avoid pulling on the drapes or pushing on the eyelids during the open-sky period. This period should be limited in duration and an earnest effort should be made to close the wound as quickly as possible.

An eyelid speculum is inserted to allow adequate exposure of the anterior globe. If the eyelid fissure is excessively small, a lateral canthotomy helps to improve the surgical exposure. The canthotomy site usually heals well postoperatively without any sutures. A single or double Flieringa ring is sutured to the episclera. The ring helps support the globe against collapse during the open-sky period and may reduce wound distortion and postoperative corneal astigmatism. Tying the sutures loosely on the ring avoids creating wound distortion. Some surgeons do not use a scleral support ring on phakic or pseudophakic eyes, since they do not distort or collapse as easily as aphakic eyes. The scleral support afforded by the Flieringa ring enhances the maintenance of the anterior chamber during PKP in all eyes, whether phakic, aphakic, or pseudophakic. My preferred method of scleral support is the McNeill-Goldman blepharostat (Fig. 17–3), which combines a double Flieringa ring withthe eyelid speculum, effectively preventing the globe from sinking or collapsing posteriorly during PKP. Theblepharostat is secured to the superficial sclera with interrupted 6-0 Vicryl or 5-0 dacron or mersilene sutures.

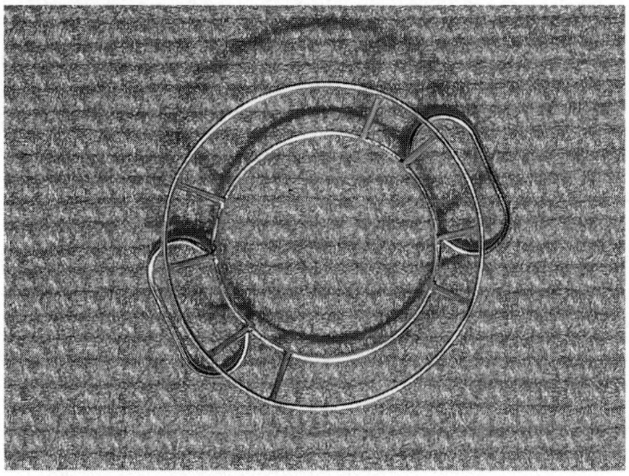

Figure 17–3. McNeill-Goldman Blepharostat composed of double scleral fixation ring and attached wire eyelid speculum.

PREPARATION OF THE DONOR CORNEA

The donor cornea should be completely prepared for transplantation *before* the recipient eye is surgically opened so that the open-sky duration is minimized. Because most surgeons use donor corneas stored in media, the standard procedure is to trephine the donor cornea from the endothelial side on a special cutting block (see section below on Trephines and Cutting Blocks). The trephined donor corneal button is left immersed in storage medium endothelial-side-up until ready for suturing to the recipient. Alternatively, when stored corneoscleral buttons are unavailable, the whole donor globe may be trephined using the anterior corneal approach. Since the advent of storage media and the subsequent reports showing better endothelial survival with the posterior punch method, the anterior approach is rarely employed.[16] An "artificial anterior chamber" device is available that allows excised corneoscleral buttons to be trephined from the anterior approach.

When trephining the donor corneal button, most surgeons use a donor button 0.25 to 0.50 mm larger in diameter than the recipient bed. When punching a donor corneoscleral button from the endothelial side, it has been demonstrated in some studies that this donor–recipient disparity is necessary to reduce postoperative hyperopia and to facilitate and ensure a waterproof wound closure.[17–21] While most studies have corroborated the theoretical advantages of reductions in hyperopia, astigmatism, and incidence of postoperative glaucoma in oversize grafts, Perl and co-workers reported no significant differences in postoperative spherical refraction and glaucoma, and they actually observed more postoperative astigmatism in oversize grafting than in same-size grafting.[20] Another presumed advantage of an oversized graft is the transfer of greater numbers of healthy donor endothelial cells to an endothelial cell–deficient recipient. On the other hand, a theoretical disadvantage of oversizing is the transfer of increased numbers of donor antigens and immunoactive Langerhans cells to the host, resulting in a higher propensity for graft rejection. In recipient eyes with high myopia (e.g., keratoconus), some surgeons use either same-size or undersize grafting to reduce the degree of postoperative myopia. In most such cases, mild oversizing (0.25 mm) of the donor (rather than undersizing or same-sizing) reduces the incidence of wound leakage and facilitates suturing. Achieving watertight closure of the wound with even a 0.25-mm disparity is noticeably more demanding than with a 0.5-mm donor oversize; same-size or undersize grafting requires even tighter suturing and occasionally greater numbers of suture bites to maintain watertightness. With the exception of eyes with excessively steep corneal curvature (such as in severe keratoconus), same-size or undersize grafts also result in noticeably shallower anterior chambers than oversize grafts and may manifest some degree of aqueous outflow impediment. Contact lenses are harder to fit postoperatively in patients with same or undersized donor buttons, as postoperatively they have much flatter corneas.

TREPHINING THE RECIPIENT CORNEA

When trephining the recipient cornea, many surgeons center the circular cut whenever possible over the pupil. Other surgeons prefer to center the trephine slightly nasally because (1) the pupil is often normally displaced nasally, and (2) a slightly inferonasal displacement of the cut conforms better to near-vision tasks. Yet other surgeons may prefer to center the trephination over the geometric center of the recipient cornea, essentially ignoring the pupillary position. The trephination may sometimes need to be grossly decentered and oversized in order to either avoid or better encompass zones of pathology, such as areas of excessive corneal thinning, overhanging glaucoma filtering blebs, foci of infection, or inferior conical apices in keratoconus or pellucid marginal degeneration. The disadvantages of large, decentered grafts include high astigmatism and problems inherently associated with the proximity of the graft–host junction to the limbus—i.e., increased risk of rejection and glaucoma. Small peripheral grafts are occasionally used to excise persistent limbal fistulas following cataract surgery or perforating injuries.[22] These small (< 3 mm diameter) penetrating grafts are particularly effective in closing persistent wound leaks that are accompanied by significant tissue loss, because the graft allows wound closure without the need for excessively tight suturing (Fig. 17–4).

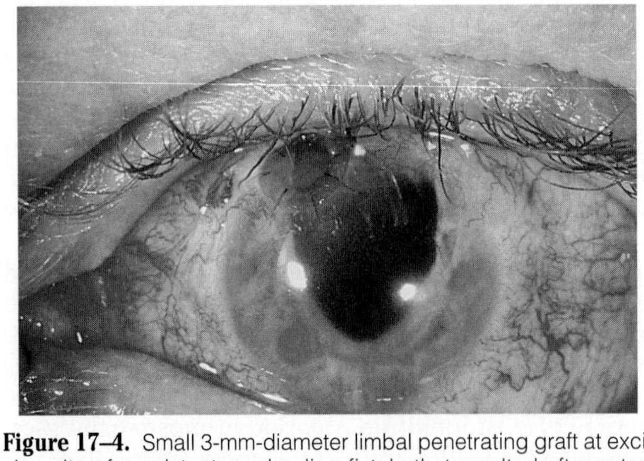

Figure 17–4. Small 3-mm-diameter limbal penetrating graft at excision site of persistent, nonhealing fistula that resulted after extracapsular cataract extraction.

The corneal surface is marked with gentle, but firm downward pressure with the trephine to delineate the size and centration of the intended circular cut. Cellulose spears are used to dry the corneal surface to improve visualization of the mark. In vascularized corneas, bleeding may obscure the trephine mark. Although mild bleeding is usually not problematic, extensive bleeding may need to be controlled with either epinephrine- or phenylephrine-soaked cellulose sponges to constrict the vessels or with either wet-field or heat cautery of the limbal feeder vessels. The graft–host junction itself should never be cauterized because excessive wound distortion, contraction, and leaks may result. Finally, whenever possible, the corneal surface should be covered with a wet cellulose sponge or a corneal shield to reduce the possibility of sustaining retinal damage from the microscope light.

TREPHINES AND CUTTING BLOCKS

Early trephines did not have disposable blades and consequently would require resharpening. As a result, after some time, the circular blades would become altered and distorted. Many improvements have since been made, including inexpensive disposable circular blades, an adjustable central coaxial obturator to reduce the chance of damage to the lens and iris from unprotected entry into the anterior chamber, suction trephines, and motorized trephines. At this time, the most commonly used trephines for use on the recipient eye are the non-suction, obturator-protected, disposable blade models. In experienced surgeons' hands, these trephines perform well. The disadvantages of these trephines include (a) inability to peer down the core of the trephine to aid in the centration and to directly view the central cornea during trephination, (b) tendency of the handle to wobble during manual to-and-fro rotary movements, (c) higher chance of obtaining beveled or tilted cuts rather than straight vertical cuts, and (d) difficulty seeing the entirety of the trephine blade under the microscope with the surgeons' fingers wrapped around the handle. The Hessburg-Barron disposable trephine (Fig. 17–5) with an outer suction ring, an inner cutting blade and no obturator allows the surgeon to (a) peer down the central core of the trephine, (b) avoid wobbly handle movements through a combination of firm suction attachment of the trephine to the cornea and a shorter handle length, (c) make straight, vertical cuts with the aid of the stable vacuum attachment regardless of eye position, and (d) have a clear, unobstructed view of the trephine tip without blockage by fingers during trephination. The suction attachment also makes this trephine use-ful on extremely hypotonous or perforated eyes. Motor-driven circular trephine devices with blade stops that do not obscure the central cornea are manufactured by several companies. Some motorized trephines also have suction attachment capabilities.

Since the 1980s, with the availability of stored corneoscleral buttons, most donor corneas are now punched

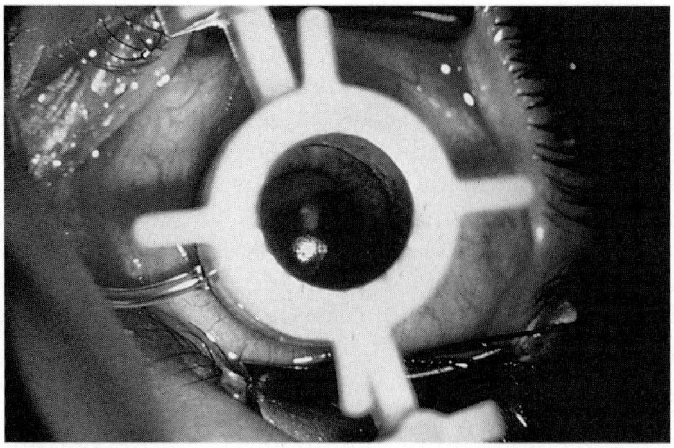

Figure 17–5. Hessburg-Barron vacuum trephine composed of a double-barrel structure, with rotatable inner circular cutting blade and coaxial outer circular suction rings. Cutting blade is turned with the 4-prong plastic handle. Two plastic stabilizing grips are also visible at a slightly oblique axis. Suction cannula is visible on left.

from the endothelial side, either with the free-hand manual method using a circular trephine onto a Teflon block or with a donor corneal cutting system consisting of a guiding shaft for the trephine blade (vertical piston assembly) and a matched Teflon cutting block consisting of a concave well that conforms to the anterior curvature of the cornea (Fig. 17–6). Some systems have incorporated a suction hole in the concave well to more completely immobilize the cornea during the punching process, and some allow the surgeon to choose the well with the best radius of curvature for the particular corneal button being prepared. Other cutting blocks mark the donor epithelial surface to facilitate suture placement at the graft–host junction. These marking systems often have matching markers for the recipient cornea.

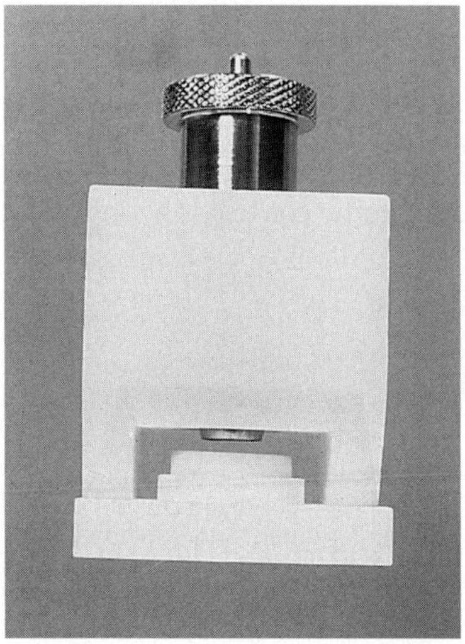

Figure 17–6. A donor cornea trephining system with vertical guiding shaft for the trephine and a Teflon cutting block on the bottom platform.

SURGICAL STEPS FOLLOWING INITIAL PREPARATION

The trephination may be performed through full-thickness cornea or instead through partial-thickness cornea followed by entry into the anterior chamber with a sharp blade. The latter method provides a certain degree of control and safety (especially in phakic eyes where trephine damage to the lens can be minimized), and may permit beveling of the recipient wound edge to allow enhanced watertightness. A beveled wound, however, may produce a higher degree of astigmatism.

In eyes with severe keratoconus, the high cone may come into contact with the obturator or trephine guard and cause the trephine to float, skate, or wobble. The obturator also flattens the cornea, leading to a smaller cut than intended in the recipient. To prevent this, one may retract the obturator higher up into the circular shaft (however, this may increase the risk of damage to the lens and iris during entry), flatten the cone by applying cautery burns just before trephination, or use an obturator-free trephine model.

After trephination, the diseased corneal button is excised with curved corneal scissors. Although a single pair of curved miniature Wescott scissors may be used for both clockwise (right-handed) and counterclockwise (left-handed) cutting, some surgeons may favor the use of separate pairs of right- and left-handed curved corneal scissors. Blunt-tip scissors should always be used for this purpose to avoid inadvertently impaling or cutting iris and lens. The posterior scissors tip should always be angled slightly anteriorly and be in full view to avoid iris and lens damage. If the posterior wound bevel is excessive, it may be trimmed with miniature Wescott or Vannas scissors. The tissue should be trimmed as a long, single, continuous strip whenever possible to avoid the formation of multiple jagged edges of stroma and Descemet's membrane. Overly enthusiastic trimming, leading to an undermining cut of the Descemet's membrane, may increase the chance of astigmatism and wound leakage. After excision of the host corneal button, it is important to ascertain that Descemet's membrane from the excised button is not retained within the eye. In highly edematous corneas, such as seen in aphakic or pseudophakic bullous keratopathy and severe Fuchs' corneal dystrophy, Descemet's membrane is easily stripped off and may inadvertently be left behind in the eye. Retention of central host Descemet's membrane may damage the new donor endothelium. The possibility of Descemet's membrane retention is completely eliminated if additional procedures besides the PKP (e.g., anterior vitrectomy, lensectomy, and IOL procedures) are done as these maneuvers necessitate working posterior to the pupillary plane. Thus, the greatest risk of inadvertent retention is in eyes with highly edematous corneas that require only PKP.

A viscoelastic substance is placed in the anterior chamber prior to suturing the donor cornea in place. Viscoelastic is valuable in protecting the donor endothelium, maintaining the anterior chamber depth, slowing minor anterior uveal bleeding, and improving the accuracy and symmetry of corneal suture placement. The viscoelastic material should be aspirated as completely as possible once the wound becomes watertight. Excessive quantities of retained viscoelastic may lead to severe intraocular pressure rises after surgery. I sometimes place patients on oral acetazolamide for 24 to 48 hours after PKP to reduce the possibility of pressure spikes in the immediate postoperative phase. In patients with a history of severe glaucoma it may be necessary to employ the least amount of viscoelastic or eschew it altogether, and instead use a combination of air and balanced-salt solution to maintain the chamber during the suturing process. In the presence of an anterior chamber IOL, however, viscoelastic is absolutely necessary to avoid IOL contact with the overlying donor endothelium.

The donor corneal button is then secured with four interrupted 10-0 nylon cardinal sutures placed 90 degrees apart. As the donor tissue is gently stretched during placement of the first two cardinal sutures (usually placed at the 12 o'clock and the 6 o'clock positions), a buttock-like groove is formed on the anterior corneal surface, giving the surgeon an excellent cue to equally distribute tissue on the right and left halves. As the remaining two cardinal sutures are placed, a four-cusp pattern is formed by the tensile folds, thus giving the surgeon excellent landmarks to accurately divide the four quadrants during placement of the rest of the sutures. Needless to say, tensions must be equal in all four sutures. Some surgeons (Dr. Walter J. Stark, personal communication) intentionally place the initial cardinal sutures at oblique axes to reduce hand and wrist contortions when suturing the 3 o'clock and 9 o'clock meridians. The corneal sutures should be placed at 60% to 90% stromal depth to reduce posterior gaping of the wound. If the cardinal sutures appear less than symmetrical or radial, the aberrant suture(s) should be removed and repositioned. The anterior graft surface should be flush with the recipient corneal surface without any override or underride. Misalignment of the anterior surfaces is much more prone to refractive errors, scarring, and delayed healing than misalignment of the endothelial surface.

Following placement of the initial cardinal sutures, wound closure may be achieved with the following suturing techniques: (1) all-interrupted 10-0 nylon sutures (16–32 total), (2) a single continuous 10-0 nylon suture (16–24 bites), (3) double-running or torque-antitorque continuous sutures (Fig. 17–7*A*) using one 10-0 and one 11-0 nylon suture (12–16 bites each), or (4) a combination of 10-0 nylon interrupted sutures and a single running 11-0 nylon suture (Fig. 17–7*B*). The all-interrupted suture technique is by far the least technically demanding and is best for use in corneas with peripheral thinning, active areas of corneal inflammation, or significant vascularization. In these clinical situations, when running sutures are used, unraveling or loosening of sutures in one meridian invariably results in loosening of the entire continuous suture. On the other hand, interrupted sutures take longer to place, and the surgeon has to contend with the onerous task of burying all the knots during the surgery, only to struggle again in the late postoperative period with the removal of stubbornly buried knots. Suture knots should be buried to avoid foreign body sensation, epithelial breaks, infection, and giant papillary conjunctivitis.[23] Knots should be buried just below the corneal surface to facilitate suture removal in the postoperative period. Argon laser burns to the buried knots may facilitate suture removal. If complete removal of a suture is not possible because of recalcitrantly buried knots, the buried fragment may be left behind without causing any problems. Running sutures take a shorter time to place. In addition, small amounts of slippage and cheesewiring of running sutures tend to reduce the meridional suture tension disparities. Postoperatively at the slit lamp, the astigmatism may be reduced further by the redistribution of meridional suture tensions with tying forceps (Fig. 17–8).[24] Although these adjustment techniques appear to indeed reduce the corneal astigmatism, the long-term stability of the refraction may be uncertain, especially after all sutures are removed. The combined running and interrupted suture method possesses the additive advantages of each individual technique and allows earlier postoperative selective removal of interrupted sutures in accordance with meridional astigmatism or focal wound healing. The presence of the running suture as a backbone prevents wound dehiscence even if the interrupted sutures are removed as early as 1 week after surgery. Early selective suture removal ostensibly allows a greater degrees of astigmatic control than in the late postoper-

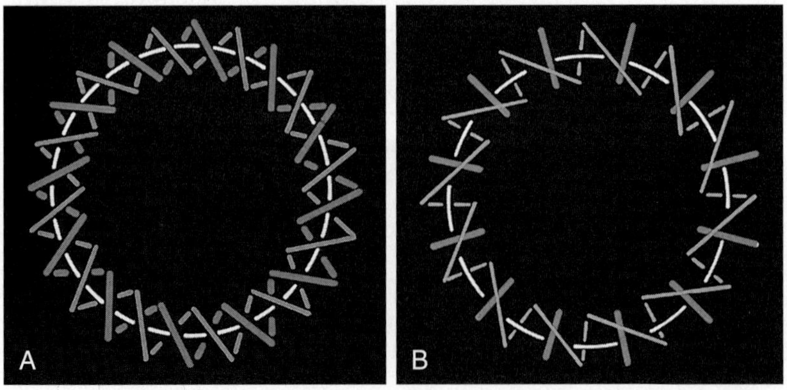

Figure 17–7. Schematic appearance of (*A*) double-running suture method and (*B*) combined running and interrupted suture method. Light suture represents 10-0 nylon, and dark suture represents 11-0 nylon.

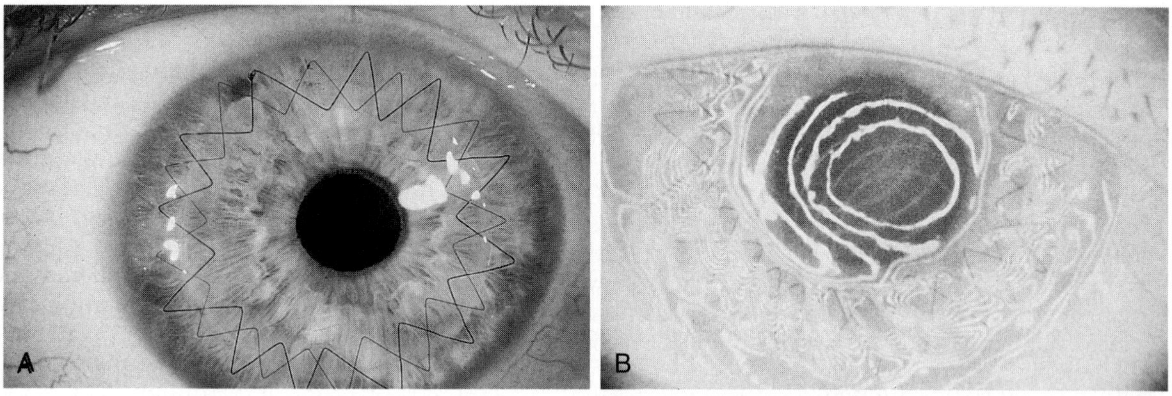

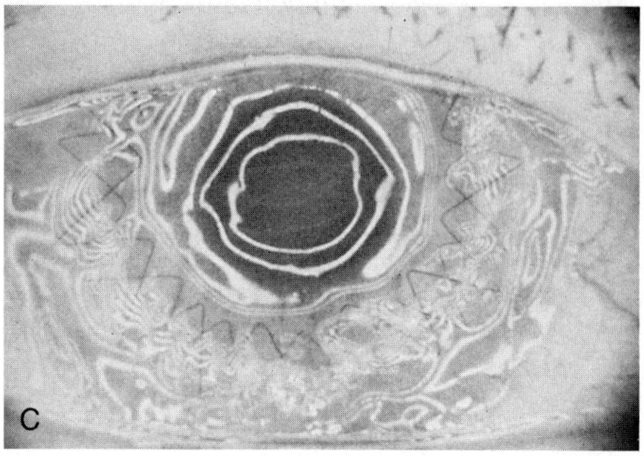

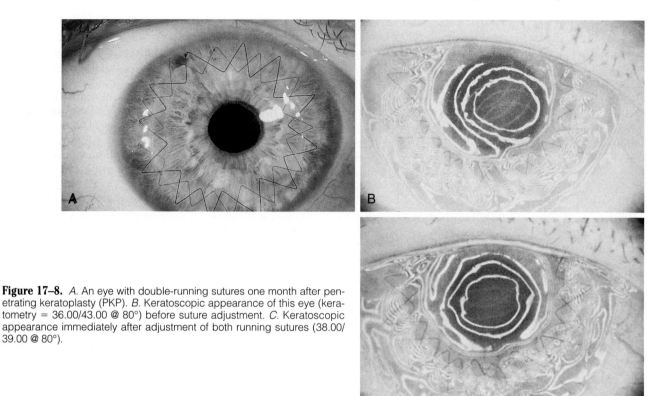

Figure 17–8. *A.* An eye with double-running sutures one month after penetrating keratoplasty (PKP). *B.* Keratoscopic appearance of this eye (keratometry = 36.00/43.00 @ 80°) before suture adjustment. *C.* Keratoscopic appearance immediately after adjustment of both running sutures (38.00/39.00 @ 80°).

ative period, when the wound healing is more established. A double-running suture combines the advantages of a single-running suture with added wound security. McNeill and Kaufman[25] reported earlier visual rehabilitation due to lower astigmatism with this technique. If the astigmatism is significant (e.g., >3–4 diopters), the 10-0 nylon running suture may be removed at 3 months (when adequate wound healing may have occurred). The double-running techniques demand more technical expertise than any of the alternative suturing techniques. Troutman has described the antitorque effects of double-continuous suturing, with the second suture applied in the reverse direction from the first, thus counteracting the torquing effects of the first suture.[26] With any suturing method, intraoperative keratoscopy or keratometry may help reduce the postoperative corneal astigmatism.

Following completion of suturing, the anterior chamber is fully reformed with balanced salt solution. Viscoelastic material is aspirated from the anterior chamber with a cannula-tipped syringe. Short-acting miotics, such as acetylcholine (Miochol) or carbachol (Miostat), may be used to constrict the pupil, especially if the pupil was dilated during the surgery. The graft–host junction is tested for watertightness either by drying the overlying surface with cellulose sponges while looking for fluid leaks, or by performing the Seidel test (both spontaneous and provocative methods) using unpreserved, anesthetic-free fluorescein (e.g., fluorescein paper strips). By raising the intraocular pressure for the provocative test, a less than secure wound may be provoked to leak. For this test, I apply steady, gentle pressure with a blunt instrument *as far away from the wound as possible,* thus avoiding leakage produced by local wound distortion from the instrument. Wound leaks may be treated with additional interrupted sutures or by readjusting the distribution of tension in the continuous suture(s). In general, edematous or "spongy" corneas, such as in bullous keratopathy or decompensated Fuchs' dystrophy, allow easier watertight wound closure than non-edematous, rigid ones, such as in corneal scarring or interstitial keratitis. A cornea that has undergone radial keratotomy may leak from the intersections of the radial incisions with the graft–host junction and may require suturing of the keratotomy incisions.

Tuberville and co-workers[27] suggested that denuding the donor corneal epithelium and its inherent antigens may reduce the incidence of immune graft rejections, but other studies have not confirmed this.[28] Leaving the epithelium intact reduces the possibility of postoperative persistent epithelial defects, infections, stromal melting, and prolonged vision deficit, and therefore appears advisable.

Subconjunctival corticosteroids and antibiotics may be injected into the inferior cul-de-sac. Gentamicin should generally be avoided because of the retinal toxicity and damage that may occur if some should seep into the wound. The subconjunctival injection provides a long-acting depot of medication while the eye is completely patched during the first 24 hours after surgery. Additional use of a corticosteroid–antibiotic combination ointment prior to patching protects and lubricates the corneal surface underneath the patch, which is helpful if the eyelids should open before the patch and shield are removed.

COMBINED PROCEDURES

Penetrating keratoplasty may be combined with other procedures, such as cataract extraction, IOL implantation/explantation/exchange, anterior vitrectomy, glaucoma filtering procedures, or retinal procedures (sometimes necessitating a temporary keratoprosthesis). The advantages of combining such procedures include convenience, reduction of anesthesia risk, and possibly a lower overall risk of CME. The disadvantages include longer operating times, a higher one-time combined surgical risk, and relatively unreliable IOL strength measurements.

Cataract extraction with IOL implantation is technically easy to perform through an open-sky PKP wound, since visibility and accessibility are excellent. The lens extraction process begins with either a "can-opener" or "scissors" capsulotomy, or a continuous-tear capsulorrhexis. This may be followed by either extracapsular nuclear expression or "in-the-bag" phacoemulsification. Both scissors capsulotomy and continuous-tear capsulorrhexis have the advantage of creating a smooth-edge capsular opening, free of tags that may inadvertently be aspirated into the suction port during lens cortical cleanup. They also allow a stable fixation in the bag for the posterior chamber IOL. When these two capsular opening methods are used in conjunction with nuclear expression, it is important to make several radial relaxing cuts along the anterior capsule edge to avoid inadvertent intracapsular delivery of the lens. In contrast, a can-opener capsulotomy, which is characterized by spoke-like radial cuts along the circular edge of the capsular opening, is not associated with this problem. Alternatively, phacoemulsification may be used to fragment the nucleus into smaller pieces that can then be removed with minimal hazard through an unrelaxed anterior lens capsular opening.

If the PKP surgeon opts to express the unfragmented whole nucleus out of the lens capsular bag, this can be accomplished easily by transmitting pressure to the vitreous by applying a gentle, steady push on the midperipheral globe with the "knee" of a muscle hook. As the resulting vitreous pressure pushes the lens anteriorly, the nucleus is prolapsed by spearing and rotating by means of an iris sweep, a Sinskey hook, or a 20-gauge disposable needle on a TB syringe. The nucleus may also be "walked" out with repeated spearing in an alternating, stepwise fashion with two hypodermic needles. Alternatively, the nucleus may be removed by irrigation with a vectis placed underneath the nucleus or by extraction with a cryoprobe. In eyes that have been subjected to chronic miotic therapy and whose pupils cannot be adequately dilated, a radial iridotomy or sphincterotomy may facilitate nucleus expression. The radial iris incision may be sutured after IOL implantation with 10-0 polypropylene sutures. If preferred, iris incisions may be avoided by using Grieshaber iris hooks to stretch open the pupil.

If the nucleus should deliver itself spontaneously after anterior capsulotomy or if the posterior lens capsule should bulge anteriorly after nucleus removal, complicating cortical cleanup and IOL implantation, a small, full-thickness pars plana incision with a sharp disposable knife is made and a 25-gauge needle is inserted through the incision to aspirate liquid vitreous. Enough liquid vitreous is removed to completely relieve the bulge of the lens capsule. The incision is left unsutured as it is small enough to self-seal on withdrawal of the aspiration needle. Intravenous mannitol may be used to reduce the vitreous volume; however, the delay in effect and the risk for use in older patients with compromised cardiovascular function make mannitol therapy relatively impractical. Alternatively, a 27-gauge needle may be passed across the anterior chamber from limbus to limbus, just anterior to the iris plane after the posterior chamber IOL is implanted (limbal skewer technique).[29] This technique will stabilize the implant, restore the anterior chamber depth, and facilitate suturing of the corneal graft. Once the nucleus has been delivered, the posterior capsule is extremely sensitive to vitreous pressure changes, as revealed by the retinal arteriolar pulsations transmitted to the capsular surface. For this reason, no undue pressure or manipulation should be exerted onto the eyelids, malar region, or the drapes. Such pressure changes are easily transmitted to the vitreous, resulting in possible capsular tear and vitreous loss. The patient should be positioned carefully to avoid any extreme Trendelenberg posturing that may further increase vitreous pressure.

Following removal of the lens nucleus, the lens cortical remnants may be removed by mechanized irrigation-aspiration methods. When using machine aspiration, it is important to realize that the irrigation-aspiration tip is working in an open system and does not have the benefits of a closed system (as in small-incision cataract surgery) in which fluid pressure buildup in the anterior chamber aids in pushing the cortical material into the aspiration port.

To facilitate implantation of the posterior chamber IOL into the capsular bag, the anterior and posterior lens capsules are separated by the injection of viscoelastic material. I prefer to use an all-PMMA, single-piece, 7.0-mm optic diameter lens without centration holes. These larger diameter lenses without holes are less likely to be affected by decentration, glare, and ghost image problems, and they easily fit through the large, open-sky wound. If the posterior lens capsule is broken, anterior vitrectomy is performed carefully through the capsular rent. The lens haptics can be inserted into the capsular bag or into the ciliary sulcus. With larger capsular tears or zonular tears, an all-PMMA (polymethyl methacrylate), open-loop anterior chamber IOL, such as the Kelman lens, may be implanted. Alternatively, a posterior chamber lens may be sutured to the iris or to the sclera.

Although a peripheral iridectomy or iridotomy is optional in quiet eyes, it is strongly recommended in eyes that may be prone to postoperative inflammation. Irides are often extremely friable in eyes with interstitial keratitis and may tear easily with the slightest manipulation (iridectomy, iris suturing, etc.).

In eyes undergoing IOL explantation or exchange, rigid anterior chamber IOLs and iris-support pupillary IOLs are usually easy to remove. Closed-loop anterior chamber IOLs, in contrast, are more difficult to remove.

The haptics need to be severed with scissors and carefully slipped out of the cocoon (peripheral iris adhesions around the haptic). Extreme care must be taken to avoid iris tears during this process. Excessive iris tear may result in serious intraoperative bleeding, pupillary eccentricity, and iridocorneal adhesions. Viscoelastic material is instilled to keep fibrin, blood, and torn iris edges from forming peripheral anterior synechiae (PAS). The PAS may progressively distort the pupil and increase immune rejection risks (by placing the avascular cornea in direct apposition to the vascular iris). Sector iridectomies are closed with 10-0 polypropylene sutures to flatten the iris plane, thus preventing the floppy iris edges at the sector iridectomy from forming PAS. Iris sphincterotomy, combined with pupillary suturing, may help with the re-centering of eccentric pupils (corectopia) caused by either acquired or congenital etiologies.

Anterior vitrectomy is sometimes necessary to avoid retinal traction and vitreous contact (or adhesion) with the graft endothelium. It also facilitates insertion of a sutured, acapsularly fixed posterior chamber IOL behind the iris. Mechanical vitrectomy can be performed either through the pupil or through the peripheral iridectomy.

The explanted IOL may be exchanged for a posterior chamber IOL sutured to the iris or sclera,[30,31] an unsutured posterior chamber IOL implanted in the ciliary sulcus (if the peripheral lens capsule is intact or if a Soemmering's ring is present), or a Kelman-style anterior chamber IOL.

Reasonably accurate predictions of IOL power can be made by using standard cataract regression formulas[13] or by using average postoperative keratometric measurements for a given PKP surgeon in standard IOL power formulas. Accurate choice of IOL power is, nevertheless, hampered by the inability to accurately predict post-PKP keratometry, axial length, and anterior chamber depth.

Glaucoma filtering and shunt procedures, when necessary, may be performed before, during (combined procedure), or subsequent to PKP. There are major advantages to having these procedures done before or in combination with PKP, so that the intraocular pressure is well-controlled after PKP, when postoperative pressure spikes are relatively common.

In patients with cloudy corneas undergoing retina and pars plana vitrectomy procedures, the diseased cornea may be temporarily replaced during surgery with a plastic keratoprosthesis to allow intraoperative visualization of the retina and vitreous cavity. The temporary keratoprostheses is then replaced with a permanent donor corneal button at the end of the retinal-vitreal procedure.

PEDIATRIC KERATOPLASTY

Corneal transplantation in the pediatric age group presents special considerations and unique problems. The development of amblyopia and nystagmus and the presence of concomitant congenital ocular abnormalities often contribute to poor postoperative vision after PKP despite a technically beautiful graft. Detailed ophthalmological examination, including measurements of visual acuity and intraocular pressure, is typically difficult and often less than reliable in younger children. Examination under anesthesia is absolutely necessary in the younger age group, but unfortunately precludes subjective visual acuity measurements and may be associated with inaccurate intraocular pressure measurements induced by anesthetic agents. With recent improvements in pediatric anesthesia and with the recognition of amblyopia as a major impediment to useful vision in congenital and childhood diseases of the anterior segment, PKPs are now performed in neonates as early as 2 weeks after birth.

Corneal grafting in children under the age of 2 years is associated with rapid corneal neovascularization, especially along the sutures, and necessitates suture removal as early as 2 weeks after PKP. The eye wall is extremely flaccid at this age and it collapses readily during surgery when the recipient cornea is excised. Other commonly encountered problems include anterior bulging of the lens-iris diaphragm (sometimes resulting in spontaneous delivery of the lens) and the propensity for development of goniosynechiae and large zones of iridocorneal adhesions. In general, the uveal tissues in infants are extremely "sticky" and are characterized by exuberant inflammatory responses, fibrinous exudation, and neovascularization. Viscoelastic substances should be freely applied to the anterior chamber, particularly into the periphery, to prevent iridocorneal adhesions from forming during the surgery. The open-sky wound should be closed as rapidly as possible to reduce the chances of spontaneous lens expulsion and PAS formation. Surgeon skill and speed are of utmost importance in this age group. A scleral support ring is crucial in most pediatric PKPs, particularly in the neonate and infant. Intravitreal pressure may be reduced by preoperative massage or ocular compression, and by use of intravenous hyperosmotic agents, such as mannitol. A small-size graft (e.g., 5.0 to 6.5 mm diameter) may reduce the degree of anterior lens-iris bulge and the chances of PAS formation. Leaving a slight bevel (rather than having a perfectly straight wound edge) in neonates and infants facilitates placement of the initial cardinal sutures by keeping the an-teriorly bulging iris away from the path of the suture needle. The small size of the eye, the thinness and floppiness of the corneal tissue, and the narrow eyelid fissures all further contribute to the complexity and difficulty of surgery.

In monocular aphakes, early fitting of the eye with a contact lens (as early as the time of PKP) may reduce the degree of amblyopia. Posterior chamber IOLs are being implanted in increasing numbers of children, thus circumventing many of the problems associated with contact lens wear. However, IOL implantation in children under the age of 2 years is often associated with exuberant intraocular inflammation and cyclitic membrane formation. Opacification of the posterior lens capsule in this age group is almost a *fait accompli,* leading many surgeons to perform primary posterior capsulotomy/ capsulorrhexis and anterior vitrectomy at the time of cataract extraction. The lens capsule is extremely tough, frequently causing continuous-tear capsulorrhexis attempts to go awry. Intraocular lens power calculations are complicated in infant eyes by inherently steep keratometric curvatures and short axial lengths. Fortunately, by the age of 2 years, most eyes are within 90% of the final adult size. Occlusive, refractive, and pharmacologic therapies are frequently necessary to stem the rapid development of amblyopia. Postoperative glaucoma and immune rejection are extremely common in the younger children, owing perhaps to the hyperactive inflammatory and immune responses. Many pediatric grafts undergo non-immune graft failure and become cloudy for idiopathic, infectious, and inflammatory reasons. Self-induced and accidental traumata are also disproportionately more common in the younger children. In consideration of the frequent, and often severe problems associated with pediatric grafts, especially in the first 2 years of life, patients should be examined very closely and frequently after PKP. Most of the time, either sedation or general anesthesia is necessary for detailed postoperative examination and suture removal. The need for younger donor corneas corresponding to recipient age also complicates tissue procurement and elective surgical scheduling. If the corneal opacity is central and small, a safer and easier alternative to PKP is an optical iridectomy, which allows the patient to see around the opacity, thus avoiding the pitfalls of PKP. The parents should be highly motivated and play a pivotal role in maintaining therapeutic compliance. Pediatricians, pediatric anesthesiologists, pediatric ophthalmologists, and, in many cases, social workers should be integral players in the care of the pediatric PKP patient.

Recent studies[32,33] have shown a relatively guarded prognosis for vision in pediatric PKPs. Graft clarity at 1 year ranged between 60% and 80%, and at 2 years averaged around 67%. Vitrectomy, lensectomy, regrafts, and postoperative complications were associated with significantly poor allograft survival. Eighteen percent of all eyes had worse vision at the time of the last follow-up than preoperatively. Sixty seven percent of the eyes had vision less than 20/200.

LAMELLAR KERATOPLASTY

Lamellar keratoplasty (LKP) consists of transplanting partial-thickness donor cornea, devoid of endothelium, Descemet's membrane, and deep stroma, onto a complementary recipient bed that has been dissected free of overlying abnormal anterior stroma. The procedure is seldom performed at present, owing mainly to recent advances and high success rates of PKPs, coupled with the technical complexity of LKPs. In fact, LKPs are currently performed mainly for optical and tectonic (restoration of structural integrity) purposes.[34,35] Optical LKPs are performed mainly for anterior stromal opacities, Bowman's layer pathology, and irregular anterior corneal surface topography. Specific clinical examples of optical indications include Salzmann's nodular degeneration with deep anterior opacities, posttraumatic or postinfectious anterior stromal scarring, and seldomly, keratoconus. Tectonic LKPs are performed mainly for corneal ectasias, perforations (Fig. 17–9), and descemetoceles, but also may be done in conjunction with lamellar keratectomy for benign anterior corneal tumors (e.g., dermoids) and pterygia. Cosmetic LKP in an eye with no visual potential is contraindicated. Better cosmesis is achievable with scleral shells and cosmetic contact lenses.

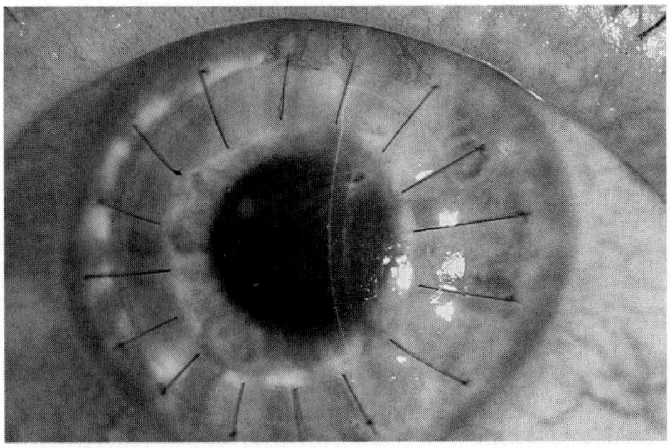

Figure 17–9. Lamellar graft performed for small corneal perforation (delineated by the narrow slit beam). Graft–host lamellar interface is also highlighted by the slit beam.

Lamellar keratoplasty has several advantages over PKP. Because the integrity of Descemet's membrane and posterior stroma is not violated, the wound strength is far superior to PKP. Therefore, it is well suited to patients who are physically active, young, or mentally retarded. The graft–host junction in PKP *never* heals to full preoperative corneal strength, and wound dehiscence may occur after seemingly inconsequential trauma even 10 years after PKP. In LKP, in contrast, not only is Descemet's membrane intact, but the graft–host junction is essentially the entire planar interface between donor and recipient cornea. Consequently, the wound strength is considerably greater with LKP. In addition, LKP surgery does not violate the intraocular structures of the eye, and is accordingly less prone to glaucoma, cataract formation, retinal detachment, CME, expulsive hemorrhage, endophthalmitis, and epithelial downgrowth. It does not involve transplantation of the endothelium; it therefore does not require donor corneas with healthy endothelium. Eyebank donor tissue rejected for PKP because of poor endothelial status or tissue deemed unsuitable for PKP because of excessive time of preservation can still be used for most LKPs. It is an ideal procedure for use in regions of the world where PKP tissue is sparse or where patients have poor access to ophthalmologists for postoperative care. Unsuccessful LKPs may always be converted in the future to PKPs, but not vice versa.

On the other hand, visual quality after LKP is often inferior to PKP, owing to haze, vascularization, blood, and particulate debris (e.g., cotton fibers from swabs, powder from gloves, and lint from cloth drapes) in the graft-host planar interface. Inadequately deep lamellar dissection of the recipient stroma may result in residual opacities. Lamellar keratoplasty is contraindicated for recipient eyes with unhealthy endothelium (PKP should be done instead), for actively infected corneas (PKP can more reliably remove deep microbial inocula), and for excision of malignant tumors. The surgical procedure is significantly more difficult than for PKP, and it is generally not within the purview of the general ophthalmologist.[34]

The preoperative evaluation of the LKP patient is similar to that of the PKP candidate; however, due to the essentially extraocular nature of LKP, considerations of glaucoma, CME, uveitis, and goniosynechiae are not as crucial. If active stromal melting of a systemic etiology (e.g., rheumatoid arthritis) is present, attention must also be directed toward instituting appropriate systemic corticosteroids and immunosuppression to arrest the underlying disease.[34]

The recipient cornea is trephined to a stromal depth appropriate to the pathology with a disposable trephine, preferably one with an obturator that can be set for the proper depth. Alternatively, a Hessberg-Barron vacuum trephine without an obturator has threaded walls allowing the surgeon to cut a predetermined depth that is linearly related to the number of turns on the trephine blade.

Peripheral ectasias are often furrow-shaped and abut the limbus. In such cases there may be a need to be dissected free-hand without the use of a circular trephine or be marked with two coaxial trephine marks to approximate a furrow-like or crescentic lamellar dissection bed.

The lamellar dissection is initiated with a sharp knife at the desired stromal depth. After establishing a plane of dissection, the remainder of the lamellar surgery may be done either with the same sharp-point knife, with a sharp-edged lamellar dissector (e.g., Crescent blade [Alcon] or Beaver 6600 blade), or with a blunt lamellar dissector (e.g., Martinez or Troutman dissectors). The extent and progress of dissection may be monitored through the overlying cornea (in which case the surface should be kept wet to improve visibility) or via direct stromal visualization with the anterior corneal flap lifted up (in which case the exposed stroma should be kept dry to prevent the fluid meniscus from obscuring the view). The blunt lamellar dissectors work best with circular, sweeping movements of the tip, while the sharp dissectors are best used with less aggressive, scratching-type movements. Injection of air into the deep stromal lamellae may facilitate separation of the interlamellar bonds, and allows safer dissection even down to Descemet's membrane.[36] If a small tear in Descemet's membrane should occur, the lamellar dissection may be gently completed with a sharp dissector. Larger perforations may necessitate conversion to a PKP. The lamellar recipient bed should be free of any irregularities and the depth of dissection should be uniform throughout, and should be meticulously irrigated with balanced salt solution to remove any traces of particulate matter that could become entrapped in the graft–host interface.

The lamellar donor cornea is usually prepared from a whole globe (either fresh, moist-chamber stored, or frozen), although some surgeons prefer to use corneal buttons (artificial anterior chambers are available to facilitate lamellar dissection of tissue-cultured corneal buttons). Lamellar dissection of the donor cornea is initiated with a sharp blade at the limbus and completed with a blunt lamellar dissector. Once an adequate area of cornea has been thus dissected, a trephine is used to punch out a circular button of anterior cornea. Because most whole globe corneas are quite edematous, the donor lamellar buttons should be dissected thicker than the recipient lamellar bed, taking into account the deturgescence of the donor tissue once it is sutured into place. I usually oversize the diameter of the donor button about 0.5 mm larger than the recipient bed, thereby reducing lateral wound tension and corneal flattening. Ready-to-use lyophilized human lamellar corneal donor tissue is commercially available and requires rehydration of the lamellar button in saline prior to use. Commercial manufacture of lyophilized tissue, capable of being stored at room temperature, began as an offshoot of epikeratoplasty (epikeratophakia) lenticule production in the 1980s. A LASIK-style automated microkeratome has been used by some surgeons for lamellar cutting of both donor and host corneal caps in LKP. If the LKP is to serve as a patch graft for a perforated cornea, care should be taken to avoid formation of a "pseudochamber." A pseudochamber results when aqueous humor gains entry into the graft–host interface through the hole in the recipient cornea, where it forms an intralamellar cistern. It may sometimes degrade visual acuity.

The suturing techniques are essentially the same as for PKP; however, I prefer to use all interrupted sutures because of the tendency toward rapid, uneven meridional healing in LKP, necessitating early, selective suture removal. Often, LKP sutures loosen as early as 1 month after surgery due to rapid wound contraction and vascularization.

Recently, posterior LKP (replacing the endothelium, Descemet's membrane, and posterior stroma) has been proposed as an alternative to PKP in endothelial disorders, such as Fuchs' dystrophy, PBK, and ABK.[37] This may reduce postoperative astigmatism and the incidence of wound dehiscence.

POSTOPERATIVE CARE

Specifics of postoperative management vary between surgeons, the indications for the keratoplasty, and the intraoperative events that may have occurred. For routine postoperative care in uncomplicated cases, the patient should be seen the day after surgery, toward the end of the first postoperative week, about 2-4 weeks after surgery, and then every 2 to 3 months over the ensuing year. After the first year, stable patients need to be followed up as infrequently as once a year, but they should be followed regularly nevertheless.

Especially the night after surgery, the patient should be warned about the symptoms of early postoperative glaucoma, such as a dull, achey ocular or periorbital pain (as opposed to scratchy, foreign-body sensation which usually connotes a more benign ocular surface discomfort). If this is accompanied by nausea and vomiting (caused by a vagal response to high intraocular pressure), the suspicion of glaucoma is further heightened. While nausea and vomiting may occasionally be seen as a sequel of general anesthesia and of narcotic analgesia, it is rarely seen purely as a result of local anesthesia by itself. I instruct patients to return to my office or the hospital to have their intraocular pressure measured, should the dull, achey pain not resolve with mild analgesics such as acetaminophen. For this reason, it is advisable to avoid prescribing stronger narcotic-type analgesics, which may mask the symptoms of a postoperative pressure spike. With very few exceptions after uncomplicated PKP, patients do not usually experience pain severe enough to need narcotics; if the pain is severe enough, it is a sign that they need to be examined by an ophthalmologist. Aspirin and nonsteroidal anti-inflammatory drugs (NSAIDs) should not be used within the first few days after surgery because of the risk of precipitating or prolonging intraocular hemorrhage. The risk of early postoperative acute glaucoma is higher in PKP than in other surgeries such as small-incision phacoemulsification, because of the more extensive nature of tissue alteration, the difficulty in completely removing all viscoelastic material from the eye, and the prevalence of preexisting inflammatory or glaucomatous disease. Pressure spikes are also likely to be more devastating in PKP than in self-sealing incision cataract surgery because of the higher risk of wound leaks and iris incarceration.

The patient is instructed to eschew vigorous physical exertion or straining for several days after PKP (unlike after small-incision cataract surgery which mandates very few restrictions). For the first postoperative month, the patient should wear a metal shield during sleep and spectacles during wake hours for protection. In PKP, mild eye trauma may easily result in severe wound dehiscence with loss of vital intraocular contents. In the long-term, the patient is encouraged to wear shatterproof polycarbonate spectacles because the PKP wound *never* heals to normal corneal strength.

All postoperative examinations should include measurements of visual acuity and intraocular pressure. Prolonged efforts at refraction, pachymetry, keratometry, and topography are seldom productive or useful before the first month. Intraocular pressure measurements may need to be performed with pneumotonometry, MacKay-Marg tonometry, Tonopen tonometry, or with the fingers, because irregular corneal mires preclude the use of the applanation tonometer. Epithelial defects are often present during the first week, but as long as they continue to diminish in size, no intervention is necessary. Persistent, nonhealing defects, on the other hand, may require the application of a bandage contact lens or collagen shield, an increase in corneal surface lubrication, or the discontinuation or reduction of topical medications that are toxic to the epithelium. In severe, recalcitrant cases, a tarsorrhaphy may need to be performed. The cornea is examined for infectious infiltrates, ulceration, wound leaks, and keratic precipitates (although rejection typically does not occur before the second week).

The anterior chamber is examined for inflammation. The presence of a hypopyon, fibrin, or large numbers of anterior chamber white cells may indicate endophthalmitis. A shallow anterior chamber may be associated with wound leak, choroidal effusions, or aqueous misdirection glaucoma.

The retina should be examined as soon as the view becomes sufficiently clear. On the first postoperative day, the posterior pole should be checked for the presence of a red reflex. Subsequently, if the view remains poor, an ultrasonic examination of the retina should be done to rule out pathology.

After removal of the bandage on the first postoperative day, topical corticosteroid drops are started. Depending on the degree of inflammation, these are prescribed between 4 times daily to as often as every hour. Severe cases may require the addition of systemic corticosteroids, given either as a single bolus or as a daily dose. Although many clinicians taper off topical corticosteroids after several months, I prefer to maintain low doses (e.g., once every other day) indefinitely. Although this is anecdotal and perhaps merely coincidental, I have seen patients who developed graft rejections within a week of stopping corticosteroids, even as late as 5 years after surgery. In phakic patients, I tend to taper the cataractogenic corticosteroids more rapidly and have less reluctance to stop them altogether in the long run. Topical antibiotics are used by many surgeons, but I personally do not employ them because there is no hard evidence that they are beneficial in the routine postoperative situation; furthermore, they may delay epithelialization and promote emergence of resistant strains. In herpetic grafts, antiviral agents should be used as long as corticosteroids are in use. Topical antivirals should be tapered rapidly to a very low dose (paralleling the topical corticosteroid dosage) within weeks to prevent epithelial toxicity. Oral acyclovir is not toxic to the corneal epithelium, and its efficacy in preventing or treating herpetic relapse has been shown.[38] Cycloplegics may be used for treating iritis, improving comfort, preventing synechiae, and increasing anterior chamber depth in phakic eyes. Cycloplegics probably should be avoided in keratoconus eyes which are more prone to developing permanent pupillary mydriasis. Ocular antihypertensive medications should be used for glaucoma and in accordance with the intraocular pressure. During the first postoperative day, oral acetazolamide may be used to reduce the possibility of a pressure spike while the eye is still bandaged. Late pressure elevation after several weeks should raise the suspicion of corticosteroid glaucoma. This may require switching to fluoromethalone (FML), loteprednol (Lotemax), or rimexolone (Vexol) eyedrops and temporarily increasing the concurrent antiglaucoma medications. Topical NSAIDs should generally be avoided, because of recent isolated reports of corneal melting putatively associated with these drugs.

The need for suture adjustment or suture removal for astigmatism should be determined by refraction, keratometry, keratoscopy, or computed tomography. Occasionally, an extremely tight suture may show telltale posterior corneal stress lines in Descemet's membrane and local compressive elevation anteriorly at the graft-host junction.

Refraction and keratometry may not only be difficult to interpret while the corneal contour is distorted, but also usually provide inconclusive information. Refractive and keratometric measurements are more reliable in corneas with simple astigmatism. With keratometry, however, multiple and non-orthogonal axes of steepness may be crudely inferred from the pattern of the mires. Computed topography, and to a certain degree keratoscopy, provide a more panoramic and comprehensive view of the corneal contour, reducing the guesswork during suture manipulation.

Selective corneal suture removal or adjustment may be begun as early as the first postoperative week, depending on the type of suture method *(vide supra)*. If possible during suture removal, the buried knot should not be pulled across the graft-host junction. A particularly bulky knot may snag the wound edges and pull them apart. Topical antibiotics should be instilled after suture removal, either as a single-dose ointment or as eye drops over several days. When removing a broken suture, the loose, exposed end should not be passed through the cornea, as this may introduce microbial organisms into the corneal stroma. When removing an infected suture (i.e., from a suture abscess), the suture itself as well as the abscess contents should be cultured. Typically, corneal contour changes after suture manipulation may not stabilize until at least 1 month; it is therefore unproductive to prescribe new spectacles or remove more sutures less than a month after suture manipulation. Astigmatic keratotomy should not be done until at least 2 months after *all* the sutures are removed, until there is a reasonable degree of certainty that the refractive error is final and stable. Contact lenses for anisometropia and high astigmatism may be used prior to removal of all sutures if wound healing considerations mandate retention of sutures for a considerably longer time. The association between contact lens wear and an increased immune rejection risk of the corneal graft is still being debated.

COMPLICATIONS OF PENETRATING KERATOPLASTY

Although wound leaks and dehiscence can occur at anytime during the postoperative period, they are more common in the early phase when the wound is relatively fresh. Minor leaks may not seep unless provoked by raising the intraocular pressure or by focally deforming the wound with an instrument. Such leaks may occasionally be successfully treated with the use of bandage contact lenses, collagen shields, and pressure patching. The use of acetazolamide reduces aqueous humor production and may help facilitate sealing of a leak. More persistent or severe cases need placement of new or additional interrupted sutures, or adjustment of the tension distribution in running sutures. Cyanoacrylate tissue adhesives may be used successfully to seal leaks; however, they may cause foreign body irritation, promote corneal vascularization, and are not yet (after 30 years of use!) approved by the U. S. Food and Drug Administration. If a wound leak is persistent or is associated with focal stromal melting or infection, a small, overlapping tectonic keratoplasty involving the graft–host junction of the PKP may be performed.[63] Traumatic wound dehiscence may occur as late as years after PKP and may take place during suture removal.

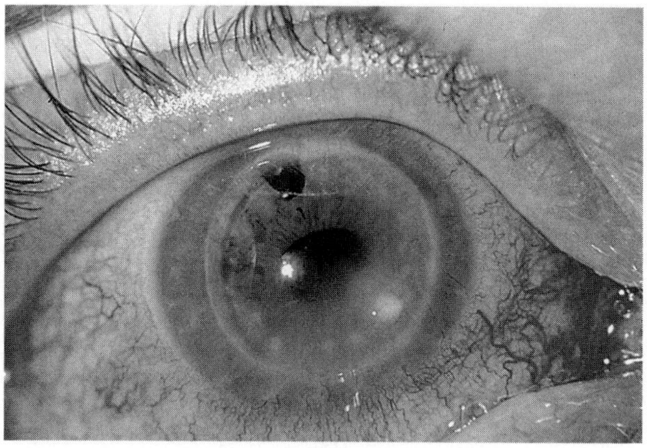

Figure 17–10. Suture abscess in graft.

Broken or loose sutures should be immediately removed or replaced. Complications include wound dehiscence, high astigmatism, vascularization along the suture track, immune rejection, and infectious suture abscesses (Fig. 17–10). Non-infectious suture infiltrates are relatively common in younger patients and are thought to be an immune or inflammatory response to the suture material. The longer the sutures are left in place, the more likely scarring will develop along suture tracks in susceptible individuals. These reactions do not cause any problems. Other suture problems and management methods are discussed in the previous section (Postoperative Care).

Persistent epithelial defects are more common in eyes with preexisting ocular surface problems such as Stevens-Johnson syndrome, ocular cicatricial pemphigoid, chemical burns, lagophthalmos, neurotrophic disease, entropion/ectropion, trichiasis, medicamentosa, and dry eye. These conditions must be adequately controlled, preferably before PKP is performed. Management methods include the use of preservative-free tears and ointments, bandage contact lenses or collagen shields, topical fibronectin or growth factors, conjunctival and stem cell transplantation, and tarsorrhaphy.[39] Persistent epithelial defects may be complicated by infection, scarring, and stromal melting.

Filamentary keratitis (Fig. 17–11) in the early postoperative period is usually self-limited and occurs in as many as 27% of PKPs.[40] These lesions do not cause any discomfort on the denervated donor cornea, but they may cause irritation and foreign body sensation on the recipient cornea. Filaments may be treated with artificial tears or 10% to 20% *N*-acetylcysteine (Mucomyst) drops, debrided with fine forceps, or be left untreated. Kaye dots are discrete, white specks in the peripheral donor corneal epithelium adjacent to the sutures and may represent a response to topographical elevation of the

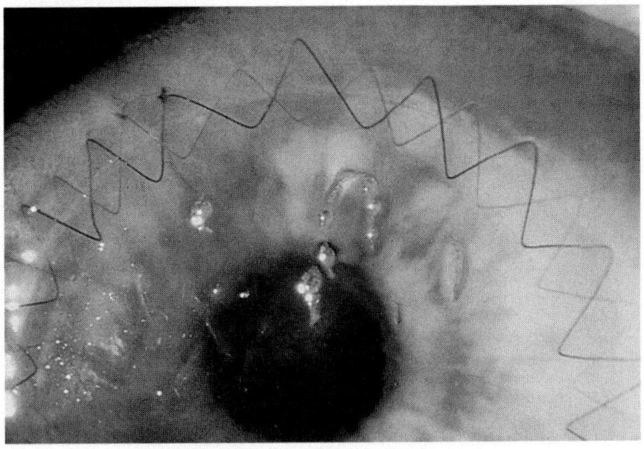

Figure 17–11. Filamentary keratitis on donor corneal epithelium 2 months after penetrating keratoplasty (PKP).

cornea in the area of wound compression by sutures.[41] Kaye dots do not stain or cause discomfort and are seen mostly in younger patients. They usually disappear within months or with suture removal and are not associated with any secondary complications.

Postoperative inflammation is more common and severe in previously operated eyes, pediatric grafts, PKPs done during the acute phase of inflammation (e.g., for a perforated cornea or during an active corneal ulcer), after intraoperative complications, and in PKPs done in eyes with keratouveitis and anterior segment neovascularization. Inflammation must be aggressively controlled with topical (and sometimes systemic or periocular) corticosteroids to reduce the possibility of synechia formation, CME, pupillary block or angle closure glaucoma, cyclitic or retrocorneal membrane formation, and immune rejection. Peripheral anterior synechiae may not only increase the risk of graft rejection but also may lead to glaucoma and corneal endothelial damage.

Postoperative corneal infection may occur as a sequel to suture abscesses, persistent epithelial defects, ocular surface problems, suture removal, contact lens wear, or inadequate excision in PKPs done for infectious keratitis. Rarely, infectious keratitis in the graft may be manifested by intrastromal crystalline deposits distributed in a "frond" or "snow-flake" pattern within a discrete stromal lamellar plane. This clinical phenomenon, known as *infectious crystalline keratopathy* (Fig. 17–12), is usually caused by low-virulence organisms (e.g., α-hemolytic streptococcus) in the setting of host immunocompromise associated with chronic corticosteroid use.[42] Infectious keratitis at the graft–host junction is especially worrisome for intraocular extension of the organisms, converting the surface infection into endophthalmitis.

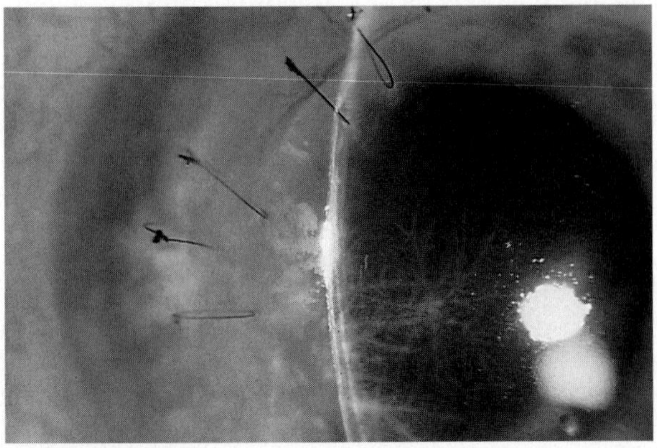

Figure 17–12. Infectious crystalline keratopathy in corneal graft, beginning in an infected suture track. Note crystalline, snowflake-like intralamellar infiltrate, containing streptococci.

Although contaminated the donor tissue is a very infrequent source of infection, the donor rim is routinely cultured at the time of PKP for in the event of clinical infection. Long-term use of corticosteroids may increase the infection risk. Endophthalmitis after PKP occurs in less than 1% of grafts and is more common in patients with positive donor rim cultures. Fibrin, hypopyon, and increased white cells and flare in the anterior chamber may be indicators of intraocular infection. Ocular pain and eyelid swelling are less reliable signs. Aspirates of aqueous humor, or better yet vitreous, may be obtained through the wound or through the pars plana. Aggressive therapy is necessary in all postoperative infections. Recurrent herpetic infection is most often seen in grafts done for herpetic keratitis, but may also occur *de novo* in grafts as a consequence of chronic corticosteroid therapy.

Primary donor failure is defined as irreversible donor corneal edema developing within the immediate postoperative period, usually within the first 2 days. It may result from poor donor preservation, unhealthy or low donor endothelial counts, surgical trauma, or idiopathic causes. Herpes simplex virus has been detected by polymerase chain reaction in donor corneal buttons in cases of primary graft failure.[43] Although the graft with primary failure may clear and deturgesce to some degree as the normal postoperative inflammation subsides and the intraocular pressure normalizes, it will not recover full clarity as would a healthy graft. Postoperative hypotony in a healthy donor cornea is often associated with a thick, but *clear* graft. It is prudent not to rush into regrafting before 2 months, as some edematous grafts (in my experience) have taken as long as 3 months to completely recover clarity and still continue to retain clarity after 12 years. Primary donor failure is relatively rare (less than 0.5% of donor corneas in most eye bank reports) and must be reported on adverse reaction forms provided by the eye bank.

Glaucoma after PKP is very common, with reported frequencies ranging from 11% to 46%, depending on the complexity of surgery, prevalence of preoperative glaucoma, previous surgery, and indications for PKP.[44–46] The recognition and treatment of postoperative glaucoma are described in other chapters of this book, and are touched upon briefly in earlier sections of this chapter.

Immune corneal graft rejection after PKP is not uncommon and is encountered in up to 12% of PKPs at the University of Michigan W. K. Kellogg Eye Center. Most of those rejections are reversible with treatment, and consequently less than 2% of the PKPs suffer from irreversible, rejection-related graft failure. It is therefore of paramount importance to be thoroughly familiar with the clinical signs of graft rejection and so be able to achieve early diagnosis and render prompt, aggressive therapy. Although the avascular cornea is indeed isolated from the immune system to a degree, the isolation is far from perfect. Immunologic communication occurs between the donor tissue and the recipient via the aqueous humor circulation and the limbal vasculature. The tears may also contain immunocompetent leukocytes. The presence of iridocorneal adhesions opens up another pathway for immunologic communication.

Each layer of the cornea could sensitize the recipient and undergo immunologic allograft rejection. Immunologic damage to the endothelial cells, however, is most damaging to the overall function of the donor cornea. Possible risk factors for corneal graft rejection include large-diameter grafts, corneal vascularization (particularly deep vessels), young recipient age, regrafting (especially for prior rejection-related graft failure), glaucoma, and active ocular inflammation.[47–49] The immunologic risks of bilateral corneal grafting, fever, or of systemic vaccinations or blood transfusions are not yet clear. Immunocompetent Langerhans cells are normally present in the peripheral one-third of the corneal epithelium. This, together with the limbal vasculature, may contribute to the propensity for large-diameter or peripherally eccentric grafts to reject. After rejection occurs, Langerhans cells begin to populate the central corneal epithelium, as well as the endothelium.

Graft rejection is a predominantly cell-mediated (delayed hypersensitivity) immunologic phenomenon. The earliest rejection takes place a minimum of about 2 weeks after PKP. This latency is related to the time necessary for the afferent and efferent moieties of the cell-mediated response to take place. Therefore, keratic precipitates that are deposited on the graft endothelium prior to this period are not likely to be rejection related, and other causes, such as herpetic disease, should be considered. The graft is never fully safe from rejection, as immune reactions have occurred as late as 20 years after PKP. In general, however, the risk of rejection is highest in the few years after grafting and subsides in the later years. At our institution, 60% of the rejections have occurred within the first 2 years after PKP. Occasionally, rejection episodes may cease completely after one or two initial episodes. This curious phenomenon may be related to the development of immunologic tolerance to the donor cornea. In the Collaborative Corneal Transplantation Study (CCTS), 62% of the 456 high-risk patients had at least one rejection episode after PKP, and median time for the first rejection was 6 months.[48]

Subjective symptoms of graft rejection could be nondescript and subtle. Those described in the CCTS were redness, photophobia, vision loss, and pain. Patients who reported a red eye were 3.1 times more likely to experience rejection. Those reporting decreased vision were 2.7 times more likely to have rejection. Photophobia and pain were statistically only weakly associated with rejection. Overall, patient-reported symptoms were neither sensitive nor specific for a rejection.[50]

Early clinical signs of graft rejection may be subtle and easily missed by the casual or neophyte observer. Iritis, especially in association with increased graft thickness,[51] may be an early sign of rejection (Fig. 17–13*A*). Iritis signifies increased intraocular inflammation and immune activity, while the increased donor corneal thickness signifies endothelial morbidity and reduced function. Kuchle and co-workers describe the use of an aqueous cell-flare meter[52] for detecting subtle iritis in the anterior chamber after PKP. Pachymetry of the graft should be performed on each postoperative visit (after 2 weeks) to monitor the thickness. If new iritis is associated with greater than 10% increase in graft thickness from the previous visit, immune rejection may exist and treatment should be instituted.

Keratic precipitates on the graft endothelium (Fig. 17–13*B*) raise the specter of endothelial rejection. These white precipitates are aggregates of immune complexes containing T-lymphocytes, macrophages, and complement. Although other diseases, such as herpetic keratouveitis, may cause keratic precipitates, it is nevertheless prudent to consider rejection in the differential diagnosis. Generally, in pure endothelial graft rejection, the precipitates are confined to the donor side of the endothelium. *It takes only one precipitate to make a diagnosis of graft rejection.* Keratic precipitates probably originate from the aqueous humor circulation, as they are often distributed in the same pattern as a Krukenberg's spindle, ostensibly following the convection currents of the aqueous humor.

Subepithelial infiltrates (SEI) are immune complexes in the superficial graft stroma (Fig. 17–13*C*) and are indistinguishable from SEI due to epidemic keratoconjunctivitis. These are a manifestation of stromal rejection and are seen in 4% of the PKPs at our institution. Although SEI are not immediately of concern as they do not constitute endothelial rejection, they are harbingers of serious rejection, including endothelial graft rejection. Therefore, some surgeons elect to treat SEIs immediately by temporarily increasing the corticosteroid dosage, to perhaps "appease and mollify" the immune system from eventually launching an all-out attack on the donor endothelium. Sometimes SEI are seen in concert with other signs of rejection.

An epithelial rejection line (Fig. 17–13*D*) consists of T-lymphocytes and other immunocompetent cells forming a continuous line on the donor corneal epithelium. These are seen in about 6% of PKPs at our institution; the true incidence may be higher if the patients are more closely followed with less time between visits. The line develops along the demarcation between host and donor epithelium, ostensibly if there is sufficient mutual immunological mismatch. Although the phenomenon itself is benign because endothelium is unaffected during its acute phase, many of the corneas with epithelial rejection eventually develop endothelial rejection. Like the SEI, epithelial rejection lines can sometimes coexist with other signs of corneal rejection. Many corneal surgeons choose to treat epithelial rejection lines with a burst of topical corticsteroids.

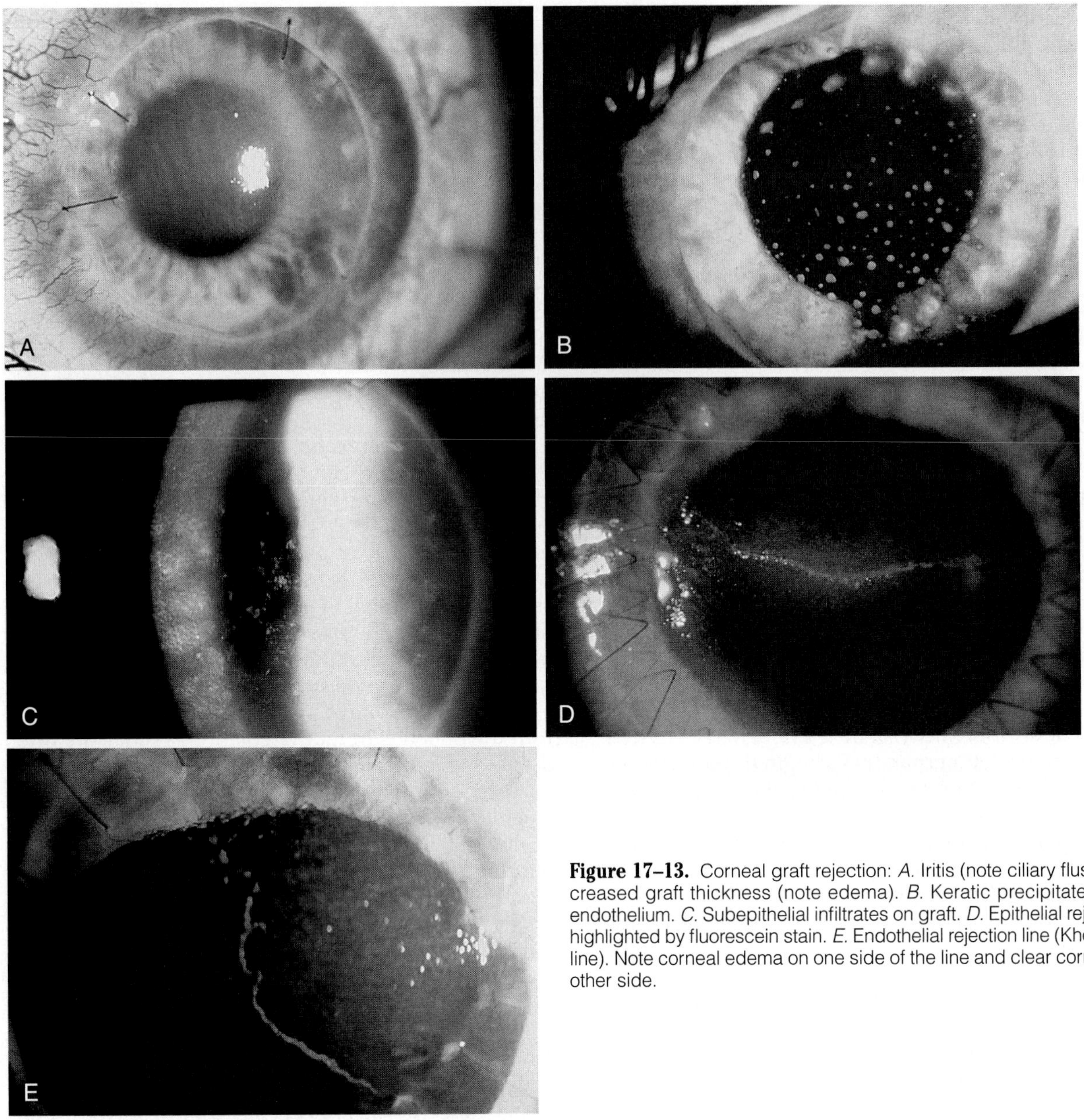

Figure 17–13. Corneal graft rejection: *A.* Iritis (note ciliary flush) and increased graft thickness (note edema). *B.* Keratic precipitates on graft endothelium. *C.* Subepithelial infiltrates on graft. *D.* Epithelial rejection line highlighted by fluorescein stain. *E.* Endothelial rejection line (Khoudadoust line). Note corneal edema on one side of the line and clear cornea on the other side.

Isolated rejection of the stroma per se is rare, but is manifested by focal or diffuse stromal infiltration, interstitial vascularization, keratocyte death, and uncommonly, stromal necrosis. More commonly, this sign is seen in conjunction with other signs of graft rejection.

The endothelial rejection line, or Khoudadoust line (Fig. 17–13*E*), is considered the hallmark of endothelial rejection. The line is composed of T-lymphocytes and other immunocompetent components, and may be analogized to keratic precipitates distributed in a shoulder-to-shoulder linear fashion. The line typically begins at one end of the endothelium and usually travels across the entire endothelial surface if left unchecked by treatment. During its migration, it leaves a swath of endothelial cell destruction behind it. The donor cornea is typically clear and compact ahead of the leading edge of destruction, and cloudy and edematous behind it. The endothelial rejection is thought to originate from the limbal circulation.

The mainstay of therapy for corneal graft rejection remains topical corticosteroids, despite a long, ongoing search for alternative treatments. Serious rejections (e.g., endothelial rejection lines) may need frequent topical therapy consisting of prednisolone acetate 1% as often as hourly around the clock. A concurrent single oral or intravenous bolus of systemic corticosteroid may be necessary to boost the therapy of particularly severe cases. Subconjunctival injections may be effective as an adjunct route of administration in severe cases or in noncompliant patients. Corneal collagen shields may be soaked in intravenous injectable corticosteroids and the medication levels reconstituted at regular intervals with topi-cal corticosteroid eye drops to provide a steady, high-concentration, depot effect. Milder rejections require less frequent instillation of corticosteroid eye drops, and nighttime doses may be replaced with ointment. Topical cyclosporine eyedrops and ointments have shown promise in some studies,[53,54] however, a large, multicenter, prospective, placebo-controlled study showed no significant efficacy of the topical route over corticosteroid.[55] However, this multicenter study protocol used concurrent application of corticosteroids in addition to the study drug. It is possible that the corticosteroids may have blunted or covered up the small beneficial effects of topical cyclosporine. Cyclosporine is a fungus-derived agent that has specific anti-T-lymphocyte actions (hence ideal for cell-mediated immunity). Other similar fungus-derived, anti-T-cell agents include sirolimus and FK-506 (tacrolimus), which are being investigated for use in corneal graft rejection. Systemic cyclosporine and FK-506 are reported to be efficacous and promising for the treatment of corneal graft rejection,[56,57] although the systemic side effects (renal and hepatic toxicity) are serious. The use of anti-T-lymphocyte, as well as anti-ICAM monoclonal antibodies may show some promise in the prevention or reversal of corneal graft rejection.[58,59] The use of HLA-A, HLA-B, and HLA-DR matching showed no significant benefits in preventing allograft failure due to rejection in a large, multicenter, prospective, double-blind study.[48] The same study showed statistically significant improvement in graft survival with ABO blood-group matching. However, some single-institution studies have shown beneficial effects of HLA matching.[60–62] As in the multicenter topical cyclosporin study mentioned above, the CCTS also allowed the use of high-dose corticosteroids in concert with the HLA matching. It is possible, therefore, that corticosteroids may have blunted whatever small beneficial effect HLA matching might have provided. Argon laser photocoagulation of corneal vessels has also been advocated for the prevention of rejection in PKP.

REFERENCES

1. Mannis MJ, Krachmer JH: Keratoplasty: A historical perspective: Surv Ophthalmol 1981;25:333.
2. Duke-Elder S, Leigh AG: Diseases of the outer eye. In Duke-Elder S, Leigh AG (eds.), System of Ophthalmology, vol VIII:648. St. Louis, CV Mosby; 1977.
3. Coster DJ: Doyne Lecture. Influences on the development of corneal transplantation. Eye 1994;8:1.
4. Zirm EK: Eine erfolgreiche totale Keratoplastik [A successful total keratoplasty]. Refract Corneal Surg 1989;5:258.
5. Waring GO III: The 50-year epidemic pseudophakic corneal edema. Arch Ophthalmol 1989;107:657.
6. Arentsen JJ, Morgan B, Green WR: Changing indications for keratoplasty. Am J Ophthalmol 1976;81:13.
7. Smith RE, McDonald HR, Nesburn AB, Minckler DS: Penetrating keratoplasty: Changing indications, 1947-1978. Arch Ophthalmol 1980;98:1226.
8. Sharif KW, Casey TA: Changing indications for penetrating keratoplasty, 1971-1990. Eye 1993;7:485.
9. Simonds RJ, Holmberg SD, Hurwitz RL, et al.: Transmission of human immunodeficiency virus type I from a seronegative organ and tissue donor. N Engl J Med 1992;326:726.
10. Pepose JS, MacRae S, Quinn TC, et al.: Serologic markers after the transplantation of corneas from donors infected with human immunodeficiency virus. Am J Ophthalmol 1987;103:798.
11. Mata B: The uses of cornea from gliomatous eyes in corneal transplantation. Acta Soc Ophthalmol Jpn 1939;43:1963.
12. McGeorge AJ, Thompson P, Elliott D, et al.: Papillary adenocarcinoma of the iris transmitted by corneal transplantation. EBAA Abstracts. Cornea 1994;13:102.
13. Soong H, Meyer RF, Sugar A: The triple procedure. Ophthalmol Clin North Am 1990;3:697.
14. Isenberg SJ, Apt L, Yoshimori R, et al.: Chemical preparation of the eye in ophthalmic surgery. IV. Comparison of povidone-iodine on the conjunctiva with a prophylactic antibiotic. Arch Ophthalmol 1985;103:1340.
15. Speaker MG, Menikoff JA: Prophylaxis of endophthalmitis with topical povidone-iodine. Ophthalmology 1991;98:1769.
16. Brightbill FS, Polack FM, Slappey T: A comparison of two methods for cutting donor corneas. Am J Ophthalmol 1973;75:500.
17. Olson RJ: Variation in corneal graft size related to trephine technique. Arch Ophthalmol 1979;97:1323.
18. Troutman RC: Astigmatic consideration in corneal graft. Ophthalmic Surg 1979;10:21.
19. Bourne WM, Davison JA, O'Fallon WM: The effects of oversize donor buttons in postoperative intraocular pressure and corneal curvature in aphakic penetrating keratoplasty. Ophthalmology 1982;89:242.
20. Perl T, Charlton KH, Binder PS: Disparate diameter grafting, astigmatism, intraocular pressure, and visual acuity. Ophthalmology 1981;88:774.
21. Olson RJ, Mattingly TP, Waltman SR, Kaufman HE: Refractive variation and donor tissue size in aphakic keratoplasty. Arch Ophthalmol 1979;97:1480.
22. Soong HK, Meyer RF, Wolter JR: Fistula excision and peripheral grafts in the treatment of persistent limbal wound leaks. Ophthalmology 1988;95:31.
23. Sugar A, Meyer RF: Giant papillary conjunctivitis after keratoplasty. Am J Ophthalmol 1981;91:239.
24. McNeill JL, Wessels IF: Adjustment of single continuous suture to control astigmatism after penetrating keratoplasty. Refract Corneal Surg 1989;5:216.
25. McNeill JL, Kaufman HE: A double running suture technique for keratoplasty: Earlier visual rehabilitation. Ophthalmic Surg 1977;8–58.
26. Troutman RC: Microsurgery of the Anterior Segment of the Eye, vol II, St. Louis: CV Mosby; 1977.
27. Tuberville AW, Foster CS, Wood TO: The effect of donor corneal epithelium removal on the incidence of allograft rejections. Ophthalmology 1983;90:1351.
28. Stulting RD, Waring GO III, Bridges WZ, Cavanaugh DH: Effect of donor epithelium on corneal transplant survival. Ophthalmology 1988;95:803.
29. McCartney DL, Gottsch JD, Stark WJ: Managing posterior pressure during pseudophakic keratoplasty. Arch Ophthalmol 1989;107:1384.
30. Soong HK, Meyer RF, Sugar A: Techniques of posterior chamber lens implantation without capsular support during penetrating keratoplasty: A review. Refract Corneal Surg 1989;5:249.
31. Schein OD, Kenyon KR, Steinert RF, et al.: A randomized trial of intraocular lens techniques with penetrating keratoplasty. Ophthalmology 1993;100:1437.
32. Dana MH, Moyes AL, Gomes JAP, et al.: The indications for and outcome in pediatric keratoplasty: A multicenter study. Ophthalmology 1995;102:1129.
33. Stulting RD, Sumers KD, Cavanagh HD, et al.: Penetrating keratoplasty in children. Ophthalmology 1984;91:1222.
34. Soong HK, Farjo AA, Katz D, et al.: Lamellar corneal patch grafts in the management of corneal melting. Cornea 2000;19:126.
35. Soong HK, Katz D, Farjo AA, et al.: Central lamellar keratoplasty for optical indications. Cornea 1999;18:249.
36. Archila EA: Deep lamellar keratoplasty dissection of host tissue with intrastromal air injection. Cornea 1984/1985;3:217.
37. Melles GRJ, Lander F, van Dooren BTH, et al.: Preliminary clinical results of posterior lamellar keratoplasty through a sclerocorneal pocket incision. Ophthalmology 2000;107:1850.
38. Herpetic Eye Disease Study (HEDS) Group: Acyclovir for the prevention of recurrent herpes simplex virus eye disease. N Engl J Med 1998;339:300.
39. Soong HK: Penetrating keratoplasty in ocular surface disease. In Krachmer JH, Mannis MJ, Holland EJ (eds.), Cornea, vol III. St. Louis, CV Mosby–Year-Book; 1997:1781.
40. Rotkis WM, Chandler JW, Forstot SL: Filamentary keratitis following penetrating keratoplasty. Ophthalmology 1982;89:946.
41. Kaye DB: Epithelial response in penetrating keratoplasty. Am J Ophthalmol 1980;89:381.
42. Meisler DM, Langston RHS, Naab TJ, et al.: Infectious crystalline keratopathy. Am J Ophthalmol 1984;97:337

43. Cockerham GC, Krafft AE, McLean IW: Herpes simplex virus in primary graft failure. Arch Ophthalmol 1997;115:586.
44. Thoft RA, Gordon JM, Dohlman CH: Glaucoma following keratoplasty. Trans Am Acad Ophthalmol Otolaryngol 1974;78:352.
45. Wood TO, West C, Kaufman HE: Control of intraocular pressure in penetrating keratoplasty. Am J Ophthalmol 1972;74:724.
46. Olson RJ, Kaufman HE: Prognostic factors of intraocular pressure after aphakic keratoplasty. Am J Ophthalmol 1978;86:510.
47. Maguire MG, Stark WJ, Gottsch JD, et al.: Risk factors for corneal graft failure and rejection in the (CCTS). Ophthalmology 1994; 101:1536.
48. The Collaborative Corneal Transplantation Studies Research Group: The Collaborative Corneal Transplantation Studies (CCTS): Arch Ophthalmol 1992;110:1392.
49. Boisjoly HM, Tourigny R, Bazin R, et al.: Risk factors of corneal graft failure. Ophthalmology 1993;100:1728.
50. Kamp MT, Fink NE, Enger C, et al.: Patient-reported symptoms associated with graft reactions in high-risk patients in the (CCTS). Cornea 1995; 14:43.
51. McDonnell PJ, Enger C, Stark WJ, Stulting D: Corneal thickness changes after high-risk penetrating keratoplasty. Arch Ophthalmol 1993;111:1374.
52. Küchle M, Nguyen NX, Naumann GOH, et al.: Aqueous flare following penetrating keratoplasty and in corneal graft rejection. Arch Ophthalmol 1994;11:354.
53. Goichot-Bonnat L, Chemla P, Pouliquen Y: Cyclosporine haut risque. II Resultats cliniques post-operatoires. J Fr Ophtalmol 1987;10:213.
54. Belin MW, Bouchard CS, Frantz S, Chmielinska J: Topical cyclosporine in high-risk corneal transplants. Ophthalmology 1989;96:1144.
55. Data on File: Sandoz Pharmaceuticals, 1990.
56. Hill JC: Systemic cyclosporine in high-risk keratoplasty. Short- versus long-term therapy. Ophthalmology 1994;101:128.
57. Dickey JB, Cassidy EM, Bouchard CS: Periocular FK-506 delays allograft rejection in rat penetrating keratoplasty. Cornea 1993;12:204.
58. Ippoliti G, Fronterre A: Usefulness of CD3 or CD6 anti-T monoclonal antibodies in the treatment of acute corneal graft rejection. Transplant Proc 1989;21:3133.
59. Guymer RH, Mandel TE: Immunosuppression using a monoclonal antibody to ICAM-1 in murine allotransplantation. Transplant Proc 1992;24:218.
60. Boisjoly HM, Roy R, Dube I, et al.: HLA-A, -B, and -DR matching in corneal transplantation. Ophthalmology 1986;93:1290.
61. Volker-Dieben HJM, Kok-van Alphen CC, Lansbergen Q, Persijn GG: The effect of prospective HLA-A and -B matching on corneal graft survival. Acta Ophthalmol 1982;60:203.
62. Sanfilippo F, McQueen JM, Vaughn WK, Foulks BN: Reduced graft rejection with good HLAA and -B matching in high risk corneal transplantation. N Engl J Med 1986;315:29.
63. Soong HK, Meyer RF, Sugar A: Small, overlapping tectonic keratoplasty involving graft-host junction of penetrating keratoplasty. Am J Ophthalmol 2000;129:465.

CHAPTER 18

Radial Keratotomy: Principles and Practice

J. JAMES ROWSEY, M.D.

Although radial keratotomy expertise is now routine for the refractive surgeon, knowledge of the nuances of this field are appropriate for all surgeons. Lans[1] noted the early effects of corneal relaxing incisions in rabbits in 1898, and Sato[2,3] described a 1.5- to 7.0-diopter correction of myopia in 1950 and 1953. Sato's radial incisions into the anterior and posterior cornea were associated with bullous keratopathy approximately 20 years after the surgery, causing justifiable reservations about these experimental techniques. Durnev and others[4-6] reevaluated Sato's technique in the early 1970s and obtained 2.65 diopters of correction $\pm$ 0.2 diopters using a 3-mm optical zone. This potential correction of myopia encouraged numerous U.S. investigators to evaluate radial keratotomy. Hoffer and colleagues reported 3.4 diopters of myopic reduction in 1981,[7] and Cowden and Bores reported 1.18 diopters of correction with a 16-incision radial keratotomy in 1982.[8,9] Our results of 5.2 diopters of correction with an 8-incision procedure have encouraged our further investigation.[10] The procedure has progressed from a 16-incision to an 8-incision and, finally, a 4-incision procedure,[11–13] with sufficiently satisfactory results to encourage further investigation.

The Prospective Evaluation of Radial Keratotomy (PERK)[14,15] collaborative study and careful follow-up of other authors demonstrated the range of potential efficacy of this procedure, predictive variables of importance, and numerous unsuspected complications.[16–20]

This chapter discusses the fundamental principles of incisional refractive surgery, corneal topography, preoperative preparation of the patient for radial keratotomy, necessary operative instrumentation, surgical technique, postoperative care, and methods of minimizing complications in radial keratotomy.

PRINCIPLES OF REFRACTIVE SURGERY

The basic caveats in keratorefractive surgery are important for an understanding of the effects anticipated with surgical procedures.[20]

1. *The normal cornea flattens over any incision.* A traumatic or surgical incision in the cornea produces flattening of the corneal tissue adjacent to the incision. As the incision fills with epithelium and collagen, and during wound healing, the surface area of the cornea is increased. A longer radius of curvature is produced in this area, thus providing permanent corneal flattening. Corneal flattening decreases the refractive power of the cornea, a valuable asset to the myopic patient. Figure 18–1 is an eye bank eye with 16 radial incisions in the cornea, each filled with tattoo dye to demonstrate the flattening of the cornea along each incision. Figure 18–2 is a corneascope photograph of a patient eye 1 year after an 8-incision radial keratotomy, demonstrating an unusual but persistent irregular

Research for this chapter was supported by The Gustavas and Louise Pfeiffer Foundation, an unrestricted grant from Research to Prevent Blindness, Inc., and the private philanthropy of the citizens of Oklahoma.

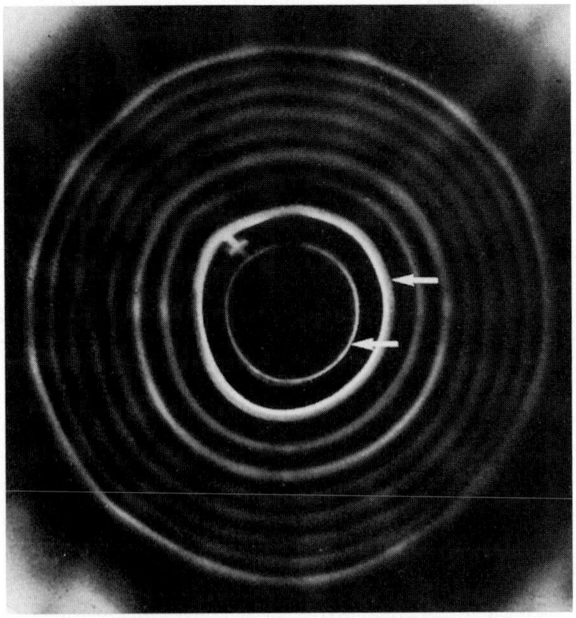

Figure 18–1. Kera corneascope photographs of a 16-incision eye bank eye radial keratotomy with tattoo in each incision, demonstrating marked corneal flattening over the incisions as shown by a wide separation of the central corneal rings (arrows).

ring pattern. Epithelium and collagen have filled each incision, flattening the center of the cornea.

2. *Radial corneal incisions flatten the adjacent cornea and the cornea 90 degrees away.* Incisions that traverse the cornea from the periphery to the center produce corneal flattening as described, but they simultaneously flatten the dome of the cornea 90 degrees from the actual incision site. This provides a unique corneal symmetrizing effect from radial incisions. A 4-incision radial keratotomy uses this propensity for flattening in two meridians. A single incision produces marked corneal flattening over the corneal dome by expansion in the center of the incision site.
3. *The corneal flattening effect increases as incisions approach the visual axis.* One of the major variables in radial keratotomy is the size of the optical zone. Smaller optical zones produce a larger magnitude of corneal flattening.[10,15] Traumatic corneal lacerations that traverse the visual axis may produce 20 diopters or more of corneal flattening when repaired. Figure 18–3 shows that the magnitude of corneal flattening with corneal incisions is greatest in the center of the cornea and diminishes as incisions approach the limbus.
4. *The cornea flattens directly over any sutured incision.* The sutured corneal incision produces an indentation vector of corneal flattening. For this reason, perforations that may require suturing are avoided in radial keratotomy. Suturing reverses the effect of the radial keratotomy and accentuates any induced corneal astigmatism.
5. *The limbal cornea flattens adjacent to loose sutures.* Circumferential limbal corneal incisions or cataract incisions produce wound gaping analogous to any other incision of the cornea. However, the circumferential or limbal corneal incision flattens the cornea directly over the incision and 180 degrees away while *steepening* the cornea 90 degrees away. Disparate refracting effects adjacent to and 90 degrees from an incision are termed "corneal coupling." The corneal coupling ratio is defined as the magnitude of the refractive effect at the surgery site: divided by the magnitude surgical effect 90 de-

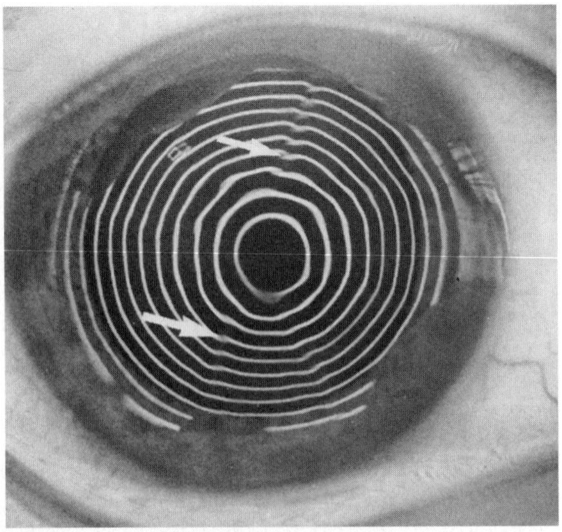

Figure 18–2. One year postoperatively, two incision sites are still visible in some patients as an uneven break in the rings on Kera corneascopy (arrows).

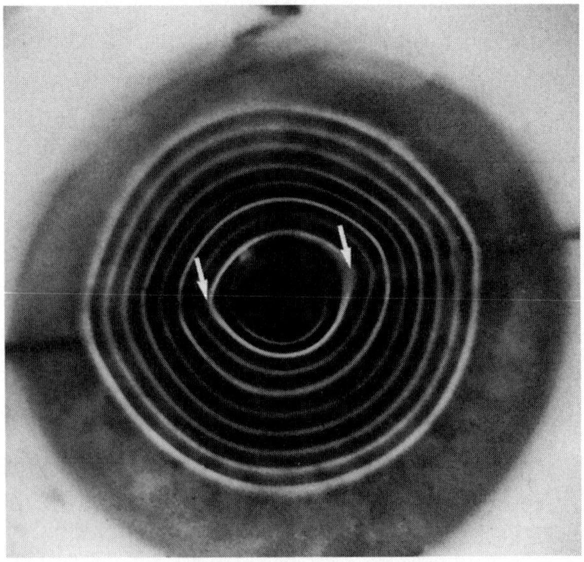

Figure 18–3. Kera corneascope photograph of a two-incision radial keratotomy in an eye bank eye, demonstrating flattening along the incisions of approximately 6 diopters and flattening 90 degrees away of approximately 3 diopters. A 3-mm optical zone is used. The central ellipse confirms flattening of the cornea along the incisions (arrows).

grees away (in diopters). Movement of the circumferential incision onto the clear cornea away from the limbus produces the astigmatic relaxing effect of tangential keratotomies. The effect of the circumferential incision should be distinguished from that of the radial corneal incision. The latter flattens the cornea both along the incision and 90 degrees away. The circumferential incision flattens the cornea in the axis of the incision and steepens the cornea 90 degrees away. The combination of radial and circumferential corneal incisions, therefore, has marked astigmatic correction potential.

6. *The limbal cornea steepens adjacent to tight sutures and steepens 180 degrees away; the cornea flattens 90 degrees away from tight sutures.* This description of the classic balloon model of Troutman[21] is easily visualized with a tight limbal compressive suture producing a vector of indentation of the cornea under the suture or flattening in this area (Fig. 18–4*A*). The cornea is steepened (Fig. 18–4*B*) anterior to the tight suture over the corneal apex and is flattened 90 degrees away. This steepening of the corneal apex anterior to the limbal sutures produces "with the rule" astigmatism (plus cylinder, at cylinder axis *90 degrees*) with routine 12-o'clock incisions.
7. *The cornea flattens overlying wedge resections.* Removal of corneal tissue in a microwedge allows for greater posterior vector compression from the sutures, and marked flattening of the cornea in the area of the wedge is observed.
8. *The cornea steepens anterior to the wedge resections or tucks.* A limbal wedge resection or tuck produces apical corneal steepening. The steepened corneal apex moves away from the area of the wedge resection (Fig. 18–4*B*).
9. *Tissue removal produces corneal flattening over the site of tissue removal.* This insight is true for wedge resections regardless of their cause, both in surgery and in trauma. Therefore, during repair of traumatic corneal lacerations, all possible tissue is preserved, with a conscious effort to remove as little tissue as possible.
10. *The cornea flattens adjacent to areas of full-thickness tissue additions to the cornea.* Wedge additions to the cornea accentuate the flattening effect seen in caveat number 1 by increasing the surface area over which the epithelium may heal. The microwedge addition technique, therefore, provides the potential for marked corneal flattening.

A basic understanding of these topographic insights is useful before radial keratotomy, relaxing incisions, or wedge resections are attempted, for the modulation of these caveats is under the control of the surgeon.

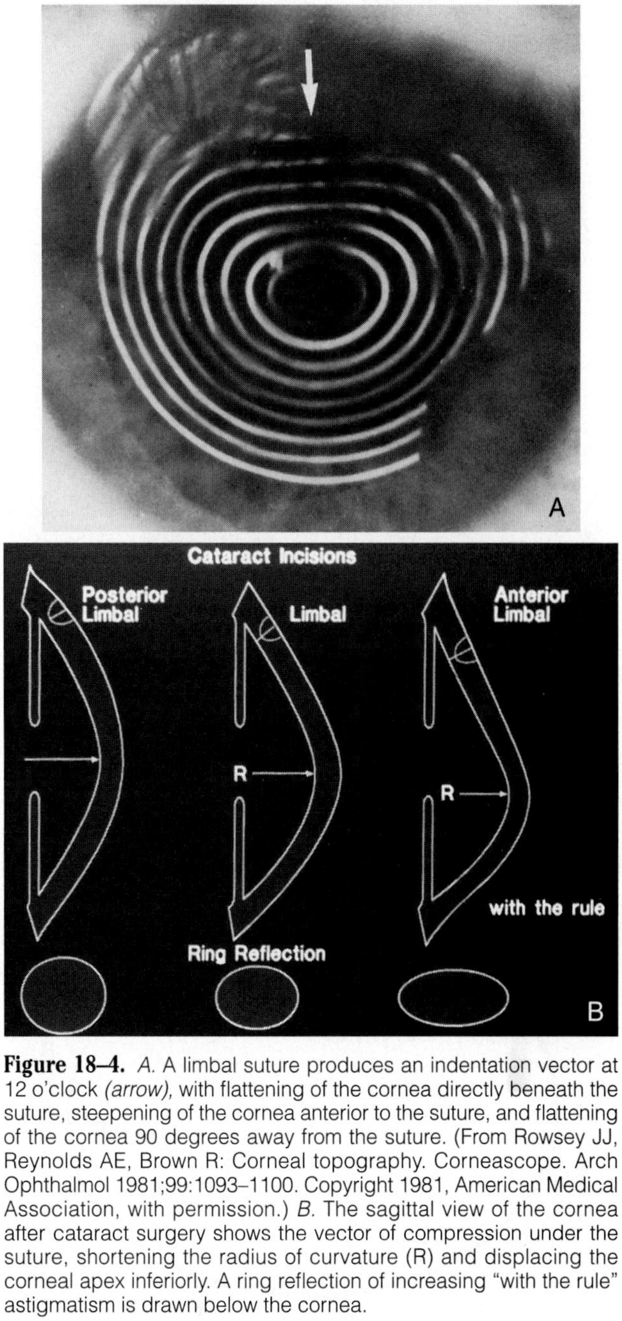

Figure 18–4. *A.* A limbal suture produces an indentation vector at 12 o'clock *(arrow)*, with flattening of the cornea directly beneath the suture, steepening of the cornea anterior to the suture, and flattening of the cornea 90 degrees away from the suture. (From Rowsey JJ, Reynolds AE, Brown R: Corneal topography. Corneascope. Arch Ophthalmol 1981;99:1093–1100. Copyright 1981, American Medical Association, with permission.) *B.* The sagittal view of the cornea after cataract surgery shows the vector of compression under the suture, shortening the radius of curvature (R) and displacing the corneal apex inferiorly. A ring reflection of increasing "with the rule" astigmatism is drawn below the cornea.

CORNEAL TOPOGRAPHY

The corneal shape, or surface topography, has been compared to a prolate ellipse,[22,24] with a short radius of curvature at the apex and flattening in all meridians (Fig. 18–5*A*). We have analyzed the corneal topography preoperatively and postoperatively in the PERK study and with the Humphrey keratometer, to determine the correlative factors in corneal shape that would allow for effective refractive change. Figure 18–5*B* and *C* presents a sagittal view of the cornea compared to an ellipse. The steep central cornea flattens in the periphery. Henslee and Rowsey[25] have previously demonstrated the reversal of this topographic shape to a flat central cornea steepening in the midperiphery after effective radial keratotomy surgery (Fig. 18–6*A* and *B*). The relationship between the central radius of curvature appears to be a significant predictive factor in radial keratotomy. Corneas that are flat in the center and flatten more toward the periphery have the greatest potential for corneal flattening in radial keratotomy. Corneas that are steep in the center and steepen toward the periphery have a resistance to the effect of radial keratotomy.

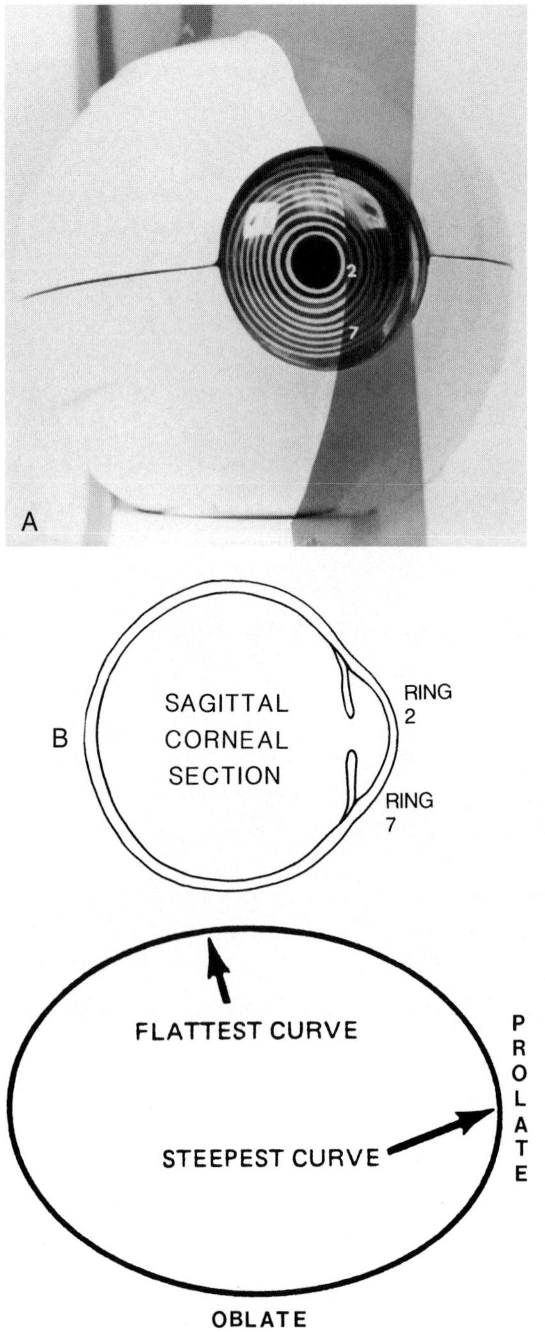

Figure 18–5. *A.* A sagittal corneal section approximates an ellipse with a steep central cornea (ring 2) and flattening toward ring 7. *B.* A sagittal plane through the cornea demonstrates the anterior–posterior relation of the central corneal rings (ring 2) and the peripheral rings of corneoscopy (rings 7–9). *C.* The cornea shape approximates an ellipse. The prolate cornea is similar to an ellipse with a steep central curvature, the spices of the ellipse. The flat side of the ellipse is the oblate side.

This is an "oblate" cornea, similar to the side of an egg in shape. The relationship between the center and the periphery of these relative corneal shapes is a greater contributor to the effectiveness of the operation than either radius of curvature individually.[26] The prolate side of an ellipse (Fig. 18–5*A*) flattens toward the periphery, whereas the oblate side (Fig. 18–5*A*) of an ellipse steepens toward the periphery. The prolate corneal shape provides the ideal candidate for radial keratotomy, whereas the oblate corneal shape frequently seen after a radial keratotomy procedure resists further central corneal flattening, and therefore produces a diminished radial keratotomy effect. Figure 18–6*A* shows the preoperative and postoperative radial keratotomy corneascope photographs emphasizing the marked corneal flattening of the center of the cornea after this surgery. Figure 18–6*C* demonstrates the preoperative and postoperative videokeratography of a radial keratotomy patient. The marked central corneal flattening is denoted by the blue center. Pattern recognition in videokeratography is important to understand the efficacy and stability of all refractive surgical procedures.

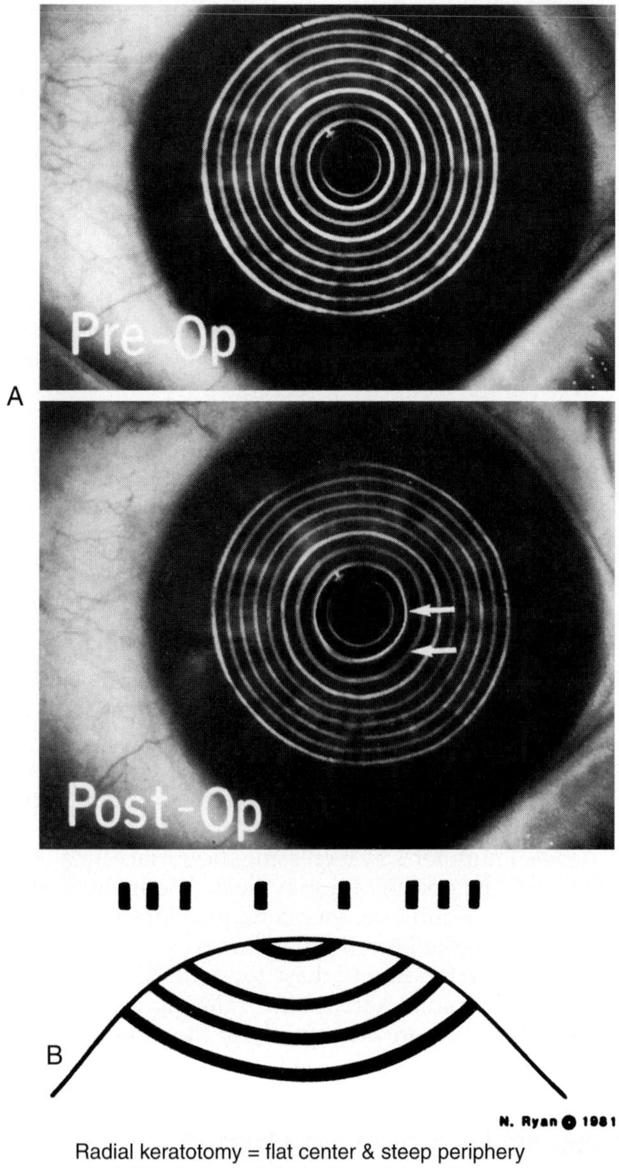

Figure 18–6. *A.* Preoperative Kera corneascope photograph of the cornea before radial keratotomy. Postoperative radial keratotomy photograph shows marked flattening of the cornea. Note the widening of the second and third rings, denoting central corneal flattening analogous to Figure 10–1. *B.* Schematic of the side view of the cornea, demonstrating marked corneal flattening after radial keratotomy.

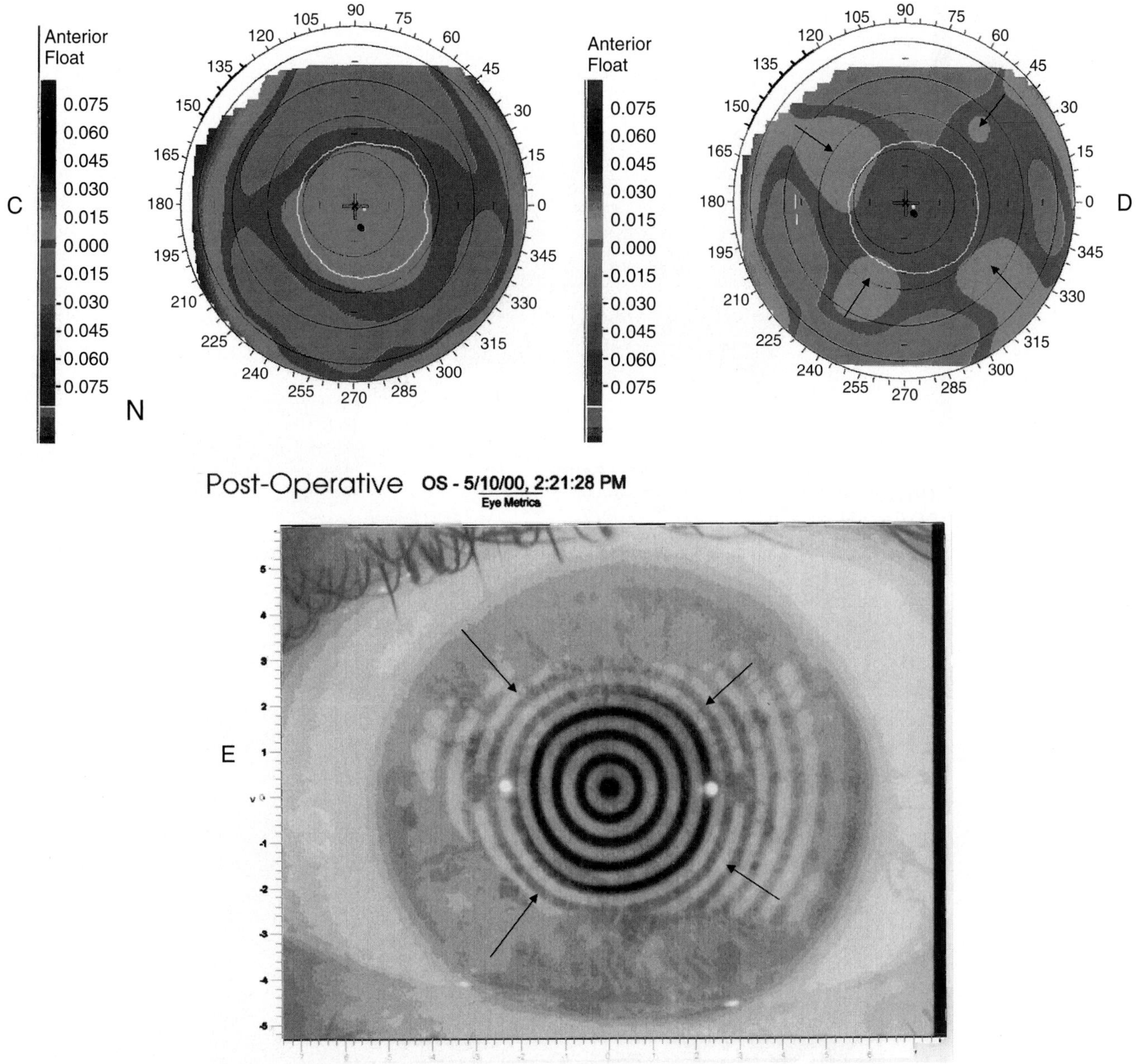

Figure 18–6 *Continued* *C.* Preoperative radial keratotomy corneal topography with an average corneal power of 42.75 diopters. The cornea is prolate with corneal flattening form the center to the periphery. *D.* Postoperative radial keratotomy corneal topography with an average corneal power of 40.45 diopters. The cornea is now oblate with a flatter cornea centrally than in the periphery. Each of 4 radial keratotomy incisions demonstrates accentuated flattening as manifested in the surface arrows. *E.* Postoperative radial keratotomy ring corneal topography from patient in Figure 18–6*D*. Note the box-like ring shapes at the arrows in the same areas as the arrows in Figure 18–6*D*. This separation of the rings produces irregular astigmatism from localized corneal flattening.

Illustration continued on following page

PREOPERATIVE PATIENT SELECTION AND PREPARATION

Radial keratotomy is reasonably effective in the −2 to −8 diopter myopic patient, depending on the patient's age. Higher levels of myopia, between −8 and −15 diopters, may be satisfactorily repaired in the 50- to 60-year-old patient with a 16-incision technique, but the outcome is less predictable. In general, patients should have a stable myopia that is nonprogressive and without signs of keratoconus. Radial keratotomy is a valuable modifying technique for undercorrected PRK and LASIK procedures.[27] Figure 18–6*D* demonstrates the videokeratograph of keratoconus with inferior corneal steepening (red), steep central cornea (over 47 diopters) and non-orthogonal axis of astigmatism (over 22 degrees off 180 degrees). Slit-lamp examination should preclude significant external disease that may contribute to subsequent corneal infection. Collagen diseases or connective tissue diseases, uncontrolled lid

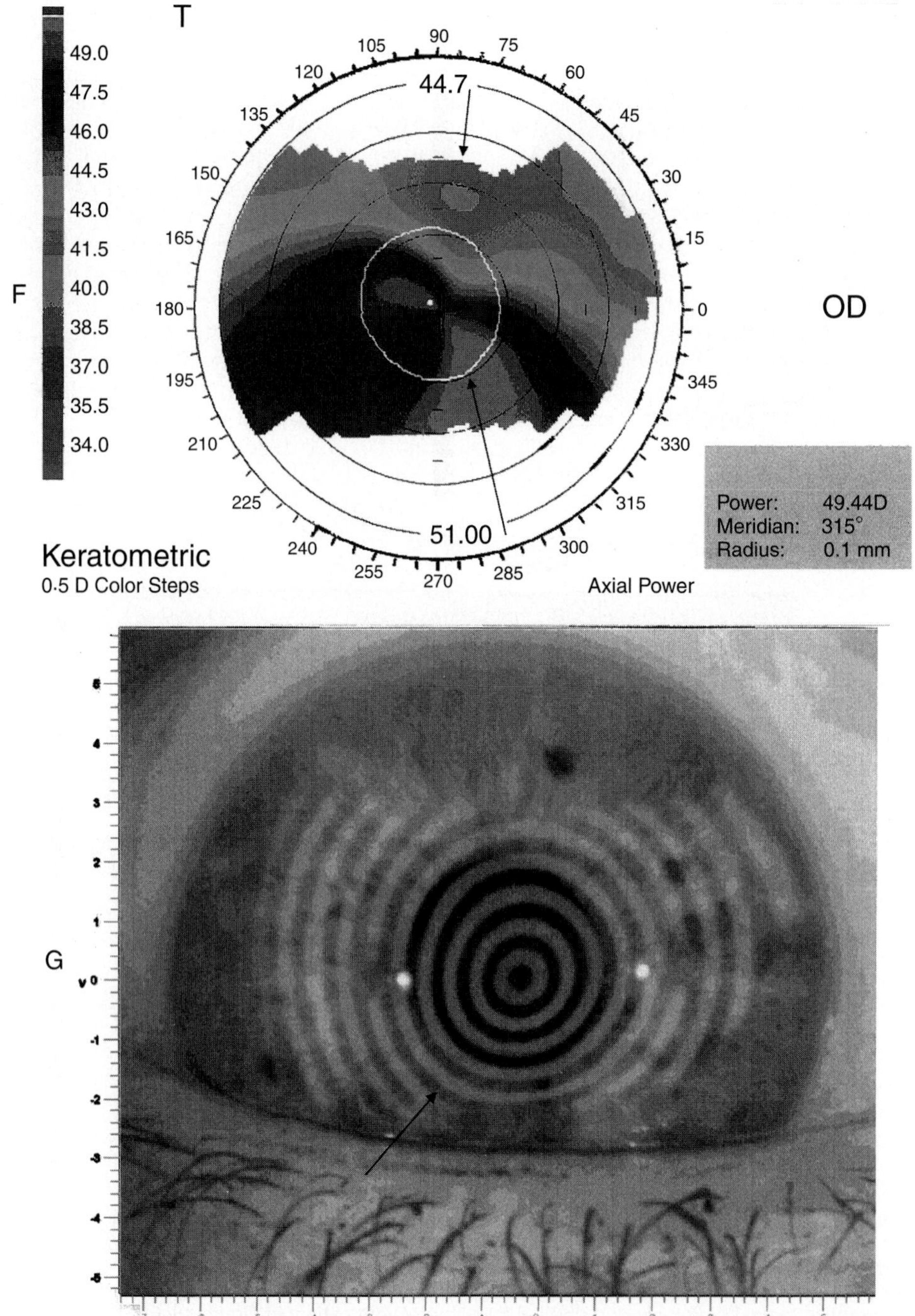

Figure 18–6 ***Continued*** *F.* Keratoconus corneal topography demonstrates inferior corneal steepening (large arrow) and is generally considered a contraindication to radial keratotomy or Lasik. Note the cornea is 51 diopters at 6 o'clock (large arrow) and 44.7 diopters superiorly (small arrow). *G.* Keratoconus ring corneal topography of Figure 18–6*F.* The rings demonstrate the path gnomonic "tear drop" shape of steepening inferiorly in the keratoconic cornea (arrow).

infections, glaucoma, or uveitis should be avoided, because the operative results on these patients may be unpredictable and surgery may complicate their underlying ocular disease process. Patients who are satisfactorily corrected with glasses or contact lenses should not be encouraged to undergo radial keratotomy. "Medical, legal and ethical considerations can almost always be resolved by doing what is in the best interest of the patient without regard for finances, personal aggrandizement, or other possible benefits to the surgeon," as emphasized by Bettman.[27]

Adequate informed consent includes (a) detailed explanation of the proposed procedure; (b) explanation of the known risks and benefits; (c) discussion of the alternatives to surgery and alternative surgeries such as surface PRK (photorefractive surgery), LASIK (laser assisted in situ keratomileusis) and the ICR (intracorneal ring); (d) review of all questions provided by the patient and open discussion of risks and benefits; and (e) adequate time between the discussion and the surgical procedure so that the patient may review the information and withdraw consent for the surgical intervention, awaiting further developments in the field.

It is especially important that patients realize that the results of the surgical procedure cannot be precisely predicted at this time. We have found it exceedingly important to explain presbyopic symptoms to patients, and this is our most difficult area of informed consent. Myopic patients realize that they may read simply by removing their glasses; overcorrecting prepresbyopic patients in the phoropter to demonstrate the incipient requirement for glasses is appropriate. A complete eye examination, including cycloplegic refraction, tonometry, external examination, slit-lamp examination, evaluation of the posterior pole and peripheral retina, and muscle balance is completed. An accurate measurement of the corneal thickness, along with endothelial evaluation, is necessary. Corneas that are thinner than 500 μm centrally and those that thin inferiorly may demonstrate early keratoconus, which should be avoided. Corneas that are thicker than 620 μm may be on the verge of corneal decompensation from endothelial dysfunction, and endothelial examination or cell counts are appropriate to preclude this possibility.

A nomogram summarizing pertinent refractive results is shown in Figure 18–7. The optical zone for each patient is reviewed. The greater the myopic refractive error, the greater the effect of a single operation; the greater the patient's age, the greater the effect of the procedure. Male patients have a greater effect with a similar optical zone procedure than do females unless topical steroids are used postoperatively; topical steroids equalize the male and female effect for a given age and operation. The PERK patients did not use steroids, whereas the University of Oklahoma and University of South Florida patients have all been placed on steroids (nomogram, Fig. 18–7). Three optical zones have been used in these two studies, 3.0, 3.5, and 4.0 mm. An optical zone smaller than 3.0 mm produces excessive glare in many patients and should be abandoned.[29] The primary predictive factors emphasized in this nomogram are preoperative myopia and patient age. The higher the preoperative myopia and/or patient age, the greater the effect of the surgical procedure. The nomogram is used by determining the patient's myopia on the left and traversing horizontally until the patient's age is observed. The average refractive change observed for the studied population is presented as the sloping regression lines. If an undercorrection is desired, a fewer number of incisions are made or a larger optical zone is chosen. It is better to undercorrect the patient, and subsequently add incisions, than to overcorrect to hyperopia. Lindstrom et al., have proposed the use of mini-RK-shortened incisions to 2.0 mm to avoid corneal instability and corneal fluctuation.[30] The primary surgical variables that may be altered include the optical zone length and number of incisions. Refractions between the current regression lines provided would infer that an intermediate optical zone marker could be used at this position. However, the data to substantiate such a recommendation are not currently available.

SURGICAL TECHNIQUE

Topical anesthesia with 0.5% proparacaine is used in all patients. Topical anesthesia is initiated approximately 5 minutes before preparation of the patient. Deep conjunctival anesthesia is obtained with 2 drops of proparacaine every 5 minutes until the visual axis is marked. Excessive anesthetic may loosen the epithelium, rolling under the blade producing shallow incisions. The eye is draped in a sterile manner after alcohol and iodine asepsis of the periocular skin has been accomplished. The visual axis marking (Fig. 18–8*A*

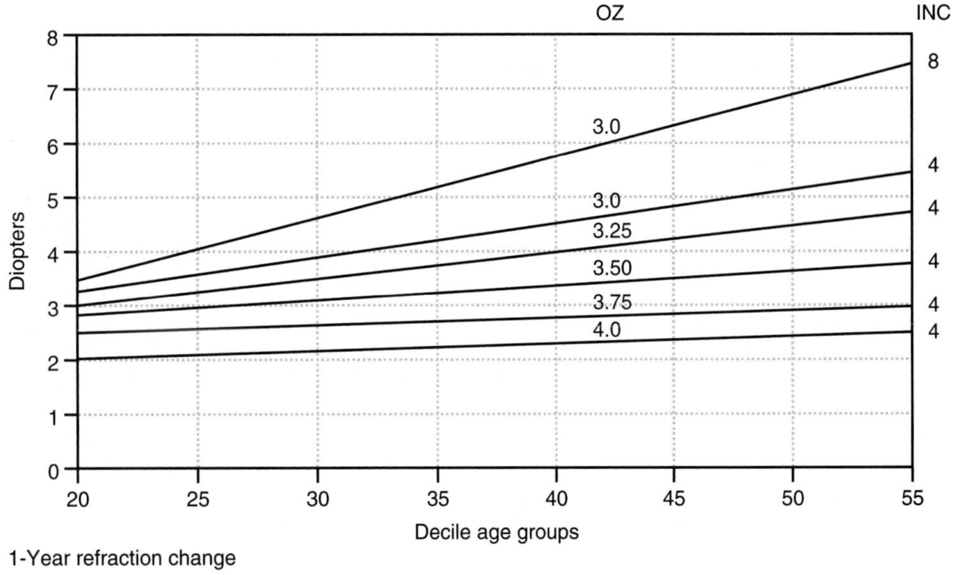

Figure 18–7. Nomogram to determine the optical zone for radial keratotomy, depending on myopia and patient's age.

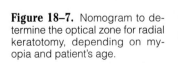

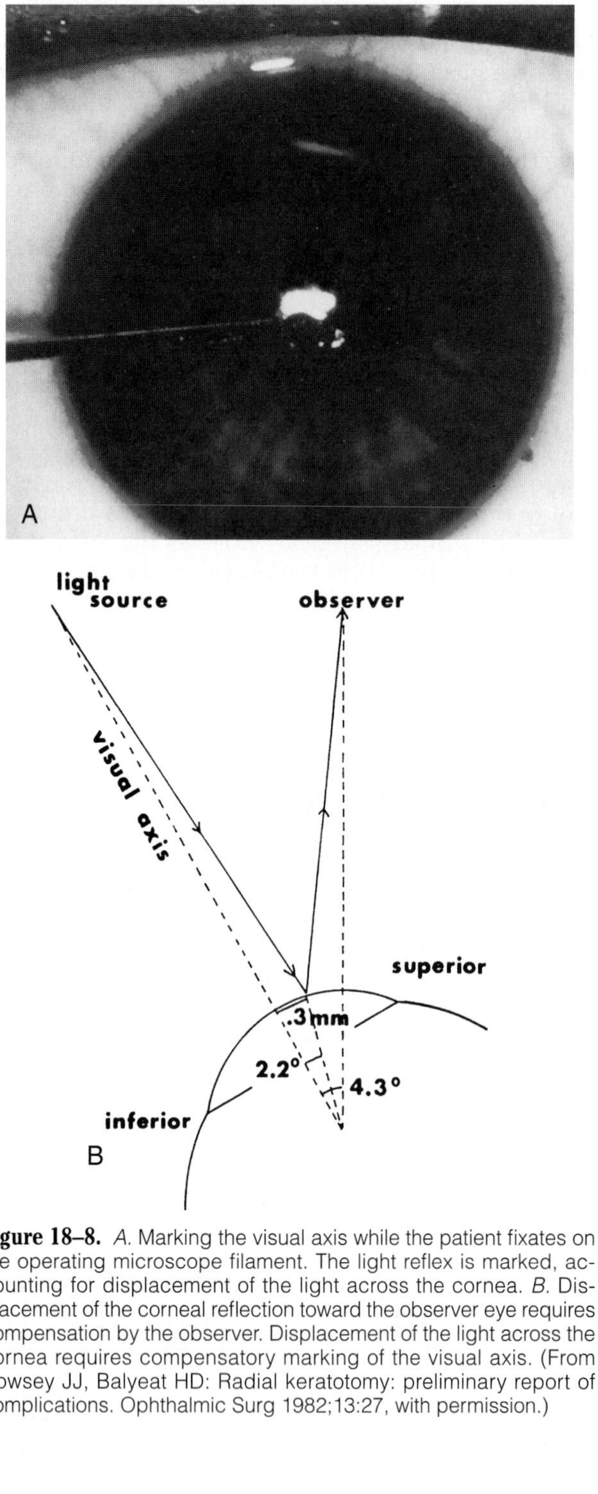

Figure 18–8. *A.* Marking the visual axis while the patient fixates on the operating microscope filament. The light reflex is marked, accounting for displacement of the light across the cornea. *B.* Displacement of the corneal reflection toward the observer eye requires compensation by the observer. Displacement of the light across the cornea requires compensatory marking of the visual axis. (From Rowsey JJ, Balyeat HD: Radial keratotomy: preliminary report of complications. Ophthalmic Surg 1982;13:27, with permission.)

and *B*) is accomplished by observing the pupil center. The visual axis and optical axis are difficult to delineate, and the "entrance pupil" or pupil projection through a round cornea is the appropriate point for marking the cornea. The virtual image of the pupil, denoted as the "entrance pupil" observed through the operating microscope will move toward the steeper side of the cornea because of the lens magnification effect on the steep cornea. This optical effect of a displaced pupil is only important in distorted corneas undergoing refractive surgery and should not confound routine myopic radial keratotomy. The patient is then directed to look away and subsequently refocus the light source to determine if a similar position is reflected from the cornea. Patients have a tendency to look away from the light source because of its irritation, and the visual axis determination should be confirmed. A Sinsky hook or 26-gauge needle may be used to lightly mark the epithelium, avoiding damage to the basement membrane or Bowman's membrane (Fig. 18–8*A*).

A trephine is selected between 3 and 4 mm (see nomogram, Fig. 18–7), and the visual axis is circumscribed with the appropriate-sized optical zone (Fig. 18–9*A* and *B*). Trephines are typically calibrated by measuring inside edge to inside edge. Radial corneal incisions, therefore, must begin on the inside edge of the corneal trephine mark, cutting across the trephine mark itself to maximize the effect of the procedure. A set of trephines is shown in Figure 18–9*A*, and the entire surgery tray in Figure 18–10 (diamond knife, coin gauge, Thornton fixation ring, ultrasonic pachymeter, irrigation canula [30-gauge], anesthetic, lid speculum, micro sponges, and syringe). We avoid a solid lid speculum, as the diamond knife may be easily chipped on this device. The Thornton fixation ring allows performing the incisions by rotating the globe or rotating the knife around the cornea. It also simultaneously allows the pressure on the globe to increase, to maximize the depth of incisions. High pressure in the eye improves corneal sectility (cutting facility) even with a diamond knife, allowing equal depth of cut in the American downhill (centrifugal), or Russian uphill (centripetal) incisions. Double cutting blades are available which allow cutting in either direction. The newest diamonds are sharpened only on the anterior inferior 200 microns, thereby avoiding invasion into the visual axis with bidirectional incisions. Pachymetry (Fig. 18–11) is completed in the central cornea and at each of four positions along the trephine mark of the cornea. The pachymeter tip is set at a tangent to the trephine marks. The visual axis normally traverses the nasal cornea, and the geometric center of the cornea is, therefore, temporal to the visual axis (Fig. 18–11*B*). The geometric center of the cornea is thinner than any other cornea position, including the nasal visual axis. The thin geometric corneal center is routinely expected for the diamond knife setting. The diamond knife is extended to 100% of the thinnest paracentral reading (Fig. 18–12). Attention to the diamond is important to avoid chipping or overextending the blade. The current gauges allow the surgeon to set the diamond within 5 μm of the desired level (Fig. 18–12). Variations in diamond knife quality and calibration have been demonstrated with the new high-magnification gauges (Fig. 18–13*A*), which allow inspection of the diamond for internal cleavage planes and chipping. The high magnification of the newer inspection tools also demonstrates any unevenness of the platforms, the poor polishing frequently associated with rough handling, and the diamond defects provided in industrial-grade compared with gem-grade diamonds (Fig. 18–13*B* and *C*). The use of these inspection tools before surgery to calibrate the micrometer handles of the newer diamonds to greater precision avoids the need for use of the gauge block during surgery. The

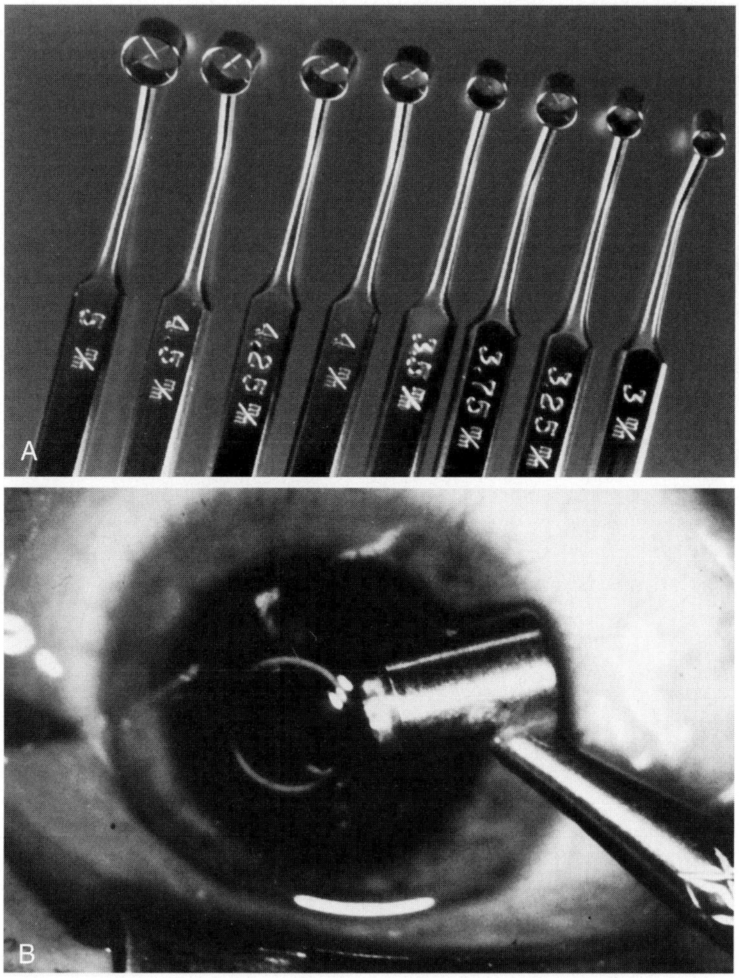

Figure 18–9. *A.* Blunt trephines are used to circumscribe the visual axis. *B.* A blunt trephine surrounds the visual axis, marking the optical zone.

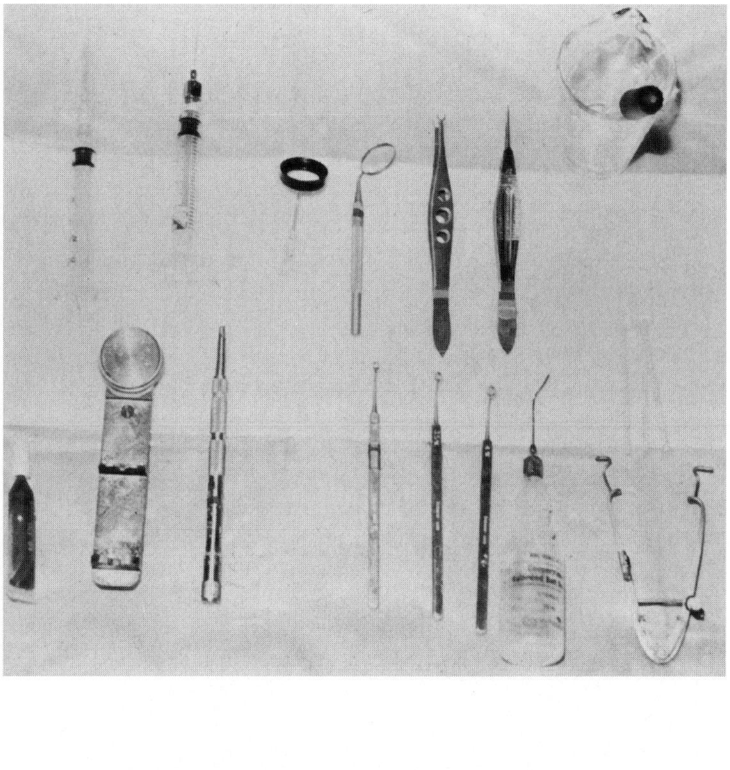

Figure 18–10. A radial keratotomy operative tray, showing the useful equipment.

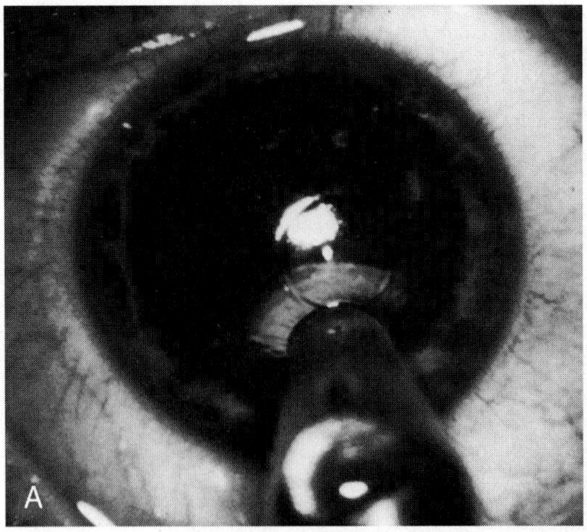

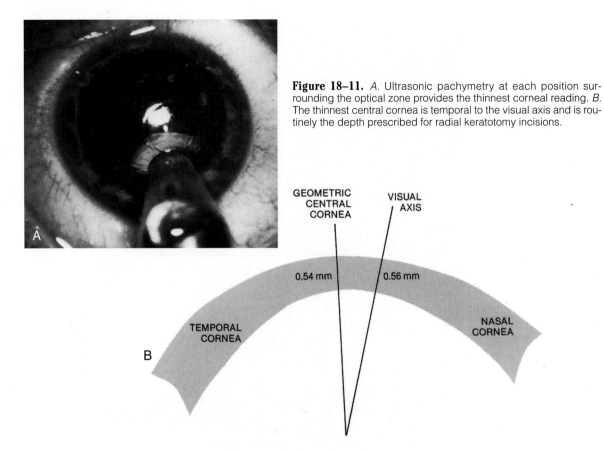

Figure 18–11. *A.* Ultrasonic pachymetry at each position surrounding the optical zone provides the thinnest corneal reading. *B.* The thinnest central cornea is temporal to the visual axis and is routinely the depth prescribed for radial keratotomy incisions.

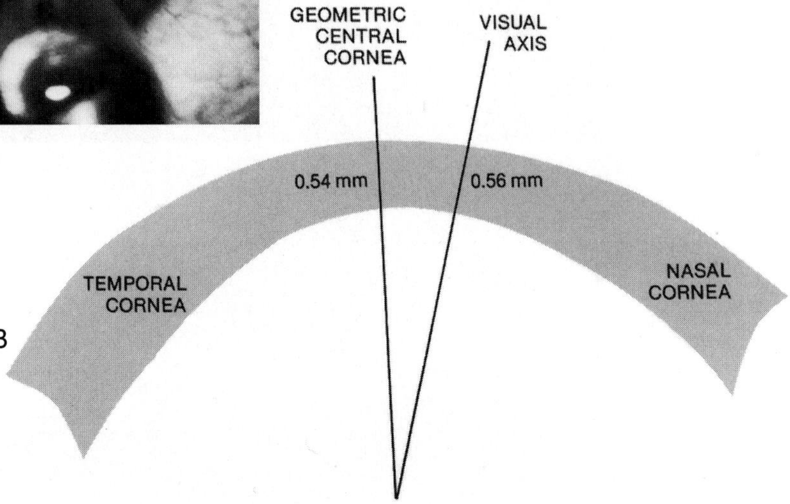

B

Figure 18–12. The diamond gauge device allows daily recalibration of the blade.

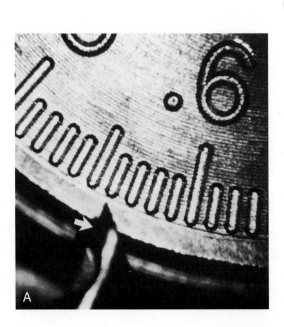

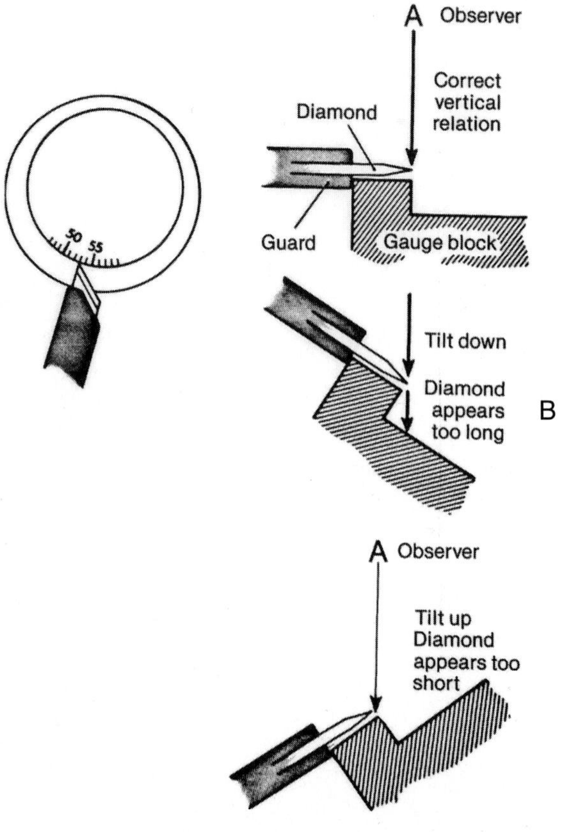

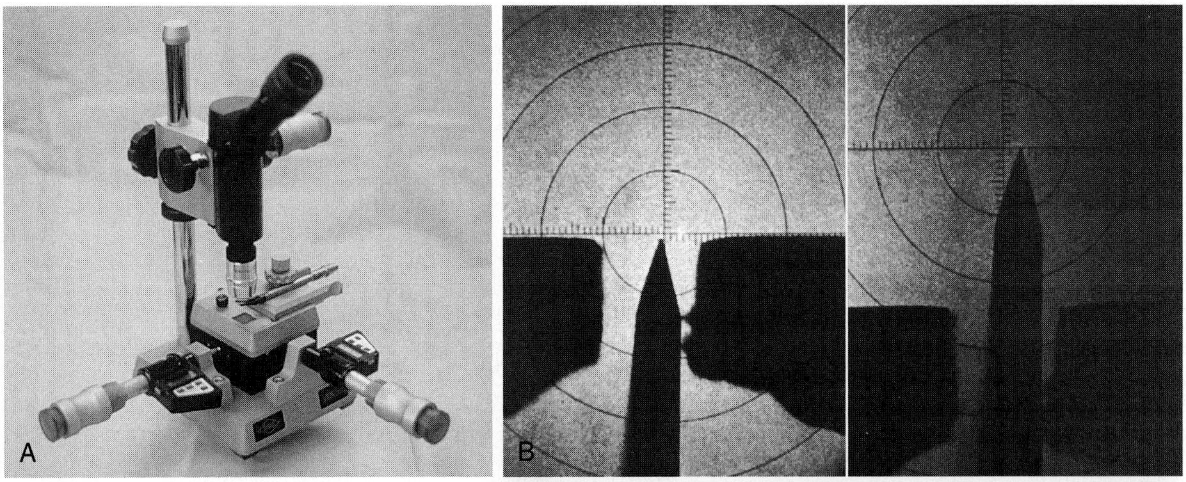

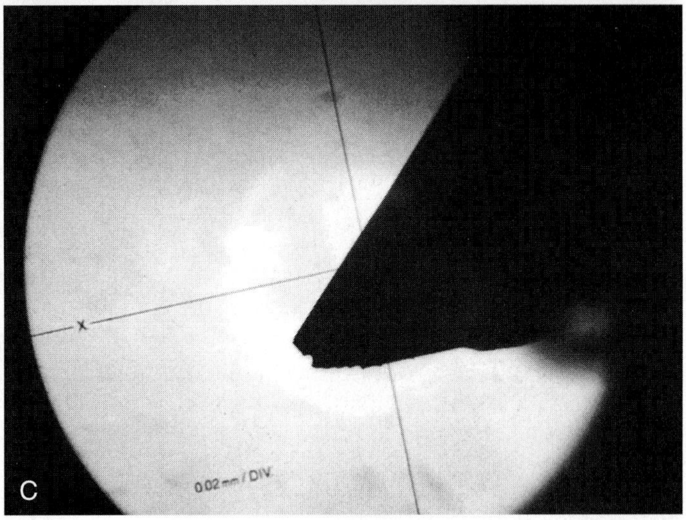

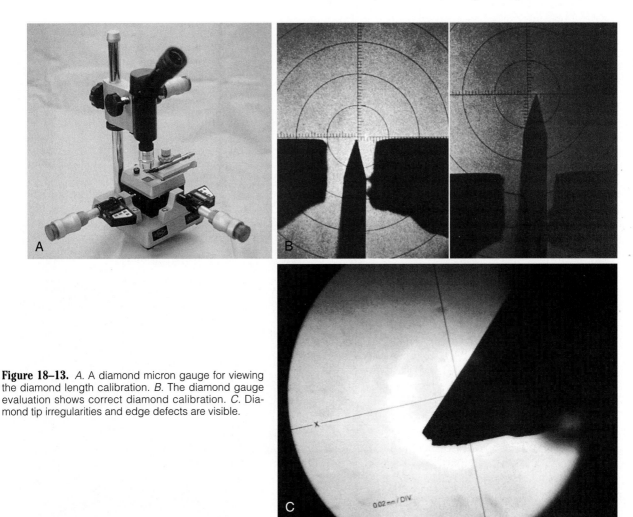

Figure 18–13. *A.* A diamond micron gauge for viewing the diamond length calibration. *B.* The diamond gauge evaluation shows correct diamond calibration. *C.* Diamond tip irregularities and edge defects are visible.

older gauge blocks have been associated with trauma to the guard of the diamond, producing variable diamond extensions in subsequent surgery, and are best avoided. The diamond knife is provided with two advance mechanisms, coarse and fine. The coarse advance destabilizes the calibration. Therefore, only the fine advance and retraction are used after the diamond micrometer handle has been calibrated.

The globe is fixed with the Thornton fixation ring (Fig. 18–14), and the intraocular pressure is increased to between 30 and 40 mm Hg. This higher intraocular pressure maximizes corneal sectility. Improved sectility improves incision depth. The trephine mark must be excised (Fig. 18–15*A*). Vertical corneal incisions maximize the flattening cornea (Fig. 18–15*B*), according to the valve rule of Eisner ("incisions through the wall of the globe produce valves whose margin of watertightness is proportional to the projection of the incision onto the wall of the globe").[32] Vertical corneal incisions, therefore, spontaneously open (see caveat number 1), whereas shelving corneal incisions spontaneously close, diminishing the effectiveness of radial keratotomy. The surgeon should, before surgery, practice producing a vertical radial corneal incision in all quadrants; this will accentuate the effect of the incisions. During the initiation of the incision, the knife should be placed at full depth through the optical zone mark, and seated for a count of 1 to 2 seconds before the incision is initiated. If peripheral movement begins before complete seating of the diamond occurs, a diminished effect will be observed.

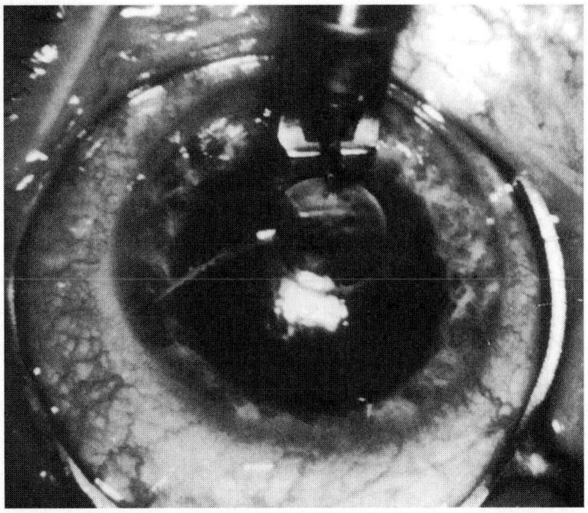

Figure 18–14. Radial corneal incisions maximize the corneal flattening effect. Adequate globe fixation is important, Thornton ring (arrow).

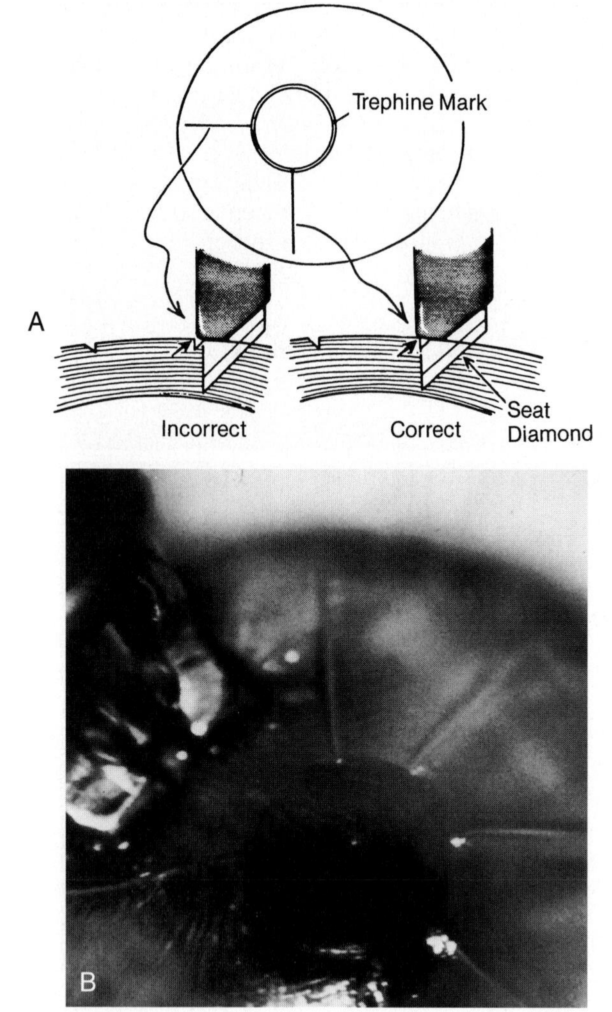

Figure 18–15. *A.* Incisions must incise the trephine mark after scating the blade *(B)* to full depth. *B.* Vertical corneal incisions maximize the corneal flattening. Oblique incisions produce shallow, self-closing valves.

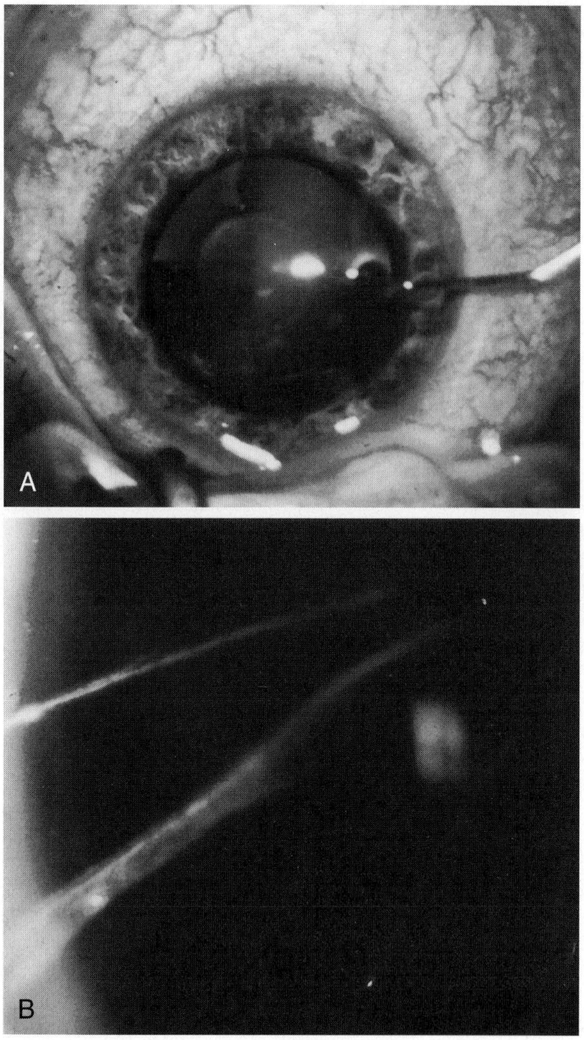

Figure 18–16. *A.* Irrigations of the incisions minimize epithelial debris. *B.* Epithelial debris (white dots) that remains in the incisions may produce glare and can be avoided by meticulous incision irrigation.

Meticulous irrigation of the incisions (Fig. 18–16*A*) at the end of the procedure prevents some of the major complications of excessive corneal scarring, epithelial ingrowth (Fig. 18–16*B*), and glare after the procedure. It is worthwhile to irrigate parallel to the incision, gently removing all epithelial debris. Descemet's membrane may be stripped from the posterior aspect of cornea if irrigation is too vigorous, so the gentle use of intraoperative saline solution or balanced salt solution along the incisions with a 30-gauge needle is warranted. The diamond knife should be carefully irrigated with saline solution and washed with alcohol or hydrogen peroxide to remove all epithelial debris before it is resterilized. If the diamond knife is steam sterilized with epithelial debris or serum on the tip, this material will harden and present as apparent dullness on subsequent surgical procedures. Inspection of the diamond knife under high magnification may demonstrate epithelial or caked debris; this may be removed by wetting the blade with alcohol and making an incision through Styrofoam. The roughened incision edge of the Styrofoam will remove most debris.

AVOIDING COMPLICATIONS AT SURGERY

Good patient rapport is required to allow the patient to relax during surgery. Before surgery we provide 5 to 10 mg of oral diazepam. If the visual axis is mismarked, incisions may traverse the visual axis, producing marked glare and decreased vision. Excessive opening of the lids with the lid speculum when the lid is not blocked may produce lid spasm and conjunctival protrusion into the operative field during the surgical procedure. A gentle wire lid speculum avoids these complications. Ptosis has been reported after radial keratotomy. Although there are other possible explanations, the ptosis may conceivably be related to squeezing against the lid speculum. Topical anesthesia may be fortified with 0.1 ml injections of 2% lidocaine near the limbus to allow for adequate fixation with the Thornton ring or two-point fixation forceps.

The patient may find the light of the microscope the most uncomfortable aspect of the procedure. It is important to diminish the light of the operating microscope from full illumination. This not only reduces patient discomfort but also decreases the possibility of macular phototoxicity. It should be recalled that correct determination of the visual axis requires the patient to fixate the bulb of the microscope, to visualize the pupil center.

It is necessary to maintain good globe fixation pressure with the surgeon's nondominant hand to avoid complications. Inadequate globe pressure may allow the diamond to push the cornea posteriorly, engaging the iris or lens on the indented Descemet's membrane, thereby producing iris atrophy or a cataract. Lack of irrigation of the incisions at the end of the procedure will produce epithelial debris and excessive corneal scarring, which is unacceptable.

If the anterior chamber is entered inadvertently, the chamber may collapse, engaging the iris or the lens on the diamond knife. Perforations are to be avoided. Microperforations, in an attempt to accentuate the effect of the operation, turn the procedure from an extraocular to an intraocular procedure, greatly increasing the risk to the patient without adding to the benefit.

POSTOPERATIVE CARE

Topical Tobradex eye drops are applied 4 times a day for 1 week and then fluorometholone (FML) is used 4 times a day for 1 month. Voltaren eye drops 4 times a day for 2 days alleviate the incision pain, and eye patching is no longer required. For the first 24 hours after surgery the patient may be irritated by a pressure patch and find the eye more comfortable without a patch. Topical steroids maximize the flattening effect of the procedure.

Patients are reevaluated 1 week postoperatively, 4 weeks, 3 months, 6 months, 1 year, 2 years, and 3 years after the surgery. No further surgery is initiated until 3 months after the initial surgical procedure.

COMPLICATIONS

The complications of radial keratotomy[10,15,33–40] should be thoroughly reviewed by the surgeon and the patient considering refractive surgery. The major problem is a *lack of predictability*.[31] For example, 1.6 diopters of greater effect may be seen with sea-level treatment compared with 6000 feet altitude.[33] We would consider a predictable operation one in which the residual ametropia misses a plano or zero refractive error by no more than 10% of the original refractive error. For example, a desirable operative result in a −2.50 myope would be plano ± 0.25 of a diopter. A −10 myope would be reasonably pleased with a refractive error of plano ± 1 diopter. This expectation is being approached in radial keratotomy but it cannot be guaranteed. *Regression* of myopic flattening occurs with wound healing as corneal scarring ensues. The flat initial cornea gradually steepens, and the initially overcorrected patient will approach emmetropia. The patient who is undercorrected in the first 1 week postoperatively will seldom obtain an emmetropic state. More recent reports, however, demonstrate *progression*, or a hyperopic shift, 1 to 10 years after the surgery. A hyperopic shift greater than 1.0 diopters may occur in over 34% of patients.[34] This suggests that a slight undercorrection, instead of overcorrection, may be preferable. PERK optical zones of 3.0, 3.5, 4.0 mm demonstrate a 0.99 diopter, 0.63 diopter, and 0.40 diopter hyperopic shift, respectively, between 1 and 10 years after surgery.[30] Clearly, further investigation is required to settle this matter.

Epithelial defects are observed in all patients postoperatively. The epithelium normally heals within 2 to 3 days after the surgery; in fact, it is frequently essentially healed within 24 hours with residual punctate epithelial staining remaining. *Recurrent erosions* may occur if Cogan's mapdot fingerprint corneal dystrophy precedes the radial keratotomy. Cogan's dystrophy is, therefore, a relative contraindication to the procedure. *Subepithelial fibrosis* indistinguishable from Cogan's dystrophy may occur after the procedure and may represent occult recurrent microepithelial erosions. *Moncreiff iron lines*[37] associated with corneal topography shift after the procedure are frequently observed, but are not associated with glare or patient complaints.

Residual blood in the incisions may be associated with subsequent *corneal vascularization* or *excessive glare* and should be avoided at the time of surgery. Vascular ingrowth with *contact lens wear* is associated with partial anoxia or decreased contact lens mobility. Contact lens fitting problems may increase, and patients should be aware that if they have been contact lens failures, they will probably not have success with a contact lens after radial keratotomy.

Perforation of the anterior chamber has been associated with localized *epithelial downgrowth, endophthalmitis,* and *cataract.* Any perforation should be reported to the patient, who is forewarned to notify us if increasing pain, redness, or decreasing vision occurs.

Early infectious keratitis *(Staphylococcus aureus)* or late incisional infections *(Pseudomonas aeruginosa)* are seen more frequently with contact lens use after surgery.[38]

Astigmatism is produced in a low magnitude correction, +0.5 to +2.00 diopters, as frequently as it is spontaneously eliminated by the symmetrization process of the procedure (15%).

Incisional *epithelial ingrowth* can be avoided by meticulous irrigation of the incisions after the procedure. Residual epithelium appears to predispose incisions to subsequent infections. Unfortunately, late incisional infections may cause endophthalmitis and demand aggressive therapy.[39] *Glare* is observed in all patients in the immediate postoperative period and may persist for up to 5 years postoperatively. This glare is associated with decreased night vision potential. Rarely patients are unable to drive at night because of the glare of oncoming headlights through the corneal incisions.

Fluctuating vision is greatest in the early postoperative period. The cornea appears to be flattest in the morning and steepens throughout the day. The overcorrected patient is hyperopic in the morning and, as the cornea steepens throughout the day, approaches emmetropia. The patient barely corrected to emmetropia in the morning develops progressive corneal steepening from morning to evening associated with progressive myopia, requiring glasses by evening for the residual myopic correction. This fluctuating vision averages 0.36 +/− 0.58 diopters from morning to evening ($p < .01$). This continued steepening of the cornea is possibly related to a progressive drop in intraocular pressure during the day.[40] Incisional instability is especially onerous when cataract surery is required. A hyperopic shift is routinely observed and intraocular lens calculations should anticipate 2.0 diopters of flattening postoperatively.[41] *Marked overcorrections* of 4 or 5 diopters may occur, but should be infrequent with the newer 4-incision procedures. Precipitation of an *esotropia,* if the patient has a heterophoria before surgery and has a sudden anisometropia after the first operation, is possible but infrequent.

Globe ruptures after radial keratotomy are still being reported 10 to 13 years postoperatively.[42] *Endothelial cell loss* appears to be between 7% and 8% with each operation, is nonprogressive, and has not been associated with endothelial decompensation with the current U.S. techniques.

SUMMARY

Radial keratotomy can reduce myopia in the −2 to −8 diopter range, depending on the patient's age.[43] New instrumentation (including diamond knives, corneascopy, ultrasonic pachymetry, and globe fixation devices), control of incision depth and wound healing, and linear regression models of predictive variables may allow greater precision of this procedure in the future. The most common complications appear to be lack of predictability, glare, and fluctuating vision. The long-term complications of this procedure are now observed as progressive effect or a hyperopic shift.

Patients must be fully informed regarding the complications already known. In addition, they must be made aware that the long-term effects of radial keratotomy are still unknown even 20 years after surgery. The surgery has a place in the treatment of myopia only in patients who have fully considered the risks and benefits of this procedure, compared to the cost, risk, and benefits of newer alternatives.

REFERENCES

1. Lans RJ: Experimentelle Untersuchungen uber Entstehung von Astigmatisms durch nicht-perforirende Corneawunden. Albrecht Von Graefes Arch Ophthalmol 1898;45:117.
2. Sato T: Treatment of conical cornea (incision of Descemet's membrane). Acta Soc Ophthalmol Jpn 1939;43:544.
3. Sato T, Aldyama K, Shibata H: A new surgical approach to myopia. Am J Ophthalmol 1953;36:823.
4. Durnev VV: Decrease of corneal refraction by anterior keratotomy method with the purpose of surgical correction of myopia of mild moderate degree. Proceedings of the First Congress of Ophthalmologists of Transcaucasia Tollisi, USSR, 1976:129.
5. Durnev VV, Ermoshin AS: Determination of dependence between length of anterior radial nonperforating incisions and cornea and their effectiveness. Transactions of the Fifth All-Union Conference of Inventors and Rationalizers in Ophthalmology Field, Moscow, USSR, 1986:106.
6. Fyodorov SN, Durnev VV: Operation of dosaged dissection of corneal circular ligament in cases of myopia of a mid degree. Ann Ophthalmol 1979;11:1885.
7. Hoffer KJ, Darin JJ, Pettit TH, et al.: UCLA clinical trial of radial keratotomy: preliminary report. Ophthalmology 1981;88:729.
8. Cowden JW, Bores LD: A clinical investigation of the surgical correction of myopia by the method of Fyodorov. Ophthalmology 1981;88:737.
9. Cowden JW: Radial keratotomy: retrospective study of cases observed at the Kresge Eye Institute for six months. Arch Ophthalmol 1982;100:578.
10. Balyeat HD: Radial keratotomy: preliminary report of complications. Ophthalmic Surg 1982;13:27.
11. Bonham RD, Hays JC, Rowsey JJ: Efficacy of four incision radial keratotomy. ARVO Abstracts. Invest Ophthalmol Vis Sci 1985; 26(Suppl):202.
12. Salz JJ, Villasenor RA, Elander R, et al.: Four-incision radial keratotomy for low to moderate myopia. Ophthalmology 1986;93:727.
13. Vaughan ER: The 4-cut radial keratotomy in low myopia. Refract Surg 1986;2:164.
14. Waring GO, Moffitt SD, Gelender H, et al.: Rationale for and design of the National Eye Institute Prospective Evaluation of Radial Keratotomy (PERK) study. Ophthalmology 1983;90:40.
15. Waring GO, Lynn MJ, Gelender H, et al.: Results of the Prospective Evaluation of Radial Keratotomy (PERK) study one year after radial keratotomy. Ophthalmology 1985;92:177.
16. Waring GO, Laibson P, Lindstrom R, et al.: Changes in refraction, keratometry and visual acuity during the first year after radial keratotomy in the PERK study. Invest Ophthalmol Vis Sci 1985;56 (Suppl):202.
17. Rowsey JJ, Balyeat HD, Rabinovitch B, et al.: Predicting the results of radial keratotomy. Ophthalmology 1983;90:642.
18. Dietz MR, Sanders DR, Marks RG: Radial keratotomy: an overview of the Kansas City study. Ophthalmology 1984;91:467.
19. Arrowsmith PN, Sanders DR, Marks RG: Visual refractive and keratometric results of radial keratotomy. Arch Ophthalmol 1983;101:873.
20. Rowsey JJ: Ten caveats in keratorefractive surgery. Ophthalmology 1983;90:147.
21. Troutman RC: Microsurgery of the anterior segment of the eye. Vol. 2, The Cornea: Optics and Surgery, St. Louis, CV Mosby; 1977:268.
22. Smith TW: Corneal topography. Doc Ophthalmol 1977;43:249.
23. Mandell RB, St. Helen R: Mathematical model of the cornea contour. Br J Physiol Optics 1977;26:183.
24. Humphrey Instruments, Model 410 Auto keratometer. Owner's manual. San Leandro, CA, Humphrey Instruments, Inc.
25. Henslee SL, Rowsey JJ: New corneal shapes in keratorefractive surgery. Ophthalmology 1983;90:245.
26. Au Y-K, Rowsey JJ: Bending moment modeling in radial keratotomy. In Spaeth GL, Katz J, Parker KW (eds.), Current Therapy in Ophthalmic Surgery. Philadelphia, BC Decker, Inc.; 1989:47.
27. Kwitko ML, Jovkar S, Yan H, Atas M. Radial keratotomy for residual myopia after photorefractive keratectomy. J Cataract Refract Surg 1998;24:315–319.
28. Bettman JW: Refractive keratoplasty: medicolegal aspects. In Sanders DR, Hofmann RF, Salz JJ (eds.), Refractive Corneal Surgery. Thorofare, N.J., Slack, Inc.; 1985:17.
29. Grimmett MR, Holland EJ: Complications of small clear-zone radial keratotomy. Ophthalmology 1996;103:1348.
30. Lindstrom RL: Minimally invasive radial keratotomy: mini-RK. J Cataract Refract Surg 1995;21:27.

31. McDonnell PJ, Nizam A, Lynn MJ, Waring GO: Morning-to-evening change in refraction, corneal curvature, and visual acuity 11 years after radial keratotomy in the prospective evaluation of radial keratotomy study. The PERK Study Group. Ophthalmology 1996;103:233.
32. Eisner G: Eye Surgery: An Introduction to Operative Technique. Berlin, Springer-Verlag; 1980.
33. Cinal A, Yasar T, Demirok A, et al.: A comparative study on the effect of radial keratotomy in patients who live at sea level and high altitude. Eye 1999;13:339–344.
34. Charpentier DY, Garcia P, Grunewald F, et al.: Refractive results of radial keratotomy after 10 years. J Refract Surg 1998;14: 646–648.
35. Rowsey JJ, Balyeat HD: Radial keratotomy: preliminary report of complications. Ophthalmic Surg 1982;13:27.
36. Rowsey JJ, Hays JC: Recent Advances in Ophthalmology, Radial Keratotomy, Vol. 7. Edinburgh, Churchill Livingstone; 1985.
37. Davis RM, Miller RA, Lindstrom RL, et al.: Corneal iron lines after radial keratotomy. J Refract Surg 1986;2:174.
38. Heidemann DG, Dunn SP, Chow CY: Early-versus late-onset infectious keratitis after radial and astigmatic keratotomy: clinical spectrum in a referral practice. J Cataract Refract Surg 1999; 25:1615–1619.
39. Erkin EF, Durak I, Ferliel S, Maden A: Keratitis complicated by endophthalmitis 3 years after astigmatic keratotomy. J Cataract Refract Surg 1998;24:1280–1282.
40. Kemp JR, Martinez CE, Klyce SD, et al.: Diurnal fluctuations in corneal topography 10 years after radial keratotomy in the Prospective Evaluation of Radial Keratotomy Study. J Cataract Refract Surg 1999;25:904–910.
41. Bardocci A, Lofoco G: Corneal topography and postoperative refraction after cataract phacoemulsification following radial keratotomy. Ophthalmic Surg Lasers 1999;30:155–159.
42. Panda A, Sharma N, Kumar A: Ruptured globe 10 years after radial keratotomy. J Refract Surg 1999;15:64–65.
43. Rowsey JJ, Morley WA: Surgical correction of moderate myopia: which method should you choose? Surv Ophthalmol 1998; 43:147–156.

CHAPTER 19

Laser in Situ Keratomileusis
SURGICAL TECHNIQUE

JONATHAN D. CARR, M.D., M.A., R. DOYLE STULTING, M.D., Ph.D., KEITH P. THOMPSON, M.D., and GEORGE O. WARING, M.D.

Laser in-situ keratomileusis (LASIK) evolved in the early 1990s as a surgical method for altering the refractive power of the cornea, to correct myopia, hyperopia, and astigmatism.[1] The LASIK procedure involves the use of a microkeratome to create a hinged flap in the cornea, underneath which an excimer laser is used to remove micron amounts of stromal tissue to correct the particular refractive error.

Microkeratomes have become increasingly sophisticated in recent years, allowing the LASIK procedure to be performed more safely by more ophthalmic surgeons than ever before. Microkeratomes vary in terms of design, but can be classified according to whether a nasal or superior hinge is created, and whether microkeratome translation is achieved manually or with automation. This chapter reports the use of the Hansatome (Bausch & Lomb, Rochester, NY) at Emory Vision in Atlanta, Georgia. The use of other microkeratomes will not be discussed.

Excimer laser technology has advanced considerably since 1996. The shape and size of laser beam delivery has been modified in a variety of ways by laser manufacturers, to overcome the beam inhomogeneity that was observed with the broad-beam lasers of the early 1990s.[2] As the size of the laser beam has been reduced by manufacturers to a slit or a spot, a need for eye trackers has emerged. Trackers have also become important in the evolution of customized laser ablation where the laser needs to align accurately, registering in the same alignment as the wavefront sensor used preoperatively to gather aberration data. This chapter will not report any specific details about one particular laser or another; general points about laser delivery will be discussed.

There is an increasing number of reports of corneal ectasia after LASIK.[3–13] Continued study of the accuracy and precision of preoperative corneal thickness measurement, whether by ultrasound or Orbscan topography (Bausch & Lomb, Salt Lake City, UT), together with better knowledge of the variability in flap thickness created by our microkeratomes, will further minimize the likelihood of ectasia after LASIK.

SURGICAL EQUIPMENT FOR LASIK

The Hansatome microkeratome is the one predominantly used at Emory Vision. The keratome consists of a suction ring and a microkeratome head (Fig. 19–1). The suction ring is placed on the ocular surface to generate suction, thereby raising the intraocular pressure. The keratome has three parts, a motorized handpiece, a pivot collar, and a microkeratome head. The microkeratome blade is inserted into the microkeratome head. The pivot collar is placed between the handpiece and the microkeratome head and is positioned to allow procedures on either the right or the left eye (Fig. 19–2). The operating room technician must reposition the pivot collar between surgery on the first and second eyes.

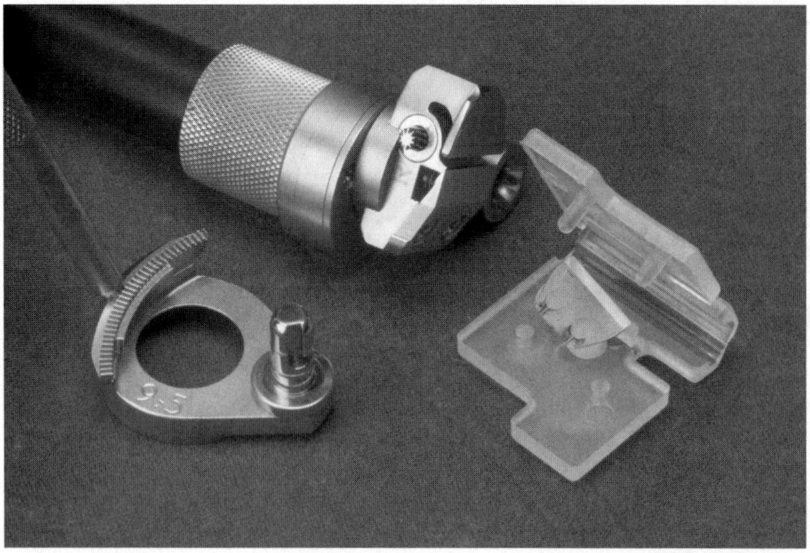

Figure 19–1. The Hansatome (Bausch & Lomb, Rochester, NY) consists of a suction ring and a microkeratome head into which a blade is inserted. (Courtesy of Ray Swords and Emory Vision.)

Meticulous maintenance and cleaning of the microkeratome is essential for complication-free surgery. The device must be assembled with great care prior to surgery to avoid inadvertent damage to the microkeratome blade. It is the surgeon's responsibility to ensure that the microkeratome is operating correctly before the start of the LASIK procedure. Emory Vision has several Hansatome microkeratomes available in the operating room. This creates the additional burden of ensuring that the serial number on the suction ring matches the serial number on the microkeratome head and the pivot collar. Failure to use equipment with matching serial numbers would increase the potential for microkeratome jams during translation across the cornea. Proponents of microkeratomes that have manual translation of the keratome head by the surgeon argue that microkeratome jams are not seen because of the lack of automation.

Several excimer lasers are available at Emory Vision including the Nidek EC-5000 (Nidek, Japan) and the Summit-Autonomous LADARVision laser (Alcon). Investigational studies of other lasers, performed under the auspices of the U.S. Food and Drug Administration (FDA), are ongoing but will not be discussed in this chapter. At the time of this writing, there are no peer-reviewed data to support the argument that one FDA-approved excimer laser achieves significantly better refractive outcomes (safety and efficacy) over any others. It is noteworthy that the data presented to the FDA by laser manufacturers when they petition for approval of their respective systems, are often eclipsed by peer-reviewed reports in the years that follow approval. This has allowed a level playing field among approved lasers in terms of results. It is anticipated, however, that as our understanding of wavefront sensing technology advances, we will have at our disposal a new metric for reporting the quality of results. This technology may allow us to discriminate among the currently available excimer lasers.

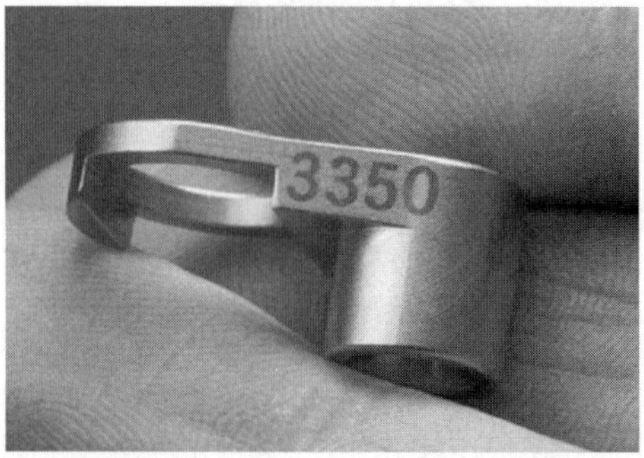

Figure 19–2. The pivot collar is positioned for either a right or left eye procedure. It must therefore be rotated 180 degrees after the first eye and before operating on the fellow eye. (Courtesy of Ray Swords and Emory Vision.)

EVOLUTION OF LASIK TECHNIQUE AT EMORY VISION

LASIK has been performed at Emory since 1994. Four of Emory's surgeons had prior experience with lamellar surgery, having performed Automated Lamellar Keratoplasty (ALK) for some years. Thus, considerable expertise was available at the beginning of the first FDA study of LASIK at Emory. A credentialing system was imposed for all surgeons who would begin performing LASIK. The system involved a didactic series of lectures on surgical technique and all elements of the surgeon's decision-making process. This was followed by multiple "wet-lab" sessions where prospective LASIK surgeons used the microkeratome to create flaps in pig corneas until proficiency was demonstrated. At this time, the entire procedure was rehearsed by the surgeon, including the correct use of the excimer laser. All surgeons completed the appropriate training require-

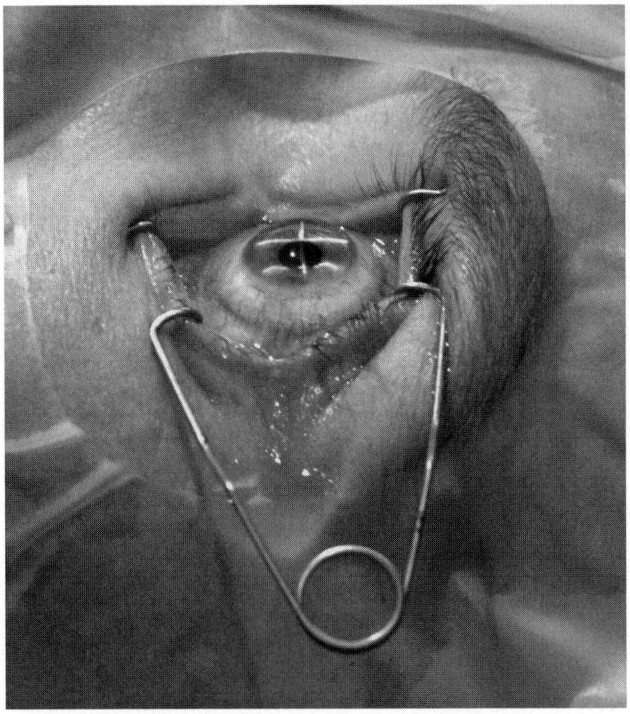

Figure 19–3. An open-bladed speculum is used predominantly at Emory. (Courtesy of Ray Swords and Emory Vision.)

ments of the laser manufacturers to allow use of the machine. Having completed the wet lab, one of the four Emory surgeons with prior lamellar surgery experience (faculty surgeons) completed an oral examination of the prospective surgeon's knowledge. Satisfactory completion of this oral examination allowed the surgeon to perform LASIK. The first ten patient procedures were typically proctored by one of the faculty LASIK surgeons. All refractive results were entered into a database that allowed active surveillance of the performance of all surgeons. All surgeries performed at Emory Vision were videotaped to allow review in the event that a surgeon had an intraoperative complication. Such review took place at periodic surgeon group meetings; this allowed the surgeons to continue to improve technique during the years that followed.

PREPARATION OF THE SURGICAL FIELD

Eyelid specula come in a variety of shapes and sizes, each having its own advantages and disadvantages. The speculum that is routinely used at Emory is the Miltex eyelid speculum (Miltex, Germany). This is an "open" bladed speculum through which the eyelashes are directly visible (Fig. 19–3). Initially, the eyelashes were draped with tape, protecting the eyelid margin during use of the microkeratome and laser treatment. Subsequently the eyelid margins were not routinely draped.

PREPARATION OF THE MICROKERATOME

Several microkeratomes have been used at Emory Vision. Prior to the Hansatome, Emory surgeons used the Automated Corneal Shaper (Bausch & Lomb, Rochester, NY) that was originally designed for automated lamellar keratoplasty. The Automated Corneal Shaper later underwent design modification with LASIK in mind.

The Hansatome allows the surgeon to select one of two flap thicknesses by assembly of either the "160" or "180" keratome head, achieving flap thicknesses of approximately 160 and 180 microns, respectively. Thin flaps are desirable in all cases because they greatly minimize the likelihood of post-LASIK ectasia, caused by leaving too little residual stromal tissue beneath the corneal flap.[14,15] Leaving as much residual corneal stromal tissue beneath the flap also preserves the opportunity for enhancement to be performed. The surgeon's enthusiasm for use of the 160 plate rather than the 180 plate is tempered by the fact that it is difficult to manipulate the thinner 160 micron flap, there is more likelihood of encountering a flap "buttonhole" in the second eye of a simultaneous bilateral procedure, and the thinner flaps are more difficult to re-lift. (Wallerstein et al.: Buttonholes in thin flaps in LASIK surgery. Paper presented at the American Society of Cataract and Refractive Surgery Annual Meeting, May 2001, San Diego, CA.) The occurrence of Bowman's layer cracks (microfolds) is likely multifactorial (Fig. 19–4). It has been hypothesized that such Bowman's layer cracks are more commonly observed with higher laser corrections because of more radical changes in corneal curvature. It has not yet been shown that routine use of a 160 micron Hansatome plate leads to more frequent Bowman's layer cracks than would be observed with use of a 180 micron plate.

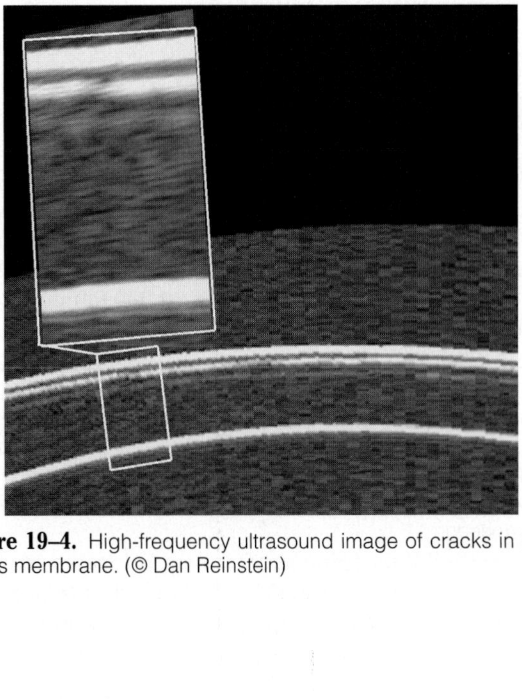

Figure 19–4. High-frequency ultrasound image of cracks in Bowman's membrane. (© Dan Reinstein)

Prior to use of the microkeratome the surgeon must specify whether the 160 or 180 plate will be used, together with the ring size. Two ring sizes are available, "8.5" and "9.5," indicating that the achieved flap diameter will be approximately 8.5 and 9.5 mm, respectively. These flap diameters are only rough guides, because the achieved flap diameter is significantly affected by the preoperative keratometry, and the sagittal depth from the ring fixation point to the apex of the cornea. As a general rule, the steeper the cornea, the larger the achieved flap diameter for a particular keratome ring.

Some surgeons will have the 9.5 ring as their "default," reserving the 8.5 ring for corneas with preoperative keratometry above 45 diopters. The reason for this is that in the unlikely event of an overcorrection where a patient is rendered hyperopic, the flap would be sufficiently large to allow for the wider area of ablation necessary for hyperopic treatments. Other surgeons argue in favor of a smaller flap for myopic corrections on the grounds that overcorrections should be unusual. Moreover, it has recently been suggested that larger flaps might have further reduction in corneal sensation than smaller flaps; this may have an effect on the likelihood of postoperative dryness during the first few months after surgery.[16] Additionally, it was recently shown that flaps with superior hinges were more likely to have reduced corneal sensation than flaps with nasal hinges (Donnenfeld et al.: The effect of hinge position on corneal sensation and dry eye signs and symptoms. Presented at the American Academy of Ophthalmology Annual Meeting, 2001, New Orleans). Whatever one's philosophy with regard to the use of the 9.5 ring as the default ring, there is broad agreement that for corneas with preoperative keratometry below 41 D, the 9.5 ring should be used in order to achieve an adequate flap size for even a myopic ablation. For corneas with preoperative keratometry above 45 D, the 8.5 ring should be selected to minimize the likelihood of getting an excessively large flap that may cleave superficial capillaries near the limbus. Surgeons should be aware that limbal capillaries would also be more likely cut by the microkeratome in corneas with smaller diameters.

CREATION OF THE FLAP

The surgeon uses two hands to place the Hansatome suction ring onto the surface of the eye. One hand holds the shaft of the suction ring, and the index finger of the other hand is in contact with the post (Fig. 19–5). The post is always oriented such that it is temporal, and the track along which the keratome translates is nasal. This is important to verify mentally, because it is easy for the surgeon to place the ring onto the eye in the orientation that it arrives from the operating room assistant. It is desirable to create a flap hinge that is located well away from a planned ablation to avoid the need to protect the hinge with a surgical sponge during laser ablation.

Once the Hansatome suction ring is located in a satisfactory position on the ocular surface, the surgeon pushes down (retropulsion) on the globe and asks the assistant to engage suction. Pressure within the tubing begins to rise and the suction ring gains purchase on the ocular surface. This pressure rise evolves over one or two seconds, accompanied by a series of "beeps." It is important for the surgeon to maintain the retropulsive maneuver during this pressure rise in order to prevent the suction ring from moving on the globe, creating a decentered flap. The number of beeps emitted by the Hansatome machine is characteristic for the ambient conditions in any given operating room. Factors contributing to the number of beeps include the vacuum setting on the Hansatome, the compliance of the conjunctiva, the anatomy of the globe, and the occurrence of air leaks below the ring when suction is applied. This is an important point because if, for example, seven beeps are heard, when four beeps might be characteristic, it becomes important for the surgeon to quickly verify that intraocular pressure is sufficiently high. This can be accomplished by asking the patient whether everything "has gone dark," whether the globe feels appropriately firm to a gloved finger, and whether the applanation of the eye is satisfactory. Some surgeons also routinely measure the achieved intraocular pressure by pneumotonometry, and this is likely the most accurate method.

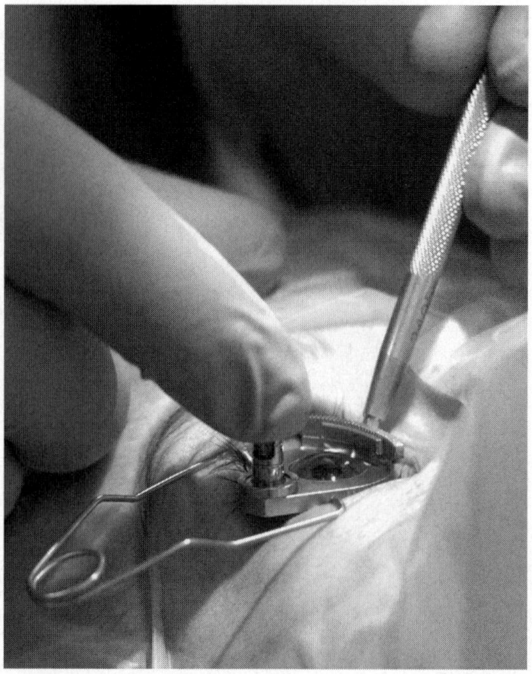

Figure 19–5. A bimanual technique is used for placement of the Hansatome suction ring on the ocular surface. (Courtesy of Ray Swords and Emory Vision.)

MANAGEMENT OF THE FLAP DURING SURGERY

After completion of microkeratome translation, the flap is picked up with non-toothed forceps, avoiding excessive manipulation, stretching, and folding. Placement of the elevated flap is easiest when the eyelid margin has either been draped or isolated with a closed blade

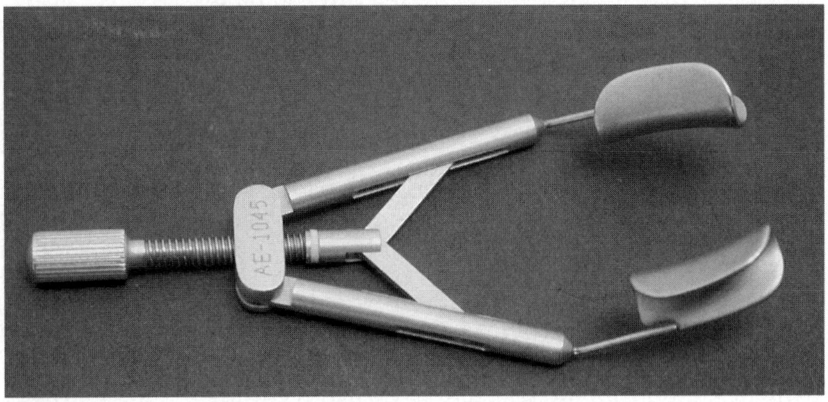

Figure 19–6. A closed blade Liebermann speculum achieves excellent exposure while keeping the eyelashes away from the operative field. (© Jonathan Carr. carr@lasereye-consultants.com and Emory Vision.)

speculum such as a Liebermann speculum (Fig. 19–6). If the eyelashes are not draped or protected with a closed blade speculum, the surgeon can "taco" fold the flap, or if sufficient space exists, place it on the superior bulbar conjunctiva.

Upon completion of laser ablation the flap is placed back in position. Technique varies here, but the guiding principles should be to avoid having the epithelial surface of the flap come into contact with the stromal bed and to minimize the possibility that debris from the fornices and ocular surface will enter the interface. The use of Merocel sponges to remove fluid from the conjunctival fornices can minimize access of material from the conjunctival surface into the stromal bed beneath the corneal flap. When replacing the corneal flap, some Emory surgeons use this irrigating cannula to "stroke" the stromal surface of the flap, moving from the superior fornix toward the center of the cornea (Fig. 19–7).

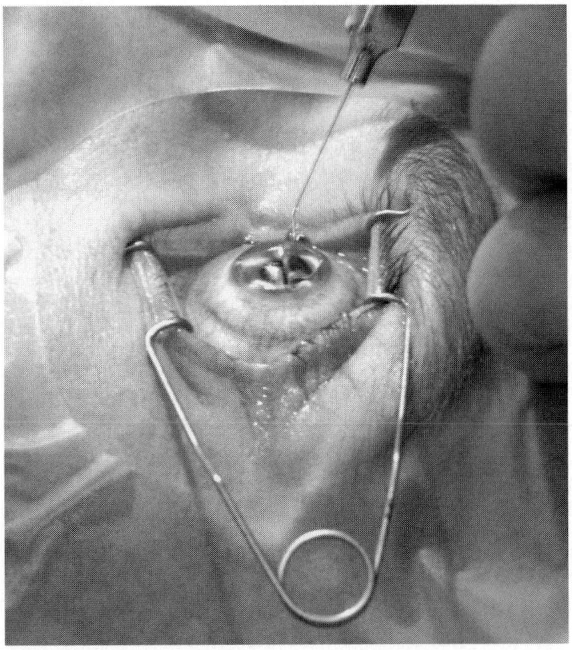

Figure 19–7. A cannula is used to gently stroke the flap back into position. (Courtesy of Ray Swords and Emory Vision.)

This has the effect of avoiding placing an instrument on the epithelial surface and then immediately into the interface. An alternative maneuver would be to place the cannula at the flap hinge on the epithelial surface and allow the flap to fall back into position.

Once the flap is back into position, the surgeon uses an irrigating cannula to direct saline solution beneath the flap to remove any debris. Emory surgeons tend to irrigate less today than was the case for the earliest LASIK surgeries performed. Excessive irrigation produces flap swelling and this may be associated with increased symptoms for the patient during the initial hours after surgery, and increased likelihood of flap slippage. Excessive irrigation also widens the "gutter" between flap edge and peripheral cornea. A moistened Merocel sponge can be used to "squeegee" fluid from the interface; this is achieved by stroking movements from the corneal vertex toward, but not reaching, the flap edge. This maneuver is performed less aggressively than in the past because surgeons irrigate less saline beneath the corneal flap. Use of a moistened Merocel at the flap edge to draw fluid from the interface by capillary action is another useful technique. This also allows the surgeon to verify that the gutter is symmetrical, indicating good flap repositioning.

RELIFTING CORNEAL FLAPS FOR ENHANCEMENT PROCEDURES

Most enhancements are performed shortly after the 3-month postoperative visit, at which time refractive stability is achieved in all but the most highly myopic eyes. Flaps can be lifted more than 1 year postoperatively, but it can be difficult. Thin flaps are also typically more difficult to relift. Lifting a corneal flap is achieved by a variety of techniques, but the initial requirement is that the flap edge be lifted at some point by dividing the corneal scar. A Sinskey hook is typically used at Emory to elevate the flap edge. Some surgeons use the operating microscope as they lift the flap edge, whereas others use the slit-lamp microscope, moving the patient to the operating microscope to complete the flap lift prior to laser retreatment. Whichever approach is adopted, it is important to minimize epithelial trauma near the flap edge because this increases the likelihood that epithelial cells will gain access to the flap interface. A retrospective multivariate analysis of risk factors for surgical flap revision showed that flap edge epithelial trauma arising during flap re-lift, while being associated with epithelial cells beneath the flap edge, did not typically require removal of epithelial cells by the surgeon.[17] Replacement of the flap after enhancement is accomplished using the same technique as for primary LASIK.

RECUTTING CORNEAL FLAPS

Extreme caution should be exercised when recutting corneal flaps. The typical situation requiring a surgeon to recut a flap is after incomplete flap preparation at the time of primary surgery. Historically, it was accepted to wait for 3 months from the time of the primary flap complication and recut with a Bausch & Lomb Automated Corneal Shaper (ACS). With the advent of the Hansatome, we hypothesize that a longer period should elapse before considering a recut. This is so because the Hansatome exerts a considerable translational force as it traverses the cornea, in rare instances leading to dissection of the original incomplete flap. The same concern would apply to many of the other keratomes currently in use in the United States. Unfortunately, no published data exist to guide the surgeon as to favorable clinical signs that would promote a successful flap recut.

EXCIMER LASER ISSUES

The use of eye trackers has greatly improved the centration of treatments, reducing the possibility of aberrations caused by decentration. From an optical perspective, because of the minified image that results from hyperopic corrections, centration of hyperopic and compound hyperopic astigmatic treatments is even more important than centration for myopic corrections. The trackers currently in use with the various approved excimer lasers differ in terms of their eye position acquisition rate, but the response times of the systems are similar. This chapter will not review in detail the particular nuances involved in use of the various excimer lasers available today. Surgeons using eye trackers should understand, however, that an incorrectly centered tracker would guarantee decentration and a poor visual result.

TROUBLESHOOTING

AVOIDING FLAP COMPLICATIONS

Incomplete Flaps

Incomplete flaps are typically the result of microkeratome jams during translation. Microkeratome jams happen as a result of erros in microkeratome assembly and maintenance. Such jams occur in the middle of forward microkeratome translation and are to be distinguished from jams that occur at the level of the superior hinge.

Buttonholes in the Flap

Flap buttonholes should be rarely observed with the Hansatome. It has been suggested that buttonholes are more likely in eyes with steep preoperative keratometry.[18] In addition, because the flap is thinner in the second eye of bilateral simultaneous LASIK procedures, there should be a greater likelihood of buttonholes in the second eye. This was confirmed in a retrospective analysis of a consecutive series of 21,000 eyes in which 32 buttonholes here identified; buttonholes were 65% more likely to occur in the second eye of bilateral simultaneous LASIK procedures ($p = 0.01$). (Wallerstein et al.: Buttonholes in thin flaps in LASIK surgery. Paper presented at the American Society of Cataract and Refractive Surgery Annual Meeting, May 2001, San Diego, CA.) To minimize the likelihood of buttonhole in the second eye, surgeons should become adept at identifying unusually thin flaps in the first eye. A thin flap in the first eye should trigger a request for a new blade for the fellow eye.

Laser ablation should be postponed in the presence of a flap buttonhole. Of the intraoperative flap complications at Emory, eyes with flap buttonholes had a greater propensity to lose best spectacle corrected visual acuity.[19] An analysis of flap buttonholes at Emory failed to demonstrate that they occur more frequently in the record of two simultaneously treated eyes. However, the low frequency of buttonhole at Emory and the relatively small sample size prevented an adequate statistical treatment of this issue.

Free Corneal Flaps

Free flaps are more likely to occur in eyes whose corneas are flat preoperatively. In these instances the surgeon will likely have selected the 9.5-mm suction ring. In flat corneas, the hinge will be relatively narrow, and inadvertent superior decentration of the suction ring will promote a narrower hinge to the point that a free flap is created.

In the presence of a free flap, laser ablation can usually proceed if sufficient stromal bed exists. The flap can be replaced without sutures, with the option of a bandage contact lens overnight. The majority of surgeons at Emory elect to secure the flap with 10-0 nylon suture, using either an interrupted or 8-bite running technique. The running suture technique should be rehearsed to competence before a surgeon contemplates its use in securing a free flap.

Prevention of free corneal flaps is the best remedy. Surgeons should meticulously place the suction ring in eyes with flat corneas and maintain retropulsion during the pressure rise to avoid the globe moving under the suction ring. This will promote a well-centered suction ring, avoiding the narrow hinge that would be created in a flat cornea with a superiorly decentered function ring.

Avoiding Epithelial Defects

As a general rule, surgeons should reduce to a minimum the likelihood of epithelial defects occurring during LASIK. This is important because it reduces the incidence of epithelial ingrowth.[17] Preoperative anesthetic drops should be instilled immediately before surgery rather than significantly in advance of surgery. Epithelial trauma at the flap edge during re-lift enhancement procedures should be kept to a minimum.

Avoiding Microkeratome Jams

As stated previously, microkeratome jams that occur early in keratome translation are often the result of contact with the lower eyelid, lashes, or a surgical drape. Recognizing and correcting inappropriate positioning of the suction ring before keratome translation is the best remedy. The most important issue concerns how to control the forward and backward movement of the keratome when a jam occurs. The initial maneuver should be a forward movement to establish whether forward translation can resume. This can be repeated if necessary. Surgeons should be aware that if they reverse keratome translation away from the jam and the keratome head moves back along the track, there can be NO forward translation thereafter. The case is over for that day.

The Hansatome can also jam at the end of forward translation at the level of the superior hinge. A multivariate analysis of hinge jams confirmed that in addition to one of the two Hansatomes (two identical Hansatomes were used to treat eyes in the study) playing a role, the level of surgeon experience and the operating room technician also played a role in the occurrence of hinge jams. (Carr: An epidemiologic investigation to identify the cause of microkeratome jams during LASIK. Paper presented at the American Society of Cataract and Refractive Surgery Annual Meeting, May 2001, San Diego, CA.) The unifying explanation for these risk factors would be that some Hansatomes are more likely than other Hansatomes to restrict the oscillating blade at the end of forward excursion; in such cases, a technician and/or surgeon might excessively tighten the handpiece on the keratome head/pivot collar complex, further restricting the oscillating blade at the level of the hinge.

A number of maneuvers can resolve a microkeratome jam at the hinge. Repeatedly activating reverse translation with the foot pedal is often all that is necessary. This maneuver can be repeated several times. If this is not successful, the surgeon can slightly unscrew the motor handpiece and repeat the reverse translation. While these events are unfolding, the surgeon should pay attention to the time that has elapsed since suction was turned on. It is important to remember that if suction is turned off and the corneal flap is still present within the keratome head, the patient should be instructed to avoid looking inferiorly. This will prevent creation of a free flap. A gentle and slow movement of the keratome/suction ring complex inferiorly usually allows the surgeon to free the corneal flap from within the keratome.

POSTOPERATIVE CONSIDERATIONS

Flap Slips

Flap slips occur with flaps created with either nasal or superior hinges. We hypothesize that they typically occur in the initial few hours after surgery rather than later in the day. If a patient does not blink enough or lubricate enough immediately after surgery, the corneal surface becomes dry. As corneal anesthesia subsides in the second hour after surgery, the eyelids begin to make fuller lid excursions, and the upper lid can engage the flap edge, producing a slip. Flap slips are associated with increased discomfort and deterioration of vision. Flap replacement after cleaning of the stromal bed with Merocel sponges and irrigation with saline allows for restoration of vision. Epithelial ingrowth is more likely to occur after flap slip, but it is usually non-progressive, not predisposing the eye to a flap revision.[17]

Flap Folds

Flap folds can be indicative of flap misalignment such as would occur in a partial flap slip. They are to be distinguished from cracks in Bowman's membrane that result from excessive manipulation of a thin corneal flap. Realignment of a slipped flap will result in resolution of flap folds within one hour. Cracks in Bowman's membrane will not resolve with further flap surgery, and therefore surgery should be avoided.

Epithelial Ingrowth

Implantation of epithelial cells into the flap interface does not, in and of itself, lead to epithelial growth. It is only when epithelial cells are in continuity with the limbal stem cells that a progressive growth of epithelial cells occurs underneath the flap. A fistula will therefore exist in cases where epithelial ingrowth is progressive. A retrospective multivariate analysis of risk factors for epithelial ingrowth identified corneal epithelial defect as the single most important risk factor that predicted the need for a flap revision.[17] Other risk factors that were associated with non-progressive epithelial ingrowth included laser enhancement procedures where the primary flap was re-lifted and postoperative flap slips. Experienced surgeons were significantly less likely to have operated on eyes with non-progressive epithelial ingrowth. The mechanism that explains the statistical findings is corneal flap edema that leads to poor apposition of flap edge to peripheral corneal bed. Epithelial cells moving centrally from the limbus are then able to move beneath the edematous flap edge where they may or may not continue to move centrally.

Epithelial ingrowth should be followed conservatively, given that most epithelial nests involute spontaneously. Progression of epithelial ingrowth centrally with poor flap edge apposition (fluorescein staining under the flap edge can be a helpful sign) are factors that should lead the surgeon to consider flap revision to remove the cells. The cells must be removed from both the stromal bed and the stromal surface of the flap before the flap is replaced. One flap revision is usually all that is required. However, recurrence of epithelial ingrowth can on rare occasions occur requiring additional flap lifts. In these rare instances, it is wise to secure the flap edge with an interrupted 10-0 nylon suture that is an appositional suture rather than a compression suture. A "2-1-1" knot can be used to allow for easier burial of the suture knot. The suture can be removed after a few days.

Diffuse Lamellar Keratitis

Much has been written about diffuse lamellar keratitis (DLK) since it was first reported by Smith and Maloney.[20] DLK can occur as a sporadic, rare event, or it can occur in the setting of an outbreak of DLK where many or all eyes treated during a surgical session develop sterile inflammation. Sporadic cases have a multifactorial etiology, whereas clusters of cases have been attributed by some to a sterile inflammatory response to *Pseudomonas* biofilm. Holland and colleagues have reported that biofilm can develop in the distilled water reservoirs of commonly used autoclaves and that minute amounts gain access to the cartridge that houses instruments during the sterilization cycle. Meticulous attention to the autoclave can reduce to almost zero the likelihood of a DLK outbreak.

Diffuse lamellar keratitis presents in the first two to three postoperative days with mild blurring of vision and a mild conjunctival hyperemia. If not identified, the sterile inflammation can rapidly progress, ultimately causing flap melting and a very poor visual outcome from surgery. When identified and treated early, DLK need not mean a poor result for the patient. There is universal agreement by surgeons that intensive topical corticosteroids are the initial mainstay of therapy. Surgeons are divided, however, as to how to manage the more aggressive cases of DLK. Some advocate flap lifting and irrigation with saline to reduce the inflammatory load beneath the flap. Others initiate systemic corticosteroid in a reducing regimen over 10 to 14 days.[21] Whatever your opinion, it is vital that this condition be treated promptly to allow a favorable visual outcome.

Our improving understanding of LASIK has allowed us to achieve outstanding results. The acceptable treatment range has been narrowed as we have come to understand the importance of mechanical stability of the cornea. Preoperative corneal thickness together with scotopic pupil size are two vital pieces of information that help determine LASIK candidacy. Work continues in the arena of wavefront-guided customized laser treatments. In this regard, the epithelium continues to undermine the true potential of custom treatments; a better knowledge of epithelial healing may allow further improvement of outcomes in our patients.

REFERENCES

1. Pallikaris IG, Papatzanaki ME, Stathi EZ, et al.: Laser in situ keratomileusis. Lasers Surg Med 1990; 10:463–468.
2. Carr JD, Thompson KP, Stulting RD, Waring GO 3rd: Ablation profilometry and outcome of LASIK. Invest Ophthalmol Vis Sci 1996;37:S62 (Abstract).
3. Chayet AS, Assil KK, Montes M, et al.: Regression and its mechanisms after laser in situ keratomileusis in moderate and high myopia. Ophthalmology 1998;105:1194–1199.
4. Geggel HS, Talley AR: Delayed onset keratectasia following laser in situ keratomileusis [see comments]. J Cataract Refract Surg 1999;25:582–586.
5. Wang Z, Chen J, Yang B: Posterior corneal surface topographic changes after laser in situ keratomileusis are related to residual corneal bed thickness. Ophthalmology 1999;106:406–409; discussion 409–410.
6. Seiler T, Quurke AW: Iatrogenic keratectasia after LASIK in a case of forme fruste keratoconus. J Cataract Refract Surg 1998;24: 1007–1009.
7. Seiler T, Koufala K, Richter G: Iatrogenic keratectasia after laser in situ keratomileusis. J Refract Surg 1998;14:312–317.
8. Holland SP, Srivannaboon S, Reinstein DZ: Avoiding serious corneal complications of laser assisted in situ keratomileusis and photorefractive keratectomy. Ophthalmology 2000;107:640–652.
9. Ozdamar A, Aras C, Ustundag C, et al.: Corneal iron ring associated with iatrogenic keratectasia after myopic laser in situ keratomileusis. J Cataract Refract Surg 2000;26:1684–1686.
10. Argento C, Cosentino MJ, Tytiun A, et al.: Corneal ectasia after laser in situ keratomileusis. J Cataract Refract Surg 2001;27: 1440–1448.
11. Pallikaris IG, Kymionis GD, Astyrakakis NI: Corneal ectasia induced by laser in situ keratomileusis. J Cataract Refract Surg 2001;27:1796–1802.
12. Seitz B, Torres F, Langenbucher A, et al.: Posterior corneal curvature changes after myopic laser in situ keratomileusis. Ophthalmology 2001;108:666–672; discussion 673.
13. Vinciguerra P, Camesasca FI: Prevention of corneal ectasia in laser in situ keratomileusis. J Refract Surg 2001;17(2 Suppl): S187–S189.
14. Reinstein DZ, Silverman RH, Sutton HF, Coleman DJ: Very high-frequency ultrasound corneal analysis identifies anatomic correlates of optical complications of lamellar refractive surgery: anatomic diagnosis in lamellar surgery. Ophthalmology 1999; 106:474–482.
15. Reinstein DZ, Silverman RH, Raevsky T, et al.: Arc-scanning very high-frequency digital ultrasound for 3D pachymetric mapping of the corneal epithelium and stroma in laser in situ keratomileusis. J Refract Surg 2000; 16:414–430.
16. Wilson SE: Laser in situ keratomileusis-induced (presumed) neurotrophic epitheliopathy. Ophthalmology 2001;108:1082–1087.
17. Carr JD, Nardone R, Stulting RD, et al.: Risk factors for epithelial ingrowth after LASIK. Invest Ophthalmol Vis Sci 1997;38:S232.
18. Gimbel HV, Penno EE, van Westenbrugge JA, et al.: Incidence and management of intraoperative and early postoperative complications in 1000 consecutive laser in situ keratomileusis cases [see comments]. Ophthalmology 1998; 105:1839–1847; discussion 1847–1848.
19. Stulting RD, Carr JD, Thompson KP, et al.: Complications of laser in situ keratomileusis for the correction of myopia. Ophthalmology 1999;106:13–20.
20. Smith RJ, Maloney RK: Diffuse lamellar keratitis. A new syndrome in lamellar refractive surgery. Ophthalmology 1998;105: 1721–1726.
21. Macaluso DC, Rich LF, MacRae S: Sterile interface keratitis after laser in situ keratomileusis: Three episodes in one patient with concomitant contact dermatitis of the eyelids. J Refract Surg 1999;15:679–682.

CHAPTER 20

Photorefractive Keratectomy

RAYMOND STEIN, M.D., F.R.C.S.(C)

Photorefractive keratectomy (PRK) was the first laser vision correction procedure adopted by ophthalmologists and patients around the globe. Today it has been generally supplanted by laser *in situ* keratomileusis (LASIK) as the predominant refractive procedure. Most notable is the fact that surface ablation either by the technique of photorefractive keratectomy or laser epithelial keratomileusis (LASEK) has greatly renewed interest. Surface ablation avoids the microkeratome related complications and decreases the chances of corneal ectasia. There are certain conditions in which a patient may be a better candidate for PRK than for LASIK. These LASIK contraindications include the following (Table 20–1): (1) epithelial basement membrane dystrophy because of the risk of epithelial ingrowth, (2) keratoconus because of the risk of corneal ectasia, (3) difficulty achieving satisfactory suction for the microkeratome cut, and (4) corneal thinning in which less than 250 μm of tissue would be left in the bed. Laser vision correction surgeons should be comfortable with the techniques of PRK and the management of potential complications.

The advancements in excimer laser technology, surgical techniques, and pharmacotherapy have improved the outcomes of PRK (Table 20–2). Intensive research in pharmacological management will continue to improve our ability to modulate wound healing.

This deals with the following aspects of PRK: preoperative assessment, operative techniques, and postoperative management.

PREOPERATIVE ASSESSMENT

Refractive errors that can be treated with PRK with a satisfactory visual outcome include myopia up to −10 diopters, astigmatism up to 6 diopters, and hyperopia up to 5 diopters.[1] The best results, with the lowest incidence of complications, occur in the lower ranges of myopia, astigmatism, and hyperopia. The higher the refractive error the greater the chance of regression and corneal haze. Conditions in which a patient may be a poor candidate for PRK are summarized in Table 20–3.

TABLE 20-1. Ocular Characteristics of Poor Candidates for LASIK Who May Be Treated with PRK

Epithelial basement membrane dystrophy
Keratoconus*
Deep-set eyes
Flat corneas < 40 D
Steep corneas > 46 D
Thin corneas that would leave a bed after LASIK with < 250 μm

*Keratoconus patients with satisfactory best corrected spectacle correction may be treated with PRK.

TABLE 20-2. Photorefractive Keratectomy Complications

Complication	1990	2002
Pain	High	Low
Visual recovery	Slow	Rapid
Central islands	High	Rare
Decentration	Occasional	Rare
Haze	High	Low
Refractive accuracy	Low	High

TABLE 20-3. Characteristics of Poor Candidates for PRK

Less than 18 years of age
Progressive myopia/unstable refractive error
Pupil size greater than 8 mm in diameter (dim illumination)
Cataracts that are visually significant
Poor spectacle visual acuity secondary to irregular astigmatism
Collagen vascular disease on immunosuppressive medication
Pregnancy
Unrealistic expectations
Unwilling to commit to post-procedure follow-up and care instructions
Advanced dry eye syndrome with central punctate keratitis

Naturally occurring myopic astigmatism is usually regular astigmatism with symmetrical steepening in the two steepest hemimeridians. The cornea should be evaluated preoperatively by computerized videokeratography to rule out asymmetric or irregular astigmatism. In the future, topographically linked ablations may allow the treatment of these forms of astigmatism.

RISKS AND RELATIVE CONTRAINDICATIONS

During pregnancy or nursing, hormonal changes could alter the refractive error. In addition, medications (sedation, pain medications, and possibly eyedrops) can be transmitted to the fetus through the mother's bloodstream or to the baby in breast milk. For these reasons, refractive surgery should not be performed on a pregnant woman or a nursing mother.

A recent study has demonstrated that there is a 13.5 times higher chance of regression in women using oral contraceptives.[2] Patients should be counseled of this apparent increased risk.

The importance of an accurate refraction cannot be overstated. If astigmatism is present, it is extremely important to determine the proper axis. If the cylinder is 15 degrees off axis, the effect from treatment may be decreased by 50%. The phoropter and the patient's head should be properly aligned during the refraction.

Computerized videokeratography has become the standard of care to rule out subtle abnormalities of the cornea. Videokeratography is used to identify early keratoconus or "keratoconus suspect," corneal warpage, and asymmetric or irregular astigmatism. Each condition has a different prognosis. Patients with keratoconus have asymmetric and/or irregular astigmatism, and the laser is not now capable of correcting this abnormality. Even if the myopia were reduced, any residual irregular astigmatism would require a rigid contact lens for correction. In addition, the correction of asymmetric astigmatism is difficult to treat with the present laser machines because more laser pulses would be required at the steeper quadrant than at the meridian 180 degrees away. Another concern in treating unrecognized keratoconus patients is the potential for litigation if keratoconus is detected postoperatively and is thought to have been caused by the laser procedure.

Patients with keratoconus and a relatively stable refractive error that can be corrected to a satisfactory level with glasses are candidates for PRK but not for LASIK. Although there is a higher incidence of regression and the need for an enhancement, the visual outcomes and patient satisfaction levels have been excellent.

Slit-lamp examination is used to rule out any significant corneal abnormalities, such as neovascularization, scarring, or keratoconus, as well as the presence of a cataract. Vascularization that involves the optical zone of the ablation can result in bleeding during the procedure and lead to an irregular ablation. Because topical steroids can cause a posterior subcapsular cataract, this type of lens opacity is extremely important to identify preoperatively as part of the baseline examination.

Because patients may be given topical steroids postoperatively, it is important to rule out glaucoma or identify the possibility of glaucoma in a patient who may be vulnerable to raised intraocular pressures with topical steroids. This is especially important in patients with the higher ranges of myopia because of the greater risk of significant corneal haze that may require a course of intensive topical steroids.

Funduscopy is a very important examination in myopic patients because they may have a retinal hole or retinal degeneration. It also rules out any optic disc or macular disease as a baseline measurement. Patients with myopic degeneration and loss of best corrected visual acuity are at higher risk for progressive visual loss because of the natural history of their disease. A patient who loses vision post–laser vision correction will generally not accept the diagnosis of progression of myopic degeneration. Surgeons should be conservative when dealing with patients with any macular disease.

Advanced keratitis sicca with diffuse superficial punctate keratopathy or corneal filaments is a contraindication for PRK. Other contraindications for the excimer laser procedure include uveitis, cataract, retinopathies, and significant lagophthalmos. In addition, patients whose pupils are large (>8 mm) in dim light are poor candidates for PRK because they are at increased risk of night glare and halos. As optical zones and transition zones of the laser ablation become larger, this complication will be less common. The larger the pupil the greater the chance that a small decentration will result in symptoms. Further, patients with active systemic connective tissue diseases (e.g., systemic lupus erythematosus, rheumatoid arthritis) are considered poor PRK candidates because of the potential for poor epithelial healing and the risk of a corneal melt. Finally, a history of keloid formation of the skin is no longer considered a contraindication to PRK. There does not appear to be an increased risk of corneal haze.

OUTCOMES AND PATIENT EXPECTATIONS

Clearly, careful patient selection and review of the risk: benefit ratio of PRK is essential. Patient education is a primary prerequisite for PRK. Knowledge and understanding of the excimer laser procedure and postoperative evaluation can be conveyed through printed information sheets and through discussion with patient counselors, the surgeon, and other patients.

Each patient should have realistic refractive outcomes expectations. Ideally, very soon after the operation the patient will be able to see at least as well without corrective lenses as he or she had been able to see with the best possible glasses or contact lenses, and to do so with no side effects. In reality, however, the outcome is usually something less than this in one or more aspects and is sometimes considerably less. It is therefore important that the patient have reasonable expectations and a clear understanding of the ways in which those expectations might not be met.

PHOTOREFRACTIVE KERATECTOMY FOLLOWING OTHER SURGICAL PROCEDURES

Photorefractive keratectomy can be performed to alter the refractive error after previous eye surgery. There is an increased risk of corneal haze when PRK is performed after penetrating keratoplasty, radial keratotomy, or LASIK. The best outcomes are after cataract surgery. In one case, a patient was referred 12 months post-cataract surgery with a −7 D refractive error from an incorrect lens power; a cataract then developed in the fellow eye. Photorefractive keratectomy was performed on the −7 D eye, resulting in a near plano refraction. The patient later underwent successful cataract surgery in the fellow eye.

Treatment of post-radial keratotomy (RK) patients requires particular caution. After RK some patients complain not only of poor vision due to undercorrection, overcorrection, or induced astigmatism but also of fluctuating vision and problems seeing at night. Photorefractive keratectomy enhancements will not improve night vision, nor can they correct vision fluctuations. Therefore the PRK surgeon should not attempt to correct the preexisting vision problems caused by the RK. Patients who have had four-incision RK, however, often do well with PRK enhancements, whereas those with 12 or more RK incisions tend to do poorly, with a high incidence of corneal haze. The source of this haze is not known, but it may be related to a dellan-like effect from the corneal contour. Generally, PRK enhancements are not recommended for patients who have had more than eight-incision RK. If the patient has had eight-incision RK and if the pre-RK refractive error was less than −6.00 D, PRK enhancement is useful. If the refractive error was greater than −6.00 D, however, there is a greater incidence of central corneal haze. Longitudinal studies indicate a fairly significant hyperopic drift in RK eyes. Therefore, performing a PRK enhancement on an RK patient who is −1 D may not be in the patient's best interest.

Photorefractive keratectomy can be used to treat anisometropia after corneal transplantation.[3] Many patients may be disappointed in their surgery despite clear grafts with 20/20 corrected vision because of induced myopia, astigmatism, or hyperopia. Safety is a concern in these patients because of an increased risk of corneal haze or of graft rejection after laser treatment. Myopic or hyperopic patients with regular astigmatism may do well; if they have irregular or asymmetric astigmatism, then an astigmatic keratotomy is preferred to create more regular astigmatism, followed by PRK enhancement. In the future, flying spot excimer laser technology, together with computerized videokeratoscopy, may be used to treat the steeper areas of the cornea to correct the irregular surface.

OPERATIVE TECHNIQUE

The calibration of the excimer laser is of utmost importance in achieving excellent visual results. Each excimer laser system will have an operators manual that outlines the calibration guidelines. Important measurements include the depth per pulse, fluence, quality of the ablation, and centration of the laser beam.

PREOPERATIVE MEDICATIONS

Our present protocol calls for eyedrops to be given approximately 20 minutes prior to laser surgery. Preoperative medications include a nonsteroidal anti-inflammatory drop such as ketorolac trimethamine 0.5% (Acular) or diclofenac sodium (Voltaren), given one drop every 10 minutes for three times. This medication has been shown to decrease postoperative pain. The use of a broad-spectrum antibiotic such as one of the fluoroquinolones, one drop every 10 minutes for three times, will decrease the chance of infection. Immediately prior to laser surgery, several drops of a topical anesthetic (proparacaine hydrochloride) are instilled into the eye.

PATIENT POSITION BENEATH THE LASER

Minimal head or body movement is important, so the patient should be positioned comfortably. The legs should not be crossed, because this may lead to an unstable body position. The neck should not be turned or twisted, because this can result in misalignment of the astigmatic axis (Fig. 20–1). The head position should be such that when the lid speculum is inserted an equal amount of sclera is visible on the inferior and superior aspects of the globe. If more sclera is showing inferiorly than superiorly, the patient's chin should be elevated (Fig. 20–2). If more sclera is visible superiorly than inferiorly the patient's chin should be depressed. The nonoperative eye is covered or taped closed for comfort and better fixation of the eye to be ablated. Typically a wire lid speculum is inserted.

COMPUTER INPUTTING

At this point in the procedure, relevant data are entered into the computer (Fig. 20–3). Depending on the laser being used and the software version, this may include

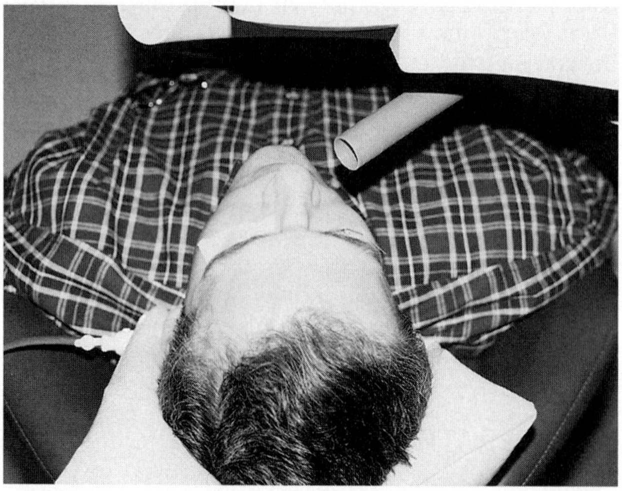

Figure 20–1. Misalignment of the head. Note that the patient's head is mildly tilted, which will result in misalignment of the astigmatic axis.

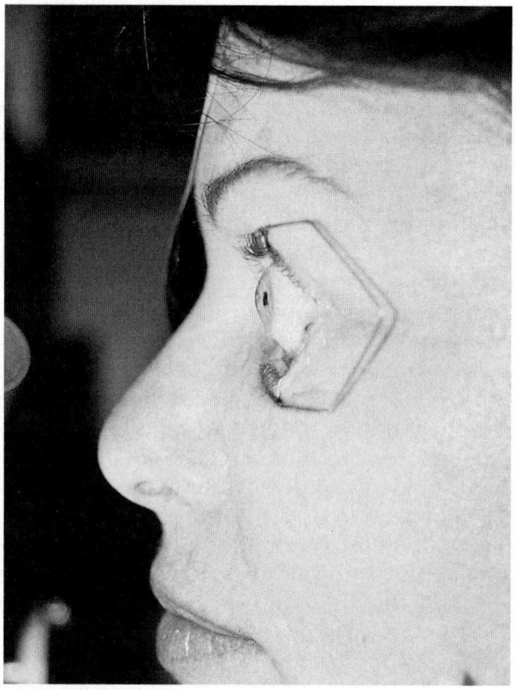

Figure 20–2. Improper eye position. Note that more sclera is visible inferiorly than superiorly. The patient needs to raise the chin so that an equal amount of sclera is visible from the limbus to the lid speculum.

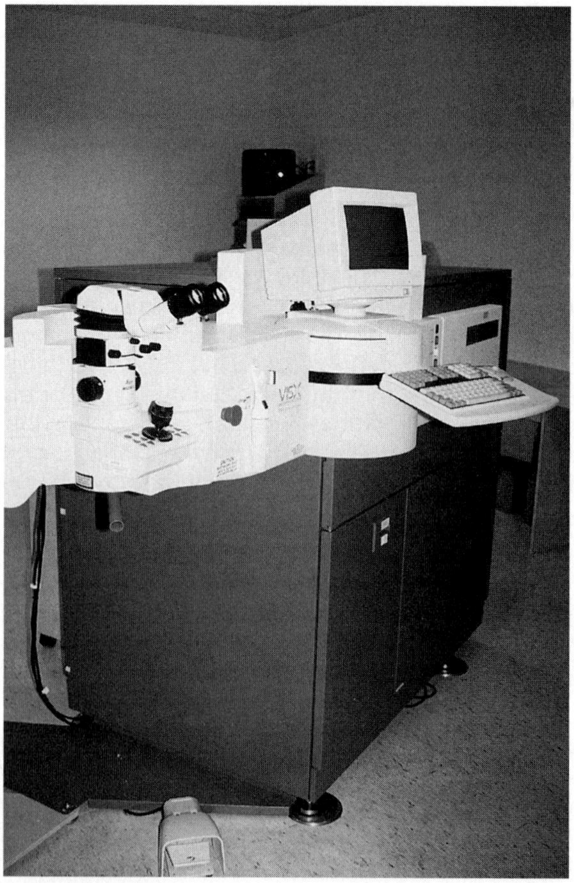

Figure 20–3. Visx Star laser with a built-in computer terminal, microscope head, joy-stick for focusing, and direct and indirect lighting system.

name, refraction, intended correction, keratometry values, epithelial removal technique, optical zone, transition zone, single pass or multipass, single zone or multizone, and anti-island correction. The surgeon should verify that the patient beneath the laser, the chart, and the entered data are consistent.

CENTRATION KEY TO GOOD PRK OUTCOMES

Centration is critical in achieving excellent visual results. Decentered ablations are best approached from a preventive standpoint because no satisfactory treatment exists. It is important to center the ablation over the pupil and not the visual axis when using a 6-mm optical zone. If a patient has a positive or negative angle kappa and the surgeon centers on the visual axis, the ablation will be decentered relative to the pupil, a situation that could result in glare and halos, especially at night. In the future if larger optical zones are used, the procedure may be centered over the visual axis.

The surgeon should focus the microscope on the surface of the cornea because this focus helps with centration. If the surgeon is focused at the level of the iris, it can be difficult to determine if the eye is tilted. It is possible to be focused in the center of the pupil, at the level of the iris, and actually be ablating the superior portion of the cornea.

Eye movement may be secondary to actual movement of the eye or due to head movement. By placing a hand on the patient's forehead the surgeon can easily discern the source of the movement. If head movement is secondary to respiratory excursions, the patient should be instructed to take shallow breaths.

There are five ways to achieve eye fixation:

1. **Self-fixation.** Most patients are able to fixate on a target light. By reducing the intensity of the operating microscope light and providing indirect illumination, patient self-fixation is easier to achieve. Occasionally, external fixation is required, but self-fixation is the most popular method. If the surgeon holds the eye, it is difficult to align the visual axis and easy to put undue pressure on one quadrant or another, thereby distorting the globe. Treating higher corrections with self-fixation is more difficult because patients have more trouble fixating as the corneal surface dries during the procedure.
2. **Fixation ring with suction.** A hand-held suction ring can be used to stabilize the globe. This device is usually large and cumbersome to use. A disposable suction speculum, designed by Dr. Neal Sher, is easier to use and provides superior alignment.
3. **Fixation ring without suction.** There are a variety of fixation rings available. A 10-mm compression ring is easy to use and effective.
4. **Forceps.** Because of an increased risk of patient discomfort, subconjunctival hemorrhage, and distortion of the globe, forceps are not widely used.
5. **Tracker.** Tracking systems have been incorporated into most of the excimer lasers. An ideal tracker must track in X, Y, and Z planes; if the laser tracks only in the X–Y plane and the patient's chin tilts up or down, alignment will be disrupted because the eye will be elevated or depressed. It is important for the laser to stop firing if there is significant eye deviation.

PREOPERATIVE SEDATION

Preoperative sedation is generally indicated only if the surgeon plans to hold the eye during ablation. Otherwise, preoperative sedation is not recommended because it would affect self-fixation.

COMMUNICATION

Patients have different perceptions of their situation and different levels of stress or anxiety. The surgeon, technician, or counselor should counsel the patient and explain what to expect during surgery. This discussion should include descriptions of what the patient might feel, see, smell, or hear during the surgical procedure. It also gives the patient information about the sequence of these events. Sensory information can lessen the stress or discomfort associated with excimer laser surgery.

Communication by the doctor and/or technician during the procedure is important because the patient needs to maintain fixation and remain motionless for a finite period of time. It is important to encourage patients during the procedure; physician communication alleviates much patient anxiety. Patients may become concerned if their sight blurs during the procedure. Reassurance during the procedure lets patients know they are doing well and keeps them informed. Some patients have panicked when their vision blurred because they thought they were losing their sight. To reduce anxiety and help ensure a good outcome, we talk the patient through the entire process.

QUIET PLEASE

For the patient to concentrate well, distractions should be kept to a minimum (i.e., nursing staff and visiting doctors should not talk during the procedure). Patients distracted by conversation may not be completely focused on the fixation light. Similarly, the surgeon may be distracted by background conversation.

EPITHELIAL REMOVAL TECHNIQUE

Different corneal tissues ablate at different rates, so the amount of tissue removed with each pulse varies. The cornea is not a homogeneous structure, and the epithelium ablates at a faster rate than the corneal stroma. Precise, quick epithelial removal is crucial to a good PRK outcome. A variety of removal techniques exist, and all have advantages and disadvantages from both the surgeon's and the patient's standpoints.

The epithelium can be removed by any of four methods:

1. **Mechanical debridement.** Mechanical epithelial removal should not take longer than 2 minutes to avoid corneal hydration changes that may affect the outcome.[5] Mechanical debridement consists of marking a 6- or 7-mm circular groove on the host corneal epithelium over the pupil, not the visual axis. A blunt spatula is typically used to scrape the epithelium from the periphery toward the center. A sponge hydrated with balanced saline and wiped across the cornea may be used to remove particles of tissue. A spatula is used to remove excess fluid. The resultant "glistening" cornea is ideal for PRK because it is uniformly moist.

   Beginning surgeons often remove the central epithelium first and then struggle with removal of the peripheral epithelium, exposing the central cornea to dehydration. This can result in overcorrection and haze. The quicker the epithelium is removed, the less chance there is for stromal dehydration.

   The epithelium may be softened by repeated instillation of drops before the procedure begins. In most virgin corneas the epithelium comes away quite easily. In patients who have had previous surgeries, such as RK, the epithelium is often found wedged between the grooves and is more difficult to remove. In any event, mechanical debridement is used by many surgeons as a satisfactory means of removing epithelium down to Bowman's layer.

   One advantage of this technique is that it is not dependent on the quality of the laser optics, as is the case in laser-scrape or transepithelial removal (discussed below). A disadvantage is that patients often prefer other techniques, such as transepithelial ablation. Typically the epithelium takes 1 to 2 days longer to heal. The surgeon should scrape from the outside in rather than inside out to avoid heaping the epithelium at the margins, which also extends the time to healing.

2. **Laser scrape technique and transepithelial laser removal.** Two laser removal approaches can be used: the laser-scrape technique and the transepithelial technique. The laser-scrape method is performed by typically removing 38 to 45 μm of tissue with a phototherapeutic keratectomy (PTK). The residual debris is mechanically removed with a spatula. This technique is relatively easy for beginning surgeons. Because the diaphragm on the laser is wide open, it is important to warn patients that the sound of the laser will be loud. If the PTK centration is not accurate, stromal ablation will be difficult to center.

   This technique is dependent on the tear film quality, so once the lid speculum is inserted, the surgeon must proceed quickly. Waiting too long will cause tear film disruption and an irregular surface. Patients with meibomitis and variable tear film quality may not be candidates for this technique. Occasionally irrigating with balanced saline and removing excess tears creates a smooth, homogeneous surface prior to laser ablation.

   Rather than using a standard depth for epithelial removal, another approach uses the blue fluorescence that appears when the laser strikes the epithelium. When the microscope light is dimmed, a blue fluorescence appears as the epithelium is ablated. Once the laser reaches the stroma, the blue fluorescence disappears, and the surgeon sees a black area. Typically, the peripheral stroma is reached before the center. When the blue fluorescence disappears, the surgeon stops and scrapes away the debris. It is not easy to observe the precise moment when the blue fluorescence disappears; we do not typically use this approach for routine cases but for enhancements, especially if haze is present.

   Although the epithelial defects made with the laser heal faster than those made by mechanical removal with a spatula, complications can occur. If the stroma is entered too deeply, a steep border between unablated and ablated stroma results. This can lead to an abnormal healing response, with peripheral arcuate haze and scarring. Although this disappears with time, it can result in progressive hyperopia in that haze and scarring in the peripheral part of ablation will steepen the central cornea. Restarting the postoperative steroid regimen is indicated in these hyperopic cases. Arcuate haze may also induce astigmatism, another indicator that steroids should be restarted.

   The pure transepithelial laser ablation technique typically uses a 6-mm optical zone. A myopic PRK of approximately 1.5 D is performed initially, followed by a PTK to ablate through the epithelium. As the ablation is performed, a blue fluorescence can be seen if the operating microscope light is turned down. When the epithelial ablation is complete and Bowman's layer is reached, the fluorescence disappears. There is a human variation of about 15 μm of epithelial thickness among individual corneas.

   Although this "no-touch" technique is popular with patients, it increases the number of factors that affect outcome; hence it takes longer to master. It is advantageous because the cornea is more uniformly moist. There is evidence that the incidence of haze is lower with this method.

3. **Alcohol technique.** Absolute alcohol is mixed with balanced salt solution to make a dilute solution of 20% and applied to a 6-mm sponge disc. It is allowed to remain on the central cornea for 2 minutes. The central epithelium can then be lifted by two blunt McPherson forceps, leaving Bowman's layer crystal clear for ablation.

   Another technique uses a 6- or 7-mm metal optical zone marker placed on the eye and a few drops of 20% alcohol placed within the marker. After 20 to 30 seconds, the alcohol is irrigated and the epithelium comes off easily. With this approach, the epithelium usually heals within 2 to 3 days with minimal transient corneal haze.

4. **Rotary brushing.** An instrument for removing the epithelium, developed by Drs. Percy Amoils and Ioannis Pallikaris, consists of a rotary brush (the Amoils brush, Innova, Toronto, Canada; Fig. 20–4) made of fine hairs that do not injure the underlying Bowman's layer. Use of this technique provides a smooth corneal surface. Brushes of different depths

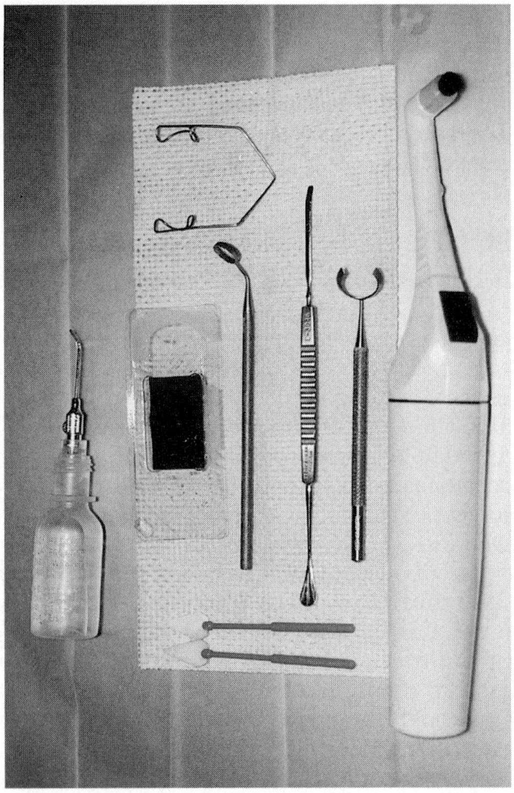

Figure 20–4. Instruments that may be used for photorefractive keratectomy (PRK): Amoils rotary brush for epithelium removal, balanced saline for irrigation of the ocular surface, wire lid speculum, optical zone marker and ink pad if using mechanical debridement, globe fixation device if patient has difficulty with self-fixation, sponges soaked with balanced saline that can be used after mechanical epithelial removal to clean the surface of the cornea prior to ablation.

(6.5 mm and 9 mm) can be used for myopic or hyperopic ablations.

This technique is easy to use, and the epithelium is removed within a few seconds. This appears to be promising, especially for hyperopic ablations, which generally require removal of 9 mm of epithelium, a procedure that is too lengthy and difficult with mechanical removal. It is important to use a rotary brush and not an oscillating brush to achieve complete epithelial removal.

A disadvantage is that patients lose fixation when the pupil is occluded with the brush, and, with the resulting eye movement, the surgeon can remove too much epithelium. Disposable sterile brushes are available that make this a very attractive technique.

OTHER ISSUES

Sometimes, outcomes, techniques, or environments can affect the choice of procedure. For example, because it excessively dried the cornea, nitrogen blowing is no longer used. Often it caused differential drying; its use resulted in a high incidence of haze but no cases of central islands.

The VISX STAR (VISX, Santa Monica, California) uses a suction tube placed about 1.25 inches away from the cornea, and all nomograms are based on this position. If the suction tube is too close to the eye, it will dehydrate the corneal surface, resulting in overcorrections. If it is too far away, fluid will accumulate, resulting in undercorrections.

Room humidity may affect outcomes. As surgeons develop their own data pool, it is important to keep as many factors as possible constant. That means keeping temperature and humidity relatively constant in the laser room. It is worthwhile having temperature and humidity gauges. A cornea that is too dry after epithelial removal and/or during laser ablation may result in haze.

CHILLED BALANCE SALINE

Dehydration appears to contribute significantly to haze. Chilled balance saline placed on the cornea following the procedure or after each of the multipass or multizone ablations cools the cornea and provides clearer postoperative corneas. Irrigating the cornea at the conclusion of the procedure removes much of the microscopic debris that has fallen onto the cornea during the ablation process and makes the patient more comfortable when wearing a bandage lens.

IMMEDIATELY AFTER THE PROCEDURE

At the end of the procedure, with the lid speculum still in place, the eye is flooded with a nonsteroidal drop, an antibiotic, and a steroid. A technician then inserts a disposable bandage contact lens and the wire speculum is removed.

POSTOPERATIVE MANAGEMENT

Excimer patients should expect vision to be blurry while the epithelium is healing. They should know that symptoms like ghosting, glare, and shadows are usually transient phenomena and will disappear.

The physician must devote substantial time during postoperative visits explaining what is happening to the patient. Issues of hygiene and the increased risk of infection during the first few postoperative days are of particular importance.

Patients also need to know that changes in vision with healing of epithelium and stroma are normal during the early postoperative course. A delay in vision recovery might affect the patient's ability to work, or may interfere with hobbies, vacation, or travel. A patient should always allow more than enough time for healing to occur before resumption of activities requiring critical vision.

With PRK, patients often observe transitory changes in visual acuity. These visual changes correspond with changes in corneal transparency and corneal topography. It is essential that the patient understand that such changes may occur, and that they are temporary. The combination of preoperative and postoperative nonsteroidal anti-inflammatory administration, together with a soft contact lens, has resulted in a major decrease in pain, such that 90% of patients are comfortable following PRK. The 10% who do experience discomfort usually have minimal to moderate discomfort overnight, which quickly resolves. Prior to the use of nonsteroidal drops, all patients had significant pain. This important breakthrough in treatment is thought to be related to the blockage of prostaglandins by the nonsteroidal anti-inflammatory drops and the protective effect of the contact lens bandage on the denuded epithelial surface.

THE FIRST POSTOPERATIVE WEEK

During the first 3 postoperative days, examinations are typically scheduled until the epithelium is healed. Nonsteroidal anti-inflammatory drops[6] are instilled a few times per day for 24 to 48 hours. A fluoroquinolone antibiotic is used five times a day for 5 days or until the epithelium becomes intact. A corticosteroid is instilled five times a day and slowly tapered (see below). A topical anesthetic (preservative free)[7] in the form of tetracaine 0.5% is given to be used, as a minimum, once at bedtime and once the following morning.

Re-epithelialization usually takes 2 to 3 days, after which the bandage contact lens is removed. If the contact lens is removed prior to epithelial healing, the patient will often experience significant pain.

STEROID COURSE

There is no universally accepted steroid regimen. Reasonable options consist of one of the following:

1. **No steroid.**[8] If during follow-up there is significant regression or haze, then steroids are started.
2. **Short steroid course.** Typically, steroids can be used four times a day for 1 week, three times a day for 1 week, two times a day for 1 week, then once a day for 1 week. If there is overcorrection, regression, or significant haze, then the steroid dosage and course can be altered.
3. **Long steroid course.** The topical steroid can be used five times a day for 1 month, four times a day for 1 month, three times a day for 1 month, twice a day for 1 month, then finally once a day for one month. This regimen may be altered if overcorrection, regression, or significant haze develops.

EFFECT OF POSTOPERATIVE STEROIDS

The use of topical steroids after photorefractive keratectomy is controversial. Studies in the low myopia range (less than 6 D) have shown no significant difference in refractive outcome or development of haze between eyes treated with steroids and those treated with artificial tears. Our own clinical experience, especially in high myopia, is that there is greater evidence of regression and haze when steroids are not used or when they are discontinued abruptly. It is hoped that better and more effective nonsteroidal modulating medications will be developed.

Disadvantages of steroid use include such adverse effects as elevated intraocular pressure, posterior subcapsular cataracts, ptosis, and reactivation of herpes simplex keratitis.

EFFECT OF NONSTEROIDAL ANTI-INFLAMMATORIES

Nonsteroidal, anti-inflammatories like diclofenac sodium (Voltaren) and ketorolac tromethamine (Acular), through inhibition of prostaglandin synthesis, produce a potent analgesic effect that is important in the early postoperative period following photorefractive surgery. The use of diclofenac has been shown to promote regression and therefore is occasionally used when dealing with an overcorrected PRK.

The use of such medications should be combined with a topical steroid to prevent accumulation of white blood cells in the cornea, which will produce corneal infiltrates in 1 of 250 eyes in which steroids are not used in conjunction with a nonsteroidal in the early postoperative period. A combination of steroids used with a nonsteroidal in the early postoperative period will dramatically decrease the incidence of sterile infiltrates.

TOPOGRAPHY

Corneal videokeratoscopy should be performed preoperatively and at 1 month postoperation, and the difference maps should be evaluated.[9] Preoperative topographies, therefore, are an essential reference from which to derive the difference map postoperatively. At 1 month, the difference will tell whether the ablation has been properly centered. This feedback allows the surgeon to monitor and improve centration techniques, especially in patients who are asymptomatic, with small pupils, and a mildly decentered ablation.

COMPLICATIONS

Clinicians must understand and recognize the potential complications of PRK. With an appreciation of the possible complications, precautions can often be taken to minimize them. In addition, the eyecare practitioner who recognizes the early symptoms and signs of these complications can initiate appropriate treatment or reassure the patient that they are benign.

Complications can be divided into the following categories[10]:

- A. Side effects of corticosteroid use
  1. Ocular hypertension
- B. Early (less than 6 weeks) complications
  1. Discomfort/pain
  2. Corneal infection/sterile infiltrates
  3. Delayed epithelial healing
  4. Pseudodendrites

C. Early or late complications
   1. Loss of best-corrected visual acuity
   2. Halo effect
   3. Central islands
   4. Decentration
   5. Recurrent corneal erosion
   6. Ocular hypertension
D. Late (greater than 6 weeks) complications
   1. Diffuse haze
   2. Arcuate or peripheral haze
E. Refractive complications
   1. Undercorrection
   2. Overcorrection
   3. Presbyopia
   4. Regression with or without haze
F. General awareness

Side Effects of Corticosteroid Use

Ocular Hypertension

Clinical Features

In a small percentage of patients, the postoperative use of steroids can result in increased intraocular pressure (IOP). Reduction or discontinuation of the steroid dose and application of beta-blockers or other glaucoma medications will typically return the IOP to normal. It is critical to monitor IOP following the PRK while the patient continues to use topical steroids. To reduce the incidence of such occurrence, fluorometholone and rimexolone (Vexol) have become more commonly used postoperative topical steroids than the more penetrating steroids, like prednisolone acetate or dexamethasone.

Other potential complications associated with the use of topical steroids include:

- Reactivation of latent herpes simplex virus, which can be treated with antiviral medications.
- Ptosis due to an effect on muscle tissue. This tends to occur more often in young women than in other patients.
- Posterior subcapsular cataracts

Management

With an elevation in IOP (greater than 23 mm Hg), add a beta-blocker (if there are no contraindications: asthma, heart block) and re-check IOP. Follow closely and if not improved, taper off steroid drops. Reduce frequency of steroid dose until IOP is controlled. Other complications resulting from the use of topical steroids are typically addressed by discontinuing steroid use.

Early (less than 6 weeks) Complications

Discomfort/Pain

Clinical Features

Patients may experience postoperative discomfort that is similar to that associated with a corneal abrasion. Ninety percent of patients report little to no discomfort after PRK and 10% of patients report discomfort or pain that resolves within 24 to 36 hours of the procedure. Most patients who have discomfort describe it as the sensation of having sand or an eyelash in their eye.

Management

The postoperative pain has been greatly reduced or eliminated by the use of nonsteroidal anti-inflammatory drugs (e.g., ketorolac tromethamine 0.5% [Acular] or diclofenac sodium 0.1% [Voltaren]) during the first few days following the PRK procedure in combination with a bandage soft contact lens. In addition, topical anesthetics without preservatives, e.g., Tetracaine minum can be used a few times per day during the first 24 hours. Irrigating the eye with balanced saline solution at the completion of the PRK procedure decreases the chances of trapped epithelial debris under the bandage lens. Systemic medication (e.g., Demerol, Tylenol with Codeine No. 3) may be used if necessary. Cold compresses applied to the lids are often helpful. In patients with a dry eye, wearing a soft contact lens during the first few days after the PRK procedure can result in some irritation or discomfort. Frequent use of preservative-free artificial tears can relieve the discomfort. Also, dry eye patients may benefit from the insertion of collagen implants or silicone punctal plugs.

Corneal Infection/Sterile Infiltrates

Clinical Features

Symptoms and Signs

Occasionally patients are asymptomatic early in the postoperative course. Pain, discharge, or redness may be present. Corneal infection and/or sterile infiltrates are rare complications and have been reported to occur, on average, in one out of every 500 cases. These corneal problems are usually recognized on the second to fourth postoperative day. A corneal infection usually involves a single white infiltrate and purulent discharge. In contrast, sterile infiltrates are frequently multiple in number without an associated discharge.

Management

To treat the complication, remove the soft contact lens and send it for bacterial culture and drug-sensitivity testing. A corneal scraping is also recommended for culture and testing. Treat as a bacterial corneal ulcer with broad-spectrum antibiotics. If the white infiltrate is small *m* less than 2 mm in size *m* consider monotherapy with a fluoroquinolone every hour during the day and taper the dose with improvement in the clinical course. If the infiltrate is greater than or equal to 2 mm, consider treating with fortified antibiotics, for example, tobramycin 15 mg/cc and cefazolin 50 mg/cc, every 30 to 60 minutes and gradually taper the dose. If there is no purulent discharge, and there are multiple infiltrates, consider cautiously adding a topical steroid to counteract a possible immune reaction secondary to the nonsteroidal anti-inflammatory drug.

Delayed Epithelial Healing

Clinical Features

Symptoms and Signs

Persistent blurred vision occurs with an epithelial defect. The epithelial defect usually has well-defined borders. The stroma may show folds secondary to edema.

Management

If the epithelial surface is not intact by 4 days postoperatively, initiate the following steps:

1. Discontinue all drops except the antibiotic and preservative-free artificial tears. Be sure the patient is not self-medicating with a topical anesthetic.
2. If the soft contact lens placed after the PRK procedure is still present, remove it and insert a new lens.
3. If the contact lens has been removed, then you may wish to reinsert another protective contact lens.
4. After the epithelium is intact, remove the protective lens and restart the topical steroid.

Pseudodendrites

Clinical Features

Symptoms

Vision may be blurred if the pseudodendrite is in the visual axis.

Management

Pseudodendrites do not represent a true complication, but rather one part of the normal healing response. Do not confuse them with a herpetic lesion. A pseudodendritic pattern may become apparent as the epithelial surface re-forms in the healing process during the third and fourth days after the laser procedure. This is a normal healing pattern and will resolve within a few days. No change in the medication is required.

EARLY AND LATE COMPLICATIONS

Loss of Best-Corrected Visual Acuity

Clinical Features

The source of blurred vision, or loss of best-corrected visual acuity, can usually be detected with the standard eye examination. Occasionally, computerized videokeratography may be necessary to detect more subtle causes for loss of visual acuity. Typical causes of loss of best-corrected visual acuity include epithelial irregularity, central islands, corneal haze, and decentered ablation.

Vision is typically very blurry immediately after the procedure, and it generally starts to improve once the epithelium has grown back, which in most cases takes 2 to 4 days. However, vision can continue to be blurry for a number of weeks. After the epithelial defect has healed, loss of best-corrected visual acuity is usually secondary to an irregular epithelium, which usually smoothes out over a few weeks. Longer term, some patients lose one to two lines of Snellen acuity in comparison to their previous best-corrected vision. With higher corrections, more variability is to be expected.

Management

If epithelial irregularity with or without superficial punctate keratitis (SPK) is noted, preservative-free artificial tears should be added. Loss of acuity from other causes should be managed as outlined in this section.

Halo Effect

Clinical Features

Halos may be experienced in the first 4 to 6 weeks following the procedure as the epithelium heals and smooths out over the complete ablation zone. Symptoms are more apt to occur at night when dilatation of the pupil allows light transmission at the edge of the ablation zone. Persistent halos rarely occur and are usually related to large pupils, small ablation zone, or a decentered ablation.

Management

With most patients, the halo effect tends to diminish with time. In the case of undercorrection, retreatment with a larger optical zone may alleviate the halos. Halos can also be minimized through the use of pilocarpine drops which constrict the pupil; or alphagan drops to decrease dilatation of the pupil.

Central Islands

Clinical Features

Central islands, small elevated areas of tissue left in the center of the ablation field, may occur following PRK.[11] Central islands may cause monocular diplopia or blurred vision. The definition of a central island is a central or pericentral area of steepening that is

- At least 1.00 D in height
- A diameter of at least 1 mm
- Measured at least 1 month postoperatively

Patients may be asymptomatic or experience qualitative visual changes. The islands may be visible as a small central shadow on retinoscopy. Diagnosis can be confirmed with computerized videokeratography showing an elevation within the central or pericentral zone. A number of reasons have been proposed to explain the cause of central islands:

- Vortex plume theory, in which the ablated debris interferes with the laser pulses
- Degradation of optics leading to reduced ablation centrally
- Epithelial hyperplasia or thickening, which has been documented through use of sophisticated ultrasound techniques
- Acoustic shockwave theory, in which each pulse produces a shockwave that leads to stromal hydration

- A theory that the flat and homogeneous laser beam profile produces central fluid accumulation at the time of the procedure, which results in decreased ablation centrally. The etiology is probably multifactorial.

Management

The prevention of central islands can be achieved by producing additional pulses to the central 2.5 mm ablation area. If central islands are noted, most disappear after a period of months. If after 10 months there is a persistent symptomatic central island, the laser can be used to vaporize the central elevation. Computerized topography is used to determine the location, width, and steepness of the central island. After mechanical epithelial removal, an ablation zone of less than 3 mm is used to flatten the island by PRK.

Decentration

Clinical Features

Decentration can occur if the laser beam is not precisely aligned with the surgeon's eyepiece prior to the procedure, or as a result of poor patient fixation. Although significant eye movement when the laser is pulsing can create decentration when a tracker is not used, the ophthalmologist has the ability to control this error by stopping the laser procedure at any point during the PRK. A small amount of eye movement typically will not affect the outcome of the procedure. Decentration of the ablation zone can cause an increase in corneal astigmatism.[12] Eyes with higher attempted correction have a greater probability of decentration of the ablated zone because these patients have greater difficulty in maintaining fixation during treatment, either because of their greater myopia or because more time is required for laser treatment.

Management

Although a number of approaches have been used to treat the effects of decentration, none is completely satisfactory. It is best to treat the residual myopia and to decenter the ablation in the opposite quadrant. A technique developed by Julian Stevens of England is to decenter a PRK in the epithelium and then obtain computerized videokeratography to document improvement in the centration. Then a PTK should be performed centrally and stopped when the blue fluorescence has disappeared (personal communication 1997). This is more of an art than a science, but the results appear encouraging. Currently, either topographically guided ablations or a masking agent may be used. Masking agents that ablate at the same rate as the corneal stroma may be used to smooth the corneal surface. By molding the collagen compound with a rigid gas-permeable lens, a smooth anterior surface is created. The laser can be used to ablate directly through the masking agent to produce a spherical central cornea.

Recurrent Corneal Erosion

Clinical Features

Symptoms and Signs

Patients may complain of pain, tearing, and photophobia. This is more common in the morning on awakening. The symptoms may resolve in an hour or persist for hours, if significant. An epithelial defect or erosion may be seen during the acute episode. Epithelial microcysts may be noted after the erosion has healed.

Management

Recurrent corneal erosions are more common with mechanical epithelial debridement than with laser transepithelial removal. The erosion tends to occur outside the laser area of ablation. Management is similar to that of a recurrent corneal erosion, with hypertonic drops and ointment. If this is not satisfactory in preventing a recurrence, a bandage soft contact lens can be tried. If this is not successful, a PTK can be performed to the eroding area. The epithelium in the area is gently removed and a PTK with an optical zone of 2 to 6 mm to encompass the erosion site is selected with a depth of 5 to 8 μm.

LATE (longer than 6 weeks) COMPLICATIONS

Diffuse Haze

Clinical Features

Corneal haze usually takes the form of a fine reticular subepithelial pattern that does not interfere with vision. Corneal clarity is graded on a scale of 0 to 4+. The haze corresponds to a corneal healing response following PRK, induced by activation and migration of keratocytes (fibroblasts) and newly synthesized collagen. The haze is first noted between 2 and 4 months; it gradually fades away by 6 to 12 months. Severe haze rarely occurs. There are some factors that may be related to increased haze: depth of ablation, laser beam homogeneity, epithelial removal method, corneal dryness during treatment, keratitis sicca, and solar exposure. Age does not seem to be an enhancing factor.

Management

If the patient has moderate or severe haze that interferes with vision, steroid drops should be increased in frequency to five times per day and gradually tapered over 2 to 3 months. Topical steroids are used to try to modulate the stromal wound healing response. The mechanism is decreased DNA synthesis, as well as lens-specific anti-anabolic effects, leading to decreased keratocyte activity and decreased collagen synthesis. Rarely, a persistent haze will require a repeat laser treatment. It is usually best to treat the haze with a "no-touch" technique using a PTK mode. Any residual refractive error can be managed in the future with a PRK. The refractive error tends to be unreliable when there is severe corneal haze.

A transepithelial or no-touch technique is preferred. In these eyes, the epithelium is often mixed with newly formed collagen, and, if all the epithelium is removed mechanically, the result is an irregular surface. It is best to use the laser on the epithelium as a masking agent to achieve a smoother surface. Unfortunately, despite use of the no-touch technique, there is an 80% recurrence of the haze with this method. The adjunctive use of mitomycin C 0.02% as a single intraoperative application for 2 minutes or as a postoperative drop three or four times a day for 1 to 4 weeks has been shown to dramatically decrease the incidence of recurrent haze.

Although decentered ablations are relatively uncommon in association with retreatment, the incidence is higher than in primary procedures. The risk is especially great with mechanical epithelial removal techniques, because the patient's view of the red fixation light is often blurred. The surgeon must be aware of this and may need to hold the eye for proper fixation.

If possible it is best to wait for resolution of the haze before retreating. Patients should be off all eye drops and have a stable refraction before an enhancement. If there is sufficient corneal thickness these patients are best treated with a LASIK enhancement to minimize the wound healing response.

Arcuate or Peripheral Haze

Clinical Features

Haze in the peripheral area of the ablation bed can lead to a hyperopic shift and/or induced astigmatism. This peripheral haze is more commonly seen with a laser epithelial ablation that was too deep. In this case, a steep transition exists between the ablated zone and the untreated area.

Management

Peripheral haze, like diffuse haze, should be managed with the frequent use of steroid drops five times per day with a gradual tapering over 2 to 3 months. This is the only situation in which steroid drops are increased when dealing with a hyperopic refractive error.

REFRACTIVE COMPLICATIONS

Undercorrection

Clinical Features

Residual myopia is a consequence of insufficient initial treatment, which is more common with higher degrees of myopia. Undercorrection may result from an excessively moist cornea during the procedure.

Management

If there is an undercorrection and the patient is not satisfied with the level of vision and is not interested in monovision, additional treatment can be performed. It is usually best to wait until the refraction is stable.

Overcorrection

Clinical Features

With overcorrection, patients may experience blurred vision when viewing close-up objects. In some cases, particularly in patients over 40 years old who are presbyopic, vision may also be blurry when viewing objects in the distance. A small amount of initial overcorrection is acceptable because some regression will often take place. Possible causes include a cornea that is too dry during the procedure and manifest preoperative refraction that did not account for accommodation.

Management

Any significant degree of hyperopia should be managed by tapering the dosage of the steroid drops over 2 to 4 weeks. A more rapid withdrawal of steroids can lead to significant haze. If regression toward myopia is not satisfactory, diclofenac eye drops or a bandage contact lens can promote epithelial hyperplasia and regression. Surgical options include hyperopic PRK, holmium laser, radiofrequency laser, or hyperopic LASIK.

Presbyopia

Clinical Features

In the case of overcorrection, presbyopic symptoms may be produced following the procedure.

Management

Reading glasses may be required, even for patients who did not require corrective lenses for reading prior to the procedure.

Regression with or without Haze

Clinical Features

Regression is more likely to occur with higher degrees of myopic and/or astigmatic correction. Factors that may lead to regression include preoperative flat keratometry, small optical zones, single zone treatment, high myopia, and steep wound edges.[13,14] Another factor that can lead to regression is secondary ultraviolet (UV) exposure. Anecdotal reports have indicated regression after intense UV exposure, and UV-related regression is most likely to occur during the first 6 postoperative months with exposure to unfiltered sunlight at high altitude, such as when skiing.

Management

If regression occurs, steroid drops should be either increased in frequency or restarted. If after a few months there is improvement in the refractive error, the steroid dose is tapered. If the eye remains undercorrected, retreatment can be performed after the steroids have been discontinued and after the refraction becomes stable. Typically, retreatment is not considered earlier than 6 months after the PRK procedure.[15] As a precaution, it is advised that patients use UV-protective sunglasses when exposed to sunlight at a high altitude during the first 6 postoperative months.

Regression without haze can be managed with a PRK enhancement that is similar in technique to a primary procedure. If there is regression with mild haze, a transepithelial approach followed by a PRK for the residual refractive error can be performed. If there is regression with severe haze, then a no-touch technique using a PTK mode should be done. Any residual refractive error can be managed later with a PRK enhancement for myopia, astigmatism, or hyperopia.

For regression, mechanical epithelial removal should be accomplished using a spatula, rotating brush, or alcohol technique. It is important to note that some patients who were plano after a primary PRK procedure and then regressed will often be hyperopic early post-enhancement. As the epithelial thickness changes, their hyperopia resolves, sometimes taking up to 4 months. This is a normal condition requiring no extra treatment. However, patients who were undercorrected after their primary procedure with a relatively stable refractive error are close to plano soon after the enhancement and tend to remain stable.

GENERAL AWARENESS

Pregnancy

If a patient becomes pregnant prior to having PRK or at any time during the first year following the procedure, the doctor must be made aware because pregnancy can affect the healing response. Also, some medications may pose a risk to an unborn or nursing child.

Eye Sensitivity

Some patients continue to experience tenderness when they rub their eyes. Such sensitivity may continue for a long time. Additionally, patients may continue to experience sensitivity to light. Such sensitivities tend to diminish with time as the healing process evolves and use of eyedrops is discontinued.

SUMMARY

A thorough understanding of the preoperative assessments, techniques, and postoperative management are essential to achieve satisfactory visual outcomes with PRK. Laser safety checks are mandatory. A well-functioning excimer laser with good optics is essential. The surgeon must avoid any decentration or global tilt, and all aspects of the technique must be performed with attention to detail. The postoperative management requires frequent follow-up visits and psychological reinforcement of a healing process that is not instantaneous. This is evolving technology. Although the results today are impressive, the complications will continue to decrease with changes in lasers, techniques, and pharmacological management.

REFERENCES

1. Stein H, Cheskes A, Stein R: The Excimer, 2nd Edition. Thorofare, N.J.: Slack, Inc.; 1998:10–64.
2. Corbett MC, O'Brart DP, Warburton FG, Marshall J: Biologic and environmental risk factors for regression after photorefractive keratectomy. Ophthalmology 1996;103:1381–91.
3. Amm M, Duncker GI, Schroder E: Excimer laser correction of high astigmatism after keratoplasty. J Cataract Refract Surg 1996;22:313–7.
4. Pallikaris I, McDonald MB, Siganos D, et al.: Tracker-assisted photorefractive keratectomy for myopia of −1 to −6 diopters. J Refract Surg 1996;12:240–7.
5. Stein H, Stein R: The Excimer Video Course. St. Louis: Medical Productions; 1994.
6. Tutton MK, Cherry PM, Raj PS, Fsadni MG: Efficacy and safety of topical diclofenac in reducing ocular pain after excimer photorefractive keratectomy. J Cataract Refract Surg 1996;22:536–41.
7. Verma S, Marshall J: Control of pain after photorefractive keratectomy. J Refract Surg 1996;12:358–64.
8. Corbett MC, O'Brart DP, Marshall J: Do topical steroids have a role following excimer laser photorefractive keratectomy? J Refract Surg 1995;11:380–7.
9. Johnson DA, Haight DH, Kelly SE, et al.: Reproducibility of videokeratographic digital subtraction maps after excimer laser photorefractive keratectomy. Ophthalmology 1996;103:1392-8.
10. Stein R, Stein H, Cheskes A: Photorefractive keratectomy. Continuing Education Manual, Bochner Eye Institute, 1999.
11. Krueger RR, Saedy NF, McDonald PJ: Clinical analysis of steep central islands after excimer laser photorefractive keratectomy. Arch Ophthalmol 1996;114:377–81.
12. Aktunc R, Aktunc T: Centration of excimer laser photorefractive keratectomy and changes in astigmatism. J Refract Surg 1996; 12:S268–71.
13. Gauthier CA, Holden BA, Epstein D, et al.: Role of epithelial hyperplasia in regression following photorefractive keratectomy. Br J Ophthalmol 1996;80:545–8.
14. Goggin M, Foley-Nolan A, Algawa K, O'Keefe M: Regression after photorefractive keratectomy for myopia. J Cataract Refract Surg 1996;22:194–6.
15. Matta CS, Piebenga LW, Deitz MR, Tauber J: Excimer retreatment for myopic photorefractive keratectomy failures. Six to 18 month follow-up. Ophthalmology 1996;103:444–51.

CHAPTER 21

Keratoprosthesis

BEYOND CORNEAL GRAFT FAILURE

CLAES H. DOHLMAN, M.D., PhD., JUAN CARLOS ABAD, M.D., ERIC J. DUDENHOEFER, M.D., and JOHN M. GRANEY

Keratoprosthesis (KPro) has been sparingly used as a last resort in severe corneal diseases during the last half century. A considerable amount of research on this topic has been conducted by several groups of investigators, however, the number of patients subjected to this procedure remains small. The long history of KPro development will not be covered here—the reader is referred to earlier extensive reviews[1,2] on the subject. Rather, this communication will focus on the use of a specific KPro of a collar button design (Dohlman-Doane Type I),[3] and its indications, surgical techniques, and follow-up.

KERATOPROSTHESIS DESIGNS

The KPro is made of polymethyl methacrylate (PMMA) and is machined as a front part and a separate back plate, which is screwed on to the stem, clamping a corneal graft. It has undergone a number of design changes since the mid-1960s. Thus the diameter of the front and the back plates, the stem diameter, the absence or presence of holes, and their diameter, in the back plate has varied. The present version (Fig. 21–1) has a front plate diameter of 7.0 mm, a stem diameter of 3.35 mm, an inter plate distance of 0.75 mm and a back plate diameter of 7.0 mm. The back plate has 8 holes of 1.3 mm size. The holes have proven of value because they facilitate nutrients from the aqueous to reach the stroma and its keratocytes. Also, the holes allow aqueous more rapidly to replace fluid that has evaporated from the corneal surface. The details of the manufacture of this KPro have been described earlier.[4]

PATIENT EVALUATION

Taking a detailed history is mandatory. This usually reveals the underlying cause of the corneal condition (disease, trauma, surgery), the duration of symptoms, whether unilateral or bilateral disease, whether episodic (herpes simplex?) or steadily progressive. Particularly important for predicting outcome is any history of glaucoma, especially following chemical burns. Severe corneal damage often makes exact pressure measurements impossible and many such patients have had their glaucoma inadequately treated. Details and dates of previous surgery (keratoplasty, cataract extraction, glaucoma shunt, retina repair, etc.) should be solicited.

Blink mechanism and tear secretion are important factors in assessing KPro prognosis. Blink rate and completeness can be estimated when the patient does not feel observed. Lagophthalmos and frank chronic exposure are extremely important to recognize when present. Tear secretion should be measured with Schirmer test. Break-up time of the tear film may have some value in assessing the health of the ocular surface.

Visual acuity should be recorded in the standard fashion. If the corneal surface is highly irregular in the presence of only moderate stromal opacities, hard contact lens refraction can be revealing. When the cornea has opacities of such severity that a keratoprosthesis may be contemplated, a standard visual field test is rarely applicable but gross projection should be assessed. Testing presence or absence of central fixation and, particularly, absence of light projection nasally, are often revealing. If nasal projection is lost, end-stage glaucoma must be suspected.

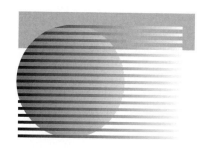

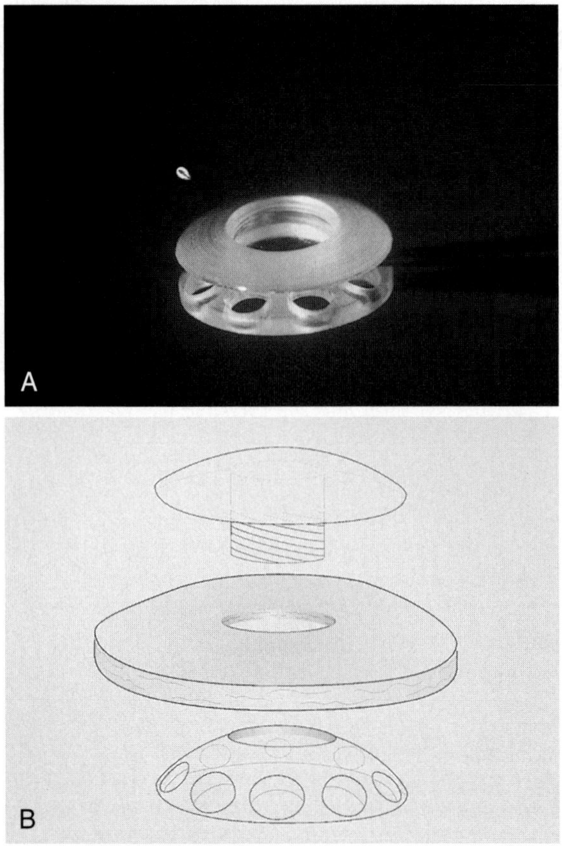

Figure 21–1. Type I collar-button KPro basics. *A.* Assembled Type I KPro. *B.* Anatomy of the KPro/cornea complex: The stem of the mushroom shaped front plate passes through a trephined central opening in the corneal graft. The back plate then screws onto the exposed threads of the stem to sandwich the cornea between front and back plates.

Slit lamp examination should routinely take note of conjunctival inflammation, surface keratinization, and fornix shortening or symblephara. Corneal opacity from scarring or edema, as well as vascularization, should be recorded and evaluated whether explaining the visual acuity. Anterior chamber reaction and the status of the iris and lens (or IOL) are important factors. The fundus is often not observable but, when it is, disc cupping has high prognostic importance and may require aqueous shunt implantation.

Recording intraocular pressure can be fraught with error. Usually, in severe corneal pathology, pneumotonometry is more reliable than the applanation technique. In addition, it is always prudent to try to estimate the intraocular pressure by digital palpation, however imprecise.

Electroretinogram (ERG) and Visual Evoked Response (VER) have not been very helpful in our hands. They can give falsely negative results, leading to the conclusion that the situation is more hopeless than it actually is.

Ultrasound examination is mandatory. A B-scan can reveal a retinal detachment, massive debris or advanced optic nerve cupping behind the opaque cornea or lens. Still a fair sized cup may not be detectable on the exam and, therefore, ultrasound is not a reliable method of diagnosing glaucoma damage. If a glaucoma shunt has been implanted previously, a B-scan ultrasonography can identify a fluid cleft over the shunt plate. This indicates patency of the shunt tube. An A-scan measurement of the axial length of the eye is also required in order to allow a KPro of the correct dioptric power to be chosen.

Finally, external photography of the eyes, pre- and postoperatively is important for the recording of the progress and outcome.

PATIENT SELECTION

This particular KPro is primarily aimed at patients who have a reasonably intact blink mechanism and tear secretion in place. Patients with heavy exposure to substantial evaporative forces may still be candidates for the procedure but would need extensive tarsorrhaphy and other lid adjustments in order to limit the exposure to the plastic surface only and not to the surrounding tissue (see below).

Autoimmune diseases such as ocular cicatricial pemphigoid, Stevens-Johnson syndrome, atopy or after very severe burns are not suitable candidates for this type of KPro. They may be helped with a through-the-lid prosthesis (Dohlman-Doane Type II) which will not be addressed here.[5]

Experience with a Type I KPro has shown that the prognosis for a good outcome is better in eyes that have experienced little intraocular inflammation in the past. This means, in practice, that a KPro in a failed graft performed in a case of corneal opacities or edema in dystrophies, degenerations, surgical or other trauma, also after bacterial or fungal keratitis, has a good five-year prognosis.[6] A history of herpetic keratitis may bring down the outlook somewhat.[7] Longstanding uveitis, whether in combination with rheumatoid disease or not, or end-stage phthisis presently constitute contraindications.

We recommend that if a standard corneal transplant has a good chance of giving longstanding good vision, this would be the preferred technique. However, if one or more graft failures have occurred within months after surgery, bringing down vision to finger counting or less, a KPro might be considered. Also, the status of the opposite eye must be factored in. A good vision in that eye makes KPro surgery unnecessary but if vision is 20/100 or below, a KPro indication for the worst eye becomes stronger. Finally, the age of the patient can be a consideration. If long-term survival of the KPro is questionable, it follows that elderly patients have a greater chance of a trouble free course than younger individuals (also see below).

SURGICAL TECHNIQUE

In preparation for the operation, the following items should be available:

1. A KPro with a dioptric power suitable for the axial length of the patient's eye (Massachusetts Eye and Ear Infirmary, Boston, MA)
2. A donor cornea in storage solution, requested from the local Eye Bank

3. A Troutman punch device (Pilling Weck Surgical, Ft. Washington, PA) able to accommodate trephine blades larger than 9.0 mm
4. Trephine blades 9.5 mm. and 9.0 mm. (Stortz # E3096 L), as well as 3.0 mm. (Accuderm Inc., Ft. Lauderdale, FL)
5. Hessberg-Barron vacuum trephine (Barron Precision Instruments, 1.L.C., Grand Blanc, MI)
6. Trephine handle, universal (Storz # E3095)
7. Adhesive patch and spanner wrench to facilitate the KPro assembly (included in the KPro package) (J.G. Machine Co., Woburn, MA)
8. Irrigation/aspiration unit, vitrector and light pipe
9. Standard keratoplasty instrument set
10. Fine bipolar cautery
11. Dexamethasone phosphate solution (4 mg/ml), Viscoelastics (optional)
12. Soft contact lens (e.g., Kontur lens, Kontur Contact Lens Co., Richmond, CA., 16.0 mm diameter, 9.8 mm base curve, plano)
13. Video (optional)
14. If needed, glaucoma valve shunt (Ahmed shunt S-2), (New World Medical Inc., Rancho Cucamonga, CA) and Tutoplast (from the same company)

PREOPERATIVE EVALUATION

Standard preoperative general medical assessment is done a few days before the surgery. The anesthesia can be general or local (retrobulbar and lid block). Since the KPro operation usually takes longer time than standard keratoplasty, we prefer general anesthesia when safe. Antibiotics intravenously (e.g., Cefazolin 1.0 g, if no allergy) at the start of surgery is recommended.

KPro ASSEMBLY

The first phase of the operation entails implantation of the KPro into a fresh corneal graft. This is conveniently carried out on a small side table. The corneal tissue is delivered from its cooled storage solution and put into the Troutman punch. Using a 9.5 mm. trephine blade the graft if punched out. It is allowed to stay in the teflon well with the endothelial side up, blotted gently centrally with a tip of a cellulose sponge and marked with a marking pen exactly centrally. The 3.0 mm. punch is then used to trephine a hole, as a central as possible (Fig. 21–2).

The KPro is brought out and the back plate is unscrewed (or the back plate may have been packaged separately). In order to stabilize the KPro during assembly, a small adhesive patch (included in the package) is attached to a stable surface, e.g., the plate of the Troutman punch. The back cover is peeled off and the patch is pressed in place. The top cover is now also peeled off, baring a brown adhesive surface. The front plate of the KPro is placed front plate down on the adhesive (Fig. 21–3). The corneal graft with its central hole is then slid

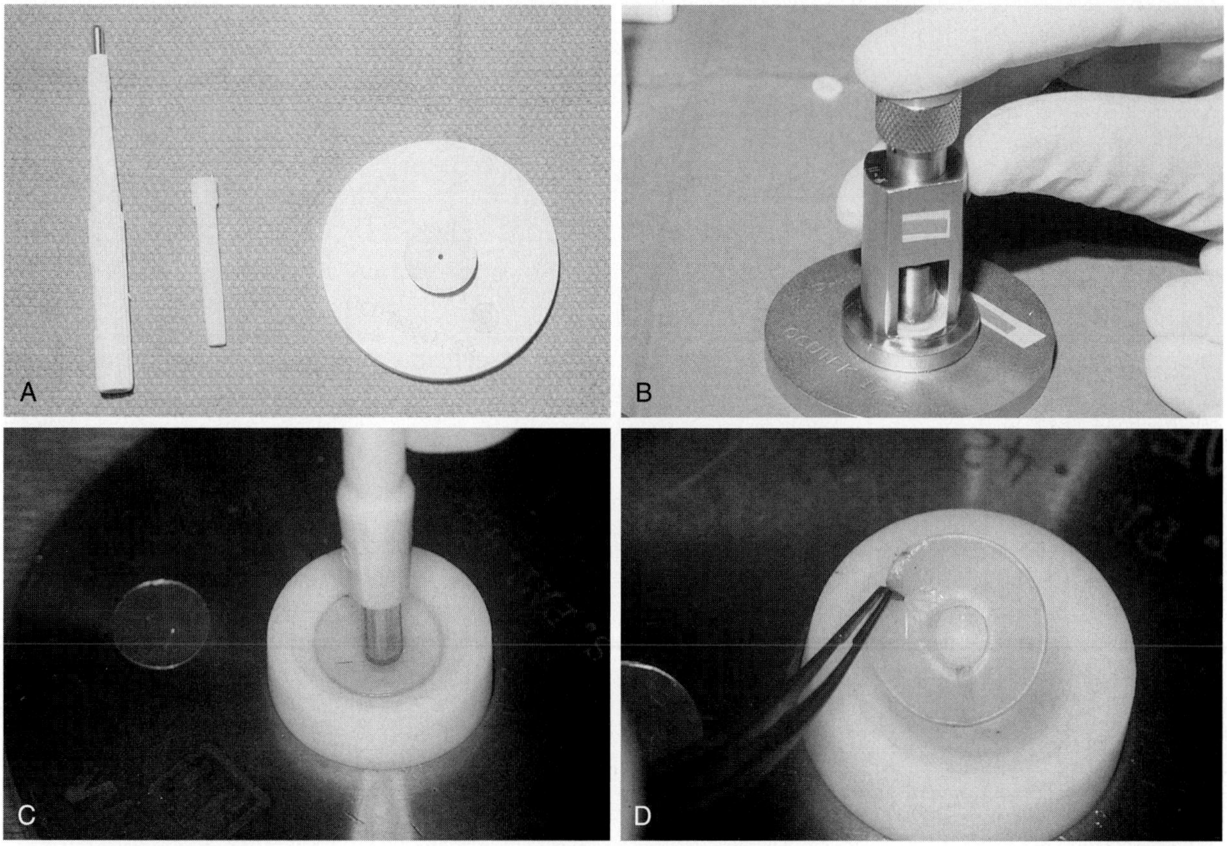

Figure 21–2. Preparation of the donor cornea. *A.* Tools for assembly (left to right): dermatologic punch, spanner wrench, Troutman punch base plate and cutting block with attached adhesive pad. *B.* A Troutman punch is used to trephine the donor corneal tissue. A 3.0 mm dermatologic punch *(C)* creates the central opening *(D)* to accommodate the KPro stem.

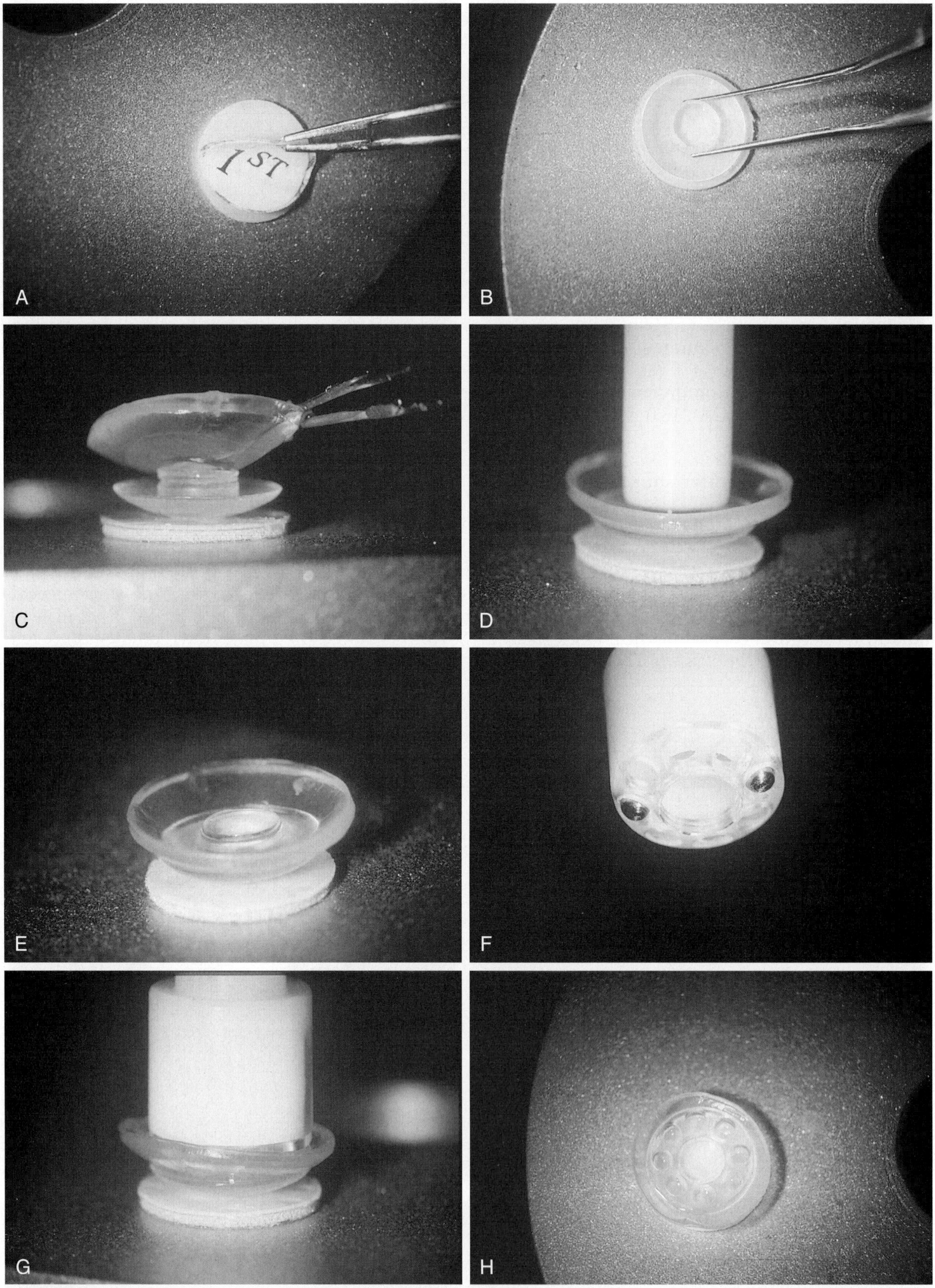

Figure 21–3. Preparation of the KPro/cornea complex. *A.* The adhesive pad is attached to the base plate and the printed top cover is removed. *B.* The KPro front part is placed face down on the adhesive surface. *C.* The donor ring is then fitted over the stem and *(D)* tamped into position using the hollow opposite end of the spanner wrench, allowing exposure of the threads *(E)*. Next, the back plate is placed, convex side out, onto the spanner wrench *(F)* and screwed onto the stem *(G)* to complete assembly *(H)*.

{ED: Call-Out "H"?}

down over the KPro stem. The back end of the thin white spanner wrench (included in the package) has a hole in its stem and it can be used to gently push down the graft against the front plate, avoiding excessive pressure. (Avoid the use of viscoelastics, that may allow the tissue to slide back over the screwthreads, making the re-screwing of the back plate more difficult). Finally, the wrench is used to pick up the back plate—the pegs into the holes—and screwed onto the stem. First the pin should be rotated *counter clockwise* against the stem until one feels a slight snap when the screw threads become engaged. Then rotate clockwise until *firm* resistance (a loosely applied back plate may become unscrewed later in the eye). It is recommended that the posterior surface of the stem be cleaned with a wet cellulose sponge. The fully assembled graft-prosthesis combination is finally removed from the patch and can now be kept in the storage solution until needed.

THE PATIENT'S EYE

The attention should now be focused on the patient's eye. A Weiner lid speculum is inserted. A vacuum trephine with a 9.0 mm. blade is chosen to incise the cornea (if suction cannot be accomplished, the cornea may have to be trephined using a handle and a disposable blade (Fig. 21–4). It is recommended that the trephining be down only half way through the cornea in order to eliminate bleeding sources before opening the eye. This is best done with fine bipolar cautery directed to the wound groove and it should be done extensively to complete dryness. Finally, the wound can be opened with a "super-blade" and excision completed with standard transplant scissors (e.g., Katzin scissors, Stortz # E 3232, and E 3233).

As the next step, the iris and the pupil should be assessed. We do not, as a rule, remove the total iris at the root since postoperative bleeding is not rare and future glare problems can be increased. If the pupil is small, or even normal, small iridotomies will expand the pupil enough not to interfere with the visual axis if the KPro should end up slightly eccentric.

If the lens is in place it should be removed in extracapsular fashion whether cataractous or not. Likewise, any IOL should be removed (a KPro with optics adjusted for pseudophakia can be used but postoperative internal reflexes make this approach impractical). If a cataract extraction has been done previously, peripheral cortical remnants, sometimes massive, often remain. If they are well encapsulated and not blocking vision, it is safest to leave them in place.

If the vitreous surface seems intact and not protruding, it is better left untouched. If broken and strands appear over the corneal rim, a moderate core vitrectomy is in order. It is particularly important to remove any speck of blood that may have originated from the corneal wound or the iris.

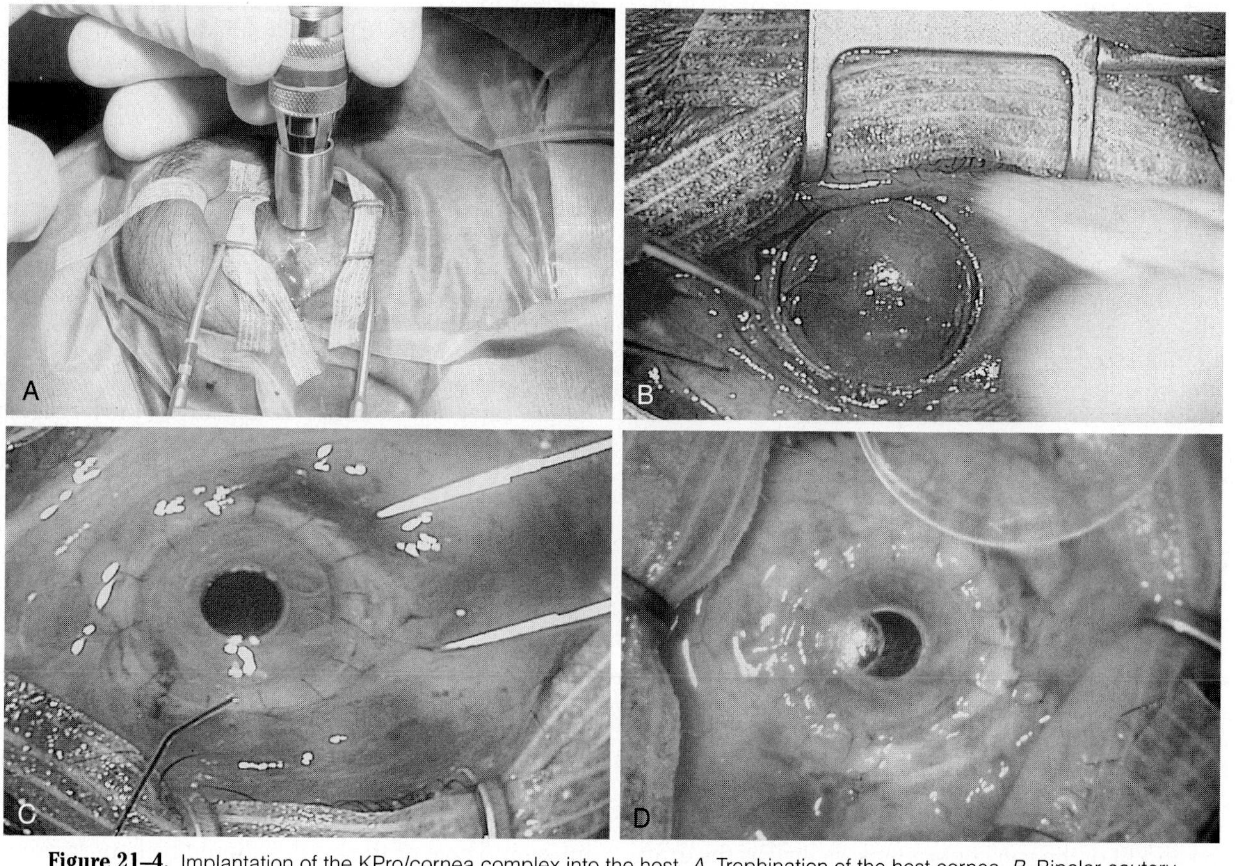

Figure 21–4. Implantation of the KPro/cornea complex into the host. *A.* Trephination of the host cornea. *B.* Bipolar cautery of wound prior to entry into the anterior chamber. *C.* Graft secured to host with 16, 10-0 nylon sutures; dexamethasone injection into the anterior chamber. *D.* Placement of soft contact lens.

It is now time to place the oversized corneal graft with its prosthesis into the patient's eye. There is no need to use viscoelastics. We recommend suturing the graft in the standard manner with sixteen 10-0 nylon interrupted sutures, burying the knots. The surgeon may now want to deepen the anterior chamber with balanced salt solution, followed by injection of 200–400 μg of dexamethasone into the anterior chamber (using a tuberculin syringe with a 30 gauge cannula). Finally, a soft contact lens is applied over the surface. A few drops of an antibiotic solution, e.g., polymyxin B/trimethoprim ophthalmic (Polytrim), are applied to the eye. A patch and a shield finalize the surgery.

Under some circumstances when prolonged postoperative soft contact wear is impractical, or when lid or blink functions are marginal, especially in a dry climate, a total conjunctival flap over the KPro is recommended.[8] This is performed at the time of the KPro implantation and a small central opening is added. The vascularized flap serves to protect the corneal tissue similar to a soft lens.

In more extreme situations of exposure, radical lateral and medial permanent tarsorrhaphies may have to be performed so that all ocular surface tissues will be covered by lids and only the plastic is exposed.

SEVERE GLAUCOMA

If the patient clearly has glaucoma that cannot be controlled, or is barely controlled medically, or present intraocular inflammation is expected to make the outflow problem worse, the addition of a glaucoma shunt is in order.[9] We suggest that an Ahmed valve shunt be implanted after the cornea is superficially trephined and vessels cauterized but before the eye is opened. The tube should be directed in such a way that it cannot end up centrally blocking the vision. If the shunt plate is placed above, 7-9 mm from the limbus, the incision into the eye should be made a millimeter outside the limbus, directed very tangentially towards 6 o'clock. Ideally, the tube should become lodged anteriorly close to the KPro back plate. If a vitrectomy is indicated, this should be done in a reasonably extensive way to avoid vitreous later moving forwards, blocking the tube. Tutoplast can be used to cover the tube and the conjunctiva is sutured back in the standard way.

POSTOPERATIVE CARE

The patient should be seen on the day following surgery. Inquiry should include pain, how much need for pain medication, if slept well, etc. Lids and lashes should be cleaned and mucus removed from the eye to improve visualization. Visual acuity and approximate intraocular pressure (finger palpation) should be recorded.

Slit lamp examination should be directed to the position and fit of the soft contact lens, as well as the graft sutures. Usually, in tight suturing, the graft periphery forms a circular groove where mucus tends to accumulate beneath the contact lens. This is harmless and this furrow gradually decreases during the period of healing.

Inflammatory reaction in the anterior chamber is important to grade. If outright fibrin is present, a sub-Tenon injection of steroids is recommended (40 mg. triamcinolone through the lower lid). Usually only cellular reaction is seen and the steroid injection can be postponed a few days. If inflammation is mild, only topical steroids (prenisolone acetate suspension 1% four times daily) are necessary.

The clarity of the vitreous usually determines the initial postoperative visual acuity. Past disease may have caused dense opacities, which can only partly be removed by open sky vitrectomy during the operation. If vitrectomy was needed even though the vitreous was relatively clear, the gel usually ends up somewhat broken-up and it may take a couple of weeks to become clear again.

The fundus should be inspected, if possible, with a 90 diopter or a 78 diopter lens, or by direct ophthalmoscopy. Usually the disc and macula have not been seen for a long time and the new view may reveal disappointing surprises. The details, especially the cup/disc ratio will need to be drawn or photographed.

MEDICATION

Our patients are usually given prescriptions for topical medications consisting of vancomycin (14 mg/ml), ofloxacin (Ocuflox 0.3% Allergan) and prednisolone acetate suspension 1%, all initially four times daily but tapered to twice daily over a month. This level of medication should then be continued *for life.* This point should be strongly stressed to the patient. Systemic antibiotics, e.g., cephalexin 500 mg twice daily for 7 to 10 days is recommended. If penicillin allergy exists, ciprofloxacin 500 mg twice daily may be substituted.

The inclusion of vancomycin deserves additional comment. Severe infection leading to endophthalmitis was, in the past, not uncommon after KPro in ocular cicatricial pemphigoid, Stevens-Johnson syndrome, atopy, and after severe chemical burns.[10] In our "graft failure category," which numerically is the largest and the category considered in this communication, we have not lost an eye to infection (we have had examples of seemingly sterile vitritis after which the original vision has eventually been restored—see below). After starting to include vancomycin in our routine prophylactic antibiotics regimen two and a half years ago, we have not had a single bacterial endophthalmitis, even in the high risk autoimmune and chemical burn groups. It, therefore, seems prudent to use vancomycin routinely in all cases, thus even in the low risk "graft failure group." Availability is a problem since vancomycin is not marketed as eye drops in the United States. It has to be specially made up in a hospital or compounding pharmacy. We prescribe four bottles of 5 ml each. Three of the bottles should be kept frozen until needed. The bottle in use should be kept in a refrigerator and should not be used for more than a two week total. The medication is expensive but it is reimbursable for patients who have insurance. Considering the potential importance of vancomycin, the cost seems a wise investment. Our patients are presently being monitored for emergence of vancomycin-resistant bacteria—none have been found yet.

If the intraocular pressure is elevated, standard glaucoma medication is added (see below).

The patient is advised to wear a metal shield during the night for protection during the first three months. Similarly, wearing glasses during the day should be encouraged.

With regard to scheduled return visits, it should be strongly emphasized to the patient how important compliance is in this respect. On an average we see the patient after one week, two weeks, one month, and then every 2 to 3 months—for life! Occurrence of complications may, of course, change this routine.

COMPLICATIONS

Loss of the Soft Contact Lens

Evaporation and irregular drying of the corneal tissue around our double-plated KPro can be disturbing problem. Dellen formation, epithelial defects, stromal thinning can occur with long-term undesirable consequences. However, a hydrophilic soft contact lens worn around-the-clock has been found to be highly protective.[11] The lens seems to diffuse the evaporative forces to allow better hydration and health of the underlying corneal tissue. Ideally, these patients should wear a lens for the rest of their lives, allowing for occasional replacements.

The corneal surface is initially quite flat postoperatively and a 16.0 mm diameter lens with a base curve of 9.8 mm is usually appropriate. However as the eye is healing and gradually assumes a more normal contour, a lens with a steeper base curve is often needed. We usually then switch to a lens with 7.0 mm base curve and 18.0 mm diameter. Also, by that time the corrective need of the eye has become more stable and a lens with the appropriate power can be chosen. If retained well, the lens can be allowed to stay in place for months without need for removal or cleaning. In a few instances, deposits accumulating on the surface necessitate lens change. More often inadvertent loss of the lens requires replacement, which adds to the overall cost.

Inflammation

This is often a serious issue in eyes that have undergone many surgical procedures. Patients with a history of substantial chronic inflammation have a worse prognosis after KPro implantation compared to those lacking such history. Particularly, autoimmune diseases such as ocular cicatricial pemphigoid, Stevens-Johnson syndrome, severe uveitis, graft-versus-host disease, advanced Sjögren's syndrome, etc., are prone to chronic low grade postoperative inflammation that can lead to the formation of a retroprosthesis membrane or an epiretinal membrane, as well as angle-closure glaucoma.

To a considerable degree such developments can be suppressed with corticosteroids. Drops of prednisolone acetate 1% 2 to 4 times daily are routine. In addition, sub-Tenon injections of 40 mg triamcinolone every 2 to 4 weeks for a total of 1 to 4 such injections have proven very helpful in cases at risk. Cases of graft failures in diseases that have not been particularly inflamed in the past, such as corneal edema following cataract extraction, rarely need sub-Tenon injections of steroids. Patients with herpes simplex infection in their history, or following bacterial or fungal infections, have a greater need for steroid treatment (plus long-term prophylaxis with systemic antivirals). Systemic medication with prednisone tablets have not been favored by us since high doses may be required, which could lead to problematic side effects.

Retroprosthesis Membrane

When thin, they can be opened with YAG laser.[12] Difficulty can arise if the membrane has been formed flush with the posterior surface of the stem, in which case laser opening can result in pock marking the plastic. If too much energy is used, the plastic can even crack. Therefore, it is recommended that the laser energy be kept lower than 2.0 mJ unless the membrane (or lens capsule) is located further posteriorly. A sub-Tenon injection of 40 mg triamcinolone is recommended afterwards. In the case of a membrane that has become very dense, and particularly if containing blood vessels, laser cannot be used. A bleeding into the vitreous can be highly troublesome and may take months to clear. In such a situation, a surgical membranectomy and vitrectomy can be performed by a retina specialist and with a three port entry and high infusion pressure to close the vessels.[13] Alternatively, the whole KPro procedure can be repeated and the membrane removed surgically open-sky.

Stromal Thinning or Melt Around the KPro

Tissue melt around the stem could happen with some frequency with earlier collar button designs and it posed a threat to the integrity of the eye.[6] Efforts to repair had usually no beneficial effect. With the present model (7.0 mm back plate with large holes) nutrition of the stroma from the aqueous seems improved and melt around the stem is now a rarity.

Another type of stromal change is the uniformed thinning without threatening leak around the stem. This seems to be an evaporative phenomenon. Again, large holes in the back plate facilitate fluid replacement from the aqueous and this complication is also now less common. In addition, permanent soft contact lens wear help protect the underlying tissue from this type of thinning. Should it still occur, the front plate ends up protruding from the tissue surface, which can be uncomfortable and potentially dangerous. This situation can be ameliorated by cutting a hole (4 or 5 mm) in the center of the soft lens and slide it over the front plate so that the lens comes to lodge *behind* the plate. This arrangement can be quite satisfactory and reduces the likelihood of lens loss.

Infectious Endophthalmitis

This is the ultimate disaster after KPro surgery. Vision can become permanently destroyed within 24 hours regardless of counter measures. Fortunately, such a calamity has not happened in any of our 79 cases of the "graft failure" group since 1990 (in contrast, devastating endophthalmitis happened not infrequently in the early cases of KPro in ocular cicatricial pemphigoid and Stevens Johnson syndrome).[10] As mentioned above, we recommend vancomycin and ofloxacin drops at least twice daily for life, also in the "graft failure" group under consideration here. Should a bacterial endophthalmitis still occur, the patient should be brought to diagnosis and treatment with the utmost speed. Aqueous tap for culture should be done promptly, followed by injection into the eye of 1.0 mg of vancomycin, 0.4 mg of amikacin, and 0.4 mg of dexamethasone. The patient should be hospitalized with intravenous and topical antibiotics.

Uveitis-Vitritis-Presumed Sterile

This is a disturbing phenomenon that can occur in this group of patients. It manifests itself as an explosive cloudiness of the vitreous with little redness of the eye and with negligible pain. For safety, we have, in all cases, treated them as suspected bacterial endophthalmitis as outlined above. The patients have been hospitalized for a few days on systemic antibiotics, followed later in the course by sub-Tenon steroid injections. No infection has been found. Invariably these cases have had a very benign course and they have all regained the vision that they had before the episode. Still, these mysterious bouts of inflammation, possibly on an immune basis, constitute a worrisome aspect of the present keratoprosthesis approach.

Glaucoma

Since the risk of severe infection—endophthalmitis—following KPro implantation has recently been brought under reasonable control, glaucoma remains the greatest problem. In the often severely diseased eyes that become candidates for a KPro, glaucoma is often preexisting. Postoperatively, especially in eyes with chronic inflammation, the intraocular pressure can over time become markedly aggravated, most likely due to a progressive angle-closure mechanism. It is, therefore, extremely important to monitor the intraocular pressure and any nerve damage postoperatively by whatever means are possible. Only finger palpation and, in some cases, a phosphene tonometer are available for pressure measurements and the possibilities for error are therefore considerable, especially if the lid skin is thickened by disease or surgery. The disc is not always clearly visible and visual field examinations can be hampered when the visual acuity is low. It is advisable to involve a glaucoma specialist in all KPro cases to share the responsibility.

The standard glaucoma drops can be expected to be effective in spite of the large plastic barrier to diffusion into the eye (for instance mydriactics affect the pupil with some time delay). Systemic carbonic anhydrase inhibitors have the expected effect but occasionally allergy to sulfa compounds restrict their use. Finally, a glaucoma valve shunt is not rarely required and the results are generally good (see above for implantation techniques).[9] Occasionally, shunt failure due to fibrosis formation around the plate occurs. In such cases, placing an additional tube between the shunt plate and nasal sinuses can bring down the pressure.[14]

CONCLUSION

For obvious reasons, the indication for a KPro must be balanced against the perceived prognosis of another standard keratoplasty in the particular clinical situation. If the latter procedure were uniformly successful, there would be no need for KPro with its still higher risks and greater demand on follow up and physician time. This is not so, but the statistical basis for decision-making is largely lacking. Outcomes of corneal regrafts are not well documented in the literature and they are certainly dependent on severity of the original corneal disease, on geographical area, health resources, etc. For instance, in one study from the U.S. on regrafts, mostly after corneal edema, three-quarters of the grafts remained clear after two years.[15] In another large study from India only 20% of regrafts for all causes survived five years.[16] An Israeli group of regrafts similarly showed a 20% survival after five years but repeat regrafts all succumbed within the same time period.[17]

Outcome after KPro is even less well documented. For the type of KPro discussed here, some trends are beginning to emerge. In a small cohort of 19 "graft failure" patients from the early part of the 1990's, 15 cases achieved a vision of 20/200 to 20/20 and the attrition was then followed. After five years, two-thirds of the patients had retained vision at that level.[6] The results are now better but long-term outcome analysis cannot yet be done.

If statistics come out in favor of KPro, why not choose this approach earlier and on a wider scale? After all, vision can become excellent through the water-clear plastic if the eye is otherwise normal. Astigmatism is not a problem. However, a KPro still carries a greater burden than standard keratoplasty. Successful outcome requires considerable patient compliance with medication (antibiotics, etc.), more frequent follow up and more demands on physician time. It should also be added that KPro involves techniques and danger signals that are different from those in standard corneal surgery and, coupled with the inevitably few initial cases, the learning curve for the surgeon tends to be slow. Both the fields of standard keratoplasty (aided by stem cell grafts, immunosup-

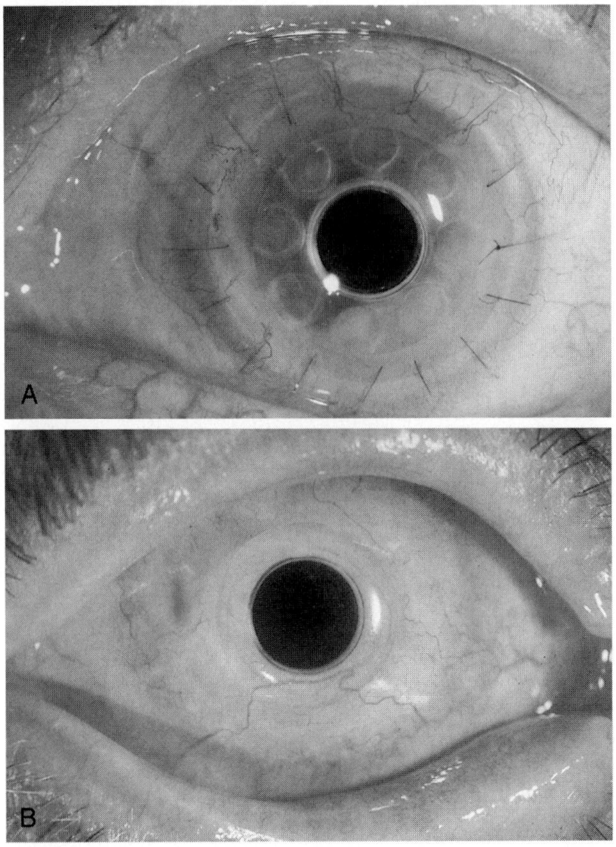

Figure 21–5. Examples of postoperative appearance in two patients. Vision is 20/25 in both instances.

pression etc.) and KPro are certainly bound to make further progress with time and the future balance between the two approaches is hard to predict. Vision in the opposite eye, age of the patient, other ocular problems, etc., must be factored in. It is reasonable to restrict KPro at present to cases where, in the surgeon's best judgement, further keratoplasty is unlikely to yield a clear graft for more than, say, a year. When successful, however, KPro can be exceedingly rewarding for the patient and the surgeon alike (Fig. 21–5).

REFERENCES

1. Mannis MJ, Dohlman CH: The artificial cornea: A brief history. *In* Mannis MD (ed). Corneal Transplantation. A history in profiles 1999;6:321.
2. Hicks C, Crawford G, Chirila T, et al.: Development and clinical assessment of an artificial cornea. Prog Retinal Eye Res 2000; 19:149–170.
3. Dohlman CH, Schneider HA, Doane MG: Prosthokeratoplasty. Am J Ophthalmol 1974;77:692.
4. Doane MG, Dohlman CH, Bearse G: Fabrication of keratoprosthesis. Cornea 1996;15:179–184.
5. Dohlman CH, Terada H: Keratoprosthesis in pemphigoid and Stevens-Johnson Syndrome. *In* Sullivan D (ed). Lacrimal Gland, Tear Film and Dry Eye Syndromes II. Basic Science and Clinical Relevance. Adv Exp Med Biol. New York: Plenum Publishing 1998; 438:1021–1025.
6. Yaghouti F, Nouri M, Al-Merjan J, et al.: Keratoprosthesis: Preoperative prognostic categories. Cornea 2001;20:19–23.
7. Crawford G: Personal communication, 2001.
8. Al-Merjan J, Sadeq N, Dohlman CH: Temporary tissue coverage in keratoprosthesis. Mid-East J Ophthalmol 2000;8:12.
9. Netland PA, Terada H, Dohlman CH: Glaucoma associated with keratoprosthesis. Ophthalmology 1998;105:751.
10. Nouri M, Terada H, Alfonso EC, et al.: Endophthalmitis after keratoprosthesis: Incidence, bacterial etiologies and risk factors. Arch Ophthalmol 2001;119:484–489.
11. Dohlman CH, Dudenhoefer EJ, Khan BF, Morneault S: Protection of the ocular surface after keratoprosthesis surgery: The role of soft contact lenses. CLAO 2002;28:72–74.
12. Bath PE, McCord RC, Cox KC: Nd:YAG laser discission of retroprosthetic membrane: a preliminary report. Cornea 1983;2:225.
13. Ray S, Khan BF, Dohlman CH, D'Amico DJ: Management of vitreoretinal complications in eyes with permanent keratoprosthesis. Arch Ophthalmol 2002;120:559.
14. Dohlman CH, Grosskreutz C, Dudenhoefer EJ, Rubin PAD: Can a glaucoma shunt be safely extended to the lacrimal sac or the ethmoid sinuses in keratoprosthesis patients? Preliminary findings. Dig J Ophthalmol 2001;7:3.
15. Patel NP, Kim T, Rapuano CJ, et al.: Indications for and outcomes of repeat penetrating keratoplasty. Ophthalmology 2000;107:719.
16. Dandona L, Naduvilath TJ, Janarthanan M, et al.: Survival analysis and visual outcome in a large series of corneal transplants in India. Br J Ophthalmol 1997;81:726.
17. Bersudsky V, Blum-Hareuveni T, Kehani U, Rumelt S: The profile of repeated corneal transplantation. Ophthalmology 2001; 108:461.

SECTION IV

George L. Spaeth, M.D.

Glaucoma

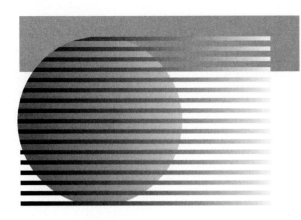

CHAPTER 22

Indications for Surgery

GEORGE L. SPAETH, M.D.

The chapter on glaucoma surgery is different from the other chapters in this text on ophthalmic surgery. It is different, because unlike cataract, melanoma, and retinal detachment (as examples), glaucoma is not a "thing." Glaucoma is not something tangible like the cornea. Thus, the very nature of glaucoma sets it apart from most other ophthalmic conditions. Additionally, the definition and the concepts regarding glaucoma have changed dramatically. In 50 years glaucoma has changed from being defined as "that situation in which the eyeball becomes hard with the consequences of that hardness," (paraphrase of Elliot) to "that condition in which the intraocular pressure is greater than 21 mm Hg," to "a characteristic optic neuropathy." Some authors now even speak of "pressure-independent glaucoma." Terminology and concepts, then, lack clarity, consistency, and consensus. The terminologies used in this chapter attempt to preserve as much as possible current usage and to eliminate ambiguities and frank contradictions (Table 22–1). For example, it seems unwise to define glaucoma as "a characteristic optic neuropathy" when a common condition presently called glaucoma has as its hallmarks pain and inflammation, and not optic neuropathy. Angle-closure glaucoma, neovascular glaucoma, and other conditions most clinicians would feel comfortable calling glaucoma do not fit into a conceptual framework in which the sole determining characteristic of "glaucoma" is the presence of an optic neuropathy.

FUNDAMENTAL PRINCIPLES OF GLAUCOMA SURGERY

The fundamental principles that apply to other surgical procedures also hold true for glaucoma. The success of the procedure is directly proportional to accuracy of preoperative diagnosis; appropriateness of the operative procedure; competence of care during the preoperative, operative, and postoperative periods; and ability of the surgeon to prevent, recognize, and correct, so far as possible, everything tending to divert the clinical course from the desired conclusion.

In at least one important aspect, however, surgery on the eye of the glaucomatous patient is different from most other types of surgery, even ophthalmic surgery. With most conditions the patient who needs surgery knows that there is an abnormality–something noticeably "wrong": a pain, a mass indicating the presence of a tumor, or poor sight. Such is not ordinarily the case with the glaucoma patient, especially in the early stages of the disease, when surgery offers the best chance of a successful result. The patient with unrecognized glaucoma is often asymptomatic. Even patients who have already been told they have glaucoma may feel completely normal. They usually believe that they "see just fine." Unlike most patients with a significant disease process, glaucoma patients often come to the doctor thinking that they are well, only to be told that they are sick.

TABLE 22–1. Terminology Related to Glaucoma

Glaucoma Suspect: A finding suggesting, but not proving, ocular tissue damage related at least in part to intraocular pressure
Pre-Glaucoma: A finding associated with the certainty that glaucoma will develop in the future
Glaucoma: Characteristic ocular tissue damage related at least in part to intraocular pressure
Risk Factors: Conditions increasing the risk of developing glaucoma
Narrow Anterior Chamber Angle: Angle configuration indicating an angle is capable of closure
Closed Anterior Chamber Angle: Presence of peripheral anterior synechiae extending anteriorly over part or all of the trabecular meshwork
Partial: Synechiae present in less than 360 degrees
Total: Synechiae present in 360 degrees

It is helpful if the surgeon can explain the findings that led to the diagnostic conclusion. Only after the surgeon has demonstrated charts documenting progressive loss of visual field, or has explained the nature and significance of a closed anterior chamber angle, can patients start to understand the need for treatment. Consider the dilemma facing patients who are told that the recommended surgery will probably make their vision worse and will not be curative, but will, at best, merely control the glaucoma. Under such circumstances the physician's and the patient's goals demand precise definition, full expression, and thorough discussion (Fig. 22–1).

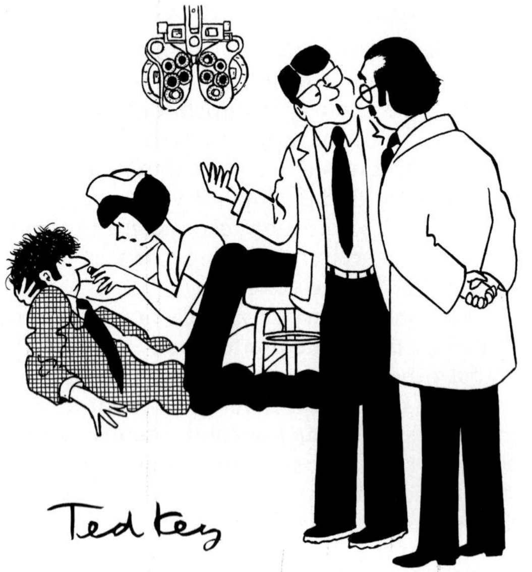

"HE THOUGHT HE JUST NEEDED NEW GLASSES, BUT WAS HE SURPRISED WHEN I TOLD HIM HE NEEDED SURGERY FOR GLAUCOMA!"

Figure 22–1. The perceptions and goals of the patient may differ from those of the physician. Communication between the two must be truthful, expressive, and sensitive.

Glaucoma patients must understand that they are already in trouble: the decision involves balancing *risk against risk and risk against benefit.* In patients with glaucoma, risk cannot be avoided. The possibility of short-term loss is usually balanced against long-term gain. The definitions of loss and gain are different for every patient. The decisions as to whether, when, and how to treat must be made only after the different factors that characterize the totality of the event have been scientifically and compassionately considered. Such consideration demands an understanding of the nature of the patient, the character of that patient's disease, and the unique interaction of these two factors over a period of time. This becomes increasingly difficult in a DRG (diagnosis-related group) society, in which patients can easily become code numbers. It also requires the ability to communicate disturbing information in such a way that patients are reassured rather than frightened. Most patients are afraid of the unknown; once they know that their doctor understands what is wrong and will guide them through the hazardous waters of illness with skill and consistency, their anxiety usually disappears. The tone in which words are said is probably more important than the specific meanings of the words themselves.

MEDICAL VERSUS SURGICAL CARE

There are many types of glaucoma; it would be surprising if the same therapeutic principles could be applied to all. Even when considering the same type of glaucoma, there is still controversy regarding the best mode of treatment. This is partially due to incomplete knowledge about the natural history of glaucoma. The variance in the degree of competence that different physicians have in using medical and surgical modes of therapy is another factor; some are better with drugs and others, with surgery. Still other considerations are the philosophical approaches of both the ophthalmologist and the patient; some have a medical bent and others, a surgical.

In a few types of glaucoma, surgery is the treatment of choice (Table 22–2). Congenital glaucoma, acute primary angle-closure glaucoma, and progressive primary open-angle glaucoma are examples, and surgery should not be considered a "last resort" in these conditions. On the other hand, there are entities, such as neovascular glaucoma, in which the results of surgery are generally so poor that medical therapy is clearly preferable where feasible (Table 22–2; see also Tables 22–11 and 22–13).

GOALS OF SURGERY IN GLAUCOMA

The primary goal of glaucoma surgery is to preserve or enhance the health of the patient. The ways to achieve preservation or enhancement of the patient's health are the preservation or enhancement of vision and relief of pain, when present. The method of accomplishing these more immediate goals is lowering the intraocular pressure (IOP). Pain and disability in glaucoma are

TABLE 22-2. Advisability of Surgical Treatment in Selected Types of Glaucoma

Condition	Usual Procedure of Choice	Alternative Procedure
Surgery Almost Always Required		
Congenital glaucoma	Goniotomy	Trabeculotomy
Phakolytic glaucoma	Cataract extraction	
Acute primary angle-closure glaucoma	Peripheral iridectomy*	Guarded filtration procedure with tightly sutured scleral flap
Pupillary block glaucomas	Peripheral iridectomy*	Synechialysis
Fellow eye of patient with primary angle-closure glaucoma	Peripheral iridectomy*	
Progressive primary open-angle glaucoma	Guarded filtration procedure or laser trabeculoplasty	Laser trabeculoplasty or standard filtering procedure
Glaucoma with 8-ball hemorrhage	Removal of clot	
Glaucoma with intraocular tumor	Enucleation	Irradiation
Failed filtration surgery	Filtering procedure with 5-fluorouracil Molteno implant	Nd:YAG cyclophotocoagulation
Surgery Often Required		
Asymptomatic narrow anterior chamber angle	Peripheral iridectomy*	
Primary open-angle glaucoma (and its variants: pigmentary glaucoma, glaucoma with exfoliation syndrome, etc.)	Laser trabeculoplasty or guarded filtration procedure†	Standard filtering procedure, or trabeculotomy
Chronic primary angle-closure glaucoma	Guarded filtration procedure with tightly sutured scleral flap	Peripheral iridectomy* or synechialysis (chamber deepening)
Glaucoma owing to posterior	Vitrectomy	Transpupillary rupture of vitreous or lens misdirection of aqueous humor extraction with vitrectomy
Secondary angle-closure glaucoma	Iridectomy*	Cyclodialysis
Noninflammatory secondary angle-closure glaucomas (Chandler's syndrome, etc.)	Guarded filtration procedure	Cyclodialysis
Inflammatory secondary angle-closure glaucomas	Molteno implant	Nd:YAG cyclophotocoagulation
Developmental glaucomas other than congenital	Guarded filtration procedure	Standard filtering procedures
Glaucomatocyclitic crisis	Guarded filtration procedure	Standard filtering procedures
Glaucoma in aphakic patients	Guarded filtration procedure or Nd:YAG cyclophotocoagulation	Molteno implant or cyclocryotherapy
Angle-cleavage glaucoma in quiet eye	Guarded filtration procedure	Standard filtering procedures
Glaucoma with traumatic hyphema	Drainage of blood	Drainage with guarded filtration procedure
Surgery Usually to Be Avoided But Not Contraindicated		
Aniridia	Guarded filtration procedure	Goniotomy
Uveitic glaucomas	Trabeculotomy	Guarded filtration procedure
Neovascular glaucoma	Molteno implant or Nd:YAG cyclophotocoagulation	Peripheral iridectomy with thermal sclerostomy or guarded filtration procedure or cyclocryotherapy
Glaucoma with Sturge-Weber syndrome	Anterior trabeculectomy	Goniotomy in infants
Glaucoma secondary to scleritis or episcleritis	None good	Filtering procedure or Nd:YAG
Ocular hypertension	Guarded filtration procedure	
Surgery Rarely Advisable		
Nonophthalmos	None good: occasionally laser iridotomy or retrobulbar chlorpromazine	Nd:YAG cyclophotocoagulation or cyclocryotherapy
Blind painful eye	Retrobulbar alcohol or enucleation	Evisceration

*Laser iridotomy is usually preferred over surgical iridectomy. (See Figure 22-37.)
†Laser trabeculoplasty is the procedure of choice for some cases of primary open-angle glaucoma.

not, however, due solely to elevated intraocular pressure or optic nerve damage. Therefore, lowering the IOP is not always an appropriate way to achieve the goals of treatment.

An overarching goal must be to avoid making the patient worse. Lowering IOP excessively, and thereby causing disability due to pain, photophobia, or double vision is not in the patient's best interest. Improving the patient's function is the goal, and this is not achieved by procedures that result in an eye that sees less well than preoperatively or is more uncomfortable.

There are two major ways to preserve or restore the visual ability of the patient with glaucoma: (1) *lowering intraocular pressure* and (2) *preventing a sudden rise in intraocular pressure.* The first method is usually achieved by correcting or circumventing blocked outflow of aqueous humor from the eye. Such blockage is the usual cause for elevated intraocular pressure, regardless of the type of glaucoma. The second technique usually involves restoration of the eye to a more normal anatomical state; the effect of peripheral iridectomy on the patient with narrow anterior chamber angles is an example.

A third goal in occasional patients is the relief of pain. Comfort usually follows restoration of pressure to a satisfactory level although glaucomatous eyes that are painful are not always painful as a result of elevated IOP. In occasional cases in which the visual ability of the eye is so poor that it is no longer of benefit to the patient, the surgeon may choose to perform surgery solely to relieve discomfort. Because every glaucoma procedure that requires penetrating surgery has been associated with sympathetic ophthalmia, the usual treatment for such painful blind eyes is enucleation or evisceration (Table 22–3). In some cases a retrobulbar injection of alcohol or chlorpromazine (25 mg) may be adequate. Though cyclodestructive procedures have been recommended and are still used for pain relief, they are rarely appropriate for this purpose.

The fourth goal of the surgeon is to avoid or correct complications. For example, the surgeon may want to perform surgery so that a high cystic bleb will be avoided, or to remedy an eye in which a complication is already present, such as a ruptured bleb.

It is essential that the surgeon realize that there is usually a series of goals to be accomplished in performing surgery. Furthermore, these goals are often quite independent of one another, and in some circumstances surgical decisions are complicated by the fact that the goals are mutually exclusive. For example, the surgeon may set as the primary goal marked lowering of the IOL. But to accomplish this it will be necessary to develop a large fistula, which will lead to the development of a large cystic bleb. Thus, a secondary goal may be to avoid creating a cystic bleb because the patient has another condition that would make such a bleb undesirable, such as a severe chronic blepharitis or the need to wear a contact lens.

In considering every case the surgeon must assess the risks and benefits, define all goals, and decide their priority (Table 22–4). *The surgeon must also be sure that the objectives of treatment and those of the patient coincide* (Fig. 22–1).

TABLE 22–3. Glaucoma Procedures Known to Have Sympathetic Ophthalmia as a Complication

Iridencleisis
Iridectomy
Trephination
Sclerectomy
Thermal sclerostomy
Guarded filtration procedure
Cyclodialysis
Cyclodiathermy

TABLE 22–4. Goals in Glaucoma Surgery

Primary Goal (Improve Quality of Life)
1. Preserve or restore visual ability
a. Maintain health of the optic nerve
b. Avoid or correct other ocular abnormality
Secondary Goal
2. Lower intraocular pressure
a. Lower mean intraocular pressure*
b. Eliminate intraocular pressure spikes
3. Correct abnormal structure†
a. Narrow or closed anterior chamber angle
4. Relieve pain
5. Avoid or correct complications, such as:
a. Flat anterior chamber
b. Hypotony
c. Bleeding
d. Failure to filter
e. Malignant glaucoma
f. Cataract
g. Cystic bleb

*The amount of intraocular pressure-lowering will vary from patient to patient.
†Other abnormal structures that need correction are pupillary block, dislocated lens, hypermature cataract, etc.

SURGICAL ANATOMY

Accurate understanding of the anatomy of the limbal area is essential for the performance of correct glaucoma surgery. Important anatomical features are shown in Figures 22–2 and 22–3.[1–5]

An important landmark in glaucoma surgery is the corneoscleral sulcus. This groove results from the difference between the radius of curvature of the scleral shell and that of the cornea. Where these two curves meet a pronounced groove, the corneoscleral sulcus, is formed. Because of the overlying conjunctiva this groove may not always be readily apparent until the conjunctiva has been reflected. The corneoscleral sulcus is of importance for two reasons: First, the conjunctiva usually terminates just anterior to this position; hence a limbus-based conjunctival flap cannot usually be dissected anterior to this

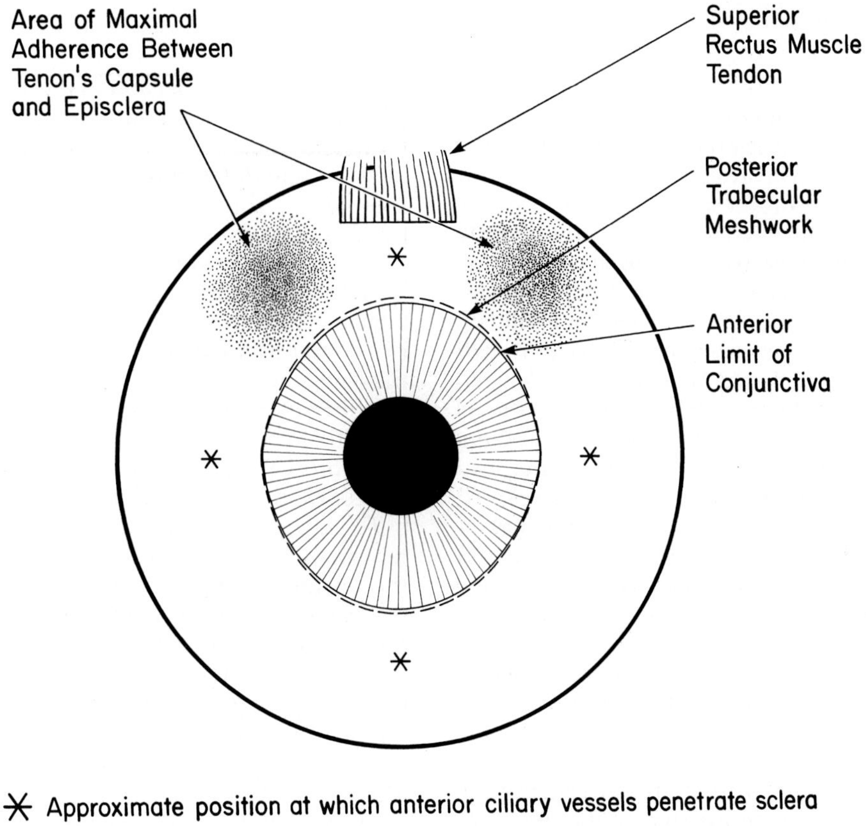

✳ Approximate position at which anterior ciliary vessels penetrate sclera

Figure 22–2. Surgeon's view of the eye, showing points of major anatomical importance (see also Figs. 22-3 and 22-4).

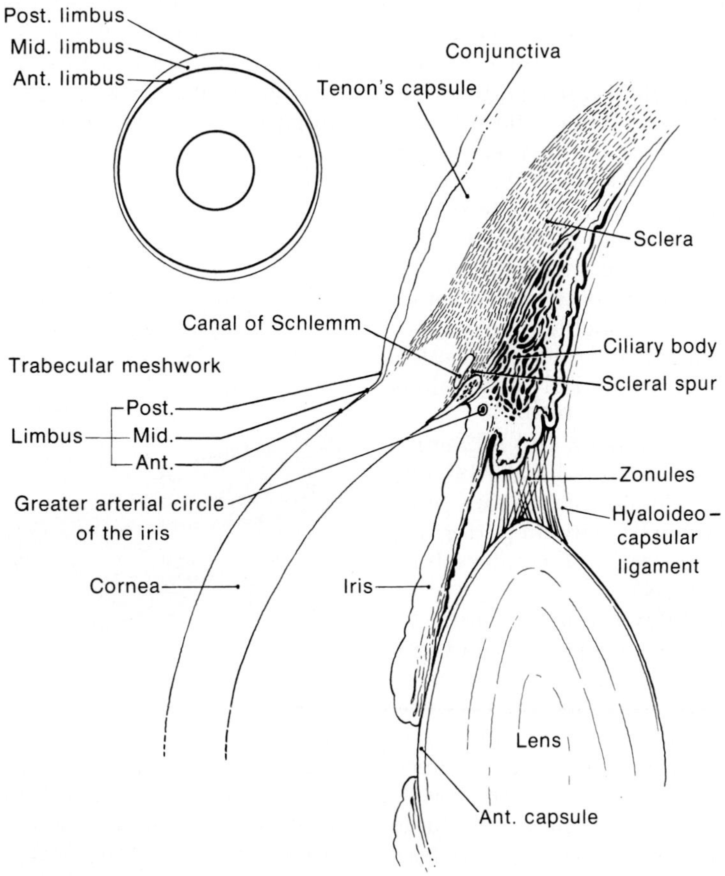

Figure 22–3. Anatomy of anterior segment of the eye. Note limbal relationships.

point. Second, in most emmetropic eyes the corneoscleral sulcus usually lies anterior to the iris root; consequently a perpendicular incision made just posterior to the corneoscleral sulcus will ordinarily enter the anterior chamber. This is an important consideration, because most glaucoma procedures require an incision into the anterior chamber. If the incision does not enter the anterior chamber but is mistakenly made into the posterior chamber or over the ciliary body, the operation will fail.

The positions of the iris insertion and the scleral spur in relation to the corneoscleral sulcus vary from eye to eye. They tend to be more anteriorly placed in patients with hyperopia and primary angle-closure glaucoma, especially when peripheral anterior synechiae are present. In contrast, they are usually more posteriorly placed in patients with myopia and those with congenital glaucoma. The relationship between internal landmarks and the surgical limbus is even more variable, because the conjunctiva may terminate posterior to, at, or anterior to the corneoscleral sulcus.

Because external and internal landmarks do not correspond exactly, the surgeon should consciously inspect the eye before making an incision; it is thus possible to determine where and how to make the incision, being sure to enter the anterior chamber. Usually the position of the iris root can be ascertained by simple inspection. Some surgeons recommend transillumination to help establish the location of the most peripheral portion of the angle recess. This technique works beautifully, but it is seldom necessary.

The position of the posterior trabecular meshwork and the point of adherence of the iris to the inner surface of the globe are two important considerations. Accurate determination of these landmarks may require gonioscopy before surgery. During the operation it may be necessary to repeat the gonioscopy if the surgeon needs to determine the exact position of the trabecular area, as is the case in goniotomy and trabeculotomy.

If the surgeon wants to avoid the trabecular area entirely, as may be the preferred approach in performing an iridectomy, then he or she must either make a perpendicular incision anterior to the corneoscleral sulcus or shelve the incision markedly anteriorly, as would be done in using a keratome.

The posterior trabecular meshwork and Schlemm's canal are, of course, anterior to the point at which the ciliary body adheres to the scleral spur. It is thus possible to excise trabecular meshwork without performing a cyclodialysis (without separating the ciliary body from the scleral spur) (Fig. 22–4).

Figure 22–2 shows the difference in curvature between the line along which the conjunctiva blends into the anterior cornea, and that of the posterior trabecular meshwork. Because the latter has a steeper curve than the former, the area separating these two differs, depending on what point on the globe is being examined. For example, at the 12 o'clock position on the limbus the conjunctival termination is usually around 2 mm anterior to the posterior trabecular meshwork. In contrast, at the 3 o'clock and 9 o'clock positions it is less than 1 mm anterior to the posterior trabecular meshwork. Therefore, it is difficult at the 3 o'clock and 9 o'clock positions to make an incision that is posterior to the surgical limbus and that the surgeon knows will enter the anterior chamber. It is even harder to be sure that such an incision will enter anterior to the posterior trabecular meshwork. The more eccentrically and the more perpendicularly the surgeon places the incision, the more likely that ciliary body will be found at its base.

Figure 22–4 shows the usual anterior termination of Tenon's capsule and episclera. This is ordinarily posterior to the point at which the conjunctiva inserts into the cornea. Consequently, by continuing the dissection of a limbus-based flap anteriorly, a flap can be developed that consists only of conjunctiva.

Tenons capsule is most adherent to the episclera at the 10:30 and 1:30 positions on the globe.

The surgeon should be aware of the position of the termination of Descemet's membrane, the anterior and the posterior trabecular meshwork, the iris root, and the major arterial iris circle; the point of penetration of the anterior ciliary vessels in relation to both the limbus (Fig. 22–2) and the four rectus muscles (Fig. 22–4); and the point at which the ciliary body is adherent to the scleral spur (Fig. 22–2). It is important to recall that the anterior uvea is normally adherent to the overlying sclera only at the point at which the scleral spur and the ciliary body come into contact. Elsewhere there is no adherence between these tissues. The implications of this are important. For example, it is possible to excise posterior trabecular meshwork without unroofing the ciliary body. Furthermore, to perform a cyclodialysis one need make the incision only a very short distance posterior to the position of the scleral spur.

It is helpful to recall that the transition from the opaque white of the sclera to the clear gray of the

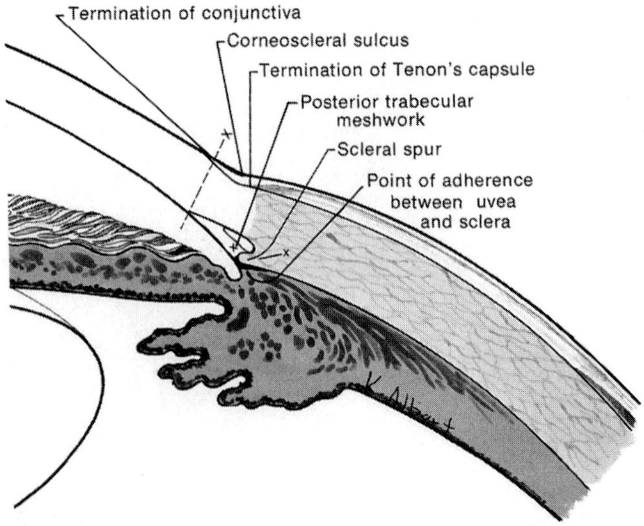

Figure 22–4. Schematic cross section of limbal area at 12 o'clock position on the globe. The corneoscleral groove (sulcus), a landmark of paramount importance, is located posterior to the termination of conjunctiva and just anterior to the termination of Tenon's capsule. A perpendicular incision (dashed line) at the corneoscleral sulcus should usually enter the anterior chamber just anterior to Schlemm's canal. Normally the uvea is adherent to the anterior uvea in only one area, a narrow ring just at the scleral spur. See also Figure 22-3.

TABLE 22–5. Factors That Influence Development of Glaucomatous Nerve Damage

I. Structural (ability of optic nerve to resist pressure damage)
  A. Heredity
  B. Race
  C. Myopia
  D. Preexisting damage to optic nerve (glaucomatous or other)
  E. Increasing age?
II. Acquired
  A. Direct effect of elevated intraocular pressure on neuron or supporting tissues
  B. Local factors
    1. Elevated episcleral venous pressure
    2. Vascular insufficiency or anomaly
    3. Vasospasm
  C. Systemic factors
    1. Cardiovascular
      a. Anemia
      b. Other factors that cause diminished oxygen-carrying capacity of blood
      c. Hypotension
      d. Low cardiac output
      e. Sedentary life-style
      f. Hematologic disorders associated with hyperviscosity
      g. Elevated episcleral venous pressure
      h. Vascular anomalies
    2. Metabolic
      a. Obesity
      b. Diabetes mellitus
      c. Vitamin deficiency
      d. Other
III. Behavioral
  A. Ability to manage one's life
  B. Ability to act in one's own best interest
  C. Accessibility to care
IV. Time*

*The duration of action and the degree of abnormality of the risk factor are of major importance. Thus a mild elevation of intraocular pressure acting for many years, or a severe elevation of intraocular pressure acting only for a few months, will both cause damage.

cornea occurs more anteriorly (that is, closer to the corneoscleral sulcus) in both the most superficial and the deepest layers of the globe. Thus the relation of Schlemm's canal and the posterior trabecular meshwork to the transition between the opaque sclera and the clear cornea will vary, depending on the depth of the scleral flap. On the surface a line dropped perpendicularly from the area of the transition will usually pass anterior to Schlemm's canal. Approximately half the way through the sclera a similar line would catch the posterior edge of Schlemm's canal (Fig. 22–4).

Incisions need to be made differently, depending on the surgeon's intent and the position of the incision on the globe. For example, let us consider the incisions at 12 o'clock. A perpendicular incision for a peripheral iridectomy should be placed at or anterior to the termination of the conjunctiva. A shelved keratome incision for iridectomy should be started 1 mm posterior to the corneoscleral sulcus. The incision for a guarded filtration procedure cannot be correctly placed unless the conjunctiva is dissected to its anterior-most position on the globe. After having made a half-thickness scleral flap, the surgeon is most likely to find Schlemm's canal immediately anterior to the point of transition from the white sclera to the clear cornea. For the ciliary body to be frozen by performing cyclocryotherapy, the tip should be placed about 2 mm posterior to the corneoscleral sulcus.

The surgeon should be familiar with the anatomical relationship between conjunctiva, Tenon's capsule, and episclera. These are discussed in detail in the subsections dealing with the development of conjunctival flaps (p. 214-216).

Pathogenesis of Optic Nerve Damage in Glaucoma

Intraocular pressure higher than the eye can tolerate is the most important of the many factors that contribute to the development of optic nerve damage in patients with glaucoma (Table 22–5).[6–10] The validity of this concept has been the cornerstone on which the entire management plan of glaucoma patients has been built during the past hundred years. The existence of other factors that contribute to optic nerve damage and the marked individual variability of response to intraocular pressure must not obscure this fundamental concept, which still is the basis of treatment for glaucoma today (Figs. 22–5 and 22–6).[10–35]

If intraocular pressure higher than the eye can tolerate is the primary factor responsible for glaucomatous dam-

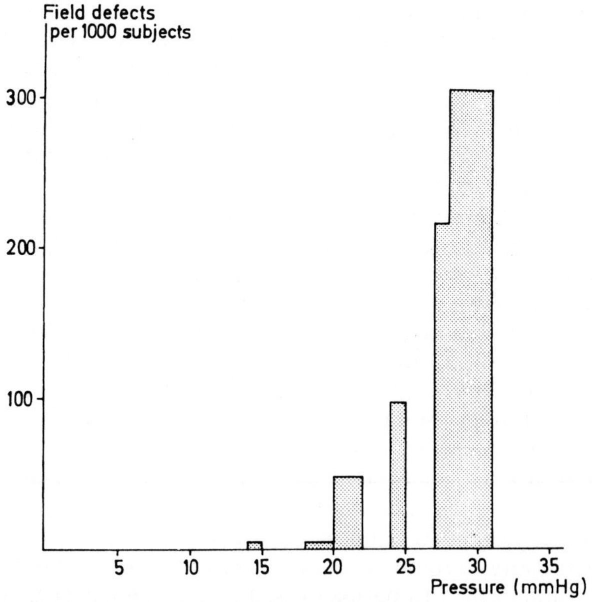

Figure 22–5. Frequency of glaucomatous optic nerve damage as manifested as a field defect in relation to intraocular pressure. There is a marked increase with rising pressure. (From Graham P: Epidemiology of chronic glaucoma. In Heilmann K, Richardson KT (eds.), Glaucoma: Conceptions of a Disease. Stuttgart: Thieme; 1978.)

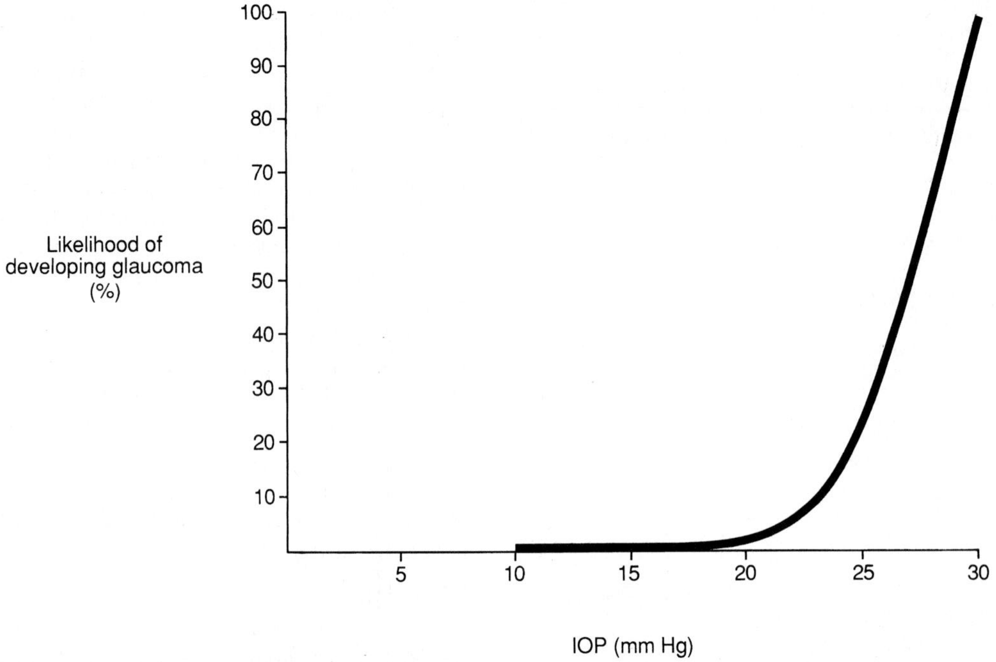

Figure 22–6. Hypothetical curve indicating relationship between intraocular pressure (IOP) and the likelihood of development of glaucomatous nerve damage. The exact position of the curve of the abscissa is not certain; it should perhaps be displaced to the right or to the left. However, it is certain that the likelihood of developing glaucomatous damage increases greatly with increasing intraocular pressure, probably in a logarithmic manner. This particular hypothetical curve suggests that optic nerve damage can be anticipated in about 50% of all people with intraocular pressure persistently above 27 mm Hg and in almost all people in whom intraocular pressure remains above 30 mm Hg.

age, then it would seem possible to study populations statistically, determine what is "normal intraocular pressure," and set a figure above which patients would develop damage. This concept has for many years been assumed to be valid. However, it is not.[6,10,35,36] Populations can be studied and *average* intraocular pressure determined (Fig. 22–7). Indeed this has been done, and average intraocular pressure found to be about 15 to 16 mm Hg, showing a slight rise with increasing age, especially in women. The standard deviation is about 3 mm Hg, suggesting that 95% of the population would be expected to have intraocular pressures ranging between 10 and 21 mm Hg. Thus, statistically speaking, people with intraocular pressure above 21 mm Hg would be expected to be sufficiently different from normal that they are abnormal. In fact, they are abnormal in the sense of not being average, but they are not necessarily abnormal in the sense of being diseased.

Careful examination of the curve of intraocular pressures shows a preponderance of people with elevated intraocular pressures. That is, the normal curve is skewed to the right (Fig. 22–7). What is relatively new information is the knowledge that has come from long-term studies that established that only a relatively small proportion of people with so-called elevated intraocular pressure, that is, intraocular pressure above 21 mm Hg, actually develop glaucomatous damage.[3,6,34,36–39] Although the precise figure is still unknown, it appears that only about 5% to 10% of those with intraocular pressures above 21 mm Hg will in fact ever develop "glaucoma," that is, glaucomatous damage to the optic nerve.[40] In the first place, most people with intraocular pressures above 21 mm Hg have intraocular pressures that range between 21 and 24 mm Hg. Thus they are within three standard deviations of normal; it is not surprising that many such people would not have deterioration of the optic nerve. But even those with intraocular pressures above 24 mm Hg will not always develop damage. However, these patients are at much greater risk, and the higher their intraocular pressures, the more likely they are to develop glaucomatous nerve damage. Clearly, factors other than intraocular pressure determine who will develop glaucomatous disease. *Within the range of 10 to 40 mm Hg, the level of intraocular pressure per se cannot be used as a meusure of presence or absence of disease.*

It appears that 27–30 mm Hg is a watershed range, most people with intraocular pressure consistently above 30 mm Hg can be expected eventually to develop glaucomatous nerve damage unless intraocular pressure is effectively lowered.[40] Saying this, however, is not the same as saying that all patients with intraocular pressure above 27 mm Hg or 30 mm Hg should be treated or that those with intraocular pressure below this range should not be treated. The decision whether or not to treat must be based an many factors other than IOP (these factors are discussed later in this chapter).

An additional and vitally important piece of information that must be considered in the pathogenesis of optic nerve damage in glaucoma is the frequency with which individuals with "low" intraocular pressures develop damage. Although the existence of "low-tension glaucoma" has been known for more than

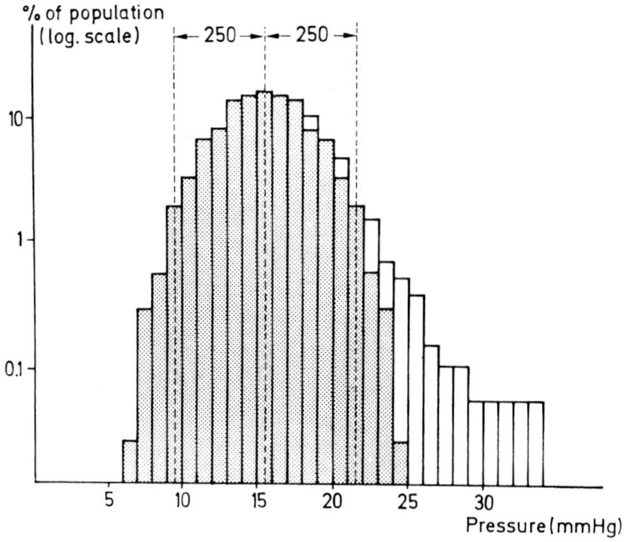

Figure 22–7. Distribution of intraocular pressures in population aged 40 to 75 years living in Ferndale, Wales, showing an excess of high intraocular pressures. A standard distribution is shown in the shaded bars. (From Graham P: Epidemiology of chronic glaucoma. In Heilmann K, Richardson KT (eds.), Glaucoma: Conceptions of a Disease. Stuttgart: Thieme; 1978.)

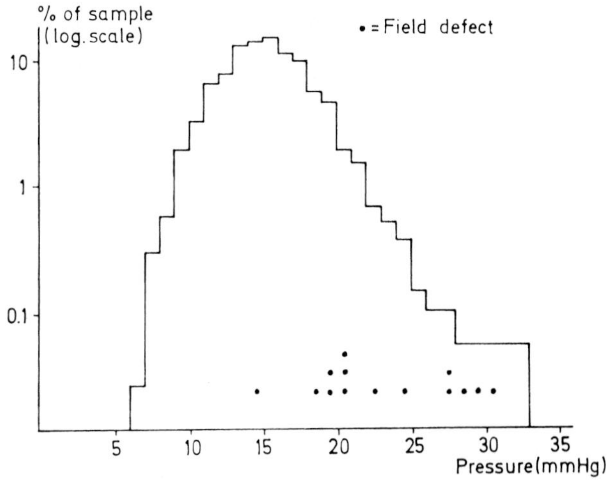

Figure 22–8. Newly discovered field defects in relation to intraocular pressure in the Ferndale (Wales) population (data of Graham and Hollows). Of the 14 patients with glaucomatous nerve damage, 7 had intraocular pressure below 22 mm Hg. (From Graham P: Epidemiology of chronic glaucoma. In Heilmann K, Richardson KT (eds.), Glaucoma: Conceptions of a Disease. Stuttgart: Thieme; 1978.)

a hundred years, it has generally been considered to be rare. This assumption is wrong.[6,10,35] If an intraocular pressure two standard deviations above the mean is taken as the dividing line between "normal" and "elevated" intraocular pressures—specifically 21 mm Hg—then one third of patients with glaucomatous nerve damage will fall in the group who have "normal" intraocular pressures (Fig. 22–8).[6] Obviously, a "normal" intraocular pressure does *not* guarantee safety from glaucoma.

In summary, then, when we recall that less than 10% of people with intraocular pressures above 21 mm Hg develop glaucomatous damage and that about one third of all people who actually have glaucomatous damage have intraocular pressures below 21 mm Hg, we see that arbitrary levels of intraocular pressure cannot be taken as adequate definitions of the presence or absence of glaucoma.

Other factors that may adversely affect the optic nerve include those listed in Table 22–5.

A schema of the pathogenesis of nerve damage in glaucoma is shown in Figure 22–9. There is evidence such that factors as glutamate may play a role in the damage to the ganglion cell. However, the therapeutic applications of this possibility are not yet available. Neuroprotective agents hold promise, but none has yet been shown to be beneficial.

Can it be said that progressive, glaucomatous-appearing damage to the optic nerve proves that IOP is too high, and that adequate lowering of the pressure would cause the progressive damage to cease? This question still cannot be answered. However, with important qualifications the answer that best serves patients is yes. That is, we should probably assume that *if the intraocular pressure is adequately lowered, glaucomatous damage will no longer occur.* Several caveats must be added to this statement (Table 22–6). First, there will be instances in which the neurons have been so badly damaged by the glaucomatous process that even if intraocular pressure is lowered to a point that would previously have allowed preservation of the health of the neurons, such mortally damaged neurons will continue to deteriorate. Furthermore, patients with glaucoma may have other causes for optic nerve damage, such as a chiasmal tumor or a meningioma pressing on the optic nerve. It is thus vitally important for the physician to be reasonably certain that causes other than intraocular pressure are not responsible for progressive nerve damage that mimics glaucoma. Third, neurons die simply because they get "old." This "preprogrammed" cell death may result in the death of around 5000 cells per year. Thus, in the healthy optic nerve such a loss of cells will not have any visual effect. However, in a person who has already lost a major portion of the optic nerve, the death of some 5000 neurons each year can result in a disturbing visual deterioration. Finally, and this is the concern that must be considered in every patient, the cause for the optic nerve deterioration is an intraocular pressure that is too high for that particular patient.

ANESTHESIA

The overwhelming majority of glaucoma procedures are best performed under local or topical anesthesia with an anesthesiologist in attendance. The reasons for this preference are listed in Table 22–7. In most cases sedation should be minimal or mild. The patient who understands what is to be done and has confidence in the surgeon may not need *any* systemic sedation. Especially in the elderly, who constitute a large percentage

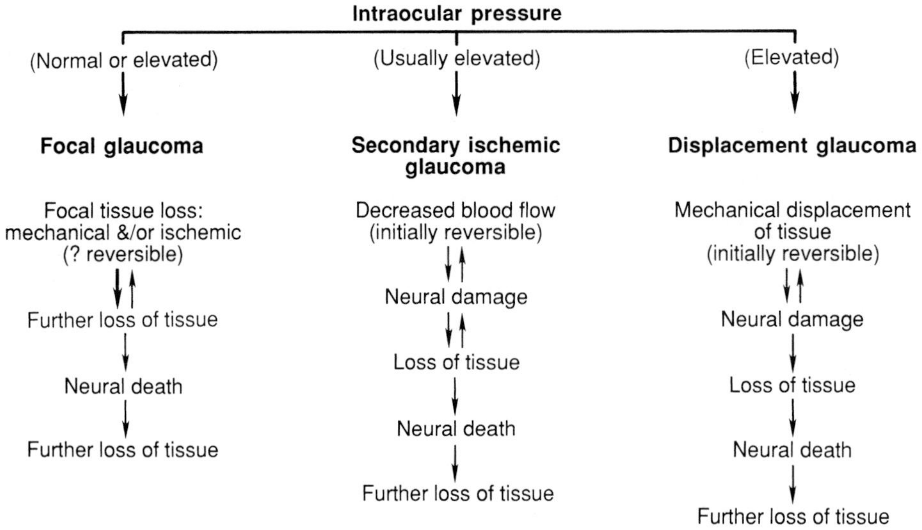

Figure 22–9. Simplified schema of the pathogenesis of optic nerve damage in glaucoma, stressing the roles of mechanical distortion of the optic nerve (displacement glaucoma) and ischemia, both caused by increased intraocular pressure.

TABLE 22–6. Causes for Progressive Optic Nerve Damage in the Patient Thought to Have Glaucoma

1. So much distortion of the optic nerve structure and so much damage to the optic neurons that the neurons are "mortally wounded"
2. A condition other than glaucoma
3. Intraocular pressure higher than the affected eye can tolerate

TABLE 22–7. Preferred Anesthesia for Glaucoma Procedures

Local

Rapid mobilization
- Allows hyphema to settle inferiorly
- More rapid recuperation of patient

Less traumatic to patient
Permits use of oral osmotic agents preoperatively
Assures minimal chance of hypotensive or hypertensive episode
Minimizes untoward reactions to anesthetic agents
Eliminates need to catheterize patient when mannitol is used
Facilitates postoperative evaluation
Less expensive than general anesthesia
Less time-consuming than general anesthesia
Fewer personnel required than with general anesthesia
Facilitates discharge on same day as surgery

Topical

Eliminates need for retrobulbar block
Eliminates possibility of retrobulbar hemorrhage
Allows maintenance of small pupil
Same advantages as for local anesthesia

General

Eliminates need for retrobulbar block
Assures most complete comfort of patient
Assures most complete and long-lasting patient cooperation
Assures most complete elimination of "positive-pressure eye"
Is usually required for infants and children, or retarded, senile, or psychotic patients

of patients who require glaucoma surgery, it is advisable to keep sedation as light as possible. Clearly the patient should not be overly anxious, apprehensive, or uncomfortable. Diazepam in small doses (4–6 mg) administered intravenously immediately before the onset of surgery provides sedation that can be accurately controlled and is usually well tolerated. In cases in which analgesia is also required, a narcotic agent may need to be added.

A retrobulbar injection is definitely not required in all cases. Under certain circumstances it is preferable to avoid this potentially complicating procedure and perform surgery using topical anesthesia alone (Tables 22–7 and 22–8). Proparacaine, 0.5%, is a suitable agent. How it is used depends on the depth of anesthesia required. For procedures such as suture removal, two or three drops are adequate. For more penetrating anesthesia the drops should be instilled every 30 to 60 seconds for 5 to 10 minutes. Ten drops over ten minutes will make procedures such as trabeculoplasty or surgical iridectomy comfortable. Tetracaine and other agents may be used, but they are likely to cause desquamation of the epithelium.

There are circumstances in which general anesthesia is preferred (Tables 22–7 and 22–8). For example, a retrobulbar block is inadvisable when repairing a wound dehiscence or when spread of infection may be a concern.

In all cases in which general anesthesia is not used, akinesia of the facial nerve is useful. A modified O'Brien block is most suitable, and should provide total paralysis of the facial muscles on the side requiring surgery.

TABLE 22–8. Preferred Anesthesia

Procedure	Method
Laser iridotomy	Few drops
Laser iridoplasty	Multiple drops
Laser trabeculoplasty	Multiple or few drops
Laser cyclophotocoagulation	Retrobulbar bupivacaine
Laser suture lysis	Multiple drops
Paracentesis	Multiple drops
Sub-Tenon's 5-fluorouracil	Multiple drops
Needling bleb	Multiple drops
Bleb blood injection	Multiple drops
Anterior chamber reformations	Multiple drops
Surgical bleb revision	Facial and retrobulbar mepivacaine with light sedation
Guarded filtration procedure; Trabeculotomy; Goniotomy; Cataract extraction; Combined cataract extraction and guarded filtration procedure	Multiple drops and subconjunctival short-acting agent or facial and retrobulbar block with mepivacaine; light sedation
Tube shunt procedure	Retrobulbar and facial nerve block with mepivacaine; light sedation
Cyclocryotherapy	Retrobulbar block with bupivacaine
Anterior segment reconstruction; Drainage of choroidal detachment; Enucleation	General anesthesia preferable, though not mandatory

The duration of the procedure and of the desired anesthetic effect will determine which anesthetic agent is chosen (Table 22–8). By and large the shortest-lasting agent expected to have a duration adequate to cover the length of the surgery should be chosen, though there are exceptions to this. Where leakage through the bleb or pain are a concern a longer-acting agent is preferred (e.g., bupivacaine).

TABLE 22–9. Factors That Influence Which Eye Should Have Surgery First

Surgery Should Usually Be Performed First on the Eye With:
Worse visual acuity
More damaged optic nerve head
Poorer control of intraocular pressure
Better visual field if field loss extends to 5 degrees of fixation
Less inflammation
Better chance of success, if there is little likelihood that patient will permit operation on the other eye

FACTORS THAT INFLUENCE WHICH EYE SHOULD HAVE SURGERY FIRST

Many patients will need glaucoma surgery on both eyes. Guidelines for determining which eye should be operated on first in such cases are included in Table 22–9. In most cases the more badly damaged eye should have surgery first, the main reason being that in the event of a bad surgical result, it is preferable to have operated on the eye of less importance to the patient. Furthermore, the general response of the patient's eyes to surgery may be learned from the first eye, enhancing the chances for success in the second eye. An additional reason for doing the more severely damaged eye first is that such an eye will tolerate higher pressures less satisfactorily than a less damaged eye. If surgery needs to be delayed for any reason, the less damaged eye can probably tolerate delay better than can the more damaged eye. Furthermore, if carbonic anhydrase inhibitors are used preoperatively, they are best stopped postoperatively, which will almost certainly allow the pressure to rise, further jeopardizing the more badly damaged eye.

There are some exceptions to operating on the worse eye first. Some patients may not be agreeable to having surgery on both eyes. In such cases the eye with the better visual potential should usually have surgery first, for the better eye is more important to the patient. There are also patients who are not likely to permit the second eye to have surgery if there is a poor result in the first eye. In such cases the surgeon should also usually do the better eye first, as it is that eye in which there is more likely to be a good result.

The second eye should have surgery as soon as the quality of the result on the first eye can be predicted with reasonable validity. This varies with the type of surgery performed (Table 22–10).

TABLE 22–10. Intraoperative Interval When Both Eyes Need Same or Similar Procedure*

Procedure	Interval
Surgical iridectomy	1 day
Guarded filtration procedure	5 days
Standard filtration procedure	7 days
Combined cataract extraction with glaucoma procedure	28 days
Goniotomy†	3 days
Trabeculotomy†	3 days
Laser iridotomy	2 weeks
Laser trabeculoplasty	2 months

*Assumes that first procedure was uncomplicated.
†Bilateral simultaneous surgery often justified with this procedure when used as therapy for congenital glaucoma.

PREOPERATIVE CARE: BASIC PRINCIPLES

A few principles are applicable to almost every patient in whom glaucoma surgery is to be done. Ideally, the intraocular pressure should be between 15 and 30 mm Hg and should be in that range for several days before surgery. If the pressure is below 10 mm Hg, the surgical technique is complicated by the softness of the eye. If it is excessively high, there tends to be more bleeding at the time of the surgery; also, rapid decompression when the globe is entered may predispose to an expulsive hemorrhage. Although lowering the intraocular pressure before surgery will not eliminate this latter possibility, allowing time for the pressure to equilibrate at a lower level before opening the eye seems like a sensible goal.

Ideally, the eye should be as quiet as feasible. Inflammation at the time of surgery predisposes to excessive bleeding and increased scarring after surgery.

The urgency with which surgery needs to be performed is primarily related to the vulnerability of the optic nerve, coupled with the rapidity with which the optic nerve is deteriorating. The vulnerability of the nerve is a function of the amount of nerve damage already present and the likelihood that the factors responsible for the damage will continue to take their toll; of these, intraocular pressure in a range that will cause continuing harm is of most concern (Table 22–5).

The absolute level of pressure is less important than the proximity to the level of pressure that caused harm in the past. For example, consider an eye with a healthy disc and with intraocular pressures consistently around 35 mm Hg; when the current intraocular pressure is 35 mm Hg there is no urgency for surgery. On the other hand, take the person whose far-advanced cupping has occurred at an intraocular pressure of about 20 mm Hg, but who now has an intraocular pressure of 35 mm Hg; in this patient surgery is urgent.

The rapidity with which damage occurs must not be underestimated. Primary open-angle glaucoma is a chronic disease, and it may have been present for many years before causing severe visual loss. Nevertheless, when vulnerability is high—as it is when field loss starts involving fixation, and pressure is rising above the level that caused the damage in the past—*sight can deteriorate rapidly,* within days or even hours. Thus the urgency with which surgery should be performed must be carefully considered. A good general rule is this: "Once the need for surgery has been agreed upon by the physician and the patient, it should be performed as soon as it can reasonably be done."

Intraocular pressures above 40 mm Hg can produce damage to the eye other than optic nerve compression. Intraocular pressure in this highly elevated range may predispose to acute anterior ischemic optic neuropathy, retinal vein occlusion, or even retinal artery occlusion.

Other factors that influence the timing of surgery are listed in Table 22–11.

Long-acting cholinesterase inhibitors should be stopped at least 2 weeks before the performance of standard filtering procedures, the guarded filtration procedure, or iridectomy. These "irreversible" parasympathomimetics predispose to increased bleeding at the time of surgery, increased postoperative inflammation, and shallow postoperative anterior chamber.* Furthermore, they make dilatation of the pupil difficult in the postoperative period. It is prudent to stop all miotics, such as pilocarpine, far enough in advance of surgery that their short-term effects will have worn off (unfortunately the long-term effects of the medication on vascularity and pupil rigidity will still be operative). Carbonic anhydrase inhibitors, topical beta-blockers, and alpha-agonists should also, theoretically, be stopped long enough before surgery designed to produce a filtering wound that their effects will have worn off; this requires 6 to 12 hours for the carbonic anhydrase inhibitors and around 2 to 4 weeks for the other agents. These agents suppress aqueous formation and may slow the rate of complete re-formation of the anterior chamber and the flow of aqueous through the fistula. Because aqueous flow appears to be essential to the development of a functioning fistula, suppression of flow may tend to predispose to surgical failure.

In actual practice, however, surgery is being performed because the intraocular pressure is too high; therefore, the theoretical advantages of stopping med-

*Because of their effect on blood pseudocholinesterase, they also may lead to complications in general anesthesia.

TABLE 22–11. Factors That Influence the Timing of all Types of Glaucoma Surgery*

Factor	Favors Delay of Surgery	Favors Proceeding with Surgery Promptly
Health of optic nerve	No apparent cupping	Advanced cupping
Visual field	Loss not approaching fixation	Loss approaching fixation†
Current level of intraocular pressure, in comparison to level at which nerve damage occurred	Lower	Higher
Absolute level of intraocular pressure	Less than 10 mm Hg	Greater than 40 mm Hg‡
Patient's ability to tolerate medications	Good	Poor
Degree of ocular inflammation	Marked	Minimal
Patient receiving long-acting cholinesterase inhibitors	Yes§	No
Patient receiving anticoagulant	Yes	No
Rapidity of rise of intraocular pressure	Slow	Sudden

*See Tables 22-9 and 22-10 for specific indications for surgery of specific types of glaucoma.
†If field defect has reached to within 5 degrees of fixation, chance of wipe-out increases.
‡The closer the intraocular pressure to systolic central retinal artery pressure, the more urgent the surgery.
§The reason for delaying is to allow the effect of the agent to wear off; this is not necessary for cyclodialysis.

TABLE 22–12. Method of Lowering Intraocular Pressure Maximally Prior to Surgery*

Agent	Route	Dose†	Time Before Surgery to Administer
Mannitol 20%	Intravenous	7 ml/kg	90 minutes
Glycerol, anhydrous‡	Oral	1 ml/kg	60 minutes
Timolol 0.5%	Eye drop	2 drops	60 minutes
Acetazolamide	Intravenous	7 mg/kg	30 minutes
Mepivacaine 0.75%	Retrobulbar block	2 ml	10 minutes
Pressure on globe	—	—	10 seconds on and 10 seconds off for 2 minutes

*This method is not advised for routine use, but should be used only in cases in which intraocular pressure is extraordinarily resistant to standard therapy.
†Dose is expressed in terms of amount per kilogram of body weight.
‡Glycerol is preferably administered in a 50% solution, in which case the dose given in this table should be doubled.

ication preoperatively are often of less concern than preventing further pressure damage. What is done in each individual case, therefore, must be determined by the ability of the optic nerve to resist pressure and the degree of effect of the agents on the intraocular pressure. One method of proceeding is to stop the long-acting agents (beta-blockers, alpha-agonists, and long-acting miotics) approximately 1 month preoperatively and control the intraocular pressure with short-acting agents such as the carbonic anhydrase inhibitors.

In extraordinary circumstances standard attempts to lower intraocular pressure may not succeed. For these cases, Table 22–12 describes a method that will provide maximum intraocular pressure–lowering potential.

INDICATIONS FOR SURGERY

PRIMARY OPEN-ANGLE GLAUCOMA

Surgery for open-angle glaucoma is indicated when there is documented or anticipated damage to the optic nerve or visual field owing to glaucoma, despite maximum tolerated medical therapy, that is developing at a rate that will diminish the patient's quality of life to the extent that the patient decides to undergo surgery in hopes that the advantages of surgery will be greater than the disadvantages (see Tables 22–13 and 22–14).

The essential consideration in determining the need for treatment or for surgery is to determine the effect of

TABLE 22–13. Risks Versus Benefits of Glaucoma Surgery*

Immediate Purposes of Surgery	
Preserve or enhance patient's quality of life	All cases
Control intraocular pressure	Most cases
Correct anterior chamber angle	Some cases
Corect anterior chamber angle and control pressure	Few cases
Risks and Benefits	**Incidence**
Guarded filtration procedure	
Risks	
Immediate risks	
Sudden, permanent loss of central vision in otherwise uncomplicated procedure	5% of cases in which visual field loss has advanced into fixation; 2% of cases in which field loss is advanced and impinges on but does not involve fixation; very rare in others
Infection	Very rare, less than 0.1%
"Malignant glaucoma" (high pressure with collapse of anterior chamber)	Rare except in a few predisposed cases
Serious bleeding inside the eye	2% of cases with advanced disease
Excessive filtration with flat anterior chamber	10%
Need for second surgery related to the first	10%
Technical problem (e.g., tear of conjunctiva)	5%
Droopy lid (temporary)	Common (occasionally permanent)
Severe blurring of vision for weeks	Usual
Late risks	
Progression of glaucoma	15%
Progression of preexisting cataract	Usual
Droopy lid	Rare
Infection	Rare: less than 0.1%, though more frequent with full-thickness filtration procedures

Continued

TABLE 22-13. Risks Versus Benefits of Glaucoma Surgery* *(Continued)*

Benefits	
Increased likelihood of maintaining vision	90%
No further progression of glaucoma	80%
Less need for medicines	80%
No need for medicines	40%
Improved vision	30%
Surgical Iridectomy	
Risks	
Immediate risks	
Decreased vision for 2 weeks	Usual
Technical problem (e.g., need for additional suture)	5%
Serious bleeding	Less than 1%
Infection	Less than 0.1%
"Malignant glaucoma"	Very rare
Late risks	
Progression of preexisting cataract	15%
Recurrent closure of angle	1%
Development of other type of glaucoma	5%
Continuing need for medication	(Depends on preoperative condition)
Benefits	
Eliminates future attacks of angle-closure glaucoma	95%
Returns anterior chamber angle toward normal	95%
Prevents "creeping angle closure"	90%
Reduces need for medicine	40%
Eliminates need for medicine	10%
Laser Iridotomy	
Risks	
Immediate risks	
Rise of intraocular pressure	Frequent
Transient blurred vision	Usual
Bleeding of significance	Very rare
Inflammation	Very rare
Retinal burn	Very rare
Late risks	
Progressive cataract	15%
Closure of iridotomy	5%
Recurrent angle closure	5%
Development of other type of glaucoma	5%
Continuing need for medications (depends on preoperative condition)	(Variable)
Benefits	
Eliminates future attacks of angle-closure glaucoma	90%
Returns anterior chamber angle toward normal	95%
Prevents "creeping angle closure"	90%
Reduces need for medicine	20%
Eliminates need for medicine	10%
Combined Cataract-Glaucoma Surgery	
Risks	
Immediate risks	
Sudden, permanent reduction of vision	5%
Temporary reduction of vision	90%
Slow recovery of vision (6 months)	20%
Need for second surgery related to first	10%
Retinal edema	20%
As per guarded filtration procedure	
Late risks	
Retinal edema	5%
Trouble with intraocular lens	5%
Failure of pressure control	15%
As per guarded filtration procedure	
Benefits	
Improvement in visual function	90%
As per trabeculectomy	

TABLE 22-13. Risks Versus Benefits of Glaucoma Surgery* *(Continued)*

Cataract Extraction Following Filtration Procedure	
Risks	
Immediate risks	
Infection or serious bleeding	Very rare, less than 0.1%
Need for second operation related to first	1%
Temporary reduction of vision	80%
Late risks	
Retinal edema and poor recovery of vision	3%
Trouble with intraocular lens	3%
Need for capsulotomy (laser)	30%
Benefits	
Improved visual function	95%

*Estimates of frequency are rough approximations based on my experience.

TABLE 22-14. Treatment Preferences

Condition	Preferred Treatment
Deterioration occurring at such a rate that visual disability is expected prior to the person's death	Filtering surgery
Deterioration occurring at a rate that may cause mild to moderate visual disability prior to the person's death	Argon laser trabeculoplasty. If ineffective, then filtering surgery
Damage present, but not expected to worsen at a rate that is likely to cause disability	Argon laser trabeculoplasty and/or medications
Damage present, but rate of deterioration not established or of great concern	Medications
Damage questionable, but risk factors a major concern	Medications or close observation
No definite damage and likelihood of visual disability occurring prior to the person's death believed to be small	Observation

the illness on the patient, that is to say, the clinical course of the disease. The intensity of intervention will vary, depending on the anticipated effect of the disease on the patient. The use of the "glaucoma graph" can be of great help in this regard (Fig. 22–10; see also the accompanying text box for a description of how to use the "Glaucoma Graph").

Condition of the Optic Nerve Head

The current management of glaucoma rests primarily on the observation of deterioration. It is hoped that in the future this system will be changed, so that management is determined primarily by lowering intraocular pressure or employing a neuroprotective agent so that there will be an improvement in the optic disc or visual field. However, this new system of management by improvement demands more meticulous examination of the patient than is currently practiced, or in many areas currently available.

Because the optic disc will often show changes before the development of detectable deterioration of the visual field, especially in the early stages of disease, documentation of disc change is of paramount importance in management, especially in glaucoma suspects or in those with early or moderately advanced glaucoma.[41–47] Proper evaluation of the nerve head is thus an essential part of the diagnostic evaluation of every case. The disc should be drawn. When possible, photographs should

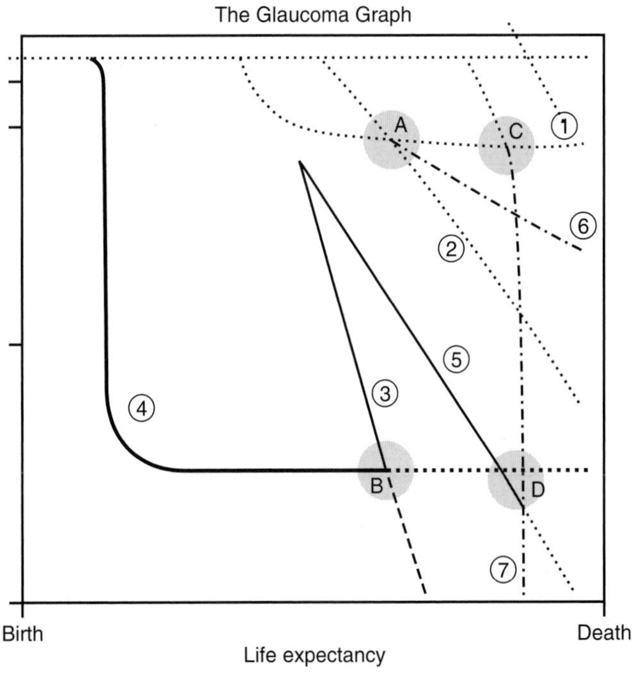

Figure 22–10. The Glaucoma Graph. (From Tasman W and Jaeger E (eds.), Wills Eye Hospital Atlas of Clinical Ophthalmology, 2nd Edition. Philadelphia: Lippincott; 2001:F3–91.)

The Glaucoma Graph

The glaucoma graph is a way of determining and understanding the clinical course of glaucoma in an individual patient.

On the y-axis of the graph is the stage of the glaucoma, and on the x-axis is the life expectancy. The slope and the curve of each of the individual lines are determined and graphed in different ways:

- **Dotted lines** indicate that the slope and the curve have been determined by plotting the results of serial studies, such as repeated disc photographs taken yearly or repeated visual field examinations.
- **Solid lines** depict the clinical course as described in the patient's history.
- **Dashed lines** are extrapolations that are presumed to represent what will happen in the future. These hypothetical, extrapolated future courses are based on the nature of the previous courses and on knowledge of what has happened since a known point in time.

Figure 22–10 shows the courses of seven different patients with different manifestations of glaucoma:

- **A patient at point "A"** has minimal glaucoma, and about one third of his or her life still to live.
- **A patient at point "B"** has advanced glaucoma and has about one third of his or her life still to live.
- **A patient at point "C"** has very early glaucoma and only a few years to live.
- **A patient at point "D"** has advanced glaucoma and only a few years to live.
- **Patient 1, considered at point "A,"** has one third of his or her life to live and is in an early stage of glaucoma. About one third of his or her life earlier, this patient was noted to have elevated pressure and was followed without treatment. No damage to the optic nerve or visual field was ever noted. It is reasonable to assume that, if the patient continues to have intraocular pressures around the same level as those noted initially, he or she will probably follow the course described by line 1, and will die without any evidence of glaucoma damage.
- **Patient 2,** also considered at **point "A,"** i.e., having minimal damage with one third of his or her life left to live. In this case, however, the patient's intraocular pressure rose continuously, and the patient was noted to develop early disc and field damage, which continued at the rate depicted by the **dashed line 2.** This patient, if untreated, would develop definite asymptomatic damage. However, the patient would have no functional loss of vision at the time of his or her death.
- **Patients 3 and 4, at point "B":** both have advanced glaucoma and one third of their lives left to live. However, **Patient 3** is deteriorating rapidly and will be blind long before he or she dies, whereas **Patient 4,** who received a blow to the eye as a child and lost vision to a steroid-induced glaucoma at that time, has had stable vision for most of his or her life, and it is reasonable to expect that it will continue to be stable.
- Patients **at points "C" and "D"** both have only a few years to live, but those at **point "C"** (like **Patients 1 and 2** at **point "A"**) have minimal damage, and those at **point "D"** (like **Patient 4** at **point "B"**) have marked damage.
- **Patient 5** started with a clinical course similar to that of **Patient 3** (advanced glaucoma and deteriorating rapidly), but around the midpoint of life, the glaucoma became less severe. Nevertheless, this patient will be blind at the time of death unless there is effective intervention. Compare **Patient 4** who at **point "D"** has the same life expectancy and the same amount of damage as **Patient 5** (only a few years to live and advanced glaucoma). **Patient 4,** however, has a stable clinical course and does not appear to need a change in therapy. In contrast, **Patient 5** needs lowering intraocular pressure urgently.
- **Patient 6,** near **point "C,"** also has only a few years of life remaining, but has glaucoma that is getting worse a little bit more slowly than that affecting **Patients 2 and 5.** However, because **Patient 6** has so little damage to start with, no treatment is necessary, even though the glaucoma is getting worse. Even without treatment, this patient will not have enough damage or visual loss due to glaucoma at the time of death that he or she will have any awareness of the disease or any limits in visual function.
- **Patient 7** at **point "C"** has only a few years left to live, but has a type of glaucoma that is progressing so rapidly that blindness will occur well before the time of death.

Using the glaucoma graph to define and characterize the nature of the clinical course helps the physician and patient to understand that:

- **Patients 1, 4, and 6** do not need any treatment at all; **Patient 1** will never develop damage, **Patient 4** has marked damage but it is not getting worse, and **Patient 6** is getting worse so slowly that the disease will not interfere with his or her life.
- **Patients 3, 5, and 7** can be seen to need treatment urgently in order to prevent them from becoming totally blind prior to the time of their deaths.
- **Patient 2:** The need for treatment is controversial. Because this patient would never develop glaucoma, perhaps he or she should not be treated at all. But since he or she would develop **some** damage, those who want to prevent any damage at all would advise therapy.

be obtained. Although now still largely investigational, quantitative image analysis with an instrument such as the Heidelberg Retina Tomograph will almost certainly provide the best documentation. In the future the evaluations should be made often enough to be reasonably sure that changes are not missed. Alterations may occur rapidly, such as the cupping that can develop within weeks in patients with congenital glaucoma or in children with secondary glaucoma. Usually, however, the changes occur slowly; in most instances it is adequate to check the disc at about 6-month intervals and repeat the disc imaging every 2 to 3 years. The level of intraocular pressure will obviously influence the frequency with which the optic nerve head needs to be evaluated: the higher the pressure, the more frequent the examination.

The appearance of the optic disc in some patients with glaucoma is so characteristic that the examiner is almost surely correct in making this diagnosis (Fig. 22–11).

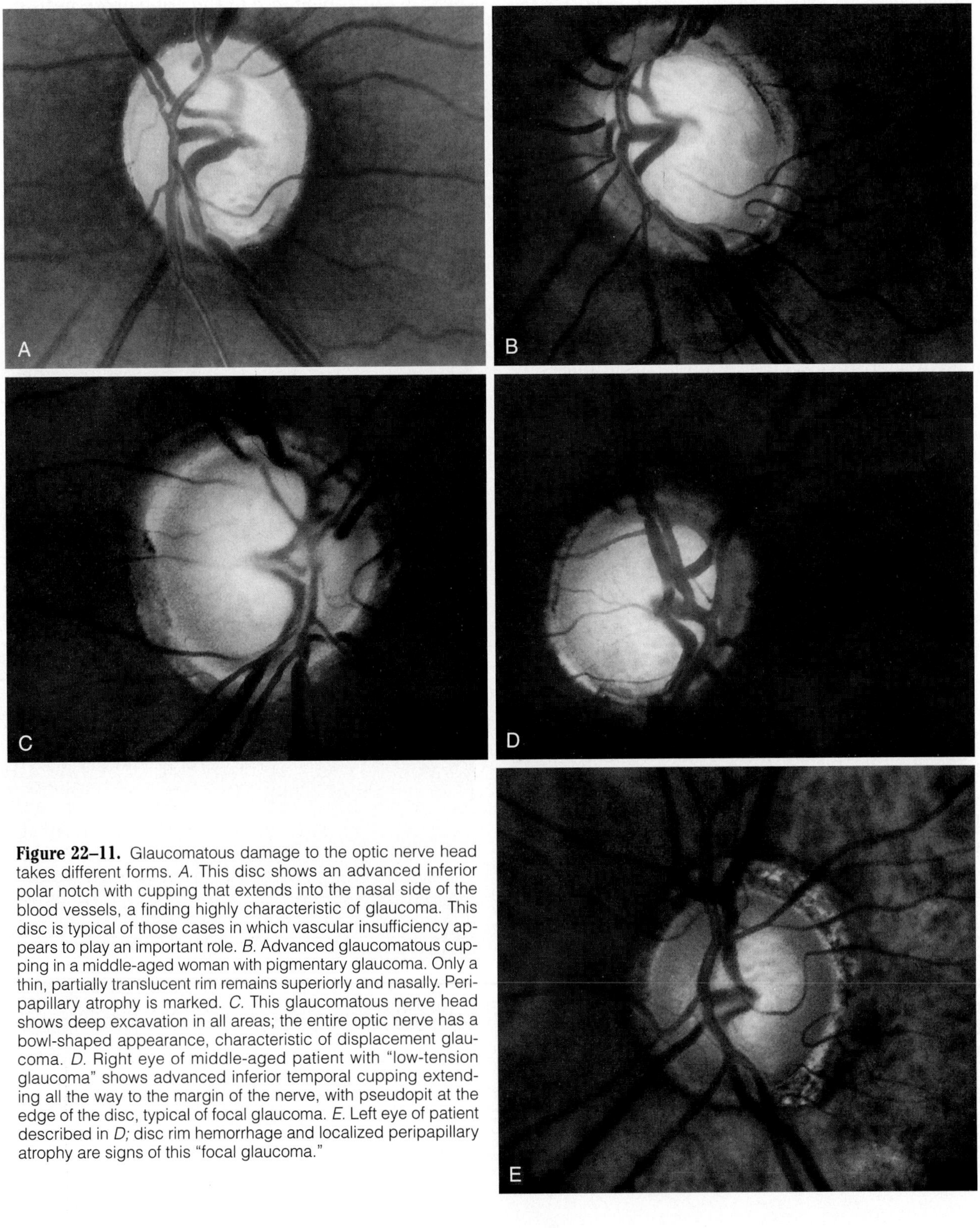

Figure 22–11. Glaucomatous damage to the optic nerve head takes different forms. *A.* This disc shows an advanced inferior polar notch with cupping that extends into the nasal side of the blood vessels, a finding highly characteristic of glaucoma. This disc is typical of those cases in which vascular insufficiency appears to play an important role. *B.* Advanced glaucomatous cupping in a middle-aged woman with pigmentary glaucoma. Only a thin, partially translucent rim remains superiorly and nasally. Peripapillary atrophy is marked. *C.* This glaucomatous nerve head shows deep excavation in all areas; the entire optic nerve has a bowl-shaped appearance, characteristic of displacement glaucoma. *D.* Right eye of middle-aged patient with "low-tension glaucoma" shows advanced inferior temporal cupping extending all the way to the margin of the nerve, with pseudopit at the edge of the disc, typical of focal glaucoma. *E.* Left eye of patient described in *D;* disc rim hemorrhage and localized peripapillary atrophy are signs of this "focal glaucoma."

However, this is not invariably the case.[48] It is generally believed that discs with large central cups, such as those with a cup–disc ratio greater than 0.8, are more sensitive to the damaging effects of elevated intraocular pressure. Some physicians also believe that myopic nerve heads or those with a posteriorly bowed lamina cribrosa are predisposed to damage.[22,42] These are not established facts, however.

Progressive narrowing of the neural rim of the optic nerve head in a patient with glaucoma is virtual proof that the glaucoma is not adequately controlled. If the rim is becoming narrower, the physician must assume that the glaucoma is getting worse, or that there is a different or additional cause for progressive cupping.[41] Although there do appear to be cases in which optic nerve damage is so marked that the neurons are "mortally wounded" (and will die no matter how low the intraocular pressure), a good working rule is to assume that the cause for progressive deterioration is intraocular pressure higher than the eye can tolerate (Table 22–6). This approach demands reasonable certainty that the deterioration is not due to causes other than glaucoma, such as compression of the chiasm by a pituitary adenoma. It also demands that the ophthalmologist and the patient be prudent in ruling out other causes of optic nerve damage, and use appropriate diagnostic tests. For example, useful tests include a sedimentation rate; measurements of optic blood flow, where appropriate; and, most important, imaging studies such as computed tomography and magnetic resonance. In the simplest terms, if the glaucoma is getting worse, this is an indication that the intraocular pressure is too high, regardless of its absolute level. Progressive deterioration of the optic nerve head must be expected unless the intraocular pressure is lowered further. Progressive cupping may occur despite intraocular pressures in the range that has been considered normal; such was the case in the person whose optic disc is shown in Figure 22–12. This middle-aged woman was never observed to have intraocular pressures above 15 mm Hg. However, during the 3 years the patient was followed, she received no treatment and had introacular pressures between 13 and 15 mm Hg; nevertheless there was progressive cupping and visual field loss. After the intraocular pressure had been lowered to the range of 10 to 12 mm Hg, deterioration stopped; there was no further damage observed in the next 10 years.

Progressive cupping may occur without detectable visual field loss. One clue that this is occurring is the presence of significant asymmetry between the optic discs, as shown in Figure 22–13. The left optic disc of this young adult with essential iris atrophy appears entirely normal when considered by itself. However, an obvious difference between the two eyes is observable when the left optic disc is compared with the right optic nerve head of the same patient. The narrowing of the optic rim of this person with persistently elevated intraocular pressure represents an acquired change.

Changes in the appearance of the optic disc need not be marked to be highly significant. Note the narrowing of the rim, the enlargement of the cup, and the deviation of the blood vessels that occurred in the 3 years separating Figure 22–14*A* and *B*. The intraocular pressure was approaching 40 mm Hg during this time. After the disc deterioration was recognized, a guarded filtration procedure was performed, after which the disc showed significant improvement (Fig. 22–14C).

Cupping is definitely reversible, especially in infants or young children.[43,44,49] A permanent improvement in the appearance of the optic nerve head is to be expected after successful treatment of early congenital glaucoma. Improvement in adults also occurs far more frequently than previously believed.[49–51] In one study one third of surgically treated patients showed reversible change. Temporary filling-in of the optic nerve has been observed. This is presumably the result of edema and should not be confused with real improvement.

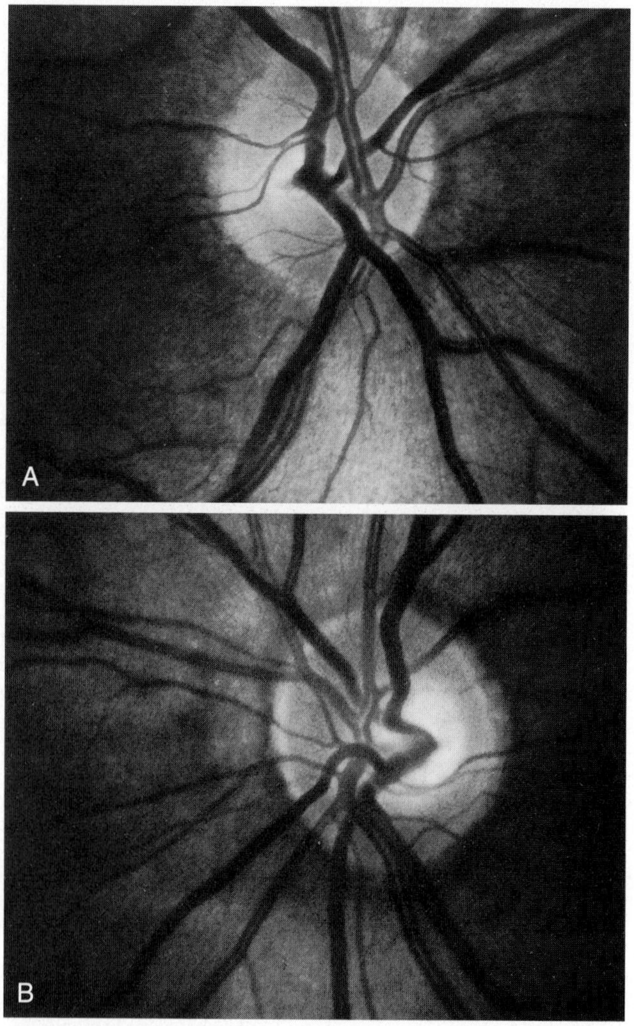

Figure 22–12. *A.* Optic disc of patient with an apparently normal right eye. *B.* Optic disc of glaucomatous left eye of same patient, showing markedly enlarged cup caused by elevation of intraocular pressure. The only clue that this disc is abnormal is asymmetry. The underlying diagnosis is glaucoma secondary to essential iris atrophy, left eye. Despite the acquired cupping, visual field loss was not detectable.

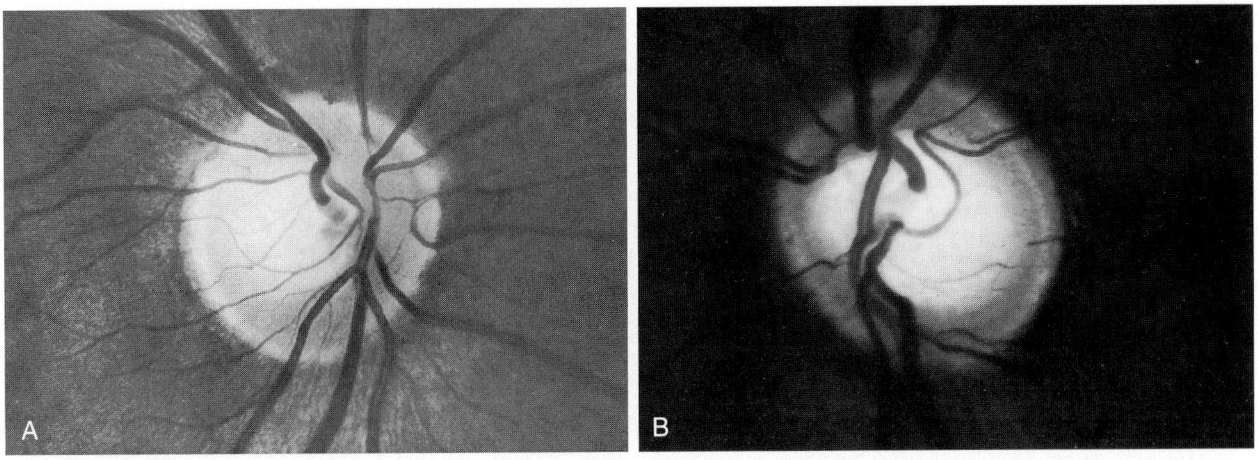

Figure 22–13. The left eye *(B)* of this young man shows a cup that is unmistakably larger than the cup in the right eye *(A)*. Furthermore, there is cupping on the nasal side of the blood vessels *(B)*. Note, however, that the entire disc in *B* is larger than the disc in *A*. The total rim area in *A* and *B* is, thus, similar. The larger cup in *B* is more a reflection of difference in disc size than of loss of tissue.

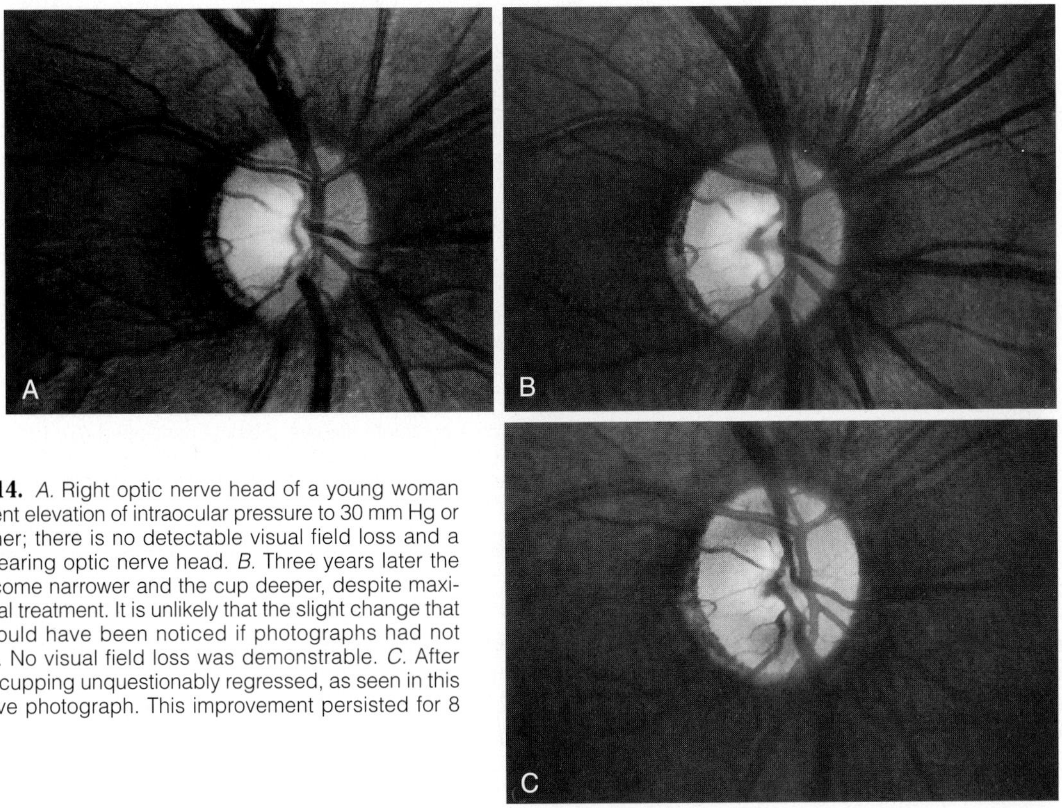

Figure 22–14. *A.* Right optic nerve head of a young woman with persistent elevation of intraocular pressure to 30 mm Hg or slightly higher; there is no detectable visual field loss and a normal-appearing optic nerve head. *B.* Three years later the rim had become narrower and the cup deeper, despite maximum medical treatment. It is unlikely that the slight change that occurred could have been noticed if photographs had not been taken. No visual field loss was demonstrable. *C.* After surgery the cupping unquestionably regressed, as seen in this postoperative photograph. This improvement persisted for 8 years.

Nature of the Visual Field

Visual field loss may occur in the absence of apparent deterioration of the optic nerve head.[7,52,53] This is uncommon in early glaucoma. But in cases with advanced cupping, progressive visual loss often occurs without the ophthalmologist's being able to note further deterioration of the optic nerve head. Consequently satisfactory management of glaucoma requires careful and frequent documentation of the visual field (Fig. 22–15).

Visual field loss in glaucoma may take various forms.[52–56] It commonly first expresses itself as an isolated scotomatous loss in the Bjerrum area, that is, within a zone approximately 10 degrees wide extending from the blind spot, becoming wider as it sweeps toward the nasal side (Fig. 22–16). The superior field is

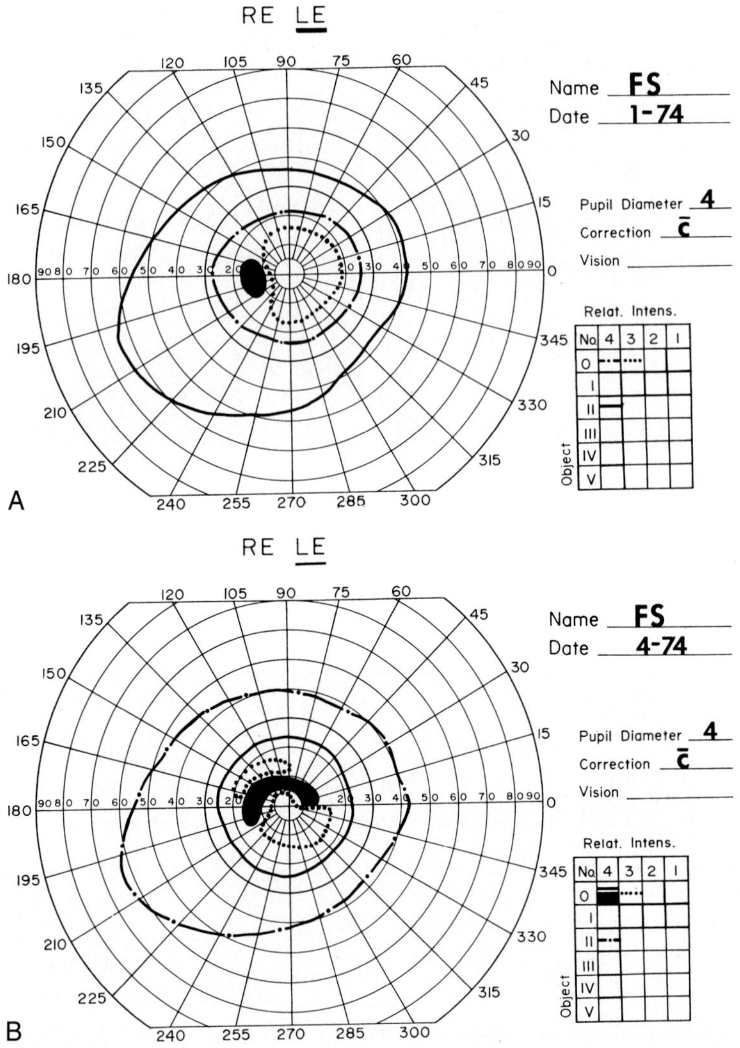

Figure 22–15. Within 3 months this middle-aged woman who had an inferior polar notch of the left eye progressed from having a normal visual field *(A)* to having a pathoglogical field in which a complete arcuate scotoma developed *(B)*. This type of change is typical of "focal glaucoma." It occurred in this patient despite her intraocular pressure's consistently being around 15 mm Hg. (Modified from Spaeth GL: The Pathogenesis of Visual Loss in Glaucoma; The Contribution of and Indications for Fluorescein Angiography. New York; Grune & Stratton, 1977.)

more often involved. Unless the visual field examination includes a specific search for such scotomas, abnormalities will be missed.[7,57] Static perimetry is of great assistance in this regard. Instruments that examine the field using computer-controlled static perimetry offer the physician the most satisfactory method of documenting the nature of the visual field and observing deterioration (Fig. 22–17).[58,59]

Artifacts that affect the visual field must be considered in interpreting repeat visual field studies. Change in the pupil size, clarity of the media, intensity of the testing light, cooperation of the patient, speed with which the object is presented, and many other factors affect the apparent visual field. It is essential that these artifacts be considered when comparing studies (Table 22–15). The surgeon is attempting to determine whether the visual field has become worse owing to progressive damage to the optic nerve. When this is the case, and when other organic causes have been ruled out, then the progressive field loss must be assumed to be glaucomatous, and by definition, the glaucoma is out of control, regardless of the level of intraocular pressure (see p. 217).

When visual field loss is so extensive that it cuts close to fixation, there is a possibility that central visual acuity will deteriorate suddenly after surgery. This phenomenon of "wipe-out" is rare but real (Fig. 22–18).[59,60] The risk must be included in the assessment of whether surgery is warranted (see Table 22–13). Completely satisfactory figures are not available, but patients must be given an estimate of the likelihood that their vision will be made immediately much worse by the surgery. If central acuity is already affected (fixation is already involved), I tell them that they have about a 10% chance of sudden visual loss; if loss cuts within 5 degrees of fixation but does not actually involve central acuity,

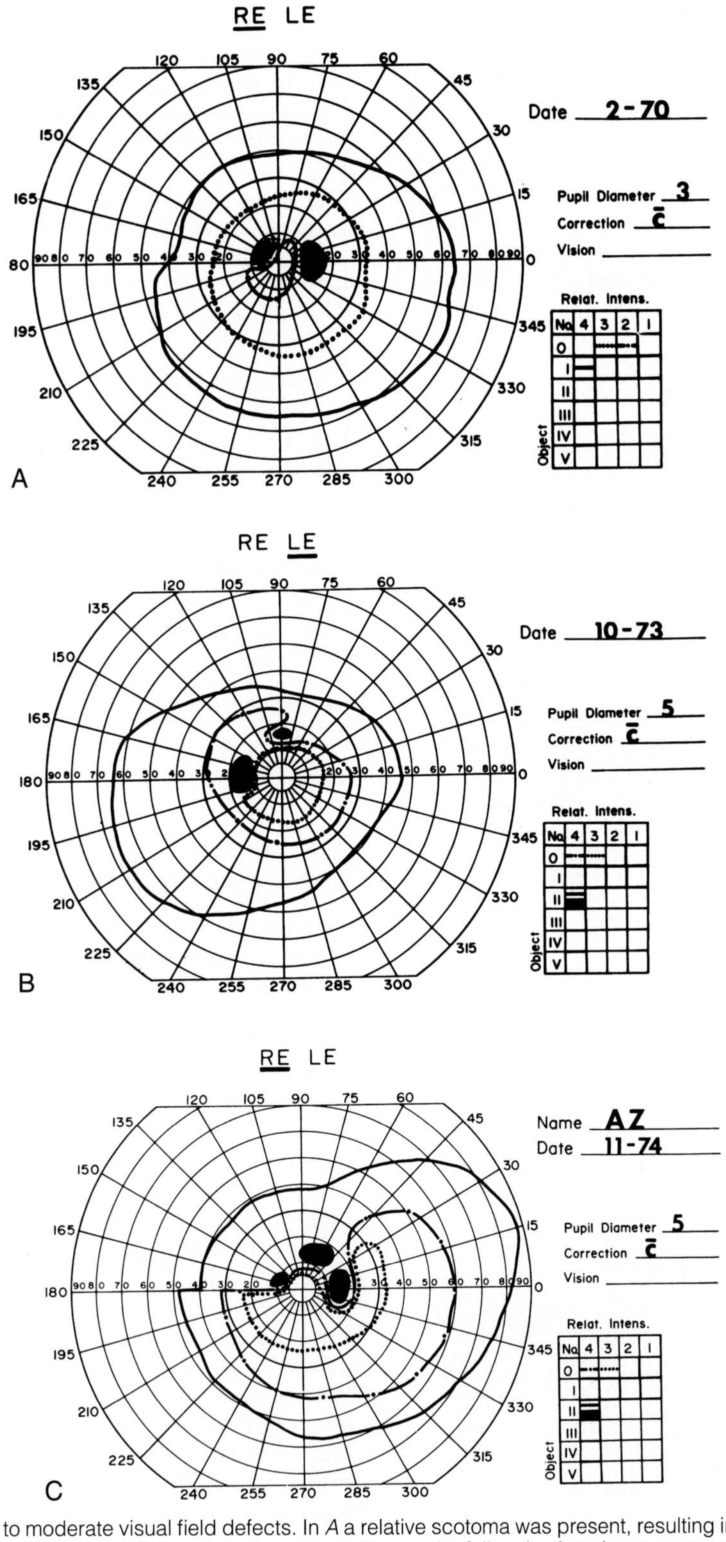

Figure 22–16. Early to moderate visual field defects. In *A* a relative scotoma was present, resulting in a superior nasal step. No absolute defect could be found. Though the isopters in *B* are quite full, a tiny but dense scotoma at 12 o'clock was detected. More advanced loss is shown in *C,* the optic disc of a young woman with a large inferior polar notch (similar to that shown in Fig. 12–15). (Modified from Spaeth GL: The Pathogenesis of Visual Loss in Glaucoma; The Contribution of and Indications for Fluorescein Angiography. New York; Grune & Stratton, 1977.)

then I tell them that the likelihood of loss is about 5%. If the visual field is tubular, not cutting into fixation, the likelihood of "wipe-out" appears to be much less. For evaluation of the visual field to be clinically meaningful, the method of examination must be sufficiently sensitive that changes that are occurring can be detected.[58] Perimeters such as the Humphrey Automated Perimeter or the Octopus offer major advantages: a built-in data bank of normative data, ease of data analysis, including quantification of change, and a high degree of reproducibility.

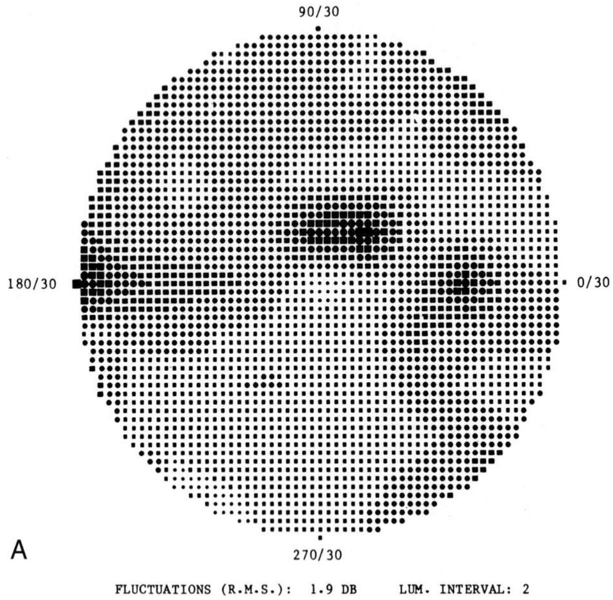

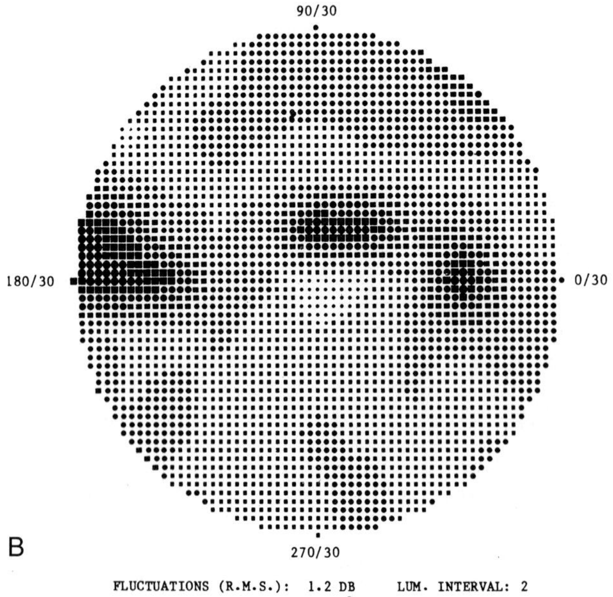

Figure 22–17. A small but clinically significant progression of the superior nasal step *(B compared with A)* was documented by Octopus computerized perimeter in this middle-aged chemist with low-tension glaucoma. Such lesser degrees of change need to be confirmed by repeated field examinations before being considered valid.

TABLE 22–15. Factors That May Make the Visual Field Deteriorate*

Decreasing Brightness or Clarity of Image on Retina
Smaller pupil
Opacities in media
Inaccurate refractive correction
Lower light intensity of object
Brighter background illumination
Smaller test object
Greater distance of patient from screen
Methods of Testing
Shorter exposure of object
More rapid motion of object
Excessively long test
Technical errors
Improper positioning of patient
Patient Factors
Lack of alertness or understanding
Fatigue or illness
Changed anatomic factors (e.g., lid droop)
Deterioration of Visual Receptors, Pathways, or Centers

*Of the four factors listed, only the last is an indication of actual worsening of the patient's disease. Furthermore, even this situation may be caused by many factors other than glaucoma.

Intraocular Pressure

The *control* of open-angle glaucoma is defined by what is happening to the optic disc and field. It is *not* defined by the level of intraocular pressure. Consequently intraocular pressure *per se* is rarely an indication for surgery in open-angle glaucoma (see p. 217).

Intraocular pressure, on the other hand, is important in deciding whether surgery should be undertaken. The reason for this is that the level of intraocular pressure helps to indicate whether disc and field changes can be anticipated; that is, intraocular pressure is a predictive indicator.

For intraocular pressure to be a valid predictive indicator, the level harmful to the patient under consideration must be established: this cannot be determined *a priori.* For although it is possible to accurately predict that in a population of 100 patients who have intraocular pressure of X mm Hg, a certain percentage will eventually develop disc and field change, one cannot predict with certainty *which* of the 100 will deteriorate and which will remain stable. Therefore, until a track record for the individual patient has been established, intraocular pressure provides nothing more than a rough guideline. With adequate evaluation and with time, it is usually possible to determine what general level of intraocular pressure is tolerated by the patient under consideration. Only after this determination has been made does intraocular pressure itself become a valid predictive indicator.

Consider individual A, whose intraocular pressure with medical treatment has ranged between 20 and 25 mm Hg for a period of 5 years, during which time there is no suggestion of deterioration of the disc or field. Patient A can be presumed to be under control (although it is not possible to say with 100% certainty that disc or field damage will not develop 5 to 10 years later even if the intraocular pressures stay in the same range). On the other hand, consider patient B, whose intraocular pressure also ranged between 20 and 25 mm Hg for 5 years, during which time there has been progressive deterioration of the optic disc or visual field. It is now established that the intraocular pressure in patient B must be lowered, and appropriate steps are taken to achieve this. The physician now sets a new level that he believes may be satisfactory, perhaps 13 to 18 mm Hg. This should be a range, not a single figure, such as "15 mm Hg." This "target range" can be estimated by using the intraocular pressure at which damage has occurred or the percentage lowering that is desired. For example, in a patient with an intraocular pressure of 40 mm Hg, the desired lowering of intraocular pressure is around 14 to 18 mm Hg, so that the final IOP is between 22 and 26 mm Hg, whereas in a patient with an IOP of 20, the goal is having IOP around 4 to 6 mm Hg so that the target range is between 14 and 16 mm Hg. If it is possible to achieve such a pressure level with medication, this course is followed and the patient is then watched to determine if deterioration occurs at that new level. *If, after pressure lowering, the disc or field improves, the new level of intraocular pressure can, with great confidence, be considered satisfactory. Such improvement in disc or field must, however, be real, and not merely a reflection of testing techniques (e.g., larger pupil, better acuity) or incorrect interpretation* (see Figs. 22–14 and 22–19). Merely because surgery has been "successful" and has lowered intraocular pressure to a range that the surgeon may have considered *a priori* to be satisfactory does not mean that the surgery will be truly successful. Achieving an intraocular pressure of, for example, 15

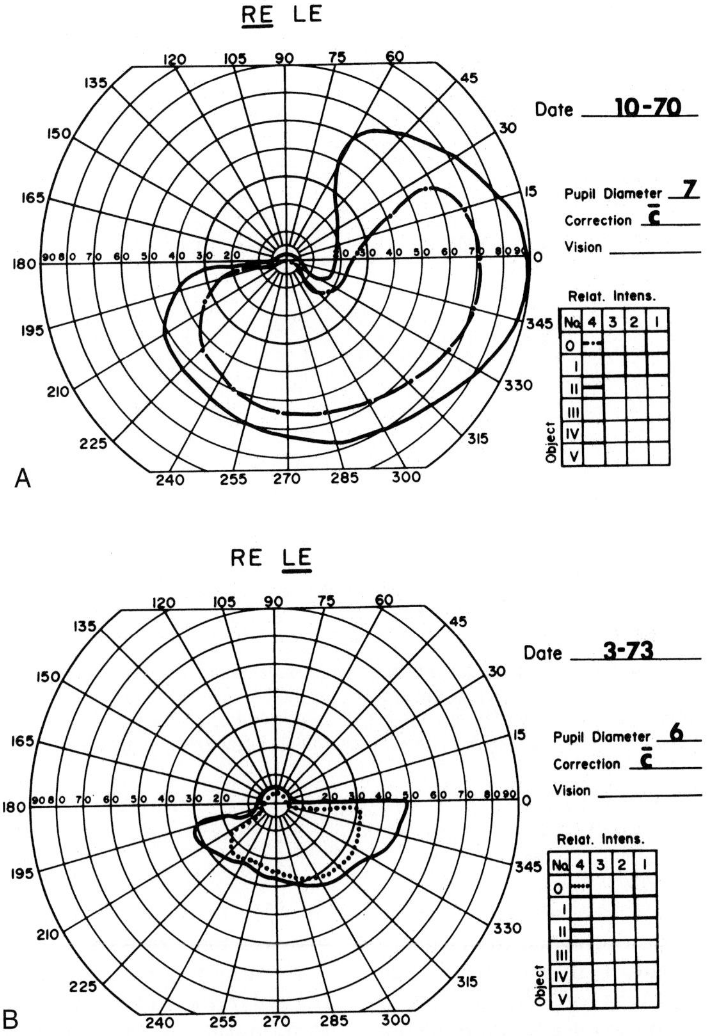

Figure 22–18. Although the extent of visual field loss in *A* is greater than in *B*, the risk for deterioration of vision after surgery is just as great, if not greater, in *B* as in *A* because of the closeness with which the field loss approaches fixation. "Wipe-out" occurs in roughly 5% of cases in which field loss reaches into fixation preoperatively. (Modified from Spaeth GL: The Pathogenesis of Visual Loss in Glaucoma; The Contribution of and Indications for Fluorescein Angiography. New York; Grune & Stratton, 1977.)

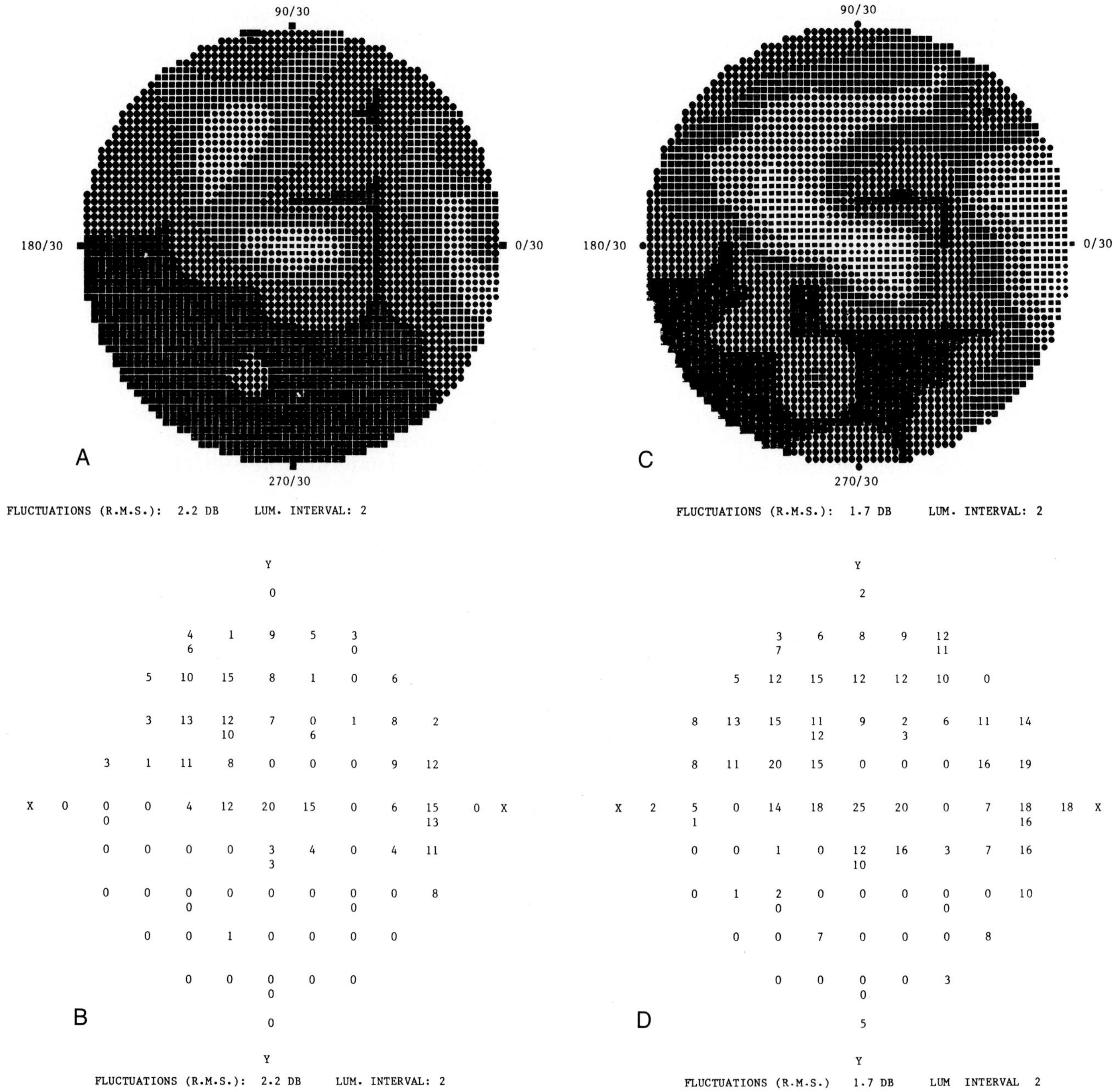

Figure 22–19. *A* and *B* represent the visual field of a woman who had demonstrated progressive glaucomatous visual field loss. The visual field, determined just before glaucoma surgery, is shown in both the gray-scale and digital modes. *C* and *D* show the same patient approximately 1 year after successful surgical lowering of intraocular pressure. Despite the advanced nature of the visual field loss, there is a significant improvement. This improvement is not the result of change in pupil size or other artifact of testing technique.

mm Hg after surgery may not be achieving control. Control is defined only in terms of the health of the optic nerve. A recent study has shown that almost 50% of patients who had surgery that was considered successful for glaucoma, and in whom the intraocular pressure had been lowered to an average of 19 mm Hg, had progressive visual field loss 5 years later; in contrast, in the same population, having surgery performed by the same surgeons with the same indications, those patients in whom the mean intraocular pressure was 14 mm Hg fared far better, with only 6% showing progressive visual loss.

Another vitally important limitation of the value of intraocular pressure in managing glaucoma is the inability to monitor it in more than the most rudimentary manner. A physician sees a patient for isolated, planned, brief moments of the patient's life, and often concludes that each such moment is representative of the vast period of time over which the patient is not being monitored. It is true that more information can be provided by "home tonometry," the practice of measuring the intraocular pressure at more frequent intervals during a patient's ordinary day. However, home tonometry by no means provides a full description of what is happening to the patient's pressure. Paradoxically, it may make it even more difficult for the patient and physician to keep in mind the truth that the matter of real concern is the patient's health, most specifically the patient's optic nerve.

It is generally accepted that when glaucoma surgery is successful it is because the mean intraocular pressure has been adequately lowered. But it may be that an additional important function of glaucoma surgery is to eliminate pressure spikes. Such a hypothesis is consistent with the observation that the patient may, before surgery, show progressive deterioration of disc and field at pressure X, and yet after surgery not show further deterioration at the same pressure level.

Summary

Shown in Figure 22–20*B* is the traditional concept of the course of glaucoma and the effect or lack of effect of treatment. Figure 22–20C depicts the "new" method of management, based on lowering intraocular pressure enough to cause an improvement in the course of the disease.

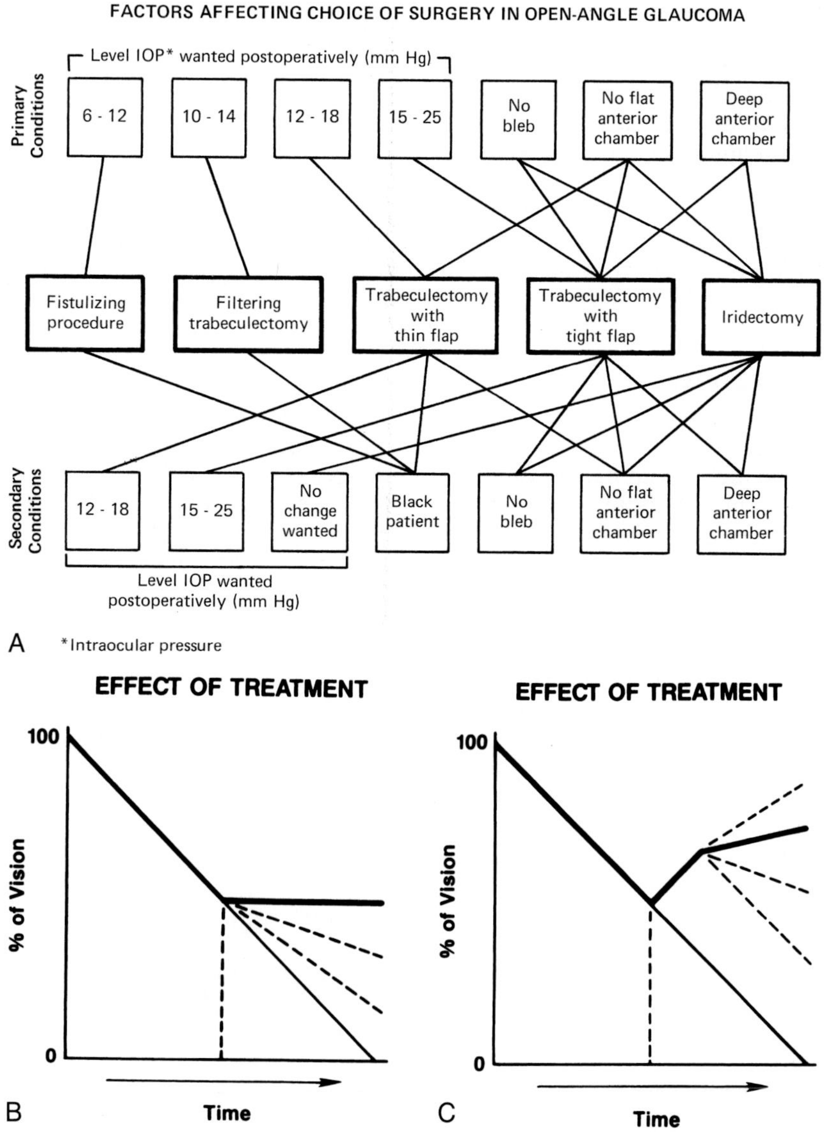

Figure 22–20. *A*. The final goals of the surgery combine with the nature of the case to determine which glaucoma surgical procedure is preferable. For example, if the goals are a postoperative intraocular pressure of around 15 mm Hg, with the least likelihood of a postoperative flat chamber, a guarded filtration procedure with a tight or a thin scleral flap is appropriate; if, on the other hand, the goal is to deepen the anterior chamber and no pressure lowering is required, then an iridectomy is indicated. *B*. Traditional concept of the effect of treatment on the clinical course of glaucoma. Treatment in some cases can make glaucoma worse, can slow the course, or can stabilize the condition, as indicated by the change in the slopes of the graph. *C*. New conception of management of glaucoma based on determination of clinical improvement in response to treatment.

The general approach to the timing of surgery in the patient with primary open-angle glaucoma has been far too aggressive in many patients and far too conservative in even more patients. Many patients will never lose functional damage, even though they have definite glaucoma. Others will rapidly become seriously handicapped. The former group do not deserve the risks of treatment. In the latter group, while we wait for definite signs of deterioration, the patient is getting worse. Especially in the early stages, when cupping can progress without detectable loss of visual field, surgery is too often delayed. When progressive disease is present, that is, when it is known that the patient's optic nerve is worsening because of glaucoma and the patient's anticipated life span is such that it is probable that visual function will be significantly affected, the best choice of treatment is usually surgery (Table 22–14). When the disease has progressed, but it is not known to be actually *progressing*, medical therapy should usually be tried, with the realization that surgery may be needed later. In those patients who have definite glaucoma, but no definite or anticipated loss, medical treatment is preferred initially. When *findings* are abnormal, such as a high intraocular pressure, medical treatment may or may not be appropriate, depending on a variety of factors (Tables 22–5 and 22–13).

PRIMARY ANGLE-CLOSURE GLAUCOMA

Indications for surgery in patients with narrow anterior chamber angles or with primary angle-closure glaucoma are still not entirely clear-cut. The reason for this uncertainty is the inability to accurately predict the future clinical course of these patients. When nerve damage is due to open-angle glaucoma, it is virtually certain that progressive deterioration will continue unless intraocular pressure is adequately lowered. However, there is little precision in prognosticating the future of many patients with narrow or partially closed anterior chamber angles. I present here an approach to the diagnosis and management of such cases that recognizes these uncertainties, but that has proved relatively satisfactory from a clinical point of view. As more knowledge is gained this approach will need revision and perhaps even major change.

The nature of the anterior chamber angle is clearly an important aspect in understanding angle-closure glaucoma. Meaningful examination of the angle by an informed person is essential. The use of gonioscopy must be mastered by anyone who wants to give patients with glaucoma satisfactory care.[61]

Nature of the Anterior Chamber Angle

The advantages of indirect gonioscopy are the remarkable ease and rapidity with which it may be done (once learned), its wide range of magnifications and illuminations, and the ability to perform indentation gonioscopy.[62] These advantages are so overwhelming that I strongly believe that gonioscopy with a lens able to be used to perform indentation gonioscopy is, by far, the examination method of choice.

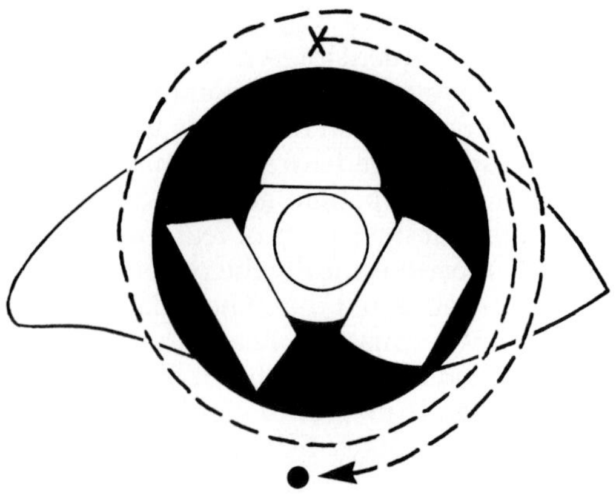

Figure 22–21. Schematic view of the Goldmann three-mirrored lens. Looking into the mirror at 12 o'clock permits good visualization of the angle at 6 o'clock. The mirror is rotated 360 degrees while the angle is viewed through the smallest mirror, permitting visualization of the entire angle.

One of the standard lenses used in indirect gonioscopy is the Goldmann three-mirrored lens. This requires a viscous substance to maintain contact between the surface of the lens and the cornea. The examiner views the angle through the smallest mirror, and rotates the lens so that the entire angle can easily be examined (Fig. 22–21). The Zeiss four-mirror lens, and similar lenses manufactured by Volk and other companies have smaller surfaces with a convexity that more accurately mimics that of the cornea. Tears provide an adequate contact material and lubrication for the lens, greatly facilitating use and eliminating the blurring effect of the viscous gonioscopic fluids (Fig. 22–22). These lenses are difficult to use because the positioning must be precise in order to obtain a satisfactory view. The lens must be held very gently against the corneal surface so that it does not distort the cornea or displace aqueous humor, which would cause distortion of the angle. Firm support for the hand holding the lens is essential. Another problem with the four-mirror lens is the fragmentation

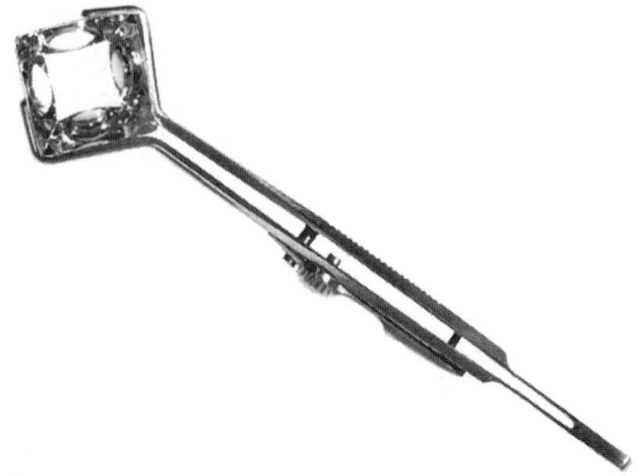

Figure 22–22. The Zeiss four-mirrored goniolens with the Ungen handle.

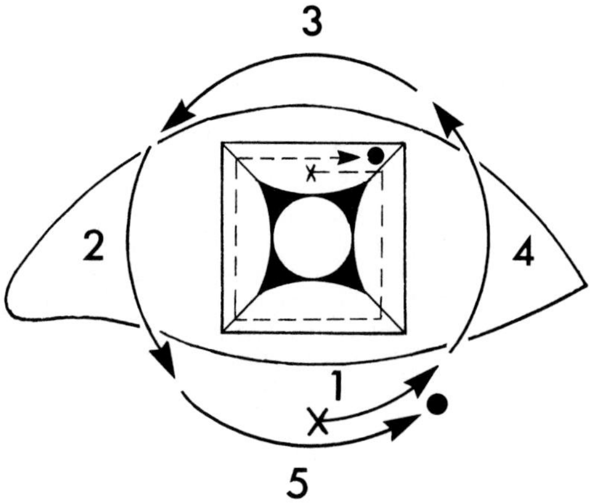

Figure 22–23. Schematic view of the Zeiss four-mirrored lens. When used with the handle shown in Figure 22–22, the mirror is not rotated; rather, the four quadrants of the angle are examined by moving the direction of gaze. If this is done in a regular clockwise manner, a fragmented view of the angle is obtained that must be reconstructed in the mind.

of the view of the angle; the observer must reconstruct the angle panorama in his or her own mind (Fig. 22–23).

The advantages of the four-mirror lens, however, are so great that its use is strongly recommended. Anyone with the dexterity required to perform ophthalmic surgery can certainly master the technique of gonioscopy using a lens such as the Zeiss.

The unique advantage of indirect gonioscopy with a lens having a small area of contact is the ability to perform Forbes' indentation gonioscopy. This is the only in-office method available for the ophthalmologist to distinguish between mere contact of the iris with the cornea and actual adhesion of the iris to the cornea. In this technique the goniolens is placed centrally on the cornea and pushed posteriorly, so that it displaces aqueous into the periphery of the anterior chamber, forcing the iris posteriorly, where it is unsupported by the lens (Fig. 22–24). If the iris is adherent to the cornea, the iris will not fall posteriorly (Fig. 22–24*C*). In contrast, when the iris is not adherent it will be displaced posteriorly, allowing visualization of the deeper angle recess (Fig. 22–24*B*).

Proper evaluation of the configuration of the anterior chamber angle requires the use of at least three descriptors: the point at which the iris is adherent to the cornea or uvea, the depth of the anterior chamber, and the curvature of the peripheral iris.[70] The Wills Eye Hospital system of grading the anterior chamber angle takes into account all three of these attributes, and has proved highly satisfactory.

The most important landmark is the posterior trabecular meshwork (Fig. 22–25). Visibility of this structure is what determines whether an anterior chamber angle is functionally open or closed, as it is through this region that the aqueous humor exits. Peripheral anterior synechiae can develop posterior to the trabecular meshwork, indicating the occurrence of an angle-closure attack. Such synechiae have no functional effect but are a definite sign of disease.

The point of contact between the iris and the inner wall of the globe should be noted (Fig. 22–26). In most eyes the iris is adherent to the anterior ciliary body, permitting visualization of all structures anterior to this. In younger people, especially those with brown eyes and most notably in black patients, the iris may normally insert more anteriorly, so that it is adherent just posterior to the scleral spur (C in Fig. 22–26). In patients with myopia the anterior chamber may be extraordinarily deep and the iris may insert more posteriorly than usual (E in Fig. 22–26). Figure 22–27 shows an eye with secondary angle closure and adherence of the iris anterior to the posterior trabecular meshwork. The angle is optically and functionally closed. Pressure gonioscopy would show that no matter how hard the central cornea is depressed, the iris cannot be displaced posteriorly beyond its current point of contact at the trabecular meshwork (Fig. 22–27).

The angle should also be graded in terms of depth of the anterior chamber. This can be measured directly in millimeters by several techniques. An easier, less exact, but clinically adequate method is to approximate anterior chamber depth in terms of angular approach to the recess (Fig. 22–28).

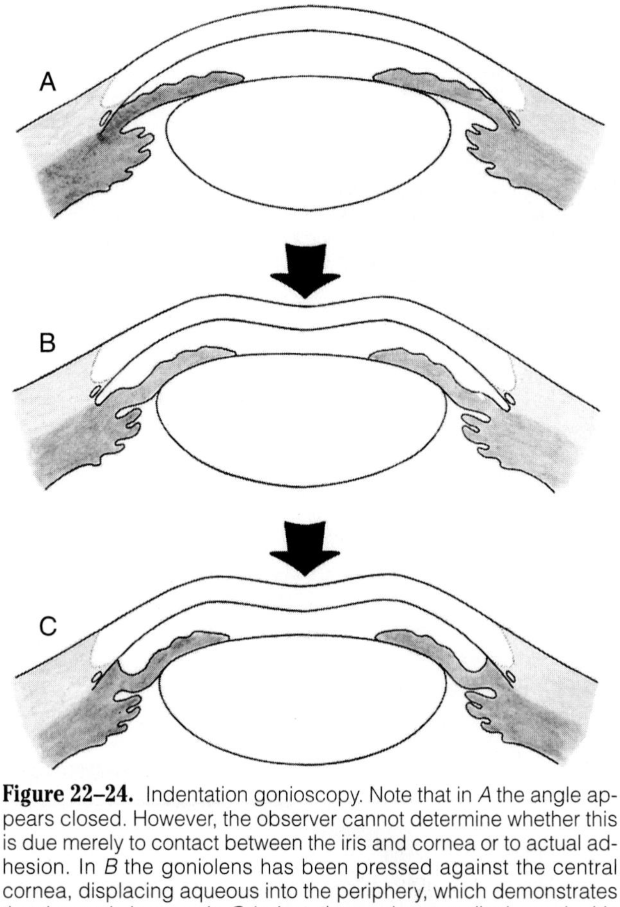

Figure 22–24. Indentation gonioscopy. Note that in *A* the angle appears closed. However, the observer cannot determine whether this is due merely to contact between the iris and cornea or to actual adhesion. In *B* the goniolens has been pressed against the central cornea, displacing aqueous into the periphery, which demonstrates that the angle is open. In *C*, indentation gonioscopy displaces the iris posteriorly, revealing peripheral anterior synechiae. (From Schwartz LW: Diagnostic evaluation of the patient. In Spaeth GL (ed.), Early Primary Open-Angle Glaucoma: Diagnosis and Management. Boston: Little, Brown; 1979:60. © Lippincott Williams & Wilkins, with permission.)

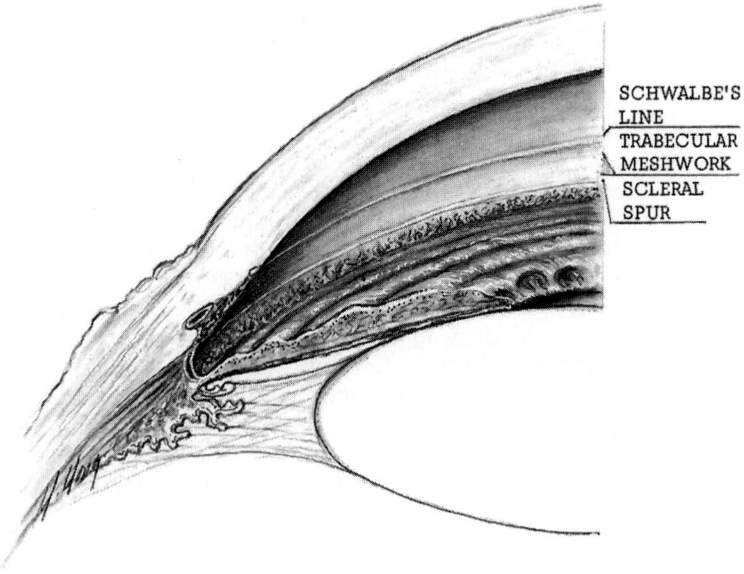

Figure 22–25. Major landmarks of the anterior chamber angle. Iris processes are fairly prominent and reach up to the scleral spur. The trabecular meshwork is not pigmented. Schwalbe's line is prominent. The angle is wide open and normal. (From Spaeth GL: The normal development of the human anterior chamber angle. A new system of descriptive grading. Trans Ophthalmol Soc UK 1971;91:709.)

Figure 22–26. Schematic drawing of five possible locations where the iris may contact the inner portion of the globe. *A* = iris insertion into or anterior to Schwalbe's line (A = anterior); *B* = iris adherent to the globe just anterior to the posterior trabecular meshwork (*B* = behind Schwalbe's line); *C* = iris arising from scleral spur; *D* = iris inserts into the anterior portion of the ciliary body (*D* = deep); *E* = iris arises from posterior portion of the ciliary body (*E* = extremely deep). *A* and *B* insertions are certainly pathologic. *C* insertion may be pathologic or normal. (From Spaeth GL: The normal development of the human anterior chamber angle. A new system of descriptive grading. Trans Ophthalmol Soc UK 1971; 91:709.)

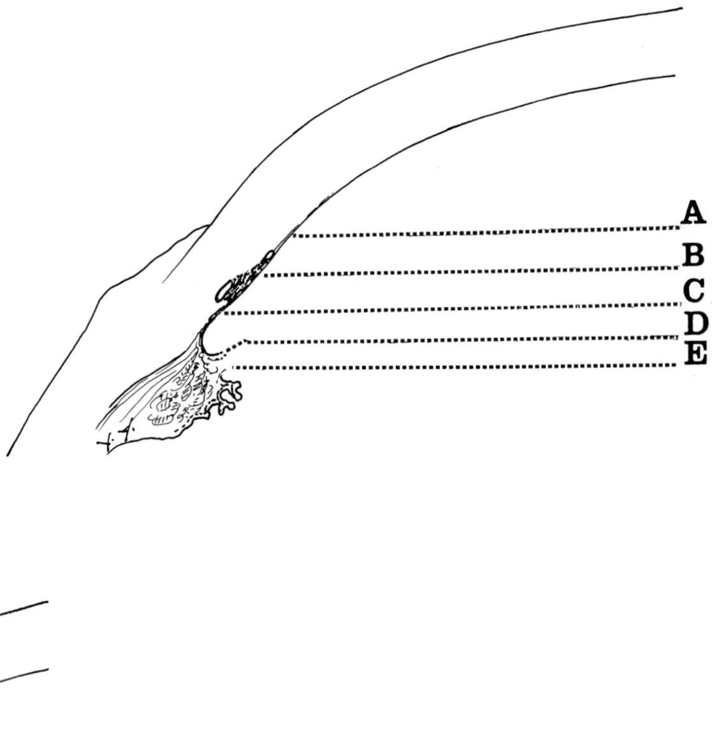

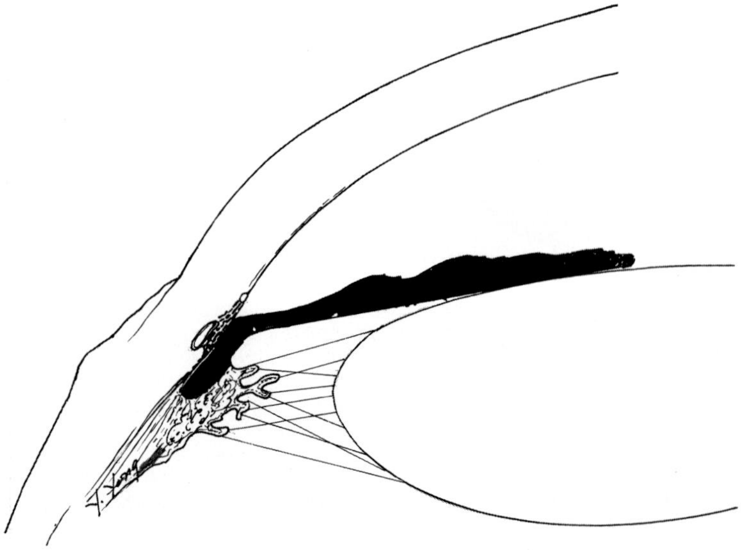

Figure 22–27. Anterior chamber angle with peripheral anterior synechia extending anterior to the posterior trabecular meshwork. This is a B insertion (see Fig. 22–26). (From Spaeth GL: The normal development of the human anterior chamber angle. A new system of descriptive grading. Trans Ophthalmol Soc UK 1971;91:709.)

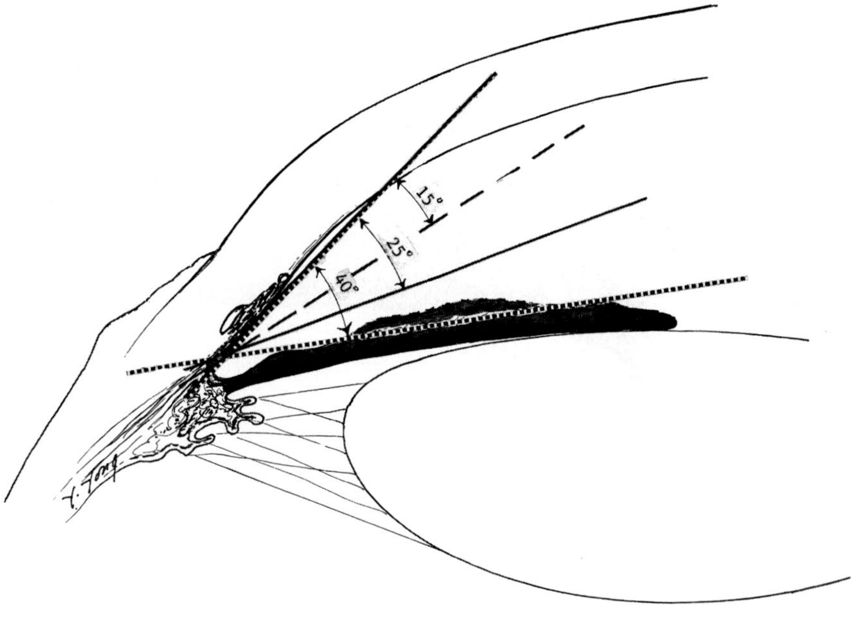

Figure 22–28. The angular width or depth of the anterior chamber recess may be estimated by constructing a tangent to the anterior surface of the iris about one third of the distance from the most peripheral portion of the iris. The angle shown has an approach of about 40 degrees. (From Spaeth GL: The normal development of the human anterior chamber angle. A new system of descriptive grading. Trans Ophthalmol Soc UK 1971; 91:709.)

The third characteristic that needs description is the peripheral curvature of the angle (Fig. 22–29). In most people there is little anterior or posterior curvature; that is, the peripheral iris is flat (f, for flat). In others, especially the elderly, the peripheral iris bends sharply and steeply anteriorly, making the angle recess shallower than one would expect on the basis of the central or even peripheral depth of the chamber. This is the appearance of the "plateau iris." "p" is the denomination for the plateau iris configuration. "p" does not mean "shallow." "p" does not mean that the iris curves convexly anteriorly. "p" refers only to the situation in which there is a sudden *change* in curvature. It is because angles can have a "c" or "p" configuration that the Van Herrick system of grading the angle is not adequate to define the nature of the angle recess itself. The only *sure* way to tell about the nature of the angle recess is to visualize it. In patients with myopia, patients with dislocated lenses, or those with aphakia, the iris falls backward, assuming a q configuration.

Figure 22–30 shows an anterior chamber angle that is clearly narrow; it is probably occludable. Without pressure gonioscopy one cannot see past the curve of peripheral iris to determine whether the iris and cornea are merely close to each other, whether they touch each other (as they do in Fig. 22–24*A*), or whether they are actually adherent (Fig. 22–24*B*). With pressure gonioscopy it is possible to see that the insertion of the iris is at the anterior ciliary body; there are no adhesions. Thus the anterior chamber angle in Figure 22–30 would be graded D-30-p; this is a shorthand way of saying that the angle is open, the anterior chamber depth is average, and there is marked anterior convexity of the iris periphery, making the angle occludable. The angle in

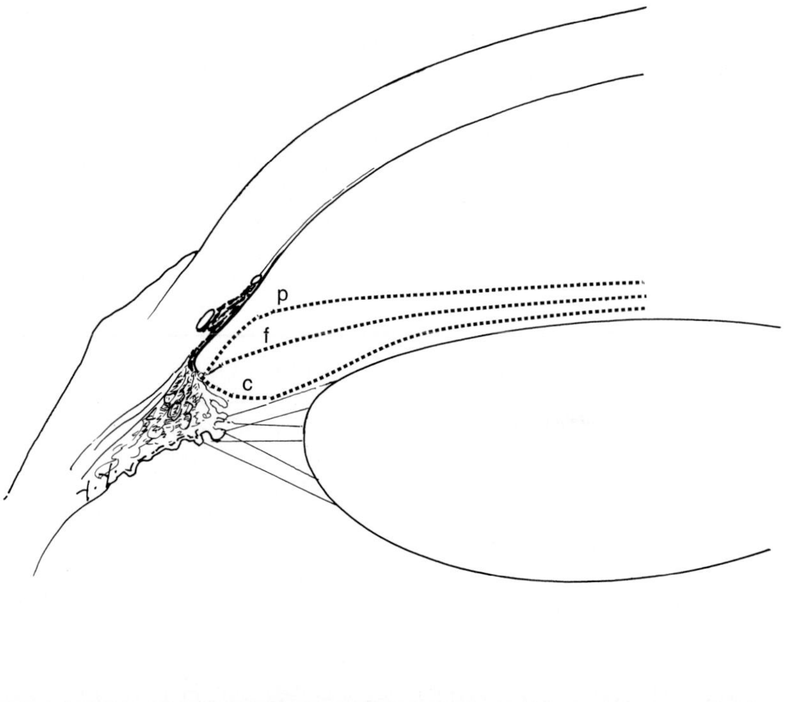

Figure 22–29. Description of the anterior chamber angle must include a comment on the curvature of the peripheral portion of the iris. It may bow steeply anteriorly *(p)*. In a more regular case there is little curvature *(f)*. In cases in which the iris has little support for the lens there may be a c configuration. (From Spaeth GL: The normal development of the human anterior chamber angle. A new system of descriptive grading. Trans Ophthalmol Soc UK 1971;91:709.)

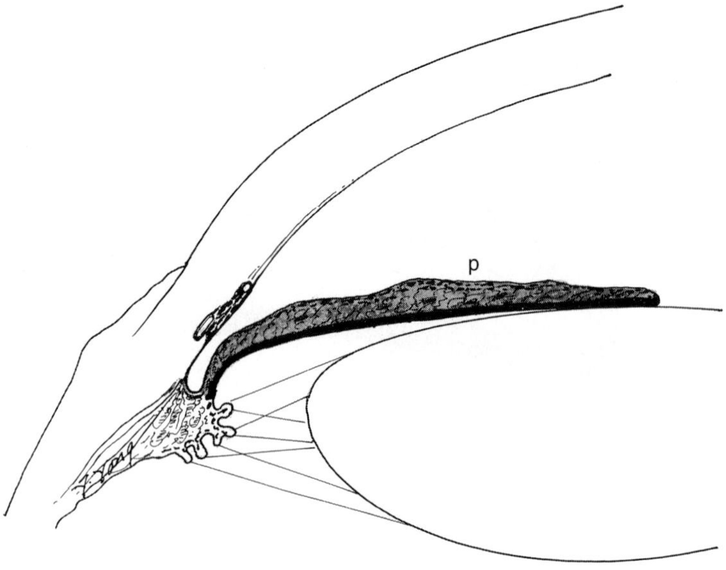

Figure 22–30. The exact nature of this angle would be difficult to determine without pressure gonioscopy. In actuality the angle is open, although the marked p-type of configuration makes visualization of the point at which the iris arises impossible. Pressure gonioscopy permits viewing of the entire angle, which would be graded D-30-p in the Wills Eye Hospital system. (From Spaeth GL: The normal development of the human anterior chamber angle. A new system of descriptive grading. Trans Ophthalmol Soc UK 1971;91: 709.)

Figure 22–27 would be a B-40-f—closed, with a deep chamber and a flat iris.

At the time of gonioscopy other aspects of the angle should be observed in addition to its configuration: such as amount, location, and nature of pigmentation; presence of inflammatory, exfoliated, or other debris; and location of any angle cleavage or cyclodialysis cleft.

History and Symptoms

The ophthalmologist should not treat "glaucoma." He or she should treat "a patient with glaucoma." It is the effect of the disease on the patient, the patient's "disease," that is of concern, not the disease itself. Therefore, because the ophthalmologist learns about the patient through history taking, the history is the single most important part of the evaluation and treatment of the patient with glaucoma.

Accurate diagnosis is important if care is to be satisfactory, and events noted in the patient's history help to establish the correct diagnosis. For example, merely because an eye has suddenly become hard and painful does not mean that the diagnosis is primary angle-closure glaucoma. It could be a sudden onset of a neovascular glaucoma, or final decompensation after chronic angle-closure glaucoma, or an acute episode of a secondary angle-closure glaucoma. Thus, when confronted with a patient with an acute glaucoma, the physician should raise the following questions: Have there been previous attacks? Is there a family history of a similar condition? What was the quality of the vision before the attack? Exactly when did the symptoms begin? What were they? Is there diabetes in the family? Is the patient a diabetic? Was there trauma to the eye? The answers to these and other questions will help the surgeon come to a better understanding of the severity of the condition, the chronicity or acuteness of the glaucoma, and the possibility of causes other than primary angle-closure glaucoma.

Of course it is well known that halos may be a sign of an angle-closure attack. Halos, however, are not diagnostic of raised intraocular pressure, but rather are highly indicative of corneal epithelial edema. Because rapid elevation of intraocular pressure is a common cause for edema of the corneal epithelium, halos do suggest the probability of angle closure and are an indication for careful gonioscopy. The halos that occur with epithelial edema are quite typical. A diffuse, hazy ring surrounds a point source of light. This hazy ring is frequently faintly colored, so that it resembles a rainbow. The halos caused by corneal epithelial edema should be distinguished from the radiating, spoke-like rays of light that are characteristic of cataract or incorrect refraction.

Severe pain in the eye is a frequent accompaniment of any condition in which there is rapid rise of intraocular pressure. It is not the level of intraocular pressure that is responsible for the pain, but the rapidity of the increase. Thus a person can have an intraocular pressure of 80 mm Hg and be asymptomatic, or a pressure of 40 and be in extreme pain. Most patients with angle-closure glaucoma do not have the fulminating attack that many clinicians have come to think of as characteristic of the disease. In fact, primary angle-closure glaucoma is asymptomatic in at least one third of cases; in most of the remainder, the symptoms are mild (Table 22–16). In cases in which episodes of angle-closure are recurrent, they tend to become less and less symptomatic. It is common to see a patient with chronic angle-closure glaucoma who has *no* ocular symptoms, and yet has an intraocular pressure of 40 mm Hg and a cupped optic disc.

Predisposing Factors

People who are predisposed to primary angle-closure glaucoma often have small anterior segments. Thus, by and large, the greater the degree of hyperopia, the greater the likelihood of angle closure. Also, increasing age, and increasing size of the crystalline lens (as in the exfoliation syndrome and with developing cataract) are associated with narrowing of the angle recess and predisposition to angle closure. Certain races have more anterior iris insertions, especially Eskimos, but also Far Eastern Asians and, to a lesser extent, black Africans. The "thinner" the iris (as in blue-eyed elderly individuals) the more likely the attack is to be acute, and the thicker the iris (as in blacks or Asians), the more likely the condition is to be chronic and insidious.

Physical findings may be prominent or almost normal in the primary angle-closure glaucomas. Elevations of intraocular pressure may be mild and transient, so that when the patient is seen in a doctor's office the eyes appear normal (although in fact they are not). Gonioscopy reveals an anterior chamber angle that was narrow enough to occlude spontaneously, or that perhaps already contained peripheral anterior synechiae. Because most primary angle-closure cases are of the intermittent or chronic variety, it is more common for the eye of a patient with primary angle-closure glaucoma to appear grossly normal most of the time than for signs to be obvious.

In the case of acute fulminating primary angle-closure glaucoma, physical findings are conspicuous: the patient is obviously having pain, the eye is bright red, the cornea is hazy, and the pupil is dilated and fixed (Table 22–17). Should the intraocular pressure spontaneously fall to normal, which is not rare, the eye will retain the signs of acute congestion and the cornea may become thicker and more edematous, but the intraocular pressure will be normal. To the inexperienced physician this may present a confusing picture (Table 22–17).

The signs of recurrent or mild attacks are quite different (Table 22–17).

TABLE 22–16. Symptoms of Primary Angle-Closure Glaucoma* and Predisposing Factors

Symptoms	Frequency of Symptom
No symptoms	One third of cases
Occasional headache	One half of cases
Episodes of smoky vision	One fourth of cases
Episodes of eyeache	Occasional
Attacks of severe pain associated with visual loss	Occasional
Episodes of visual loss	Rare
Awareness of loss of field	Rare
Predisposing Factors	
Small anterior segment	
Nanophthalmos	
Hyperopia	
Positive family history	
Elderly	
Male gender	
Far Eastern Asian origin	
Black African origin	
Increasing size of lens	
Triggering event†	

*Includes any conditions that cause sudden elevation of intraocular pressure, especially those that are recurrent: e.g., acute primary angle-closure glaucoma, chronic primary angle-closure glaucoma, uveitic glaucoma, the Posner-Schlossman syndrome.

†Anxiety, stress, or any cause for pupillary dilatation.

TABLE 22–17. Signs of Primary Angle-Closure Glaucoma*

Sign	Frequency
At Time of Acute Attack	
High intraocular pressure (above 40 mm Hg)	Always
Closed anterior chamber angle	Always
Signs that patient is having pain	Usual
Reduced vision	Usual
Red eye	Usual
Corneal epithelial edema	Usual
Dilated pupil	Usual
Abnormal optic disc	
Hyperemic and edematous	Usual
Blanched	Rare
Retinal hemorrhages	Common
One Day After Acute Attack Has Abated	
Low intraocular pressure (below 20 mm Hg)	Usual
Occludable anterior chamber angle	Always
Red eye	Often
Corneal epithelial edema	Occasional
Corneal thickening	Usual
Anterior uveitis	Usual
Oval, less reactive pupil	Usual
Anterior capsular lens opacity	Usual
Disc hyperemia and edema	Usual
Two Months or More After Acute Attack	
Normal intraocular pressure	Usual
Occludable anterior chamber angle	Always
Peripheral anterior synechiae	Often
Pupil irregularity	Usual
Localized iris atrophy	Frequent
Flat pallor of the disc	Often
Increased pigmentation of posterior trabecular meshwork	Often
Peripheral visual field contraction	Often
At Time of Recurrent, Mildly Symptomatic, or Asymptomatic Attack	
High intraocular pressure (above 30 mm Hg)	Always
Closed anterior chamber angle	Always
Peripheral anterior synechiae	Often
Pupillary irregularity	Usual
Corneal epithelial edema	Occasional
Cupped optic nerve	Often
Iris atrophy	Occasional
Glaukomflecken	Occasional
Between Episodes of Recurrent Angle Closure	
Mild elevation of intraocular pressure (20–40 mm Hg)	Usual
Occludable anterior chamber angle	Always
Peripheral anterior synechiae	Often
Pupillary irregularities	Usual
Optic nerve cupping	Often
Iris atrophy	Occasional

*Includes other causes for acute or intermittent elevation of intraocular pressure. If the cornea is hazy, anhydrous glycerin should be instilled topically so that the angle and the fundus can be examined adequately.

It is important to examine the fundus at the time the patient is first seen. The cornea can usually be cleared by instillation of topical anhydrous glycerin. Some patients will be treated with miotics after the attack and not come to iridectomy; there will be an understandable reluctance to dilate the pupil in these cases after the attack has quieted. The physician usually has the best chance to examine the fundus, then, at the time the patient is first seen.

Mechanisms of Angle Closure

There appear to be five mechanisms by which angle closure develops: (1) pupillary block, (2) angle jamming, (3) anterior displacement of the iris, (4) aqueous misdirection, and (5) blocking tissue (Table 22–18). Pupillary block is the mechanism in the overwhelming majority of cases of primary angle-closure glaucoma. It is enhanced by atrophy and flaccidity of the iris in the elderly, allowing the higher pressure in the posterior chamber to bulge the periphery of the iris anteriorly, which leads to angle closure. Factors such as partial dilatation of the pupil and anterior position of the lens increase the degree of pupillary block and predispose to the development of primary angle closure (Fig. 22–31*A* and *B*). Other causes of aqueous obstruction at the plane of the iris lead to secondary angle-closure glaucoma (Fig. 22–31*C* and *D*).

Wide dilatation of the pupil may jam the iris into the angle even in cases in which pupillary block does not play a role (Fig. 22–32). This is most frequently seen in patients with anterior insertion of the iris or a plateau iris (C insertion or S configuration).

Ocular inflammation can cause the ciliary body to swell, with consequent rotation of the root of the iris anteriorly (Fig. 22–33). The inflamed tissue under such circumstances is more likely to be sticky, predisposing to the adherence of the tissue should swelling be so marked that angle closure actually develops. Anterior displacement of the peripheral iris may also occur in other conditions that move the ciliary body anteriorly: the use of miotics, ciliary body or choroidal "detachment," interference with outflow of the vortex veins, and compression of the globe by a tumor or encircling band. A central retinal vein occlusion can also lead to shallowing of the anterior chamber.

In some instances the anterior surface of the iris is pulled anteriorly into the angle, covering the recess. This occurs in neovascular glaucoma, in which neovascular membrane "zippers up" the angle (Fig. 22–34). In the iris atrophy group of glaucomas, all of which appear to have secondary angle closure as the cause for pressure elevation, a similar mechanism is at work.

Each of the three types of angle closure must be treated differently. Pupillary block is cured by creating a communication between the anterior and posterior chambers (Fig. 22–35*A* and *B*); angle jamming is corrected by contracting the pupil; and ciliary body swelling is relieved by suppressing the inflammation or eliminating the mechanical cause for the anterior displacement of the iris diaphragm.

TABLE 22–18. Classification and Therapy of Glaucomas in Which Narrowness or Closure of the Angle is a Factor

Type of Glaucoma	Therapy
Pupillary Block	
Narrow, occludable, but open angle	Nd:YAG laser iridotomy
Primary angle-closure glaucoma	
Acute	Medicines to lower intraocular pressure; Nd:YAG laser iridotomy
Chronic	Nd:YAG laser iridotomy with medications or guarded filtration procedure
Fellow eye of patient with angle-closure glaucoma in other eye	Nd:YAG laser iridotomy
Secondary pupillary block	Nd:YAG laser iridotomy or surgical iridectomy
Plateau Iris Glaucoma (angle jamming)	
	Pilocarpine or argon laser iridoplasty
Anterior Displacement of Iris	
Miotic-induced	Stop miotic and give cycloplegic
Ciliary body swelling	Steroids
Compression	
Scleral band	Cut band
Tumor	Irradiation or other antitumor therapy
Secondary Angle-Closure Glaucomas (other than those above)	
Malignant glaucoma	Atropine, phenylephrine, acetazolamide; rupture of hyaloid face, vitrectomy or lensectomy if needed
Tumor	Irradiation or enucleation
Neovascular	Panretinal photocoagulation, atropine, steroids, and later guarded filtration procedure if eye quiets; tube-shunt procedure if good visual potential, or, rarely, cyclophotocoagulation

Provocative Tests

The anterior chamber becomes shallower with increasing age. About 10% of people over 80 years of age have anterior chamber angles that appear narrow enough to occlude.[32] However, angle-closure glaucoma is an uncommon disease in Caucasians; certainly 10% of people over 80 years of age do not develop it. The ophthalmologist is thus left with a dilemma; how can one distinguish between the eye (with a narrow anterior chamber angle) that is going to proceed to angle closure and the eye (that has a similar narrow anterior chamber angle) that will *not* develop angle-closure glaucoma? A variety

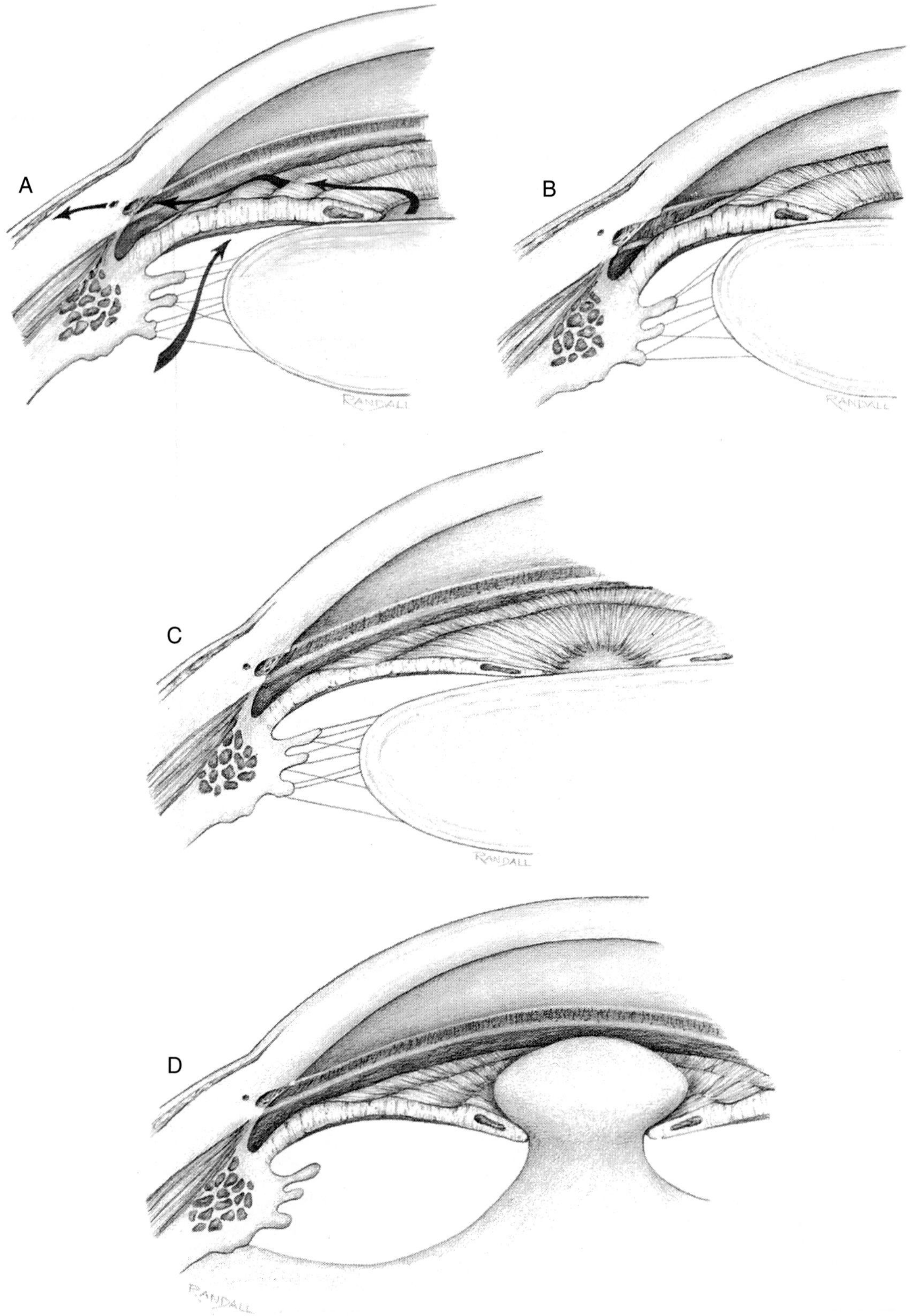

Figure 22–31. *A.* Normal, wide-open anterior chamber angle showing direction of flow of aqueous humor. This angle would be graded D-40-f in the Wills Eye Hospital system. *B.* A slightly narrow but open anterior chamber angle (D-20-p). *C.* There is anterior bowing of the periphery of the iris caused by posterior synechiae between the pupillary margin and the anterior surface of the lens. The anterior chamber is deep, but there is an iris bombé (D-30-p). *D.* Pupillary block may also be induced by constriction of the pupil around a knuckle of vitreous.

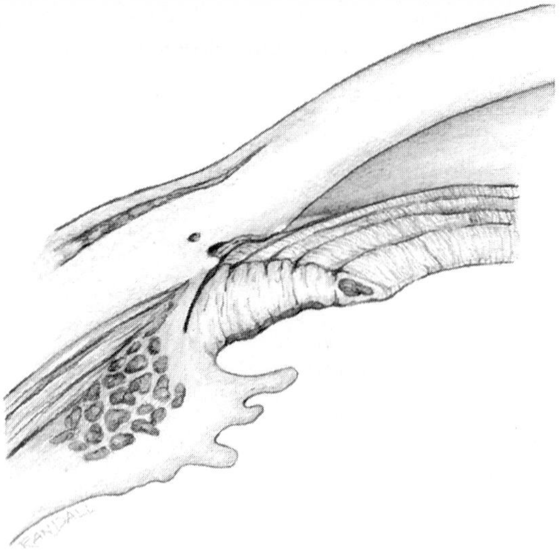

Figure 22–32. Wide dilatation of the pupil may cause the iris to become jammed into the angle recess in a predisposed patient. This is not a common mechanism for angle closure. It is more common in those with an anteriorly inserted iris root and those with a flaccid iris.

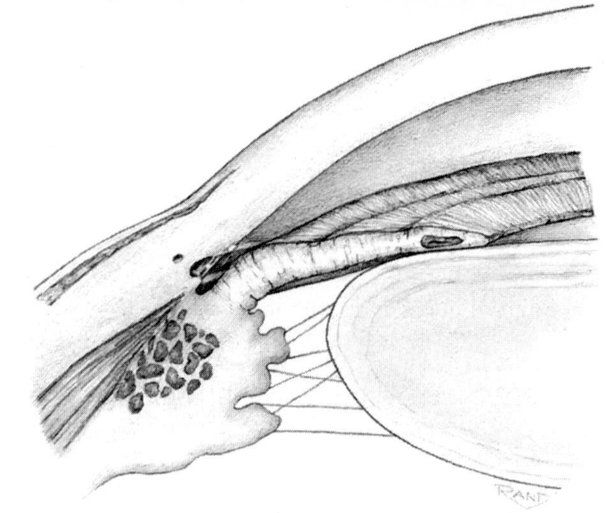

Figure 22–33. Inflammation of the ciliary body and the root of the iris may cause the iris to rotate anteriorly toward the angle recess, predisposing to peripheral anterior synechia and a secondary angle-closure glaucoma.

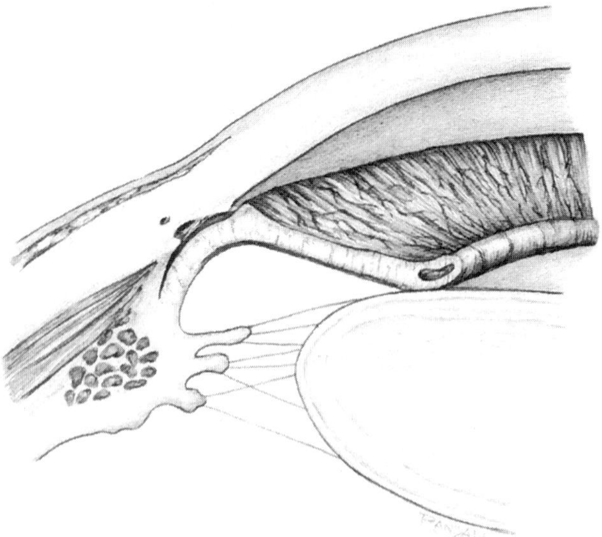

Figure 22–34. Neovascularization of the iris and angle recess often leads to broad-based peripheral anterior synechiae that completely close the anterior chamber angle.

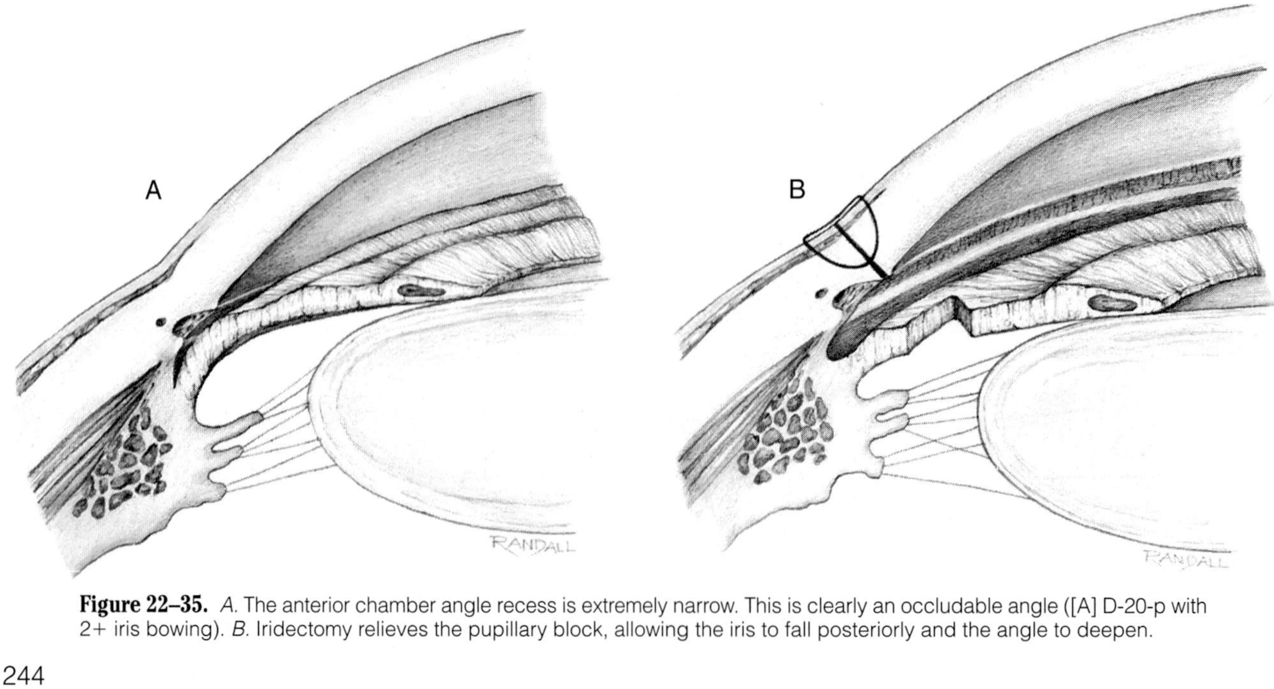

Figure 22–35. *A.* The anterior chamber angle recess is extremely narrow. This is clearly an occludable angle ([A] D-20-p with 2+ iris bowing). *B.* Iridectomy relieves the pupillary block, allowing the iris to fall posteriorly and the angle to deepen.

of "provocative tests" have been developed in an effort to answer this question. Unfortunately, with the exception of the darkroom test, they are of little or no value.

The fact that one can cause intraocular pressure to rise and the angle to close in response to instillation of a cycloplegic or a mydriatic agent does not provide the ophthalmologist with information of much value, for the changes that occur spontaneously in the eye are not mimicked by those caused by cycloplegics or mydriatics. Cyclopegics not only dilate the pupil but also cause a deepening of the anterior chamber (the opposite of the case shown in Figure 22–33). Thus false-negative results are common; that is, that the angle does not close or the intraocular pressure rise in response to dilatation of the pupil by a cycloplegic agent cannot be taken as an indication that a person with a narrow anterior chamber angle will not spontaneously develop an angle-closure glaucoma. Nor does a rise in pressure secondary to use of a cycloplegic signal angle closure; cycloplegics cause increased pressure by interfering with aqueous outflow even in wide-open angles. In a patient with unstable open-angle glaucoma, cycloplegics can induce a pressure increase of 20 mm Hg or more *without* causing angle closure. Thus a rise in intraocular pressure in response to administration of a cycloplegic such as tropicamide (Mydriacyl) is *not* proof of angle closure (false-positive test).

Nor does the instillation of a mydriatic agent such as phenylephrine mimic normal physiology. Under normal circumstances, when the dilator muscle of the iris contracts, the sphincter muscle relaxes, permitting dilatation of the pupil. However, when a mydriatic agent is instilled the dilator muscle is stimulated to contract at the same time that the sphincter muscle is still contracting; this causes an increase in the degree of pupillary block and, consequently, predisposes the subject to angle-closure glaucoma (Fig. 22–36). Thus, although it is clear that one can induce angle-closure glaucoma by dilating the pupil with a mydriatic agent, such an occurrence does not mimic an episode of spontaneous angle-closure glaucoma. In addition, most mydriatic agents cause such wide dilatation of the pupil that they induce a second mechanism of angle closure, specifically angle jamming (Fig. 22–32). Such extreme dilatation of the pupil is rare in a physiological setting.

Classification

The mechanisms of angle-closure glaucoma have been discussed. Classification can be helpful in deciding on a logical therapeutic approach; both are given in Table 22–18.

Treatment

A plan of management is shown in Table 22–19. The initial step in treatment is diagnosis. The next consideration is the urgency of treatment. Important factors are (a) the absolute level of intraocular pressure; (b) the rapidity with which the intraocular pressure has risen; (c) additional considerations that describe the health of the eye itself, such as degree of inflammation, appearance of the optic disc, and state of the retinal vessels; and (d) the general condition of the patient.

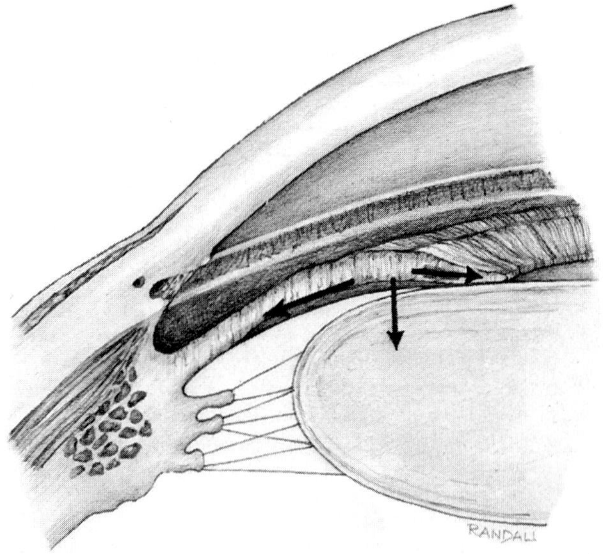

Figure 22–36. The arrow pointing to the right indicates the direction of pull of the iris sphincter; the arrow pointing to the left is the direction of force exerted by the iris dilator. The resultant vector of force is posterior. Thus simultaneous stimulation of the dilator and the sphincter muscle causes the iris to be apposed more tightly against the anterior surface of the lens.

If the intraocular pressure exceeds the systolic pressure in the arteries that supply the retina, blindness can develop in minutes. As systolic pressure in the central retinal artery is often around 70 mm Hg, intraocular pressures above this constitute a dire emergency. If the retinal arteries are collapsed and the disc is pale, the pressure must be lowered immediately. If the retinal vessels pulsate, indicating that the pressure is between the diastolic and the systolic levels, then there is more urgency than if the retinal vessels appear unaffected. If the disc shows advanced glaucomatous cupping, it is unlikely that the eye will tolerate pressure as satisfactorily as it would if the disc were healthy.

If treatment is urgent, such as in the eye with an intraocular pressure of 80 mm Hg and collapsed retinal arteries, a paracentesis may be performed. This is rarely appropriate in a patient with primary angle-closure glaucoma. When intraocular pressure is in the 60–80 mm Hg range, the approach is to administer eyedrops (topical beta-blockers, topical pilocarpine 1%–2%, and a topical alpha-agonist plus a topical steroid) and to give acetazolamide 500 mg intravenously (see Table 22–18). All of the eyedrops are instilled twice, about 5 minutes apart. Intraocular pressure should be checked 30 to 60 minutes later, and if pressure has not already started to fall markedly, an osmotic agent should be given. If the patient has a history of prostatic or cardiovascular disease, the treatment of choice is glycerol, 1 ml/kg of body weight. If the patient is nauseated or already in the hospital, or if it is convenient to administer medications intravenously, mannitol 20% in an IV drip (7 ml/kg body weight) is appropriate. The infusion should be completed within 45 to 60 minutes.

TABLE 22–19. Treatment Algorithm for Primary Angle-Closure Glaucoma

Diagnose Correctly

1. Primary relative pupillary block (vs. secondary angle-closures)
   a. Chamber depth should be shallow and symmetrical in the two eyes
   b. No neovascularization of the iris or angle
   c. A or (A) angle iris insertion
   d. Angle of fellow eye should be occludable
2. Acute
   a. No peripheral anterior synechiae
   b. No optic nerve cupping
   c. No edema present—epithelial edema when intraocular pressure elevated; stromal edema when intraocular pressure low
3. Chronic
   a. Peripheral anterior synechiae present
   b. Optic nerve cupping present and usually asymmetric

Decide on Urgency of Treatment*

1. Extremely urgent
   a. Intraocular pressure over 80 mm Hg
   b. Retinal arteries blanched
   c. Severe pain
2. Urgent
   a. Intraocular pressure 60–80 mm Hg
   b. Retinal artery pulsations or cupped optic nerve
   c. Often severe pain
3. Moderately urgent
   a. Intraocular pressure 40–60 mm Hg
   b. Questionable cupping of optic nerve
   c. Moderate pain
4. Little urgency
   a. Intraocular pressure <40 mm Hg
   b. Cornea clear
   c. No cupping
   d. No pain

Treatment

1. Extremely urgent
   a. On day of attack—immediately
      - Consider paracentesis
      - Administer topical beta-blocker and steroid; give intravenous acetazolamide (500 cc for 70 kg adult); (repeat all drops 5 minutes later: pilocarpine, beta-blocker, alpha-agonist, and topical corticosteroid)
      - Give intravenous mannitol 25% as intravenous push 50 mL
   b. 1 hour post-attack
      - If intraocular pressure not 20 mm Hg lower
        –Repeat medications
        –Clear cornea with glycerine and attempt Nd:YAG peripheral iridotomy or argon iridoplasty
      - If intraocular pressure has fallen more than 20 mm Hg
        –Recheck in 1 hour
   c. 2 hours post-attack
      - If intraocular pressure has not fallen 20 mm Hg
        –Prepare patient for surgical iridotomy or guarded filtration procedure
      - If intraocular pressure has fallen to 40 mm Hg
        –Recheck in 1 hour
   d. 3 hours post-attack
      - If intraocular pressure rising
        –Treat as at 2 hours post-attack
      - If intraocular pressure falling further
        –Recheck in 1 hour
   e. 4 hours post-attack
      - If intraocular pressure rising
        –Admit for intravenous mannitol and surgery
      - If intraocular pressure lower than the intraocular pressure in the other eye
        –Consider the attack broken and discharge patient on oral carbonic anhydrous inhibitors, topical beta-blockers, alpha-agonists, and steroids
        –See patient next day

If after 2 hours intraocular pressure has still not fallen, administration of the medication should be repeated and preparation of the patient for surgery considered (Table 22–19). If the cornea is clear, a neodymium:YAG iridotomy can be attempted. If that fails, an argon laser iridoplasty is appropriate to try. If after another hour or two the intraocular pressure is still elevated, a surgical iridectomy or guarded filtration procedure is usually necessary.

In cases of less urgency, such as when the eye is painful and inflamed but the intraocular pressure is only 40 mm Hg, it is probably adequate to administer a topical beta-blocker, carbonic anhydrase inhibitor, alpha-agonist, pilocarpine, and topical steroid and monitor the effect. If the pressure has not fallen within an hour, oral acetazolamide may need to be used as well.

When there are signs that an angle-closure attack has occurred but the intraocular pressure has fallen, treatment needs to be directed at maintaining a small pupil and eliminating inflammation. Thus topical steroids and weak pilocarpine are the agents of choice.

The next decision involves what type of surgery needs to be done. The factors affecting this decision include the level of intraocular pressure achieved with medical treatment, the percentage of the anterior chamber angle involved with peripheral anterior synechiae, the response of the angle to the administration of pilocarpine, the status of the disc and visual field, the patient's ease of access to medical care, the personality and life expectancy of the patient, and the wishes of the patient. A semiquantitative schema call help put these factors into perspective (Fig. 22–37*A*).

In the simplest terms, three major considerations need to be considered: (1) the possible risk to the patient's eye should another attack occur, (2) the psychological anxiety that is an inevitable component of

TABLE 22–19. Treatment Algorithm for Primary Angle-Closure Glaucoma *(Continued)*

f. Day 1 post-attack
- Perform Nd:YAG laser peripheral iridotomy on fellow eye.
- If intraocular pressure in the involved eye below 15 mm Hg
  - –Stop oral carbonic anhydrous inhibitor
  - –Continue beta-blockers and steroids.
- If intraocular pressure above 15 mm Hg
  - –Attack probably is not broken
  - –Continue all medications and recheck next day
- If intraocular pressure over 40 mm Hg
  - –Treat as at time of initial attack
  - –Plan to proceed with guarded filtration procedure if disc cupped
  - –Proceed with peripheral iridotomy if disc normal

2. Urgent
   a. Treat as for "Extremely urgent," but do not consider paracentesis.
3. Moderately urgent
   a. Treat as per urgent, except allow more time before deciding to proceed with laser iridotomy on the involved eye. It is better to allow the eye to become quiet, the iris less congested, and the cornea clearer before proceeding. Also, allow more time before deciding to proceed with surgical peripheral iridectomy or guarded filtration procedure if those options appear necessary.
4. Little urgency
   a. 1 hour day post-attack—initial R_x
   - Administer topical pilocarpine 1% or 2%, beta-blocker, alpha-agonist, and carbonic anhydrous inhibitor.
   - Repeat all four drops 5 minutes later.
   - If intraocular pressure less than 20 mm Hg, watch carefully.
   - If intraocular pressure above 20 mm Hg, repeat drops once.

   b. 2 hours post-attack
   - If intraocular pressure below intraocular pressure of other eye
     - –Consider attack broken
     - –Discharge patient on topical beta-blockers and carbonic anhydrous inhibitors
     - –Prescribe steroids 4 times daily if eye inflamed.

   c. Day 1 post-attack
   - Check intraocular pressure, angle, and disc in both eyes
   - If intraocular pressure less than 20 mm Hg and cornea clear and pupil small
     - –Perform peripheral iridotomy in involved eye
   - If intraocular pressure 20–40 mm Hg or pupil large or cornea not clear
     - –Perform peripheral iridotomy in fellow eye
     - –Increase treatment to use topical beta-blockers, alpha-agonists, carbonic anhydrous inhibitors
     - –Consider performing iridoplasty in involved eye

   d. Day 2 post-attack
   - If intraocular pressure below 20 mm Hg
     - –Perform peripheral iridotomy in fellow eye
     - –Reduce medications to topical beta-blocker and steroids if needed in involved eye.
   - If intraocular pressure above 20 mm Hg
     - –Attempt peripheral iridotomy; if unsuccessful, perform iridoplasty in involved eye

   e. Day 4 post-attack
   - If intraocular pressure below 20 mm Hg
     - –Stop topical steroids and perform peripheral iridotomy if not already done in involved eye
   - If intraocular pressure above 20 mm Hg
     - –Patient will probably need surgical peripheral iridotomy or guarded filtration procedure.

*The clarity of the cornea and the degree of pain are indicators of the rapidity with which the attack has occurred. The greater the corneal edema and pain, the more acute the attack. When there is no edema or pain, the intraocular pressure has been elevated before or for at least 1 week. When intraocular pressure falls, the cornea usually becomes more edematous. The degree of optic nerve damage is a rough measure of the chronicity and severity of previous attacks. The amount of nerve damage in each eye should be compared in this regard.

knowing that a subsequent attack can occur, and (3) the cost, inconvenience, and risk of the surgery itself.

A variety of studies suggest that approximately 50% of patients having had an attack of primary angle-closure glaucoma in one eye will have an attack in the other eye within 5 years.[63,64] The damage that may be caused by the attack of primary angle-closure glaucoma should be recalled. Peripheral anterior synechiae develop in most eyes in which an angle-closure attack persists for longer than 3 days. Of more concern, however, is the development of cataract and the damage to the optic nerve that may occur. If the pressure elevation is extreme and the rise rapid, the attack can leave a previously normal eye with little or no visual function. It is my clinical impression that recovery of vision after most attacks of acute angle-closure glaucoma is seldom complete. Considering these matters together allows us to conclude that approximately 50% of patients who have had an attack of acute primary angle-closure glaucoma in one eye can expect to lose a significant amount of vision in the other eye within the next 5 years, unless intervention is effective.

Another factor is the psychological effect of knowing that sight might be lost at any time. Although some patients handle this uncertainty with equanimity, others are incapacitated by the anxiety. The extent of the psychological damage to patients faced with such a terrible prospect is difficult to evaluate, and it may be overlooked by ophthalmologists, who tend to be more deeply involved with the health of their patients' eyes than with the health of the entire patient.

Finally, it should be kept in mind that the risks of surgery are far less than the risk of an attack of acute glaucoma.

In conclusion, then, surgery on the involved eye is usually indicated in patients who have had an attack of acute primary angle-closure glaucoma. Similarly, the patient should also have surgery on the fellow eye as well.

A	**Iridotomy Preferred** ◄	———	► **Iridotomy Deferred**
History indicative of angle-closure glaucoma	Definite		Questionable
Narrowness of anterior chamber angle	Adhesions present	Occludable	Narrow but ? occludable
Life expectancy	>20 years		<5 years
Ease of access to treatment	Difficult		Easy
Likelihood patient will care for himself well	Poor		Excellent
Response to pilocarpine	Angle and anterior chamber become shallow	No change	Angle definitely deepens

B	**Trabeculectomy Preferred** ◄	———	► **Iridotomy Preferred**
Extent of damage to optic nerve (disc/field)	Advanced	Mild	None
Intraocular pressure on therapy	>40 mmHg		≤15 mmHg
Degrees angle closed by adhesions (anterior to trabecular meshwork)	360°		0°
Anticipated quality of follow-up care	Poor		Excellent

Figure 22–37. *A.* Factors that determine the choice of treatment in patients with narrow anterior chamber angles. *B.* Factors that affect whether the guarded filtration technique or iridectomy should be performed in patients with primary angle-closure glaucoma.

There are a few specific situations in which surgery appears to be either unnecessary or, at best, avoided. For example, in the patient who has had a devastating attack with massive iris atrophy as the result, a peripheral iridectomy may not be necessary because the degree of atrophy may permit adequate communication between the posterior and the anterior chambers. If, after the attack, the pressure rapidly falls to normal and gonioscopy shows that the anterior chamber deepens remarkably in response to pilocarpine 1% twice daily, then the urgency for surgery decreases. In such a patient, should there be extenuating circumstances such as a morbid fear of surgery or far advanced visual field loss, then probably medical treatment is preferable. If one is considering surgery on the second eye, the experience on the first eye can be a valuable guide. If a significant complication occurred during the first procedure, and the cause could not be determined in order to prevent its occurring during a second operation, the surgeon must expect a similar complication to develop in the second eye.

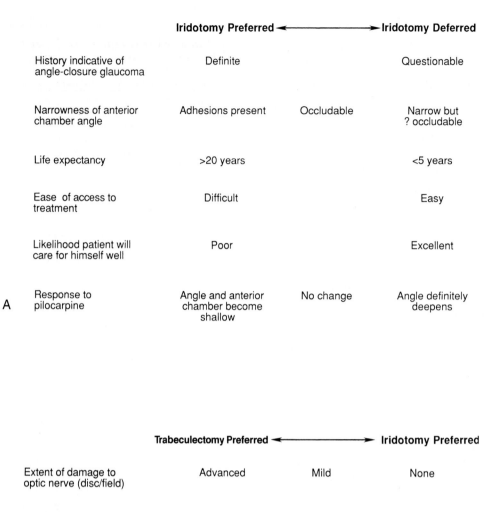

The choice of procedure is the next decision. Unless the angle appears to be totally closed with adhesions *and* the optic nerve is already damaged, the treatment of choice in the involved eye is always an Nd:YAG iridotomy. In the fellow eye the preferred treatment is also virtually always an Nd:YAG iridotomy. If significant optic nerve damage has already occurred, or if the angle closure is greater than 50% and it is not likely that the patient will be able to be followed closely, then a guarded filtration procedure with a very tightly sutured scleral flap is appropriate. Atropine and phenylephrine need to be used postoperatively in such cases and the sutures gradually released over 1- to 2-week period, which will minimize the likelihood of flat anterior chamber and malignant glaucoma. If the intraocular pressure does not fall, the optic nerve shows no signs of glaucoma damage, and the laser iridotomy and iridoplasty are unsuccessful, then a surgical iridectomy is appropriate. This is best done through clear cornea. The anterior chamber is reformed and a goniosynechiolysis considered if the peripheral chamber does not become deeper at the time of surgery. Other factors that enter into the choice of surgery are the nature of the patient, the quality of follow-up care, the access to care, and the response to medical treatment.

In summary, if the anterior chamber angle is believed to be occludable, or if there are signs of previous occlusion of the anterior chamber angle, an Nd:YAG laser iridotomy is usually the treatment of choice. There are special reasons to try to avoid surgery that opens the eye, as indicated in Table 22–20. If the patient has a narrow anterior chamber angle with an elevated intraocular pressure and no optic nerve damage, then the usual treatment is an Nd:YAG peripheral iridotomy. If optic nerve damage is present, the usual treatment is a guarded filtration procedure or tightly sutured scleral flap. Angle-closure glaucoma is a serious disease with devastating short-term and long-term effects, but with proper treatment, most patients do well.

GLAUCOMA IN INFANTS

Glaucoma occurs only rarely in infants.[65] It will be dealt with here only briefly. The surgery and long-term management of glaucoma in infants is best accomplished in referral centers that have specialized facilities and personnel. Correct diagnosis is vital. None of the common diagnostic findings is, by itself, pathognomonic. The differential diagnosis of the most common symptoms and signs is given in Table 22–21. Despite the rarity of congenital glaucoma, infants with tearing and photophobia and cloudy or large eyes should be assumed to have congenital glaucoma, and the appropriate diagnostic tests should be undertaken promptly.

TABLE 22-20. Special Indications for Trying to Avoid Surgery that Opens the Eye

Active external infection
Bleeding disorder (argon pretreatment)
Predisposition to malignant glaucoma
Complication at time of previous surgery
Nanophthalmos

TABLE 22-21. Glaucoma in Infants: Differential Diagnosis of Signs and Symptoms

Elevated Intraocular Pressure
Spurious determination, owing to squeezing, ketamine, etc.
Corneal Enlargement
Megalocornea
Corneal Haziness
Trauma
Mesodermal dysgenesis
Keratitis
Congenital hereditary corneal edema
Congenital dystrophy of the cornea
Cystinosis
Familial plasma lecithin–cholesterol acyl transferase deficiency
Generalized gangliosidosis
Glycogenoses
Hurler's syndrome
Ichthyosis
Maroteaux-Lamy syndrome
Morquio's syndrome
Mucolipidosis
Osteogenesis imperfecta
Scheie's syndrome
Trisomy 18
Photophobia
Albinism
Cone dysfunction syndrome
Cystinosis
Down's syndrome
Keratosis follicularis spinulosa decalvans
Lowe's syndrome
Menke's disease
Phenylketonuria
Porphyria
Tryptophanemia
Xeroderma pigmentosum
Tearing
Congenital absence of lacrimal puncta
Cystinosis
Dacryocystitis
Englemann's disease
Prophyria

Cupping of the optic disc develops rapidly in infants. Irreversible damage may occur in a period as short as 1 month. Thus, when infantile glaucoma is suspected, efforts should be made to reach a diagnosis within 1 week.

As with other forms of glaucoma, the diagnosis is most certain when a constellation of findings is characteristic. As in adults, a variety of forms of glaucoma occur in infants (Table 22–22). Associated ocular or systemic abnormalities should be sought because the glaucoma may be part of a more global condition.

TABLE 22–22. Classification of Glaucoma in Infants

Genetically Related Glaucoma

Infantile or primary congenital glaucoma—trabeculodysgenesis
Glaucoma with associated anomaly or disease
1. Phakomatoses
   - Encephalotrigeminal hemangioma (Sturge-Weber syndrome)
   - Neurofibromatosis (von Recklinghausen's disease)
   - Oculodermal melanocytosis (nevus of Ota)
   - Retinocerebellar angiomatosis (von Hippel-Lindau disease)
   - Tuberous sclerosis (Bourneville's disease)
2. Mesodermal anomalies
   - Axenfeld's syndrome
   - Peter's anomaly
   - Rieger's syndrome
3. Metabolic disease or syndrome
   - Amyloidosis
   - Hallermann-Streiff syndrome
   - Homocystinuria
   - Hurler's syndrome
   - Lawford's syndrome
   - Lowe's syndrome
   - Marfan's syndrome
   - Pierre Robin's syndrome
   - Refsum's disease
   - Rubenstein's syndrome
   - Weill-Marchesani syndrome
4. Aniridia
   - Aniridia
   - Aniridia with Wilms' tumor
5. Gene defects
   - Trisomy 13
   - Trisomy 18
   - Chromosome 18 deletion
6. Nonhereditary
   - Trauma
   - Inflammations
   - Rubella syndrome
   - Tumors
   - Vascular problems

Modified from Shaffer RN, Weiss DI: Congenital and Pediatric Glaucomas. St. Louis: CV Mosby; 1970:8–9.

Congenital Glaucoma (Trabeculodysgenesis)

Congenital glaucoma is the traditional phrase applied to the glaucoma that occurs in infants in whom other systemic or ocular abnormalities are absent. That is, it is the "primary" glaucoma of infants. The adjective "congenital" is a poor one and probably should no longer be used. Although in some instances the condition is noted at birth, in most infants it does not become apparent until several months later. In some cases its onset may not occur until early adolescence.

The basic cause of the disease appears to be an anomaly of the angle structures that results in interference with aqueous outflow.[66,67] In the great majority of cases a delicate incision into the covering of the angle recess (a goniotomy) is adequate to lower intraocular pressure.[18]

The diagnosis of congenital glaucoma is based in large part on the same criterion used to diagnose other types of glaucoma: evidence of damage to the optic nerve caused by elevated intraocular pressure. Because an accurate assessment of intraocular pressure is difficult in infants, and visual field examination is obviously rudimentary at best, the appearance of the optic nerve takes on added importance.

The intraocular pressure of the anesthetized infant may be misleading. If taken in the early stages of anesthesia or when the infant is in a light plane, the intraocular pressure tends to be spuriously high. If determined when the infant is fully anesthetized, the intraocular pressure is lower than it would be in the unanesthetized subject. This effect of sedation or incomplete relaxation must be kept in mind when intraocular pressure is measured in the infant. The small size of the infant cornea also makes measurement with a Schiøtz tonometer imprecise. The hand-held applanation tonometers are recommended; the Tonopen is especially helpful and accurate in infants. It is not highly accurate, however, when intraocular pressures are above 30 mm Hg. If intraocular pressure is 4 mm Hg or higher in one eye than in the other, or if the level when determined with the infant in a deeply sedated, intubated condition is above 25 mm Hg, it is likely that the intraocular pressure is abnormal.

The optic nerve heads of the infant's two eyes should be symmetrical and normal in appearance.[68] Asymmetry is highly suggestive of glaucoma. Cupping occurs rapidly and resembles that seen in the "hyperbaric" type of primary open-angle glaucoma; that is, there is progressive enlargement of the cup, usually in a concentric manner but occasionally in a pattern of increasingly large ovals. The appearance of the discs should be drawn or photographs obtained at each examination.

Corneal changes, when present, are strong indicators of pathology, but they may be absent in the earlier stages of the disease. Thus corneal enlargement, edema, and tears in Descemet's membrane should be looked for, but their absence does not mean absence of glaucoma. Their presence does not necessarily mean a glaucoma, either (Table 22–20).

Gonioscopy in the infant is of often little diagnostic value. In the first place, because this type of examination is so rarely done in infants and there is no standard for determining what is "normal," most ophthalmologists have never seen a normal infant angle; consequently they cannot distinguish between the normal and the pathological. Second, the angle of the infant with congenital glaucoma does not present a pathognomonic picture. For example, although an apparently imperforate sheet spreading over the whole angle recess is typical of congenital glaucoma, this so-called Barkan's membrane is present in almost all infant angles, though to a lesser extent.[32]

When the question of congenital glaucoma arises, an attempt should be made to perform an adequate examination of the unanesthetized infant. The use of

Richardson's infant diagnostic Koeppe lens is helpful, more for fundus examination than for the less essential gonioscopy. After this, an examination under full anesthesia is usually required promptly. Infants tend to tolerate the inhalation anesthetic agents well, without developing liver damage. Therefore, in centers properly equipped and staffed to provide care for infants, there is little risk from the anesthesia itself.

Accurate determination of the axial length of the eye with A-scan ultrasound will help in both diagnosis and management. Globes that are longer than normal, especially when different from the other eye, are highly suspicious. Globes that elongate more rapidly than normal are almost certainly actively glaucomatous.

If intraocular pressure is marginal and the disc changes are suspicious but not definite, repeat anesthesia examination 2 to 4 weeks later should usually make the diagnosis clear. If corneal diameters and axial lengths remain unchanged, intraocular pressure is roughly the same, and, most important, the discs have not changed for the worse, usually it is best to defer any surgery and reexamine the infant again 1 month later. A third examination without change is strongly indicative that glaucoma is not present. Nevertheless, close follow-up is in order, as marginal cases can become frankly glaucomatous many months later.

If the initial examination is diagnostic, or if on subsequent examination an enlargement of the cup is noted or the intraocular pressure is unquestionably high, surgery should be performed during the same anesthetic experience. If the angle can be well seen, goniotomy is the procedure of choice. If the surgeon is not a skilled gonioscopist and is not fully familiar with the technique of goniotomy, a trabeculotomy should be done.

Repeat anesthetic examinations should be made 1 month after surgery, at which time goniotomy or trabeculotomy can be repeated if necessary.

If further surgery is required, the infant should again be reexamined 1 month later. If three goniotomies or two guarded filtration procedures have failed, then a guarded filtration procedure, with or without antimetabolites, is usually the treatment of choice. My preference in the Caucasian patient is to use no antimetabolite, and in a black or Asian patient to use 5-fluorouracil. Filtering procedures are not the initial choice because they are more traumatizing, and have no higher success rate than a goniotomy or a guarded filtration procedure.

In most children with congenital glaucoma it is possible, with modern surgical techniques, to control the intraocular pressure satisfactorily. However, visual results are often still poor. The proper management of these infants includes early refraction and appropriate correction to prevent the amblyopia that is a routine part of the condition. Contact lenses have been tried in some centers with moderate success. A pediatric ophthalmologist should be part of the team that provides the ongoing management of these cases. When a guarded filtration procedure has become necessary and has failed, then a tube-shunt procedure is usually indicated.

SECONDARY GLAUCOMAS

The secondary glaucomas constitute a heterogeneous group of conditions in which intraocular pressure is elevated owing to a mechanism different from that in either primary angle-closure or primary open-angle glaucoma. In most instances the basic mechanism is interference with outflow.

Obstruction of aqueous flow in the secondary glaucomas occurs in different locations. A classification of the secondary glaucomas is given in Table 22–23.

The goal of medical and surgical therapy in the treatment of the secondary glaucomas is the same as in the primary glaucomas: to preserve the sight of the eye by preventing damage to the optic nerve caused by intraocular pressure higher than the eye can tolerate. However, several aspects of the secondary glaucomas are so different from the primary glaucomas that the specifics of management differ markedly.

In the primary glaucomas intraocular pressure rises progressively, causing progressive deterioration of the optic nerve, whereas in the secondary glaucomas the cause for pressure elevation is often transient. A second major difference is the reaction to surgery. In contrast to the primary glaucomas, for which surgery is usually successful, in many of the secondary glaucomas operative procedures have a discouragingly poor outcome, often resulting in further complications such as neovascular glaucoma, the Sturge-Weber syndrome, and uveitis.

TABLE 22–23. Classification of Secondary Glaucomas

Aqueous Block
In vitreous (aqueous misdirection syndrome)
At anterior face of vitreous (aqueous misdirection syndrome)
At pupil
1. Iris adhesions to lens, pseudophakos, vitreous, or any membrane; "air block"
At angle recess
1. Epithelial ingrowth
2. Fibrinous membrane
3. Neovascular membrane
4. Iris
5. Angle cleavage
6. Extension of Descemet's membrane
7. Tumor or cyst
In trabeculum
1. Pigment
2. Inflammatory debris
3. Exfoliated material
4. Red blood cells or ghost cells
5. Mucopolysaccharide (due to steroids?)
In sclera
1. Episcleritis
2. Obstruction of extraocular veins
Aqueous hypersecretion
Iridocyclitis

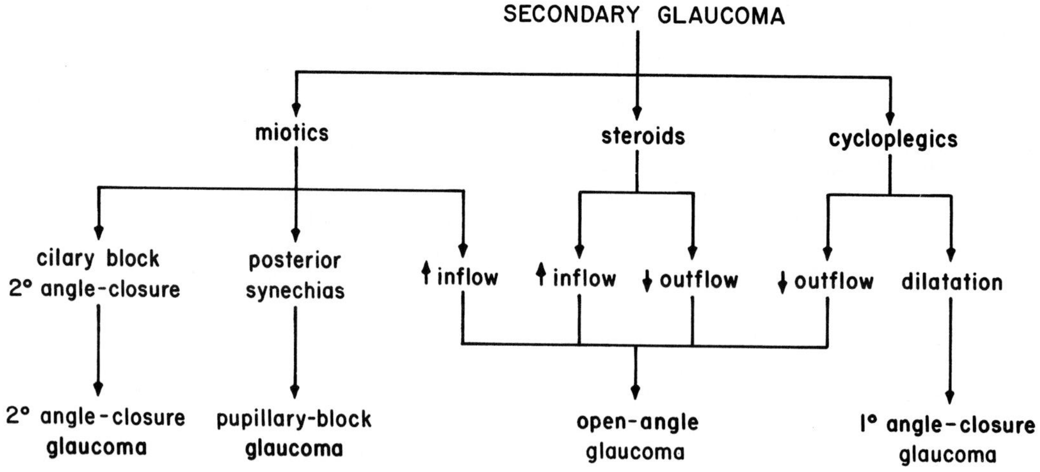

Figure 22–38. This flowsheet demonstrates how a patient with a secondary glaucoma may change from having one mechanism responsible for the pressure elevation to having another in response to treatment.

As the clinical course of a secondary glaucoma evolves, the cause for the elevated intraocular pressure may change. This often complicates therapy significantly. For example, a patient with uveitis may initially have a rise in pressure because of a trabeculopathy; as the uveitis clears through treatment with corticosteroids, the pressure may remain elevated because of the topical steroids themselves, even though the trabecular meshwork is no longer inflamed; later, inflammatory synechiae may close the angle so that the patient develops a secondary angle-closure glaucoma. Thus, in such a case, the treatment in the early stages of the disease would be corticosteroids, in the secondary stages elimination of the corticosteroids, and in the third stage aqueous suppressants or surgery designed to increase aqueous outflow. Some of these problems are shown in the therapeutic flowsheet in Figure 22–38.

The surgeon confronted with a patient with secondary glaucoma should proceed as follows in planning therapy:

1. Properly diagnose the underlying entity.
2. Determine the mechanism for elevation of the intraocular pressure.
3. Direct therapy first at the primary condition and then at the secondary elevation of intraocular pressure.
4. Recall that preservation of the health of the optic nerve is paramount and that proper monitoring demands repeated evaluation of the disc and field.

The only diagnostic test that will be mentioned here is the use of intravenous fluorescein to define the location of aqueous block. This simple test can provide invaluable information. Sodium fluorescein for injection (2.5 to 5.0 ml) is injected intravenously through the arm. The room should be dark. The eye is observed, using the finely focused, maximally intense beam of the slit lamp, noting the pattern of entry of fluorescein. Fluorescein should seep around the pupil gradually, first being visible about 30 seconds after injection. No fluorescein should be seen posterior to the posterior chamber; that is, fluorescein should not be noted behind the lens or anterior vitreous face. In many instances this simple test will establish whether a secondary glaucoma is caused by aqueous misdirection into the vitreous cavity or aqueous sequestration in the posterior chamber. When the eye is markedly inflamed, the iris vessels become permeable to fluorescein and the leakage that occurs on this account must be distinguished from flow that originates in the ciliary body.

The appropriate surgical procedure for each type of secondary glaucoma can be established logically by thoughtful consideration of the patient (Table 22–23).

In summary, surgery to control intraocular pressure in patients with secondary glaucoma is indicated when, despite medical therapy, the intraocular pressure is sufficiently elevated that it is causing or is anticipated to cause damage to the optic nerve at a rate that will interfere with the patient's way of life. The surgery is directed toward the elimination of the cause for the elevated intraocular pressure. The risk of the surgery should be balanced not only against the potential benefit but also against the risk of not performing surgery. This latter point should not be forgotten. Thus, for instance, although there is a moderate risk associated with cyclophotocoagulation in a diabetic whose intraocular pressure is 50 mm Hg owing to a complete closure of the anterior chamber by peripheral anterior synechiae related to a neovascular glaucoma, the risk of *not* performing cyclophotocoagulation is higher.

REFERENCES

1. Chandler PA, Grant WM: Lectures on Glaucoma. Philadelphia: Lea & Febiger; 1965.
2. McLean JM: Atlas of Glaucoma Surgery. St. Louis: CV Mosby; 1967:17.
3. Swan KC: Iridectomy for closed- (narrow) angle glaucoma. Am J Ophthalmol 1966;61:601.
4. Duke-Elder WS, Wybar KC (eds.): System of Ophthalmology, Vol. II: The Anatomy of the Visual System. St. Louis: CV Mosby; 1961:186–215;420.

5. Last RJ (ed.): Eugene Wolff's Anatomy of the Eye and Orbit, 6th Edition. Philadelphia: WB Saunders; 1968:59.
6. Hollows FC, Graham PA: The Ferndale Glaucoma Survey. In Hunt LB (ed.), Glaucoma: Epidemiology, Early Diagnosis and Some Aspects of Treatment. London: Williams & Wilkins; 1966.
7. Armaly M: Ocular pressure and visual fields. A ten-year follow-up study. Arch Ophthalmol 1969;81:25.
8. Schappert-Kimmijser J: A five-year follow-up of subjects with intra-ocular pressure of 23–30 mm Hg without anomalies of optic nerve and visual field typical for glaucoma at first investigation. Ophthalmologica 1971;162:289.
9. Davanger M: Intraocular pressure in normal eyes and in eyes with glaucoma simplex. Acta Ophthalmol 1965;43:299.
10. Spaeth GL: Low tension glaucoma: Its diagnosis and management. In Documenta Ophthalmologica Proceedings, Series 22, Glaucoma Symposium, Diagnosis and Therapy, Amsterdam, 1979, Greve EL (ed.). The Hague: Junk Publishers; 1980:263–88.
11. Becker B: Diabetes mellitus and primary open-angle glaucoma. Trans Am Acad Ophthalmol Otolaryngol 1971;75:239.
12. Becker B, Kolker A, Roth D: Glaucoma family study. Am J Ophthalmol 1960;50:557.
13. Bertelsen TI: The relationship between thrombosis in the retinal veins and primary glaucoma. Acta Ophthalmol 1961:39:603.
14. Drance SM: Some factors involved in the production of low-tension glaucoma. Br J Ophthalmol 1972;56:229.
15. Werner EB, Drance SM: The interrelationship of intraocular pressure and other risk factors in the development of optic nerve excavation and nerve fiber bundle field defects. Perspect Ophthalmol 1977;1:153.
16. Francois J, Heintz-DeBree C: Personal research on the heredity of chronic simple glaucoma. Am J Ophthalmol 1966;62:1067.
17. Hansen E, Sellevold OJ: Pseudoexfoliation of the lens capsule. III. Ocular tension in eyes with pseudoexfoliation. Acta Ophthalmol 1970;48:446.
18. Harrington DO: The pathogenesis of the glaucoma field; clinical evidence that circulatory insufficiency in the optic nerve is the primary cause of visual field loss in glaucoma. Am J Ophthalmol 1959;47:177.
19. Hitchings RA, Spaeth GL: Chronic retinal vein occlusion in glaucoma. Br J Ophthalmol 1976;60:694.
20. Kass MA, Kolker AE, Becker B: Prognostic factors in glaucomatous visual field loss. Arch Ophthalmol 1976;94:1274.
21. Kellerman L, Posner A: The value of heredity in the detection and study of glaucoma. Am J Ophthalmol 1955;40:681.
22. Knapp A: Glaucoma in myopic eyes. Trans Am Ophthalmol Soc 1925;23:61.
23. Layden WE, Shaffer RN: The exfoliation syndrome. Am Acad Ophthalmol Otolaryngol 1974;78:326.
24. Lichter PR: Pigmentary glaucoma—current concepts. Trans Am Acad Ophthalmol Otolaryngol 1974;78:309.
25. Lowe RF: Primary angle-closure glaucoma: Family histories and anterior chamber depths. Br J Ophthalmol 1967;48:191.
26. Moller HV: Excessive myopia and glaucoma. Arch Ophthalmol 1948;26:185.
27. Podos SM, Becker B, Morton WR: High myopia and primary open-angle glaucoma. Am J Ophthalmol 1966;62:1308.
28. Phojanpelto PE, Hurskainen L: Studies on relatives of patients with pseudo-exfoliation of the lens capsules. Acta Ophthalmol 1972;50:255.
29. Reese AB, McGavic JS: Relation of field contraction to blood pressure in chronic primary glaucoma. Arch Ophthalmol 1942;27: 845.
30. Safir A, Paulsen EP, Klaymen J, et al. (eds.): Ocular abnormalities in juvenile diabetics: Frequent occurrence of abnormally high tensions. Arch Ophthalmol 1966;76:557.
31. Spaeth GL: Visual loss in glaucoma clinic. I. Sociological considerations. Invest Ophthalmol 1970;9:73.
32. Spaeth GL: The normal development of the human anterior chamber angle. A new system of descriptive grading. Trans Ophthalmol Soc UK 1971;91:709.
33. Sugar HS: Pigmentary glaucoma: A 25 year review. Am J Ophthalmol 1966;62:499.
34. Wilensky JT, Podos SM, Becker B: Prognostic indicators in ocular hypertension. Arch Ophthalmol 1974;91:200.
35. Levene RZ: Review: Low-tension glaucoma: A critical review and new material. Surv Ophthalmol 1980;24:621.
36. Bankes JLK, Perkins ES, Tsolakis S, et al.: Bedford Glaucoma Survey. Br Med J 1968;1:791.
37. Linnér E, Strömberg U: Ocular hypertension: A five year study of the total population in a Swedish town, and subsequent discussions. In Leydhecker W (ed.), Glaucoma: Tutzing Symposium. Basel: S. Karger;1967:187.
38. Norskøv K: Routine tonometry in ophthalmic practice. I. Primary screening and further examinations for diagnostic purposes. Acta Ophthalmol 1970;48:838.
39. Perkins ES: Recent advances in the treatment of glaucoma. Trans Ophthalmol Soc UK 1966;86:199.
40. Spaeth GL: Ocular hypertension: Reasons for abandonment of the term. In Spaeth GL (ed.), Early Primary Open-Angle Glaucoma: Diagnosis and Management. Boston: Little, Brown; 1979:37–49.
41. Spaeth GL: Appearances of the optic disc in glaucoma: A pathogenetic classification. In New Orleans Academy of Ophthalmology: Symposium on Glaucoma. St. Louis: CV Mosby; 1981:114–153.
42. Chandler PA, Grant WM: Lectures on Glaucoma. Philadelphia: Lea & Febiger;1965:11.
43. Hetherington J Jr, Shaffer RN, Hoskins HD: The disc in congenital glaucoma. In Etienne R, Paterson GD (eds.), International Glaucoma Symposium, Albi. Marseille: Diffusion Générale de Librairie;1975:127–43.
44. Quigley HA: The pathogenesis of reversible cupping in congenital glaucoma. Am J Ophthalmol 1977;84:358.
45. Read RM, Spaeth GL: The practical clinical appraisal of the optic disc in glaucoma: The natural history of cup progression and some specific disc-field correlations. Trans Am Acad Ophthalmol Otolaryngol 1974;78:255.
46. Hitchings RA, Spaeth GL: The optic disc in glaucoma: Classification. Br J Ophthalmol 1976;60:778.
47. Kolker AE, Hetherington J Jr: Becker and Shaffer's Diagnosis and Therapy of the Glaucomas. 3rd Edition. St. Louis: CV Mosby; 1970:131,161.
48. Spaeth GL: Morphological damage of the optic nerve. In Heilmann K, Richardson KT (eds.), Glaucoma: Conceptions of a Disease. Pathogenesis, Diagnosis, Therapy. Philadelphia: WB Saunders, 1978:138–56.
49. Spaeth GL, Fernandes E, Hitchings RA: The pathogenesis of transient or permanent improvement in the appearance of the optic disc following glaucoma surgery. In Documenta Ophthalmologica Proceedings, Series 22, Glaucoma Symposium, Diagnosis and Therapy. Amsterdam, 1979, Greve EL (ed.). The Hague: Junk Publishers;1980:111–26.
50. Pederson JE, Herschler J: Reversal of glaucomatous cupping in adults. Arch Ophthalmol 1982;100:426.
51. Greenidge KC, Spaeth GL, Traverso CE: Change in appearance of the optic disc associated with lowering of intraocular pressure. Ophthalmology 1985;92:897.
52. Drance SM: The early field defects in glaucoma. Invest Ophthalmol 1969;8:84.
53. Werner EB, Drance SM: Early visual field disturbances in glaucoma. Arch Ophthalmol 1977;95:1173.
54. Aulhorn E, Harms H: Early visual field defects in glaucoma. In Leydhecker W (ed.), Glaucoma: Tutzing Symposium. Basel: S. Karger; 1967:151.
55. Peter LC: Principles and Practice of Perimetry. Philadelphia: Lea & Febiger;1938:14, 186.
56. Drance SM, Anderson D: Automatic Perimetry in Glaucoma: A Practical Guide. Orlando, Fla: Grune & Stratton; 1985.
57. Caprioli J, Sears M, Miller JM: Patterns of early visual field loss in open-angle glaucoma. Am J Ophthalmol 1987;103:512.
58. Whalen WR, Spaeth GL: Computerized Visual Fields: What They Are and How to Use Them. Thorofare, N.J.: Slack, Inc.; 1985.
59. Gloor B, Stürmer J, Vökt B: Was hat die automatisierte Perimetrie mit den Octopus für neue Kenntnisse über glaukomatöse Gesichtsfeldveränderungen gebracht? Klin Monatsbl Augenheilk 1984;184:249.
60. Kolker AE: Visual prognosis in advanced glaucoma: A comparison of medical and surgical therapy for retention of vision in 101 eyes with advanced glaucoma. Trans Am Ophthalmol Soc 1977;75:539.

61. Spaeth GL: Primary angle-closure glaucoma: Methodology of diagnosis and management of patients with glaucomatous disease. In New Orleans Academy of Ophthalmology: Symposium on Glaucoma. St. Louis: CV Mosby; 1981:203–20.
62. Spaeth GL: Gonioscopy: Uses old and new. The inheritance of occludable angles. Ophthalmology 1978;85:222.
63. Benedikt O: Prophylaktische Iridektomie nach Winkelblockglaukom am Partnerauge. Klin Monatsbl Augenheilk 1970;156:80.
64. Snow JT: Value of prophylactic peripheral iridectomy on the second eye in angle-closure glaucoma. Trans Ophthalmol Soc UK 1977;97:189.
65. Shaffer RN, Weiss DI: Congenital and Pediatric Glaucomas. St. Louis: CV Mosby; 1970.
66. Shaffer RN, Hoskins HD: Goniotomy in the treatment of isolated trabeculodysgenesis (primary congenital (infantile) developmental glaucoma). Trans Ophthalmol Soc UK 1983;103:581.
67. Jerndal T: Goniodysgenesis and hereditary juvenile glaucoma. Acta Ophthalmol, Suppl 107, Copenhagen: Munksgaard; 1970.
68. Richardson KT: Optic cup asymmetry in normal newborn infants. Invest Ophthalmol 1968;7:138.
69. Spaeth GL: The management of patients with cataract and glaucoma. Ophthalmic Surg 1980;11:780.
70. Stewart RH, Loftis MD: Combined cataract extraction and thermal sclerostomy versus combined cataract extraction and traceculectomy. Ophthalmic Surg 1976;7:93.

CHAPTER 23

Limbus-Based Conjunctival Flap

GÜNTHER K. KRIEGLSTEIN, M.D.

The initial incision through the conjunctiva for a limbus-based flap can be placed in the supranasal or in the supratemporal quadrant or at the 12 o'clock position, in front of the superior rectus muscle insertion. If another perilimbal procedure, i.e., cataract, is foreseeable one should aim for the supratemporal or supranasal option of the flap location (Fig. 23–1). Conjunctival incision and flap preparation at the 12 o'clock position renders better exposure of the surgical field and an easier technique. The curvilinear conjunctival incision should be approximately 8 mm posterior to the limbus, extending about 3 clock hours, meticulously keeping the distance to the limbus constant (Fig. 23–1).

The following descriptions and illustrations apply to a conjunctival flap created at the 12 o'clock position. A 4-0 black silk bridal suture is placed with as much care as possible posterior through the tendon of the muscle. The muscle itself has to be strictly avoided because of the risk of instantaneous subconjunctival hemorrhage and unnecessary complication of surgery. The conjunctiva is grasped with toothed forceps, gently tented in front of the bridle suture (Fig. 23–2) and pulled slightly downward, with the superior muscle tonus as counteraction. The bite of the forceps should include only conjunctiva. Initial incision of the conjunctiva together with the Tenon's capsule increases the risk of bleeding from episcleral vessels. Opening of the conjunctiva is accomplished using a blunt-tipped pair of scissors, with the blades of the scissors held perpendicular to the globe to obtain a limbus-parallel opening after release of the forceps (Fig. 23–2). The resulting conjunctival hole is extended to either side for a distance of about 6-8 mm to produce an incision of 3 clock hours at appropriate distance to the limbus.

The Tenon's capsule is apparent within the opening of the epibulbar conjunctiva. While the limbus-based conjunctiva is held back with the base of a triangular cotton sponge, thereby avoiding stretch on the corneolimbal junction, Tenon's capsule is gently grasped with the tooth-tipped forceps, lifted, and incised with scissors close to the posterior conjunctival wound edge (Fig. 23–3). The scissors used for the conjunctiva are used here, and in the same perpendicular position. Separate opening of the conjunctiva and the Tenon's capsule minimizes the risk of bleeding and creates a better basis for partial dissection of the Tenon's tissue, an optional step that depends on the requirements of the individual case. The hole in the Tenon's capsule is enlarged to both sides, parallel to the posterior conjunctival wound (Fig. 23–4), after which the desired area of the Tenon's tissue is resected.

Preparing the flap at its base, the corneolimbal junction, requires cutting adhesions of Tenon's tissue to the sclerolimbal junction. For this purpose the limbus-based conjunctival flap is reflected to the cornea and held gently in place with a cotton sponge (Fig. 23–5). Fusion of the Tenon's capsule with the sclerolimbal junction creates a space that can be entered with a small, sharp-tipped pair of scissors, the blades of which are held parallel to the limbus, so one blade can enter this space for cutting (Fig. 23–5). This phase of flap preparation requires great care to avoid trauma to the insertion of the conjunctiva at the corneolimbal junction which would result in formation of a "buttonhole." During this episcleral and limbal preparation, the conjunctiva should not be held with sharp instruments, and major stretching forces on the wound edges should also be avoided. The inevitable minor bleeding from the episcleral field are best treated with low-voltage bipolar cautery. Wound closure of a limbus-based conjunctival flap is crucial for the long-term efficacy and morphology of the filtering bleb.

I prefer layer-by-layer wound closure of Tenon's capsule and the conjunctiva. Tenon's is best sutured with

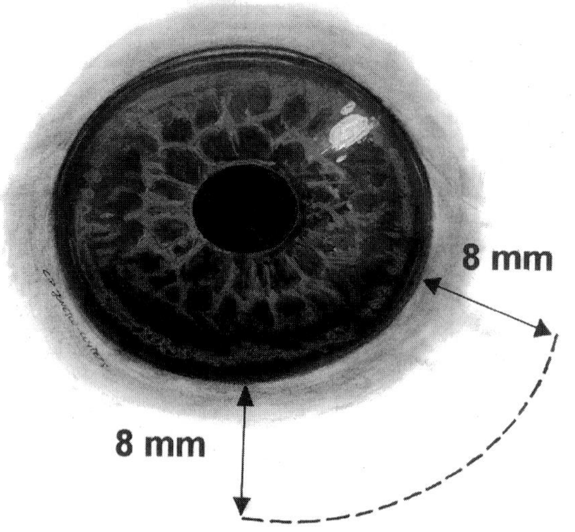

Figure 23–1. Preparation of a limbus-based conjunctival flap. The initial, curved conjunctival incision should follow an equal distance to the limbus for about 8 mm.

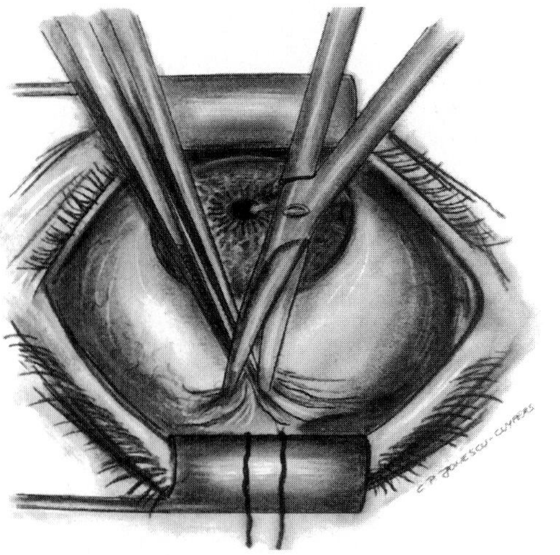

Figure 23–2. The conjunctiva is lifted from the globe in appropriate distance to the limbus and incised posterior to the bite of the forceps and anterior to the upper rectus muscle bridle suture.

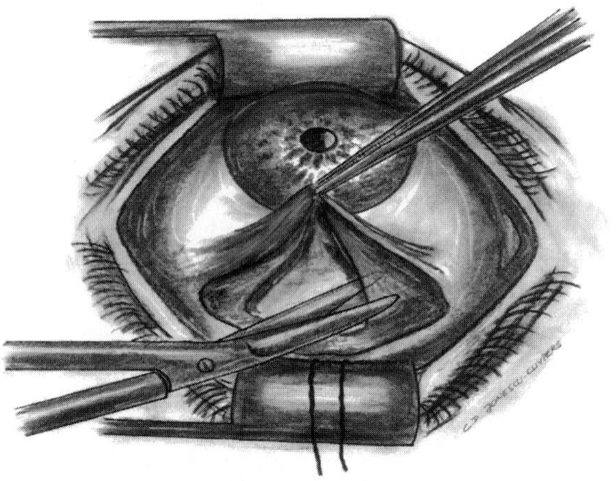

Figure 23–4. The incision of Tenon's capsule is extended to both sides of the initial opening following conjunctival incision somewhat anteriorly.

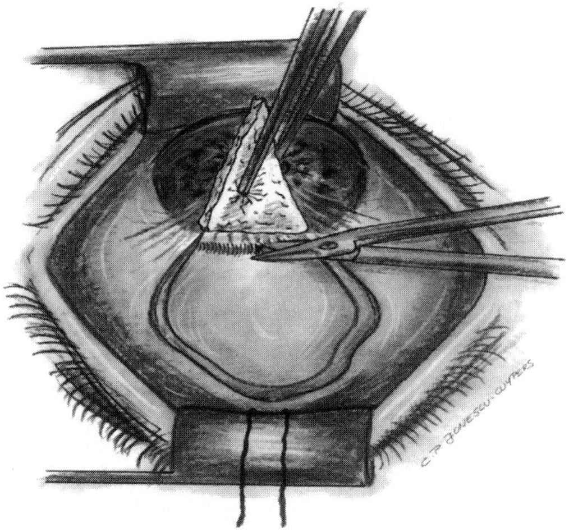

Figure 23–5. The fusion of Tenon's capsule with the episcleral tissue 0.5 mm behind the conjunctival insertion at the limbus is separated with a small Vannas scissors.

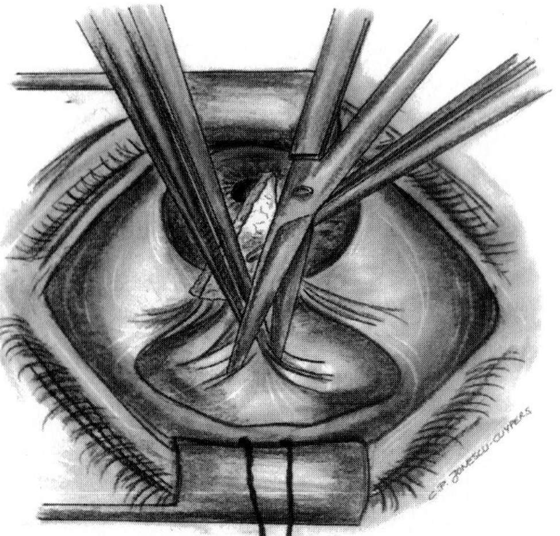

Figure 23–3. After completion of the conjunctival incision, Tenon's capsule is opened in similar fashion.

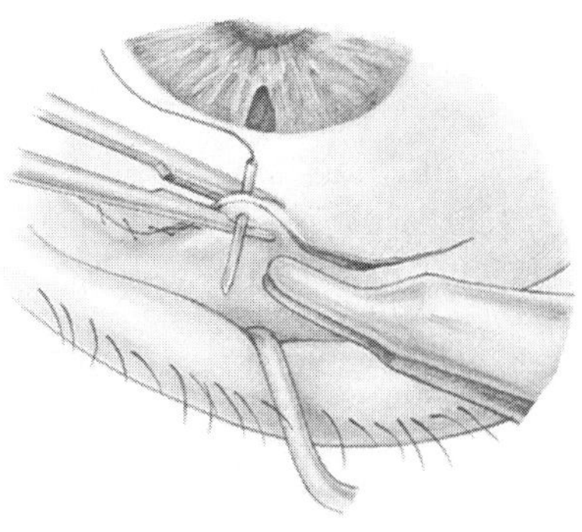

Figure 23–6. The conjunctiva is closed with closely spaced running, unlocked sutures. The final suture is securely tied.

8-0 or 9-0 running Vicryl. For the conjunctival suture, absorbable 8-0 Vicryl is in common use. The needle used should be very sharp and rounded, to reduce trauma to the conjunctiva. The forceps used for holding wound edges must be untoothed, and the bite of the forceps to the tissue should be very soft. The right-handed surgeon usually starts wound closure from the right side, beginning with a single knot and continuing with a running suture technique (Fig. 23–6). The smooth-tipped forceps should be used to hold the wound edges in the proper position so that the needle can pass through the anterior and posterior wound lip without changing its position in the needle-holder. The needle is guided through the conjunctival wound lips very close to the edges because watertight conjunctival wound healing requires a closure of epithelium to epithelium. It is easier to accomplish the correct wound alignment when the lid speculum is released somewhat to reduce traction on the conjunctival fornix during wound closure. The end of the thread on both knots of the running suture should be cut short to the knot, to diminish suture-related ocular irritation.

In most instances, the conjunctiva is best closed with a two-layer approach, approximating Tenon's capsule to Tenon's capsule, and independently closing conjunctiva superficial to Tenon's capsule. Closure of Tenon's capsule results in covering the filtering area or the implanted device with tissue that is thick and strong, providing a safe cover for what lies underneath. Additionally, approximating Tenon's results in less traction on the conjunctival edges of the conjunctival incision, decreasing the likelihood of "cheese-wiring" and dehiscence of the conjunctiva. Excision of Tenon's capsule has been recommended by some, but it was shown by Kapetansky not to result in lower intraocular pressure, and such excision increases the likelihood of postoperative complication. It is not recommended except in those individuals in which the Tenon's capsule is so inflamed that it mechanically interferes with closure.

A two-layer conjunctival closure technique is performed as follows: The needle should not be a cutting-type needle but should have a sharp point with a round cross-section (taper point) so that it will cause the smallest hole in the tissue through which it is being placed. This is especially important when closing the conjunctiva itself. The preferred suture is 8-0 or 9-0 Vicryl. The edge of the conjunctiva attached to the limbus is lifted with a non-toothed forceps (such as a Hoskin's forceps) and held on stretch. It is essential that the tissue be put on stretch, so there will be no folds in the conjunctiva. If there are folds, the needle going through Tenon's may also go through conjunctiva, causing a buttonhole. Once the conjunctiva is on stretch, it can be held in place by meticulously placing the needle through the very edge of the conjunctiva and lifting it up towards the operating microscope. The free edge of Tenon's capsule attached to the limbus (part of the Tenon's–conjunctival flap) is then grasped with a non-toothed forceps at the extreme right end of the incision (for a right-handed person) and the needle is placed through Tenon's capsule (Fig. 23–7). The non-toothed forceps is then used to grasp the free edge of the conjunctiva superiorly. The free edge often retracts beneath the lid, so it is helpful to use a retractor to hold the upper lid back. The cut edge of the conjunctiva is grasped with a non-toothed forceps and lifted toward the microscope and then toward the head of the patient, away from the limbus. This action is performed quite vigorously, exposing the underlying Tenon's capsule. Tenon's capsule is then hooked with the needle that has gone through the inferior edge of Tenon's capsule, so that the Tenon's capsule will not retract superiorly when the conjunctiva is released. The conjunctiva is released and the Hoskins forceps used to grasp the superior Tenon's capsule. This is pulled up toward the operating microscope and anteriorly toward the limbus until it is possible to see the cut edge of conjunctiva superiorly. The needle is then passed through Tenon's capsule, exiting as close to the cut edge of the superior conjunctiva as possible. This first bite is then securely tied. Additional bites are taken in Tenon's capsule with the same technique, locking each suture. For a conjunctival incision of approximately 6 to 8 mm in width, four bites in Tenon's capsule are usually adequate. This portion of the closure need not be watertight. The closeness of the sutures depends on the thickness of Tenon's capsule and the desire of the surgeon to have a very secure closure at that level.

After the closure of Tenon's capsule is complete, that is, when the left side has been reached for a right-

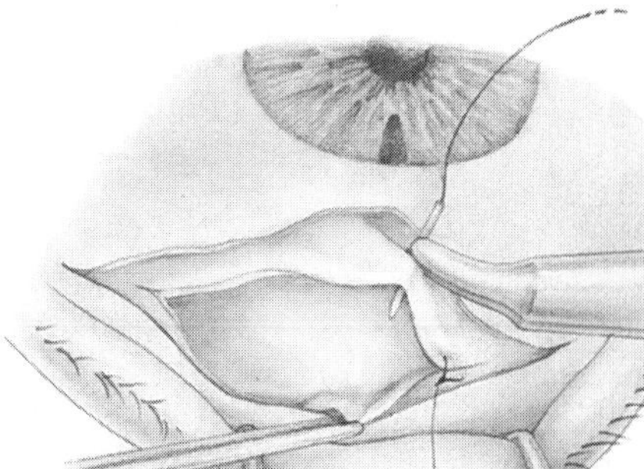

Figure 23–7. The superior edge of Tenon's capsule tends to retract up under the lid and must be looked for. It can be hooked over the needle and pulled inferiorly. Sutures are locked.

handed person, the needle is exteriorized, starting at the Tenon's capsule side, and exiting through the conjunctiva. Exteriorization is done at the extreme left edge of the incision (Fig. 23–8). The conjunctiva is then grasped with a non-toothed forceps such as a Hoskins forceps and lifted toward the operating microscope. Again, it is essential that the conjunctiva be placed on stretch. There is a great tendency not to lift the tissue with sufficient vigor, and if it is not lifted high enough, the edges cannot be seen well and the closure is less likely to be satisfactory. The non-cutting needle wedged onto the suture is then placed through the edge of the conjunctiva that is attached to the limbus, approximately 1 mm from the cut edge. The forceps is then used to lift the superior edge of the conjunctiva, again placing the tissue on stretch. With this technique, it is usually not difficult to find the conjunctiva when Tenon's capsule has been closed properly. The conjunctiva is elevated well above the Tenon's capsule, and the needle goes from the underside to the outerside of the conjunctiva, approximately 2 or 3 mm posterior to the cut edge of the conjunctiva. The suture is pulled up and the two edges of the conjunctiva are held together immediately beside the needle, either at the left edge, or deep to the needle (Fig. 23–9). If the tissue is held vertically, that is, at the edge of the needle, it is important not to include more than 2 or 3 mm of tissue in the forceps; if more tissue is grasped, there is a chance that the edge of the forceps will buttonhole the conjunctiva.

A second suture is then placed very close to the first bite in the conjunctiva, no more than 1 mm from the first. The goal of the conjunctival closure is to obtain a watertight closure. After the needle has passed through both of the cut edges, about 1 mm from the inferior edge and about 2 to 3 mm from the superior edge the suture is pulled so that the cut edges of the conjunctiva are firmly approximated. If this is done properly, the suture is buried in the edge of the conjunctiva and the suture becomes invisible. The assistant, using a forceps such as an angled tying forceps, then grasps the suture approximately 1 to 3 cm above the eye, and pulls the suture firmly toward the left side of the incision. This keeps the suture taut, so that as subsequent sutures are placed it will not loosen. Additional bites are then placed in the two edges of the conjunctiva until the entire conjunctival incision has been closed. Again, it is essential to lift the conjunctiva firmly so as to be sure that the needle goes through conjunctiva alone and not through Tenon's capsule. If Tenon's capsule is incorporated within the cut edges of the conjunctiva, it may produce a "Tenon's wick," which allows aqueous humor to leak through the conjunctiva. Finally, the suture can either be tied on itself or secured to the end that was used to tie the first suture in Tenon's capsule.

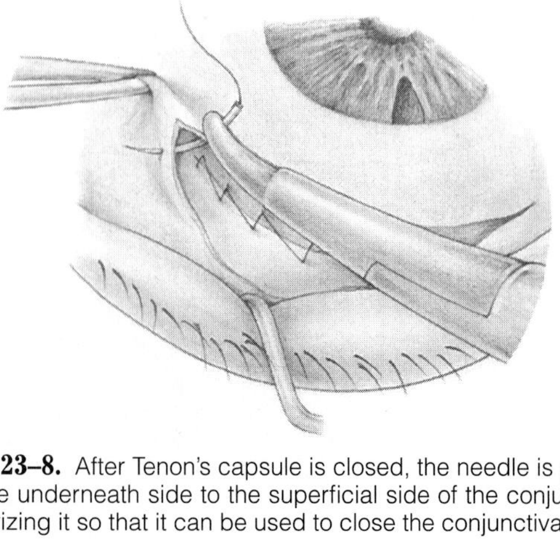

Figure 23–8. After Tenon's capsule is closed, the needle is placed from the underneath side to the superficial side of the conjunctiva, exteriorizing it so that it can be used to close the conjunctiva.

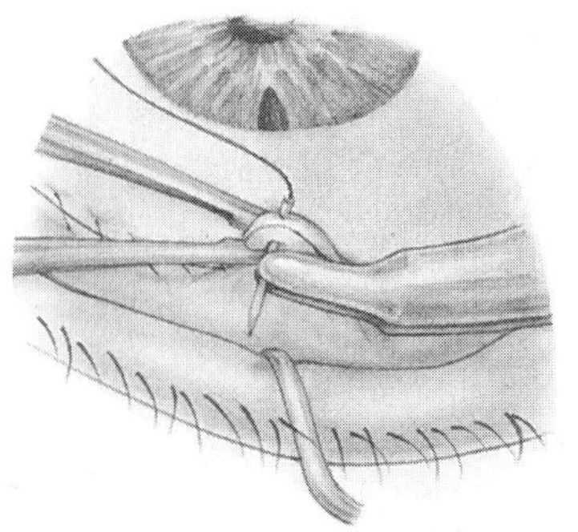

Figure 23–9. After the needle has passed through the tissue, it is lifted away from the globe rather firmly, with the underlying tissue put on stretch. A blunt forceps then grasps this underlying tissue firmly, as close to the needle as possible. This will hold the needle firmly in place, permitting the surgeon to release the end of the needle containing the suture without having to change the position of the needle.

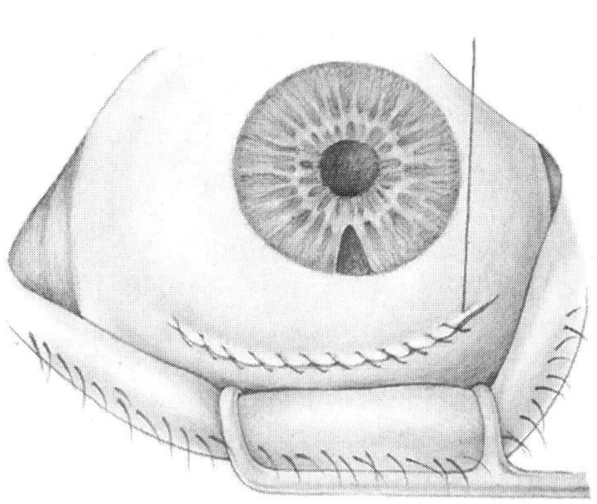

Figure 23–10. The closure of the conjunctiva should be watertight.

It is essential to use an absorbable suture in the Tenon's capsule portion of the two-layer closure. Though it is my preference, it is not essential to use an absorbable suture in the conjunctival portion of the closure. Some surgeons prefer to use a 10-0 nylon, especially when utilizing antimetabolites.

If a guarded filtration procedure has been performed, the tightness of the conjunctival closure should be checked after the closure is complete by filling the anterior chamber and seeing a high bleb develop (Fig. 23–10). The conjunctival surfaces are checked with sponges to make sure there is no leakage through the cut edges and that there are no buttonholes.

REFERENCES

1. Agbeja AM, Dutton GN: Conjunctival incisions for trabeculectomy and their relationship to the type of bleb formation—A preliminary study. Eye 1987;24:176–7.
2. Brinker P, Kessing SV: Limbus-based versus fornix-based conjunctival flap in glaucoma filtering surgery. Acta Ophthalmol 1992;70:641–4.
3. Chew PT, Watson PG, Chee CK: Vascular changes over trabeculectomy blebs. Eye 1994;8:389–93.
4. Freedman J: Flap selection in glaucoma filtration surgery. Ann Ophthalmol 1987;19:449–50.
5. Grehn F, Mauthe S, Pfeiffer N: Limbus-based versus fornix-based conjunctival flap in filtering surgery. A randomized prospective study. Int Ophthalmol 1989;13:139–43.
6. Kapetansky F: Trabeculectomy or trabeculectomy plus tenonectomy: a comparative study. J Glaucoma 1980;2:451-3.
7. Kaushik NC: Limbal- vs fornix-based conjunctival trabeculectomy flaps. Am J Ophthalmol 1988;105:219–20.
8. Kahn AM, Jilani FA: Comparative results of limbal based versus fornix based conjunctival flaps for trabeculectomy. Indian J Ophthalmol 1992;40:41–3.
9. Luntz MH: Limbal- vs fornix-based conjunctival trabeculectomy flaps. Am J Ophthalmol 1988;105:100–1.
10. Murchison JJ, Shields MB: Limbal-based vs fornix-based conjunctival flaps in combined extracapsular cataract surgery and glaucoma filtering procedure. Am J Ophthalmol 1990;109: 709–15.
11. Reichert R, Stewart W, Shields MB: Limbus-based versus fornix-based conjunctival flaps in trabeculectomy. Ophthalmic Surg 1987;18:672–6.
12. Schuhmann G, Hesse W, Faschinger C, et al.: Limbus-based flap versus fornix-based flap in goniotrepanation. Klin Mbl Augenheilkd 1986;189:407–8.
13. Traverso CE, Tomey KF, Antonios S: Limbal- vs fornix-based conjunctival trabeculectomy flaps. Am J Ophthalmol 1987;104:28–32.

CHAPTER 24

Fornix-Based Conjunctival Flaps for Filtering Surgery

REBECCA HEAPS WARD, M.D. and MICHAEL A. KASS, M.D.

SURGICAL TECHNIQUES

CONJUNCTIVAL FLAPS

The development of a conjunctival flap is an integral part of many glaucoma procedures. Even techniques that are designed to lower intraocular pressure without gross filtration require cutting the conjunctiva to reach the sclera. A conjunctival flap can be raised from either the limbus or the fornix (Table 24-1). Anatomical considerations are illustrated in Figures 24-2 and 24-4.

COMPARISON OF FORNIX-BASED FLAPS WITH LIMBUS-BASED FLAPS

There have been multiple comparisons of fornix-based to limbus-based conjunctival flaps for glaucoma filtration surgery. Studies done without antimetabolites found equal success rates for *trabeculectomy* performed with either limbus or fornix-based conjunctival flaps.[1–5] Two studies demonstrated better intraocular pressure control in the first 2 days postoperatively with limbus-based flaps but equal long-term intraocular pressure with the two-flap techniques.[6,7] In studies where antimetabolites were used, the success rates of limbus and fornix flaps have been comparable.[8–11]

Fornix-based conjunctival flaps have a number of advantages over limbus-based flaps for filtering surgery. The fornix flap is an easier technique to perform, allows for better visualization of the limbal area, permits less handling of the flap with decreased risk of buttonholing the conjunctiva, requires less suture material for closure, and avoids posterior conjunctival scarring that might limit posterior flow of aqueous humor.[1,2,4,12–15] Although fornix-based flaps are generally thought to be faster and easier to perform without a skilled assistant, one prospective study found that the difference in time to perform the two procedures was not as great as had been anticipated. The average time was 55 minutes for the guarded filtration procedure with limbus-based flaps and 44 minutes for the guarded filtration procedure with fornix-based flaps.[3] Fornix-based flaps may be preferable in a number of situations, including combined cataract extraction and *trabeculectomy*[2,8,9,11,14] and reoperations where scar tissue may limit exposure of the limbus.[1–3,15,16]

A study by Agbeja and Dutton[17] compared the appearance of the blebs after fornix-based versus limbus-based conjunctival flaps. Operations with fornix-based flaps produced diffuse blebs with a normal vascular pattern. Operations with limbus-based flaps were more likely to produce cystic blebs. Low-lying, diffuse blebs are preferable to large, cystic blebs because they are more comfortable for the patient, they facilitate tear film distribution on the cornea, and they may be at lower risk for bleb leak.

One disadvantage of fornix-based flaps over limbus-based flaps in the guarded filtration procedure is difficulty cauterizing posterior sources of bleeding. Other disadvantages include more frequent spontaneous

TABLE 24–1. Indications for the Various Types of Conjunctival Flaps in Glaucoma Surgery

Type of Procedure or Diagnosis	Preferred Approach	Alternative Approach
Peripheral iridectomy for neglected primary angle-closure, chronic angle-closure, or combined mechanism glaucoma	Clear cornea	Guarded filtration procedure with tightly sutured scleral flap
Peripheral iridectomy for primary angle-closure glaucoma	Small fornix-based flap	Clear cornea
Peripheral iridectomy for the fellow eye	Small fornix-based flap	Clear cornea
Guarded filtration procedure with a tightly sutured scleral flap	High limbus-based flap	Large fornix-based flap
Guarded filtration procedure with scleral flap intended to leak	High limbus-based flap	—
All standard filtration procedures	High limbus-based flap	—
All reoperations of standard filtration procedures and guarded filtration procedure	High limbus-based flap*	—
Cataract extraction without combined glaucoma procedure†	Clear cornea	Small fornix-based flap
Cataract extraction with cyclodialysis	Fornix-based flap	Clear cornea
Cataract extraction with guarded filtration or other filtration procedure	Fornix-based flap	Large limbus-based flap

*Incision should usually be made at the same site as the primary incision.
†Patient under consideration has definite glaucoma, but glaucoma procedure not considered necessary at the time of cataract extraction.

leaks at the limbus in the early postoperative period and greater risk of leaks with digital massage, antimetabolites, and scleral flap suture lysis.

TECHNIQUE FOR CREATING A FORNIX-BASED CONJUNCTIVAL FLAP

Elevation of the conjunctiva from the limbus may first be performed with anesthetic from the retrobulbar injection or balanced salt solution injected with a 30-gauge needle a distance away from the proposed surgical site. This can delineate areas of scarring if there is a question of access to the limbus at the proposed surgical site. This elevation approach is especially useful if the patient has had previous surgery, trauma, or inflammatory disease.

Blunt-tipped scissors[12,13] or a sharp knife[9] and smooth forceps are first used to fashion a peritomy of approximately 2 clock hours. The conjunctiva is incised from the cornea as far anteriorly as possible (Fig. 24–1). Unnecessary handling of conjunctiva is avoided, especially if antimetabolites are to be used (Fig. 24–2). The incision is made in either the superonasal or superotemporal quadrant to preserve a scar-free quadrant should further filtering surgery become necessary.[6,12–14] A relaxing incision at one end of the peritomy may be made if necessary to facilitate exposure of the sclera,[13,14,18] although this approach may make it more difficult to create a watertight closure at the end of the procedure (Fig. 24–3).[12]

The conjunctiva is grasped gently with smooth forceps at the cut edge and blunt scissors[12] are used to tunnel under Tenon's capsule to form a potential space for aqueous humor filtration (Fig. 24–4). Sharp dissection of episcleral adhesions may be necessary with a blade or with sharp scissors. Care should be taken to avoid the rectus muscles and the anterior ciliary vessels during the posterior dissection. Adequate posterior and posterolateral blunt dissection should be performed to encourage the formation of a diffuse, broad, low-lying bleb.[11,12]

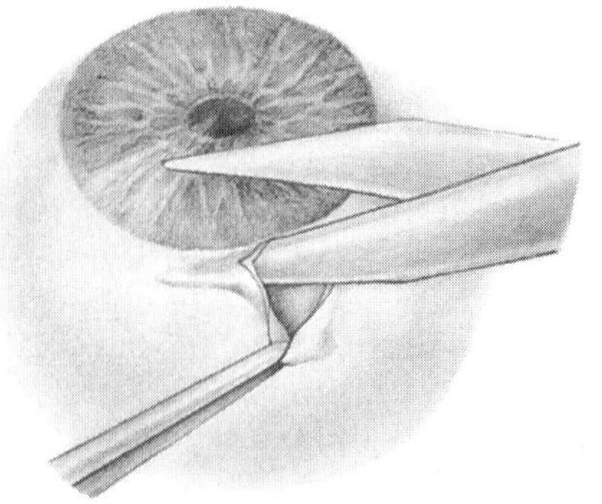

Figure 24–1. The incision is widened, with the surgeon making sure that the forceps puts the tissue on good stretch; the scissors cuts inferiorly so that there will be no remnant of conjunctiva left on the globe.

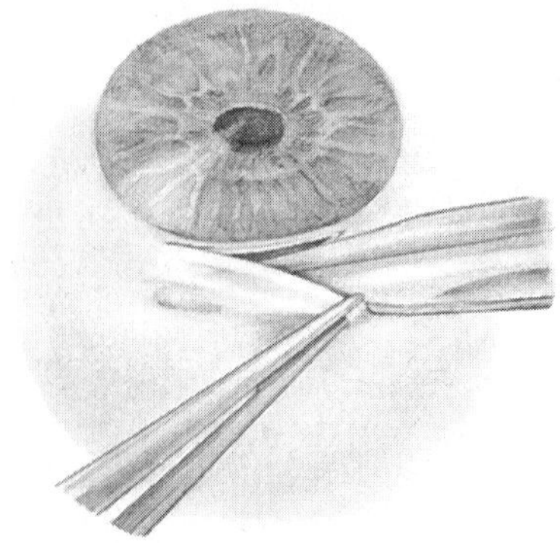

Figure 24–2. Tissue is separated from the globe by inserting the scissors with tips closed and then spreading them bluntly.

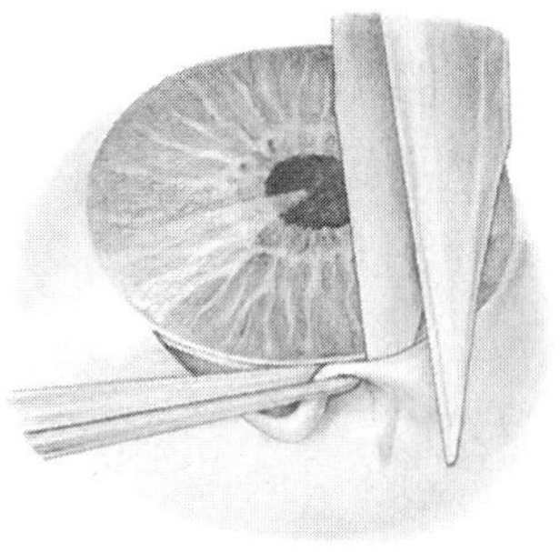

Figure 24–3. A radial cut at the edge of the peritomy can improve visualization of the sclera and permit a tight closure of the conjunctiva.

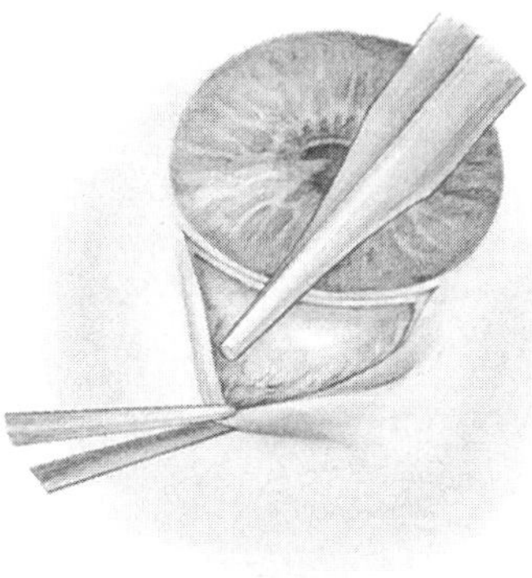

Figure 24–4. Blunt dissection is continued until the sclera is adequately cleaned. Bleeding from the cut conjunctival vessels is almost inevitable and usually exceed that which occurs when raising a limbus-based flap.

TECHNIQUE FOR CLOSING A FORNIX-BASED CONJUNCTIVAL FLAP

The advent of the antimetabolite era has changed the approach to closure of fornix-based conjunctival flaps in *trabeculectomy.* Loose reapproximation of conjunctiva to the limbus is not adequate and often leads to leaks with attendant choroidal detachment and shallow anterior chamber postoperatively. New suturing techniques[8,9,11,18] are being employed to permit safe use of antimetabolites and fornix-based conjunctival flaps in *trabeculectomy* and combined procedures.

TWO WING SUTURES

In placing wing sutures, 8.0 or 9.0 polygalactin suture is used to take a firm bite of the cornea inferolateral to the edge of the peritomy (Fig. 24–5). One anterior-lateral edge of cut conjunctiva from the peritomy is then stretched tightly across the peripheral cornea and secured with an interrupted suture to the cornea (Fig. 24–6). The same procedure is performed at the opposite end of the peritomy. The peripheral corneal epithelium may be debrided to facilitate adhesion of the conjunctiva to the peripheral cornea. Interrupted single[12] or mattress[13] 10.0 nylon or polygalactin sutures may be used to close gapes or obvious areas of leakage at the conjunctival edge. The wound should be tested by injection of balanced salt solution through a paracentesis to detect leaks.

RUNNING VERTICAL MATTRESS SUTURES

The fornix conjunctival flap can be closed with a 9-0 nylon suture and a VAS-100 needle as described by Wise.[9] This needle has a small cutting tip on a tapered needle. The needle is passed lateral to the peritomy through peripheral cornea to anchor the suture. The suture is tied and the free end is trimmed on the knot. The second bite begins in cornea adjacent to the first bite, and emerges through the free edge of the conjunctiva. A running vertical mattress suture attaching the edge of the conjunctiva to the peripheral cornea every 2 mm is then continued along the full length of the peritomy for

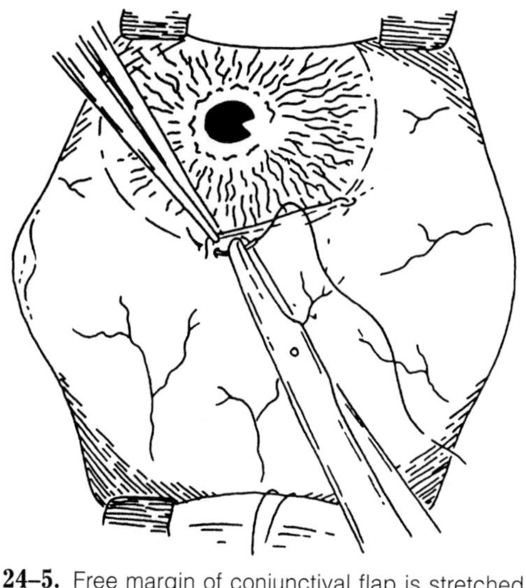

Figure 24–5. Free margin of conjunctival flap is stretched tightly over peripheral cornea with single sutures at either end of peritomy in the guarded filtration procedure with fornix-based conjunctival flap. (From Reichert R, Stewart W, Shields MB: Limbus-based versus fornix-based conjunctival flaps in trabeculectomy. Ophthalmic Surg 18:672–676,1987, with permission.)

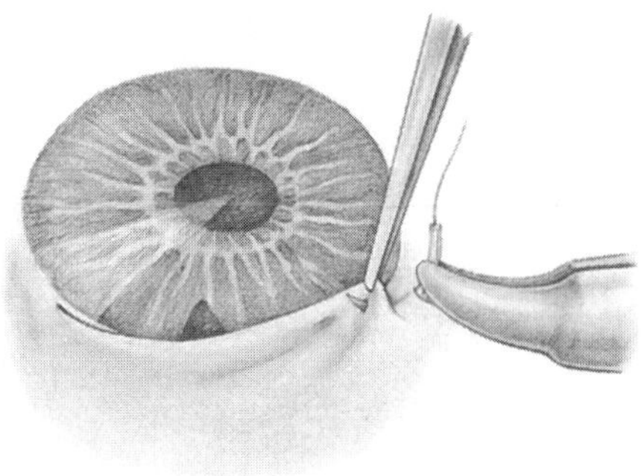

Figure 24–6. The cut edge of a fornix-based flap is pulled inferiorly and secured with a 10–0 nylon suture.

TABLE 24–2. Studies on Conjunctival Flaps for Trabeculectomy

Primary Author	Reference	Flap	No. Eyes	Combined Procedure	Mitomycin C Used	Success Rate (%)	IOP Defining Success	Complications	Follow-Up Months
Shuster	1	Limbus	18	No	No	94	21	4 eyes in the fornix group had positive	17
		Fornix	19			89		Seidel tests in first 3 days	
Luntz	2	Fornix	83	No	No	91.5	21	50% of patients on aqueous humor	1967–79
			10	Yes		100		suppressants postoperatively	
Traverso	3	Limbus	20	No	No	76	15	Temporary positive Seidel test:	8
		Fornix	20			71		2/20 limbus and 6/20 fornix group	
Murchison	6	Limbus	22	Yes	No	100	15	All but 6 on topical aqueous humor	1.5
		Fornix	25	ECCE		100		suppressants postoperatively	
Joos	8	Fornix	74	Yes	Yes	85	15	3 hypotony, 5 wound leaks, 5 hyphema,	12
				ECCE				1 endophthalmitis	
Wise	9	Fornix	316	No	50%	91	19	12% positive Seidel test in first month,	2–18
					Patients			1 endophthalmitis	
Megevand	10	Limbus	50	No	Yes	88	21	3 blebitis, 5 hypotony, 1 maculopathy	12
Lederer	11	Fornix	51	Yes	Yes	95	15	11% bleb leaks, 9% hypotony,	
				Phaco				9% cystoid macular edema	12
Agbeja	17	Fornix	10	No	No	100	"Adequate"	None	6
		Limbus	20			100			
Reichert	7	Limbus	20	No	No	90	21	Each group 1 choroidal drainage,	14
		Fornix	20			90		fornix 1 wound repair	
Stewart	5	Limbus	15	Yes	No	100	16	Limbus group: 1 suprachoroidal hemor-	6
		Fornix	16	Phaco		100		rhage, 4 bleb leaks. Fornix group:	
								1 hyphema, 1 bleb leak.	

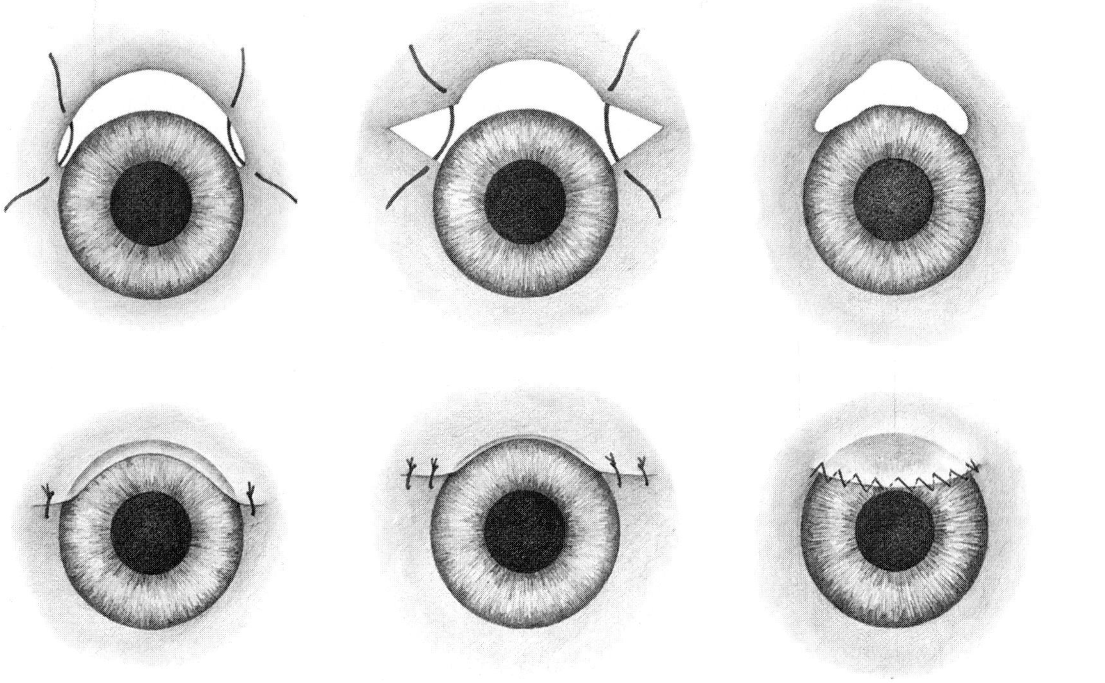

Figure 24–7. Methods of closing fornix-based flaps. *Left (top and bottom)*, Flap in which there is a small overlap of tissue. *Middle*, The use of relaxing incisions *(top)* has made it easier to approximate the conjunctiva back to its proper position *(bottom)*. *Right (top)*, Here tissue such as a failed bleb was excised. When this is done, the conjunctiva usually needs to be sutured into the cornea if the surgeon wants to cover the limbus tightly *(bottom)*.

a watertight closure. The suture is completed with a bite through cornea lateral to the end of the peritomy, and the knot is buried. The suture is stretched taut along the conjunctival edge to seal the conjunctiva to the peripheral cornea before the knot is tied.[9]

CENTRAL HORIZONTAL MATTRESS STITCH WITH LATERAL PURSE-STRINGS

For placing the central mattress suture, 10-0 nylon or polygalactin suture is passed horizontally through the cornea parallel to the limbus.[8] The suture bite is 1 mm anterior to the limbus, and in front of the scleral flap. The suture is then passed through the conjunctiva near the edge of the peritomy and back down through the conjunctiva as a horizontal mattress stitch and tied.

In placing the lateral purse-string, a bite is taken into clear cornea lateral to the lateral edge of the peritomy.[8] Conjunctiva is pulled taut across the limbus and impaled on the needle. An interrupted stitch secures the conjunctiva in place. This suture can then be run posteriorly to close a relaxing incision if necessary (Fig. 24–7).

COMPLICATIONS

Common complications of both limbus-based and fornix-based conjunctival flaps include episcleral bleeding, hyphema, conjunctival wound leaks with or without hypotony, corneal surface irregularities, and serous choroidal detachments (Table 24–2). With imprecise conjunctival closure, bleb leaks can lead to hypotony with decreased visual acuity secondary to astigmatism or maculopathy. Less frequent but more serious complications of filtering surgery include suprachoroidal hemorrhage and endophthalmitis. Reoperation may be necessary to lower intraocular pressure if the bleb scars and intraocular pressure rises leading to progression of optic nerve damage. No difference has been demonstrated between fornix-based and limbus-based conjunctival flaps in the rate or nature of complications except for wound leak in the early postoperative period.[3–6,8–11,17]

REFERENCES

1. Shuster JN, Krupin T, Kolker AE, Becker B: Limbus- v fornix-based conjunctival flap in trabeculectomy: A long-term randomized study. Arch Ophthalmol 1984;102:361.
2. Luntz MH: Trabeculectomy using a fornix-based conjunctival flap and tightly sutured scleral flap. Ophthalmology 1980;87:985–9.
3. Traverso CE, Tomey KF, Antonios S: Limbal- vs fornix-based conjunctival trabeculectomy flaps. Am J Ophthalmol 1987;104:28–32.
4. Luntz MH, Freedman J: The fornix-based conjunctival flap in glaucoma filtration surgery. Ophthalmic Surg 1980;11:516–21.
5. Stewart WC, Crinkley CM, Carlson AN: Fornix- vs. limbus-based flaps in combined phacoemulsification and trabeculectomy. Doc Ophthalmol 1994;88:141–51.
6. Murchison JF Jr, Shields MB: Limbal-based vs fornix-based conjunctival flaps in combined extracapsular cataract surgery and glaucoma filtering procedure. Am J Ophthalmol 1990;109:709–15.

7. Reichert R, Stewart W, Shields MB: Limbus-based versus fornix-based conjunctival flaps in trabeculectomy. Ophthalmic Surg 1987;18:672–6.
8. Joos KM, Bueche MJ, Palmberg PF, et al.: One-year follow-up results of combined mitomycin C trabeculectomy and extracapsular cataract extraction. Ophthalmology 1995;102:76–83.
9. Wise JB: Mitomycin-compatible suture technique for fornix-based conjunctival flaps in glaucoma filtration surgery. Arch Ophthalmol 1993;111:992–7.
10. Megevand GS, Salmon JF, Scholtz RP, Murray ADN: The effect of reducing the exposure time of mitomycin C in glaucoma filtering surgery. Ophthalmology 1995;102:84–90.
11. Lederer CM Jr: Combined cataract extraction with intraocular lens implant and mitomycin-augmented trabeculectomy. Ophthalmology 1996;103:1025–34.
12. Thomas JV: Filtering operation with scleral flap. In Thomas JV, Belcher CD, Simmons RJ (eds.), Glaucoma Surgery. St. Louis: Mosby-Year Book; 1992:29–41.
13. Hoskins HD, Kass MA: Becker-Shaffer's Diagnosis and Therapy of the Glaucomas, 6th Edition. St. Louis: CV Mosby; 1989:554–6.
14. Spaeth GL: Glaucoma surgery. In Spaeth GL (ed.), Ophthalmic Surgery: Principles and Practice. Philadelphia: WB Saunders; 1990:271–3.
15. Epstein DL, Allingham RR, Schuman JS: Chandler and Grant's Glaucoma, 4th Edition. Baltimore: Williams & Wilkins; 1997: 518–20.
16. Shields MB: Textbook of Glaucoma, 3rd Edition. Baltimore: Williams & Wilkins; 1992:578–80.
17. Agbeja AM, Dutton GN: Conjunctival incisions for trabeculectomy and their relationship to the type of bleb formation—a preliminary study. Eye 1987;1:738–43.
18. Liss RP, Scholes GN, Crandall AS: Glaucoma filtration surgery: New horizontal mattress closure of conjunctival incision. Ophthalmic Surg 1991;22:298–300.

CHAPTER 25

Primary Guarded Filtration Procedure Without Antimetabolite

ROGER A. HITCHINGS, F.R.C.S., F.R.C.Ophth. and
WENDY A. FRANKS, M.B., B.Chir., F.R.C.S., F.R.C.Ophth.

This chapter looks at the role for and the results that can be obtained from filtration surgery for glaucoma, without the use of antiproliferative agents. The principles of surgery are presented and standard surgical techniques are described. Factors that adversely affect outcome are discussed.

HISTORY OF THE DEVELOPMENT OF FILTRATION SURGERY

Glaucoma operations devised to lower intraocular pressure depended for their success on making a new permanent track for the aqueous humor to leave the eye. This fistula had to remain open despite wound healing, which starts in response to surgical injury.

The first approaches dating to the early years of the 20th century involved removal of a piece of full-thickness limbal sclera (see Shields[1] for a review). The most recent variants were the posterior lip sclerectomy described by Iliff and Haas in 1962,[2] and the mechanical removal of the sclera by trephination described independently by Elliott and Fergus[3,4] and later placed posteriorly to minimize the risk of infection (limboscleral trephination).[5] A third approach used cautery to effect retraction of the wound edges (thermal sclerostomy).[6,7] With all of these procedures, the normal healing response would appear to have been overcome by the flow of aqueous from the anterior chamber. These "full-thickness" operations produced low intraocular pressures, often with transconjunctival fluid flow (sweating).

The bulk outflow of aqueous humor from the anterior chamber that occurred after the full-thickness procedures produced an unacceptably high incidence of problems in the immediate postoperative period. Additionally the conjunctiva overlying the fistula tended to atrophy with time, with the risk of late endophthalmitis.

PRINCIPLES OF MODERN FILTRATION SURGERY

To reduce complications the "guarded sclerostomy" operation was devised.[8,9] Both of the originators referred to the operation as a "trabeculectomy." The reduction in immediate postoperative complications was spectacular and the guarded sclerostomy in one form or another became the "gold standard" for glaucoma surgery.

However because the operation avoided bulk outflow, it risked successful wound healing and a consequent resistance to the passage of aqueous through the coats of the eye, with a subsequent increase in intraocular pressure.

The term *trabeculectomy* was used as it was believed that aqueous humor drained circumferentially from the anterior chamber to the canal of Schlemm.[9] This is now known not to be the case, and there is no correlation between successful surgery and the presence or absence of Schlemm's canal, or trabecular meshwork, in the excised tissue.[10,11] Experimental and fluorescein studies have shown that aqueous reaches the subconjunctival space by percolating both around[12] and through the lamellar scleral flap[13] and is absorbed by lymphatic vessels and aqueous veins.[14] In modern practice the tissue excised is peripheral cornea, and the operation should, strictly speaking, be called *guarded corneostomy;* however, *guarded filtration procedure* is the preferred term.

The object of the operation is to create a full-thickness hole in the peripheral cornea and cover it with a lamellar corneoscleral flap. This flap is sutured into position tightly enough to create resistance to bulk outflow of aqueous in the immediate postoperative period and to prevent hypotony with shallowing of the anterior chamber. The flap is covered with conjunctiva to absorb aqueous percolating into the subconjunctival space. An iridectomy is performed to prevent occlusion of the ostium by this tissue.

PREPARATION FOR SURGERY

CONSENT

The necessity of performing an operation when there is no prospect of improvement in symptoms requires careful explanation. It is essential that the patient have a realistic expectation of the outcome of surgery. As well as informed consent concerning the potentially serious and blinding complications, more common potential problems such as ptosis[15] and bleb discomfort should be discussed.

OCULAR ASSESSMENT PREOPERATIVELY

Chronic lid margin infections should be treated preoperatively with topical broad-spectrum antibiotics and, in severe cases, with oral tetracycline. Cystic blebs are a common outcome in eyes with tear film instability secondary to chronic lid disease, with a likelihood of increased ocular discomfort after surgery.

Long-term use of topical medications also prejudices the long-range outcome of glaucoma surgery.[16-19] The effect due in part to the preservative that is a standard part of almost all typical medications used to treat glaucoma, but some antiglaucoma drugs, notably sympathomimetics, cause inflammation in their own right.[20] Treatment with topical beta-antagonists for 3 years does not affect outcome, but the addition of a second drug, pilocarpine, does. The addition of a third drug, for example a sympathomimetic, lowers the success rate still further.[21]

If the intraocular pressure is greater than 40 mm Hg preoperatively, uncontrolled with eye drops or systemic carbonic anhydrase inhibitors, then intravenous mannitol 1 mg/kg should be given 1 hour before surgery, provided the patient has good renal function.[22]

Preoperative steroids significantly increase the success rate[23,24] and should be considered for patients with chronically red eyes secondary to blepharitis or prolonged eye drops use.

ANESTHESIA

Choice of technique depends on the experience of the surgeon, stoicism of the patient, and ocular factors likely to make the surgery prolonged and difficult, such as palpebral aperture and previous conjunctival surgery.

Topical anesthesia is appropriate for experienced surgeons undertaking simple cases, but is not advised if there is difficult exposure or previous conjunctival surgery.

Local infiltration with 2% lignocaine injected temporal to the operation site and directed over the area of the scleral flap provides adequate anesthesia[25] for most cases but may be difficult to achieve in cases with poor exposure because of a small palpebral aperture.

Sub-Tenon's anesthesia is popular and provides both good anesthesia and akinesia, but it has been associated with local subconjunctival haemorrhage. Cautery to the incision site is usually necessary. An advantage is that antibiotics and corticosteroids may be given through the same site at the end of surgery.

Peribulbar and retrobulbar anesthesia are not suitable for cases with advanced optic disc cupping, because intraocular pressure spikes are likely and they increase the risk of postoperative central visual field loss.[26–28] Addition of adrenaline may further increase the intraocular pressure.[29]

General anesthesia lowers intraocular pressure and is useful when preoperative intraocular pressure is difficult to control medically. It is also the preferred option for the novice surgeon or restless patient.

SURGICAL PROCEDURE

CORNEAL TRACTION SUTURE

Superior rectus sutures are likely to be complicated by subconjunctival haemorrhage. A better means of fixing the eye in down-gaze during surgery is with a corneal traction suture (Fig. 25–1). Using silk suture material, pass the needle along a track in the peripheral cornea superiorly, 1 mm anterior to the limbus, employing as long a track as possible at 90% corneal depth. The end

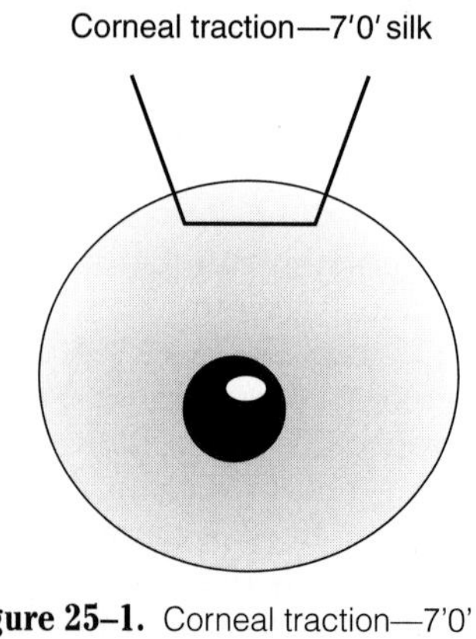

Figure 25–1. Corneal traction—7'0' silk.

of the suture can be clipped to the drape below the lower lid.

In prominent eyes with good exposure, a traction suture may not be necessary. Topical adrenaline blanches the conjunctiva prior to surgery to minimise haemorrhage.

CONJUNCTIVAL FLAPS

Conjunctival flaps may be either limbal based (the incision as far back in the fornix as possible) or fornix based (the conjunctiva is dissected from the limbus).[30–34] The design of the conjunctival flaps is described in Chapters 23 and 24. Any bleeding points should be cauterized immediately to prevent blood from spreading into the subconjunctival space. Blunt dissection clears episcleral adhesions.

We prefer fornix-based flaps because they can be created quickly and have less associated hemorrhage. Most important, they allow easier access to perform a very anterior full-thickness block. Their main disadvantage is that fornix-based flaps require very careful suturing to avoid postoperative leaks. Limbal-based flaps ease secure closure with suturing, but they are associated with more bleeding and potential damage to the superior rectus muscle.

SCLERAL DISSECTION

The scleral flap should be sited in the upper 180 degrees above the limbus. Sclerostomies in the lower 180 degrees have a higher risk of postoperative infection.[35] Placing the flap at the 12 o'clock position, is ideal, because this leaves room on either side should the operation ever need to be repeated.[36–38] Small-size punch sclerostomies increase this advantage.[36]

The shape and size of the scleral flap have no influence on outcome, although there is a suggestion that thin scleral flaps are associated with a lower postoperative intraocular pressure.[37] We recommend use of a scleral pocketknife to produce a scleral flap 3 mm × 3 mm (Fig. 25–2). A partial-thickness scleral groove is made 3 mm posterior to the limbus and a scleral pocket dissected into the peripheral cornea. The sides of the flap are then opened with a blade or scissors. To help reduce the risk of wound leaks, particularly when a fornix-based conjunctival flap has been used, the sides of the scleral flap should not be extended as far anteriorly into the peripheral cornea as the central dissection. Unsutured scleral tunnels have been advocated, but they provide less scope for postoperative manipulation of drainage.[39,40]

PARACENTESIS

To accomplish the optimal paracentesis, an oblique track reduces the risk of lens damage, and an inferotemporal approach facilitates re-formation of the anterior chamber postoperatively if shallowing occurs. If a hemorrhage occurs during surgery, a viscoelastic substance can be injected through the paracentesis for tamponade.

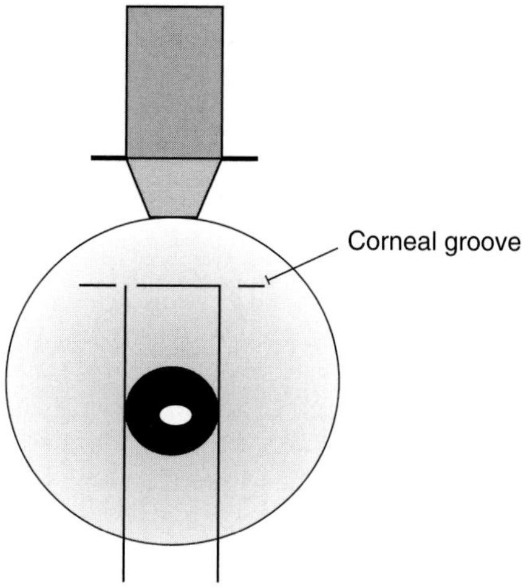

Figure 25–2. Scleral flap dissection with pocket knife.

PREPLACED SCLERAL FLAP SUTURES

There are many ways of using releasable sutures[41,42]; we favor pre-placement of releasable sutures (Figs. 25–3 and 25–4) to allow the eye to be closed quickly and thus reduce the amount of time the eye is hypotonous. Placement is easier in a firm eye prior to deep block dissection.

Two corneal grooves are made on either side of the scleral flap for placement of releasable suture loops so that postoperatively the epithelium covers the suture, reducing the risk of suture irritation and infection. Two 10-0 nylon sutures are preplaced prior to dissecting the scleral block (Fig. 25–4).

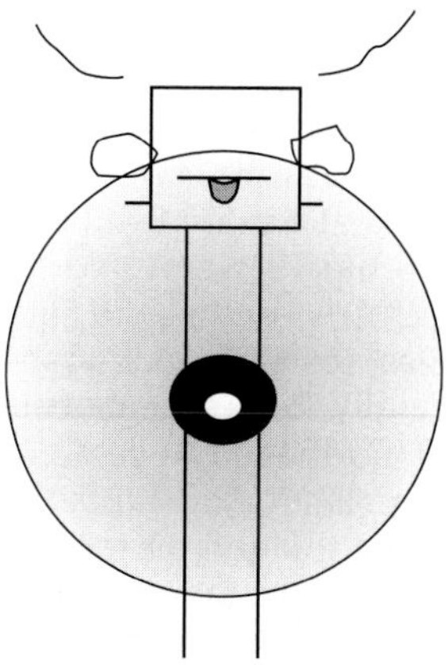

Figure 25–3. Deep pocket dissection with punch (preplaced releasable sutures).

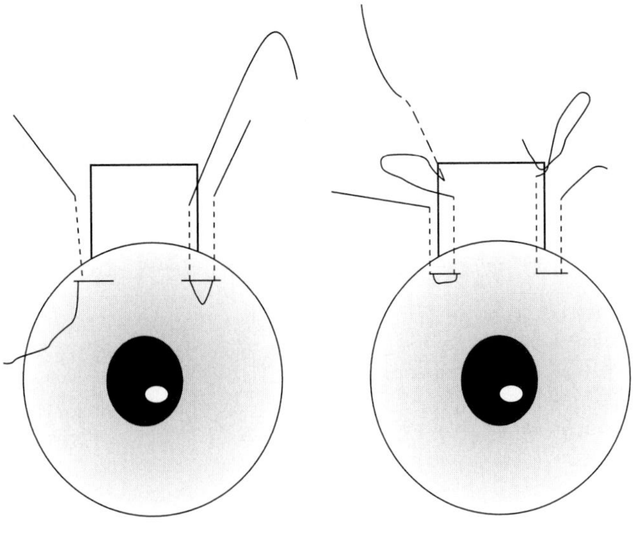

Figure 25–4. Releasable suture technique.

DEEP BLOCK

An incision is made in clear cornea 3 mm in length and as far anteriorly as possible, and a punch is used to remove a full-thickness block of tissue. As an alternative to using a punch, a sharp blade can be used to excise a rectangular block of tissue, but care must be taken that the sides of the block are vertical. Too large a block may cause weakening of the wound and changes in corneal topography[43]; too small, and it may become blocked by iris or other tissue. The advantage of using a punch is that it ensures a full-thickness block and the procedure is quick.[36]

PERIPHERAL IRIDECTOMY

The iridectomy is peripheral, but not basal, so that trauma to blood vessels in the anterior chamber angle is avoided. The iridectomy should be large enough to minimize the risk of iris tissue occluding the deep block, but not so large that the patient runs the risk of monocular diplopia. In practice, then, an iridectomy that involves the outer one-third to one-half of the radius of the iris, that is two clock hours in width at the base, and that is sited so that it lies behind the upper eyelid will suffice. The iris should be inspected before being cut, and any visible iris vessels should be cauterized. The iris should be fixed at a point just beneath the anterior edge of the deep block and pulled through centrifugally; the "tented" iris can then be cut with sharp scissors and the edges washed back into the anterior chamber. Bleeding usually stops spontaneously. Tamponade of persistent haemorrhage can be accomplished by injection of a viscoelastic substance into the anterior chamber. Excessive traction on the iris root can cause bleeding from vessels in the anterior chamber angle. These vessels are difficult to cauterize and it may take some time before the bleeding stops spontaneously.

The integrity of the wound must be checked after balanced salt solution is injected through the paracentesis to form the anterior chamber fully. Pressure applied to the posterior margin of the scleral flap should cause a bleb to form. Subconjunctival corticosteroids and antibiotics should be given on completion of surgery.

POSTOPERATIVE MANAGEMENT

Intensive postoperative management is crucial to the success of the operation. Topical corticosteroids should be applied as frequently as every 2 hours for the first 2 weeks, reducing to 4 times daily for a further 6 weeks, and then tapering over a period of 3 months.

The beneficial effects of postoperative topical steroids have been demonstrated by Spaeth and co-workers, who showed that eyes treated with topical steroids had significantly lower intraocular pressures than those not treated.[44] Others have confirmed these findings.[45,46] A topical antibiotic is used for the same period.

In eyes with an unusual amount of inflammation or where a hyphema has occurred, postoperative cycloplegia with cyclopentolate twice daily is prescribed. If the intraocular pressure is high on the first postoperative day, the bleb can be massaged by pressing on the posterior margin of the scleral flap.[47] Releasable sutures are not removed at this stage unless drainage cannot be achieved by massage.

Subconjunctival steroids can be given, as an alternative to antiproliferatives, in the area of the bleb postoperatively to reduce inflammation and to break down adhesion between the conjunctival and scleral flaps. Over the next few weeks if the bleb drains but the pressure is higher than desired, the releasable sutures can be removed one at a time. If the intraocular pressure is satisfactory the releasable sutures are not removed unless proud of the epithelium.

RESULTS

Guarded sclerostomy was quickly accepted by ophthalmologists because of reduced postoperative complications. The initial popularity of the operation was followed by many review papers assessing the intraocular pressure control at varying periods after surgery and quoting success rates of 75% to 95%,[48–53] where success was defined as an intraocular pressure within the normal range. It was suggested that intraocular pressures in the postoperative period could predict long-term success.[54,55] In eyes without "risk factors" for failure (see below) the mean intraocular pressure after surgery was 15 mm Hg, whatever the preoperative pressure had been,[48] suggesting that the healing response could reset resistance to flow at a surprisingly constant level.

Because the reason for glaucoma surgery is to prevent visual loss, this should be the measured outcome.[55–58] Long-term follow-up studies that assessed the percentage of eyes in groups of patients undergoing fistulizing surgery revealed that the proportion continuing to lose visual field was inversely proportional to the mean postoperative intraocular pressure, with the mean intraocular pressures in the different studies ranging from 14.5 to 19.0 mm Hg.[59] Few studies to date have managed to show success in terms of visual outcome, although recent assessments of change after surgery in normal tension glaucoma have attempted to do so.[60–62] It remains easier to use postoperative intraocular pressure as a proxy, equating success with pressures at least within the normal range and preferably in the low or mid teens.

RISK FACTORS FOR FAILURE

Glaucoma surgery can fail, i.e., the intraocular pressure rises above the norm (21 mm Hg) at any time after the operation. A review of the histology of conjunctival and episcleral tissues removed at re-operation at different stages after the original surgery revealed two different pictures: "early failure," occurring within the first 3 months, and "late failure," seen at any point beyond 3 months.[63] The former exhibited an acute inflammatory response; the latter, an acellular response with deposition of collagen and ground substance. These changes are mirrored by the timing of "failure" after surgery, most failures occurring within the first 3 months (after the acute inflammatory response),[16] after which a gradual attrition of success rates continues.[18,45,50]

Risk factor inducing early failure include the following:

- Those which prime conjunctival and episcleral fibroblasts
- Prior conjunctival surgery
- Chronic conjunctival inflammation
- Those which produce abnormal aqueous, stimulating fibroblast activity
- Prior intraocular surgery
- Concurrent ocular inflammation
- An inherent tendency for an increased response in the untreated conjunctiva
- Youth
- Black race

A similar response can be triggered by subsequent events such as intraocular surgery or bleb infections.

Factors inducing late failure are less clear. Here the process appears to be deposition of ground substance and collagen sheets producing a flat scar of cystic elevation without overt signs of inflammation. The process would seem to be continuous and due to slow replication of fibroblasts. There is a tendency for the rate of failure to increase with time.[49,52,59]

FUTURE OF FILTRATION SURGERY

Guarded fistulizing surgery remains the "gold standard" for glaucoma, although nonpenetrating surgery is gaining popularity with some surgeons. Antiproliferative treatment has greatly improved the success rate in eyes at risk of failure, as described. The advantages of nonpenetrating surgery are fewer postoperative complications both early and late, with less risk of postoperative anterior chamber shallowing, hypotony, and hyphema.[64–66] Also, because the blebs formed are very shallow, there is no postoperative tear film disturbance. The main disadvantages are difficult surgical technique and poorer intraocular pressure control. Long-term studies are required to compare the effectiveness of the variants[67] of the operation with conventional surgery.

CONCLUSION

This chapter emphasizes the seminal role for the guarded filtration surgery in glaucoma. By restricting fluid flow in the immediate postoperative period postoperative wound healing is the main reason for failure to control intraocular pressure. Some preoperative and postoperative risk factors for failure can be avoided without the need to suppress the healing response with antimetabolites.

REFERENCES

1. Shields MB: Filtering surgery. In Textbook of Glaucoma, 3rd Edition. Baltimore: Williams & Wilkins;1992:577–611.
2. Iliff CE, Haas J: Posterior lip sclerectomy. Am J Ophthalmol 1962;54:688–92.
3. Elliott RH: A preliminary note on a new operative procedure for the establishment of a filtering cicatrix in the treatment of glaucoma. Ophthalmoscope 1909;7:807.
4. Fergus F: Treatment of glaucoma by trephining. Br Med J 1909;2:983.
5. Sugar H: Limboscleral trephination. Arch Ophthalmol 1961;85: 703–6.
6. Preziosi C: The electrocautery in the treatment of glaucoma. Br J Ophthalmol 1924;8:414.
7. Scheie HG: Retraction of scleral wound edges as a fistulising procedure for glaucoma. Am J Ophthalmol 1958;45:220.
8. Sugar H: Experimental trabeculectomy in glaucoma. Am J Ophthalmol 1961;51:623.
9. Cairns JE: Trabeculectomy. Preliminary report of a new method. Am J Ophthalmol 1968;5:673–7.
10. Schmitt H: Histological examination of discs obtained by goniotrephining with scleral flap. Klin Monastsbl Augenheilk 1975;167:372–81.
11. Taylor H: A histologic survey of trabeculectomy. Am J Ophthalmol 1976;82:733–7.
12. Benedikt OP: Demonstration of the mode of action of trabeculectomy. Klin Monatsbl Augenheilk 1975;167:679–82.

13. Shields M, Bradbury M, Shelburne J, Bell S: The permeability of the outer layers of the limbus and anterior sclera. Invest Ophthalmol Vis Sci 1977;16:866–70.
14. Benedikt OP: Demonstration of aqueous outflow patterns of normal and glaucomatous human eyes through the injection of fluorescein sodium into the anterior chamber. Graefes Arch Clin Exp Ophthalmol 1976;199:45–54.
15. Sung MS, Shin DH, Spoor TC: Incidence of ptosis following trabeculectomy, a comparative study Korean J Ophthalmol 1996; 10:97–103.
16. Lavin MJ, Wormald RPL, Migdal CS, Hitchings RA: The influence of prior therapy on the success of trabeculectomy. Arch Ophthalmol 1990;108:11543–8.
17. Broadway D, Grierson I, Hitchings R: the effect of topical antiglaucomatous medications on the cell profile of the conjunctiva. Current Opin Ophthalmol 1993;4:51–7.
18. Broadway D, Grierson I, Hitchings R: Topical antiglaucomatous therapy; adverse effects of the conjunctiva and implications for filtration surgery. J Glaucoma 1995;4:136–48.
19. Broadway DC, Grierson I, O'Brien C, Hitchings RA: Adverse effects of topical antiglaucoma medication. II. The outcome of filtration surgery. Arch Ophthalmol 1994;112:1446–54.
20. Wright P: Adverse reactions to guanethidine eye drops (letter). Br J Ophthalmol 1987;71:323.
21. Broadway D, Hitchings R: Conjunctival damage induced by long-term topical anti-glaucoma therapy (letter; comment). Acta Ophthalmol Scand 1996;74:97.
22. O'Keefe M, Naibul M: The use of mannitol in intraocular surgery. Ophthalmic Surg 1983;14:55–6.
23. Giangiacomo J, Dueker DK, Adelstein E: The effect of preoperative subconjunctival triamcinolone administration on glaucoma filtration. I. Trabeculectomy following subconjunctival triamcinolone.
24. Broadway DC, Grierson I, Sturmer J, Hitchings RA: Reversal of topical antiglaucoma medication effects on the conjunctiva. Arch Ophthalmol 1996;114:262–7.
25. Noureddin BN, Jeffrey M, Franks WA, Hitchings RA: Conjunctival changes after subconjunctival lignocaine. Eye 1993;7:457–60.
26. Morgan JE, Chandra A: Intraocular pressure after peribulbar anaesthesia—Is the Honan balloon necessary. Br J Ophthalmol 1995;79:46–9.
27. O'Donoghue E, Batterby M, Lavy T: Effect on intraocular pressure of local anaesthesia in eyes undergoing surgery. Br J Ophthalmol 1994;78:605–7.
28. Bowman R, Liu C, Sarkies N: Intraocular pressure changes after peribulbar injections with and without ocular compression. Br J Ophthalmol 1996;80:394–7.
29. Gjotterberg M, Ingemansson SU: Effect on intraocular pressure of retrobulbar injection of xylocaine with and without adrenaline. Acta Ophthalmol 1977;55:709–16.
30. Brincker P, Kessing SV: Limbus-based versus fornix-based conjunctival flap in glaucoma filtering surgery. Acta Ophthalmol Copenh 1992;70:641–4.
31. Traverso CE, Tomey KF, Antonius S: Limbal-based versus fornix-based conjunctival trabeculectomy flaps. Am J Ophthalmol 1987;104:28–32.
32. Grehn F, Mauthe S, Pfeiffer N: Limbus-based versus Fornix-based conjunctival flap in filtering surgery. A randomised prospective study. Int Ophthalmol 1989;13:139–43.
33. Murchison JF Jr, Shields MB: Limbal-based versus fornix-based conjunctival flaps in combined extracapsular cataract surgery and glaucoma filtering procedure. Am J Ophthalmol 1990;109: 709–15.
34. Reichart R, Stewart W, Shields MB: Limbus-based versus fornix-based conjunctival flaps in trabeculectomy. Ophthalmic Surg 1987;18:672–6.
35. Caronia RM, Liebmann JM, Freidman R, et al.: Trabeculectomy at the inferior limbus. Arch Ophthalmol 1996;114:387–91.
36. Suzuku R: Trabeculectomy with a Kelly Descemet membrane punch. Ophthalmologica 1997;211:93–4.
37. Vernon SA, Spencer AF: Intraocular pressure control following microtrabeculectomy. Eye 1995;9:299–303.
38. Ophir A: Minitrabeculectomy without radial incisions. Am J Ophthalmol 1999;127:212–3.
39. Lai JSM, Lam DSC: Trabeculectomy using a sutureless scleral tunnel technique —A preliminary study. J Glaucoma 1999;8:188–92.
40. Schumer RA, Odrich SA: A scleral tunnel incision for trabeculectomy. Am J Ophthalmol 1995;120:528–30.
41. Jacob P, Thomas R, Mahajan A, et al.: Releasable suture technique for trabeculectomy. Indian J Ophthalmol 1993;41:81–2.
42. Kolker AE, Kass MA, Rait JL: Trabeculectomy with releasable sutures. Arch Ophthalmol 1994;112:62–6.
43. Claridge KG, Galbratih JK, Karmel V, Bates AK: The effect of trabeculectomy on refraction, keratometry and corneal topography. Eye 1995;9:292–8.
44. Roth SM, Spaeth GL, Starita RJ, et al.: The effects of postoperative corticosteroids on trabeculectomy and the clinical course of glaucoma: Five year follow-up study. Ophthalmic Surg 1991;22:724–9.
45. Miller MH, Grierson I, Unger WG, Hitchings RA: The effect of topical dexamethasone and preoperative beta irradiation on a model of glaucoma fistulising surgery in the rabbit. Ophthalmic Surg 1990;21:44–54.
46. Fechner PU, Wichman W: Retarded corneo-scleral wound healing associated with high preoperative doses of systemic steroids in glaucoma surgery. Refract Corneal Surg 1991;7:174–6.
47. Traverso CE, Greenidge KC, Spaeth GL, Wilson RP: Focal pressure: A new method to encourage filtration after trabeculectomy. Ophthalmic Surg 1984;15:62–5.
48. Jay JL, Murray SB: Characteristics of reduction of intraocular pressure after trabeculectomy. Br J Ophthalmol 1980;64:432–5.
49. Mills KB: Trabeculectomy; a retrospective long term follow up of 444 cases. Br J Ophthalmol 1981;65:790–5.
50. Watson PG, Jakeman C, Ozturk M, et al.: The complications of trabeculectomy (a 20 year follow-up). Eye 1990;4:425–38.
51. Migdal C, Gregory W, Hitchings R: Long term functional outcome after early surgery compared with laser and medicine in open angle glaucoma. Ophthalmology 1994;101:1651–6.
52. Chen TC, Wilensky JT, Viana MA: Long term follow-up of initially successful trabeculectomy. Ophthalmology 1997;104:1120–5.
53. Robinson DI, Lertsumitkul S, Billson FA, Robinson LP: Long-term intraocular pressure control by trabeculectomy: A ten year life table. Aust NZ J Ophthalmol 1993;21:79–85.
54. Downes SM, Misson GP, Jones HS, O'Neill EC: The predictive value of post-operative intraocular pressures following trabeculectomy. Eye 1994;8:394–7.
55. Bayer AU, Erb C, Ferrari F, et al.: The Tubingen Glaucoma Study. Glaucoma filtering surgery—A retrospective long-term follow-up of 254 eyes with glaucoma. German J Ophthalmol 1995;4: 289–93.
56. Hitchings RA: Outcome measures for glaucoma treatment. Br J Ophthalmol 1997;81:427.
57. Zimmerman TJ, Karunaratna N, Fechtner RD: Glaucoma: Outcomeology. (Part I). (editorial). J Glaucoma 1996;5:152–5.
58. Zimmerman TJ, Karunaratna N, Fechtner RD: Glaucoma: Outcomeology. (Part II). (editorial) J Glaucoma 1996;5:152–5.
59. Palmberg P: Epidemiology of POAG and rationale for therapy. Glaucoma Abstracts 1989;6:10–23.
60. Koseki N, Araie M, Shirato S, Yamamoto S: Effect of trabeculectomy on visual field performance in central 30 degrees field in progressive normal-tension glaucoma. Ophthalmology 1997;104: 197–201.
61. Bhandari A, Crabbe DP, Poinoosawmy D, et al.: Effect of surgery on visual field progression in normal tension glaucoma. Ophthalmology 1997;104:1131–7.
62. Collaborative Normal-Tension Glaucoma Study Group: Comparison of glaucomatous progression between untreated patients with normal-tension glaucoma and patients with therapeutically reduced intraocular pressures. Am J Ophthalmol 1998;126:487–97.
63. Hitchings RA, Grierson I: Clinico-pathological correlation in eyes with failed fistulising surgery. Trans Ophthalmol Soc 1983;103: 84–8.
64. Mermoud A, Schnyder CC, Sickenberg M, et al.: Comparison of deep sclerectomy with collagen implant in open angle glaucoma. Br J Ophthalmol 1999;83:6–11.
65. Sourdille P, Santiago PY, Villan F, et al.: Reticulated hyaluronic acid implant in non-perforating trabecular surgery. J Cataract Refract Surg 1999;25:322–9.
66. Bechetoille A: External trabeculectomy with aspiration: Surgical technique. J Fr Ophtalmol 1999;22:781–6.
67. Stegmann R, Pienaar A, Miller D: Viscocanalostomy for open angle glaucoma in black African patients. J Cataract Refract Surg 1999;25:316–22.

CHAPTER 26

Guarded Filtration Procedure with 5-Fluorouracil

RICHARD K. PARRISH II, M.D. and STEVEN J. GEDDE, M.D.

The goal of glaucoma filtering surgery is to create a permanent flow of aqueous humor from the anterior chamber to the subconjunctival space, which results in the formation of a filtering bleb and the reduction of intraocular pressure. Bleb failure most often results from excessive healing from fibroblast proliferation and subconjunctival fibrosis.[1] Therefore, glaucoma filtering surgery differs from other surgical procedures in that inhibition of wound healing is desirable to achieve surgical success. Considerable attention has been directed to pharmacological techniques to interfere with wound healing. 5-Fluorouracil (5-FU) was identified as a potent inhibitor of fibroblast proliferation and modulates wound healing through this mechanism.

5-FU is a pyrimidine analogue that inhibits proliferating cells by acting selectively on the S (synthesis) phase of the cell cycle[2,3]; it is a chemotherapeutic agent that is frequently employed in the treatment of breast and colon cancers.[2] The drug was first used in ocular therapy for the treatment of proliferative vitreoretinopathy.[4] It was subsequently investigated as an adjunct in glaucoma filtering surgery. In animal studies 5-FU demonstrated a decidedly positive effect in filtering bleb survival.[5] A pilot study in humans suggested that it was beneficial in glaucoma patients with poor surgical prognosis owing to aphakia, previously failed filtering surgery, or neovascular glaucoma.[6–8] These promising results led to a multicenter, randomized clinical trial that provided validation for the use of 5-FU in glaucoma filtering surgery.[9–11]

INDICATIONS

Adjunctive use of 5-FU is indicated in glaucomatous eyes with poor surgical prognoses. In the Fluorouracil Filtering Surgery Study (FFSS), eyes with aphakia, pseudophakia, or previously failed filtering surgery underwent a guarded filtration procedure with or without postoperative subconjunctival 5-FU injections. This study demonstrated a statistically significant enhancement of intraocular pressure control and avoidance of reoperation for pressure control in the 5-FU group compared with the standard treatment group at 1-year, 3-year, and 5-year follow-up.[9–11] Other clinical studies have suggested a beneficial effect of 5-FU on surgical outcome in other glaucomas at high risk for failure of filtering surgery, including neovascular glaucoma,[6–8,12–14] inflammatory glaucoma,[12–16] and juvenile glaucoma.[13,14] Other groups in which 5-FU may improve surgical success are young patients (age less than 40 years)[17] and black patients,[18] who exhibit an exuberant healing response after glaucoma surgery. Adjunctive 5-FU may also be useful after needing revision of failing filtering blebs.[19,20]

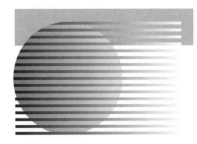

Based on encouraging results in eyes with poor surgical prognoses, interest has grown in the use of 5-FU for cases not traditionally considered high risk (Table 26–1). The need for extremely low intraocular pressures, as in normal-tension glaucoma and advanced primary open-angle glaucoma, may also be an indication for 5-FU, even in the absence of risk factors for fail-

TABLE 26–1. Indications for Use of 5-Fluorouracil

- Aphakia/pseudophakia
- Failed filtering surgery
- Neovascular glaucoma
- Inflammatory glaucoma
- Juvenile glaucoma
- Young age (<40 years)
- Black race
- Following needling revision of a failing filtering bleb
- Need for a very low intraocular pressure

ure of filtering surgery.[21] Low-dose postoperative 5-FU has been shown to improve the success rate in uncomplicated primary guarded filtration procedures.[22,23]

CONTRAINDICATIONS

The potential risks of using 5-FU must be considered along with its benefits (Table 26–2). Because of an increased risk of serious postoperative corneal complications, postoperative subconjunctival 5-FU should be avoided in patients with preexisting corneal and conjunctival disease, such as severe keratitis sicca, bullous keratopathy, or limbal stem cell deficiency. Similarly, caution is warranted with the administration of 5-FU in patients with abnormalities of lid function or lid position, including lagophthalmos, entropion, and ectropion. Use of 5-FU is not advised in pregnant or nursing women, young children, or any patient contemplating pregnancy within the subsequent few months, male or female, because of possible adverse effects on development.

SURGICAL TECHNIQUE

POSTOPERATIVE SUBCONJUNCTIVAL INJECTION

Subconjunctival injections of 5-FU may be administered in an undiluted (50 mg/ml) or diluted (10 mg/ml) concentration (Table 26–3). A standard dose of 5 mg (0.1 ml of the 50 mg/ml solution or 0.5 ml of the 10 mg/ml solution) is drawn into a tuberculin syringe. The syringe plunger is withdrawn to produce a small air bubble in the barrel of the syringe. The tuberculin needle is then replaced by a smaller, ⅝", 30-gauge needle for the actual subconjunctival injection. The air bubble is expressed into the needle's protective cap. A drop of proparacaine is administered, and a cotton-tipped applicator soaked in 4% topical lidocaine is applied to the planned injection site to provide adequate anesthesia. The injection is given 180 degrees from the guarded filtration site and approximately 5 mm from the limbus, preferably with the aid of some magnification (slit lamp or loupes) so that conjunctival blood vessels may be avoided. The needle is advanced into the subconjunctival space, and 5-FU is injected slowly. A slow injection of 5-FU seems to lessen patient discomfort and facilitate spreading. Sterile balanced salt solution is used to wash away any excess 5-FU from the conjunctival sac and cornea immediately following injection. The 5-FU vial, needles, and syringe should be disposed of in accordance with environmental regulations.

In the FFSS, 5-FU was injected subconjunctivally at a dose of 5 mg twice a day during postoperative days 1 through 7, and 5 mg once a day during postoperative days 8 through 14 (total dose 105 mg).[9] However, subsequent reports have suggested that lower doses produce comparable intraocular pressure control with fewer side effects.[12–14] Many ophthalmologists inject 5 mg of 5-FU once daily during the first postoperative week and three times total, during the second week (total dose 50 mg). Others have initiated injections at the first clinical signs of bleb failure, including flattening of the bleb, an increase in vascularity, or elevation of intraocular pressure. The optimum dose will depend on the results of further clinical trials. The best amount given probably varies among patients and depends on the risk factors present that predispose to bleb failure.

Before each postoperative subconjunctival injection, a careful slit-lamp examination must be performed; this examination includes Seidel testing of the wound and bleb. Injections are typically withheld in the presence of a large corneal epithelial defect, conjunctival wound leak or "buttonhole," or overfiltration with hypotony,

TABLE 26–2. Contraindications for Use of 5-Fluorouracil

- Preexisting corneal and conjunctival disease (e.g., severe keratitis sicca, bullous keratopathy, limbal stem cell deficiency)
- Abnormalities of lid function or lid position (e.g., lagophthalmos, entropion, ectropion)
- Pregnant or nursing women
- Young children
- Patient (male or female) contemplating pregnancy

TABLE 26–3. Steps in Postoperative 5-Fluorouracil Injections

1. Draw 5 mg of 5-FU into a tuberculin syringe.
2. Replace the tuberculin needle with a 30-gauge needle.
3. Instill a drop of proparacaine, and apply a cotton-tipped applicator soaked in lidocaine to the planned injection site.
4. Advance the needle into the subconjunctival space 180 degrees from the trabeculectomy site approximately 5 mm from the limbus.
5. Slowly inject the 5-FU.
6. Wash away any excess 5-FU from the conjunctival sac and cornea with balanced salt solution.
7. Discard the 5-FU vial, needles, and syringe in accordance with environmental regulations.

TABLE 26–4. Reasons to Withhold Postoperative 5-Fluorouracil Injections

- Corneal epithelial defect
- Conjunctival wound leak or "buttonhole"
- Overfiltration with hypotony, anterior chamber shallowing, or "kissing" choroidal detachments

anterior chamber shallowing or "kissing" choroidal detachments (Table 26–4). Although daily injections are inconvenient, the ability to withhold 5-FU doses when there is clinical evidence of toxicity or excessive filtration allows for a desirable level of control.

INTRAOPERATIVE APPLICATION

The intraoperative application of 5-FU has been reported.[18,24–27] With this technique, a cellulose sponge soaked in 50 mg/ml of 5-FU is placed under the scleral and conjunctival flap for 5 minutes. The sponge is then removed, and the area is copiously irrigated with balanced salt solution to remove any residual 5-FU before the eye is entered. The advantages of direct intraoperative application of 5-FU include reduced corneal toxicity, immediate exposure of the target tissue to a maximum concentration of drug, and ease of administration compared with repeated subconjunctival injections. Recent cell culture work has demonstrated prolonged inhibition of human ocular fibroblast proliferation after a single 5-FU exposure.[28] Several investigators have shown good outcomes using this technique.[18,24–27]

COMPLICATIONS

CORNEAL EPITHELIAL TOXICITY

Among the complications associated with the use of 5-FU (Table 26–5), corneal epithelial toxicity is the most common. It usually becomes manifest as punctate epithelial erosions, filaments, and corneal epithelial defects. Severe corneal complications, including sterile and bacterial ulceration, corneal keratinization, and striate melanokeratosis, have also been reported in patients with preexisting corneal abnormalities who received postoperative 5-FU.[29,30] The drug nonselectively inhibits cell replication in dividing cells, and corneal toxicity is a direct result of its antiproliferative effect on corneal epithelial cells.

Corneal side effects associated with the use of 5-FU appear to be dose related. Adjusting the dose of 5-FU according to the clinical response can reduce the incidence and severity of corneal complications.[12] Punctate epithelial erosions usually precede the development of a frank epithelial defect and are a sign of early corneal toxicity. Corneal epithelial defects are best managed by withholding additional 5-FU injections, which can then be reinstituted when the epithelium has healed.

TABLE 26–5. Complications Associated with 5-Fluorouracil

- Corneal epithelial toxicity
- Conjunctival wound leaks
- Suprachoroidal hemorrhage
- Late-onset bleb leaks
- Late-onset bleb-related endophthalmitis

CONJUNCTIVAL WOUND LEAKS

Because 5-FU inhibits wound healing, conjunctival wound leaks and buttonholes are more problematic when adjunctive antifibrosis therapy is used. Conjunctival wound leaks occurred more frequently in the 5-FU group than in the standard treatment group in the FFSS.[9] Persistent aqueous leaks can jeopardize the formation of a filtering bleb during the postoperative period. Conjunctival leaks may also result in hypotony and anterior chamber shallowing with their attendant complications.

Certain modifications in surgical technique become especially important when wound healing is pharmacologically impaired. A corneal traction suture is an effective alternative to a superior rectus bridle suture to enhance surgical exposure, and it eliminates the risk of postoperative aqueous leaks through the bridle suture needle tracts. A limbus-based conjuctival flap is preferred to a fornix-based flap because it allows greater security of wound closure. Because the filtering bleb may become thin-walled when 5-FU is used, a tenonectomy generally should not be performed. Careful dissection of the conjunctival flap is critical, so buttonholes may be avoided.

Subconjunctival injection of balanced salt solution may facilitate elevation of the conjunctiva and permit identification of areas of scarring in difficult cases. Meticulous closure of the wound, and of any conjunctival buttonholes, is imperative. A two-layer closure of Tenon's capsule and conjunctiva separately helps ensure the fluid-tight integrity of the wound. A tapered microvascular needle should be used, because it creates a needle tract that is only slightly larger than the suture itself and the needle tract is filled by the suture. Subconjunctival injections at the conclusion of the case should be given 180 degrees from the filtering site through a 30-gauge needle. This serves to reduce the risk of postoperative aqueous leaks through the needle tract. Postoperative subconjunctival 5-FU injections should be withheld in the presence of a conjunctival wound leak.

LATE-ONSET BLEB-RELATED ENDOPHTHALMITIS

The blebs produced after filtering surgery with 5-FU are often thin-walled, avascular, and cytic, and they are prone to develop late-onset leaks and bleb-related endophthalmitis. The incidence of late bleb-related endophthalmitis after a guarded filtration procedure with

5-FU appears to be higher than filtering surgery without adjunctive 5-FU, especially when the surgery is performed from below.[31]

Filtering surgery in the inferior quadrants should be avoided if at all possible. The value of chronic antibiotic prophylaxis in the setting of a late-onset bleb leak or a thin walled, ischemic bleb remains to be determined.[31] Any patient with a filtering bleb should be instructed to seek immediate medical attention for the development of redness, pain, photophobia, or decreased vision. Early treatment of bleb infections appears to be associated with an improved prognosis for visual recovery and preservation of bleb function.[31]

REFERENCES

1. Skuta GL, Parrish RK II: Wound healing in glaucoma filtering surgery. Surv Ophthalmol 1987;32:149–70
2. Falck FY, Skuta GL, Klein TB: Mitomycin versus 5-fluorouracil antimetabolite therapy for glaucoma filtration surgery. Semin Ophthalmol 1992;7:97–109.
3. Tahery MM, Lee DA: Review: Pharmacologic control of wound healing in glaucoma filtration surgery. J Ocul Pharmacol 1989;5:155–79
4. Blumenkranz MS, Ophir A, Claflin AJ, Hajek A: Fluorouracil for the treatment of massive periretinal proliferation. Am J Ophthalmol 1982;94:458–67.
5. Gressel MG, Parrish RK II, Folberg R: 5-Fluorouracil and glaucoma filtering surgery: I. An animal model. Ophthalmology 1984;91:378–83.
6. Heuer DK, Parrish RK II, Gressel MG, et al.: 5-Fluorouracil and glaucoma filtering surgery. II. A pilot study. Ophthalmology 1984;91:384–93.
7. Heuer DK, Parrish RK II, Gressel MG, et al.: 5-Fluorouracil and glaucoma filtering surgery. III. Intermediate follow-up of a pilot study. Ophthalmology 1986;93:1537–46.
8. Rockwood EJ, Parrish RK II, Heuer DK, et al.: Glaucoma filtering surgery with 5-fluorouracil. Ophthalmology 1987;94:1071–8
9. The Fluorouracil Filtering Surgery Study Group: Fluorouracil filtering study one-year follow-up. Am J Ophthalmo 1989;108: 626–35.
10. The Fluorouracil Filtering Surgery Study Group: Three-year follow-up of the fluorouracil filtering surgery study. Am J Ophthalmol 1993;115:82–92.
11. The Fluorouracil Filtering Surgery Study Group: Five-year follow-up of the fluorouracil filtering surgery study. Am J Ophthalmol. 1996;121:349–66.
12. Weinreb RN: Adjusting the dose of 5-fluorouracil after filtration surgery to minimize side effects. Ophthalmology 1987;94:564–70.
13. Ruderman JM, Welch DB, Smith MF, Shoch DE: A randomized study of 5-fluorouracil and filtration surgery. Am J Ophthalmol 1987;104:218–24.
14. Rabowsky JH, Ruderman JM: Low-dose 5-fluorouracil and glaucoma filtration surgery. Ophthalmic Surg 1989;20:347–49.
15. Jampel HD, Jabs DA, Quigley HA: Trabeculectomy with 5-fluorouracil for adult inflammatory glaucoma. Am J Ophthalmol 1990;109:168–73.
16. Patitsas CJ, Rockwood EJ, Meisler DM, Lowder CY: Glaucoma filtering surgery with postoperative 5-fluorouracil in patients with intraocular inflammatory disease. Ophthalmology 1992;99:594–9.
17. Whiteside-Michel J, Liebman JM, Ritch R: Initial 5-fluorouracil trabeculectomy in young patients. Ophthalmology 1992;99:7–13.
18. Egbert PR, Williams AS, Singh K, et al.: A prospective trial of intraoperative fluorouracil during trabeculectomy in a black population. Am J Ophthalmol 1993;116:612–16.
19. Ewing RH, Stamper RL: Needle revision with and without 5-fluorouracil for the treatment of failed filtering blebs. Am J Ophthalmol 1990;110:254–9.
20. Shin DH, Juzych MS, Khatana AK, et al.: Needling revision of failed filtering blebs with adjunctive 5-fluorouracil. Ophthalmic Surg 1993;24:242–8.
21. Wilson RP, Steinmann WL: Use of trabeculectomy with postoperative 5-fluorouracil in patients requiring extremely low intraocular pressure levels to limit further glaucomatous progression. Ophthalmology 1991;98:47-52.
22. Liebmann JM, Ritch R, Marmor M, et al.: Initial 5-fluorouracil trabeculectomy in uncomplicated glaucoma. Ophthalmology 1991;98:1036–41.
23. Goldenfeld M, Krupin T, Ruderman JM, et al.: 5-Fluorouracil in initial trabeculectomy. A prospective, randomized, multicenter study. Ophthalmology 1994;101:1024–9.
24. Smith MF, Sherwood MB, Doyle JW, Khaw PT: Results of intraoperative 5-fluorouracil supplementation on trabeculectomy for open angle glaucoma. Am J Ophthalmol 1992;114:737–41.
25. Dietze PJ, Feldman RM, Gross RL: Intraoperative application of 5-fluorouracil during trabeculectomy. Ophthalmic Surg 1992;23: 662–5.
26. Lanigan L, Sturmer J, Baez KA, et al.: Single intraoperative applications of 5-fluorouracil during filtration surgery: Early results. Br J Ophthalmol 1994;78:33–7.
27. Mora JS, Nguyen N, Iwach AG, et al.: Trabeculectomy with intraoperative sponge 5-fluorouracil. Ophthalmology 1996;103:963–70.
28. Khaw PT, Sherwood MB, MacKay SLD, et al.: Five minute treatments with fluorouracil, floxuridine, and mitomycin have long-term effects on human Tenon's capsule fibroblasts. Arch Ophthalmol 1992;110:1150–4.
29. Knapp A, Heuer DK, Stern GA, Driebe WT Jr: Serious corneal complications of glaucoma filtering surgery with postoperative 5-fluorouracil. Am J Ophthalmol 1987;103:183–7.
30. Petersen MR, Skuta GL, Phelan MJ, Stanley SA: Striate melanokeratosis following trabeculectomy with 5-fluorouracil. Arch Ophthalmol 1990;108:1216–17.
31. Wolner B, Liebmann JM, Sassani JW, et al.: Late bleb-related endophthalmitis after trabeculectomy with adjunctive 5-fluorouracil. Ophthalmology 1991;98:1053–60.

CHAPTER 27

Guarded Filtration Procedure with Mitomycin C

TETSUYA YAMAMOTO, M.D. and YOSHIAKI KITAZAWA, M.D., Ph.D.

The adjunctive use of mitomycin C in glaucoma filtering surgery was pioneered by C.W. Chen,[1,2] who performed a guarded filtration procedure with mitomycin C in the early 1980s. Chen, who was the first to report favorable results in 1983, had the idea of using the agent as an adjunct to glaucoma filtering surgery based on his experience watching pterygium surgery when he studied ophthalmology in Tokyo. In Japan, mitomycin C has been used as an adjunct to pterygium surgery to suppress its recurrence since the 1960s. Chen's discovery was neglected until Palmer[3] and Kitazawa and associates[4] independently rediscovered the effectiveness of mitomycin C in 1991. Since then, the adjunctive use of mitomycin C has rapidly spread worldwide.[5-10]

MITOMYCIN C

Mitomycin C is an anticancer agent isolated from *Streptomyces caespitosus* (Fig. 27–1) and has very potent antifibrotic activity. The ID_{50} of conjunctival fibroblast proliferation was reported to be 2×10^{-3} mg/l or some $\frac{1}{300}$ of that for 5-fluorouracil.[11] Mitomycin C has both a urethane and a quinone group, in addition to an aziridine ring. These structural characteristics are essential for the antiproliferative effects of mitomycin C. Its primary mechanism for suppression of cell proliferation is an inhibitory action on DNA synthesis via formation of crosslinks to the double helix of DNA. In this regard, the mechanism of action is slightly different from that of 5-fluorouracil, which acts mainly through competitive inhibition of a precursor of DNA.

APPLICATION OF MITOMYCIN C

Several methods have been reported regarding the use of mitomycin C as an adjunctive treatment to glaucoma filtering surgery.[1–4,12–21] The reports are divided into two categories: intraoperative use and pre- or postoperative use. The intraoperative method is the most widely accepted mode of administration and should be used in most cases. The dosage of mitomycin C transferred to the target ocular tissues, i.e., the sclera and the conjunctiva, is approximately one-sixth the total dose administered intraoperatively.[22] In addition, after copious irrigation only about 10% of the agent remains on the ocular surface.[23]

The current method of mitomycin C administration is a short-duration application of the agent with surgical sponges followed by copious irrigation. However, the methods vary among surgeons. Application time ranges from 30 seconds to 5 minutes and the drug concentration varies from 0.004% to 0.05%. Our method of mitomycin C application is as follows: 2 mg of mitomycin C is dissolved in 5 ml of distilled water; small pieces of surgical absorbent sponge are soaked in 0.1 to 0.2 mg (0.25–0.5 ml) of the 0.04% mitomycin solution; the sponges are placed on the exposed ocular tissues for 3 to 5 minutes after the scleral flap has been prepared but before the limbal block has been excised. After application of the mitomycin C, the sponges are removed and the wound is irrigated with 250 ml of physiological saline; many surgeons use smaller amounts of irrigating fluid, some as little as 5 ml.[4,15] When perforation of the anterior chamber occurs or a large buttonhole is created before mitomycin C administration, its use should

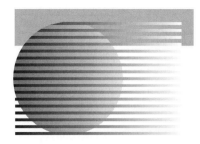

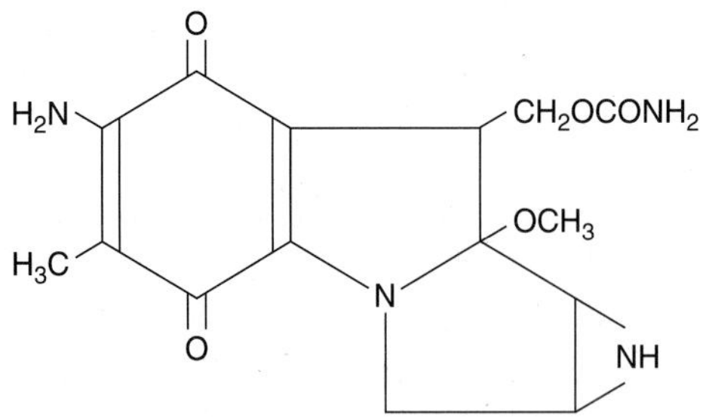

Figure 27–1. Chemical structure of mitomycin C.

be avoided. Postoperative 5-fluorouracil is preferable in such a case.

It is absolutely essential that the irrigating fluid be collected and appropriately handled. Mitomycin C is a potential carcinogen, and the patient, the surgeon, and the nurses need to be protected from its harmful effects. The collected fluid is disposed of in a container used for toxic materials; also, all sponges, gloves or other disposables contaminated with mitomycin are placed in the same toxic waste container. Contaminated instruments are meticulously rinsed.

INDICATION FOR MITOMYCIN C

The indication for adjunctive mitomycin C in a filtration procedure is a subject for controversy among glaucoma specialists. Each patient should be considered on an individual basis. Adjunctive use of mitomycin C should be limited in cases where there is a severe threat to visual function and where medical treatment fails to maintain intraocular pressure at a desirable level. Generally speaking, mitomycin C is indicated in eyes with empirically known risk factors for failed filters. Also, in most cases, eyes that need lower levels of intraocular pressure require mitomycin C or its equivalent.

SURGICAL TECHNIQUE MODIFIED FOR GUARDED FILTRATION PROCEDURE WITH MITOMYCIN C

The antiproliferative guarded filtration procedure is, in a sense, entirely different from the conventional guarded filtration procedure. Surgeons should understand the characteristics of the surgery and the postoperative course and modify the surgical technique accordingly. Antiproliferative surgery commonly causes postoperative overfiltration, which may lead to several complications such as shallow anterior chamber, prolonged hypotony,[24] wound leakage, and choroidal detachment unless measures are taken to prevent them.[9] Thus preventive methods for overfiltration are of great value in avoiding worsening of visual outcome while achieving better intraocular pressure control. Anesthesia and preoperative care for patients undergoing a guarded filtration procedure with adjunctive mitomycin C is similar to that for a conventional guarded filtration procedure.

PREPARATION OF THE CONJUNCTIVAL FLAP

Both limbal-based and fornix-based conjunctival flaps can be used, although the limbal-based flap is preferable because postoperative overfiltration is less likely. It is important to not make a buttonhole in the conjunctival flap. Thus, the surgeon as well as the assistant should pay great attention to the conjunctiva. The best way is to avoid touching the conjunctiva as long as possible.

PREPARATION OF THE SCLERAL FLAP

For the mitomycin guarded filtration procedure the half-layer scleral flap should be made neatly and sutured tightly at the time of operation. Then, to obtain appropriate filtration, the sutures can be cut by laser suture lysis at some time postoperatively. This approach can greatly diminish postoperative complications caused by overfiltration. The thickness of the scleral flap is about half that of the scleral thickness, and it should be even. Specifically, the flap should be made thicker than that made in surgery without antimetabolites.

SCLERAL FLAP SUTURE

The scleral flap should be sutured snugly with black 10-0 monofilament nylon. In most cases 4 to 6 stitches are enough to produce a tight suture. Black color is preferable because of the possible need for future suture lysis. If the scleral flap is closed tightly, the necessity of doing laser suture lysis increases, and may lead to an increased chance of postlaser hypotony in some cases. In contast, if the scleral flap is too loose, additional sutures may need to be placed to correct overfiltration associated with a variety of well-known sequelae. Thus, the number of the sutures and their tightness should be adjusted during the operation. Injection of balanced salt solution into the anterior chamber permits intraoperative observation of pressure change and seepage of fluid at the edge of the scleral flap.

CONJUNCTIVAL FLAP SUTURE

The conjunctiva must be sutured meticulously to prevent aqueous leakage between the lips of the flap. Before the operation is completed, the conjunctiva should be explored again for an inadvertent buttonhole formation by gently touching and compressing the globe with a dry sponge.

POSTOPERATIVE CARE

In cases of guarded filtration procedure with mitomycin C, postoperative care is of utmost importance in obtaining the best surgical outcome. The goal is to create appropriate filtration and to maintain intraocular pressure at 6 to 12 mm Hg during the early postoperative period. When early postoperative intraocular pressure is higher than 10 to 12 mm Hg, laser suture lysis is indicated, but in most cases we wait until the 7th postoperative day to perform laser suture lysis. This delay reduces the incidence of overfiltration resulting from early laser suture lysis. Ocular hypotensive agents may need to be used to avoid early suture lysis.

Overfiltration during the early postoperative period should be managed with a pressure bandage or megasoft contact lens. When overfiltration is due to an insufficient number of sutures in the scleral flap, it is usually necessary to take down the scleral flap and close it more tightly by placing additional sutures (see Chapter 39 Shallow or Flat Anterior Chamber).

REFERENCES

1. Chen CW: Enhanced intraocular pressure controlling effectiveness of trabeculectomy by local application of mitomycin-C. Trans Asia Pacific Acad Ophthalmol 1983;9:172.
2. Chen CW, Huang HT, Shen MM: Enhancement of IOP control effect of trabeculectomy by local application of anticancer drug. In Acta XXV Concilium Ophthalmologicum (Rome) 1986. Amsterdam, Kugler & Ghedini; 1987:1487.
3. Palmer SS: Mitomycin as adjunct chemotherapy with trabeculectomy. Ophthalmology 1991;98:317.
4. Kitazawa Y, Kawase K, Matsushita H, et al.: Trabeculectomy with mitomycin. A comparative study with fluorouracil. Arch Ophthalmol 1991;109:1693.
5. Azuara-Blanco A, Wilson RP, Spaeth GL, et al.: Filtration procedures supplemented with mitomycin C in the management of childhood glaucoma. Br J Ophthalmol 1999;83:151.
6. Beatty S, Potamitis T, Kheterpal S, et al.: Trabeculectomy augmented with mitomycin C: Application under the scleral flap. Br J Ophthalmol 1998;82:397.
7. Cheung JC, Wright MM, Muradi S, et al.: Intermediate-term outcome of variable dose mitomycin C filtering surgery. Ophthalmology 1997;104:143.
8. Nuijts RMMA, Vernimmen RC, Webers CA: Mitomycin C primary trabeculectomy in primary glaucoma of white patients. J Glaucoma 1997;6:293.
9. Perkins TW, Gangnon R, Ladd W, et al.: Trabeculectomy with mitomycin C: Intermediate-term results. J Glaucoma 1998;7:230.
10. Scott IU, Greenfield DS, Schiffman J, et al.: Outcomes of primary trabeculectomy with the use of adjunctive mitomycin. Arch Ophthalmol 1998;116:286.
11. Yamamoto T, Varani J, Soong HK, et al.: Effects of 5-fluorouracil and mitomycin C on cultured rabbit subconjunctival fibroblasts. Ophthalmology 1990;97:1204.
12. Ichien K, Yamamoto T, Kitazawa Y, et al.: Mitomycin C dissolved in a reversible thermosetting gel: Tissue concentrations in the rabbit eye. Br J Ophthalmol 1997;81:72.
13. Kim YY, Sexton RM, Shin DH, et al.: Outcomes of primary phakic trabeculectomies without versus with 0.5- to 1-minute versus 3- to 5-minute mitomycin C. Am J Ophthalmol 1998;126:755.
14. Kitazawa Y, Suemori-Matsushita H, Yamamoto T, et al.: Low-dose and high-dose mitomycin trabeculectomy as an initial surgery in primary open-angle glaucoma. Ophthalmology 1993;100:1624.
15. Kitazawa Y, Yamamoto T, Sawda A, et al.: Surgery for refractory glaucoma. Aust NZ J Ophthalmol 1996;24:327.
16. Mermoud A, Salmon JF, Murray ADN: Trabeculectomy with mitomycin C for refractory glaucoma in blacks. Am J Ophthalmol 1993;116:72.
17. Nuyts RMMA, Greve EL, Geijssen HC, et al.: Treatment of hypotonous maculopathy after trabeculectomy with mitomycin C. Am J Ophthalmol 1994;118:322.
18. Sanders SP, Cantor LB, Dobler AA, et al.: Mitomycin C in higher risk trabeculectomy: A prospective comparison of 0.2- to 0.4-mg/cc doses. J Glaucoma 1999;8:193.
19. Singh K, Egbert PR, Byrd S, et al.: Trabeculectomy with intraoperative 5-fluorouracil vs mitomycin C. Am J Ophthalmol 1997;123:48.
20. Skuta GL, Beeson CC, Higginbotham EJ, et al.: Intraoperative mitomycin versus postoperative 5-fluorouracil in high-risk glaucoma filtering surgery. Ophthalmology 1992;99:438.
21. Smith MF, Doyle JW, Nguyen QH, et al.: Results of intraoperative 5-fluorouracil or lower dose mitomycin-C administration on initial trabeculectomy surgery. J Glaucoma 1997;6:104.
22. Yamamoto T, Kitazawa Y: Residual mitomycin C dosage in surgical sponges removed at the time of trabeculectomy. Am J Ophthalmol 1994;117:672.
23. Kawase K, Matsushita H, Yamamoto T, et al.: Mitomycin concentration in rabbit and human ocular tissues after topical administration. Ophthalmology 1992;99:203.
24. Suer IJ, Greenfield DS, Miller MP, et al.: Hypotony maculopathy after filtering surgery with mitomycin C. Incidence and treatment. Ophthalmology 1997;104:207.

CHAPTER 28

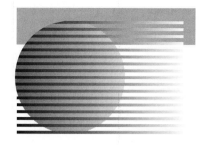

Laser Suture Lysis

GEORGE L. SPAETH, M.D.

Surgery for glaucoma that relies on filtration through the sclera has been practiced for over 100 years. One of the challenges is to get enough aqueous humor to flow through the sclerostomy that the procedure works to control the pressure, and at the same time to maintain enough resistance to the outflow of that aqueous humor that the anterior chamber does not collapse. Initially the surgery was performed by making a full-thickness hole. A major problem with this was the high frequency of flat anterior chambers, hypotony, and the extremely disturbing complications associated with hypotony (see Chapter 40, Low Postoperative Intraocular Pressure). When "trabeculectomy" was introduced, physicians were quick to switch from full-thickness procedures to a method that at least partially controlled the flow of aqueous. Other authors suggested different methods of limiting aqueous outflow, such as putting a suture across a guarded filtration procedure in order to decrease flow, at least temporarily. This led to the phrase "guarded filtration procedure," which is now the preferred name because a "trabeculectomy" does not work by being a "trabeculectomy" but rather by producing filtration.

As glaucoma surgery has evolved, most surgeons now use some type of method for controlling the amount of aqueous flow in the postoperative period and so prevent the complications of hypotony and excessive outflow.

HOW TO INCREASE AQUEOUS FLOW AFTER A GUARDED FILTRATION PROCEDURE

There are three basic methods for altering the amount of aqueous flow after filtration surgery: (1) compression on the incision, (2) releasing a releasable suture (which can be removed following the surgery), and (3) cutting a previously placed suture postoperatively, either with a sharp-edged instrument or with a laser.

COMPRESSION (CARLO TRAVERSO MANEUVER)

It is useful to distort the edge of the scleral flap to encourage filtration after a guarded filtration procedure. The indications for doing this are an intraocular pressure higher than believed ideal (see below) and a desire to increase the amount of aqueous flowing through the sclerostomy. This maneuver is not to be confused with what is often called "digital ocular compression," which some surgeons use on a long-term basis to encourage filtration. The purpose of the Carlo Traverso maneuver (CTM) is solely to disrupt the incision during the time of healing to try to prevent the sclerostomy from closing.

Before the surgeon performs the CTM, the eye is gonioscoped to make sure that iris or vitreous is not

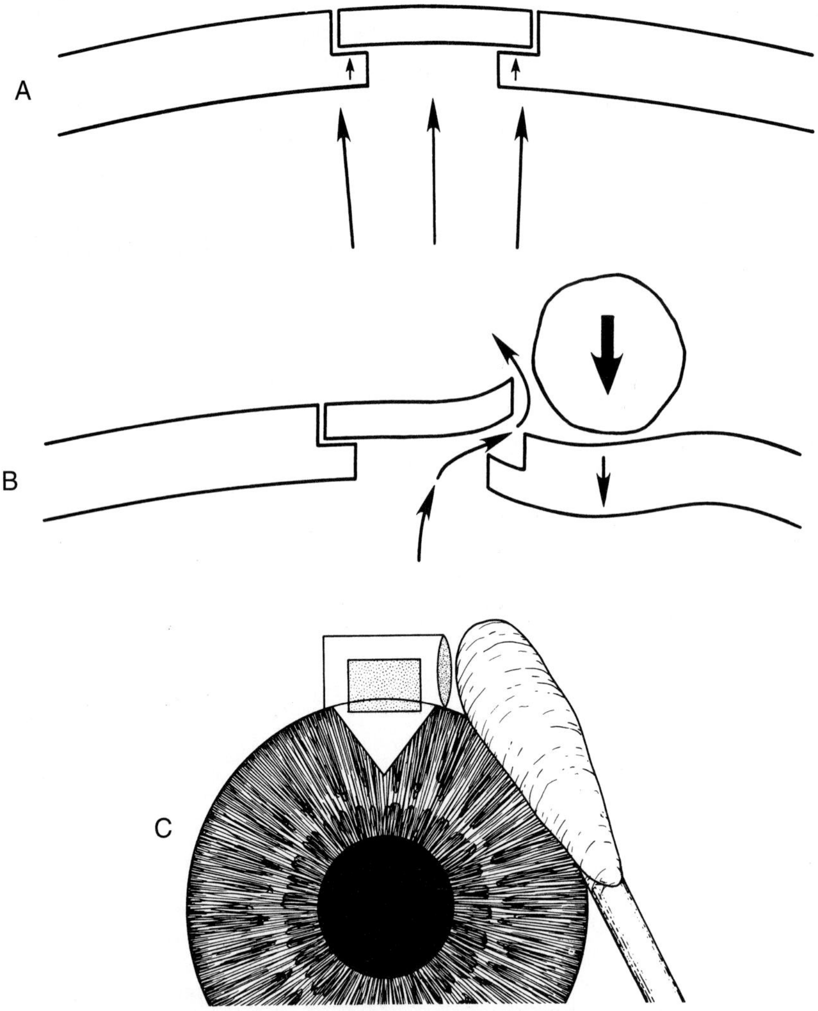

Figure 28–1. The Carlo Traverso maneuver. *A.* With a guarded procedure, increasing the pressure inside the eye is not a good way to cause increasing filtration. *B.* Deforming the sclera adjacent to the radial groove allows exodus of aqueous humor. *C.* Schematic depiction of method of performing a Carlo Traverso maneuver.

occluding the sclerostomy. In such a case pressing on the eye will probably only increase the severity of the iris or vitreous prolapse. If blood or a clot occludes the sclerostomy, however, CTM is not contraindicated. In fact, such occlusion is frequently an indication for performing a CTM.

Before a CTM, the eye must be well anesthetized with topical anesthetic. The patient is seated at the slit lamp and asked to look down. An applicator is saturated with topical anesthetic. The cotton swab end of the applicator is placed just temporal to the temporal radial groove of the sclerostomy, directly on the conjunctiva, and the conjunctiva and underlying sclera are depressed under direct visualization (Fig. 28–1). If the sclerostomy is disrupted, the conjunctiva adjacent to the swab will immediately become elevated and the intraocular pressure will fall. The anterior chamber may or may not become shallower. If there is no effect after pressing on the temporal radial groove of the scleral flap, then the patient is asked to blink, and the applicator is placed just nasal to the nasal radial groove of the scleral flap. Again, to disrupt the junction between the scleral flap and the underlying sclera, the applicator is pressed against the sclera. If this disruption occurs, the conjunctiva will be seen to balloon quickly. If there is no apparent effect from this method, the intraocular pressure has to be checked to make sure that, indeed, it has not been lowered, and the procedure is repeated on the temporal side, but with more vigorous compression. If no success, then it is repeated on the nasal side, again with more vigorous compression. After the CTM has been seen to be successful, the intraocular pressure is measured, and the result will determine whether the pressure has been lowered adequately. For example, if the target pressure is around 15 mm Hg and the intraocular pressure prior to CTM was 30 mm Hg, and the pressure following CTM is 25 mm Hg, then the CTM is repeated until the pressure comes down to around 15 mm Hg.

If the pressure falls, but the bleb does not become elevated, then it is essential to check the conjunctiva carefully with fluorescein. The most likely explanation for the absence of the development of a filtering bleb is that there is a hole in the conjunctiva and the aqueous is seeping out through the conjunctiva.

The goal is to develop a bleb but not to cause the anterior chamber to become shallow.

If the CTM fails to produce a bleb and to lower the intraocular pressure, and if the sclerostomy has been seen by prior gonioscopy not to be occluded with iris or vitreous, then the incision must have been sutured so tightly that it is not possible to disrupt the incision. This indicates that the surgery intended to produce filtration was not performed properly. At the time of the surgery the incision should be tested to make sure that pressure on the edge of the incision disrupts the incision, allowing aqueous to exit. If the CTM fails, then it is quite certain that the guarded filtration procedure will fail. At that point it is usually necessary to cut a suture or to release a suture to ensure that filtration will occur.

Once the CTM has been tried and failed, and it is decided that filtration is necessary, then an appropriate suture is cut or released. If this is not associated with immediate development of a bleb and the lowering of intraocular pressure, the CTM is then repeated. This should result in the development of a bleb and a lowering of intraocular pressure. If the CTM again fails, gonioscopy is repeated and, if the sclerostomy is open, and it is determined that a low intraocular pressure is in fact essential, then an additional suture is cut or released and the CTM again repeated.

RELEASING A RELEASABLE SUTURE

Releasable sutures can be of great value. There are a variety of methods, but the following is the author's favorite. This is described for use with a corneoscleral incision such as that used during a combined cataract-glaucoma operation. It applies equally well to a scleral-scleral incision such as that used during a guarded filtration procedure.

The method is illustrated in detail in Figure 28–2*A*. The needle enters at point 1, in the sclera, crosses the incision, and exits on the opposite side of the incision at point 2. A loop approximately 2 inches long is made. The needle enters the sclera at point 3, passes the desired distance in sclera or cornea, and exits at point 4. With a limbus-based flap, the reflection of the conjunctiva would be between point 3 and point 4. Thus the needle would go under the insertion of the conjunctiva at the corneoscleral sulcus and would emerge on the corneal side. In most instances the surgeon wishes to bury the suture so that the cut end does not irritate the eye or the patient. This is done by making the loop, again about 2 inches long, and entering the cornea at point 5, approximately a quarter of a millimeter from point 4. Point 5 should be close enough to point 4 that a large loop does not result when a suture is pulled tight. On the other hand, point 5 should be far enough from point 4 that the suture remains on the surface and is thus able to be easily grasped at that point for subsequent removal. After the needle enters the cornea at point 5, it passes intracorneally for a distance of approximately 1 cm, exiting the cornea at point 6.

The releasable suture is tied in the following fashion (Fig. 28–2*B*): End C is pulled up so that loop B, between points 2 and 3, is approximately 2 to 3 mm long. End C (with the needle on it) is then released. The trailing end of the suture, A in Figure 28–2, is grasped by a tying forceps, and four throws are placed around another tying forceps. The second tying forceps is then used to grasp the end of loop B. The tying forceps in the left hand holding end A is pulled toward point 5, and suture loop B in the right-hand tying forceps, is pulled away from point 5. This results in a single knot that pulls the incision closed. This is a slip knot, and it can be pulled to the tightness desired. After the slip knot

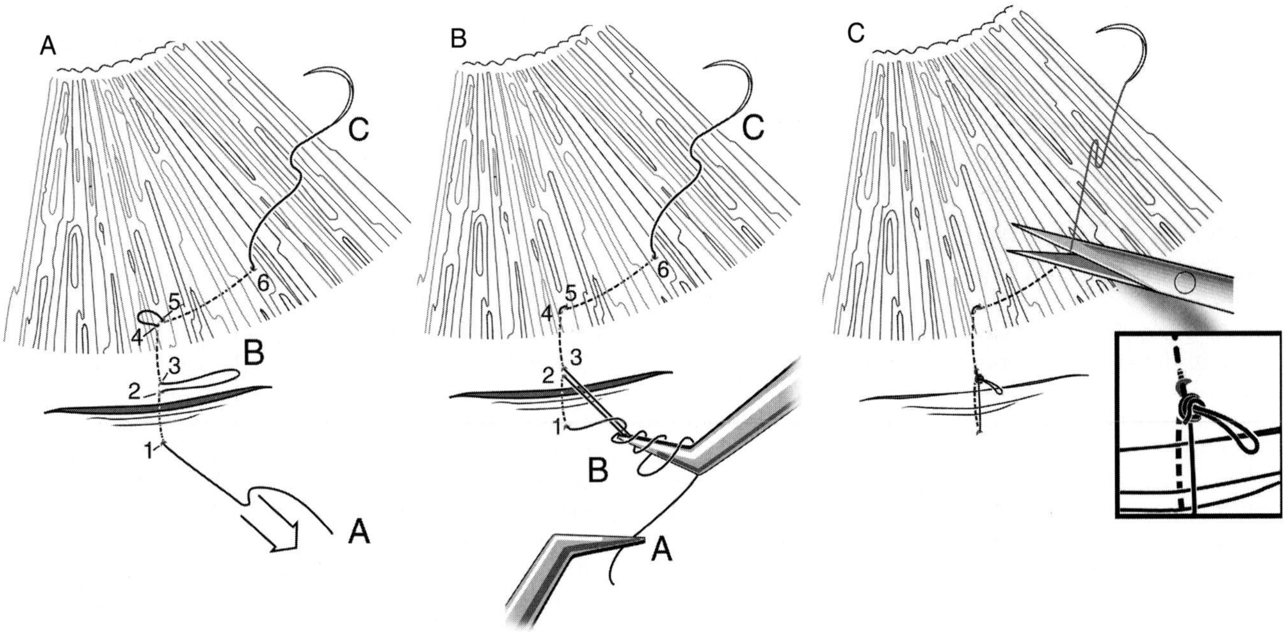

Figure 28–2. One method of placing a releasable suture.

has been tied, the trailing end, A, is cut with a scissors, leaving an approximately 1–3 mm end (Fig. 28–2C). The leading edge of the suture, C, is cut directly at point 6, without leaving any suture extruding. Before this is cut the leading edge, C, is pulled gently to make sure that there is no elevation of the loop between points 4 and 5. The suture must be cut flush with the cornea in order to avoid a corneal foreign-body sensation.

The suture is then released by grasping the loop between points 4 and 5 with a jeweler's forceps, and pulling away from point 1. Thus, if the suture were placed at the 12 o'clock position at the corneoscleral sulcus, the loop between points 4 and 5 would be grasped and pulled directly down toward the lower lid. The pull is made slowly and constantly in order not to break the suture.

TECHNIQUE OF SUTURE CUTTING WITH A LASER

Laser suture lysis can be done using an argon, diode, or krypton laser. A lens must be used to compress the suture. The Hoskins lens or the Ritch compression lens are both excellent. The settings are similar to those used with an argon laser trabeculoplasty. Specifically, the duration is 0.1 seconds, and the power approximately 500 mW. The spot size needs to be around 100 microns to facilitate the laser cutting. If the conjunctiva is hemorrhagic, then the argon laser should not be used. A diode or krypton laser with similar settings is much preferred.

The technique is simple. After compression of the suture with the lens, heat is directly applied to the suture under direct visualization. The suture can be seen to break apart when the cutting is complete.

The complications of laser suture lysis are a coring of the conjunctiva, or the development of excessive filtration. It is important to make sure that the tissue is well compressed, and that the conjunctiva is clear to avoid making a hole in the conjunctiva with the laser. Following the instructions just given will decrease the likelihood of overfiltration. Only one suture should be cut at a time, and the pressure should be checked after the release of the individual suture.

WHEN TO RELEASE OR CUT SUTURES

Suture release is timed to avoid an intraocular pressure that will damage the nerve on a short-term basis and to avoid making the patient worse by causing a flat anterior chamber or other complications associated with suture release

The expected effect from releasing a suture depends first on resistance to outflow. This resistance is based on the amount of flow through the edge of the scleral flap prior to placing the suture; the amount of aqueous production; the resistance to outflow through the sclera provided by the superficial tissues, specifically the Tenon's conjunctival flap; and the amount of aqueous flow through the edge of the scleral flap prior to closure of the scleral flap of the suture.

1. *The amount of flow through the edge of the scleral flap prior to placing the suture:* Sutures that are used to close large gaps through which there is so much leakage of aqueous that the chamber becomes flat should not be cut until the surface tissues have healed considerably. Ideally, they will not be cut at all. The operating surgeon should indicate in the operating note and on the patient's chart which sutures those are so that physicians following the patient postoperatively know which sutures should not be cut.
2. *The amount of aqueous humor the patient is producing:* The amount of aqueous humor produced by an eye is a rough measure of the health of the eye. Eyes with uveitis, following severe trauma, or with far-advanced glaucoma do not produce much aqueous humor. Thus, chambers will become flat unless there is only minimal outflow through the cut edge of the scleral flap. The surgeon performing the surgery should have an idea about this and design the scleral flap appropriately. Cutting or releasing sutures in such eyes is far more hazardous than in healthier eyes making more copious amounts of aqueous humor.
3. *Resistance provided by the Tenon's-conjunctival flap:* The resistance provided by the Tenon's conjunctival flap varies markedly from individual to individual. In older patients this tissue is frequently thin and provides little resistance. In fact it may be so thin that it is difficult to close the flap without leaving small holes in the conjunctiva. In such individuals it is essential to use a taper point needle rather than a cutting needle so that multiple small perforations are not made at the edge of the conjunctiva. Such perforations will predispose to leakage through the conjunctiva and decrease the resistance of the flap. In younger patients and especially those who have had previous surgery so that the tissue is thick, the resistance provided by a watertight Tenon's conjunctival closure can be great. Prior to pulling a releasable suture or cutting a suture with a laser, the surgeon should have an idea of the likely resistance of the covering tissue. Where such resistance is believed minimal either because the tissue is very thin or, most obviously, there is a leak through the conjunctiva, the surgeon must realize that releasing the suture is more hazardous than when there is a conjunctival-Tenon's flap likely to provide good resistance to outflow.
4. *The amount of aqueous flow through the edge of the scleral flap prior to closing the scleral flap of the suture:* This should be known and documented. For example, a large gap may exist through which there is gross flow, associated with immediate flattening of the anterior chamber. Let us say that that large gap is closed with one tightly placed suture so that there is no flow through that portion of the scleral flap. In this case when that suture is cut, there will again be marked flow of aqueous through the scleral flap. Unless there has been a marked healing of the surface tissue so that there is now no resistance of those

tissues, the chamber will again become flat. In contrast, if there is minimal leakage through the incision prior to placing the suture, there will be minimal leakage through the incision when the suture is released.

Further, the expected effect from releasing a suture relates to the repetitiousness and intensity of the postoperative healing/scarring process. Where this occurs slowly, the effect of the suture release will be greater than where this occurs rapidly. Factors that increase the repetitiousness of healing/scarring include: (1) intensity of inflammation, (2) irritating substances such as blood or absorbable sutures, (3) younger age, and (4) possibly, increased pigmentation of the skin. Factors that tend to be associated with slower healing include: (1) increasing age, (2) use of healing retarding agents such as corticosteroids and antimetabolites. Of these agents, corticosteroids are the least effective, 5-fluorouracil in the middle, and mitomycin C most effective. This is only a very rough guideline, as it depends on how much of the substance is used for how long, how frequently, etc. Many surgeons believe that the use of corticosteroids every 2 or perhaps even every 1 hour is more effective than less frequent use, say 4 times daily. There is some intuitive logic in this, but there is no supporting evidence.

The duration of effect of the topical corticosteroids is roughly 6 to 12 hours. There is a dose–effect relationship with 5-fluorouracil: a near-maximal effect appears to be obtained by using 0.1 ml subconjunctivally every other day for 2 weeks. It is possible that using 0.3 ml every 4 to 7 days may give a similar effect, but this has not been established. There is also a dose-effect relationship with mitomycin C, but again the methods of applying it and rinsing it off are so highly variable that it is hard to say that there is a dose-effect relationship; the details of this are not very well known. It appears that one minute's administration of 0.4 mg/mL mitomycin achieves near maximal saturation of the sclera.

These comments also have ramifications for the timing of suture cutting. The following cautions should be kept in mind: (1) Releasing a suture when no antimetabolite has been used is usually ineffective beyond 7 days after surgery. (2) Where 5-fluorouracil 5-FU has been employed, suture release is usually ineffective later than about 2 weeks after the use of the 5-FU. (3) The effect of mitomycin C characteristically lasts at least 1 month, and may last 6 months or even longer.

Finally, special considerations are required in releasing sutures in patients in whom intraocular pressure is elevated or who have a flat anterior chamber. For example, in a patient with a stage 7 disc who has gotten worse with pressures in the mid-teens and a postoperative pressure of 50 mm Hg, releasing a suture would likely be quickly damaging. In contrast, in a patient whose preoperative pressure was 50 mm Hg and in whom the rate of glaucoma damage has been slow and who has a stage 3 or 4 optic nerve, a postoperative pressure of 50 mm Hg is of minimal concern. Similarly, in a patient with a deep anterior chamber, myopia, and a clear lens, excessive filtration has far less effect than in a patient who is hyperopic, has a shallow anterior chamber, and already has a moderate, visually significant cataract. In deciding whether to release the suture or not, the surgeon must judge the significance of leaving the suture in place and having an elevated pressure versus removing the suture and introducing a complication. This decision depends strictly on the specific situation.

SPECIFIC RECOMMENDATIONS

1. Preoperatively, pick a specific peak pressure above which you do not wish the intraocular pressure to rise in the postoperative period and record it. Determine an ideal goal of intraocular pressure postoperatively. This is the "surgical" intraocular pressure goal.
2. Intraoperatively, titrate leakage to achieve the desired amount of filtration, taking into account the patient's propensity to heal, the amount of aqueous likely to be produced, and the desired postoperative intraocular pressure.
3. At the time of surgery, determine which suture you wish to have released in which order and record this information.
4. Postoperative care

   Day of surgery: Check intraocular pressure approximately 2 hours postoperatively. If it is above the goal intraocular pressure, perform CTM gently. If the intraocular pressure falls, record the new level. If it does not fall, do nothing. If the intraocular pressure is above peak levels, perform CTM vigorously. If it falls, either do nothing or recheck in 2 hours depending upon the surgeon's anxiety level regarding tolerance of nerve. If the intraocular pressure does not fall, use medications: beta-blocker, topical carbonic anhydrase inhibitor, systemic carbonic anhydrase inhibitor, or alpha-agonist, in that order. Avoid prostaglandin analogs and miotics. Recheck the patient one day postoperatively.

   First postoperative day: If the intraocular pressure is above the set goal, perform CTM. If it falls below the goal, do nothing. If the intraocular pressure is below the permissible peak, do nothing or start glaucoma medications and recheck in 1 to 2 days. Prior to therapy of any kind, the first step is to decide upon the diagnosis. Thus if the intraocular pressure is elevated, the first step is to determine why its elevated. This demands estimating the depth of the anterior chamber, the height of the bleb, and the presence or absence of leakage through the conjunctiva, and determining if the pressure is elevated gonioscopically. A CTM should never be performed until gonioscopy has been done to determine whether or not the iris is incarcerated or there is another reason why it would be inappropriate to perform a CTM.

   Second postoperative visit (day 3 or 4): If the intraocular pressure is above the surgical goal, perform CTM. If the intraocular pressure falls, leave it alone. If the pressure does not fall, remove the releasable suture or cut one suture. Recheck the pressure. If it has fallen, do nothing. If it has not fallen, perform CTM. If the intraocular pressure has not fallen below the surgical goal, remove the second releasable suture or cut the second suture. After the second suture is cut, perform CTM. If the intraocular pressure has not fallen to a satisfactory level, usually do not cut further sutures at that point but leave them alone. Or if the intraocular pressure is above the surgical goal, put the patient on medications and recheck in around 3 days. If the patient is predisposed to flat anterior chamber and malignant glaucoma, that is, if the patient is a high hyperope or has primary angle-closure glaucoma, do **not** cut the suture at this visit but defer suture cutting until the next visit, at one week.

One week postoperative visit: If the intraocular pressure is above the surgical goal, cut all remaining sutures. If the surgical goal cannot be achieved, the surgery has probably failed. Resume medical therapy or consider surgical approaches such as needling, open sclerostomy, etc., depending upon gonioscopic and other findings.

If 5-FU was administered during surgery, usually delay cutting or releasing sutures by doubling the number of days listed in the above recommendations. Thus it is desirable to try to avoid releasing sutures prior to 6 days. If mitomycin C was employed, it is advisable, by and large, to quadruple the days listed in the above recommendations. That is, try not to cut or release sutures for 12 days, and be aware that cutting sutures in these patients may have an effect up to 6 months later.

CHAPTER 29

Coincident Cataract and Glaucoma Surgery

THOMAS W. SAMUELSON, M.D.

Indications
Anesthesia
Preoperative Considerations
Surgical Technique
Postoperative Care
Pupil Management

The management of coincident cataract and glaucoma presents common and challenging decisions for the ophthalmic surgeon. Technological advances in the last decade have revolutionized the glaucoma combined procedure.[1] Traditionally, the management of coincident cataract and glaucoma generally involved sequential surgery, that is, initial glaucoma surgery followed by cataract extraction months later when the intraocular pressure was controlled and the bleb had matured. The rationale for the sequential approach was based on the poor success rate of combined extracapsular cataract extraction (10 mm scleral incision) and glaucoma filtration surgery. The advantage of the sequential approach is the high success rate of primary filtration surgery. The disadvantages are that the patient is faced with at least two operations, prolonged poor vision, and the risk of bleb failure after the cataract operation. With current techniques for combined cataract and glaucoma surgery, most patients will require just one procedure. Based on the success of small-incision phacoemulsification and guarded filtration surgery with antimetabolites, most glaucoma surgeons now prefer the combined procedure rather than sequential surgery. With the small-incision combined glaucoma surgery techniques described in this chapter, if subsequent filtration surgery becomes necessary, there is ample virgin superior limbus available to permit the second procedure. Most patients, however, will achieve adequate pressure control after modern combined surgery.[2] Finally, with recent advances in glaucoma therapeutics and the increased popularity of clear corneal phacoemulsification, the option of performing phacoemulsification initially, followed by filtration surgery later if needed has become more common. With the addition of topical carbonic anhydrase inhibitors, selective alpha-2 agonists, and prostaglandins to the list of available medical treatment options, more patients with glaucoma can be successfully managed medically. Cataract extraction alone often results in a modest reduction in intraocular pressure. Therefore, in selected patients with early to moderate glaucoma,[3] cataract extraction employing a conjunctiva sparing approach, may be a viable treatment option.

The success of modern combined small-incision phacoemulsification and glaucoma filtration procedure with mitomycin approaches the success of glaucoma filtration alone.[4] Because the glaucoma combined procedure provides rapid visual rehabilitation and satisfactory intraocular pressure control in most patients,[2,4] it has become a gratifying operation for both surgeons and their patients.

INDICATIONS

The basic indications for coincident cataract and glaucoma surgery are uncontrolled glaucoma that requires surgery in a patient with visually significant cataract, or the need for cataract extraction in a patient with advanced or poorly controlled glaucoma. The mere coexistence of glaucoma and cataract is not in itself an indication for combined cataract and glaucoma surgery.[5] In fact, mild glaucoma that is controlled well on minimal medication is usually best managed by cataract extraction without the glaucoma filtration procedure. In these instances, it is wise to perform the cataract extraction using a conjunctival sparing approach such as a clear corneal or temporal limbal incision. Any conjunctival incision should be sutured closed to minimize conjunctival retraction and scarring. If the glaucoma later

TABLE 29–1. Options for Surgical Management of Coincident Cataract and Glaucoma*

Trabeculectomy First; Cataract Extraction Later	Combined Cataract Extraction–Trabeculectomy†	Cataract Extraction First; Trabeculectomy Later if Needed‡
• Consider if employing large-incision 10–11 mm extracapsular cataract extraction	• Most cases of true glaucoma requiring two or more medications	• Mild glaucoma, well-controlled intraocular pressure with additional medical options available
• Consider if marked inflammation noted preoperatively	• Far advanced glaucoma	• Untreated or medically controlled ocular hypertension with additional medical options available
• May be safest approach for very high risk eyes, i.e., monocular patient with preoperative intraocular pressure >50 mm Hg	• Patients on MTMT or patients intolerant to medications	
	• Patients poorly compliant with medications	
	• Low target intraocular pressure	

*Assumes visually significant cataract.
†Small-incision approach.
‡Conjunctival Sparing Technique—Preferably Clear Cornea.
MTMT = maximally tolerated medical therapy.

becomes uncontrolled or nonresponsive to medical therapy, a glaucoma filtration procedure can be readily performed. Small-incision cataract extraction techniques have made the "cataract extraction first, GFP later if necessary" approach more feasible, especially if an effort is made to conserve conjunctiva (Table 29–1).[3]

The goal of coincident cataract and glaucoma surgery varies from patient to patient. For example, a patient with advanced, but nonprogressive glaucoma whose intraocular pressure is well controlled with minimal medication, may require a functional filtration bleb for a short time to prevent further optic nerve damage. In such cases, once the eye has recovered from surgery, the intraoperative pressure is often easier to control. In such patients, it is possible to avoid the problems associated with a long-term bleb that is filtering copiously and still get the patient through the surgery without further loss. Conversely, a patient with progressive glaucoma and poorly controlled intraocular pressure requires a long-term filtration bleb to achieve adequate pressure. Thus, management of individual patients will differ according to the specific goals of treatment.

ANESTHESIA

Combined cataract and glaucoma procedures are generally performed under retrobulbar or peribulbar anesthesia. Prior to the retrobulbar block, a combination of agents with ultra-short-acting sedative and amnesiac properties such as methohexitol 20 to 30 mg (Brevitol, Jones Medical), midazolam HCl 1 mg (Versed, Roche Laboratories), or alfentanil 250 μg (Alfenta, Janssen Pharmaceutica Inc.) may be given intravenously to reduce anxiety and pain. This combination of medications provides several minutes of deep sedation during which the block can be given without pain or patient awareness. The retrobulbar block consists of 2% xylocaine (Lidocaine, Astra) without epinephrine. Hyaluronidase (Wydase, Wyeth-Ayerst) is generally not necessary. In most cases, bupivacaine HCL (Marcaine, Sanofi Winthrop) 0.75 is not needed, but it may be used if the anticipated surgical time is to be longer than 1 hour. Within minutes after administration of the block, the patient is aware and able to cooperate with the surgeon. During the procedure only light sedation or none at all will be required. It is important to control the patient's systemic blood pressure during the surgery for many reasons, but primarily to reduce the risk of suprachoroidal hemorrhage. After administration of the peribulbar or retrobulbar block, it is helpful to apply pressure to the globe for several minutes, using digital compression over a closed eyelid or a mechanical device such as a Honan balloon. This pressure serves to prevent bleeding into the retrobulbar space, it facilitates diffusion of the anesthetic solution into the orbital tissues, and it softens the eye, making the surgery safer.[5] The Honan device has been shown to be safe when used for this purpose. In one series of more than 1,000 cataract extractions, no cases of optic atrophy or central retinal artery occlusion were reported.[6] The risk of applying external compression to eyes with badly damaged optic nerves is not clear. It is therefore advisable to limit the magnitude and duration of ocular compression to 20 to 30 mm Hg and 5 to 10 minutes in such patients.

For patients with markedly elevated intraocular pressure, preoperative administration of intravenous mannitol will minimize the abrupt change in intraocular pressure following the incision. The need for mannitol to suppress intraocular pressure is infrequent, however, and depends on the clinical circumstance and the general health of the patient, especially from a cardiopulmonary prospective. Osmotic agents like mannitol are preferred over aqueous suppressants because they dehydrate the vitreous, thereby reducing vitreous volume and softening the eye. Conversely, aqueous suppressants retard aqueous production during the early perioperative period. At least theoretically, reduced aqueous outflow through the new filter could exacerbate hypotony and bleb fibrosis.

PREOPERATIVE CONSIDERATIONS

The preoperative clinical examination is extremely important. The conjunctiva should be examined carefully. Topical steroids should be administered if the conjunctiva is inflamed as described by Broadway[7] (see Chapter 25).

Additional preoperative considerations include documentation of the pupillary response to pharmacologic dilatation. If dilatation is poor and pupil manipulation is anticipated, the patient should be informed of the likely need for pupil stretch or iris manipulation, which may result in anisocoria or pupillary distortion. This precaution is particularly important for younger patients with light irides in whom the cosmetic effect of anisocoria or irregular pupillary contour will be more apparent. Finally, patients should be educated preoperatively about the intense character of the postoperative period, which will require frequent doctor visits and prolonged visual recovery, beyond that expected for standard cataract surgery in non-glaucomatous eyes. Finally, the surgeon should carefully examine the eye for the presence of exfoliative material, which can be associated with a more aggressive postoperative inflammatory response, weakened zonular fibers, and poor pharmacologic dilation.[8,9]

SURGICAL TECHNIQUE

Small-incision cataract extraction techniques have vastly improved the glaucoma combined procedure. The entire procedure can be performed through essentially the same types of conjunctival and scleral incisions used in standard filtration surgery. Because only 3.5 mm of the superior limbus is involved in the incision, if additional filtration surgery becomes necessary, adequate space in the adjacent superior limbus is available.

Current techniques for combined glaucoma surgery using small-incision phacoemulsification will be described here. Other techniques, such as a standard extracapsular (see Chapter 8) or intracapsular extraction may be preferable in some cases, as in eyes with extremely dense nuclei or compromised zonular integrity. Surgeons should either be competent in these other techniques or refer specific cases.[5,10]

A limbus-based conjunctival flap is preferred. One of the significant advantages of combined surgery with small incision phacoemulsification techniques is that only 3.5 mm of limbal exposure is needed, and the extent of conjunctival dissection is thus quite limited. Creation of a limbus-based conjunctival flap is easily accomplished using the Spaeth, three-layer technique.[5] The advantages of a limbus-based approach include fewer wound leaks and enhanced safety if antimetabolites are employed. Additionally, the limbus-based approach results in a higher bleb with greater separation of the conjunctiva and the sclera, theoretically decreasing the likelihood that these two raw surgical surfaces will scar together. Moreover, a limbus-based flap facilitates postoperative massage techniques such as the Carlo Traverso maneuver (CTM).[11] When performed in a patient with a limbus-based conjunctival flap, CTM results in prompt elevation of the bleb. Conversely, the same technique performed in the presence of a fornix-based flap may result in a rush of aqueous down the anterior surface of the cornea and can predispose to a persistent bleb leak. The disadvantages of a limbus-based flap are that it is a slightly more demanding technique for which a competent surgical assistant may be required. Many surgeons prefer a fornix-based conjunctival flap because of the more diffuse and posterior bleb formation with such an approach.[12,13] For descriptions of limbus-based and fornix-based flaps, see Chapters 23 and 24.

A preferred technique for combined cataract and glaucoma surgery is to mimic a standard trabeculectomy (guarded filtration procedure).[14–16] The globe is immobilized with a 4-0 nylon suture beneath the tendon of the superior rectus muscle. A Lester forceps is passed beneath the upper eyelid, which is simultaneously lifted from the globe by elevation of the lid speculum with a second instrument. Alternatively, the globe may be infraducted by a second instrument such as a muscle hook, exposing the region 8 to 10 mm posterior to the superior limbus. The jaws of the Lester forceps are held closed as the forceps is passed beneath the upper eyelid, reducing the possibility of conjunctival tear from the teeth of the forceps. The superior rectus tendon is then grasped 9 to 10 mm posterior to the limbus. The rectus suture should be placed accurately and efficiently on the first pass. Repeated attempts may traumatize the conjunctiva or create a hematoma. The conjunctival dissection is then initiated 8 to 10 mm posterior to the limbus. It is important that the conjunctival incision be far enough posterior.

The conjunctival incision is identical to that of a standard guarded filtration procedure. The dissection is carried anteriorly until Tenon's layer is disinserted approximately 1 mm posterior to the conjunctival insertion. The disinsertion of Tenon's layer provides an excellent landmark and generally indicates that the dissection is adequately anterior. It is vital that the conjunctival insertion at the limbus remain intact. The surgeon should be continuously aware of the fragility of the conjunctiva, avoiding unnecessary handling of the conjunctiva, especially with toothed forceps. Whenever possible, Tenon's tissue, rather than conjunctiva should be grasped to mobilize the conjunctiva and prevent "buttonhole" formation. To control bleeding, cautery should be used judiciously yet without reservation. Blood within the bleb is highly undesirable because it may obstruct filtration or contribute to inflammation and bleb fibrosis.

The role of antimetabolites in combined cataract and glaucoma surgery is determined by the goals of the procedure. For example, antimetabolites may be most appropriate for patients in whom a long-term bleb is desired. Antimetabolites may be less appropriate for the patient with mild glaucoma in whom the goal of surgery is perioperative intraocular pressure control. Mitomycin C (MMC), if employed, is applied to the proposed filtration site following dissection of the con-

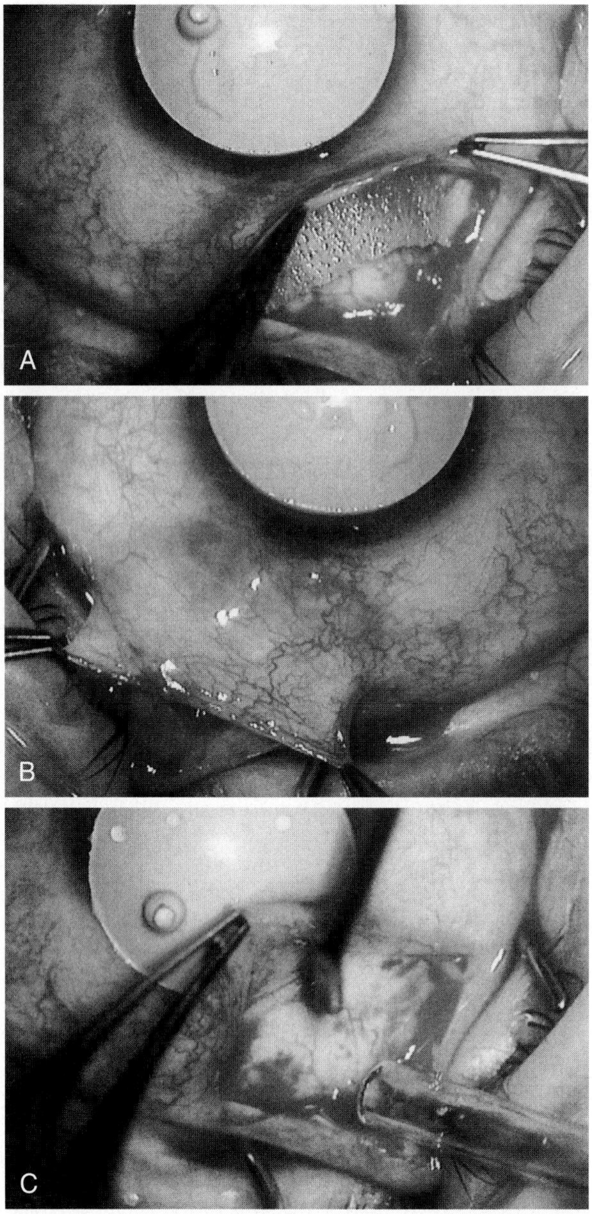

Figure 29–1. *A.* The antimetabolite is applied to the proposed filtration site between uncut sclera and the conjunctival flap. *B.* The posterior edge of the conjunctival incision is protected from exposure to the antimetabolite. *C.* After application of the antimetabolite, the entire surgical site is irrigated with copious balanced salt and the diluent is removed with a suction catheter. (From Samuelson TW: Management of coincident cataract and glaucoma. Curr Opin Ophthalmol 1993;4:90–6. Copyright Rapid Science Publishers.)

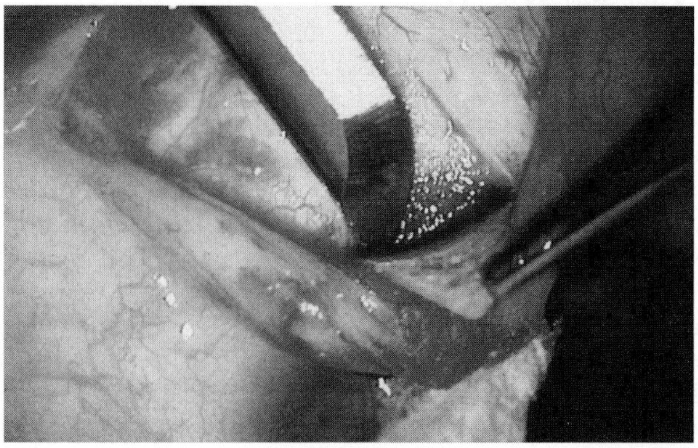

Figure 29–2. A 3.5-mm scleral flap is dissected. The dissection is carried anteriorly well into clear cornea. (From Samuelson TW: Management of coincident glaucoma and cataract. Curr Opin Ophthalmol 1995;6:14–21. Copyright Rapid Science Publishers.)

junctival flap (Fig. 29–1*A*) (see Chapter 27). The conjunctival incision must be protected from MMC exposure (Fig. 29–1*B*). After MMC application the pledget is removed from the subconjunctival space and the site is irrigated with balanced salt solution (Fig. 29–1*C*). The irrigating fluid and mitomycin pledget are collected and discarded as hazardous waste. A modified triangular scleral flap 3.5 mm based at the limbus is then dissected (Fig. 29–2). The scleral flap is identical to that used in standard guarded filtration procedure. Alternatively, some surgeons modify the scleral flap in combined glaucoma surgery to mimic the scleral tunnel approach of standard cataract surgery. The scleral flap is partial thickness and dissected anteriorly into clear cornea. The most posterior portion of the scleral flap is made slightly thicker than the remainder of the flap to serve as a secure handle for flap manipulation during the procedure (Fig. 29–3). For sclera of normal thickness, the depth of the flap should be at least one-half thickness. However, for sclera that is thinned from previous surgery, inflammation, or high myopia, the scleral flap should be greater than one-half the thickness of the sclera. It is better to cut too deep than too shallow when beginning the flap dissection. The flap is thinned appropriately as the dissection progresses anteriorly into clear cornea. A paracentesis tract is then performed using a 25-gauge sharp needle. A needle track is preferred over a stab incision for re-formation of the anterior chamber due to the self-sealing nature of such a paracentesis. When the anterior chamber is re-formed through a self-sealing needle tract paracentesis, the only exit site for the fluid is through the sclerostomy. As such, digital palpation during reformation can accurately assess the degree of filtration. Conversely, if the anterior chamber is reformed through a

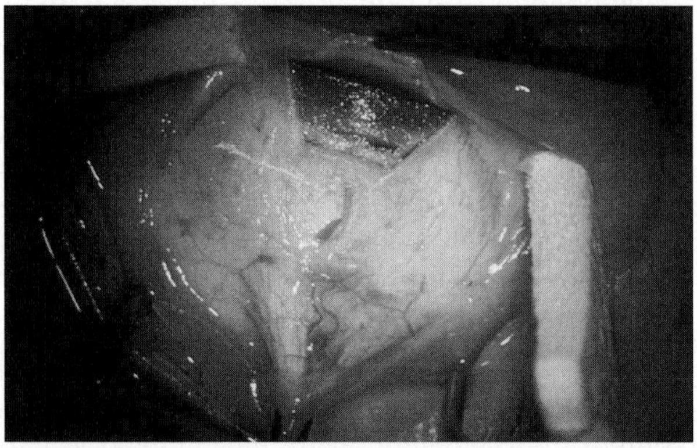

Figure 29–3. If a 5.5-mm polymethyl methacrylate intraocular lens is used, the scleral flap is larger, measuring 5 mm at the limbus. (From Samuelson TW: Management of coincident glaucoma and cataract. Curr Opin Ophthalmol 1995;6:14–21. Copyright Rapid Science Publishers.)

stab incision, the area of least resistance is back through the stab incision, and filtration through the sclerostomy is not adequately tested. After the needle track paracentesis a stab incision is created with a No. 75 blade to facilitate two-handed phacoemulsification.

The anterior chamber is then entered with a keratome beneath the scleral flap, and viscoelastic material is placed in the anterior chamber. A continuous-tear capsulectomy of approximately 5 mm in diameter is made, after which hydrodissection is performed with balanced salt solution on an irrigating cannula. Hydrodissection is perhaps the most crucial step for endocapsular phacoemulsification. It is essential that the lens nucleus rotate freely within the capsule. It is preferable that the nuclear/cortical attachments are severed with the hydrodissection rather than during mechanical attempts at rotating the nucleus with a nucleus rotator. If the torsional force inherent in nucleus rotation is used to break nuclear/cortical attachments, such force may be transmitted to the zonular apparatus, which could result in zonular dialysis. If supracapsular phacoemulsification is employed, hydrodissection is used to completely subluxate the nucleus from the capsular bag. After hydrodissection, the lens nucleus is emulsified using endocapsular or supracapsular phacoemulsification according to the preference of the individual surgeon. Before proceeding, the surgeon must perform meticulous aspiration and irrigation of all cortical material. The foldable lens implant is then placed in the capsular bag. To constrict the pupil and thereby facilitate completion of a peripheral iridectomy, a cholinergic agent such as acetylcholine (Miochol, Ciba-Vision) or carbachol (Miostat, Alcon) is instilled into the anterior chamber. Finally, the residual viscoelastic material is evacuated from the eye through the aspiration irrigation cannula.

After insertion of the intraocular lens, the surgeon must attend to the trabecular block excision. An incision has already been made with the keratome into the anterior chamber beneath the scleral flap. A Kelly Descemet's punch is now used to complete the trabecular block excision (Fig. 29–4*A*). One effective technique is to decenter the block excision toward one side of the wound as described by Wilson.[17] The block is usually decentered to the left side of the scleral flap. That is, temporally, for the left eye and nasally for the right eye. By decentering the block, the surgeon can more accurately predict the subsequent flow of aqueous and make a rational strategic plan regarding the sequence of suture release or suture lysis. For the right-handed surgeon, decentration of the block toward the left side provides a forehand stitch for the closure of the scleral flap over the sclerostomy. Finally, decentration of the block to one side promotes a greater amount of filtration in one region over another. In general, the two most important factors ensuring patency of the filtration fistula are adequate bulk aqueous flow and retardation of the healing process. If the block excision is placed centrally beneath the flap, flow will be random in all directions, and it is possible that the lack of concentrated flow will result in increased fibrosis. If the flow is directed in one region, there is a greater likelihood that the fistula will remain patent. Moreover, if suture lysis becomes necessary postoperatively, it is clear which suture should be cut. Finally, if the block is decentered toward one side, the size of the sclerostomy can be smaller than if the block is not decentered. Theoretically, against-the-rule astigmatism will be reduced if the sclerostomy is relatively small. Conversely, if there is a large central block, the superior limbus may be weakened, and the patient is at risk for against-the-rule astigmatism. It is critical that the trabecular block excision be performed far enough anteriorly to avoid incising the vascularized structures of the angle, such as the scleral spur or the ciliary processes.

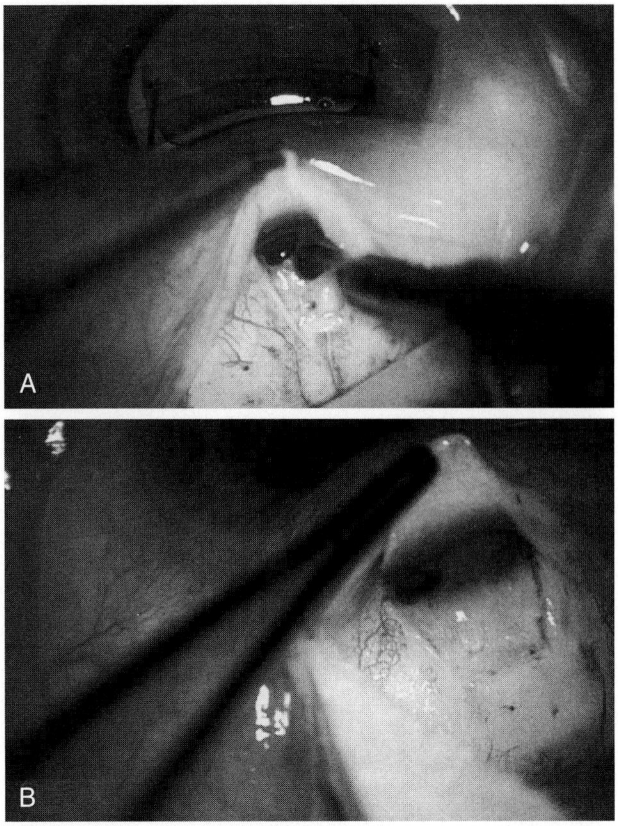

Figure 29–4. *A.* After placement of the foldable intraocular lens, a trabecular block excision is performed utilizing a Kelly Descemet's punch. A peripheral iridectomy is then performed. *B.* The sclerostomy is then carefully inspected to be certain that there is no bleeding or internal obstruction to filtration. (From Samuelson TW: Management of coincident glaucoma and cataract. Curr Opin Ophthalmol 1996;7:53–8. Copyright Rapid Science Publishers.)

After completion of the sclerostomy, a peripheral iridectomy is performed. Some surgeons have elected to omit the peripheral iridectomy in combined glaucoma surgery, but there are several advantages to performing a peripheral iridectomy in this setting. Glaucoma patients are prone to perioperative ocular inflammation. A peripheral iridectomy is safe, easy to perform, and will decrease the likelihood of pseudophakic pupillary block or migration of the iris into the sclerostomy site. When performing the iridectomy the surgeon should grasp the iris with a fine-toothed forceps and withdraw it through the wound and incise it rather than inserting the scissors into the sclerostomy. In this process, as the iris is pulled out of the wound toward the microscope, the ciliary processes will fall back into place and will not be cut with the iridectomy. This is particularly important in hyperopic eyes with shallow anterior chamber depth.

After the trabecular block excision and iridectomy, the sclerostomy site should be examined carefully to ensure that it is entirely free of debris such as blood, cortex, iris, vitreous, or Descemet's membrane (Fig. 29–4*B*). The scleral flap is then closed with interrupted 10-0 nylon sutures (Fig. 29–5). The apical suture is placed initially. The anterior chamber is then re-formed. At this point, the flow through the sclerostomy should be abundant. If flow is not adequate, the surgeon should explore the sclerostomy to rule out internal obstruction. A second scleral flap suture is then placed parallel to the limbus over the sclerostomy site. It is important that this suture is placed far enough anteriorly, as most of the filtration will be taking place near the limbus. The anterior chamber is again re-formed through the needle tract paracentesis. Filtration is assessed in three ways: First, the anterior chamber should maintain normal depth. Visualization of a deep chamber alone is inadequate to gauge filtration. Many eyes maintain a formed chamber intraoperatively despite profound hypotony. Therefore, the eye should be digitally palpated during re-formation. The eye should become firm, but not hard and then should soften slightly over the first several seconds after irrigation is discontinued. Finally, a surgical spear (sponge) should be placed in all regions around the scleral flap to observe for "passive flow," that is spontaneous aqueous flow without external pressure on the globe. If antimetabolites have been employed, it is desirable to have very little, if any, passive flow. However, it should be possible to produce flow readily by applying gentle pressure adjacent to the filtration site. This is the "active filtration test." An important truism in filtration surgery is that it is much easier to increase filtration postoperatively than it is to slow it down. Therefore, filtration surgery should be performed by creating a leaky fistula and controlling the filtration in a reversible fashion. This is accomplished with releasable sutures or argon laser suture lysis. The "active flow test" is intended to simulate the effect of eyelid activity on the filtration site. With normal blinking the filtration site is constantly "massaged" postoperatively. If there is considerable filtration on passive testing, then there is a substantial risk for overfiltration and hypotony. If the filtration proves to be inadequate postoperatively, suture lysis can be performed to augment flow.[17,18]

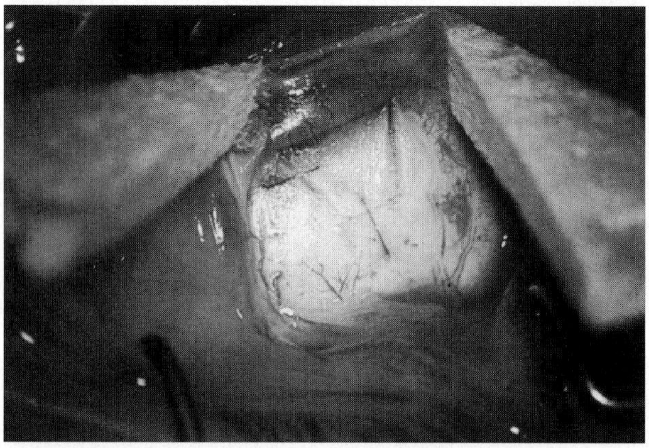

Figure 29–5. The scleral flap is closed with interrupted 10-0 nylon sutures. It is anticipated that 30% to 40% of patients will require argon laser suture lysis in the first 2 or 3 postoperative weeks to augment filtration. (From Samuelson TW: Management of coincident glaucoma and cataract. Curr Opin Ophthalmol 1996;7:53–8. Copyright Rapid Science Publishers.)

Prior to the antimetabolite era, it was critical that abundant aqueous flow be maintained from the start to ensure patency of the fistula. Indeed, before the introduction of suture lysis and antimetabolites, it was considered desirable to have early postoperative hypotony and a partially shallow anterior chamber. Early hypotony was considered necessary to achieve ultimate pressure goals. Thankfully, with antimetabolites and suture lysis, the surgeon can control early postoperative filtration, avoid profound hypotony, and "titrate" filtration based on the individual response to surgery. When antimetabolites are not used, a tightly closed scleral flap may rapidly fibrose, resulting in failure of the procedure. Without antimetabolites like MMC, the delicate balance between adequate flow to ensure patency of the fistula and overfiltration with subsequent hypotony is precarious.

One of the advantages of using intraoperative MMC is the option of closing the scleral flap more tightly to titrate the intraocular pressure to the desired range. Mitomycin C will retard wound healing during the early postoperative course when aqueous production may be reduced by the lingering effects of pharmacologic aqueous suppression. When aqueous production has improved, suture lysis may be performed to enhance outflow.

A complete discussion regarding the use of antimetabolites in filtration surgery is beyond the scope of this chapter. Mitomycin C is an extremely powerful agent that must be respected and used cautiously. It has been proved to be effective in standard filtration surgery, but the role of MMC in combined cataract and glaucoma surgery is less clear and remains controversial.[2,19–24] Many surgeons believe the potential benefits of mitomycin in conjunction with meticulous surgical techniques outweigh the risks; others disagree.

Closure of the conjunctival-Tenon's flap is performed in two layers.[5,25] This technique provides a watertight incision minimizing the chance of wound leak. With proper technique, wound leaks should be exceedingly uncommon after filtration surgery in primary eyes. This is true even if antimetabolites are used. The notion that wound leaks are to be accepted as common is dangerous; a surgeon who frequently encounters wound leaks should seriously evaluate his or her surgical technique. Initially Tenon's layer is closed with an absorbable suture such as 8-0 Vicryl in a running, locking fashion. The conjunctival layer is then closed with a running, non-locking 8-0 Vicryl suture. A vascular needle is preferred to minimize the risk of wound leaks through the needle tracks. An absorbable suture is fa-

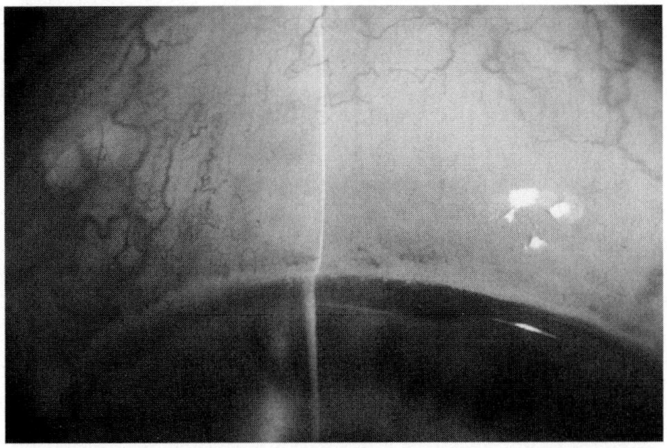

Figure 29–6. A diffuse filtration bleb is present on postoperative day 1. With a limbal based conjunctival flap, wound leaks are rare. (From Samuelson TW: Management of coincident glaucoma and cataract. Curr Opin Ophthalmol 1996;7:53–8. Copyright Rapid Science Publishers.)

vored over a longer lasting or permanent suture such as nylon or prolene, both of which require removal a few months following surgery. Removing nylon sutures from high in the superior fornix is tedious. Also, if the suture remains in place it becomes a nidus for mucus, which theoretically increases the risk of bleb infection. Wound separation from premature dissolution of an absorbable Vicryl suture is extremely rare. A diffuse, low lying, minimally vascular bleb is preferable.[6] Such blebs are more comfortable for the patient and less prone to late leaks than focal, very thin, and ischemic blebs.

POSTOPERATIVE CARE

Diligent postoperative care after any filtration procedure is vital to the success of the operation. In fact, postoperative care will determine the outcome of surgery in many cases. Patients should be educated regarding their role in the important postoperative period. All glaucoma medications should be discontinued. If the patient was taking oral carbonic anhydrase inhibitors preoperatively, then the fellow eye should be monitored carefully for increased intraocular pressure. Aggressive topical steroid use, for example every 2 hours while awake, is recommended during the first postoperative week. Topical antibiotics are instilled for 1 week after the procedure.

Topical steroid administration is continued for 3 to 4 months postoperatively. Tapering of the steroid dose is based on the amount of inflammation in and around the bleb, not intraocular inflammation, which generally subsides long before the bleb becomes quiet. Inflammatory intraocular lens deposits have been shown to peak at approximately 3 months after cataract extraction in high-risk eyes.[26,27] Therefore, the topical steroids are continued for at least 3 months unless the eye and the bleb are unusually quiet. Topical steroids may be tapered more rapidly in hypotonus eyes. Cycloplegia and mydriatic agents are used in the event of hypotony, shallow anterior chamber, and prominent inflammation or fibrin formation. However, these agents are not necessary on a routine basis.

The early postoperative period is critical. It is during this time that procedures often fail and complications are most common. If the intraocular pressure is higher than the mid-teens during the first postoperative week, focal pressure is applied adjacent to the filtration site with a cotton-tip applicator (CTM) to augment filtration.[11] This maneuver separates the flap edges, releasing aqueous from the anterior chamber through the filtration site. In most cases, the CTM pressure will instantaneously inflate the bleb, lowering the intraocular pressure. This technique is favored over releasing aqueous through the clear corneal paracentesis tract, because it encourages outflow through the sclerostomy site and can dislodge fibrin or other debris that may be limiting outflow. Not uncommonly, a single CTM procedure will bring the pressure into the favorable range. Finally, if the intraocular pressure is not lowered with CTM, gonioscopy should be performed. If the internal sclerostomy is patent, it may be assumed that the resistance to outflow is related to a tight scleral flap or conjunctival fibrosis. Argon laser suture lysis should then be considered. If suture lysis is planned on a given postoperative visit, CTM should not be performed because it is easier to lyse the suture when the eye is firm and the suture is under tension. The surgeon should resist the temptation to perform argon laser suture lysis too early. It is not uncommon for retained viscoelastic material to cause elevation of intraocular pressure during the early postoperative period. The intraocular pressure often falls as the viscoelastic material clears the eye. If antimetabolites have not been used, the schedule for releasing sutures is accelerated (Table 29–2). The schedule of postoperative visits is individualized according to each patient's progress. Typically, however, patients are seen at least 2 to 4 times during the first 2 postoperative weeks. During each visit the surgeon should record the visual acuity, intraocular pressure, bleb appearance, and chamber depth. The bleb appearance should reflect the intraocular pressure. For example, if the intraocular pressure is very low, one would expect to see an exuberant bleb. Any discrepancy between bleb appearance and intraocular pressure should warrant examination for a bleb leak. The entire bleb and wound should be painted with flourescein and examined for a Seidel test, using a flourescein-impregnated "strip" to paint the surface of the conjunctiva and then inspecting meticulously as the slit lamp into the blue filter in front of the brightest illuminating beam.

The importance of performing "controlled" filtration surgery to avoid hypotony cannot be overemphasized. The risk to hypotonus eyes is substantial. Flat chambers, choroidal effusions, suprachoroidal hemorrhage, and hypotonus maculopathy are risks associated with overfiltration. The risk of hypotonus maculopathy is greatest in young myopic patients.[28] Overfiltration in the early postoperative period may be exacerbated by decreased aqueous production by a ciliary body that is recovering from years of chronic aqueous suppression,

TABLE 29–2. Postoperative Titration of Intraocular Pressure, Timing of Suture Release, Suture Lysis*

Week 1	Weeks 2–3	Weeks 4–6	Beyond Week 6
Suture lysis uncommon—CTM recommended	Suture lysis most common	Less effect	Effect of suture lysis not predictable
Consider suture lysis if markedly elevated intraocular pressure and low target intraocular pressure	Suture lysis earlier for low target intraocular pressure—advanced glaucoma; later for mild glaucoma or higher target intraocular pressure		
Consider suture lysis if markedly elevated intraocular pressure and pronounced conjunctival inflammation			

*The timing for suture lysis is accelerated if antimetabolites have not been utilized.

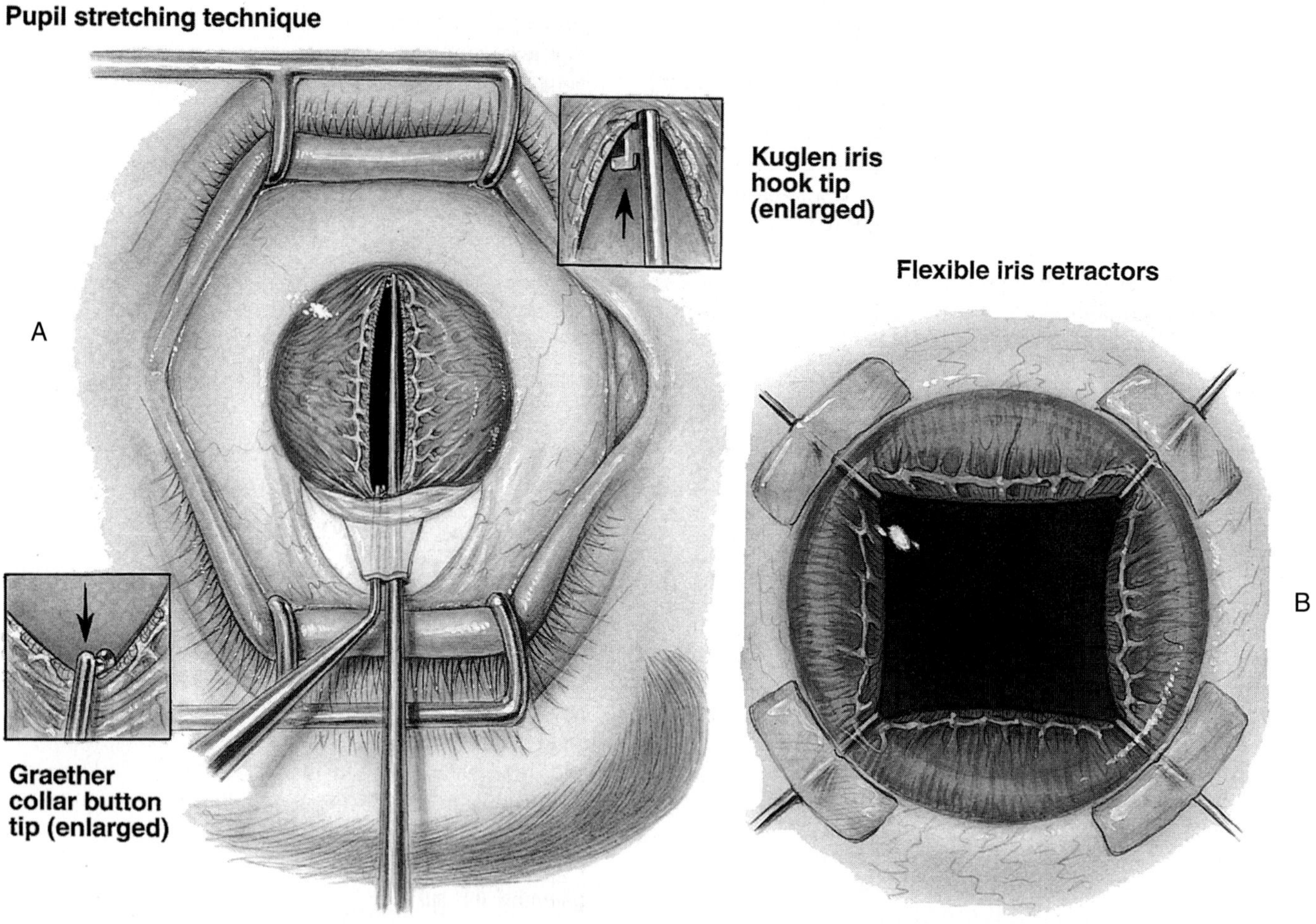

Figure 29–7. *A.* The pupil is stretched by a simultaneous push-pull technique with a Kuglen hook and a Graether collar button. The pupillary sphincter is stretched in the vertical and horizontal meridian. *B.* When pupillary stretch provides inadequate visualization, flexible iris retraction hooks (Greishaber and Company, Langhorne, PA) may be utilized. (From Samuelson TW, Lindquist TD: Combined small-incision phacoemulsification, intraocular lens implantation, and trabeculectomy. Ophthalmic Surgery. Update 2, Section E. page I-E-15, with permission.)

as well as from perioperative inflammation. Postoperative outflow should be titrated based on the individual response to surgery. With controlled glaucoma filtration surgery the scleral flap is closed more tightly, but in a "reversible" fashion. This approach limits filtration in the early postoperative period, decreasing the likelihood of hypotony. Once adequate aqueous production is established, manifest by a deep chamber and stable or rising intraocular pressure, the surgeon may augment filtration by performing suture lysis or release. The ability to titrate filtration and avoid early perioperative hypotony has greatly enhanced the safety of filtration surgery. Patients have faster visual rehabilitation when the intraocular is in the physiological range. For example an intraocular pressure of 18 mm Hg on postoperative day 1 is much more desirable than a pressure of 2 mm Hg. With CTM and judicious suture lysis the target intraocular pressure can be achieved. Moreover, it is common for the intraocular pressure to fall spontaneously over the first postoperative week as residual viscoelastic material clears the eye.

Finally, part of the routine postoperative regimen should include discussion to educate patients of the potential hazards of blebs such as late leaks or late bleb infections. It is generally helpful to provide the patient with an educational brochure describing the benefits of early and aggressive treatment for bleb-related conjunctivitis and blebitis.

PUPIL MANAGEMENT

Perhaps the single most challenging aspect of combined cataract and glaucoma surgery is cataract extraction in the presence of poor pharmacologic pupillary dilatation. Chronic miotic therapy frequently reduces the pupillary response to mydriatic agents. Additionally, conditions such as pseudoexfoliation or chronic inflammation may further limit dilatation of the pupil. A variety of techniques to enhance pupillary dilatation have been described. Traditionally, the most common technique has involved incisional iris surgery such as sector iridectomy or multiple small sphincterotomies. While incisional iris surgery adequately enhances visualization of the lens during phacoemulsification, the cut edges of the iris may be drawn into the phacoemulsification port during lens removal. This may result in significant iris trauma and postoperative inflammation. Therefore, most surgeons now prefer non-incisional techniques to enlarge the pupil such as sphincter stretching or, when necessary, use of iris retraction hooks. In eyes with poor dilatation, exposure can be significantly improved with a simultaneous push–pull technique of sphincter stretching by means of two instruments such as a Kuglen hook or a Graether "collar button" (Fig. 29–7*A*). The sphincter is stretched first in the vertical direction, then in the horizontal meridian. The sphincter is stretched to the point of minute tears in the pupillary margin which are typically seen as small, very focal hemorrhages in the iris sphincter. Additional viscoelastic material is then instilled into the anterior chamber to mechanically expand the pupil. This technique provides an additional 2 or 3 mm of pupillary dilatation. When stretching techniques are inadequate, flexible iris retraction hooks (Greishaber and Company, Langhorne, PA) are applied (Fig. 29–7*B*). The pupil stretch technique is simple, fast, effective, and avoids incisional iris surgery, while resulting in a round pupil postoperatively.[29–31] However, it is not as reliable as the use of hooks.

REFERENCES

1. Samuelson TW: Evolving techniques and changing indications for combined cataract extraction and trabeculectomy. Curr Opin Ophthalmol 1995;6:1–2.
2. Munden P, Alward W: Combined phacoemulsification, posterior chamber intraocular lens implantation and trabeculectomy with mitomycin C. Am J Ophthalmol 1995;119:20–9.
3. Shingleton B, Gamell L, O'Donoghue M, et al.: Long-term changes in intraocular pressure after clear corneal phacoemulsification: Normal patients versus glaucoma suspect and glaucoma patients. J Cataract Refract Surg 1999;4:885–90.
4. Stewart W, Crinkley C, Carlson A: Results of combined phacoemulsification and trabeculectomy in patients with elevated preoperative intraocular pressures. J Glaucoma 1995;4:164–9.
5. Spaeth GL: Ophthalmic surgery: Principles and practice. 2nd Edition. Philadelphia: WB Saunders; 1990.
6. Thomas JV, Savage JA, Albuquerque M: Surgical management of coexisting glaucoma and cataract. In Thomas JV, Belcher CD III, Simmons RJ (eds.), Glaucoma Surgery. St. Louis: Mosby-Year Book; 1992.
7. Broadway DC, Sturmer J, Grierson I, et al.: Reversal of the adverse effect of topical anti-glaucoma medication on the conjunctiva prior to trabeculectomy. Invest Ophthal Vis Sci 1994;35 (Suppl):1914.
8. Kuchle M, Vinores S, Mahlow J, et al.: Blood–aqueous barrier in pseudoexfoliation syndrome: Evaluation by immunohistochemical staining of endogenous albumin. Graefe's Arch Clin Exp Ophthalmol 1996;234:12–8.
9. Kuchle M, Nguyen N, Hannappel E, et al.: The blood–aqueous barrier in eyes with pseudoexfoliation syndrome. Ophthalmic Res 1995;27(Suppl):136–42.
10. Samuelson TW, Lindquist TD: Small incision phacoemulsification, intraocular lens implantation, and trabeculectomy. In Lindquist TD, Lindstrom RL (eds.), Ophthalmic Surg. St. Louis: CV Mosby; 1994.
11. Traverso CE, Greenidge KC, Spaeth GL, et al.: Focal pressure: A new method to encourage filtration after trabeculectomy. Ophthalmol Surg 1984;15:62.
12. Berestka JS, Brown SVL: Limbus based versus fornix based conjunctival flaps in combined phacoemulsification and mitomycin-c trabeculectomy surgery. Ophthalmology 1997;104;2:187–96.
13. Lederer CM: Combined cataract extraction with intraocular lens implant and mitomycin-c–augmented trabeculectomy. Ophthalmology 1996;103:1025–34.
14. Samuelson TW: Management of coincident glaucoma and cataract. Curr Opin Ophthalmol 1995;6:14–21.
15. Samuelson TW: Management of coincident glaucoma and cataract. Curr Opin Ophthalmol 1996;7:53–8.
16. Samuelson TW: Management of coincident cataract and glaucoma. Curr Opin Ophthalmol 1993;4:90–6.
17. Wilson RP, Steinmann WC: Use of trabeculectomy with postoperative 5-fluorouracil in patients requiring extremely low intraocular pressure levels to limit further glaucoma progression. Ophthalmology 1991;98:1047–52.
18. Hoskins DH, Migliazzo C: Management of failing filtration blebs with the Argon laser. Ophthalmic Surg 1984;15:731.
19. Joos K, Bueche M, Palmberg P, et al.: One-year follow-up results of combined mitomycin C trabeculectomy and extracapsular cataract extraction. Ophthalmology 1995;102:76–83.
20. Wong PC, Ruderman JM, Krupin T, et al.: 5-Fluorouracil after primary combined filtration surgery. Am J Ophthalmol 1994;117: 149–54.

21. O'Grady JM, Juzych MS, Shin DH, et al.: Trabeculectomy, phacoemulsification, and posterior chamber lens implantation with and without 5-fluorouracil. Am J Ophthalmol 1993;116:594–9.
22. Shin DH, Hughes BA, Song MS, et al.: Primary glaucoma triple procedure with or without adjunctive mitomycin. Ophthalmology 1996;103:1925–33.
23. Cohen JS, Graff LJ, Novack GD, et al.: A placebo-controlled, double-masked evaluation of mitomycin-c in combined glaucoma and cataract procedures. Ophthalmology 1996;103:1934–42.
24. Gandolfi SA, Vecchi M: 5-Fluorouracil in combined trabeculectomy and clear-cornea phacoemulsification with posterior chamber intraocular lens implantation. Ophthalmology 1997;104:181–6.
25. Samuelson TW, Lindstrom RL: Combined glaucoma filtration surgery and phacoemulsification. Semin Ophthalmol 1992;7:279–85.
26. Carlson D, Barad J, Parsons M: Reduced vision secondary to pigmented cellular membranes on silicone intraocular lenses. Am J Ophthalmol 1995;120:462–70.
27. Shah S, Spalton D: Natural history of cellular deposits on the anterior intraocular lens surface. J Cataract Refract Surg 1995;21:466–71.
28. Stamper RL, McMenemy M, Lieberman MF: Hypotonous maculopathy after trabeculectomy with subconjunctival 5-fluorouracil. Am J Ophthalmol 1992;114:544–53.
29. Dinsmore S: Modified stretch technique for small pupil phacoemulsification with topical anesthesia. J Cataract Refract Surg 1996;22:27–30.
30. Shepherd DM: The pupil stretch technique for miotic pupils in cataract surgery. Ophthalmic Surg 1993;24:851–2.
31. Miller KM, Keener GT: Stretch pupilloplasty for small pupil phacoemulsification. Am J Ophthalmol 1994;117:107–8.

CHAPTER 30

Aqueous Shunts

TROY M. TANJI, M.D. and DALE K. HEUER, M.D.

Aqueous shunting procedures may be useful in eyes with glaucoma when conventional filtering surgery has failed, is unlikely to succeed, is technically difficult, or is more prone to complications. Initially, shunts had to be imported or assembled from encircling bands and nasolacrimal tubes.[1–3] Numerous devices are now commercially available, and the emphasis in this chapter will be on those currently enjoying wide application, specifically the Ahmed (New World Medical, Rancho Cucamonga, CA), Baerveldt (Pharmacia, Kalamazoo, MI), Krupin (Hood Laboratories, Pembroke, MA), and Molteno (IOP, Costa Mesa, CA) implants.

A shunt consists of a silicone tube connected to an equatorial explant (or explants) of varying shapes and sizes (Table 30–1). The tube allows aqueous to pass from the anterior or posterior chamber through its lumen to the potential space surrounding the explant(s). The aqueous creates a bleb within the fibrous capsule that encapsulates the episcleral explant(s).[4,5] The fluid then passively diffuses out of the bleb, draining into the overlying circulation.[4,6,7] The posterior location of the explant allows filtration to occur away from the limbus, at which the conjunctiva is often scarred by previous surgery.

Clinical studies of aqueous shunts have reported success rates ranging from 25% to 100% in glaucomas with poor prognoses, including a variety of primary and secondary open-angle glaucomas and angle-closure glaucomas, as well as glaucomas of childhood.[8–22] Intermediate-term results with single- and double-plate Molteno implants demonstrate gradual decline in success rates over time.[16,23,24] Five-year life-table success rates in a pilot study of single-plate Molteno implants had declined to only 46% in glaucomas in aphakia/pseudophakia and 25% to 26% in other poor-prognosis glaucomas.[16] Although double-plate implants fared better, their life-table success rates also declined over time in a randomized study of single- versus double-plate Molteno implantation for glaucomas in aphakia/pseudophakia: 80% vs 96% at 6 months; 55% versus 86% at 12 months; 46% versus 82% at 18 months; and 46% versus 71% at 24 months.[23] With the larger surface area implants such as the double-plate Molteno and the 350-mm^2 Baerveldt, the authors generally anticipate an intermediate-term success rate of 70-85% in most non-neovascular glaucomas and 50-70% in neovascular glaucomas.[25]

Intraocular pressure control with single-plate Molteno implantation was comparable to guarded filtration procedures (GFPs) with 5-fluorouracil in one study, while another study comparing predominantly single-plate Molteno implantation and GFPs with mitomycin C reported higher success rates with the latter approach.[26,27] Aqueous shunting procedures only infrequently achieve intraocular pressures in the low teens; consequently, a GFP with an antifibrotic agent is generally preferred in patients in whom a low target pressure has been established.

Shunting procedures have also been reported to be roughly comparable (except for the need for fewer medications) to transscleral Nd:YAG laser cyclophotocoagulation in patients aged 40 years and older (in younger patients, shunting procedures were more frequently successful).[28] However, a more recent study suggests that shunting procedures are preferable in neovascular glaucomas.[29] Aqueous shunts may be particularly advantageous in patients for whom surgical procedures are indicated for both glaucoma and concomitant ocular diseases, such as patients undergoing simultaneous shunting procedures and penetrating keratoplasty and/or vitreoretinal surgery.[15,20]

TABLE 30–1. Characteristics of Aqueous Shunting Devices

Device	Valved/Non-Valved	Planar Surface Area (mm^3)*
Single-plate Molteno implant†[68]	Non-valved	129
Double-plate Molteno implant†[68]	Non-valved	257
Pediatric single-plate Molteno implant[68]	Non-valved	74
ACTSEB (No. 20 band)	Non-valved	302
ACTSEB (No. 31 band)	Non-valved	339
ACTSEB (No. 220 band)	Non-valved	452
Long Krupin-Denver valve to 180° (No. 220 band)[69]	Valved	226
Long Krupin-Denver valve to disk implant	Valved	184
Baerveldt implant	Non-valved	250 or 350
Ahmed S-2	Valved	184
Ahmed B-1 (biplate)	Valved	364
Ahmed S-3	Valved	96

ACTSEB = anterior chamber tube shunt to encircling band.
*Assuming an equatorial globe diameter of 24 mm.[70]
†Available with an inverted V-shaped ridge on the top surface of the plate that separates the top plate surface (only the proximal plate of double-plate implants) into two compartments; implantation with Tenon's capsule drawn tightly over the plate surface is thought to limit initial aqueous flow to the smaller proximal compartment, thereby reducing initial hypotony, even with one-stage installation without tube occlusion.[71]

PREOPERATIVE CARE

Careful inspection of the anterior segment should be performed preoperatively for surgical planning. Sufficient corneal clarity must be present to allow proper placement of the intraocular segment of the tube. Anterior chamber depth should be assessed to determine if sufficient space between the cornea and iris is present for tube placement. If the anterior chamber depth is not sufficient, the surgeon should perform posterior vitrectomy with particular attention to meticulous removal of the vitreous base to allow pars plana insertion of the tube into the posterior chamber.[30] The presence of vitreous at the pupillary plane or within the anterior chamber should also be noted as it may block the tube, preventing its function; in such eyes, anterior or preferably posterior vitrectomy should be performed before tube insertion.

Most glaucoma medications are continued until the time of surgery. Long-acting cholinesterase inhibitors should be discontinued a few weeks preoperatively if possible to reduce the risk of increased intraoperative bleeding and postoperative inflammation. If a ligated non-valved implant is planned, patients are informed that glaucoma medications will probably be continued after surgery until the tube opens.

The type and size of glaucoma implant should be selected preoperatively; however, which specific device provides the best intraocular pressure control with the fewest complications has not been established. Short- to intermediate-term results with the Baerveldt, Krupin, and Ahmed implants have been favorable, however long-term follow-up studies of these devices are not available given their relatively recent introduction.[22,31–33] Longer-term clinical experience with the Molteno implant has been reported.[16,19] Valved implants are designed to provide immediate reduction of intraocular pressure with less risk of early postoperative hypotony. To reduce the risk of early postoperative hypotony, non-valved implants are installed with temporary closure of the shunt tube (or occasionally in two-stage procedures), such that pressure reduction is usually delayed for a few weeks until the tube spontaneously opens or is surgically opened (or inserted in the case of two-stage procedures). Therefore, the urgency of intraocular pressure lowering must be taken into account when selecting the type of implant and the surgical technique.

The long-term intraocular pressure needs of the eye must also be considered when selecting an implant. The Molteno and Baerveldt implants are available with varying explant surface areas, to which a shunt's ability to lower intraocular pressure has been related.[4,7,23,34] However, an upper limit to the relationship probably exists, as the life-table success rates with the 350-mm^2 and 500-mm^2 Baerveldt implants were comparable; furthermore, higher rates of complication, such as choroidal effusions, were also observed with the larger implants.[33] Thus the medium-sized explants such as the double-plate Molteno or 350-mm^2 Baerveldt implant are used in most cases as they provide the best compromise between intraocular pressure control and complications. Shunts with smaller explants (possibly even the pediatric Molteno implant) may be appropriate in eyes in which aqueous hyposecretion is suspected, such as eyes with a history of cyclodestruction or chronic uveitis.[35] Larger plates, such as the previously available 425-mm^2 and 500-mm^2 Baerveldt implants, are no longer manufactured.

ANESTHESIA

Local anesthesia is usually sufficient for installation of aqueous shunts. A retrobulbar block is usually administered to produce both anesthesia and akinesia. A facial nerve block may be given if eyelid akinesia is also desired. Topical anesthesia alone can also be considered, although patient discomfort may be encountered when the rectus muscles are manipulated or when the explant is inserted into its equatorial position. Peribulbar infusion of an anesthetic solution into the sub-Tenon's space with a cannula can be used to alleviate any discomfort encountered intraoperatively. When lengthy combined procedures are planned, general anesthesia may be preferable.

SURGICAL TECHNIQUE

The superior temporal quadrant is the preferred location for a glaucoma implant. Except for Molteno implants, installation into the nasal quadrants is less desirable because of the more limited orbital space and more problematic intraoperative exposure. Motility disturbances have been reported with all of the devices, but they appear to be more frequent with the larger implants and with implantation in the superonasal quadrant.[21,36–40]

A fornix-based conjunctival flap is preferred by the authors for installation of glaucoma implants, as it avoids placement of a wound posteriorly where dehiscence might expose the shunt tube or equatorial explant. Furthermore, the often-scarred limbal conjunctiva can more easily be elevated with this approach, affording better limbal access and exposure, which are particularly important as clear visualization of the limbus is critical for accurate tube placement. The fornix-based conjunctival flap is created with radial relaxing incisions approximately 90° apart with blunt Wescott scissors (Fig. 30–1). In eyes with severely scarred conjunctiva, a Beaver blade may be used to start the anterior limbal aspect of the conjunctival flap, as well as to establish the correct plane of dissection between fibrotic Tenon's capsule and episclera. Blunt Wescott or Stevens scissors are then used to open Tenon's capsule posteriorly. The adjacent rectus muscles are identified and, for the Baerveldt and possibly Krupin implants, isolated with muscle hooks; (Fig. 30–2), and the underlying and intervening sclera is inspected for ectatic areas that might complicate implantation or suturing of the equatorial explant. Application of mitomycin C to the equatorial episcleral and Tenon's capsule has been advocated by a few investigators,[41,42] but its benefit was not confirmed by another recent study.[43] Because the role of antifibrotic agents in aqueous shunting surgery has not been well defined, specifically lacking clinical trials demonstrating improved success rates without substantially higher complications rates, the authors do not favor their use.

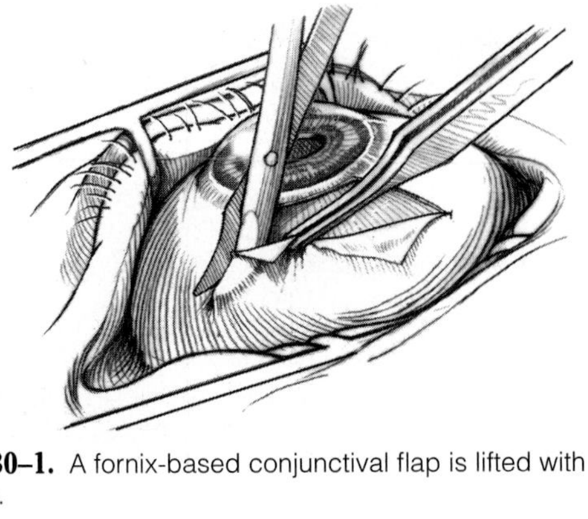

Figure 30–1. A fornix-based conjunctival flap is lifted with Wescott scissors.

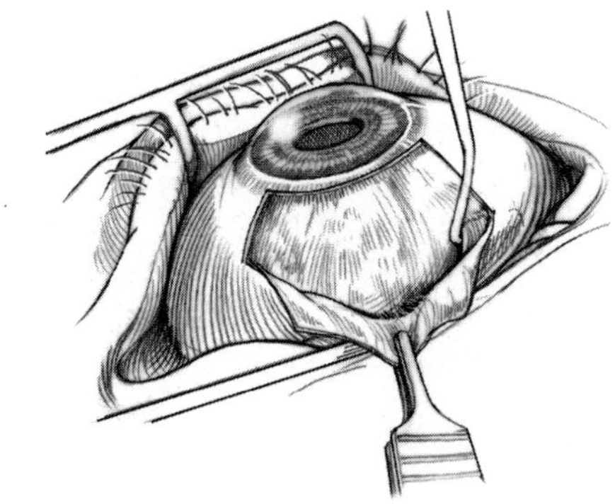

Figure 30–2. The adjacent rectus muscles are identified (and isolated with muscle hooks for the Baerveldt and Krupin implants). The underlying and intervening sclera is inspected for ectatic areas.

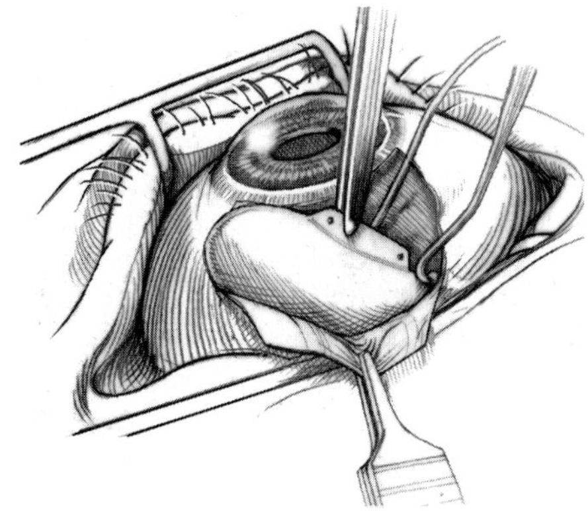

Figure 30–3. After the implant is inspected, the explant is placed into position on sclera. Muscle hooks are helpful in manuvering the Baerveldt and Krupin plates under the adjacent rectus muscles.

The implant should be inspected before installation. Balanced salt solution is irrigated through the tube to demonstrate flow. After the explant(s) is (are) in the appropriate position(s), it (they) should be relatively stable even before sutures are placed. If an explant springs forward or to one side, further dissection of Tenon's capsule should be performed or the explant should be repositioned relative to the rectus muscles (Fig. 30–3). The anterior edge of the plate is securely fixed to the sclera approximately 8 mm (Ahmed implants) to 10 mm (Baerveldt, Krupin, and Molteno implants) posterior to the limbus, typically with non-absorbable sutures, such as 8-0 nylon (Fig. 30–4). The appropriateness of the explant position should be confirmed with calipers before and after suture placement. The implants have holes (Ahmed, Baerveldt, and Molteno implants) or a fixation ridge (Krupin implant) along the anterior portion of the explant for suture placement. Once in place, the sutures are rotated to bury their knots within the explant fixation holes or under the explant to reduce the risk of ero-

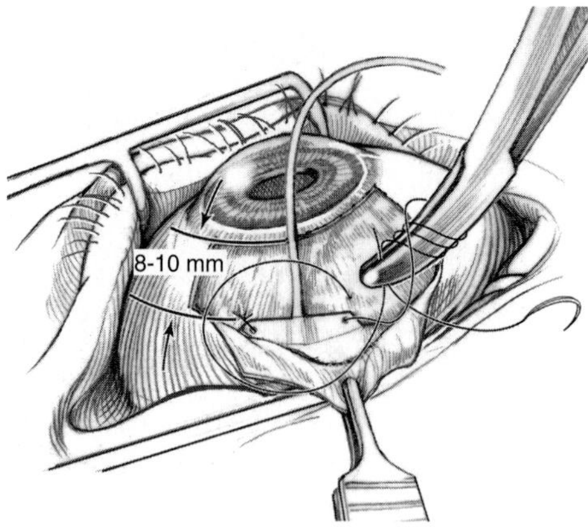

Figure 30–4. The anterior edge of the explant is secured to sclera with nonabsorbable sutures 8 to 10 mm from the limbus.

sion through the conjunctiva. Secure fixation of the explant to the underlying sclera should be confirmed to reduce the risk of substantial migration of the explant and its tube further into or out of the anterior chamber postoperatively. Equatorial placement of the explant reduces the risk of extrusion as it is posterior to the action of the eyelids, and appropriate positioning relative to the rectus muscle insertions also seems to reduce the risk of strabismus.

Before insertion into the eye, the tube must be shortened to the desired length and, in non-valved implants, the tube lumen must be occluded (techniques for which will be discussed later in this chapter). The intraocular portion of the tube should be approximately 2 mm in length. This allows the tube to remain in the eye should the implant migrate posteriorly, yet keeps it short enough to reduce the risk of either corneal or iris touch. When the tube is shortened for insertion, an anterior bevel is also placed on its end to reduce the risk of iris incarceration into its lumen, which can block aqueous outflow. Similarly, a posterior bevel is used when the tube is inserted through the pars plana into the posterior chamber. A sharp bevel also facilitates tube insertion through its scleral tract. When trimming the tube, it is better to err in favor of leaving the tube too long, after which it can be shortened further, rather than initially cutting it too short and having to lengthen the tube or replace the entire shunt device.

The limbal and peripheral corneal epithelium is removed to promote the sealing of conjunctiva to the limbus and to reduce the risk of wound dehiscence and possible epithelial ingrowth. A 23-gauge needle is used to create the fistula for the tube as it provides a tight seal. With non-valved implants, some surgeons have advocated the use of a larger needle for the sclerotomy as it allows aqueous to leak around the tube to provide some lowering of the intraocular pressure postoperatively until the tube ligature spontaneously opens or is surgically opened. Proper placement and orientation of the limbal tract are critical, as it determines the tube's position within the eye. The tract is usually started at the mid-limbus in phakic eyes or the posterior limbus in aphakic and pseudophakic eyes, so that the replaced conjunctiva covers its entry site (Fig. 30–5*A*). The needle should enter the eye just anterior to iris insertion and be directed parallel to the plane of the iris (Fig. 30–5*B*). The shortened, beveled tube is then inserted through the sclerostomy (Fig. 30–6*A*). A correctly placed tube should lie anterior to the iris and posterior to the cornea (Fig. 30–6*B*). A malpositioned tube may cause complications, such as iritis or corneal decompensation, therefore proper placement should be achieved intraoperatively. Additional sclerostomies can be placed adjacent to the previous tract if necessary until appropriate positioning is obtained.

With the tube in the eye, the extraocular portion of the tube is secured to episclera to reduce the chance of shifting before the fibrous capsule surrounds it (Fig.

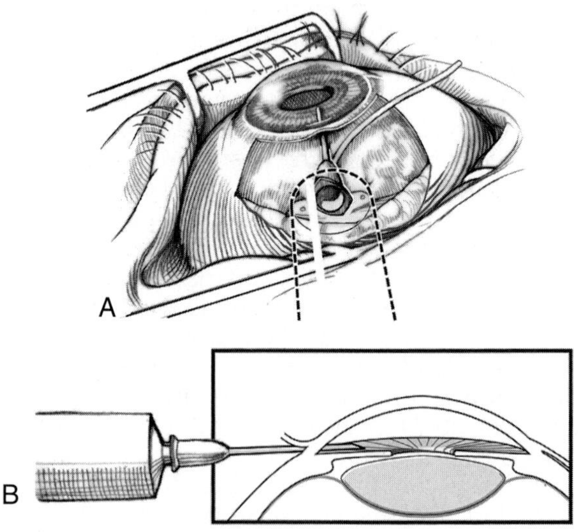

Figure 30–5. *A.* 22- or 23-gauge needle is used to create the fistula for tube placement into the anterior chamber. *B.* The fistula created should enter the anterior chamber just anterior to iris insertion and be directed parallel to the iris plane.

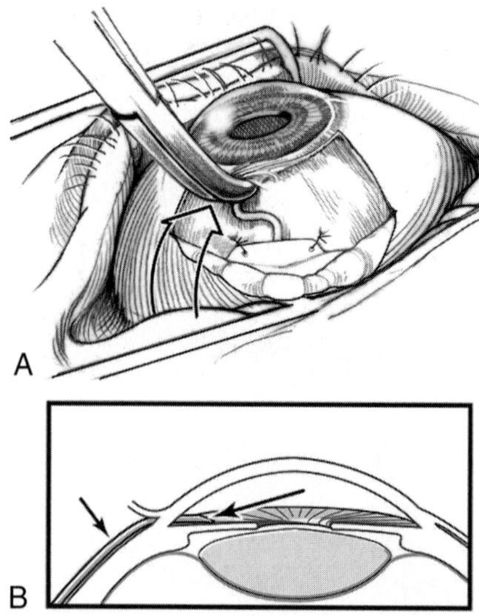

Figure 30–6. *A.* The shortened and anterior beveled tube within the anterior chamber. *B.* A properly positioned tube should lie anterior to the iris and posterior to the cornea.

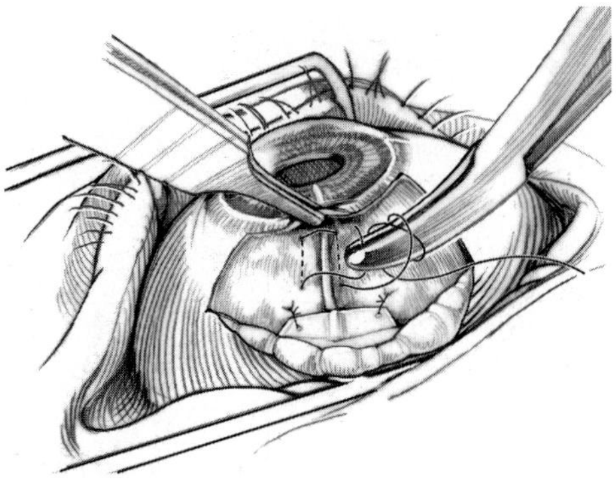

Figure 30–7. The extraocular portion of the tube is secured to episclera with an absorbable suture.

30–7). An absorbable suture, such as 7-0 or 8-0 polyglactin, is sufficient for this purpose. To avoid erosion and extrusion of the tube through conjunctiva, a donor patch graft is placed over the subconjunctival portion of the tube. Alternatively, a scleral flap can be dissected parallel to the tube and flapped over the tube; if the sclera adjacent to the tube is unsuitable for such a flap, a lamellar autograft can be harvested from elsewhere on the globe. Another technique involves dissection of a lamellar scleral flap, similar to a trabeculectomy flap, under which the tube is inserted into the anterior chamber. However, we do not advocate this approach because dissection of the flap can be technically difficult in eyes that have had multiple previous procedures; furthermore, placement of the tube through full-thickness limbal tissue probably provides greater stability of the tube tip within the anterior chamber. A variety of allogeneic grafting materials have been used recently with good success. Donor sclera, pericardium, and fascia lata are currently commercially available.[44–46] We prefer to use one of the processed donor materials that have been sterilized to avoid the possible transmission of infectious diseases. These products can be routinely available in the operating room for urgent situations as each has a long shelf life. Implantation of the grafting material is similar regardless of the material employed.

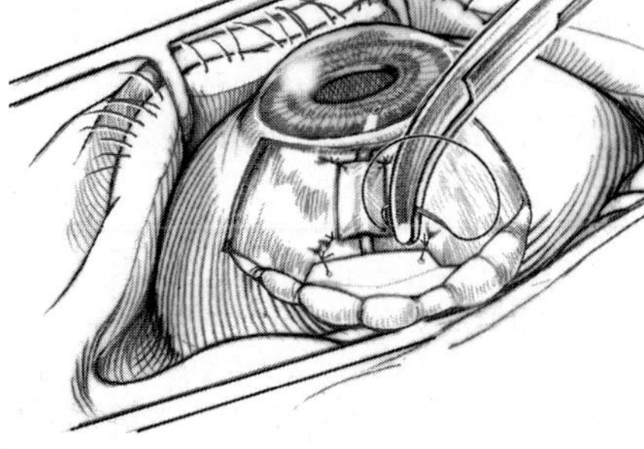

Figure 30–8. A donor patch graph is placed and secured over the extraocular portion of the tube to prevent erosion through overlying conjunctiva.

The graft is shaped free-hand to cover the scleral fistula site(s) and the anterior, subconjunctival portion of the tube. Particular attention should be made to cover the tube's entry into the eye, as erosion commonly occurs at that site. Secured tightly across the limbus, the graft may also help reduce unwanted leakage of aqueous humor during the early postoperative period. An interrupted 7-0 or 8-0 polyglactin absorbable suture placed at each corner through episclera is sufficient to fix the graft (Fig. 30–8). (Over the ensuing weeks, host fibroblasts will colonize the graft, incorporating it into host tissue to form a watertight seal around the tube.) The conjunctival flap is then closed with a combination of mattress sutures at the limbal corners and running sutures along the relaxing incisions, both with 7-0 or 8-0 polyglactin (Fig. 30–9). In cases in which a valved implant has been used, the relaxing incisions may be closed with 8-0 polyglactin on a BV-130 taper-point needle (rather than the typical spatula needle) to increase the likelihood of a watertight closure.

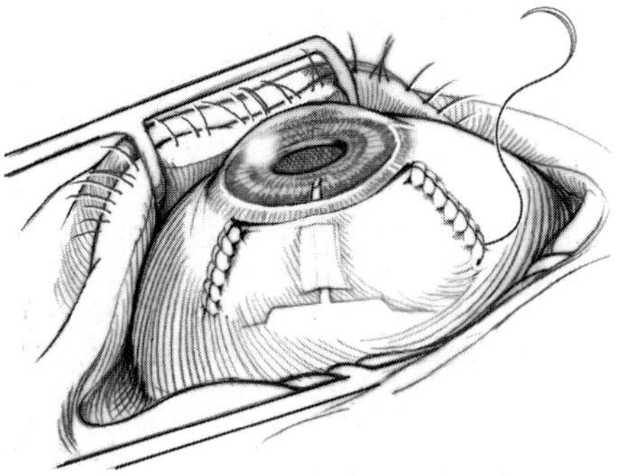

Figure 30–9. The conjunctival flap is closed with a combination of absorbable mattress sutures and running absorbable sutures.

A limbal paracentesis incision is created temporally to facilitate anterior chamber access, if needed postoperatively. Subconjunctival antibiotic and corticosteroid injections are administered at the conclusion of surgery. Atropine 1% ophthalmic solution is applied for cycloplegia, and the eye is patched and shielded before the patient leaves the surgical suite.

MODIFICATIONS OF THE SURGICAL TECHNIQUE

MANAGEMENT OF EARLY POSTOPERATIVE HYPOTONY WITH NON-VALVED IMPLANTS

Installation of a non-valved glaucoma implant without temporary occlusion invariably leads to early postoperative hypotony. Consequently, single-stage installation of the non-valved implants usually includes temporary occlusion of the tube.[47] This allows formation of a fibrous capsule around the equatorial explant to provide the necessary resistance to aqueous outflow. Continuation of glaucoma medications moderates the intraocular pressure during the early postoperative period until flow through the tube begins. Two-stage installation can also be performed, with the explant initially implanted without tube insertion. This allows the fibrous capsule to form around the plate before the tube is inserted into the eye, typically 4 to 6 weeks later. This may be the safest approach with respect to minimizing the risk of early postoperative hypotony; however, two sessions in the operating room are required.[48]

For temporary occlusion of the tube, a ligature with an absorbable suture (e.g., 7-0 or 8-0 polyglactin) is tightened securely around the tube to close its lumen. Complete closure is confirmed by attempting to irrigate fluid through the tube after placement of the ligature (Fig. 30–10). If there is any flow, another ligature must be placed, because hypotony can occur if the tube is not totally occluded.[48,49] This suture is usually placed 1 to 2 mm from the tube–explant junction (at approximately the anticipated posterior border of the donor patch graft) to allow easy localization should it be necessary to find it postoperatively. Polyglactin sutures typically dissolve 3 to 5 weeks postoperatively, allowing spontaneous opening of the tube. Releasable ligatures with the end of the suture buried in the cornea or subconjunctival space have also been described.[50] However, consistent occlusion of the tube is often difficult with the releasable knots; therefore, we prefer to use a permanent square knot. Tying off the intraocular portion of the tube with a black nylon suture has also been described. The ligature can be cut later with a laser to permit flow.[51]

An unacceptably high intraocular pressure in a patient on maximal medications may favor initiating flow through the implant before spontaneous release of the ligature. Release of the ligature by incisional surgery or laser applications is possible; however, placement of a subconjunctival, extraluminal "ripcord" during surgery is much more convenient and predictable.[52] The ripcord is a relatively large-caliber suture, such as a 4-0 or 5-0 nylon or polypropylene, placed alongside the tube and incorporated within the ligating suture. After the tube has been inserted into the eye, the tube is secured to the underlying sclera with mattress sutures, so that postoperative removal of the ripcord does not pull the tube tip out of the anterior chamber. The free end of the ripcord is positioned in the interpalpebral or inferotemporal subconjunctival space and stabilized, if necessary, with an interrupted 7-0 or 8-0 polyglactin suture. To reduce the risk of creating a potential tract from within the potential space around the explant along the course of the "ripcord" suture, to the hole created in the conjunctiva and Tenon's capsule, the explant end of the ripcord is trimmed just anterior to the explant. This will permit removal the ripcord postoperatively. The donor patch graft is then placed, and the conjunctiva closed (Fig. 30–11). If early initiation of flow through the shunt tube is desired (or after the ligature has spontaneously dissolved), the ripcord is removed at the slit lamp with Vannas scissors to dissect the overlying conjunctiva and forceps to remove the ripcord suture. After its removal, flow through the tube occurs, with lowering of the intraocular pressure and formation of a bleb over the plate (occasionally flow through the tube is still delayed, presumably due to elasticity of the ligature). If the intraocular pressure is lower than desired, viscoelastic material can be injected to reinflate the anterior chamber and retard flow through the shunt tube. Variations of this technique include intraluminal placement of the ripcord, use of absorbable sutures, and externalization of the free end of the ripcord through the conjunctiva into the inferior fornix.[53,54]

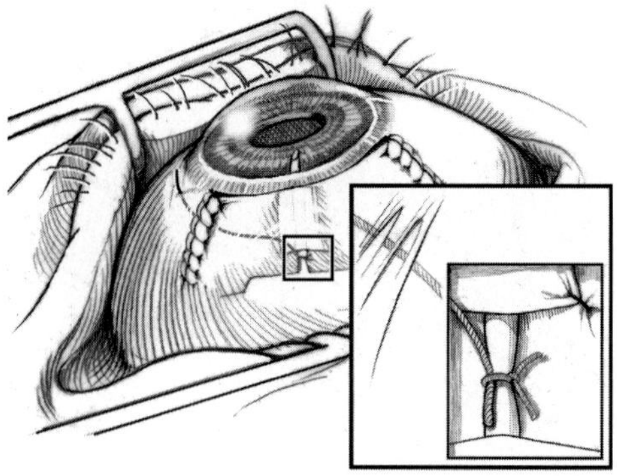

Figure 30–11. A "ripcord" suture may be placed adjacent to the tube and within the ligature suture for initiation of early flow through the tube before spontaneous release of the ligature suture occurs. (See text for further description.)

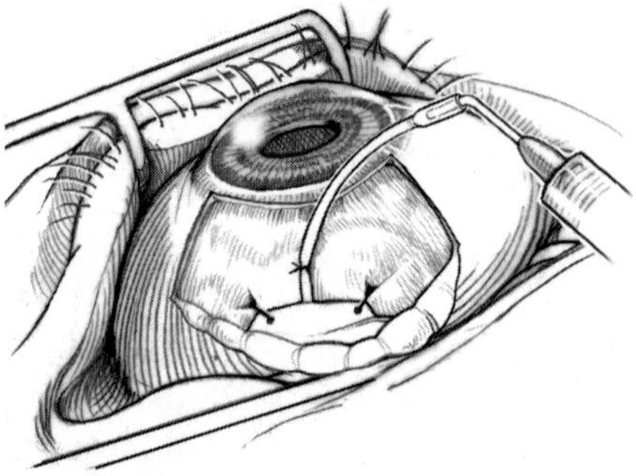

Figure 30–10. For temporary occlusion of non-valved implants, an absorbable suture is used to ligate the tube, usually 1 to 2 millimeters from the tube–explant junction. Total occlusion of the tube is confirmed by attempting irrigation of the tube with fluid.

MANAGEMENT OF POSTOPERATIVE INTRAOCULAR PRESSURE WITH A LIGATED, NON-VALVED IMPLANT

Because non-valved glaucoma implants are installed in two stages or with their tubes occluded to avoid early postoperative hypotony, intraocular pressure control can be problematic until flow occurs; however, moderately elevated intraocular pressure is preferable to hypotony, particularly in patients with extremely high preoperative pressures, in whom the risk of choroidal hemorrhage[55] or other complications is substantial. In addition to the use of glaucoma medications, a variety of modifi-

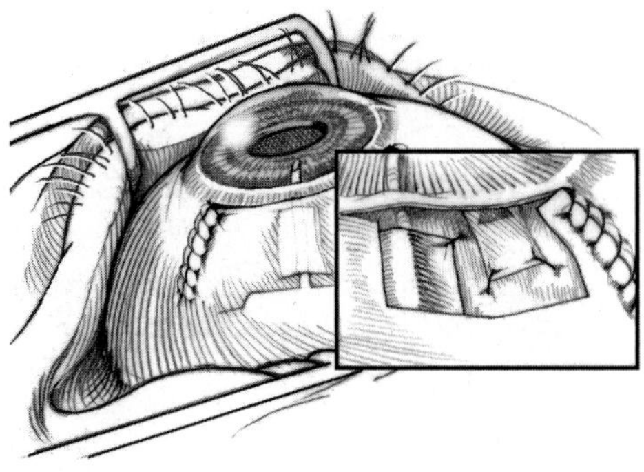

Figure 30–12. A glaucoma filtering procedure can provide early postoperative pressure control when performed simultaneously with a ligated, non-valved implant.

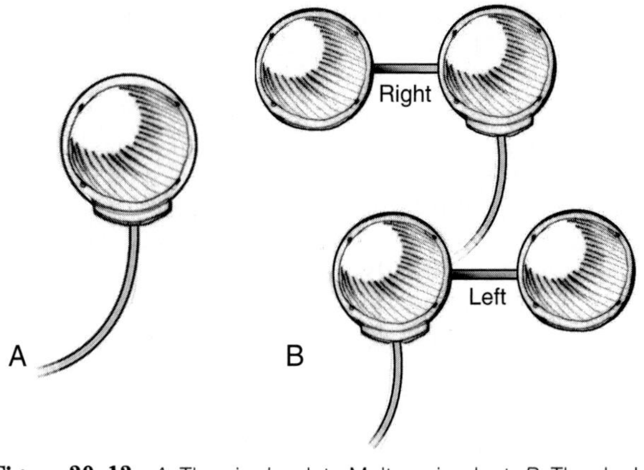

Figure 30–13. *A.* The single-plate Molteno implant. *B.* The double-plate Molteno implant.

cations to the installed tube have been suggested to control intraocular pressure until the shunt functions. These include use of a larger needle for the sclerostomy, creation of slits in the tube anterior to the ligature, and partial ligature (incomplete lumen occlusion) of the tube.[56] All of these methods allow some aqueous flow immediately after surgery to lower pressure; unfortunately, they are unpredictable and unreliable.

Other surgeons have advocated simultaneously performing GFPs to control intraocular pressure. No antifibrotic agent is used at the GFP site, so the filter usually scars closed within a few weeks, just as the shunt is about ready to function (Fig. 30–12). This combined surgery may be considered in eyes with extremely fragile nerves in which a substantial pressure spike could cause "snuff." Eyes with extremely high preoperative pressures, as in the case of severe neovascular glaucoma, may also benefit from a "bridge" GFP with the shunt procedure. Similarly, a GFP can be performed with the first stage of a two-staged installation, after which the tube insertion can be performed if the GFP ceases to provide adequate control of the intraocular pressure. Otherwise, the first stage of a planned two-stage procedure usually has no effect on pressure because it is an extraocular procedure. Predictable pressure lowering usually occurs during the second stage with tube insertion. It should be considered in fragile eyes with extensive damage and in patients at high risk for choroidal hemorrhage, such as patients with aphakic, vitrectomized eyes or with glaucoma associated with the Sturge-Weber syndrome, elevated episcleral venous pressure, or nanophthalmos.[57]

The Molteno Implant

The Molteno implant was the first commercially available, non-valved glaucoma implant to gain widespread use. The single-plate Molteno consists of a circular polypropylene explant with a 13-mm diameter (Fig. 30–13*A*). The episcleral plate, with a planar surface area of approximately 130 mm^2, is connected to the silicone tube that is inserted into the eye. The double-plate Molteno, with twice the surface area, is probably a better choice for most patients[23,34]; however, its two plates, which are connected by a 10-mm segment of silicone tubing, require twice the amount of conjunctival dissection for installation into adjacent quadrants. A "pediatric" Molteno with an approximately 74-mm^2 planar surface area plate is also available and may be useful in eyes with severely compromised aqueous inflow, such as eyes with chronic uveitis or that have undergone multiple cyclodestructive procedures.[35]

The double-plate Molteno is available in a right and left eye configuration (Fig. 30–13*B*). Each was designed for installation with the a plate in each of the superior quadrants, with the tube inserted superonasally. However, conjunctival or limbal scarring, limbal access (such as in a patient with deep-set eyes or a prominent brow or nose), or anterior chamber depth may favor tube insertion from the superotemporal quadrant; in such an instance, a left eye implant is used in the right eye and vice versa.

Installation of the double-plate Molteno implant begins with dissection of a fornix-based conjunctival flap in two adjacent quadrants. Posterior Tenon's capsule is opened and the superior rectus muscle is isolated with a muscle hook. Attachments between the muscle and episclera are lysed with the aid of a second muscle hook, which is slid posteriorly while the muscle insertion is secured with the first muscle hook. As shown in Figure 30–14, one of the Molteno plates is then passed under the superior rectus muscle (preferably the plate destined for the superonasal quadrant is passed under the superior rectus muscle from temporal to nasal to

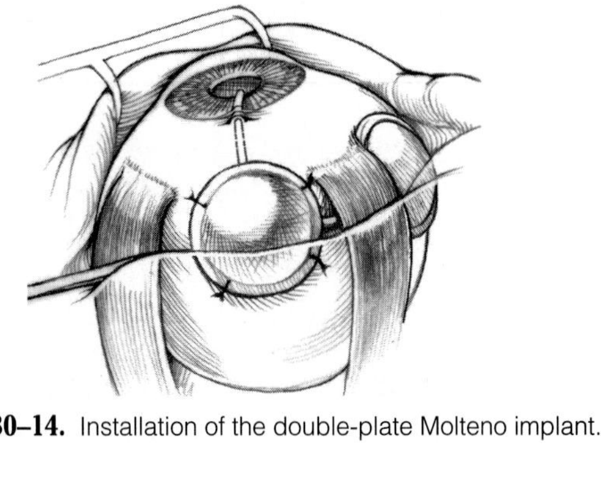

Figure 30–14. Installation of the double-plate Molteno implant.

reduce the risk of damage to the superior oblique muscle). Because of the difficulty of that maneuver and possible attendant trauma to the superior rectus muscle, many surgeons prefer to place the interplate tube over the rectus muscle. With either approach, each plate is secured to the globe approximately 10 mm posterior to the limbus and the tube installed as previously described. Space availability around the globe may dictate the actual location of the two plates. The relatively small size of the Molteno plates allows a plate to be installed in any of the four quadrants as necessary.

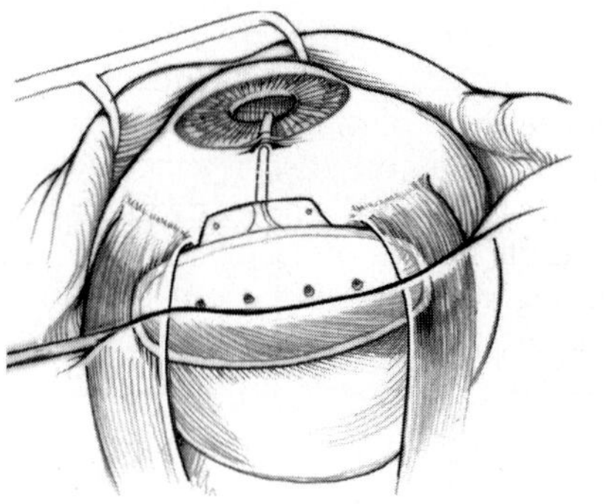

Figure 30–16. Installation of the Baerveldt glaucoma implant.

The Baerveldt Implant

The Baerveldt implant, a non-valved glaucoma device, is available with two different explant sizes of approximately 250 mm^2 and 350 mm^2 (Fig. 30–15). Each consists of an oblong silicone explant connected to a silicone tube. A pars plana model is also available for placement into the posterior chamber.[30,58] The Baerveldt implant has the advantage of affording a relatively large equatorial explant surface area with only one quadrant dissection for installation. In a recent study that compared the 350-mm^2 size to the then available 500-mm^2 implant, similar rates of success were found. The larger explant more frequently controlled intraocular pressure without medications, but it was associated with a higher rate of some complications, such as choroidal effusions.[33] The 350-mm^2 size therefore appears to offer a reasonable balance between intraocular pressure reduction and fewer postoperative complications.

Installation of the Baerveldt implant is similar to that described previously. This implant may be used in any of the four quadrants, however reports of an acquired Brown's syndrome when placed into the superior nasal quadrant have made installation there less desirable.[21,36] After the conjunctival flap has been dissected in the selected quadrant and the posterior Tenon's capsule opened, the two adjacent rectus muscles are identified and isolated with muscle hooks. Blunt dissection of attachments between the muscles and episclera is performed by sliding another muscle hook posteriorly with the muscle still secured anteriorly with the first muscle hook. The use of two muscle hooks to open the appropriate space by lifting the muscle slightly off of the globe posteriorly facilitates placement of the implant's lateral wings under the rectus muscles, posterior to their insertion (Fig. 30–16). The plate is fixed to the sclera 10 mm posterior to the limbus, and the tube is then inserted into the eye with a ligature as previously described.

The Krupin Implant

The Krupin implant is an oval Silastic disk with a planar surface area of approximately 184 mm^2 (Fig. 30–17). The explant end of its tube consists of a Silastic tube with horizontal and vertical slits, which restrict aqueous flow, thereby allowing installation of the device in one stage without tube ligature, but with less risk of immediate hypotony. Intermediate-term results have been favorable; however, the slits in the Silastic tube do not always prevent postoperative hypotony.[31,32]

Installation of the Krupin implant is similar to that of the non-valved Molteno and Baerveldt implants, except that, because of the presence of the valve slits, a tube ligature is not generally employed. A cannula is provided already connected to the tube to allow irrigation with balanced salt solution and thereby confirm that the valve slits allow flow. It may be necessary to compress the valve end with smooth forceps to ensure that each of the four quadrants of the valve moves independently; this is especially important if the implant has been sterilized in the autoclave (as was the case early after its commercial introduction), which may cause the edges of the slits to adhere to one another. Al-

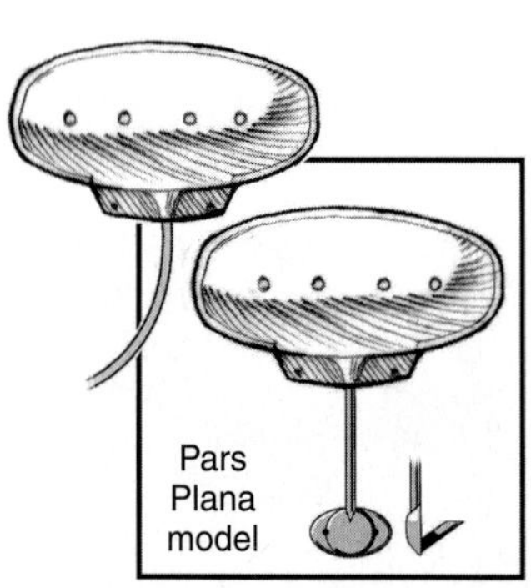

Figure 30–15. The Baerveldt glaucoma implant.

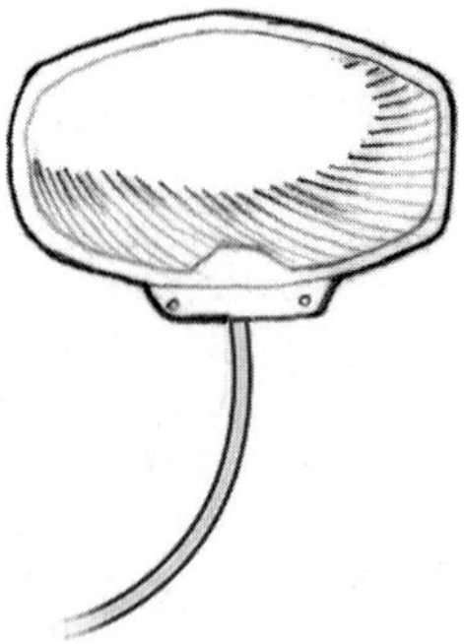

Figure 30–17. The Krupin implant.

though the extent to which the Krupin implant is inserted under the adjacent rectus muscles is not as great as the Baerveldt implant, it is still important to identify the muscles to ensure that the explant is secured posterior to their points of insertion, and not mistakenly over their bellies more posteriorly. The implant should be secured approximately 10 mm posterior to the limbus, preferably with one nonabsorbable suture on each side of the tube through the implant's fixation ridge.

The Ahmed Implant

The Ahmed implant (model S2) consists of a rectangular polypropylene explant with a planar surface area of approximately 184 mm^2 (Fig. 30–18). Each implant has two layers of a thin silicone membrane through which aqueous flows before entering the plate. These membranes restrict aqueous flow, which reduces the risk of postoperative hypotony and allows implantation without tube closure for aqueous drainage immediately after surgery. Short-term results with this device have been favorable, but in some cases the implants required intracameral irrigation of the tube postoperatively to relieve apparent blockage.[20,22,59]

Installation of the Ahmed implant is similar to that described previously. It is critical to "prime" the implant with balanced salt solution to break the surface tension between the two silicone sheets; otherwise the tube will not drain postoperatively. To be doubly sure that this step has been performed, it is the authors' practice to routinely irrigate balanced salt solution through the device before securing the explant to the globe and again just before inserting the tube into the anterior chamber. The Ahmed implant should also be installed with the anterior edge of the plate positioned approximately 8 mm from the limbus rather than the 10 mm employed for the other commercially available devices (Fig. 30–19). Studies have shown that its longer design may abut the optic nerve if the explant is placed more posteriorly.[60] With the recently available double-plate Ahmed B-1 model, the interplate tube can be disconnected, thereby allowing placement of the interconnecting tube under the superior (or other) rectus muscle without passing one of the plates under the muscle.

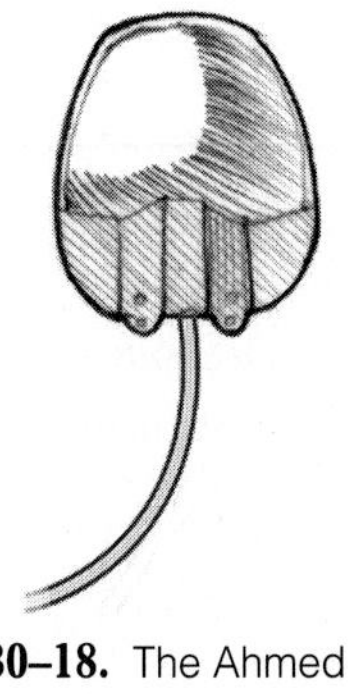

Figure 30–18. The Ahmed implant.

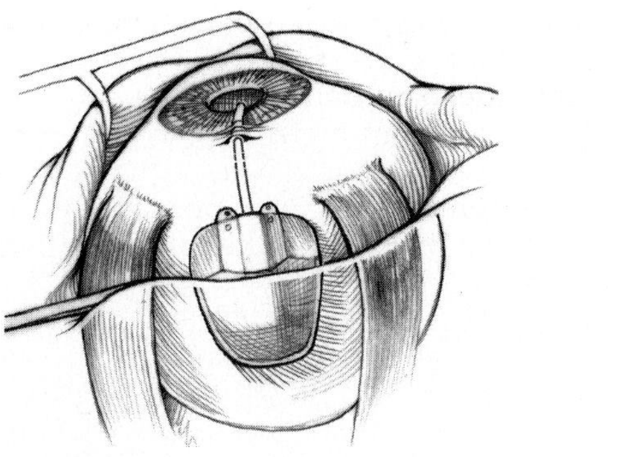

Figure 30–19. Installation of the Ahmed implant.

POSTOPERATIVE CARE

If the patient has advanced glaucomatous damage, examination an hour or two after surgery is recommended. The anterior chamber depth should be noted and the intraocular pressure measured, because anterior chamber manipulations with tube insertion may cause increased pressure postoperatively. If the intraocular pressure is high, aqueous can be released at the slit lamp through a paracentesis site (we routinely create a paracentesis tract temporally just anterior to the limbus to facilitate this maneuver) and glaucoma medications reinstituted immediately. The patient is discharged after his/her IOP has stabilized at an acceptable level. Patients are instructed to wear protective eyewear at all times, with activity restrictions similar to those after GFPs.

A topical antibiotic, cycloplegic agent, and corticosteroid are administered postoperatively. Our usual regimen consists of prednisolone phosphate 1% hourly during the waking hours, atropine 1% twice daily, and a fluoroquinolone antibiotic four times daily. If a single-staged non-valved glaucoma implant was performed, preoperative glaucoma medications are continued until the implant begins functioning, and topical steroids may be limited to four to six times daily for the first 10 to 14 days to allow more rapid encapsulation of the explant, particularly in patients in whom early initiation of flow is likely. Topical miotics are discontinued to minimize inflammation.

Patients are seen the day after surgery, within a week postoperatively, and thereafter as the clinical situation dictates. Attention should be paid to detection of early postoperative infection, proper conjunctival healing, good intraocular tube position, control of intraocular inflammation, and maintenance of the intraocular pressure at an acceptable level. Weekly visits are recommended for patients with ligated tubes until proper function occurs and intraocular pressure is adequately lowered. Timing of the ligature release varies and mainly depends on the size and type of absorbable suture used. A 7-0 or 8-0 polyglactin ligature will usually release spontaneously 3 to 5 weeks after surgery. As discussed earlier, placement of a ripcord allows the option of opening the tube at the slit lamp earlier. Whenever possible, removal is delayed for at least 10 to 14 days af-

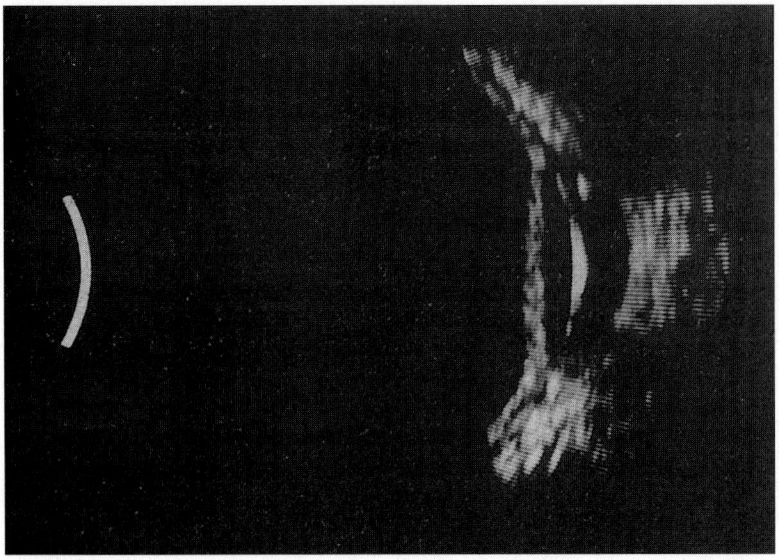

Figure 30–20. B-scan ultrasound demonstrating an expanded capsule around a functioning glaucoma drainage explant. (From Minckler D, Heuer D, Hasty B, et al.: Clinical experience with the single-plate Molteno implant in complicated glaucomas. Ophthalmology 1988; 95:1181.)

ter surgery to allow formation of the fibrous capsule around the equatorial explant. Earlier opening increases the risk of hypotony and its associated complications.

With the tube open and functioning, an elevated bleb overlying the plate should be present. If a bleb or the explant is not visible at the slit lamp, ultrasonography may used to detect the presence or absence of a bleb (Fig. 30–20).[61,62] The decrease in intraocular pressure is often associated with increased intraocular inflammation that can be controlled with frequent topical corticosteroids. Cycloplegia should also be continued as the drop in pressure can be associated with choroidal effusion and anterior chamber shallowing.

A hypertensive phase may be encountered 1 month after the initiation of aqueous flow through the aqueous shunt, as can also be seen with encapsulated blebs after GFPs (Fig. 30–21). This rise in intraocular pressure may be related to several factors, including: increased aqueous inflow as the eye recovers from surgery and as complete washout of the glaucoma medications occurs; thickening of the fibrous capsule surrounding the plate and reduction of flow out of the bleb; and, in susceptible patients, corticosteroid effect. There is usually a gradual decline in pressure over the ensuing months. Addition of glaucoma medications can be considered to maintain an acceptable pressure level during this phase, which is usually self-limiting. Switching from topical prednisolone or dexamethasone to topical rimexolone or fluorometholone acetate may also be considered. The hypertensive phase usually resolves over the ensuing few months, after which it may be possible to discontinue or reduce glaucoma medications.

The frequency of late postoperative visits is gradually reduced, as after GFPs. At each visit, particular attention should be paid to the proper position and patency of the tube. Corneal endothelial damage due to direct mechanical injury can lead to corneal decompensation over the long term.[8,18,63] A posteriorly directed tube can irritate the iris, causing chronic uveitis and cataract formation in phakic eyes. The subconjunctival portion of the tube should be covered by conjunctiva and the donor patch graft. An exposed tube requires urgent repair in the operating room before frank infection (or potentially epithelial ingrowth) occurs.[64] Finally, a bleb should be present over the explant, indicating a functioning shunt.

If an unexpected rise in intraocular pressure occurs during the late postoperative period with a previously functioning glaucoma implant, the same systematic examination should be performed. The intraocular opening of the tube is inspected as blood, fibrin, vitreous, or iris may occlude the tube lumen. Ultrasound can be used to locate a tube that cannot be visualized at the

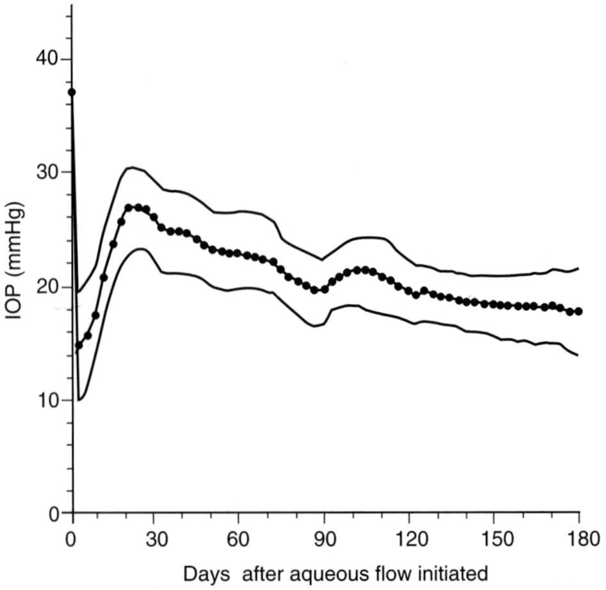

Figure 30–21. Composite intraocular pressure profile (mean interpolated pressure ± 95% confidence limits) in single-plate Molteno implant patients who were successful in the intermediate term, demonstrating "hypertensive phase" common to aqueous shunting procedures. (Modified from Minckler D, Heuer D, Hasty B, et al.: Clinical experience with the single-plate Molteno implant in complicated glaucomas. Ophthalmology 1988;95:1181.).

slit-lamp.[65] An argon or Nd:YAG laser can be used to clear the blockage. Intracameral injection of tissue plasminogen activator has also been used to dissolve fibrin and blood clots.[66] Pushing on the bleb of a non-valved implant can also help dislodge any debris from the tube. Irrigation of the tube in the clinic with a cannula has successfully restored function of valved implants.[22,67] A return trip to the operating room may be needed to reestablish patency with repositioning of the tube.

Next, an elevated bleb over the plate is sought. If the bleb or the explant is not visible at the slit lamp, ultrasonography is used to detect a bleb. If neither intraocular tube blockage nor a bleb is present, obstruction of the tube elsewhere or of the valve must be present. Thorough exploration in the operating room may be both diagnostic and therapeutic. In cases of blocked valved implants, surgical removal of the valve can restore flow and function of the implant.

A higher than desired intraocular pressure in eyes with a functioning shunt is thought to be due to excessive capsular fibrosis around the explant that limits diffusion of aqueous humor. The addition of glaucoma medications may provide additional pressure lowering. However, even with glaucoma medications, shunts infrequently achieve an intraocular pressure level below the mid-teens. The placement of additional shunts or application of cyclodestructive treatment may be considered in an eye with a functioning implant not providing adequate control of intraocular pressure.

REFERENCES

1. Schocket S, Lakhanpal V, Richards R: Anterior chamber tube shunt to an encircling band in the treatment of neovascular glaucoma. Ophthalmology 1982;89:1188.
2. Sherwood M, Joseph N, Hitchings R: Surgery for refractory glaucoma. Results and complications with a modified Schocket technique. Arch Ophthalmol 1987;105:562.
3. Sidoti P, Minckler D, Baerveldt G, et al.: Aqueous tube shunt to a pre-existing episcleral encircling element in the treatment of complicated glaucomas. Ophthalmology 1994;101:1036.
4. Minckler D, Shammas A, Wilcox M, et al.: Experimental studies of aqueous filtration using the Molteno implant. Trans Am Ophthalmol Soc 1987;85:368.
5. Rubin B, Chan C-C, Burnier M, et al.: Histopathologic study of the Molteno glaucoma implant in three patients. Am J Ophthalmol 1990;110:371.
6. Prata JJ, Mérmoud A, LaBree L, et al.: In vitro and in vivo flow characteristics of glaucoma drainage implants. Ophthalmology 1995;102:894.
7. Wilcox M, Minckler D, Ogden T: Pathophysiology of artificial aqueous drainage in primate eyes with Molteno implants. J Glaucoma 1994;3:140.
8. Beebe W, Starita R, Fellman R, et al.: The use of Molteno implant and anterior chamber tube shunt to encircling band for the treatment of glaucoma in keratoplasty patients. Ophthalmology 1990;97:1414.
9. Costa V, Katz L, Cohen E, et al.: Glaucoma associated with epithelial downgrowth controlled with Molteno tube shunts. Ophthalmic Surg 1992;23:797.
10. Fish L, Heuer D, Baerveldt G, et al.: Molteno implantation for secondary glaucomas associated with advanced epithelial ingrowth. Ophthalmology 1990;97:557.
11. Freedman J, Rubin B: Molteno implants as a treatment for refractory glaucoma in black patients. Arch Ophthalmol 1991;109:1417.
12. Hill R, Heuer D, Baerveldt G, et al.: Molteno implantation for glaucoma in young patients. Ophthalmology 1991;98:1042.
13. Hill R, Nguyen Q, Baerveldt G, et al.: Trabeculectomy and Molteno implantation for glaucomas associated with uveitis. Ophthalmology 1993;100:903.
14. Lieberman M, Ewing R: Drainage implant surgery for refractory glaucoma. Int Ophthalmol Clin 1990;30:198–208.
15. Lloyd M, Heuer D, Baerveldt G, et al.: Combined Molteno implantation and pars plana vitrectomy for neovascular glaucomas. Ophthalmology 1991;98:1401.
16. Lloyd M, Sedlak T, Heuer D, et al: Clinical experience with the single-plate Molteno implant in complicated glaucomas: update of a pilot study. Ophthalmology 1992;99:679.
17. Lloyd M, Baerveldt G, Heuer D, et al.: Initial clinical experience with the Baerveldt implant in complicated glaucomas. Ophthalmology 1994;101:640.
18. McDonnell P, Robin J, Schanzlin D, et al.: Molteno implant for control of glaucoma in eyes after penetrating keratoplasty. Ophthalmology 1988;95:364.
19. Molteno A: The use of drainage implants in resistant cases of glaucoma. Late results of 110 operations. Trans Ophthalmol Soc NZ 1983;35:94.
20. Coleman A, Mondino B, Wilson M, et al.: Clinical experience with the Ahmed glaucoma valve implant in eyes with prior or concurrent penetrating keratoplasties. Am J Ophthalmol 1997;123:54.
21. Hodkin M, Goldblatt W, Burgoyne C, et al.: Early clinical experience with the Baerveldt implant in complicated glaucomas. Am J Ophthalmol 1995;120:32.
22. Coleman A, Hill R, Wilson M, et al.: Initial clinical experience with the Ahmed glaucoma valve implant. Am J Ophthalmol 1995;120:23.
23. Heuer D, Lloyd M, Abrams D, et al.: Which is better? One or two? A randomized clinical trial of single-plate versus double-plate Molteno implantation for glaucomas in aphakia and pseudophakia. Ophthalmology 1992;99:1512.
24. Mills R, Reynolds A, Emond M, et al.: Long-term survival of Molteno glaucoma drainage devices. Ophthalmology 1996;103:295.
25. Krishna R, Godfrey DG, Bundenz DL, et al.: Intermediate-term outcomes of 350-mm^2 Baerveldt glaucoma implants. Ophthalmology 2001;108:621.
26. El Sayyad F, Helal M, Elsherif Z, et al: Molteno implant versus trabeculectomy with adjunctive intraoperative mitomycin-C in high-risk glaucoma patients. J Glaucoma 1995;4:80.
27. Bluestein E, Stewart W: Trabeculectomy with 5-fluorouracil vs single-plate Molteno implantation. Ophthalmic Surg 1993;24:669.
28. Noureddin B, Wilson-Holt N, Lavin M, et al.: Advanced uncontrolled glaucoma. Nd:YAG cyclophotocoagulation or tube surgery. Ophthalmology 1992;99:430.
29. Eid T, Katz L, Spaeth G, et al.: Tube-shunt surgery versus neodymium:YAG cyclophotocoagulation in the management of neovascular glaucoma. Ophthalmology 1997;104:1692.
30. Varma R, Heuer D, Lundy D, et al.: Pars plana Baerveldt tube insertion with vitrectomy in glaucomas associated with pseudophakia and aphakia. Am J Ophthalmol 1995;119:401.
31. The Krupin Eye Valve Filtering Surgery Study Group: Krupin eye valve with disk for filtration surgery. Ophthalmology 1994; 101:651.
32. Fellenbaum P, Almeida A, Minckler D, et al.: Krupin disk implantation for complicated glaucomas. Ophthalmology 1994;101:1178.
33. Lloyd M, Baerveldt G, Fellenbaum P, et al.: Intermediate-term results of a randomized clinical trial of the 350- versus the 500-mm^2 Baerveldt implant. Ophthalmology 1994;101:1456.
34. Molteno A: The optimal design of drainage implants for glaucoma. Trans Ophthalmol Soc NZ 1981;33:39.
35. Wellemeyer M, Price F: Molteno implants in patients with previous cyclocryotherapy. Ophthalmic Surg 1993;24:395.
36. Ball S, Ellis GJ, Herrington R, et al.: Brown's superior oblique tendon syndrome after Baerveldt glaucoma implant [letter]. Arch Ophthalmol 1992;110:1368.
37. Cardakli U, Perkins T: Recalcitrant diplopia after implantation of Krupin valve with disk. Ophthalmic Surg 1994;25:256.
38. Prata JJ, Minckler DS, Green RL: Pseudo-Brown's syndrome as a complication of glaucoma drainage implant surgery. Ophthalmic Surg 1993;24:608.
39. Smith S, Starita R, Fellman R, et al.: Early clinical experience with the Baerveldt 350-mm^2 glaucoma implant and associated extraocular muscle imbalance. Ophthalmology 1993;100:914.
40. Frank J, Perkins T, Kushner B: Ocular motility defects in patients with the Krupin valve implant. Ophthalmic Surg 1995;26:228.

41. Susanna RJ, Nicolela M, Takahashi W: Mitomycin C as adjunctive therapy with glaucoma implant surgery. Ophthalmic Surg 1994;25:458.
42. Perkins T, Çardakli U, Eisele J, et al.: Adjunctive mitomycin C in Molteno implant surgery. Ophthalmology 1995;102:91.
43. Lee D, Shin D, Birt C, et al.: The effect of adjunctive mitomycin C in Molteno implant surgery. Ophthalmology 1997;104:2126.
44. Freedman J: Scleral patch grafts with Molteno setons. Ophthalmic Surg 1987;18:532.
45. Tanji T, Lundy D, Minckler D, et al.: Fascia lata patch graft in glaucoma tube surgery. Ophthalmology 1996;103:1309.
46. Brandt J: Patch grafts of dehydrated cadaveric dura mater for tube-shunt glaucoma surgery. Arch Ophthalmol 1993;111:1436.
47. Hoare Nairne J, Sherwood D, Jacob JSH, et al.: Single stage insertion of the Molteno tube for glaucoma and modifications to reduce postoperative hypotony. Br J Ophthalmol 1988;72:846.
48. Molteno A, Van Biljon G, Ancker E: Two-stage insertion of glaucoma drainage implants. Trans Ophthalmol Soc NZ 1979;31:17.
49. Melamed S, Cahane M, Gutman I, et al.: Postoperative complications after Molteno implant surgery. Am J Ophthalmol 1991; 111:319.
50. El-Sayyad F, El-Maghraby A, Helal M, et al.: The use of releasable sutures in Molteno glaucoma implant procedures to reduce postoperative hypotony. Ophthalmic Surg 1991;22:82.
51. Liebmann J, Ritch R: Intraocular suture ligature to reduce hypotony following Molteno seton implantation. Ophthalmic Surg 1992;23:51.
52. Kooner K, Goode S: Removable ligature during Molteno implant procedure [letter]. Am J Ophthalmol 1992;114:102.
53. Ball S, Herrington R: Long-term retention of chromic occlusion suture in glaucoma seton tubes [letter]. Arch Ophthalmol 1993; 111:169.
54. Egbert P, Liebermann M: Internal suture occlusion of the Molteno glaucoma implant for the prevention of postoperative hypotony. Ophthalmic Surg 1989;20:53.
55. The Fluorouracil Filtering Surgery Study Group: Risk factors for suprachoroidal hemorrhage after filtering surgery. Am J Ophthalmol 1992;113:501.
56. Brooks S, Dacey M, Lee M, et al.: Modification of the glaucoma drainage implant to prevent early postoperative hypertension and hypotony: a laboratory study. Ophthalmic Surg 1994;25: 311.
57. Budenz DL, Sakamoto D, Eliezer R, et al.: Two-staged Baerveldt glaucoma implant for childhood glaucoma associated with Sturge-Weber syndrome. Ophthalmology 2000;107:2105.
58. Luttrell JK, Avery RL, Baerveldt G, Easley KA: Initial experience with pneumatically stented Baerveldt implant modified for pars plana insertion for complicated glaucoma. Ophthalmology 2000;107:143.
59. Coleman A, Smyth R, Wilson M, et al.: Initial clinical experience with the Ahmed glaucoma valve implant in pediatric patients. Arch Ophthalmol 1997;115:186.
60. Leen M, Witkop G, George D: Anatomic considerations in the implantation of the Ahmed glaucoma valve [letter]. Arch Ophthalmol 1996;114:223.
61. Lloyd M, Minckler D, Heuer D, et al.: Echographic evaluation of glaucoma shunts. Ophthalmology 1993;100:919.
62. Minckler D, Heuer D, Hasty B, et al.: Clinical experience with the single-plate Molteno implant in complicated glaucomas. Ophthalmology 1988;95:1181.
63. McDermott M, Swendris R, Shin D, et al.: Corneal endothelial cell counts after Molteno implantation. Am J Ophthalmol 1993;115:93.
64. Gedde SJ, Scott IU, Tabandeh H, et al.: Late endophthalmitis associated with glaucoma drainage implants. Ophthalmology 2001;108:1323.
65. Crichton A, McWhae J, Reimer J: Ultrasound biomicroscopy for the assessment of Molteno tube position. Ophthalmic Surg 1994;25:633.
66. Lundy D, Sidoti P, Winarko T, et al.: Intracameral tissue plasminogen activator after glaucoma surgery. Indications, effectiveness, and complications. Ophthalmology 1996;103:274.
67. Krawitz P: Treatment of distal occlusion of Krupin eye valve with disk using cannular flush. Ophthalmic Surg 1994;25:102.
68. Peart D, Molteno A, Minckler D: Implantation of the Molteno drain. In Minckler DS, Van Buskirk EM (eds.), Glaucoma. In Wright K W (editor-in-chief), Ryan S J (consultant): Color Atlas of Ophthalmic Surgery, p 163. Philadelphia, JB Lippincott; 1992.
69. Krupin T, Ritch R, Camras C, et al.: A long Krupin-Denver valve implant to a 180° scleral explant for glaucoma surgery. Ophthalmology 1988;95:1174.
70. Hogan M, Alvarado J, Weddell J: Histology of the human eye: an atlas and textbook. Philadelphia, WB Saunders; 1971: 50.
71. Molteno A: The dual chamber single plate implant—its use in neovascular glaucoma. Aust NZ J Ophthalmol 1990;18:431.

CHAPTER 31

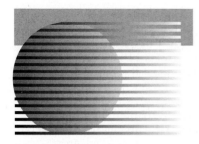

Argon Laser Trabeculoplasty: What it is and How it Works

CARLO E. TRAVERSO, M.D.

Laser trabeculoplasty (LTP) is most frequently performed using the argon laser (ALT), although other types of thermal-effect lasers have proved to be equivalent. The treatment consists in targeting the trabecular meshwork with laser applications via a goniolens. The procedure lowers the intraocular pressure, causing increased outflow facility. The precise mechanism of action is not established; accepted theories include: scarring at the site of the laser impact with subsequent tightening of the trabecular beams around it; activation of endothelial cells; release of endothelin; or changes in the extracellular matrix. Thermal laser effects on the trabecular meshwork are influenced by the energy density and the focus of the laser beam. Photocoagulation occurs independent of the wavelength and the exposure time as long as the threshold for thermal effect is reached. Theoretically, the coagulation of areas larger than planned can have adverse effects. Because one of the established methods to obtain experimentally a sustained intraocular pressure increase in primates is to treat excessively the trabecular meshwork with a thermal laser, improper or excessive applications are to be avoided.

In recent years selective targeting of the trabecular meshwork was proposed using a Q-switched 532-nm Nd:Yag laser. The advantages of selective laser trabeculoplasty (SLT) are the minimal, if any, disturbance of the trabecular anatomy, damage of a subpopulation of trabecular meshwork cells only, the possibility of treating eyes where argon laser trabeculoplasty has failed, and the possibility of repeating the treatment without the risk of damaging the functioning part of the meshwork.

INDICATIONS AND SELECTION OF CANDIDATES

Ophthalmologists planning to perform laser trabeculoplasty must be proficient with indirect gonioscopy and perfectly familiar with angle landmarks. Laser trabeculoplasty is indicated in primary open-angle glaucoma (POAG), exfoliative glaucoma, and pigmentary glaucoma when a lower intraocular pressure is advisable. Secondary glaucomas, both open and closed angle, and primary angle-closure glaucoma are contraindications for LTP. Juvenile glaucomas or glaucomas associated with angle dysgenesis or malformations do not respond well to laser trabeculoplasty. The trabecular meshwork must be visible with a Goldmann-type indirect goniolens. If the angle approach is narrow, peripheral laser iridoplasty (see Chapter 32, Laser Peripheral Iridoplasty) can be applied to stretch the iris and flatten the peripheral bowing, allowing for better visualization of the trabecular meshwork.

There appears to be a relationship between the hydrodynamic effect of ALT and the amount of pigment present in the meshwork, as well as with age: lesser-pigmented and younger patients respond the least. In pseudoexfoliation the initial effect is usually larger than in POAG; however, failures can occur earlier. The effect in pigmentary glaucoma is controversial, because good results are observed together with higher failure rates.

Overall, an average 25% intraocular pressure decrease from baseline can be expected. Such effect, however, appears to fade with time, with roughly 50% of the eyes still controlled after 5 years, and only 20% after 10 years. The role of LTP has changed during the last decade, owing to the results of prospective clinical trials and to the retrospective analysis of long-term data on a large number of patients. When introduced, it was to be applied only when patients were ready for a filtering operation, hoping to avoid surgery. With the acceptance of the concept of individualized target intraocular pressures, LTP is considered one way to lower the intraocular pressure. In some environments it is fully acceptable to perform LTP prior to use of intraocular pressure-lowering medication. As discussed later, LTP is now widely considered to be as effective as medications for the initial treatment of POAG. From the point of view of the financial resources used for managing glaucoma, primary LTP theoretically has a substantial cost over medications.

PATIENT PREPARATION AND TREATMENT TECHNIQUE

Candidates should be fully informed of the realistic intraocular pressure-lowering goal of treatment and possible complications. Everything likely to be felt or seen during the procedure should be explained in detail. The patient must be sitting comfortably at the laser slit lamp; topical anesthesia is applied. It is crucial to use a well-focused round spot of the appropriate diameter, usually 50 microns. Unless perfectly focused, the laser beam strikes an area larger than necessary and with less efficiency. The oculars of the slit lamp must be focused. A clean, unscratched, laser coated goniolens is placed with gonioscopy fluid over the eye. It is crucial to focus the laser beam accurately on the anterior portion of the meshwork; posterior treatments are equally effective, but they cause more formation of peripheral anterior synechiae and more postoperative inflammation.

Typical settings using a thermal-effect laser like argon on eyes with a moderate degree of pigment are: spot size, 50 microns; exposure time, 0.1 second; number of applications, 12 to 20 per quadrant. Initial power is 400 mW, with adjustment to obtain a slight blanching of the treated area. When the laser beam is well focused, if the meshwork has little pigment, so as to require power above 1000 mW, the intraocular pressure response is likely to be poor. Vapor bubble indicate excessive energy and should be avoided. Treatment is started at the 6 o'clock position of the angle, i.e., through the mirror at the 12 o'clock position. The goniomirror is then slowly rotated to expose progressively the other quadrants. Although excessive treatment is harmful, the lower threshold or the least number of applications still capable of effectively decreasing the intraocular pressure is not known. Either 360 or 180 degrees of the circumference can be treated. The advantage of treating only half of the circumference is a lower risk of postoperative intraocular pressure spikes; this is preferable for treating severely damaged optic nerves and/or when an intraocular pressure rise occurred after the treatment of the first eye or the first session of the same eye.

To perform SLT a frequency-doubled Q-switched Nd:YAG 532 nm laser with a fixed spot size of 400 microns and a fixed duration of 3 nanoseconds is used. Since no visible effect on the trabecular meshwork is expected, there are no visual clues.

Several drugs are effective in preventing or attenuating intraocular pressure spikes. Topical apraclonidine, brimonidine, pilocarpine, and oral acetazolamide can be used, depending on the individual patient. In patients with severe optic nerve damage such preventive measures are always advisable, and can be applied more liberally when the intraocular pressure cannot be checked during the first few hours after treatment.

Laser trabeculoplasty is effective in lowering the intraocular pressure long-term. Predictors of a better effect on intraocular pressure are a favorable outcome in the first eye, older age, and heavier trabecular pigmentation. The efficacy is limited in pseudophakia and after filtration surgery. It is important to clarify with patients that all antiglaucoma medications in use will probably be needed after the trabeculoplasty and that a decrease in the number of medications is not the rule. It is also relevant to explain that the effect on the intraocular pressure might fade with time and that it is more likely to last longer in those cases where the initial effect was larger and lasted at least one year.

In elderly patients with POAG who have well-defined pigment in the meshwork an average 20% to 25% decrease of intraocular pressure from baseline is expected. Individual variations are large, however, and if the target intraocular pressure is not reached within 4 to 6 weeks, further pressure lowering from the LTP is unlikely and other means of lowering the intraocular pressure must be considered. Visual field loss after trabeculoplasty can be seen when the LTP has a sizable effect on the intraocular pressure without reaching the stated target; we are then tempted not to proceed with further steps until deterioration is recorded.

PROSPECTIVE CLINICAL TRIALS

Data from controlled clinical trials comparing trabeculoplasty with medical and/or surgical treatment have attempted to clarify some clinically relevant points. The Glaucoma Laser Trial (GLT), the Advanced Glaucoma Intervention Study (AGIS) and the Collaborative Initial Glaucoma Treatment Study (CIGTS) addressed the outcome of ALT. These studies are very complex and data cannot always be easily extrapolated into the management of individual patients. A couple of points, however, are clear: early intraocular pressure spikes are not rare, and up to 12% of those treated can reach an intraocular pressure of at least 10 mm Hg (GLT); laser trabeculoplasty showed to be effective and safe in lowering IOP (GLT, CIGTS, AGIS).

The final status (i.e., intraocular pressure, visual field, disc, need for medication, need for surgery at median follow up of 7 years) of patients initially treated with ALT was similar or better than the final status of patients initially treated with medications (AGIS). Black patients may be better treated with LTP prior to trabeculectomy.

COMPLICATIONS

INCREASE OF INTRAOCULAR PRESSURE

An acute pressure spike is observed frequently but is rarely persistent. Patients with advanced disease and those in whom the postoperative intraocular pressure cannot be checked within a few hours should be given additional medications as outlined earlier. Staging the treatment in two sessions, treating 180 degrees of the angle each time, reduces the occurrence of this complication. A patient having an intraocular pressure spike in one eye is more likely to develop one in the fellow eye. Late progressive intraocular pressure rise is more common with longer follow-up, and can involve up to 80% of the cases 10 years after treatment.

TREATMENT OF AREAS AWAY FROM THE TRABECULAR MESHWORK

Angle features that can be mistaken as pigmented trabecular meshwork include: the ciliary band pigment over Schwalb's line and Sampaolesi's line.

TREATMENT OF INCORRECT ANGLE STRUCTURES

Laser trabeculoplasty should be aimed at the trabecular meshwork. In the case of chronic angle closure, a pigment line may be present on Schwalbe's line or anterior to it. This line can mimick a pigmented trabecular meshwork. Treatment aimed at such line of pigment will not be effective and may even be detrimental.

PERIPHERAL ANTERIOR SYNECHIAE

Peripheral Anterior Synechiae will develop in some patients. These are usually tent-like, tiny, and not clinically significant. Comparative studies have shown that treating the anterior rather than the posterior portion of the meshwork yields significantly fewer peripheral anterior synechiae.

VISUAL FIELD LOSS

Acute intraocular pressure elevation after treatment can cause visual field loss, which can be relevant in patients with advanced damage. The surgeon has to be especially prudent when the scotomas are close to fixation. Further visual field loss is also expected to occur if the target surgical pressure was not reached, even though the intraocular pressure was lowered to some extent. Patients should consider laser trabeculoplasty as an additional means of achieving the intraocular pressure level considered clinically safe, and to proceed with the planned therapeutic stepladder if that level is not obtained.

UVEITIS

Mild anterior uveitis is observed in all patients treated; only rarely is it severe. It is advisable, however, to prescribe for all patients a topical steroid or non-steroidal anti-inflammatory for up to one week. Again, aiming the laser to the posterior meshwork increases the degree of postoperative inflammation. Laser trabeculoplasty is not indicated in patients with a history of uveitis.

CORNEAL DAMAGE

Any laser treatment of the anterior segment has the potential to damage the corneal endothelium. In patients with normal endothelium, LTP is not associated with endothelial cell damage; its effects, if any, on sick corneas is not established. Transient epithelial burns can be observed and are more likely when higher power settings are used. No specific treatment is needed.

HYPHEMA

Hyphema is a rare postoperative complication. It can also occur at the time of treatment, probably as a consequence of a suction effect from the goniolens.

SYNCOPE

Syncope is not related to the laser effect but to the globe manipulation with a goniolens; it is more likely to occur in younger males.

EFFECT ON FILTRATION SURGERY

The classical treatment algorithm for POAG included laser trabeculoplasty as a step to be attempted before resorting to filtration surgery. A higher occurrence of cystic blebs and higher failures of trabeculectomy post-LTP has been suggested. Results are difficult to interpret, however, because stratification is not available for number and duration of topical treatment or for other conditions. Non-pretreating filtration procedures, especially deep sclerectomy, are claimed to be less effective and more difficult to perform in eyes previously treated with laser trabeculoplasty. Controlled, prospective, randomized data are not available.

RETREATMENT

Laser trabeculoplasty can be repeated. The effect on intraocular pressure to be expected is modest and not significant if the initial effect from the first treatment was poor. One drawback of retreatment is that patients may continue to have unsafe intraocular pressure levels while waiting for the final result. I discourage retreatment when the glaucoma damage is advanced and the target intraocular pressure is unlikely to be reached. As mentioned earlier, excessive treatment of the trabecular meshwork has been demonstrated to decrease outflow facility. Because membrane growing over the trabecular meshwork has been reported in failed eyes, the indication for treatment has been called into question.

SUGGESTED READINGS

1. The Glaucoma Laser Trial Research Group: The glaucoma laser trial (GLT). I. Acute effects of argon laser trabeculoplasty on intraocular pressure. Arch Ophthalmol 1989;107:1135–42.
2. The Glaucoma Laser Trial Research Group: The glaucoma laser trial (GLT) and glaucoma laser trial follow-up study: 7. Results. Am J Ophthalmol 1995;120:718–31.
3. Katz LJ: Argon laser trabeculoplasty. Current Med 1992;1:103–10.
4. Latina MA, Sibayan SA, Shin DH, et al.: Q-switched 532-nm Nd:YAG laser trabeculoplasty (selective laser trabeculoplasty). A multicenter, pilot, clinical study. Ophthalmology 1998;105:2082–90.
5. Reiss GR, Wilensky JT, Higginbotham EJ: Laser trabeculoplasty. Major review. Surv Ophthalmol 1991;35:407–28.
6. Schwartz AL, Van Veldhuisen P, Gaasterland D, et al.: The Advanced Glaucoma Intervention Study (AGIS): 5. Encapsulated bleb after initial trabeculectomy. Am J Ophthalmol 1999;127:8–19.
7. The AGIS Investigators: The Advanced Glaucoma Intervention Study, 6: Effect of cataract on visual field and visual acuity. Arch Ophthalmol 2000;118:1639–52.
8. Janz NK, Wren PA, Lichter PR, et al.: The Collaborative Initial Glaucoma Treatment Study: Interim quality of life findings after initial medical or surgical treatment of glaucoma. Ophthamol 2001; 108:1954–65.

CHAPTER 32

Laser Peripheral Iridoplasty

GEORGE L. SPAETH, M.D.

Laser iridoplasty is a method of causing iris tissue to contract, the goal being to pull the iris out of the anterior chamber angle, hoping to open the angle recess.

INDICATIONS

The primary indication for iridoplasty is angle closure associated with the plateau iris syndrome.[1,2] It may also be used in primary angle-closure glaucoma, especially where peripheral iridotomy fails to open the anterior chamber angle.[3,4] Iridoplasty has also been suggested for angle closure associated with neovascularization of the iris, but beneficial effects are controversial.

Laser iridoplasty is not indicated where peripheral anterior synechiae are well established, especially when they are of inflammatory origin. Thus, the procedure is not appropriate for patients with peripheral anterior adhesions secondary to uveitis, old trauma, or the various iridocorneal endothelial syndromes.

The duration of effect on angle configuration of iridoplasty varies; it has been reported that it has only a temporary deepening effect on the anterior chamber angle. In some patients, however, the beneficial effect appears to be long lasting, so that the anterior chamber angle stays open without the need to repeat the procedure.

PREPARATION OF PATIENT

Appropriate diagnosis is essential. Pilocarpine, 1% in blue-eyed individuals or 2% in brown-eyed individuals, is instilled twice 30 to 60 minutes prior to the iridoplasty to constrict the pupil and put the iris on stretch, bringing the peripheral iris into visible position, and deepen the anterior chamber. Additional pilocarpine helps lower the intraocular pressure and prevent a pressure spike. The eye is anesthetized with 5 instillations of a topical anesthetic, given over a period of 5 minutes. The patient is asked to keep the eye closed between instillations of the eye drops. Prevention of a pressure spike following the iridoplasty is appropriate, and can usually be achieved by instillation of one drop of apraclonidine or brimonidine prior to the procedure. Other aqueous suppressants such as a topical carbonic anhydrase inhibitor or beta-blocker may be used. The prostaglandin analogs are avoided.

TECHNIQUE

A contact lens may or may not be used. The lens has the advantage of holding the lids apart and partially fixating the eye. It has the disadvantage of introducing a slight risk of corneal abrasion, and it makes the procedure slightly more threatening to the patient. An argon laser[2] or a diode laser[5] may be used. The spot size should be between 250 and 500 microns, with the power between 200 and 500 mW. The duration of application is set at 0.2 seconds. The oculars are adjusted for the operating surgeon.

With the patient comfortably seated at the laser, and the eye appropriately prepared, the surgeon should inspect the iris carefully for areas of pigmentation at the periphery. The application should be placed as close to the iris periphery as possible; specifically, it should be between ~0.5 and 1 mm from the iris root. It is usually difficult to apply the laser beam any more peripherally than that. Additionally, the application should be placed, if possible, in pigmented areas. Even in the blue iris, clusters of pigment are usually visible. Patients should be instructed to direct their gaze so that any laser energy that might penetrate through the iris will not fall directly on the macula. Thus, unless the laser beam is coming in from the temporal side, the direction of gaze should never be in the primary position, that is, never straight ahead. This is especially important in lightly pigmented irides and in cases where a contact lens is not used to help focus the rays of light on the iris surface.

The first application is placed with the power at a relatively low level such as 200 mW. Power is applied until the iris is noted to shrink. If this occurs quickly, the application is stopped, even if it has not proceeded for 0.2 seconds. If no contraction of the iris is noted, the full duration of application is allowed. If no reaction is noted even after 0.2 seconds, the power is gradually increased until the application of power is associated with a definite shrinkage of tissue, that is, contraction of the iris. The surgeon will note that the peripheral edge of the area of application, that is the edge closest to the angle recess, should contract away from the angle recess toward the pupil. The iris on the central side of the application, that is, toward the pupil, will contract away from the pupil toward the iris periphery. Thus, there is usually some focal enlargement of the pupil in the direction of the area of the iris being treated by the laser beam. Once it has been determined, on the basis of trial and error, what power and what duration of laser energy results in a visible contraction of the iris, those settings are then used to continue the treatment. Additional spots are selected, approximately one half clock hour away from the previous application and further burns are made. All applications are to be made as far in the periphery as is possible. Applications are made, proceeding circumferentially around the periphery of the iris until 20 to 25 applications have been placed. It may be necessary to adjust the power or the duration depending upon the differential reactivity of the iris in different areas. If the contraction is extremely brisk, the power should be reduced, and if there is no reaction, the power should be increased. To ensure that there is minimal burning and maximal contraction, the spot size should not be less than 200 microns in diameter. The smaller the spot size the more the energy will penetrate into the iris and the less it will affect the surface of the iris. At the end of the procedure the peripheral iris should have been pulled noticeably away from the angle recess toward the pupil.

At the end of the procedure a drop of an intraocular pressure–lowering agent such as apraclonidine or brimonidine is instilled, and the angle is examined gonioscopically. The degree to which the procedure has succeeded in the primary goal of opening the anterior chamber angle should be able to be determined immediately.

POSTOPERATIVE CARE

Because many patients undergoing iridoplasty have either inflamed eyes or have been using pilocarpine, there are considerable risks for developing posterior synechiae. Because there may be a risk associated with dilatation, the prevention of posterior synechiae relies primarily on vigorous application of anti-inflammatory agents. A potent agent such as prednisolone 1% should be used postoperatively at least four times daily for about 1 week. If the intraocular pressure measurement 1 hour after the iridoplasty reveals no evidence of immediate pressure elevation, it will not be necessary to check the pressure for a week or more. If the iridoplasty has been performed for elevated intraocular pressure associated with angle closure, then the patient needs to be examined carefully at hourly intervals until the effect of the iridoplasty on the elevated intraocular pressure as well as on the anterior chamber angle can be determined.

At the first postoperative visit, generally 1 week after the iridoplasty, the surgeon must examine the eye with great care to determine whether any posterior adhesions between the iris and the lens are developing, to measure the intraocular pressure, to assess the amount of postoperative inflammation present, and to determine the nature of the anterior chamber angle. If adhesions between the lens and iris are forming, then the need for dilatation must be carefully assessed. Because the usual indication for iridoplasty is plateau iris, and because affected patients are at risk for developing angle closure with dilatation, dilatation needs to be performed with caution after an iridoplasty. One drop of ½% tropicamide is an appropriate agent because its reversal with pilocarpine will not cause as great an increase in relative pupillary block as will reversal of dilatation secondary to phenylephrine. Meticulous gonioscopy must be performed prior to dilatation to determine the effect of the iridoplasty on the anterior chamber angle. After dilatation the intraocular pressure is carefully monitored and the angle is again examined.

Even when it does not appear that posterior adhesions are developing, dilatation is appropriate not just to prevent such posterior adhesions, but also for determining the effect of the iridoplasty.

REFERENCES

1. Ritch R: Argon laser peripheral iridoplasty: An overview. J Glaucoma 1992;100:919–23.
2. Sassani JW, Ritch R, McCormick S, et al.: Histopathology of argon laser peripheral iridoplasty. Ophthalmic Surg 1993;24:740–5.
3. Robin AL, Pollack IP: Argon laser peripheral iridotomy in the treatment of primary angle closure glaucoma. Arch Ophthalmol 1982;100:919–23.
4. Lam DSC, Lai JSM, Tham CCY: Immediate argon laser peripheral iridoplasty (ALPI) as treatment of acute attack of primary angle closure glaucoma (PACG): A preliminary study. Ophthalmology 1998;105:2231–6.
5. Lai JSM, Tham CCY, Chua JKH, Lam DSC: Immediate diode laser peripheral iridoplasty as treatment of acute attack of primary angle closure glaucoma: A preliminary study. J Glaucoma 2001;10: 89–94.

CHAPTER 33

Neodymium:YAG Laser Iridotomy

GEORGE L. SPAETH, M.D.

Iridotomy performed with an neodymium:YAG laser offers considerable advantages over that performed with an argon laser. The Nd:YAG laser produces an iridotomy with a highly localized explosion. In contrast, the argon laser burns a hole in the iris with a beam that is not so precisely focused. As a result, tissues posterior to the iris receive considerable laser light, putting them at risk. It is common, for example, to see a small lens opacity posterior to an argon laser iridotomy. Retinal burns have also been reported. Such complications can be eliminated with a properly performed Nd:YAG laser iridotomy.

PREPARATION OF THE PATIENT

The primary concern with laser iridotomy is development of a ghost image. If the probability of this developing is explained to the patient preoperatively and the patient understands the reasons for it and its harmless nature, the development of a ghost image will not be disturbing. Surgeons should not mislead themselves or their patients into believing that it is possible to perform an iridotomy without the development of a ghost image. Even when the iridotomy is placed close to the 12 o'clock position and is covered by the upper lid, a ghost image may develop. The probable cause is refraction of light through the tear film at the edge of the upper lid, which apparently can have a prismatic effect, bending the light superiorly and allowing it to enter the iridotomy. The possible development of a crescentic inferior ghost image should be described to the patient as being a result of light coming through the "new pupil." The peripheral nature of the ghost image should be explained. The patient will then come to understand that by concentrating on an image directly in the visual axis, stimulation of the retina by light coming from the periphery will not be disturbing. In contrast, when the patient becomes conscious of objects in the periphery and awareness of the peripheral vision will bother the central vision. It is often helpful to point out to the patient that some people do one-eyed tasks, such as aiming a rifle or looking through the barrel of a microscope with only the involved eye open, but that many keep both eyes open, and "turn off" the uninvolved eye in the brain. Thus, even if the patient should notice a ghost image postoperatively, it will only be bothersome if he or she allows it to dominate. But if this capacity to adapt is explained to the patient in detail preoperatively the physician can prevent long and defensive postoperative discussions arising from the patient's distress that he or she was not warned that a ghost image might develop.

Bleeding from the iridotomy is virtually never a problem in patients who do not have some predisposition to bleeding, as from taking aspirin or another medication that alters clotting. If bleeding is anticipated, it may be advisable to pretreat the area of the iris with an argon laser to cauterize the blood vessels and decrease the likelihood of bleeding at the time of Nd:YAG iridotomy.

A rise in intraocular pressure may occur after an iridotomy with a Nd:YAG laser or an argon laser. The likelihood of a pressure rise is related to the amount of tissue dispersed by the iridotomy, the amount of inflammation caused by the procedure, and the capacity of the aqueous outflow channels of the eye to handle such trauma. Where the intraocular pressure is normal and there are no predisposing factors, the likelihood of a pressure spike being a problem is close to zero. Where the intraocular pressure is already elevated, the iris is

TABLE 33–1. Medication Designed to Prevent Postoperative Intraocular Pressure Rise

Optic Disc	Nature of the Iris	Ease of Aqueous Outflow	Suggested Medication
Normal	Blue, thin	Normal	None required
Normal	Blue	Abnormal	1 drop alpha-agonist preoperatively
Normal	Brown, thick	Normal	1 drop alpha-agonist preoperatively and postoperatively; 1 drop topical carbonic anhydrase inhibitor preoperatively
Abnormal	Brown, thick	Abnormal	1 drop alpha-agonist, 1 drop topical beta-blocker, and oral carbonic anhydrase inhibitor preoperatively and postoperatively
Abnormal	Blue, thin	Normal	1 drop alpha-agonist and topical carbonic anhydrous inhibitor preoperatively and postoperatively

difficult to penetrate, and the outflow channels are already compromised, as in patients with a severe expression of the pseudoexfoliation syndrome, significant increases in pressure after iridotomy are the rule and should be expected. The likelihood of an intraocular pressure rise after iridotomy can be lessened by keeping the iridotomy as small as possible and by using ocular hypotensive agents appropriately. Some guidelines for this are shown in Table 33–1. Where the optic nerve is already seriously damaged, efforts to prevent a postoperative pressure rise must be especially intense.

Where medication is believed appropriate it should be given approximately 30 minutes before the performance of the iridotomy, and where believed appropriate postoperatively, it should be given after the eye has been irrigated and the irritation caused by the goniolens has abated. Where an Nd:YAG laser iridotomy is being performed for primary angle-closure glaucoma, it is essential that the pupil be small, preferably around 2 mm. This control is most easily achieved by instilling pilocarpine once or twice preoperatively. It usually takes from 30 minutes to 1 hour for this medication to have its maximum effect; therefore the surgeon must be prepared to wait, and to monitor the pupil until the pupil is small enough. In a blue-eyed patient, one drop of 1% pilocarpine twice is usually adequate. In a brown-eyed patient, the concentration of the pilocarpine usually needs to be stronger, usually around 2%. Especially where 2% pilocarpine has been used, the patient should be forewarned that the pilocarpine will make things dark and may cause mild discomfort in the eye, best described as "brow ache." There are some patients in whom the use of pilocarpine is best avoided. Preoperative miosis with pilocarpine is not advisable for (1) patients with sensitivity to pilocarpine, (2) those with myopia greater than 4 diopters, (3) patients with pigment dispersion syndrome, (4) unaccompanied, one-eyed patients, (5) those with a retinal tear or detachment. Without pilocarpine, the pupil can usually be made sufficiently miotic by relying on the consensual pupillary reaction caused by shining a bright light in the fellow eye. Whatever method is employed, having the pupil miotic and the iris "on stretch" is essential to the optimal performance of an Nd:YAG iridotomy.

PREOPERATIVE ANESTHESIA

In most cases one drop of a topical anesthetic such as proparacaine is usually adequate. This anesthetizes the cornea to allow asymptomatic placement of the contact lens. However, in highly apprehensive patients or those with a low pain threshold, it is advisable to instill one drop of a topical anesthetic every 5 minutes for a total of 6 instillations. This result in a more profound degree of anesthesia and a more comfortable patient.

TECHNIQUE

Before proceeding with the iridotomy, the surgeon should check the laser to make sure it is working satisfactorily. The patient is prepared fully, including obtaining a fully informed consent. The patient is seated comfortably at the laser and the laser settings are adjusted. The oculars on the laser are checked to make absolutely sure that they are set for the refractive error of the surgeon. This is essential! If the laser has not been used recently, a test firing on a piece of paper will assure that the focus is correct and that the explosion will occur where it should. Suggested settings are shown in Table 33–2. However, the power of lasers varies considerably, and settings must be adjusted for the particular laser being used.

The patient is asked to lean forward to ensure the proper height for application of the laser beam. The surgeon's chair is adjusted appropriately. An armrest is helpful with most instruments to allow the contact lens to be held comfortably with the surgeon's arm firmly supported.

The magnification of the biomicroscope is set at a high level. The illuminating slit beam is sufficiently narrow to illuminate a band approximately 3 mm wide on the iris. It is usually best placed so that it is not offset either to the right or the left.

With the patient fully prepared and in the proper position, the contact lens is placed on the anesthetized eye. I prefer the CGI 1.4 lens manufactured specifically for laser iridotomy by the Lasag Company (Bern, Switzerland). Whatever lens is chosen it must have a magnifying power great enough to allow accurate concentration of the beam.

TABLE 33-2. Settings for Performing Nd:YAG Peripheral Iridotomy

1. Oculars adjusted to surgeon's refractive error
2. Mode: multimode
3. Duration: Q switch
4. Power: 18 mJ*
5. Offset: 0†

*With lasers capable of multiple firings of the laser in response to one application of power, this total energy is usually achieved by using a run of three bursts with a power of 6 mJ.
†For the technique described, it is best to have the point of laser power application exactly parfocal with the observer's gaze. Thus, no offset is employed.

Looking through the microscope, the surgeon focuses on the anterior surface of the iris. The iris is carefully inspected for a crypt or an area that appears thin. The iridotomy is best placed between the 11 o'clock and 1 o'clock positions to keep it under the eyelid. It is sometimes useful to avoid the 12 o'clock position to decrease the likelihood that bubble formation will obscure the surgeon's view. This is not a major problem, and if it appears that the 12 o'clock position is optimal, then the iridotomy should be performed there. The surgeon then identifies a site as far in the periphery of the iris as possible. Where an arcus is present it may be necessary to move slightly less peripherally. However, ideally the iridotomy should be so far in the periphery that it is almost out of sight. It is rare that it is necessary to have the iridotomy placed more than 1 mm from the iris root. In cases of iridotomy for pupillary block, as might be the case in a secondary glaucoma following implantation of an anterior chamber lens, the siting of the iridotomy is totally different. Here one looks for the area of greatest iris bowing. In such cases, and only in such cases, is it advisable to place the iridotomy anywhere except in the far superior periphery. In pupillary block, however, the iridotomy is often best performed about 4 mm from the periphery. It is virtually always preferable to perform multiple iridotomies in different areas, say at 12, 3, 6, and 9 o'clock, to have the best chance of relieving the pupillary block completely. Finally, with secondary angle closures related to occlusion of the pupil, the iridotomy should be ~0.5 mm in size to lessen the likelihood that it will close postoperatively. This is not a problem in an eye with primary angle-closure related to pupillary block.

Once an appropriate site for the iridotomy has been selected the surgeon focuses meticulously on the anterior surface of the iris until he or she is absolutely certain that the focus is perfect. At that point the joystick is advanced ever so slightly so that the focus moves into the anterior stroma of the iris. At that point the laser is activated. If all the settings are correct and the focus is correct, one application of power is usually enough to penetrate a thin iris, such as occurs in blue-eyed or hazel-eyed patients, especially when elderly. In patients of black African or Asiatic descent, the dark brown iris tends to be much thicker and the first application may make only a crater in the anterior stroma. The surgeon rapidly completes the iridotomy by repeated applications of power, focusing each application slightly more deeply into the stroma until the posterior pigment epithelium becomes apparent, at which point one burst virtually always causes penetration of the iris.

It is clear that the iris has been penetrated when there is a sudden gush of aqueous from the posterior to the anterior chamber, accompanied by multiple pigmented particles. It is usually unnecessary to enlarge the iris once penetration has occurred. This is especially true if the peripheral iris bowing present prior to penetration rapidly disappears and the plane of the iris becomes flat. If there is any question, however, one or two additional applications of power can be applied to the remaining posterior pigment epithelium.

If bleeding occurs, pushing the contact lens firmly against the eye will raise the intraocular pressure and stop the bleeding. Maintaining this pressure for approximately 30 seconds will generally prevent any further bleeding. If the blood has obscured the surgeon's view, the patient is informed that the iridotomy will be completed in about an hour. By that time the view should again be satisfactory and the iridotomy can be completed as if no further bleeding has occurred. In the extremely rare situation in which bleeding continues, it may be helpful to apply heat with an argon laser. Renewed efforts should also be made to question the patient about medications that may be predisposing to a clotting abnormality, or any family history of a clotting abnormality. If the patient is not taking aspirin or similar medication, it is appropriate to refer the patient for a workup for a blood dyscrasia.

I often invite the individual accompanying the patient to look through an observer tube in order to witness the performance of the iridotomy. This is instuctional and helps to "demistify" the procedure.

After the surgeon is sure that the iridotomy is complete, the patient to is so informed and the eye is irrigated. If it was planned beforehand, additional medication is promptly instilled after the eye has been irrigated. If the procedure is more difficult than anticipated additional hypotensive medication is usually appropriate. Many surgeons instill a drop of a topical corticosteroid at the conclusion of the surgery.

Once the eye is irrigated and any medications have been instilled, the patient is asked to keep the eye closed for the next half hour. If the patient does not do so, there is much greater likelihood that superficial punctate keratitis or a corneal epithelial defect will develop, both of which can be markedly symptomatic.

Approximately 45 to 60 minutes postoperatively, the intraocular pressure must be checked. If it has not risen more than 5 mm Hg above the preoperative level, it is extremely unlikely that there will be difficulty controlling intraocular pressure postoperatively. If the pressure rise is greater than 10 mm Hg, additional therapy will generally be necessary, especially if the optic nerve shows glaucoma damage.

POSTOPERATIVE CARE

At discharge, the patient is told that there is no limitation whatsoever on activity. If pilocarpine has been instilled, however, the surgeon should remind the patient that vision will be dark and mildly blurred for approximately 12 hours. Even if pilocarpine has not been used, the patient should be advised that vision will be mildly blurred for a day or two, but that within the limits of visual ability, he or she may resume previous activities. A topical corticosteroid is used in the eye 4 times a day for 1 week, and no longer. The prescription must be marked "not refillable," and the patient should understand that the medication must not be used for more than 1 week.

The patient is asked to return for a follow-up examination 1 to 4 weeks later. A routine examination is then performed, including measurement of visual acuity and intraocular pressure, as well as a slit-lamp examination. With the slit lamp, it should be possible to see the open iridotomy far in the periphery of the iris. Because the pupil will be larger and the iridotomy will be more peripheral than at the time of surgery, it may be difficult to see. Gonioscopy of the affected eye should reveal a significant deepening of the angle in comparison with both the preoperative appearance, and the other, unoperated, eye.

At the first postoperative visit it is often appropriate to proceed with iridotomy of the other eye. To begin, dilate the operated eye with one drop of 2.5% phenylephrine or tropicamide ½%, after informing the patient of the purpose of the dilatation and the minimal but potential risk of increasing the intraocular pressure. At the time the drop is placed in the operated eye, pilocarpine can be placed in the unoperated eye to prepare it for the peripheral iridotomy. After approximately 1 hour, the intraocular pressure and the anterior chamber angle of the operated eye should be checked to make sure that the angle is still open and that there has been no significant pressure rise in response to dilatation. This confirms that the peripheral iridotomy has done its job and both the physician and the patient feel comfortable with proceeding with Nd:YAG laser peripheral iridotomy of the other eye.

If at the first postoperative visit the angle has not deepened, then the surgeon must determine whether this is due to an incomplete iridotomy or another cause, such as the plateau iris syndrome. If it is certain that the iridotomy is open, it may be helpful to obtain an ultrasound biomicroscopy to see if the characteristic cyst and position of the ciliary body of the plateau iris syndrome may account for the anterior position of the peripheral iris. The patient should be informed that the iridotomy may not have done its job, and that it is necessary to perform further tests with a weak mydriatic to rule out the plateau iris syndrome. After the patient understands, then one drop of 2.5% phenylephrine is instilled in the operated eye and the intraocular pressure is checked 30 minutes, 1 hour, and even 2 hours later. Gonioscopy is repeated. If no pressure rise occurs, then it is probable that the iridotomy has in fact done its job and a plateau iris syndrome is unlikely. In such a situation it is appropriate to proceed with a peripheral iridotomy on the other eye.

In contrast, if the pressure rises in response to dilatation and it is certain that the iridotomy is open, then the diagnosis is the plateau iris syndrome and a treatment decision must be made. In most cases the appropriate next step is laser iridoplasty (see Chapter 32). Some surgeons prefer to use pilocarpine long term, but rarely should this be the first line of therapy. In fact, long-term pilocarpine is usually employed only in those rare situations where an argon laser iridoplasty does not deepen the angle and prevent a pressure rise in response to dilatation.

If the iridotomy is not open, then the patient is informed and the procedure is repeated with appropriate modifications. For example, if pilocarpine was not used at the original operation, the advantage of using it, at this point for more complete constriction of the pupil is explained to the patient. The procedure is then performed in essentially the same manner as before, and the surgeon again watches for the gush of aqueous carrying pigment debris from the posterior chamber into the anterior chamber.

SUMMARY

Neodymium:YAG laser peripheral iridotomy is a beautiful procedure, remarkably safe and effective. It requires good instrumentation and meticulous attention to focusing. Despite its safety, however, it has potential for producing significant side effects and a fully informed patient consent is necessary. The complications listed in Table 33–3 can be avoided or made extremely unlikely by appropriate attention to detail: obtaining a fully informed consent, making sure that the contact lens is inserted properly and the eye kept closed for a full 30 minutes after the iridotomy, obtaining a proper history about the potential for bleeding, and for any problem that may be caused by instillation of pilocarpine.

TABLE 33–3. Problems Associated with Nd:YAG Laser Iridotomy

Problem	Frequency
Postoperative pressure spike	Rare*
Postoperative ghost image	Not uncommon
Corneal abrasion or superficial punctate keratitis	Not rare if proper precautions not taken
Inconsequential bleeding of the anterior chamber	Around 5%
Clinically significant bleeding from the anterior chamber	Extremely rare
Failure to deepen anterior chamber angle owing to presence of plateau iris syndrome	Less than 1%
Posterior vitreous detachment	Extremely rare

*When appropriate medication is given, as indicated in Table 33–1.

CHAPTER 34

Argon Laser Peripheral Iridotomy

RONALD L. GROSS, M.D.

In certain instances the argon laser may be the preferred instrument for performing a peripheral iridotomy, because its thermal effect cauterizes vessels (Table 34–1). In most instances, however, the neodymium:YAG laser is the preferred instrument.[1–3]

The argon laser can be used to decrease the risk of bleeding, as in patients on anticoagulant therapy such as warfarin (Coumadin) or perhaps even aspirin, by pretreating an area of the iris prior to performing an Nd:YAG iridotomy. This may also allow obtaining a larger final iridotomy. Some surgeons have recommended an area of patent iridotomy of at least 150 microns.[4,5] In patients in whom an Nd:YAG peripheral iridotomy has not resulted in a large enough opening, the argon laser can remove adjacent tissue and increase the area of the iridotomy. The argon laser, however, is generally less desirable for performing peripheral iridotomy than the Nd:YAG laser (Table 34–2).

Where available, the surgeon may wish to use the green wavelength of the argon laser, because the blue–green wavelength is more completely absorbed by the lutien pigment of the macula, which may predispose to a detrimental effect.

PREOPERATIVE PREPARATION

Pretreatment with an anti-glaucoma agent may be appropriate, especially in patients in whom a postoperative pressure rise would be of potential concern, such as those who have a damaged optic nerve. The alpha-agonists, apraclonidine ½% or 1%, and brimonidine 0.2% appear to be effective agents in most patients in preventing postoperative pressure rises without causing undue systemic side effects.[6–10] The pupil should be constricted with a miotic agent to put the iris on tension and to thin the iris stroma as much as possible prior to the procedure. Topical anesthetic is usually adequate.

TECHNIQUE

The surgeon checks to make sure that the oculars of the biomicroscope are appropriate for his or her specific refractive error. An Abraham lens or similar laser lens should be used. This stabilizes the eye, provides a heat sink to prevent damage to the corneal epithelium, and permits additional focusing of the argon laser beam by the +66 diopter button, quadrupling the power density of the laser on the iris at the point of focus. The iridotomy is performed superiorly, away from the 12 o'clock position in order to avoid aqueous vapor bubbles. A position as far peripheral as possible is chosen, preferably within an iris crypt. The anterior chamber overlying the iris should be formed to avoid damaging the corneal endothelium.[11–14]

There are two general techniques for the performance of an iridotomy (Table 34–3). The first involves selecting a site and treating that single location repeatedly until a full-thickness defect of the desired size is obtained. A 50-micron spot size, 0.1 second duration, and approximately 1.0 W of power are reasonable initial settings, with focus in the deepest portion of the crypt and progressive application of the laser spots. Laser applications are continued with as precise a focus as possible along the sides and bottom of the defect until a puff of iris pigment epithelium is seen with flow of aqueous and iris pigment epithelial debris from the posterior chamber through the iridotomy into the anterior chamber. The iridotomy can then be enlarged as necessary by treating the edges of the opening.

TABLE 34–1. Indications for Argon Laser Peripheral Iridotomy

1. Perceived need for iridotomy
2. Tendency to bleeding by patient
   a. Neovascularization of iris
   b. Hyperemia of iris
   c. Anticoagulated patient
3. Perceived need for large peripheral iridotomy

TABLE 34–2. Problems with Argon Laser Peripheral Iridotomy

1. Success strongly related to iris color and structure
2. Produces inflammation
3. Predisposes to posterior synechiae
4. Predisposes to pupil distortion
5. May damage lens or retina
6. Likely to cause elevation of intraocular pressure

TABLE 34–3. Suggested Later Settings for Argon Laser Peripheral Iridotomy

Blue iris	
Size:	50 microns
Power:	1.5–2.0 W
Duration:	0.2–0.5 sec
Brown iris	
Size:	50 microns
Power:	1.0–1.5 W
Duration:	0.01–0.05 sec
"Drumhead" technique	
Size:	100–200 microns
Power:	0.1–0.5 W
Duration:	0.2–0.5 sec

The second technique involves tensing the iris by performing surrounding "drumhead" applications to put the iris on additional stretch, potentially allowing easier penetration of the iris stroma. Methods to accomplish this include surrounding the chosen site circumferentially or placing single burns on each side of the site approximately 150 to 250 microns away. These spot sizes tend to be larger, in the 100 to 200 micron spot size, of longer duration, and of lower power, such that they do not actually disrupt tissue, but rather cause contraction of the tissue, putting the site to be treated on stretch. The opening is then obtained using the single site method previously described.

The presence of a transillumination defect is not adequate evidence of a patent iridotomy (Fig. 34–1); there must be direct visualization of the anterior lens capsule (Fig. 34–2). To obtain the best possible focus, it is important to have the direction of the laser beam perpendicular to the tissue being treated. Because the iris is convex, if the eye is in the frontal plane, the application of the laser energy is more tangential. For that reason, it is often helpful to have the patient infraduct the eye to bring the area of treatment more into a plane perpendicular to the laser energy. In addition, because an area slightly medial or lateral to the 12 o'clock position is being treated, it is helpful to have the patient look in the opposite downward direction to bring the iris into a perpendicular plane. For example, in the right eye, if the superotemporal peripheral iris is to be treated at the 11 o'clock position, it is helpful to have the patient look down toward his/her left shoulder to bring that area of iris into the correct position.

Because of the intrinsic properties of the argon laser, the ability for it to penetrate the iris is variable. For that reason, if the initial settings are not adequate to allow penetration because of iris color, these should be modified. Specifically, in a dark brown iris, in which there is marked absorption of thermal energy, the duration of energy delivery should be decreased to 0.01 to 0.05 seconds.[15] This allows the thermal energy to reside for a shorter period of time on the iris surface and thus decrease thermal absorption. As a result of this, in most cases, it is also necessary to increase the power to allow adequate cutting. The increase should be large enough to obtain adequate effect.

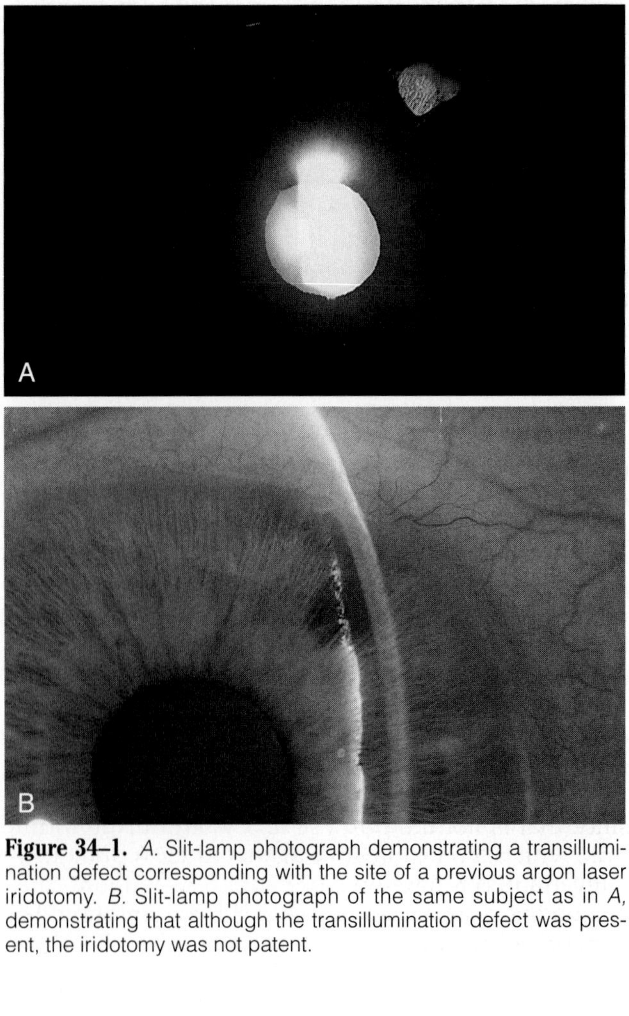

Figure 34–1. *A.* Slit-lamp photograph demonstrating a transillumination defect corresponding with the site of a previous argon laser iridotomy. *B.* Slit-lamp photograph of the same subject as in *A*, demonstrating that although the transillumination defect was present, the iridotomy was not patent.

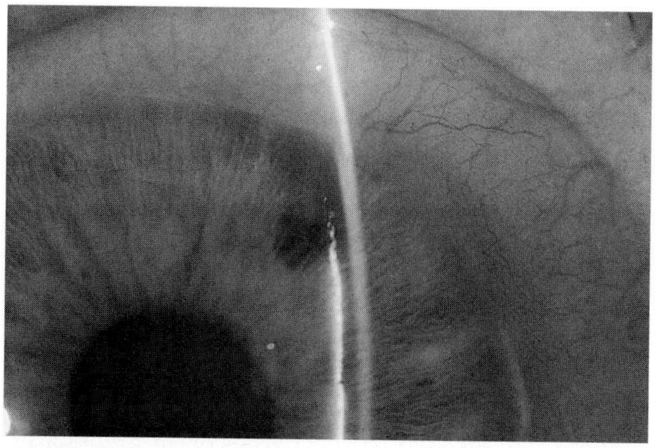

Figure 34–2. Slit-lamp photograph of the same subject as in Figure 34–1 following reopening of the iridotomy, with patency confirmed by direct visualization of the anterior lens capsule.

Conversely, in the light blue iris, because of less absorption of thermal energy, the duration of laser burn should be increased to 0.2 seconds and the power increased to 1.5 to 2.0 W to allow adequate tissue removal.

The application of the laser should be continued until the iridotomy is complete. It is important not to apply the laser bursts too rapidly as this may result in heating of the overlying aqueous and damage to the adjacent corneal endothelium. This will become manifest as an opacification of the endothelium, which makes further performance of the iridotomy more difficult and which causes endothelial damage.[13] The deeper the anterior chamber overlying the site, the more rapid the applications can be. The end point of laser application is a patent iridotomy as signaled by a gush of aqueous humor into the anterior chamber and visualization of the anterior lens capsule. However, when, despite the changes in power and duration there does not appear to be any additional iris ablation, such as with charring of the tissue in a dark brown iris, the procedure should be terminated and an alternative site, session, or method of iridotomy considered. In some instances, excessive debris from the iridotomy can also obscure the site of the iridotomy, in which case applications should be discontinued until proper visualization is possible, either in the same session or a different one. If a bubble forms, it may be possible to burst it by focusing on its surface.

If the argon laser is used prior to Nd:YAG peripheral iridotomy, either to increase the final size of the iridotomy or to prevent bleeding, the settings are those with the drumhead technique. However, the applications are made directly onto the area of the anticipated Nd:YAG laser iridotomy and should be applied in an overlapping configuration to a diameter of approximately 100 to 200 microns. Again, settings should be adjusted so that there is no disruption of the iris tissue, since that is not the purpose and would disperse debris, which would have no benefit but could potentially exacerbate a postoperative pressure rise. The area of anticipated treatment should be confluently treated with this technique.

POSTOPERATIVE CARE

Following completion of the iridotomy it is helpful to irrigate the gonioscopic solution from the eye. Any necessary topical medications are then instilled. In general, a single drop of alpha-agonist is enough to prevent pressure rise.[16] The intraocular pressure is checked approximately 1 hour after the procedure to identify a possible rise of intraocular pressure.

The complications of argon laser iridotomy are essentially the same as with any laser iridotomy procedure, although there is a greater incidence of pupillary distortion than with surgical or Nd:YAG iridotomy. This distortion results from the thermal contraction of iris tissue which may occur. At the first postoperative visit, once the patentcy of the iridotomy has been confirmed, it is vitally important to dilate the pupil. Dilatation allows an improved ability to assess the posterior segment, because presumably this has not been performed prior to the laser procedure due to the potential for acute angle closure; dilatation also helps minimize the formation of posterior synechiae, to which the eye is predisposed because of the debris and inflammation associated with the laser surgery. In general, topical corticosteroids are used for several days following the procedure to minimize postoperative inflammation. Additionally, the patient's anti-glaucoma regimen (if any) should be continued until the full effect of the iridotomy has been assessed. Assessment should include repeat gonioscopy to allow the determination of the effect of the iridotomy on the filtration angle. Over the first several months, close follow-up is needed to monitor the opening. Should closure occur, it can usually easily be reversed by additional laser application to the iris pigment epithelium. Should closure recur, an additional or alternative method of iridotomy is usually effective and should be performed.

Although there has been concern about long-term complications of laser iridotomy, primarily intraocular pressure elevation, cataract formation, and retinal damage, these have been largely ameliorated with greater experience and proper technique.[2,5,15,17,18]

REFERENCES

1. Del Priore LV, Robin AL, Pollack IP: Neodymium:YAG and argon laser iridotomy. Long term follow-up in prospective, randomized clinical trial. Ophthalmology 1988;95:1207.
2. Moster MR, Schwartz LW, Spaeth GL, et al.: Laser iridectomy: A controlled study comparing argon and neodymium:YAG. Ophthalmology 1986;93:20–4.
3. Robin AL, Pollack IP: A comparison of Nd:YAG and argon laser iridotomies. Ophthalmology 1984;91:1011.
4. Fleck BW: How large must an iridotomy be? Br J Ophthalmol 1990;74:583.
5. Morsman CD: Acute glaucoma in the presence of patent neodymium:YAG laser iridotomies. Acta Ophthalmol 1991;69:68.
6. Barnebey HS, Robin AL, Zimmerman TJ, et al.: The efficacy of brimonidine in decreasing elevations in intraocular pressure after laser trabeculoplasty. Ophthalmology 1993;100:1083.
7. Davis R, Spaeth GL, Clevenger CE, et al.: Brimonidine in the prevention of intraocular pressure following argon laser trabeculoplasty. Arch Ophthalmol 1993;111:1387.
8. Krupin T, Stak T, Feitl MR: Apraclonidine pretreatment decreases the acute intraocular pressure rise after laser trabeculoplasty or iridotomy. J Glaucoma 1992;1:79.

9. Robin AL: The role of apraclonidine hydrochloride in laser therapy for glaucoma. Trans Am Ophthalmol Soc 1989;87:729.
10. Vocci MJ, Robin AL, Wahl JC, et al.: Reformulation and drop size of apraclonidine hydrochloride. Am J Ophthalmol 1992;113:154.
11. Jeng S, Lee JS, Huang SC: Corneal decompensation after argon laser iridectomy—a delayed complication. Ophthalmic Surg 1991;22:565.
12. Schwartz AL, Martin NF, Weber PA: Corneal decompensation after argon laser iridectomy. Arch Ophthalmol 1988;106:1572.
13. Wilhelmus KR: Corneal edema following argon laser iridotomy. Ophthalmic Surg 1992;23:533.
14. Zabel RW, MacDonal IM, Mintsioulis G: Corneal endothelial decompensation after argon laser iridotomy. Can J Ophthalmol 1991;26:367.
15. Ritch R, Palmberg P: Argon laser iridectomy in densely pigmented irides. Am J Ophthalmol 1982;94:800.
16. Birt CM, Shin DH, Reed SY, et al.: One vs. two doses of 1.0% apraclonidine for prophylaxis of intraocular pressure spike after argon laser trabeculoplasty. Can J Ophthalmol 1995;30:266.
17. Maltzman BA, Agin M: Argon peripheral iridotomy and cataract formation. Ann Ophthalmol 1988;20:28.
18. Robin AL, Pollack IP: Argon laser peripheral iridotomies in the treatment of primary angle closure glaucoma: Long term follow up. Arch Ophthalmol 1982;100:919.

CHAPTER 35

Incisional Iridectomy

GEORGE L. SPAETH, M.D.

The purposes for which an iridectomy are performed are listed in Table 35–1. The primary indication for iridectomy is elimination of pupillary block. When this is the case one needs only to make a hole in the iris so that there will be constant communication between the posterior and anterior chambers. Other indications for iridectomy are related to the purpose for which the primary surgery is being performed. Neodymium:YAG laser iridotomy is now the usual procedure of choice when an "iridectomy" is indicated. However, there are still instances when laser iridotomy is inadvisable (as in eyes with flat anterior chambers) or impossible (as in eyes with cloudy corneas). Consequently surgical iridectomy is still an important procedure that ophthalmologists should be able to perform.

One should try to avoid an iridectomy when repairing a traumatized eye. If the iris is still viable, iridectomy should not be performed, because any procedure that traumatizes the uvea may predispose to sympathetic ophthalmia.

ANESTHESIA

Most iridectomies can be performed with local anesthesia, with a facial nerve block and topical anesthesia being used. Retrobulbar anesthesia is usually not needed and should be avoided, especially if the intraocular pressure is high and the surgery is required on an emergency basis, as would be the case in uncontrolled primary angle-closure glaucoma. Under such circumstances the development of a retrobulbar hemorrhage would cause the further problem of controlling intraocular pressure, and would almost certainly make it necessary to cancel surgery, resulting in a delay that could cause permanent loss of vision. In addition, a retrobulbar block may cause other complications of concern. Proparacaine 0.5% should be given topically for 10 minutes before the surgery. One drop every 30 seconds or so results in highly satisfactory anesthesia in virtually every case.

PREOPERATIVE CARE

The eye should be as quiet as possible, ideally without any internal or external inflammatory reaction. However, it is not always possible to achieve a totally quiet eye. Furthermore, the need to lower intraocular pressure may be so urgent that one cannot wait for the eye to quiet. But the principle remains valid; surgical results are better in uninflamed eyes. (This argues for the performance of iridectomy early in the course of primary angle-closure glaucoma, ideally before an attack of acute congestive angle closure has occurred. It is also a reason for performing an iridectomy on the fellow eye at the time the eye that has had the attack of glaucoma is being brought into condition for surgery.)

The timing of the surgery, then, largely depends on the degree of inflammation and the degree of difficulty involved in controlling the intraocular pressure. The greater these two factors are, the longer the preparation for surgery.

Topical corticosteroids such as prednisolone acetate 1% should be used as needed. These can be used as frequently as every hour. The steroids are used only dur-

*Indications for surgery, including timing of surgery and choice of procedure, have been discussed in detail earlier in this chapter, in the section dealing with primary angle-closure glaucoma.

TABLE 35–1. Reasons to Consider Performing Surgical Iridectomy

I. Removal of tissue
   A. Biopsy for diagnostic purposes
   B. Excision
      1. Tumor
      2. Necrotic or nonviable tissue
      3. Optical improvement
II. Elimination or prevention of block of aqueous by the iris
   A. Occludable angle
   B. Primary angle-closure glaucoma
   C. Secondary angle-closure glaucoma caused by pupillary block
      1. Dislocated lens
      2. Posterior synechiae tolens or vitreous
   D. In association with other surgery
      1. Cataract extraction
      2. Keratoplasty
      3. Glaucoma filtering procedures
III. Contraindications to laser iridotomy
   A. Cloudy cornea
   B. Flat anterior chamber
IV. In association with chamber-deepening procedures and synechialysis

ing preparation for surgery and in the immediate post-operative period; the surgeon need not be concerned about the development of a steroid-induced glaucoma in these circumstances. However, should treatment lasting more than 2 weeks be required, the chance of this occurring should be kept in mind.

When the pupil is miotic it is easy to perform an iridectomy limited to the periphery. Consequently, if the surgeon is attempting to create a cosmetically satisfactory iridectomy, the pupil should be small. In the quiet eye with a normal intraocular pressure, pilocarpine 1% instilled four times during the day before surgery and 2 hours before surgery is entirely adequate. More intensive treatment with pilocarpine is seldom necessary and may be counter-productive. If the pupil will not constrict to a satisfactory dimension with this treatment, it is unlikely that more vigorous therapy will accomplish anything more than increasing the degree of inflammation in the eye and inducing symptoms of parasympathomimetic overdosage in the patient.

Appropriate medication in the eye not receiving surgery should be ordered. If it is a "fellow eye" of a patient who has had an angle-closure attack in the first eye, probably pilocarpine 0.5% twice daily is adequate for a blue-eyed patient and 1% twice daily for a patient with a brown iris. Control of intraocular pressure before surgery has been discussed in detail (pp. 315-316) (see Chapter 33). The basic principles are to keep the pupil miotic with moderate amounts of pilocarpine and to control intraocular pressure with aqueous suppressants (beta-blockers and carbonic anhydrase inhibitors) or osmotic agents.

Intraocular pressure should ideally be between 15 and 30 mm Hg at the time surgery is started. Pressure above 30 mm Hg may predispose to malignant glaucoma or expulsive hemorrhage. Pressure below 15 mm Hg makes spontaneous prolapse of the iris more difficult and complicates the surgery.

If all medical measures to lower intraocular pressure have failed (Table 22–12), a paracentesis immediately before the surgery may be required.

Patients should be told that after surgery their vision will be different. This is not the same as saying that their visual acuity will be worse. In the overwhelming majority of cases, especially when performing surgery on a quiet eye with a clear lens, a properly performed iridectomy will not result in a decrease in visual acuity. In fact, under such circumstances it may not even predispose to more rapid progression of cataract. However, the presence of the iridectomy itself may introduce symptoms, especially if it is not completely covered by the upper lid. When a cataract is already present, the patient should understand that surgery will probably hasten its development.

The patient should also understand the purpose of the surgery. In the secondary angle-closure glaucomas, such as aphakic pupillary block glaucoma, one purpose of an iridectomy is to lower intraocular pressure by eliminating the pupillary block. However, in the primary angle-closure glaucomas the purpose is quite different; it is to prevent or eliminate the cause for progressive closure of the anterior chamber angle. Thus patients should not be told that iridectomy will "control the glaucoma," as they will interpret this as meaning that the surgery will control intraocular pressure. Rather, the surgeon should explain that although the surgery is highly successful in preventing the progression of angle closure, medications for controlling intraocular pressure may still be needed in the postoperative period. Furthermore, although the iridectomy may cure the angle closure, it will not prevent the patient from developing elevated intraocular pressure owing to another mechanism, such as primary open-angle glaucoma.

TECHNIQUE

Adherence to several principles will help to assure that an iridectomy is performed effectively and safely. An iridectomy consists of five steps: (1) incision into the eye, (2) exteriorization of a portion of the iris, (3) excision of a portion of the iris, (4) return of the remainder of the iris to its normal position within the eye, and (5) closure of the incision.

A superior rectus muscle bridle suture is placed as shown in Figures 35–1 and 35–2.

INCISION

The nature of the incision will largely determine how the iris prolapses and how the incision heals. If the surgeon believes that surgery requiring development of a conjunctival flap may later be required, it may be advisable to make the incision through the clear cornea,

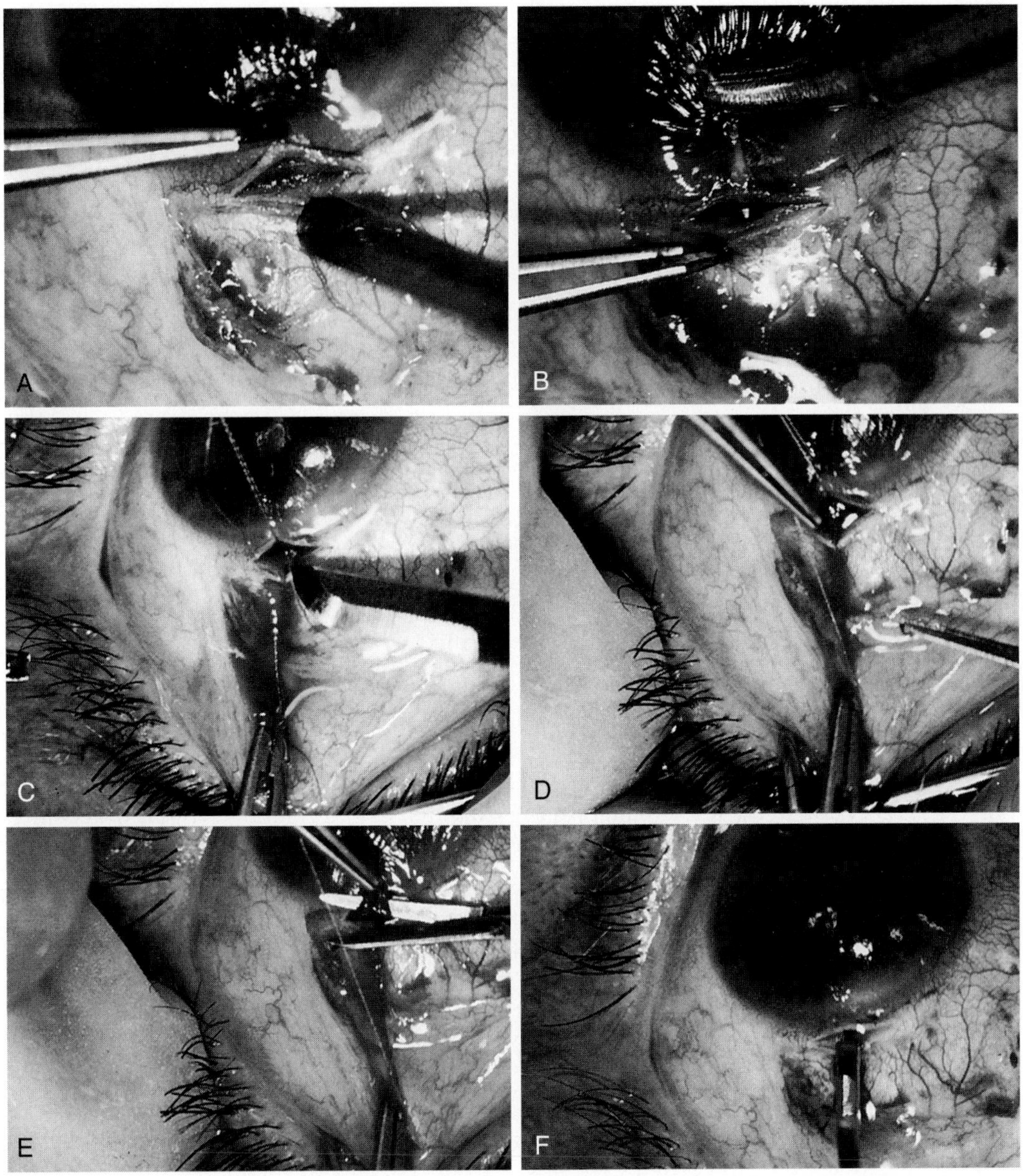

Figure 35–1. Peripheral iridectomy with a fornix-based flap and limbal incisions. *A.* Incision is made through two-thirds the thickness of the sclera directly at the corneoscleral sulcus. *B.* An 9–0 white virgin silk suture is placed in such a way that it will be able to be retracted from the depths of the incision (see Fig. 35–6). *C.* The suture is looped and used to retract the edges of the incision superiorly and inferiorly. The incision is completed, permitting prolapse of a small knuckle of iris. *D.* The iris is grasped with a fine-toothed forceps. *E.* Iris is pulled over the blade of the DeWecker scissors; after the position of the iris is noted the blades are closed and the tissue is excised. *F.* The tip of an irrigator is placed just inside the incision, with care taken to ensure that it does not enter the anterior chamber. Remnants of the pigment epithelium are flushed away, and the iris is permitted to return to its proper position so that the pupil is completely round.

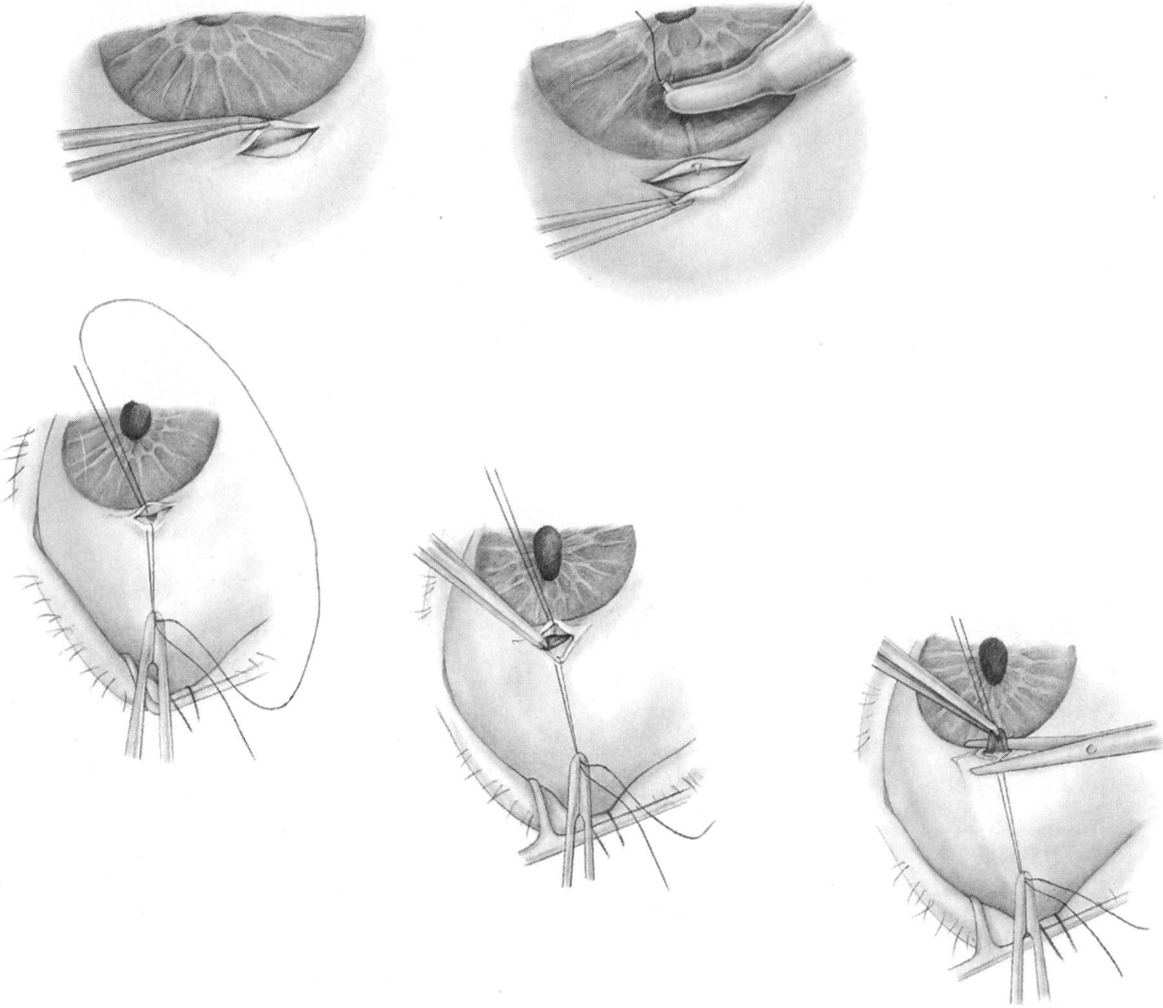

Figure 35–2. Technique described in Figure 35–1 is shown schematically.

anterior to the insertion of the conjunctiva (Fig. 35–3). Other indications for clear corneal incision are extensive peripheral anterior synechiae and the wish to minimize bleeding by avoiding incision through the sclera or conjunctiva.

In most cases, however, it is preferable to place the incision more posteriorly and to use a conjunctival flap (Fig. 35–4). Such an incision traumatizes the corneal endothelium more peripherally, usually allows easier prolapse of the iris, and can be closed with a suture that is then covered with conjunctiva. Although leakage through the incision after an iridectomy is rare, it does occur in about 1 percent of cases; if such a leak occurs underneath a conjunctival flap, the seriousness of the complication is less than it would be if such a flap were not present.[1]

The incision for a peripheral iridectomy being performed for primary angle-closure glaucoma should usually be at 12 o'clock, so that the iridectomy will be hidden under the upper lid. This will assure the best cosmetic and functional result. Other factors may make positioning the iridectomy elsewhere preferable. For example, an optical iridectomy should create an opening as close to the visual axis as possible.

The incision should be large enough to allow the iris to prolapse easily. This usually requires an incision that is about 2 mm wide at its base. It is better to have the incision slightly larger than required rather than smaller, as both prolapse and reposition of the iris are more easily accomplished with a large incision. It is simple to close an incision with fine suture, and the trauma to the eye will be less when the incision is slightly too large than when it is too small.

Before placement of a preplaced suture, and before entry into the anterior chamber, a paracentesis should be performed.

Preplacement of a suture after the incision has been made approximately one-half to two-thirds of the way through the tissue facilitates both the completion of the incision in a safe manner and the prolapse of the iris. This technique is illustrated in Figures 35–5 and 35–6. The suture used should be strong enough to be used for traction; 8–0 white virgin silk and 9–0 nylon are both suitable.

A perpendicular incision will facilitate prolapse of the iris. However, such incisions are more likely to open in response to pressure on the globe or to increased intraocular pressure. Thus they should be

A

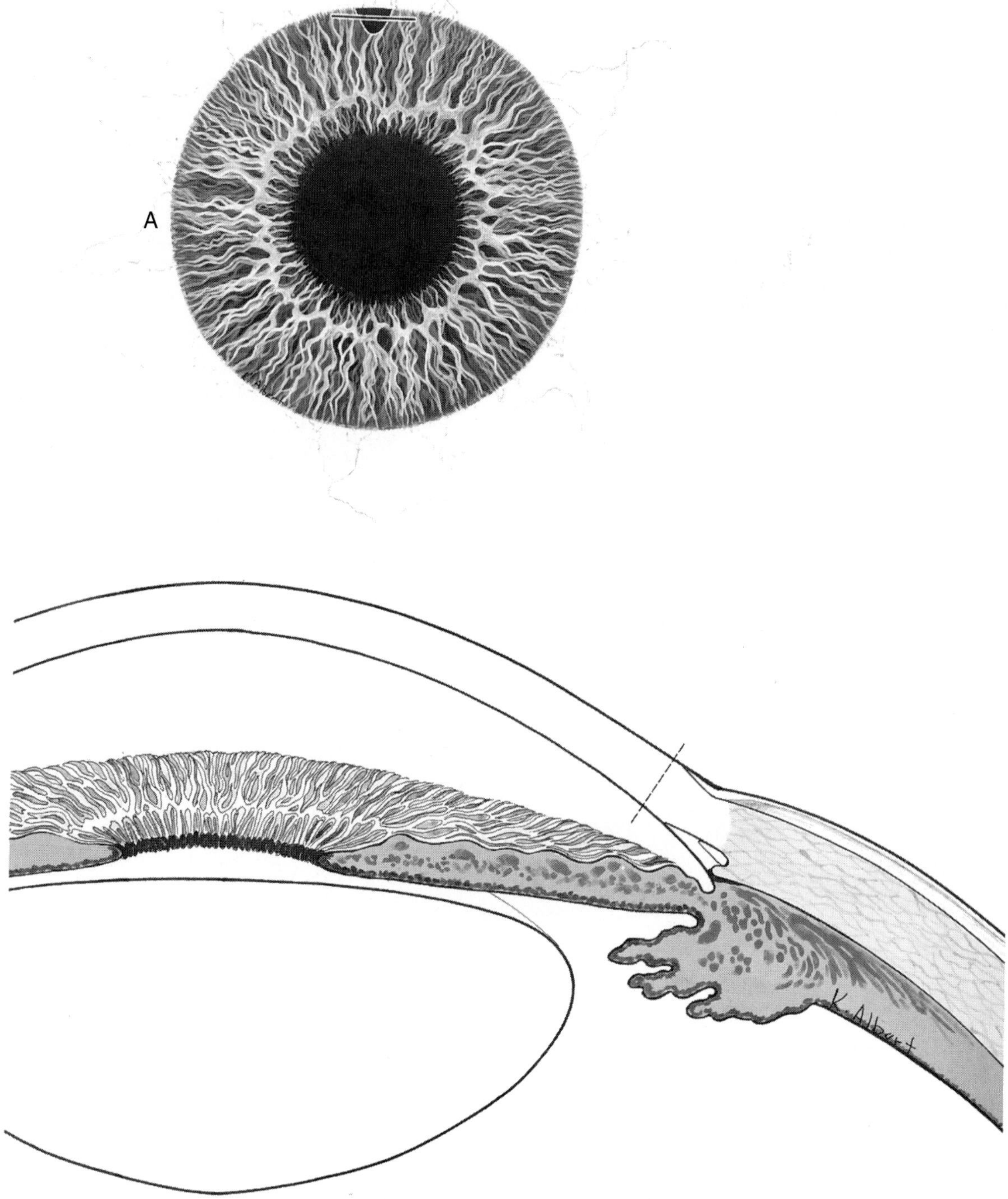

B

Figure 35–3. If the surgeon wants to preserve the conjunctiva, an iridectomy may be done through an incision made in clear cornea *(A)*. Entry into the anterior chamber is around Schwalbe's line (dashed line in *B*). The incision must not be shelved anteriorly.

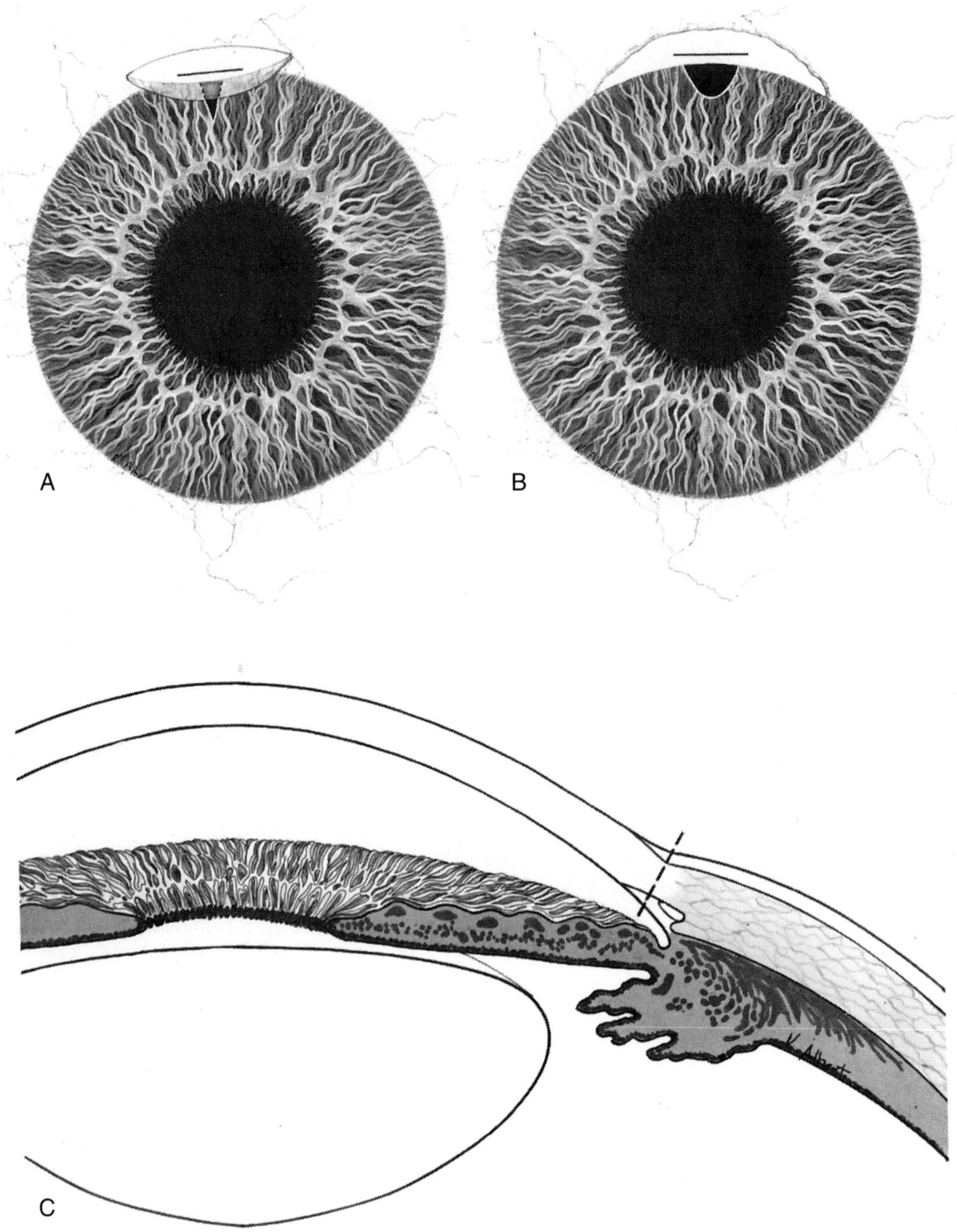

Figure 35–4. *A*. Usual location for placing the incision for a peripheral iridectomy. A small limbus-based incision has been developed. *B*. A peritomy provides adequate clearing of the conjunctiva, permitting proper placement of the incision for an iridectomy. *C*. A perpendicular incision through the corneoscleral sulcus usually enters the anterior chamber through the anterior trabecular meshwork.

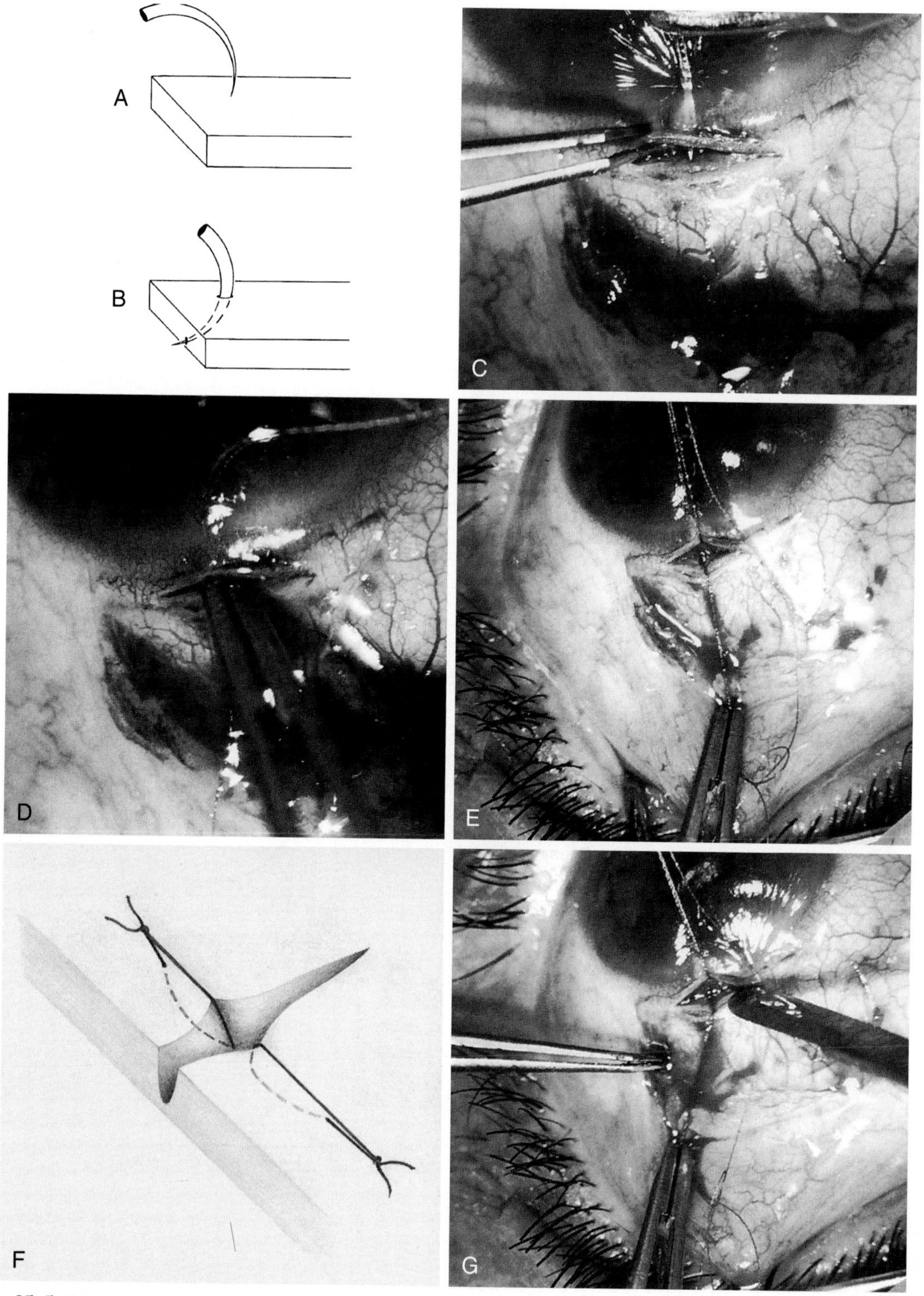

Figure 35–5. Method of placement of preplaced suture. The suture is placed more superficially than the depth of the incision and then retracted from the incision to form two loops that may be used to provide gentle retraction and excellent visualization of the depth of the incision.

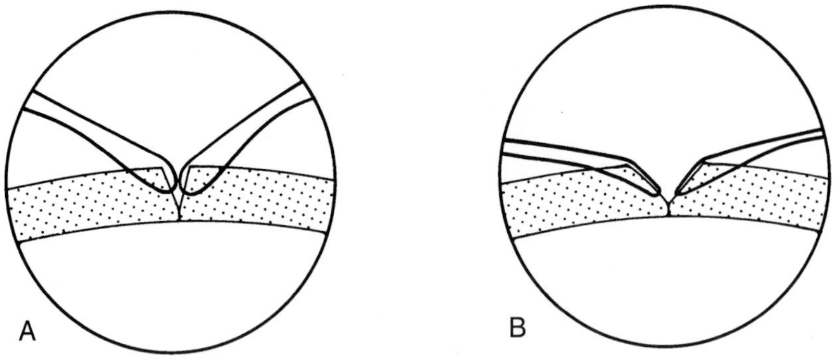

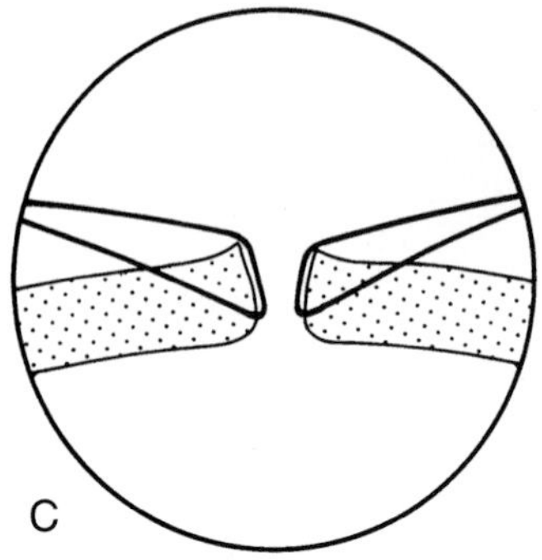

Figure 35–6. The use of a preplaced suture facilitates performance of an iridectomy. In *A* the sutures have been placed through an incision made in the cornea and looped to the sides. In *B* the traction on the sutures provides good visualization of the base of the incision. After the incision has been completed *(C)*, traction pulls the edges of the incision apart, facilitating prolapse of the iris.

closed with a fine suture, which may cause temporary astigmatism.

Incisions can also be shelved anteriorly or posteriorly. The major advantage of a shelved incision is the large overlap of the edges, which helps to assure tight closure. On the other hand, the iris is less likely to prolapse with such incisions, and closure is a bit more difficult in that the surfaces tend to slide on each other, complicating attempts to achieve exact apposition (Fig. 35–7).

EXTERIORIZATION OF IRIS

The iris prolapses from the anterior chamber through the incision because the pressure in the posterior chamber exceeds that in the anterior chamber. The surgeon, therefore, should be careful to assure maintenance of this pressure gradient (see Table 22–24). Before making the incision, the surgeon should have in mind the exact approach to the iridectomy, for once the anterior chamber has been opened no time should be wasted. The surgeon must not hesitate or debate because the gradient between the posterior and anterior chamber will be lost, as will the opportunity to achieve spontaneous iris prolapse. If the iris is penetrated, it will be far more difficult to prolapse. Such penetration can result from catching the iris on the tip of the knife at the time the incision is made. Factors that increase the likelihood of this complication include (1) the presence of peripheral synechiae; (2) a peripherally placed incision; (3) an extremely shallow anterior chamber; and (4) use of an extraordinarily sharp knife, especially if the tip of the blade is pointed.

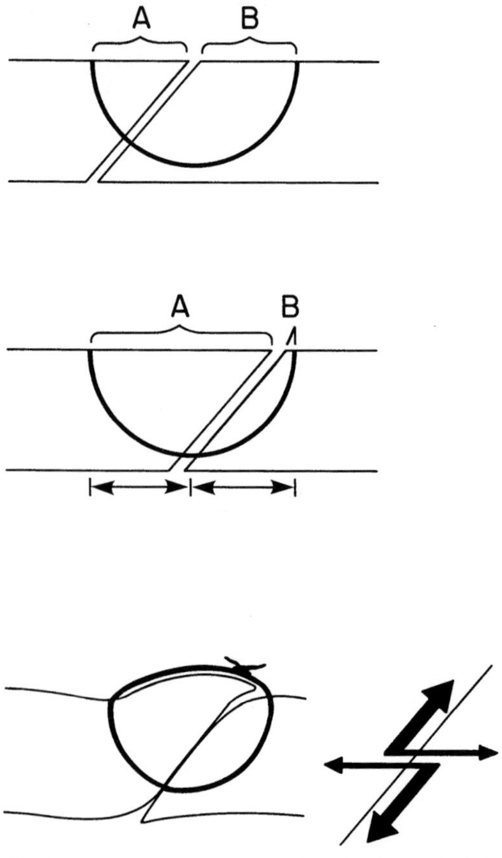

Figure 35–7. A shelved incision must be closed precisely if the tissue is not to be distorted. (Modified from Eisner G.: Augenchiurugie. Berlin: Springer-Verlag, 1978.)

TABLE 35–2. Factors that Predispose to Failure of Iris to Prolapse

1. Loss of posterior chamber pressure gradient
   a. Intraocular pressure below 15 mm Hg preoperatively
   b. Surgery performed too slowly
   c. Large pupil
   d. Penetration of iris
2. Anterior position of incision
3. Shelved incision
4. Peripheral anterior synechiae
5. Fibrosed iris

Other factors that affect how the iris prolapses include the size of the pupil and the texture of the iris, especially in its peripheral portions (Table 35–2). A small pupil assists prolapse of the iris. If it has not been possible to reduce the pupil to a diameter of 2 mm before surgery, acetylcholine can be applied after the corneal incision has been made. Clearly the iris cannot prolapse if the incision is made where the iris is adherent to the inner edge of the incision. Furthermore, the closer the incision is to the anterior extent of the adhesion, the less likely it is that spontaneous prolapse will occur. The ideal location for the incision is usually about 2 mm anterior to the base of the iris, or, if peripheral anterior synechiae are present, 2 mm anterior to the point of contact between the iris and the corneal endothelium. The shallower the anterior chamber, the more corneal the incision should be; the deeper the chamber, the more peripheral the incision.

It is usually easier to prolapse the iris through a limbal incision than through a clear-corneal incision. However, a properly placed, swiftly performed corneal incision will be followed by satisfactory spontaneous prolapse of the iris in virtually every instance. Prolapse can be facilitated by gentle traction on the two loops of the preplaced suture.

EXCISION OF IRIS

Within a few seconds after the iris has appeared in the depths of the incision, it should be grasped by a smooth or fine-toothed forceps; I prefer the Barraquer colibri 0.12-mm toothed forceps. If the iris prolapses only slightly, remaining in the depths of the incision, the forceps should be held so that it opens and closes in an axis parallel to the axis of the incision. Once the iris has been grasped, there is no longer a need to proceed rapidly.

With a limbal incision the iris is grasped as anteriorly as possible and lifted posteriorly (Fig. 35–8*A*). When the incision has been more anteriorly placed, the surgeon grasps the iris more posteriorly, lifting it anteriorly (Fig. 35–8*B*). These motions are designed to keep the iridectomy as basal as possible *without* tearing it from its root. The former goal is desirable for cosmetic reasons, and the latter, to prevent unnecessary bleeding.

After the iris has been lifted high enough that the pigment epithelial layer is exteriorized, the excision is performed. I use the micro DeWecker scissors. The iridectomy will be wide and peripheral if the axis of the blade is held parallel to the incision (Figs. 35–9 and 35–10). It will be narrower and more pointed if the scissors are held at right angles to the incision. The blades should be flush with the cornea, and the iris tissue should be deep in the crotch of the V made by the blades, as shown in the inset of Figure 35–9. If the tissue is near the tips of the blades, it will often slip out, failing to be cleanly cut and leaving a ragged iridectomy quite different from the one planned.

The position of the pupillary margin should be checked before the actual excision of tissue. If the surgeon wants the iridectomy to be peripheral, it is necessary to ensure that the pupillary margin has not prolapsed. If, on the other hand, a sector iridectomy is the goal, the pupillary margin needs to be exteriorized. With a sector iridectomy the scissors should be held at right angles to the incision, to avoid removing an excessive amount of iris.

After the blades have been closed the surgeon cautiously lifts the forceps containing the iris. This is done slowly, with the remainder of the iris through the cornea being observed to be sure that the excision has been complete and that the iris is not pulled away with the forceps. The excised iris is inspected to determine if the posterior pigment epithelium has been included. A dark smudge should be produced when the iris is rubbed against the drapes.

REPOSITIONING OF IRIS

Up to this point the anterior chamber should remain formed. The incision is presently blocked by iris. The tip of a No. 21 irrigator is placed into the incision, but not *through* the incision or through the iridectomy itself (Fig. 35–11*A*). A gentle stream of balanced salt solution flushes remaining pigment epithelium away; irrigation is continued as long as pigment continues to be seen. The stream of balanced salt solution also flushes the iris back into the anterior chamber. If the irrigator is placed through the iridectomy itself, the fluid will enter the posterior chamber, forcing the iris out of the eye rather than aiding in its repositioning.

After the iris is released from the incision it can be returned to its proper position by the surgeon's gently stroking the cornea with a blunt instrument, thus "pulling" the apex of the iridectomy inferiorly (Fig. 35–12). If this maneuver does not result in return of the iris to its preoperative condition, the internal edges of the incision can be made to gape by depressing the area of the incision with a blunt instrument, such as the heel of the irrigator tip or a muscle hook (Fig. 35–11*B*). This may release the iris when it is caught in the incision. If it does not, and if the iris sphincter is still functional, a small amount of acetylcholine can be introduced through the previously placed paracentesis track, caution being taken not to deepen the anterior chamber ex-

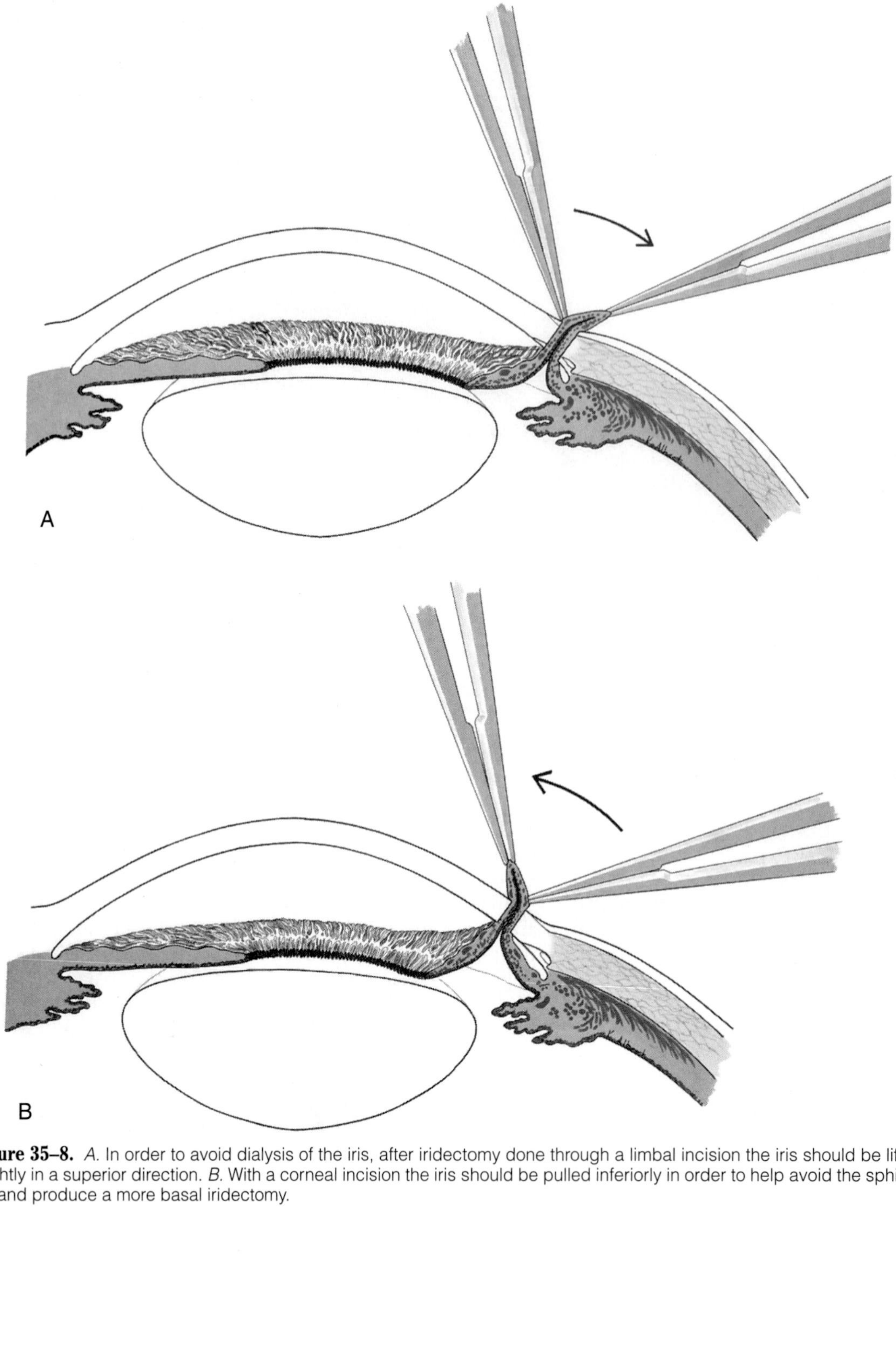

Figure 35–8. *A.* In order to avoid dialysis of the iris, after iridectomy done through a limbal incision the iris should be lifted slightly in a superior direction. *B.* With a corneal incision the iris should be pulled inferiorly in order to help avoid the sphincter and produce a more basal iridectomy.

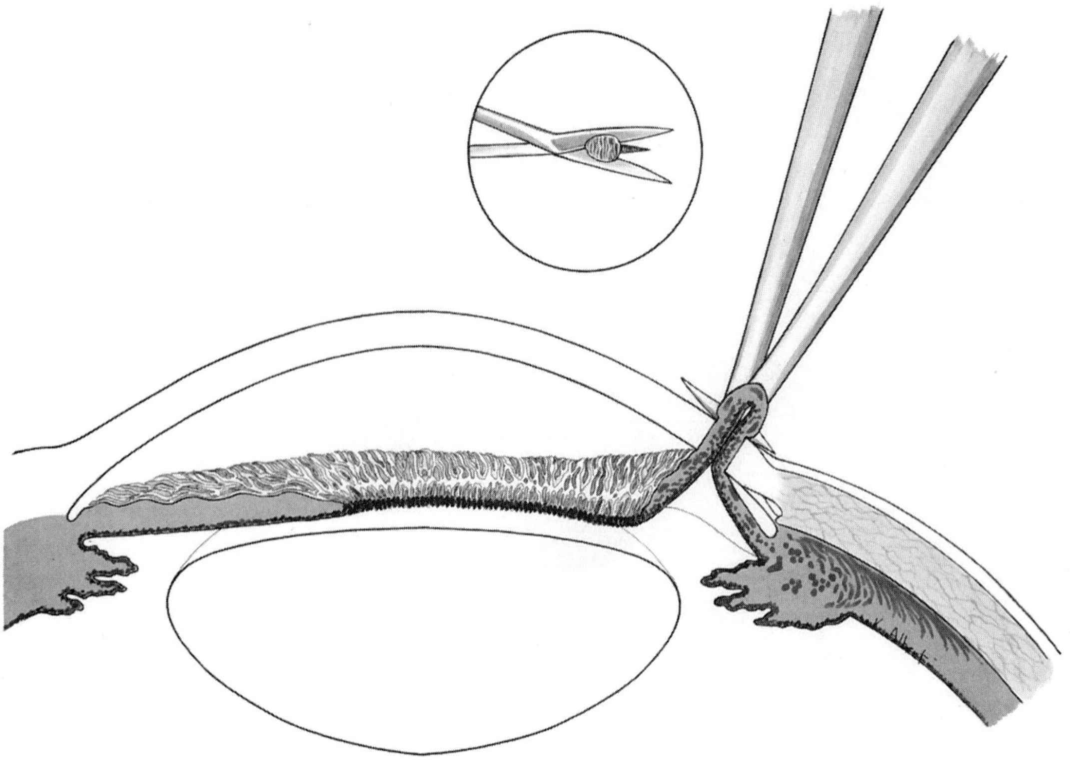

Figure 35–9. The iris scissors should be held flush with the cornea. The axis of the scissors will determine the shape of the iridectomy; if the goal is to keep the iridectomy as peripheral as possible, the axis should be held parallel to the incision (see Fig. 35–3). The inset shows how the iris should be cut in the crotch of the blades, not at the tips.

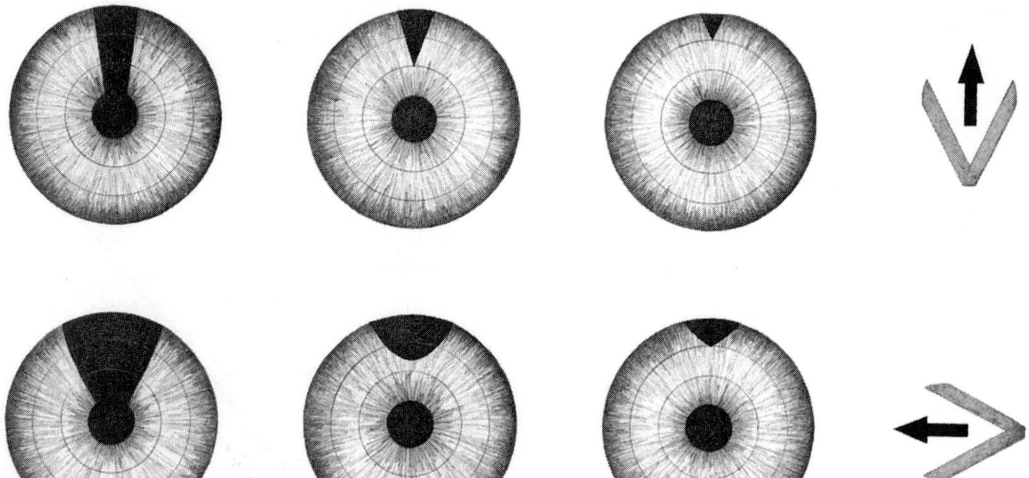

Figure 35–10. The position in which the scissors is held and the point at which the iris is grasped determine the final shape of the iridectomy performed. In *A, B,* and *C,* the scissors are held so that the cut is made at right angles to a tangent to the limbus. In *D, E,* and *F,* the axis of the scissors is meridional. To obtain iridectomies of the shape of those shown in *A* and *D,* the iris is grasped close to the pupillary margin (about 2 mm from the edge of the pupil). Iridectomies of the shape of those shown in *B* and *E* are a consequence of grasping the iris 2 mm anterior to its base. The most peripheral iridectomies (*C* and *F*) result from grasping the iris just anterior to its root.

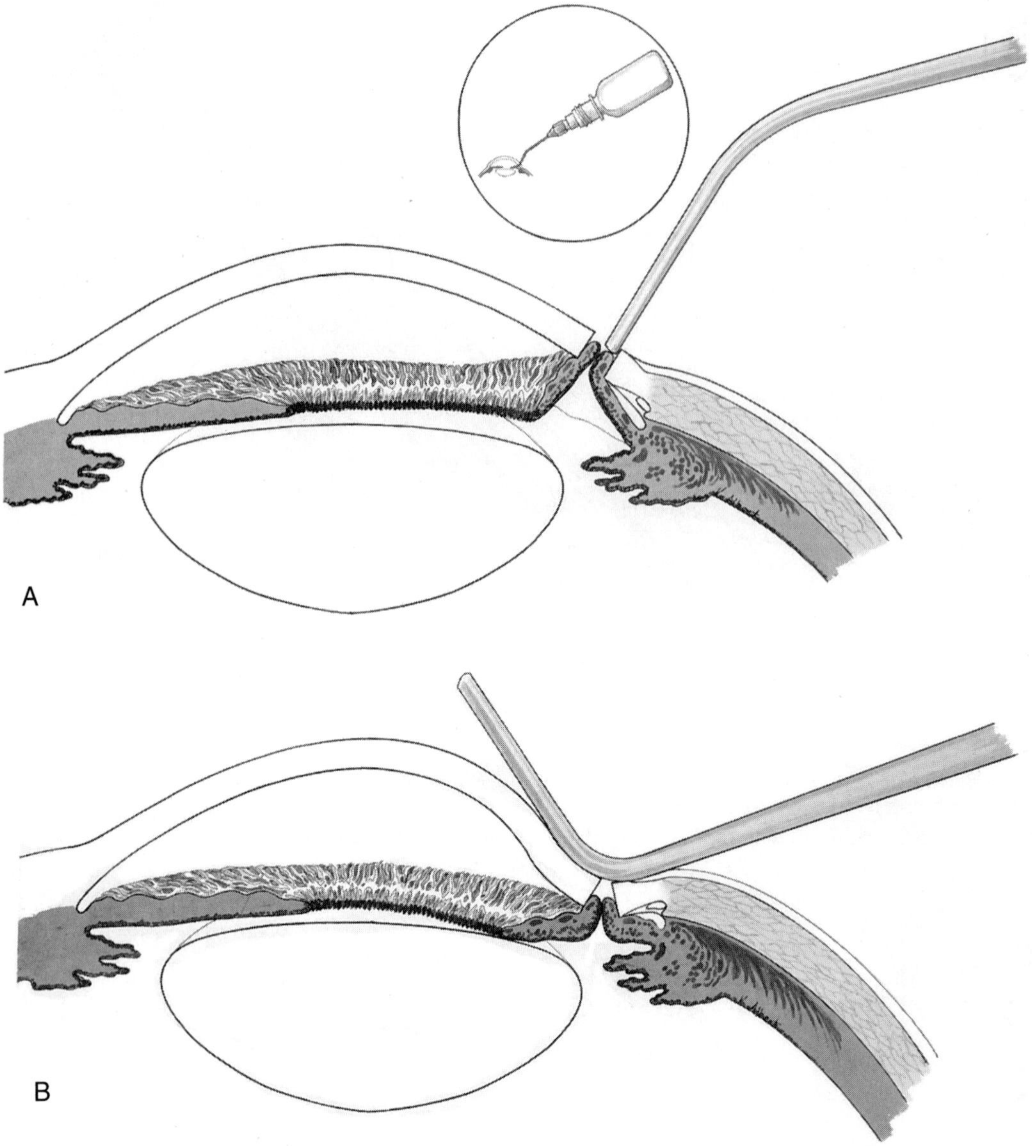

Figure 35–11. *A.* After iridectomy the iris may be repositioned by gentle irrigation. The tip of the irrigator should not be placed through the incision into the anterior chamber. *B.* Pressure on the incision causes the internal edges to gape, releasing the iris and facilitating its return to a normal position within the anterior chamber.

cessively. If the iris sphincter is dead, as is frequently the case after a severe attack of acute glaucoma, this maneuver will fail. Pressure on the posterior lip of the iris will release aqueous from the posterior chamber, almost certainly allowing the iris to fall back. The chamber will simultaneously collapse, which is of no concern when the surgeon has previously made a paracentesis, for the chamber can easily be re-formed at the end of the operation.

CLOSURE OF THE INCISION

At this point the preplaced suture can be tied tightly enough to close the incision but not so securely that it induces astigmatism. Additional sutures may be needed. If a conjunctival flap has been raised, it may be closed as described before, with a fine suture or with the wet-field cautery. If the incision is corneal, its knot is buried.

After closure is completed the surgeon may want to re-form the anterior chamber so that it is deeper than preoperatively. This is done by introducing balanced salt solution through the previously placed paracentesis track. A finger should monitor the intraocular pressure so that it does not rise excessively. Forceful deepening of the chamber may open peripheral anterior synechiae. Also, some surgeons have recommended mechanical separation of adhesions with an instrument such as a Barraquer sweep.

A small air bubble may be introduced and used as an internal probe to attempt to separate the iris from the cornea. The bubble is chased around the anterior chamber by applying external pressure on the cornea with a muscle hook or similar instrument; the eye must be soft for this maneuver to succeed.

At the end of the procedure the anterior chamber should be deep, the pupil round, the incision securely closed, and the intraocular pressure approximately 10 to 20 mm Hg. If a sector iridectomy has been performed, the pupil cannot be round, but the iris must have been returned to its proper plane.

A drop of pilocarpine 1% may be instilled, but this is usually unnecessary. In the routine case there is no reason to instill a cycloplegic at the time of surgery. Unless the patient is predisposed to a malignant glaucoma there is certainly no indication for atropine. The problem of the blurring produced by the medication far exceeds the need for its use. If inflammation is unusually severe, periocular corticosteroids may be given. An example would be betamethasone (Celestone), 3 mg. An antibiotic-corticosteroid ointment is then instilled and a patch applied. The only purpose for the patch is to protect the eye until the facial block has worn off. Figures 35–1 and 35–2 show the technique.

POSTOPERATIVE CARE

After the surgery there should be no limitation the patient's activity other than the precautions to be taken because of the sedation given. Attention should be paid to the general health of the patient, especially if extensive doses of carbonic anhydrase inhibitors and osmotic agents have been given. Serum electrolytes should be carefully monitored in such cases, and fluids should be encouraged to restore normal hydration.

The patch may be removed from the operated eye as soon as the facial block has worn off. An antibiotic-corticosteroid drop may be used for several days or a week.

A cycloplegic agent is routinely used to prevent posterior synechiae and to assure adequacy of the iridectomy. Tropicamide 1% once or twice daily for 1 or 2 weeks is usually adequate. The intraocular pressure should be checked after dilatation. Topical corticosteroids may be used to control the inflammatory response. If the anterior chamber of an eye that has had an iridectomy for primary angle-closure glaucoma is not deeper than the unoperated eye, the possibility of malignant glaucoma must be kept in mind. If the chamber becomes shallower and intraocular pressure rises, atropine 1% and phenylephrine 10% should be used in repeated doses until the pupil is maximally dilated; an osmotic agent should be given to shrink the vitreous and a carbonic anhydrase inhibitor administered to reduce the amount of aqueous that is being secreted into the vitreous cavity. When iridectomies are performed in the manner described in this chapter, the development of malignant glaucoma is extraordinarily rare.

Intraocular pressure may be measured with an applanation tonometer during the first few days, especially in patients in whom there has been a need to use medications to control the intraocular pressure preoperatively. Patients who have an iridectomy performed for long-standing chronic angle-closure glaucoma, or for a combined-mechanism glaucoma in which angle closure is superimposed on an open-angle glaucoma mechanism, will almost certainly have an elevated intraocular pressure after the surgery. This may not become apparent until the second or third postoperative day. In the immediate postoperative period the intraocular pressure should be controlled with the use of epinephrine and, if needed, a beta-blocker or a carbonic

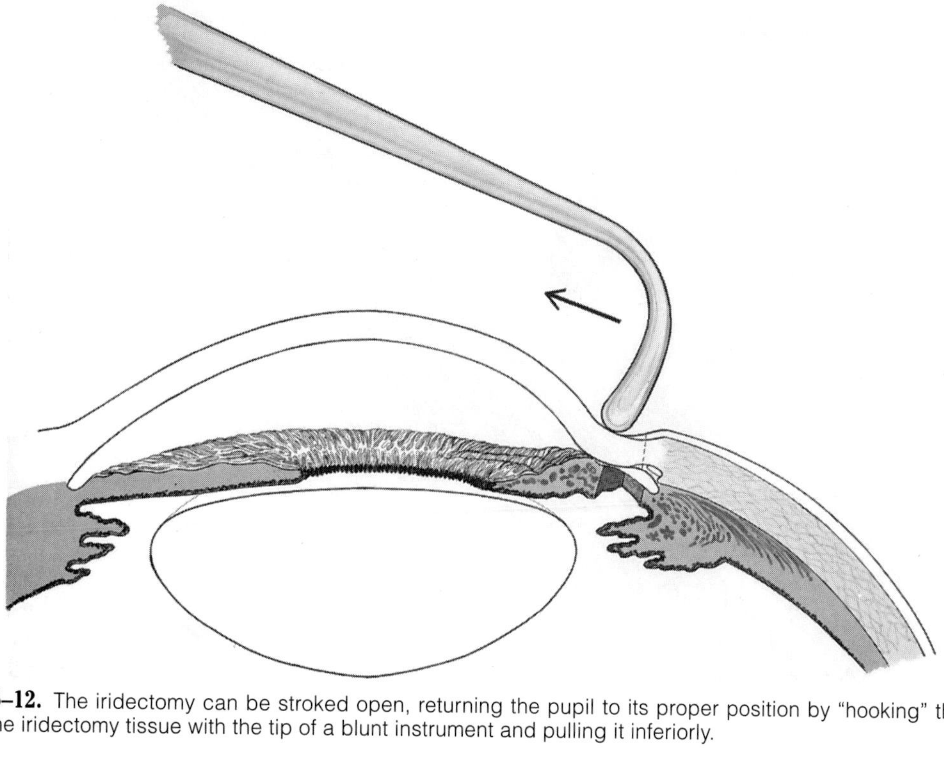

Figure 35–12. The iridectomy can be stroked open, returning the pupil to its proper position by "hooking" the inferior apex of the iridectomy tissue with the tip of a blunt instrument and pulling it inferiorly.

anhydrase inhibitor. Miotics should be avoided, as their use predisposes to posterior synechiae. Intraocular pressure should be carefully watched in the postoperative period, as optic nerve deterioration can occur if pressure remains high.

Evaluations should ordinarily be made 1 week and 1 month postoperatively. If all is in order at these visits, the patient should again be seen approximately 6 months later and then at yearly intervals. All patients should have baseline visual fields determined after the surgery. Photographs of the optic disc may also be taken, but are not essential.

Occasionally there is slight bleeding into the anterior chamber. This can be ignored unless it is so extensive that it causes pressure elevation; anterior chamber washout may be appropriate in such cases.

REFERENCE

1. Murphy M, Spaeth GL: Iridectomy as treatment for angle-closure glaucoma. II. Differential diagnosis of glaucoma associated with narrow angles. Arch Ophthalmol 1974;91:114.

CHAPTER 36

Cyclophotocoagulation

ROSARIO BRANCATO, M.D. and ROBERTO G. CARASSA, M.D.

Surgical procedures for glaucoma treatment, aimed at lowering intraocular pressure, are directed either at improving aqueous outflow or at reducing aqueous production. In the first category, laser trabeculoplasty, goniotomy, trabeculotomy, and filtering surgery are widely employed in most cases of glaucoma, with a high success rate. However, not all eyes respond well to outflow procedures, even with the adjunctive use of antimetabolites. In these cases, techniques aimed at reducing aqueous inflow are indicated. Cyclophotocoagulation is such a procedure, reducing intraocular pressure by selective destruction of the ciliary body by means of laser energy. The operation can be carried out using three different approaches. The *transscleral* technique, in which the energy is transmitted through the sclera to the ciliary body, the *transpupillary* technique where laser energy is directed toward all visible ciliary processes seen through the pupil or through iridectomies, and the *intraocular* technique which is performed during intraocular surgery using an endolaser to coagulate the visualized ciliary processes.

HISTORY

TRANSSCLERAL CYCLOPHOTOCOAGULATION

Weekers et al.[1] in 1961 were the first to use light energy for cyclodestruction. Using transscleral applications of the xenon arc they photocoagulated the ciliary body in rabbit and human eyes, thus lowering intraocular pressure. Although no clear advantage of this technique was demonstrated over cyclocryotherapy research into the use of light energy continued. In 1969 Smith et al.[2] and Vucicevic et al.[3] reported the first applications of laser energy for transscleral cyclophotocoagulation. Subsequently Beckman and co-workers described a procedure using the ruby laser in 1972[4] and the neodymium:glass laser in 1973.[5] In 1984[6] Beckman and co-workers reported a 10-year clinical experience of cyclophotocoagulation using ruby laser. Success—that is, intraocular pressure between 5 and 22 mm Hg—was achieved in 62% of the eyes, with the highest rate (86%) in eyes with glaucoma in aphakia. Hypotony occurred in 17% of cases and phthisis in 7%. The difficulty in obtaining a ruby laser limited the diffusion of the technique. In 1985 Beckman et al.[7] and Wilensky et al.[8] evaluated the Nd:YAG laser, showing its utility for transscleral cycloablation, and in 1987 Brancato et al.[9] first suggested its use for contact application through an optic fiber. Since then, Nd:YAG cyclophotocoagulation has gained acceptance and clinical experience is encouraging. In 1990 the introduction of the diode laser in ophthalmology aroused interest for its application in transscleral cycloablation, and several experimental studies were carried out.[10–12] In 1992 the first clinical trials of diode laser transscleral cyclophotocoagulation (TCP) were reported: Hennis et al.,[13] using the noncontact technique, and Carassa et al.[14] and Gaasterland et al.,[15] using the contact technique, achieved good intraocular pressure reduction. The Krypton laser was also proposed for contact TCP by Immonen et al.[16] in 1993. In a subsequent 6-month clinical trial they reported its efficacy in controlling refractory glaucomatous eyes.[17]

TRANSPUPILLARY CYCLOPHOTOCOAGULATION

Lee and Pomerantzeff in 1971[18] first described the use of transpupillary cyclophotocoagulation with an argon laser. The low success rate of the procedure, shown by Shields in 1985,[19] which is related to the limited number of ciliary processes that can be visualized and treated, restricts its acceptance as glaucoma therapy.

INTRAOCULAR CYCLOPHOTOCOAGULATION

The intraocular technique was first described by Shields et al. in 1985.[20] Using an argon laser optic fiber connected to an endoscope, they showed that precise photocoagulation of the ciliary processes could be achieved in monkey eyes. A subsequent clinical trial showed the efficacy of the treatment in lowering intraoperative pressure in glaucomatous eyes.[21] In 1992, a diode laser attached to an endoscope with television monitor was used for intraocular cyclophotocoagulation, with promising results.[22]

TRANSSCLERAL CYCLOPHOTOCOAGULATION

The transscleral approach for cyclophotocoagulation is the most widely used, thanks to its easy applicability and noninvasiveness. The ciliary body is ablated using a laser beam transmitted through the overlying conjunctiva and sclera. Laser energy can be transmitted indirectly through the air (noncontact transscleral cyclophotocoagulation, NCTCP; Fig. 36–1) or directly through a fiberoptic placed in contact on the eyeball (contact transscleral cyclophotocoagulation, CTCP; Fig. 36–2). The energy absorption by melanin induces thermal coagulation and disruption of the ciliary epithelium and of the associated vessels, as demonstrated in animal and human eyes. Noncontact TCP using continuous-wave Nd:YAG laser produces blanching and shrinkage on the surface of the ciliary processes, as seen by macroscopic examination. Histologically there is separation of the pigmented and nonpigmented ciliary epithelial layers from the underlying stroma, with blisterlike space formation. Fibrin and inflammatory cells are visible between the ciliary epithelium and the stroma, and coagulation necrosis with vascular damage and hemorrhage is evident.[23–27] Four to eight weeks after the treatment, atrophy of the ciliary processes is obtained.[23,28,29] In rabbit eyes the ciliary epithelium and vessels may subsequently partially regenerate, producing new tissue that may not be functional.[28] The short-pulsed Nd:YAG laser produces a more explosive lesion than the continuous-wave system, mostly damaging the pigment epithelium with blister formation.[30]

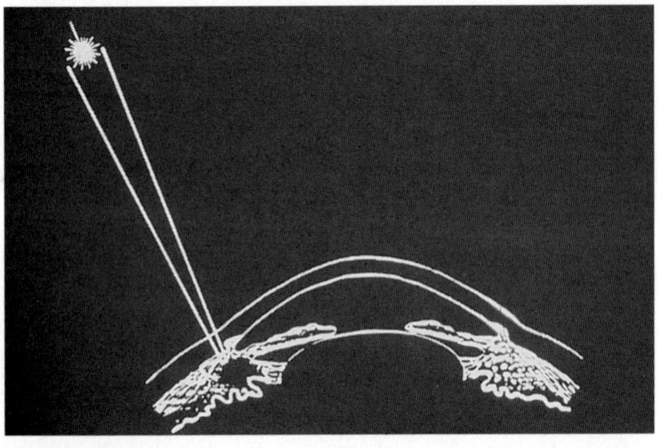

Figure 36–1. Noncontact transscleral cyclophotocoagulation: schematic view.

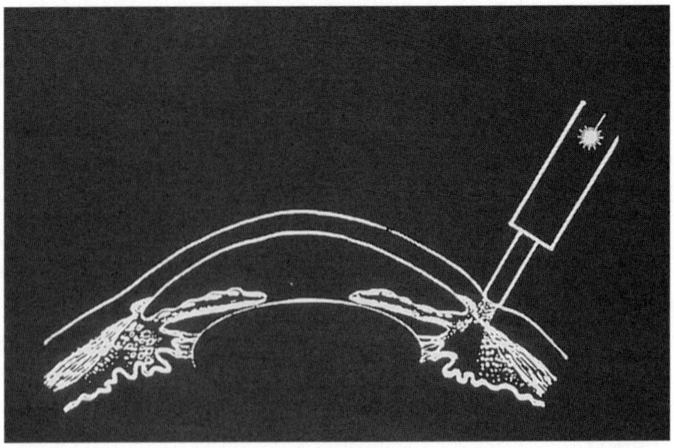

Figure 36–2. Contact transscleral cyclophotocoagulation: schematic view.

The ciliary body disruption seen after Nd:YAG CTCP is similar to that induced by continuous-wave NCTCP. Nevertheless, the longer exposure time in CTCP results more in thermal damage to the stroma with coagulative necrosis of the ciliary nonpigmented and pigmented epithelia, rather than to the blister formation seen with NCTCP.[31,32] There is no clear evidence of damage to the sclera, although areas of compression and hypercellularity were found.[33] High energy or limbal probe positioning induced peripheral iris and lens changes.[34]

The effect on tissue is similar with either the Nd:YAG or the diode laser, although the latter causes more damage to the ciliary pigmented structures (Fig. 36–3). The long exposure time combined with the shorter wavelength results in deep coagulation necrosis of the pigmented epithelium, wide disorganization of the collagen in the stroma, and intravascular coagulation in the ciliary vessels (Fig. 36–4). The diode laser needs less energy to produce ciliary body thermal coagulation (1.2 J versus 4 J for the Nd:YAG laser).[11,12,35–38]

Transscleral photocoagulation is a "blind" procedure because the ablative energy is directed toward an invisible target whose position can only be estimated from data obtained experimentally in human autopsy eyes. Exact beam focusing for NCTCP was thus suggested as

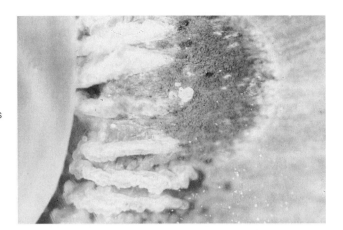

Figure 36–3. Macroscopic evidence of ciliary body lesion 11 months after diode laser CTCP.

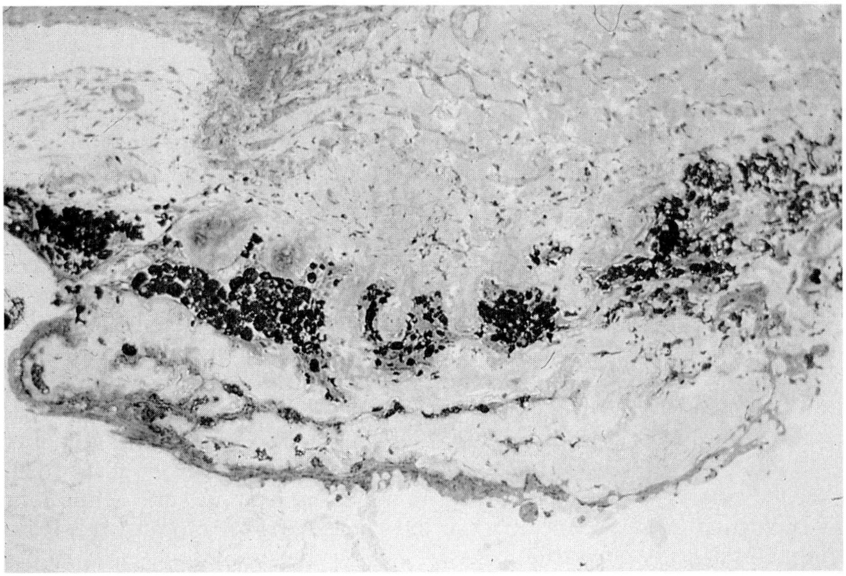

Figure 36–4. Histologic appearance of the lesion in Figure 36–3.

being 1 to 1.5 mm posterior to the limbus,[23,26,38,39] and the optimal location for the center of the probe in CTCP was 1.5 to 2 mm posterior of the corneolimbal junction.[34,40,41] The introduction of ultrasound biomicroscopy,[42] which gives sharp images of the entire ciliary body in real time (Fig. 36–5),[43] has aroused interest for its applications in TCP.[44] The system can locate the exact treatment site in each eye to be operated, and it can also detect early changes after the procedure.[45,46] A study meant to define the frequency distribution of the distance between the corneolimbal junction and the projection of the ciliary body on the ocular surface in living eyes showed that, in most cases, treatment 1.5 mm from the limbus would correctly reach the ciliary processes.[47] The real significance of ultrasound biomicroscopy examinations for TCP remains to be fully assessed.

EQUIPMENT

The treatment requires wavelengths that are strongly transmitted through the sclera in order to obtain good energy levels at the ciliary body and to reduce scleral absorption with consequent damage. Vogel et al.[48]

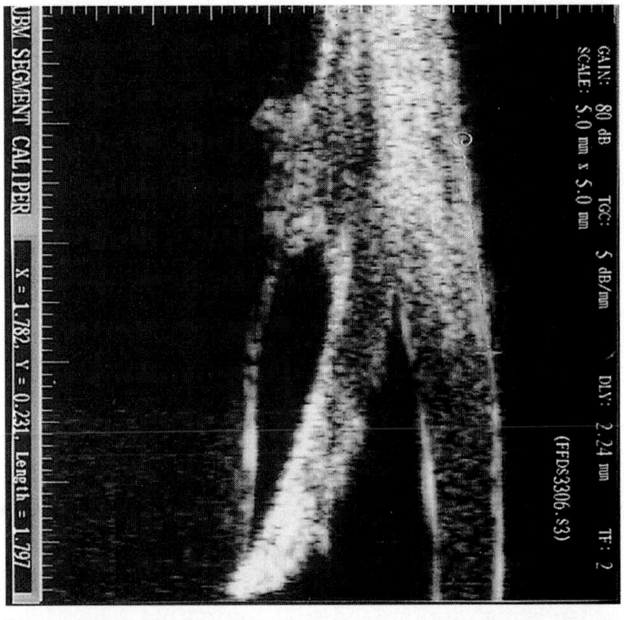

Figure 36–5. Ultrasound biomicroscopic image of the eye: the ciliary body is evident, and its location with respect to the limbus can be calculated.

showed that scleral transmission ranges from 6% at 442 nm to 35% at 804 nm and 53% at 1064 nm. Thus the Nd:YAG laser (1064 nm) and the diode laser (810 nm) are both suitable for transscleral applications. The diode laser has several advantages over the Nd:YAG laser. Its 810 nm wavelength is better absorbed by melanin, and the system is portable and less expensive.[11] However, macroscopic and histopathologic examination showed similar ciliary body thermal lesions after Nd:YAG and diode laser cyclophotocoagulation. As yet, no clinical trials have compared the clinical effectiveness of treatment with those two lasers. Either continuous-wave or pulsed laser systems are employed. A continuous-wave laser allows long and sustained energy delivery while a pulsed laser system transmits light energy at short pre-set time intervals.

The krypton laser was evaluated for CTCP with promising results.[16,17]

NONCONTACT TRANSSCLERAL CYCLOPHOTOCOAGULATION

Both NCTCP and CTCP require specialized techniques and equipment. In NCTCP, laser energy is transmitted through the air from a slit-lamp delivery system. The procedure can be carried out using either a pulsed Nd:YAG laser such as the Microruptor II (H.S. Meridian, Inc., Mason, OH), or a continuous-wave model such as the Microruptor III, or a diode laser such as the DC3000 (Nidek, Inc., Palo Alto, CA), the Microlase (Keeler Instruments, Broomall, PA), or the Oculight SLX (Iris Medical, Mountain View, CA).

The laser beam needs to be focused inside the ciliary body. This is done with the Nd:YAG laser by focusing the HeNe beam on the conjunctiva overlying the ciliary body and selecting the maximum offset (9), thus providing a 3.6 mm posterior separation between the HeNe and the therapeutic beam,[38] and with the diode laser by defocusing the beam 1 mm toward the ciliary body.[13,49]

PATIENT PREPARATION

All preoperative medications are continued. Peribulbar or retrobulbar anesthesia is essential and may be obtained by injecting a mixture of 2% lidocaine, 0.75% bupivacaine, and hyaluronidase. The lids are held open manually, with a wire speculum, or using a specific contact lens.[50] The patient is then placed in an upright position at the laser slit lamp.

TECHNIQUE

The Nd:YAG laser (Table 36–1) should be set at 4 to 8 J energy, which achieves significant intraocular pressure reduction,[26,51–58] and offset to its maximum (9). In one prospective randomized trial comparing 4 J and 8 J treatment, intraocular pressure control was significantly better using 8 J energy with no difference in side effects.[59] The diode laser (Table 36–2) should be set at 1500 to 2000 mW power output, 1 second time duration (thus producing 1.5 to 2 J spots), and 100 to 400 micron spot size.[13,49]

TABLE 36–1. Technique for Nd:YAG Laser Noncontact Cyclophotocoagulation

Energy	4–8 J
Focus	Offset 9
Spot position	1–2 mm from limbus
Laser beam	Parallel to visual axis
Number of spots	30–40

TABLE 36–2. Technique for Diode Laser Noncontact Cyclophotocoagulation

Power	1.5–2 W
Duration	1 second
Spot size	100–400 microns
Focus	Spot defocused 1 mm toward ciliary body
Spot position	1–2 mm from limbus
Laser beam	Parallel to visual axis
Number of spots	30–40

The eye can be kept in primary position because no significant differences were found between applying laser energy parallel to the visual axis or perpendicular to the sclera.[38] The beam is focused on the conjunctiva 1 to 2 mm posterior to the limbus.[26,52,53,57] The distance can be measured using a caliper and a marking pencil,[26,51,54,60] or the slit beam of the biomicroscope. In the latter case the laser spots should be placed in the middle of a 3-mm-long slit beam, projected perpendicular to the limbus.[60] A special contact lens has been designed to facilitate laser spot positioning.[50]

Thirty to forty applications, evenly spaced over 360 degrees, are placed in a single session,[26,51,52,54,61–63] usually sparing the 3 o'clock and 9 o'clock positions to avoid damage to the posterior ciliary arteries.[62,64] One prospective randomized study comparing 180 degree and 360 degree treatment found that the latter gave a better risk-to-benefit ratio.[65] Using the diode laser, each spot should be defocused 1 mm toward the ciliary body. It is mandatory to keep a diagram of the treatment, specifically noting the laser settings used.

POSTOPERATIVE TREATMENT

Because the treated eye is anesthetized, it should be patched for the day to avoid accidental lesions. Topical combinations of steroids and antibiotics together with cyclopentolate are prescribed and tapered as the inflammation subsides. Current glaucoma medication should be continued, with the exception of miotics, and adjusted according to the intraocular pressure. This needs to be checked after 1 hour and again at 1 day. Control visits should be scheduled 1 week and 1 month after the treatment.

RETREATMENT

After 1 to 4 weeks all eyes showing an inadequate response to the treatment should be retreated. All parameters used for the initial treatment are maintained but half as many spots are made.[35] Multiple retreatments can be done, although the risk of hypotony and phthisis increases.

CLINICAL TRIALS

Neodymium:YAG-NCTCP significantly reduced intraocular pressure in refractory glaucomatous eyes with an average decrease of 44% to 68%. Intraocular pressure below 22 mm Hg was obtained in 46% to 87% of the cases with 21% to 48% requiring multiple treatments.[26,51–58,62,63,66,67] In one long-term follow-up study on 500 patients intraocular pressure control was satisfactory in 62% of the cases with only one treatment.[68] Diode-NCTCP was similarly efficient for glaucoma treatment, reducing intraocular pressure below 21 mm Hg in 56% to 70% of the eyes.[13,24,49,69] Several studies aimed at defining the relationship between success and demographic or clinical characteristics. One study found that white patients had better control than black patients, but age, preoperative intraocular pressure level, and gender were not related to the outcome.[57] Neovascular glaucomas had the worst response in one study,[70] while good intraocular pressure control was obtained in eyes with penetrating keratoplasty[64,71,72] and in inflammatory glaucomas.[73]

COMPLICATIONS

The most common complications affecting all patients after Nd:YAG-NCTCP are mild pain lasting less than 1 day (although severe pain has been reported in as many as 13.5% of cases),[52] mild uveitis, easily dominated by topical steroids within the first postoperative weeks, and transient conjunctival burns and edema.[2,54,62] Visual loss, usually within 1 or 2 lines of Snellen visual acuity, occurs in up to 39% of the cases,[52,53,57,58,66,67,74] neovascular glaucomas being the most affected.[67] Hypotony has an incidence of up to 26%,[66,67,75,76] while phthisis bulbi, the most serious complication, occurred in 10.7% of eyes in one series.[63] Numerous uncommon complications have been reported such as vitreous hemorrhage, suprachoroidal serous effusion, cystoid macular edema, focal scleral thinning, and malignant glaucoma.[70,75,77,78] One very worrying complication is sympathetic ophthalmia, which has been reported in five cases treated with Nd:YAG-NCTCP.[79–82] All eyes had had previous multiple penetrating surgery and all were treated with multiple high doses of energy. One eye had had previous incisional surgery with iris incarceration. The relationship between cyclophotocoagulation and sympathetic ophthalmia is still uncertain.

Diode-NCTCP showed complications similar to the Nd:YAG procedure, although no phthisis bulbi was observed. It should be noted, however, that experience with this technique is limited.

CONTACT TRANSSCLERAL CYCLOPHOTOCOAGULATION

In CTCP light energy is directly transmitted to the globe by means of a fiberoptic ending in a hand-held probe that is positioned in contact with the ocular surface (Fig. 36–6). The contact technique has several advantages over the non-contact technique. The reduced light backscattering and the greater scleral transmission[48] allows the use of significantly less energy. Arbitrary beam defocusing is not necessary. The longer exposure time results in a predominantly coagulative necrosis of the ciliary processes as opposed to the blister formation with NCTCP.[26,31,34,38] The use of specifically designed, hand-held probes improves precision by allowing easy spot location and by avoiding eye movement.[41] The procedure can be carried out in remote locations, as the laser system is portable and needs no slit lamp. The supine position means treatment can be done under general anesthesia.

The procedure is carried out using either a Nd:YAG laser or a diode laser. All systems are portable. The commercially available Nd:YAG lasers are the SLT (Surgical Laser Technologies, Montgomeryville, PA; Fig. 36–7), the

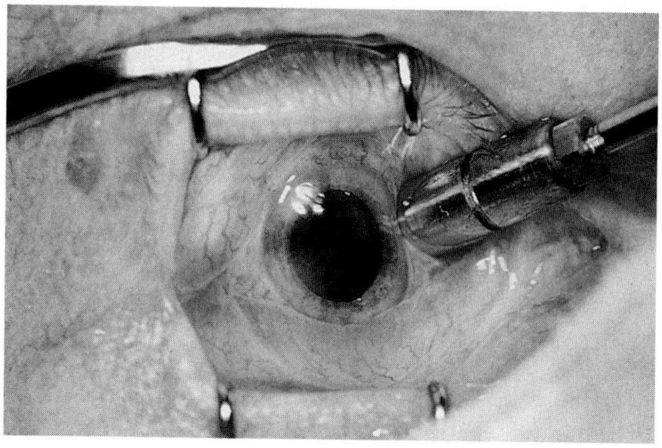

Figure 36–6. Contact TCP treatment.

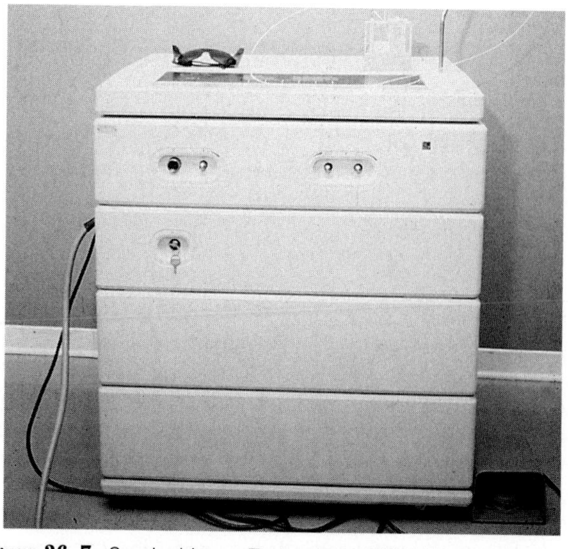

Figure 36–7. Surgical Laser Technology CW-Nd:YAG laser. Courtesy of Surgical Laser Technologies, Montgomeryville, PA.

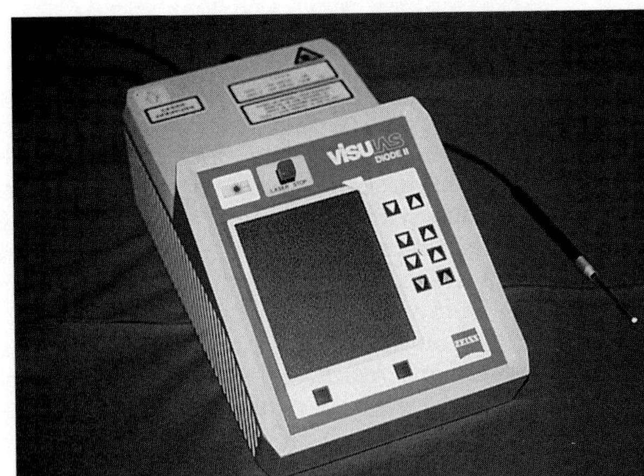

Figure 36–8. VISULAS II by Zeiss, Germany.

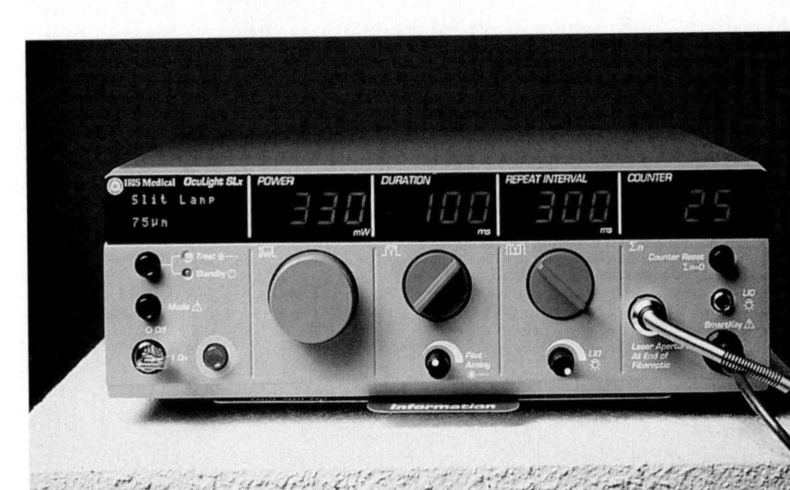

Figure 36–9. OCULIGHT SLX by IRIS Medical, Mountain View, CA.

Microruptor III (H.S. Meridian, Inc., Mason, OH), and the Emerald Crystal Focus, whereas the diode lasers are the VISULAS II (Zeiss, Germany; Fig. 36–8), the OCULIGHT SLX (IRIS Medical, Mountain View, CA; Fig. 36–9), and the DC-3000 (Nidek Inc., Palo Alto, CA). All systems are coupled with an optic fiber ending either in a sapphire probe (SLT, Microruptor III, Emerald), in a specifically designed focusing bare quartz tip (OCULIGHT SLX G-probe), or in a specifically designed optical focusing tip (VISULAS II). These tips ensure less energy dispersion and easy positioning of their centers 1.5 mm posterior to the limbus, where treatment is needed (Figs. 36–10 and 36–11).

TECHNIQUE

The Nd:YAG laser (Table 36–3) is set at 4 to 7 W of power and 0.5 to 0.7 seconds duration[83–85]; the diode laser (Table 36–4) is set at 1.75 to 2.6 W and 1.5 to 2.5 seconds.[54,86] The difference is partly related to the different size in the optic fiber used. Considering the delicacy of optic fibers and sapphire probes, a fiber transmission check must always be made to verify the total energy being delivered by the system.[86] The probe is then placed in contact with the conjunctiva, positioning its center 1.5 mm posterior to the surgical limbus. This can be easily achieved using the specifically designed tips which, being 3 mm in diameter, should be placed with

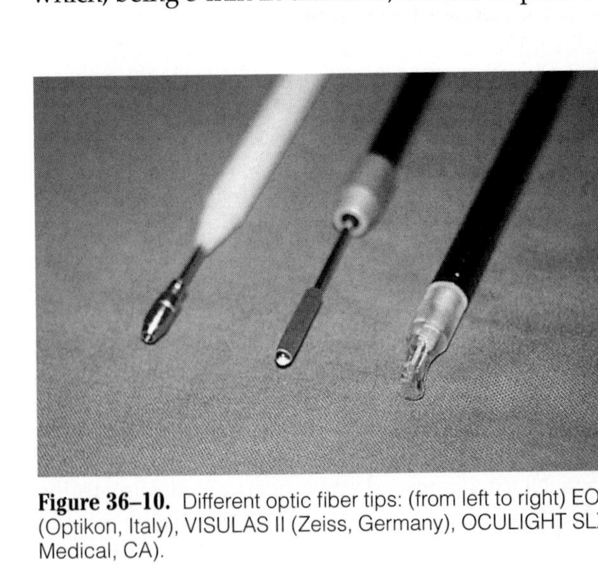

Figure 36–10. Different optic fiber tips: (from left to right) EOS3000 (Optikon, Italy), VISULAS II (Zeiss, Germany), OCULIGHT SLX (IRIS Medical, CA).

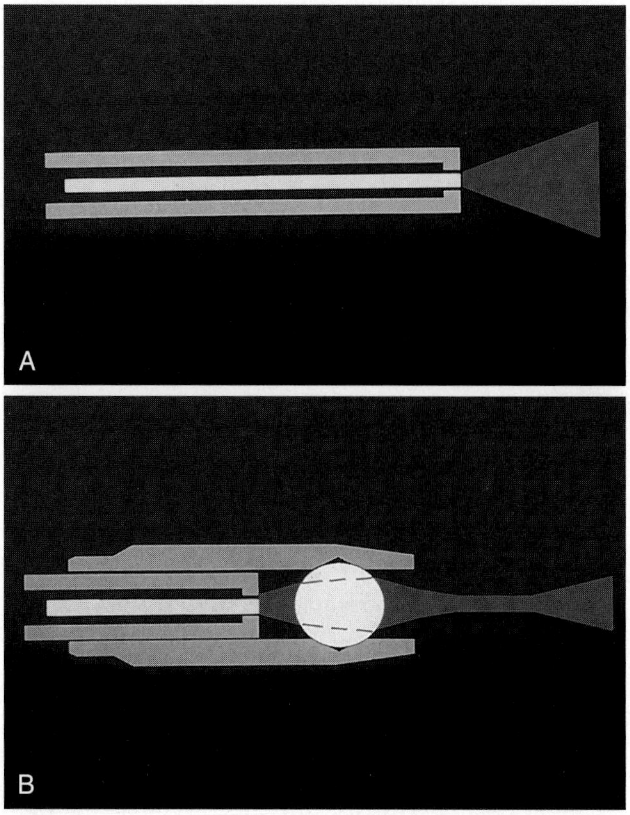

Figure 36–11. Schematic view of probes ending with the bare quartz fiber *(A)*, or with an optical-focused tip *(B)*.

their margins at the edge of the limbus.[54,86] In all other cases calipers are needed. Particular care should be taken to keep the probe perpendicular to the scleral surface: an orientation as little as 15 degrees off the perpendicular reduces the photocoagulative effect.[87] A firm indentation is always needed in order to increase the energy transmission through the sclera[48] and to avoid eye movement. From 16 to 40 spots (Nd:YAG laser) or 16 to 20 spots (diode laser) are applied over 360 degrees, sparing the 3 o'clock and 9 o'clock positions.[83–88] A "pop," caused by tissue disruption, can sometimes be heard, especially with the diode laser, because of the greater melanin absorption of its wavelength. This is a signal of overtreatment, and can be used to assess the correct energy level . By raising or lowering the power output in small increments, as in a "bracketing" strategy, the energy level just below the one causing the "pop" can then be used throughout treatment.[86,88]

TABLE 36–3. Technique for Nd:YAG Laser Contact Cyclophotocoagulation

Power	4–7 W
Duration	0.5–0.7 seconds
Probe position	1.5 mm from limbus
Probe orientation	Perpendicular to scleral surface
Number of spots	16–40

TABLE 36–4. Technique for Diode Laser Contact Cyclophotocoagulation

Power	1.75–2.6 W
Duration	1.5–2.5 seconds
Probe position	1.5 mm from limbus
Probe orientation	Perpendicular to scleral surface
Number of spots	16–20

RETREATMENT

Retreatments are indicated in eyes where the intraocular pressure is still uncontrolled 1 to 4 weeks after the primary procedure. The CTCP procedure can be repeated using the same parameters, but delivering no more than 16 to 20 spots over 360 degrees in order to reduce the risk of hypotony and phthisis bulbi.[35,83,86] Retreatments can be repeated, although each time the risk of major side effects increases. Postoperative care is exactly the same as for NCTCP.

CLINICAL TRIALS

Contact TCP with the Nd:YAG and the diode laser is effective in reducing intraocular pressure in refractory glaucomatous eyes. With the Nd:YAG laser, intraocular pressure below 22 mm Hg was achieved in 41% to 62% of the eyes, with pressure reduction ranging from 24% to 48%, and with 11% to 57% of the cases requiring multiple treatments.[83–85,89–91] Schuman et al. presented the largest series on 140 eyes followed up to 36 months, with a success rate (intraocular pressure < 22 mm Hg) of 65%, with 27% of the cases requiring multiple procedures, and a mean pressure reduction of 46.8%.[85] Diode laser CTCP was found successful in pilot studies aimed at evaluating the technique: an intraocular pressure < 21 mm Hg was achieved with 1 or more treatments in 72% of the eyes after 20.7 months of follow-up, with a mean pressure reduction of 47.4%.[86] These results were confirmed in the long-term follow-up report (up to 54 months) where the success rate was 69%.[92] Another study[88] showed a success rate (intraocular pressure <22 mm Hg or 20% pressure reduction) of 72% at 1 year and 52% at 2 years, with only one treatment in 93% of the cases. These good results have been confirmed in all subsequent clinical trials: intraocular pressures below 20 to 22 mm Hg were achieved in 50% to 84.9% of the cases, with 28% to 70% requiring retreatments.[93–99] Bloom and co-workers presented the largest series of cases treated with diode laser CTCP: on 210 eyes followed for a mean of 10 months (range 3 to 30 months), 66% achieved a final pressure below 22 mm Hg with 49% requiring multiple treatments (mean 1.75, range 2 to 5 treatments). Mean final intraocular pressure was 20.1 mm Hg, and total medical therapy was reduced from 2.3 to 1.7 treatments.[93] Two studies were aimed at comparing Nd:YAG CTCP with diode CTCP. In one randomized controlled trial on 95 eyes followed for a mean of 10.4 months the same results were achieved with both treatments,[100] although diode laser CTCP was shown more successful in a retrospective analysis on 39 eyes with 3-year follow-up.[101]

COMPLICATIONS

With Nd:YAG and diode CTCP minimal to mild postoperative pain is reported, and mild uveitis easily controlled with steroids. Anterior chamber inflammation graded 3 to 4+ was described in 10% of the cases in one study.[85] No intraocular pressure spikes greater than 8 mm Hg were detected, although pressure increases higher than baseline within a few hours from the treatment occur in up to 30% of eyes.[88] Conjunctival and scleral damage were reported with the use of probes ending with the bare quartz fiber coupled with either Nd:YAG or diode lasers: transient conjunctival lesions were reported in 33% of cases[88] (Fig. 36–12), and scleral perforation in two cases.[102,103] These complications were never reported with optical-focused tips,[86,92] probably owing to their 3 mm diameter and to the lower energy density in the contact area. In fact, dark scleral spots were described when a focusing tip was used (Fig. 36–13),[104] but ultrasound biomicroscopy excluded the presence of tissue thinning, suggesting a reactive focal hyperpigmentation. Hypotony or phthisis was reported in 10% of the eyes treated with the Nd:YAG laser,[85] whereas after diode laser CTCP, hypotony was found in 1.4% to 3.7% of eyes[86,88,92] and phthisis in 0.5% to 2%.[92,93,96] A visual acuity reduction of 2 or more lines was reported in 27% to 47% of eyes treated with the Nd:YAG laser,[85,90] and in 32% to 38% treated with the diode laser.[86,88,92,93,96–98] Complete loss of visual acuity during the follow-up period occurred in up to 18% of the cases.[85,94] This is definitely the major complication in all cyclodestructive procedures, including CTCP. The cause is still unclear, although hypotony, cystoid macular edema, and neovascular glaucoma appear to be the major risk factors. One study reported that visual loss was less after CTCP than after NCTCP.[84] Other, less frequent complications such as choroidal detachment, vitreous hemorrhage, and malignant glaucoma were reported.[86,89,91,105,106] Sympathetic ophthalmia was also described after Nd:YAG CTCP as in NCTCP, but in only two cases. One eye with previous penetrating surgery, developed the disease 18 months after CTCP,[81] and another eye with neovascular glaucoma secondary to Coats disease developed sympathetic ophthalmia after three CTCP sessions conducted within 5 weeks.[7] The cause-and-effect relationship between the disease and the procedure is not established. High energy levels or frequent multiple retreatments may be involved. Sympathetic ophthalmia has never been reported after diode cyclophotocoagulation (either NCTCP or CTCP). This may reflect either the relatively limited experience with this technique or the more coagulative and less disruptive effect of diode CTCP compared to Nd:YAG CTCP, on account of the different wavelength and the longer exposure time in the diode procedure.

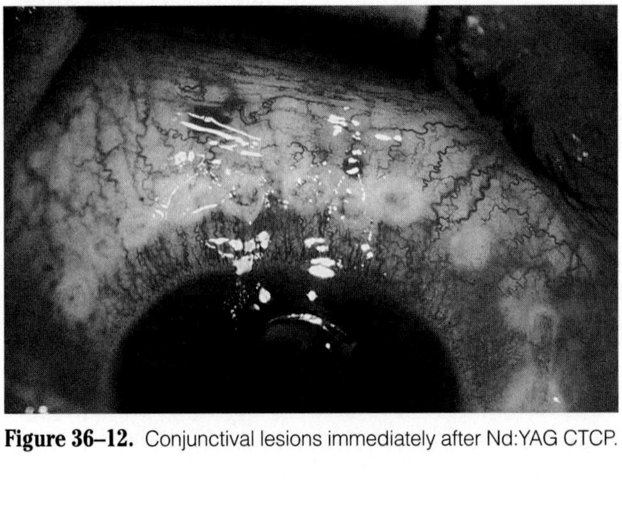

Figure 36–12. Conjunctival lesions immediately after Nd:YAG CTCP.

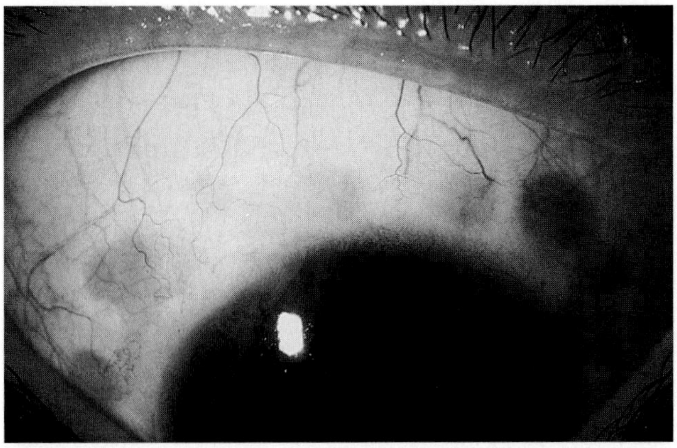

Figure 36–13. Dark scleral spots 8 months after diode laser CTCP.

TRANSPUPILLARY CYCLOPHOTOCOAGULATION

Direct photocoagulation of the ciliary processes is a tempting approach since the laser effects on the target tissue can be checked visually. Transpupillary cyclophotocoagulation can be achieved using an argon laser beam focused on the ciliary processes visualized by indirect gonioscopy. Although the procedure is applicable for large iridectomies (Fig. 36–14) or in eyes with very wide mydriasis, it is seldom effective in reducing IOP. This may be due either to the small number of ciliary processes that can be visualized and treated, or to the inadequate coagulation which only involves the anterior tip of the ciliary ridge.[19]

The treatment can be attempted in eyes where at least 25% of the ciliary processes can be treated, as in eyes with large or multiple iridectomies, in aniridic eyes (either congenital or traumatic), or in eyes with wide mydriasis (as secondary to neovascular iris retraction).[18,19,107,108]

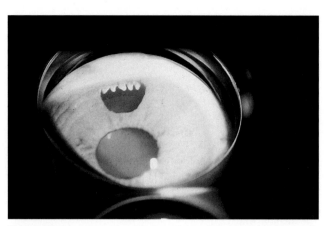

Figure 36–14. Direct visualization of the ciliary processes through an iridectomy for transpupillary cyclophotocoagulation.

EQUIPMENT

The procedure is carried out using an argon laser and a contact Goldmann-type goniolens. Laser settings are 50 to 100 micron spot size, 0.1 second duration, and 700 to 1500 mW power level.

PATIENT PREPARATION

No specific preparation is needed apart from a superficial anesthesia. The use of mydriatic drops depends on the clinical picture: mydriasis in fact can often worsen visualization of the ciliary processes through an iridectomy.

TECHNIQUE

The gonioscopic lens should be placed on the eye, and the aiming beam focused on a ciliary process. The power level should be set to obtain a concave brown burn, often associated with pigment dispersion and bubble formation. All visible processes in all their portions should be coagulated. This usually requires three to four applications per process.

POSTOPERATIVE TREATMENT

All preoperative medications are continued with the addition of a topical steroid, which is tapered as the inflammation subsides. Ocular hypotensive drugs are adjusted in relation to the intraocular pressure.

CLINICAL TRIALS

Results of transpupillary cyclophotocoagulation are unpredictable. In one series only 4 of 16 eyes had controlled intraocular pressure[19] while in another study 15 of 22 eyes had a mean pressure reduction of 50%.[18,107,109] In a later study 6 of 27 patients reached an intraocular pressure below 22 mm Hg but 18 eyes (50%) had an increase in pressure over preoperative levels within 1 month after the procedure and required conventional surgery.[110] Finally, in a recent study, transpupillary cyclophotocoagulation was successfully performed in a traumatic aniridic eye.[108]

INTRAOCULAR CYCLOPHOTOCOAGULATION

In the intraocular technique an endolaser inserted into the eyeball is used to photocoagulate the ciliary processes. One advantage of this approach is that direct control of the treatment is possible by visualization of the target tissue. It is, however, an invasive procedure, limited by the need for aphakia and extensive vitrectomy. Ciliary processes can be visualized *transpupillarily* using scleral depression. In such a case, a transparent cornea and a dilated pupil are required.[20,21] To overcome this limitation, the *endoscopic* technique was introduced[20,21] by which the ciliary processes are visualized through an endoscope inserted in the eye. A diode laser attached to an endoscope with television visualization of the ciliary body has also been used for cycloablation.[22]

EQUIPMENT

An argon or a diode laser endophotocoagulator, commonly used for intraoperative retinal photocoagulation, is employed. Settings are 1000 mW power and 0.2 second duration for the argon laser and 200 to 300 mW power and 1 to 2 seconds duration for the diode laser. For transpupillary visualization a scleral indentator is needed, and an endoscope is necessary for endoscopic visualization.

TECHNIQUE

In aphakic eyes, after anterior vitrectomy, the endolaser is inserted through the pars plana cannula. In eyes with a clear cornea and wide mydriasis a scleral indentation is made to bring the processes into view. Alternatively, they can be visualized through a microendoscope inserted in the eye. The endolaser is then positioned 0.5 to 3 mm from each ciliary process and 1 to 5 applications per process are delivered over 180 degrees. The power level should be set to produce a white reaction and shallow tissue disruption.

CLINICAL TRIALS

Clinical experience with intraocular cyclophotocoagulation is limited. The transpupillary visualization technique, used on 60 eyes, achieved intraocular pressures below 22 mm Hg in 76% to 78% of the cases.[111,112] In one trial 17% of the eyes needed a second treatment.[112] The endoscopic visualization technique, in one study, was evaluated in 10 eyes, 7 of which reached an intraocular pressure between 2 and 21 mm Hg.[22] The largest series was presented by Chen and co-workers on 68 eyes followed for a mean of 12.9 months. The survival analysis showed a success rate (intraocular pressure <21 mm Hg) of 94% at 1 year and 82% at 2 years.[113] In a recent study the procedure was also evaluated for the treatment of pedriatic glaucoma on 10 eyes of 8 children. At 3 years of follow-up, 20% of the eyes that received a single treatment of endolaser had an intraocular pressure below 22 mm Hg with or without adjunctive medical therapy.[114]

COMPLICATIONS

Hypotony, retinal dialysis, vitreous hemorrhage, transient choroidal detachment, and decreased visual acuity have been reported.[111,112] In one study on endoscopic cyclophotocoagulation, 2 of 10 eyes developed hypotony with retinal detachment.[22]

CONCLUSIONS

Cyclodestructive procedures are indicated in the management of some refractory glaucomas. These are all eyes in which intraocular pressure cannot be controlled despite maximum tolerated medical therapy, traditional laser (iridotomy or laser trabeculoplasty) and incisional surgery, including cases where either laser or incisional surgery cannot be performed or is likely to fail. The adjunctive use of antimetabolites during filtration surgery greatly improved the success rate for many of these eyes. Nevertheless neovascular glaucomas, active uveitic glaucomas, and glaucomas associated with penetrating keratoplasty, to name a few, still have a very poor prognosis.

Cyclophotocoagulation may be effective in lowering intraocular pressure in these eyes. Compared with other cycloablative surgeries, such as cyclocryotherapy, ultrasound, or microwave therapy, cyclophotocoagulation is associated with fewer side effects. The incidence of visual loss and phthisis bulbi is lower with this procedure. The transscleral technique is the most widely used because it is not invasive and gives a good result. The contact mode, delivering less energy, causes less inflammation, and seems less likely to lead to visual acuity reduction, hypotony, and phthisis bulbi. Various wavelength have been tested. The Nd:YAG laser was widely employed, but recently the diode laser has become an effective alternative, its main advantage over Nd:YAG being better melanin absorption with a consequently greater coagulative effect on the ciliary body. Together with the fact that less energy is required, this offers the potential advantage of reducing complications. Diode laser units are also portable and cheaper. Although no large controlled trials have been done to assess the best procedure for cyclophotocoagulation, it appears that the contact transscleral technique with diode laser is the best choice. Research is still needed to develop systems that reduce intraocular pressure more predictably, thus extending the role of cyclophotocoagulation in glaucoma therapy.

REFERENCES

1. Weekers R, Lavergne G, Watillon M, et al.: Effects of photocoagulation of ciliary body upon ocular tension. Am J Ophthalmol 1961;52:156.
2. Smith RS, Stein MN: Ocular hazards of transscleral laser radiation: II intraocular injury produced by ruby and neodymium lasers. Am J Ophthalmol 1969;67:100.
3. Vucicevic ZM, Tsou KZ, Nazarian IH, et al.: A cytochemical approach to the laser coagulation of the ciliary body. Bibl Ophthalmol 1969;79:467.
4. Beckman H, Kinoshita A, Rota AN, et al.: Transscleral ruby laser irradiation of the ciliary body in the treatment of intractable glaucoma. Trans Am Acad Ophthalmol Otolaryngol 1972;46:423.
5. Beckman H, Sugar HS: Neodymium laser cyclocoagulation. Arch Ophthalmol 1973;90:27.
6. Beckman H, Waeltermann J: Transscleral ruby laser cyclocoagulation. Am J Ophthalmol 1984;98:788.
7. Beckman H: Transscleral laser cyclocoagulation. Trans New Orleans Acad Ophthalmol 1985;33:158.
8. Wilensky JT, Welch D, Mirolovich M: Transscleral cyclocoagulation using a neodymium:YAG laser. Ophthalmic Surg 1985;16:95.
9. Brancato R, Leoni G, Trabucchi E, et al.: Transscleral contact cyclophotocoagulation with CW Nd:YAG laser: experimental study on rabbit eyes. Int J Tissue React 1987;6:493.
10. Schuman JS, Jacobson JJ, Puliafito CA, et al.: Experimental use of semiconductor diode laser in contact transscleral cyclophotocoagulation in rabbits. Arch Ophthalmol 1990;108:1152.
11. Brancato R, Leoni G, Trabucchi G, et al.: Histopathology of continuous wave neodymium:yttrium aluminum garnet and diode laser contact transscleral lesions in rabbit ciliary body. A comparative study. Invest Ophthalmol Vis Sci 1991;32:1586.
12. Assia EI, Hennis HL, Stewart WC: A comparison of neodymium: yttrium aluminum garnet and diode laser transscleral cyclophotocoagulation and cyclocryotherapy. Invest Ophthalmol Vis Sci 1991;32:2774.
13. Hennis HL, Steward WC: Semiconductor diode laser transscleral cyclophotocoagulation in patients with glaucoma. Am J Ophthalmol 1992;113:81.
14. Carassa RG, Trabucchi G, Bettin P, et al.: Contact transscleral cyclophotocoagulation (CTCP) with diode laser: a pilot clinical study. Invest Ophthalmol Vis Sci 1992;33(Suppl):1019.
15. Gaasterland DE, Abrams DA, Belcher CD, et al.: A multicentric study of contact diode laser transscleral cyclophotocoagulation in glaucoma patients. Invest Ophthalmol Vis Sci 1992;33(Suppl):1019.
16. Immonen I, Suomalainen VP, Kivela T, et al.: Energy levels needed for cyclophotocoagulation: a comparison of transscleral contact cw-YAG and Krypton lasers in rabbit eyes. Ophthalmic Surg 1993;24:530.
17. Immonen IJ, Puska P, Raitta C: Transscleral contact Krypton laser cyclophotocoagulation for treatment of glaucoma. Ophthalmology 1994;101:876.
18. Lee PF, Pomerantzeff O: Transpupillary cyclophotocoagulation of rabbit eyes: an experimental approach to glaucoma surgery. Am J Ophthalmol 1971;71:911.
19. Shields MB: Cyclodestructive surgery for glaucoma: past, present and future. Trans Am Ophthalmol Soc 1985;83:285.
20. Shields MB, Chandler DB, Hickingbotham C, et al.: Intraocular cyclophotocoagulation. Histopathologic evaluation in primates. Arch Ophthalmol 1985;103:1731.
21. Shields MB: Intraocular cyclophotocoagulation. Trans Ophthalmol Soc UK 1986;105:237.
22. Uram M: Ophthalmic laser microendoscope ciliary process ablation in the management of neovascular glaucoma. Ophthalmology 1992;99:1823.
23. Fankhauser F, van der Zypen E, Kwasniewska S, et al.: Transscleral cyclophotocoagulation using a neodymium:YAG laser. Ophthalmic Surg 1986;17:94.
24. Hampton C, Shields MB, Miller KN, et al.: Evaluation of a protocol for transscleral neodymium:YAG cyclophotocoagulation in 100 consecutive patients. Ophthalmology 1989;96(Suppl):92.
25. Wilensky JT, Welch D, Mirolovich M: Transscleral cyclophotocoagulation using a neodymium:YAG laser. Ophthalmic Surg 1991;16:95.

26. Blasini M, Simmons R, Shields MB: The early tissue response to transscleral neodymium:YAG cyclophotocoagulation. Invest Ophthalmol Vis Sci 1989;30(Suppl):280.
27. Nasisse MP, McGahan MC, Shields MB, et al.: Inflammatory effects of continuous-wave neodymium:yttrium aluminum garnet laser cyclophotocoagulation. Invest Ophthalmol Vis Sci 1992;33:2216.
28. England C, van der Zypen E, Fankhauser F, et al.: Ultrastructure of the rabbit ciliary body following transscleral cyclophotocoagulation with the free-running Nd:YAG laser: preliminary findings. Laser Ophthalmol 1986;1:61.
29. Gross RL, Smith JA, Font RL, et al.: Transscleral Nd:YAG laser cycloablation in rabbits. Invest Ophthalmol Vis Sci 1986;27 (Suppl):253.
30. Schubert HD: Noncontact and contact pars plana transscleral neodymium:YAG laser cyclophotocoagulation in postmortem eyes. Ophthalmology 1989;96:1471.
31. Schubert HD, Federman JL: The role of inflammation in CW Nd:YAG contact transscleral photocoagulation and cryopexy. Invest Ophthalmol Vis Sci 1989;30:543.
32. Latina MA, Patel S, de Kater AW, et al.: Transscleral cyclophotocoagulation using a contact laser probe: a histologic and clinical study in rabbits. Laser Surg Med 1989;9:437.
33. Schubert HD, Federman JL: A comparison of CW Nd:YAG contact transscleral cyclophotocoagulation with cyclocryopexy. Invest Ophthalmol Vis Sci 1989;30:536.
34. Allingham RR, de Kater AW, Hsu J, et al.: Probe placement and power levels in contact transscleral neodymium:YAG laser cyclophotocoagulation. Arch Ophthalmol 1990;108:738.
35. Schuman JS, Puliafito CA: Laser cyclophotocoagulation. Int Ophthalmol Clin 1990;30:111.
36. Monsour M, Kane H, Gaasterland D: Transscleral cyclophotocoagulation in human autopsy eyes: contact diode compared to noncontact Nd:YAG laser. Invest Ophthalmol Vis Sci 1992;33 (Suppl):1018.
37. Schuman JS, Noecker RJ, Puliafito CA, et al.: Energy levels and probe placement in contact transscleral semiconductor diode laser cyclophotocoagulation in human cadaver eyes. Arch Ophthalmol 1991;109:1534.
38. Hardten DR, Brown JD: Transscleral neodymium:YAG cyclophotocoagulation: comparison of 180-degree and 360-degree initial treatments. Ophthalmic Surg 1993;24:181.
39. Hennis HL, Assia E, Steward W, et al.: Transscleral cyclophotocoagulation using semiconductor diode laser in cadaver eyes. Ophthalmic Surg 1991;22:274.
40. Brancato R, Leoni G, Trabucchi G, et al.: Probe placement and energy levels in CW Nd:YAG contact transscleral cyclophotocoagulation. Arch Ophthalmol 1990;108:679.
41. Brancato R, Trabucchi G, Verdi M, et al.: Diode and Nd:YAG laser contact transscleral cyclophotocoagulation (CTCP) on human eye: a comparative histopathologic study on the lesions produced using a new fiber optic probe. Ophthalmic Surg 1994;25:607.
42. Pavlin CJ, Sherar MD, Foster FS: Subsurface ultrasound microscopic imaging of the intact eye. Ophthalmology 1990;97:244.
43. Pavlin CJ, Harasiewicz K, Sherar MD, et al.: Clinical use of ultrasound biomicroscopy. Ophthalmology 1991;98:287.
44. Brancato R, Carassa RG: Value of ultrasound biomicroscopy for ciliodestructive procedures. Curr Opin Ophthalmol 1996;7:87.
45. Pavlin CJ, Macken P, Trope GE, et al.: Ultrasound biomicroscopy imaging of the effects of YAG laser cycloablation in postmortem eyes and living patients. Ophthalmology 1995;102:334.
46. Carassa RG, Brancato R, Trabucchi G, et al.: Ultrasound biomicroscopy and pathologic examination of eyes treated with contact transscleral cyclophotocoagulation. Invest Ophthalmol Vis Sci 1995;36(Suppl):564.
47. Fiori M, Carassa RG, Bettin P, et al.: Localization of ciliary body by ultrasound biomicroscopy for transscleral cyclophotocoagulation. Invest Ophthalmol Vis Sci 1995;36(Suppl):564.
48. Vogel A, Dlugos C, Nuffer R, et al.: Optical properties of human sclera and their significance for transscleral use. Laser in Surg and Med 1991;11:331.
49. Kida K, Kuwayama Y, Takeuchi R, et al.: Non-contact transscleral semi-conductor diode laser cyclophotocoagulation for refractory glaucoma. Invest Ophthalmol Vis Sci 1992;33(Suppl):1267.
50. Shields MB, Blasini M, Simmons R: A contact lens for transscleral Nd:YAG cyclophotocoagulation. Am J Ophthalmol 1989;108:457.
51. Crymes BM, Gross RL: Laser placement in noncontact Nd:YAG cyclophotocoagulation. Am J Ophthalmol 1990;11:670.
52. Hawkins TA, Steward WC: One year results of semiconductor transscleral cyclophotocoagulation in glaucoma patients. Arch Ophthalmol 1993;111:488.
53. Kalenak JW, Parkinson JM, Kass MA, et al.: Transscleral neodymium:YAG laser cyclocoagulation for uncontrolled glaucoma. Ophthalmic Surg 1990;21:345.
54. Klapper RM, Wandel T, Donnenfeld E, et al.: Transscleral neodymium:YAG thermal cyclophotocoagulation in refractory glaucoma. A preliminary report. Ophthalmology 1988;95:719.
55. Noureddin BN, Wilson-Holt N, Lavin M, et al.: Advanced uncontrolled glaucoma. Nd:YAG cyclophotocoagulation or tube surgery. Ophthalmology 1992;99:430.
56. Schubert HD: Cyclophotocoagulation: how far posterior is the ciliary body? Ophthalmology 1989;96:139.
57. Simmons RB, Shields MB, Blasini M, et al.: Transscleral Nd:YAG laser cyclophotocoagulation with a contact lens. Am J Ophthalmol 1991;112:671.
58. Wright MM, Grajewski AL, Feuer WJ: Nd:YAG cyclophotocoagulation: outcome of treatment for uncontrolled glaucoma. Ophthalmic Surg 1991;22:279.
59. Shields MB, Wilkerson MH, Echelman DA: A comparison of two energy levels for noncontact transscleral neodymium:YAG cyclophotocoagulation. Arch Ophthalmol 1993;111:484.
60. Fiore PM, Latina MA: A technique for precise placement of laser applications in transscleral Nd:YAG cyclophotocoagulation. Am J Ophthalmol 1989;107:292.
61. Badeeb O, Trope GE, Mortimer C: Short-term effects of neodymium-YAG transscleral cyclophotocoagulation in patients with uncontrolled glaucoma. Br J Ophthalmol 1988;72:615.
62. Balazsi G: Noncontact thermal mode Nd:YAG laser transscleral cyclocoagulation in the treatment of glaucoma. Ophthalmology 1991;98:1858.
63. Trope GE, Ma S: Mid-term effects of neodymium:YAG transscleral cyclophotocoagulation in glaucoma. Ophthalmology 1990;97:73.
64. Chen J, Chon RA, Lin SC, et al.: Endoscopic photocoagulation of the ciliary body for treatment of refractory glaucomas. Am J Ophthalmol 1997;124:787.
65. Hardten DR, Brown JD: Malignant glaucoma after Nd:YAG cyclophotocoagulation. Am J Ophthalmol 1991;111:245.
66. Cyril MN, Beckman H, Czedik C: Nd:YAG laser transscleral cyclocoagulation treatment for severe glaucoma. Invest Ophthalmol Vis Sci 1985;26(Suppl):157.
67. Schwartz LW, Moster MR: Neodymium:YAG laser transscleral cyclodiathermy. Ophthalmic Laser Ther 1986;1:135.
68. Shields MB, Shields SE: Noncontact transscleral Nd:YAG cyclophotocoagulation: a long-term follow-up study of 500 patients. Trans Am Ophthalmol Soc 1994;92:271.
69. Hampton C, Shields MB: Transscleral neodymium:YAG cyclophotocoagulation. A histologic study of human autopsy eyes. Arch Ophthalmol 1988;106:1121.
70. Devenyi RG, Trope GE, Hunter WH, et al.: Neodymium:YAG transscleral cyclocoagulation in human eyes. Ophthalmology 1987;94:1519.
71. Thofts RA, Gordon JM, Dohlman CH: Glaucoma following keratoplasty. Trans Am Acad Ophthalmol Otolaryngol 1974;78:352.
72. Threlkeld AB, Shields MB: Non-contact transscleral Nd:YAG cyclophotocoagulation for glaucoma after penetrating keratoplasty. Am J Ophthalmol 1995;120:569.
73. Zaidman GW, Wandel T: Transscleral YAG laser photocoagulation for uncontrolled glaucoma in corneal patients. Cornea 1988;7:112.
74. Al Ghamdi S, al Obeidan S, Tomey KF, et al.: Transscleral neodymium:YAG laser cyclophotocoagulation for end-stage glaucoma, refractory glaucoma, and painful blind eyes. Ophthalmic Surg 1993;24:526.
75. Maus M, Katz LJ: Choroidal detachment, flat anterior chamber and hypotony as complications of Nd:YAG laser cyclophotocoagulation. Ophthalmology 1990;97:69.
76. Levy NS, Bonney RC: Transscleral YAG cyclocoagulation of the ciliary body for persistently high IOP following penetrating keratoplasty. Cornea 1989;8:178.

77. Fiore PM, Melamed S, Krug JH Jr: Focal scleral thinning after transscleral Nd:YAG cyclophotocoagulation. Ophthalmic Surg 1989;20:215.
78. Hamard P, Kopel J, Valtot F, et al.: Traitement des glaucomes refractaires par cyclophotocoagulation au laser semiconducteur a diode. J Fr Ophtalmol 1995;18:447.
79. Edward DP, Brown SVL, Higginbotham E, et al.: Sympathetic ophthalmia following neodymium:YAG cyclotherapy. Ophthalmic Surg 1989;20:544.
80. Brown SVL, Higginbotham E, Tessler H: Sympathetic ophthalmia following Nd:YAG cyclotherapy. Ophthalmic Surg 1990;21:736.
81. Lam S, Tessler HH, Lam BL, et al.: High incidence of sympathetic ophthalmia after contact and noncontact neodymium:YAG cyclotherapy. Ophthalmology 1992;99:1818.
82. Pastor SA, Iwach A, Nozik RA, et al.: Presumed sympathetic ophthalmia following Nd:YAG transscleral cyclophotocoagulation. J Glaucoma 1993;2:30.
83. Brancato R, Leoni G, Trabucchi G, et al.: Contact transscleral cyclophotocoagulation with Nd:YAG laser in uncontrolled glaucoma. Ophthalmic Surg 1989;20:547.
84. Schuman JS, Puliafito CA, Allingham RR, et al.: Contact transscleral continuous wave neodymium:YAG laser cyclophotocoagulation. Ophthalmology 1990;97:571.
85. Schuman JS, Bellows AR, Shingleton BJ, et al.: Contact transscleral Nd:YAG laser cyclophotocoagulation. Midterm results. Ophthalmology 1992;99:1089.
86. Brancato R, Carassa RG, Bettin P, et al.: Contact transscleral cyclophotocoagulation with diode laser in refractory glaucoma. Eur J Ophthalmol 1995;1:32.
87. Bloom M, Weber PA: Probe orientation in contact Nd:YAG laser cyclophotocoagulation. Ophthalmic Surg 1992;23:364.
88. Kosoko O, Gaasterland DE, Pollack IP, et al.: Long-term outcome of initial ciliary ablation with contact diode laser transscleral cyclophotocoagulation for severe glaucoma. Ophthalmology 1996;103:1294.
89. Kermani O, Mons B, Kirchhof B, et al.: Contact cw Nd:YAG laser cyclophotocoagulation for treatment of refractory glaucoma. Ger J Ophthalmol 1992;1:74.
90. Seah SK, Jap A, Min G: Contact transscleral cyclophotocoagulation for end stage glaucoma. Ann Acad Med Singapore 1994;23:18.
91. Kopel J, Valtot F, Poirier C, et al.: Traitement des glaucomes refractaires par cyclophotocoagulation au laser Nd:YAG. J Fr Ophtalmol 1995;18:13.
92. Carassa RG, Brancato R, Bettin P, et al.: Contact transscleral cyclophotocoagulation (CTCP) with diode laser: a long-term follow-up study. Invest Ophthalmol Vis Sci 1996;37(Suppl):261.
93. Bloom PA, Tsai JC, Sharma K, et al.: "Cyclodiode." Trans-scleral diode laser cyclophotocoagulation in the treatment of advanced refractory glaucoma. Ophthalmology 1997;104:1508.
94. Bock CJ, Freedman SF, Buckley EG, et al.: Transscleral diode laser cyclophotocoagulation for refractory pediatric glaucomas. J Pediatr Ophthalmol Strabismus 1997;34:235.
95. Schlote T, Kreutzer B, Kriegerowski M, et al.: Diode laser cyclophotocoagulation in treatment of therapy refractory glaucoma. Klin Monatsbl Augenheilkd 1997;211:250.
96. Yap-Veloso MI, Simmons RB, Echelman DA, et al.: Intraocular pressure control after contact transscleral diode cyclophotocoagulation in eyes with intractable glaucoma. J Glaucoma 1998;7:319.
97. Threlkeld AB, Johnson MH: Contact transscleral diode cyclophotocoagulation for refractory glaucoma. J Glaucoma 1999;8:3.
98. Spencer AF, Vernon SA: "Cyclodiode": results of a standard protocol. Br J Ophthalmol 1999;83:311.
99. Rebolleda G, Munoz FJ, Murube J: Audible pops during cyclodiode procedures. J Glaucoma 1999;8:177.
100. Youn J, Cox TA, Herndon LW, et al.: A clinical comparison of transscleral cyclophotocoagulation with neodymium:YAG and semiconductor diode lasers. Am J Ophthalmol 1998;126:640.
101. Oguri A, Takahashi E, Tomita G, et al.: Transscleral cyclophotocoagulation with the diode laser for neovascular glaucoma.Ophthalmic Surg Lasers 1998;29:722.
102. Gaasterland DE, Pollack IP: Initial experience with a new method of laser transscleral cyclophotocoagulation for ciliary ablation in severe glaucoma. Trans Am Ophthalmol Soc 1992;90:225.
103. Beadles KA, Smith MF: Inadvertent sclerostomy during transscleral Nd:YAG cyclophotocoagulation. Am J Ophthalmol 1994; 118:669.
104. Verdi M, Carassa RG, Bettin P, et al.: Does diode laser contact transscleral cyclophotocoagulation produce sclera thinning? An ultrasound biomicroscopical in vivo study on human eyes. Invest Ophthalmol Vis Sci 1995;36:S565.
105. Azuara-Blanco A, Dua HS: Malignant glaucoma after diode laser cyclophotocoagulation. Am J Ophthalmol 1999;127:467.
106. Werner A, Vick HP, Guthoff R: Cyclophotocoagulation with the diode laser. Study of long-term results. Ophthalmologe 1998;95:176.
107. Lee PF: Argon laser photocoagulation of the ciliary processes in cases of aphakic glaucoma. Arch Ophthalmol 1979;97:2135.
108. Kim DD, Moster MR: Transpupillary argon laser cyclophotocoagulation in the treatment of traumatic glaucoma. Glaucoma 1999;8:340.
109. Lee PF, Shihab Z, Eberle M: Partial ciliary process laser photocoagulation in the management of glaucoma. Lasers Surg Med 1980;1:85.
110. Shields S, Steward WC, Shields MB: Transpupillary argon laser cyclophotocoagulation in the treatment of glaucoma. Ophthalmic Surg 1988;19:171.
111. Patel A, Thompson JT, Michaels RG, et al.: Endolaser treatment of the ciliary body for uncontrolled glaucoma. Ophthalmology 1986;93:825.
112. Zarbin MA, Michels RS, DeBistros S, et al.: Endolaser treatment of the ciliary body for severe glaucoma. Ophthalmology 1988;95:1639.
113. Cohen EJ, Schwartz LW, Luskind RD, et al.: Neodymium:YAG laser transscleral cyclophotocoagulation for glaucoma after penetrating keratoplasty. Ophthalmic Surg 1989;20:713.
114. Plager DA, Neely DE: Intermediate-term results of endoscopic diode laser cyclophotocoagulation for pediatric glaucoma. J AAPOS 1999;3:131.

CHAPTER 37

Cyclocryotherapy

GEORGE L. SPAETH, M.D.

Cyclocryotherapy causes necrosis of the secretory cells of the ciliary epithelium; this reduces inflow of aqueous humor and lowers intraocular pressure. This destruction of tissue is also the explanation for the side effects and complications of cyclocryotherapy, as well as for its beneficial actions.

INDICATIONS

Cyclocryotherapy has played an important part in the management of patients with glaucoma in the past. However, since the advent of neodymium:YAG laser cyclophotocoagulation, cyclocryotherapy is seldom used. Where neodymium:YAG laser cyclophotocoagulation is not available, cyclocryotherapy still plays an important role in the management of patients with glaucoma.

The ideal candidate for cyclocryotherapy is an elderly patient (over 65 years of age) with an aphakic condition, advanced visual damage, previous failures with other glaucoma procedures, and poor likelihood of success with other procedures. Specific indications are the presence of neovascular glaucoma with secondary angle closure, other secondary angle-closure glaucoma, aphakic glaucomas, or inflammatory glaucomas. Cyclocryotherapy is not usually indicated in young people unless vision is seriously threatened by the glaucoma and other types of glaucoma surgery do not have a reasonable chance of succeeding.

Approximately 80 percent of cases will have successful regulation of intraocular pressure; the incidence of serious complications is at least 5 percent.

The presence of the crystalline lens within the eye is not an absolute contraindication to cyclocryotherapy. However, the likelihood of cataract developing is sufficiently high that I select cyclocryotherapy in phakic patients only when the likelihood of another procedure's succeeding is negligible.

In active neovascular glaucoma, cyclocryotherapy is a useful procedure when neodymium:YAG laser cyclophotocoagulation is not available.

When a patient wants to retain his eye despite an absolute glaucoma, cyclocryotherapy combined with a retrobulbar alcohol block may relieve pain yet preserve the globe.

Before performing a cyclocryotherapeutic procedure the surgeon should inform the patient that the procedure is a destructive one and that even when properly performed, it may result in loss of the eye in a small percentage of cases. The patient is also told that he can expect pain immediately after the procedure; this pain can vary from mild to excruciating, and is usually severe. In rare cases the pain persists for such a long time that the patient is unable to tolerate it. When this occurs, the cause is usually subchoroidal hemorrhage, which can be treated successfully. The cause for the persistent decrease in vision may be persistent uveitis, anterior chamber or vitreous hemorrhage, progressive cataract, or macular edema. Macular edema is probably rare except in cases in which excessive hypotony has developed.

ANESTHESIA

The conjunctiva is anesthetized with topical proparacaine 0.5% instilled several times over a period of 5 minutes. A retrobulbar block using 3 ml of a long-acting injectable anesthetic agent usually provides adequate anesthesia of the globe. In extremely apprehensive patients or those likely to squeeze the lids shut tightly during the procedure, a block of the facial nerve may be helpful. General anesthesia is seldom necessary.

TABLE 37–1. Complications of Retrobulbar Block with Absolute Alcohol

Pain
Swelling
Persistent anesthesia of periorbital region
Ptosis
Strabismus owing to extraocular muscle palsy
Failure to relieve pain

When the primary indication for performing cyclocryotherapy is relief of pain, retrobulbar alcohol should be used. In such circumstances 0.5 to 1.0 ml of anesthetic agent is injected first, followed by 1 ml of absolute alcohol, injected through the same needle. The alcohol should be injected slowly. The needle is then flushed with 0.25 ml of anesthetic.

Patients to be treated with retrobulbar alcohol should be warned of the potential complications (Table 37–1). When the goal of the cyclocryotherapy is to control intraocular pressure, but in addition the surgeon hopes to minimize pain in the immediate postoperative period, a reduced concentration of alcohol can be administered. In such circumstances administration of 2 ml of anesthetic agent followed by 0.5 ml of alcohol injected through the same needle will often be associated with decreased pain and will not necessarily have a deleterious effect on the postoperative vision. In patients in whom visual acuity is normal and the sole purpose of the cyclocryotherapy is to control intraocular pressure, the simultaneous use of alcohol with the retrobulbar injection is probably inadvisable.

PREOPERATIVE TREATMENT

Pretreatment with steroids and prostaglandin inhibitors may reduce the postoperative inflammation and rise in pressure. A potent topical steroid such as prednisolone acetate 1% may be used every hour for four doses, and aspirin, two 5-gr tablets (one 4 hours and one a half hour preoperatively), may be taken. Atropine may be given preoperatively.

The degree of pain after cyclocryotherapy may be severe. This may be associated with nausea, vomiting, or even shock. If these complications cannot be adequately managed in an outpatient setting, the patient is probably best hospitalized. The great majority of patients treated on the Glaucoma Service of the Wills Eye Hospital are hospitalized on the first day of treatment and are usually discharged from the hospital 2 days later. Cyclocryotherapy need not be performed in the operating room.

SURGICAL TECHNIQUE

The use of a speculum to separate the lids facilitates the procedure slightly but is not essential.

Cryotherapy instruments are clearly not identical; even those designed to have a tip capable of reaching temperatures as low as −70° or −80° C have some variance. The size of the tip, the shape of the probe, the rapidity with which the cold temperature is achieved, the absolute level of temperature reached, and the rate of thaw all vary from instrument to instrument, and each of these factors influences the nature of the damage caused to the eye by the freezing. In the Glaucoma Service of the Wills Eye Hospital equal success has not been obtained with all instruments. The following technique refers to the portable Kryo-Med, manufactured by Cryomedics Inc. Other machines undoubtedly can be used with equal success. However, the program outlined here applies to the Kryo-Med instrument.

The valve is adjusted so that the pressure of nitrous oxide is 600 pounds per square inch. This results in a temperature of −80° C at the tip of the probe. The machine is tested before giving the retrobulbar anesthetic block. After adequate anesthesia has been achieved the probe is applied to the conjunctiva 3 mm posterior to the limbus at the 12 o'clock position on the globe. The foot pedal is pressed to activate the freezing. The development of the iceball is watched. After approximately 45 seconds the first iceball will reach its maximum size. The probe is pushed moderately firmly against the globe so that the entire globe is depressed several millimeters into the orbit.

After the iceball has reached its maximum size, or starts to reach into the edge of the cornea the freezing is stopped. If the probe has been placed too close to the cornea, so that it appears that a larger iceball can be achieved, but only by having the iceball extend into the cornea further, then the freezing should be stopped and the probe placed more posteriorly, further away from the limbus. The freezing is then reactivated. After the iceball has reached its maximum, freezing is continued for an additional 15 seconds. The total freezing time, then, is usually between 45 seconds and 1 minute.

Eight applications are made. The initial site of application is at the 12 o'clock position. The second application is at 3 o'clock, the third application at 6 o'clock, the fourth at 9 o'clock, the fifth at 1:30, the sixth at 4:30, the seventh at 7:30, and the eighth and final application at the 10:30 position. The duration of freezing is approximately the same for each application. However, as subsequent applications are made, the rapidity with which the iceball is produced appears to increase. Consequently the last several applications may require less time than the first few.

The iceball that develops from the technique described is usually large enough to freeze almost the entire circumference of the globe posterior to the limbus. An area of approximately 2 mm between each application site will not be involved.

It is not usually necessary to irrigate the tip of the probe in order to hasten warming and permit more rapid removal of the probe from the globe. However, one must be certain that the probe is not adherent to the globe before it is pulled away.

Immediately after the freezing treatment the intraocular pressure of the globe should be determined, as a precipitous increase is not infrequent. If the intraocular pressure has increased to a level suggesting that the optic nerve will be damaged, immediate steps to lower the pressure need to be instituted. Intravenous acetazolamide, so helpful in patients with acute-angle glaucoma, is seldom adequate in these cases, and intravenous mannitol or another osmotic agent in appropriate doses usually needs to be administered immediately. An even more rapidly effective technique is to perform a paracentesis. The effect of this is usually only temporary, but it relieves the urgent problem. Even if the intraocular pressure is not in a range suggesting that further optic nerve damage will occur, osmotic agents should almost always be given as a routine part of the postoperative care of patients with cyclocryotherapy.

POSTOPERATIVE CARE

The three major complications after cyclocryotherapy are pain, transient elevation of intraocular pressure, and late but persistent hypotony. The pain can be excruciating. Some patients have stated that the discomfort caused by cyclocryotherapy exceeds that associated with childbirth or the passage of a renal stone. Other patients have remarkably less pain. Pretreatment with steroids and aspirin appears to decrease the postoperative reaction, including the amount of discomfort. Aspirin, two tablets every 4 hours, is prescribed as a standing order. For patients who suffer from gastrointestinal distress caused by aspirin, the buffered product may be used. A more potent analgesic such as propoxyphene (Darvon) every 4 hours is often required. Some patients may require a narcotic agent. The pain first becomes noticeable as the retrobulbar anesthesia wears off approximately 8 to 12 hours after the procedure. If a short-acting anesthetic agent is used, the pain will reach its peak about 6 hours postoperatively. It is for this reason that the long-acting agents bupivacaine and etidocaine are so strongly preferred. By 18 hours postoperatively the pain usually starts to wane. In most cases the discomfort is mild 24 hours after the freezing, unless a complication has occurred. In about a fourth of the cases some pain will persist for up to 1 week in variable and unpredictable amounts. A dull ache may last for months. Most patients will have no significant persisting discomfort. Aspirin is usually continued for approximately 1 week, both for reduction of the inflammatory response caused by the freezing and for relief of pain.

In rare cases the pain caused by a cryotherapeutic procedure may be excruciating, and may continue to be intolerable. It is a mistake to assume that this severe discomfort is necessarily related to elevation of intraocular pressure. Rather, it is usually a sign of a suprachoroidal hemorrhage, which is apparently a response to the tissue destruction. Ultrasound examination should be performed to verify this. Drainage of the hemorrhage usually results in immediate relief of the severe pain, though a moderate ache usually persists. When hemorrhage is suspected and pain persists the drainage should be done promptly; organization of a clot may have occurred, but even if it has, partial removal of the blood is still helpful.

Although the *intraocular pressure* may fall immediately in response to cyclocryotherapy, usually it rises several hours after the freezing. This is such a routine occurrence that a full dose of an osmotic agent such as mannitol 20%, 7 mm/kg body weight, is ordered routinely 1½ hours after performance of the cyclocryotherapy. The oral agents may be used, but tend to cause nausea at a time when the patient is already uncomfortable. Intraocular pressure is checked approximately 4 to 6 hours after the procedure, and osmotic agents are repeated as appropriate. In cases in which the optic nerve is already seriously damaged and the goal of the cyclocryotherapy is to preserve vision, attention to this intraocular pressure rise must be especially vigilant.

Intraocular pressure usually remains elevated for approximately 24 hours. During this period it may also be helpful to use a carbonic anhydrase inhibitor in addition to the osmotic agent, in order to keep the intraocular pressure within a satisfactory level. The intraocular pressure should have started to fall by 36 hours after performance of the cyclocryotherapy. It often reaches its lowest point about 3 days after the procedure. This low pressure level will persist for 1 to 3 weeks before a gradual rise again occurs; the intraocular pressure stabilizes somewhere around 1 month after the cyclocryotherapy. The postoperative course and the intraocular pressure will be related to the extent of postoperative course and the intraocular pressure will be related to the extent of postoperative uveitis and choroidal detachment; the former is always present and the latter is seen in most cases, and often persists for months or years.

Approximately 60 per cent of cases other than neovascular glaucoma will have a satisfactory reduction of intraocular pressure. Nevertheless, intraocular pressure must be carefully monitored during this period and appropriate medications ordered to regulate the intraocular pressure.

If intraocular pressure has not fallen by 48 hours postoperatively, it is unlikely that the response to the surgery will be adequate. Topical glaucoma medications are not usually used during the first few days, although timolol 0.5% every 12 hours may be added. After the second day, if it appears that the control of intraocular pressure will not be satisfactory, osmotic agents should be stopped and the patient's pressure controlled if possible with tolerable doses of carbonic anhydrase inhibitors and topical timolol. Epinephrine hydrochloride twice daily may be added. Pilocarpine and other miotics should be avoided in the inflammatory glaucomas; even in the noninflammatory aphakic glaucomas pilocarpine usually has little beneficial effect on the intraocular pressure until the uveitic reaction produced by the freezing has abated.

If after 3 days the intraocular pressure is so high that the surgeon believes that permanent damage to the optic nerve is imminent, the cyclocryotherapy may be repeated, using four to eight applications. Preparation of the patient and postoperative care are essentially the same after a reoperation as for the first procedure.

If the intraocular pressure is not brought under control even after the second cyclocryotherapy, the situation is serious. The surgeon has few viable options. Standard filtration procedures are doomed to failure because of the extreme inflammatory response secondary to the tissue destruction. The likelihood of excessive bleeding and the certainty of failure for response to a standard cyclodialysis are so great as to contraindicate that procedure. The results of the third cyclocryotherapy are highly unpredictable, ranging from no effect on intraocular pressure to the condition of phthisis bulbi. Probably the best coarse is to pull out all the stops of medical therapy and try to regulate the intraocular pressure with drugs without making the patient too ill. If this is not possible, the patient is presented with the unpleasant choice of losing his vision as a result of the continued elevation of pressure, gambling with a repeat cyclocryotherapy, or, usually most appropriate, having a shunt procedure such as a Molteno implant.

TABLE 37–2. Complications of Cyclocryotherapy

1. Inflammation
2. Rise of intraocular pressure
3. Pain
   a. Secondary to uveitis
   b. Secondary to suprachoroidal hemorrhage
4. Reduced vision
   a. Secondary to uveitis
   b. Secondary to hypotony
   c. Secondary to intraocular hemorrhage
5. Intraocular bleeding
6. Cataract
7. Hypotony
   a. Secondary to excessive tissue destruction
   b. Secondary to ciliary and choroidal detachment
8. Scleral staphyloma
9. Anterior segment necrosis
10. Phthisis bulbi

Strong anti-inflammatory medications, such as atropine and prednisolone acetate, are given frequently in the immediately postoperative period and are continued in a four-times-a-day dosage for 2 to 3 weeks postoperatively. As the inflammation regresses, the dosages should be tapered. Because the inflammation persists for months, it may be necessary to continue anti-inflammatory therapy for a prolonged period. In such cases an agent less likely to cause elevation, such as fluorometholone, may be beneficial. Prednisolone acetate or fluorometholone with or without atropine may have to be continued for many months. The more inflamed the eye before the cryotherapy, the more likely it is that inflammation after the procedure will prove a problem. Systemic or periocular steroids may help in some cases.

Bleeding into the anterior chamber or the vitreous may occur. So long as the globe does not become hypotonous, this blood is usually absorbed rapidly from the anterior chamber and more gradually, but satisfactorily, from the vitreous. However, if the eye is hypotonous, this adjustment will not occur, and treatment is required. Treatment of the eye with hypotony is conservative, although anti-inflammatory compounds may need to be used for a longer period of time than when this complication has not occurred.

Total anterior segment necrosis may occur. However, this is extremely rare, even in cases in which cyclocryotherapy has been applied over 360 degrees at one sitting. It is probably more common in patients in whom there is already an embarrassed circulation, such as diabetics. There is probably no effective treatment, although administration of topical corticosteroids and antiprostaglandin inhibitors is logical therapy.

Cataract is an expected outcome of cyclocryotherapy in the phakic patient.

Hypotony is the most dreaded complication, as there is no effective treatment. Unfortunately performing "small" cryotherapies is not the solution to the problem. Inadequate treatment causes severe uveitis but inadequate decrease of inflow, with consequent elevation of pressure in some cases. We have found initial treatment of 360 degrees a satisfactory approach, with fewer

TABLE 37–3. Comparison of Cyclodestructive Procedures

Factor	Cyclocryotherapy	Transscleral Neodymium:YAG	Therapeutic Ultrasound
Cost	Low	Moderate	High
Special equipment	No	Yes	Yes
Availability	Great	Good	Low
Portability of equipment	Easy	Easy	No
Experience in technique	Much	Moderate	Small
Morbidity	High	Low	Moderate
Ease of performance	Easy	Easy	Hard
Effectiveness	Good	Good	Fair
Serious complications	Frequent	Rare	Common
Postoperative inflammation			
External	Marked	Mild	Marked
Internal	Marked	Moderate	Mild

complications and greater success than is achieved when treating only 180 degrees.

The success rate of cyclocryotherapy appears to be lower and the rate of complications higher in patients with neovascular glaucoma than in those with most other conditions, although literature provides disparate findings in this regard. However, surgeon and patient alike should be aware that the success rate in these cases is probably only about 50 percent. Nevertheless, the surgeon is encouraged to be aggressive in these cases. The health of the disc is difficult to evaluate because of the neovascularity. Blindness can occur rapidly as a result of the glaucoma, even when pressure elevation is moderate.

In summary, as with cyclodialysis, cyclocryotherapy often works either too poorly or too well. Although cyclocryotherapy does have some success, the high incidence of serious complications that develop as a result of the procedure is discouraging (Table 37–2). I now almost never use cyclocryotherapy, preferring methods to develop filtration, or, when a cyclodestructive procedure is appropriate, a neodymium:YAG cyclophotocoagulation (Table 37–3). Cyclocryotherapy is included in this text because cyclophotocoagulation is not yet available everywhere.

Cyclophotocoagulation. This procedure is described in detail in the following section on laser surgery.

CHAPTER 38

Trabeculotomy

RONALD L. FELLMAN, M.D.

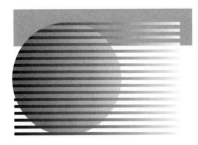

Rather than divert aqueous humor externally as in trabeculectomy, trabeculotomy ab externo is designed to interiorize a maldeveloped or dysfunctional iridocorneal angle, thereby decreasing resistance and increasing outflow through natural channels (Fig. 38–1). Allen and Burian first described trabeculotomy ab externo in 1960,[1] followed by Smith[2] in 1962. Harms[3,4] improved the technique by popularizing the identification of Schlemm's canal under a scleral flap with microsurgical techniques. Lynn[5] and others[6] designed metal trabeculotomes to improve the microsurgical opening of Schlemm's canal. Trabeculotomy is most commonly used in the management of pediatric glaucomas, but it still holds a place in the treatment of adult glaucomas.

The goal of trabeculotomy is to increase outflow by cleaving the site of greatest outflow resistance, the inner wall of Schlemm's canal and adjacent trabecular meshwork. This is accomplished with either a rigid metal trabeculotome (Fig. 38–2 *A* and *B*) or a flexible suture trabeculotome (Fig. 38–3 *A, B,* and *C*). Standard rigid metal trabeculotomes have a number of limitations. Often, they do not fit the curvature of the eye, preventing proper canalization of Schlemm's canal. This leads to the creation of unwanted passages, unnecessary cyclodialyses, premature entry into the anterior chamber, excessive bleeding, and a false assurance of actual probing of Schlemm's canal. With standard rigid trabeculotomes, it is difficult to know with 100% accuracy that the surgeon is actually in Schlemm's canal before entering the anterior chamber. To avoid these problems, to locate Schlemm's canal unequivocally, and to reduce multiple anesthetics, a modification of Redmond Smith's original method of filamentary trabeculotomy was investigated[7] and later improved upon.[8] The entire circumference of the chamber angle is opened in a single operation, and at the same time the exact location of Schlemm's canal is verified. The surgeon should be facile with both rigid and flexible trabeculotomes.

EVALUATION OF THE PEDIATRIC PATIENT

Trabeculotomy is most commonly performed in the pediatric age group. This group requires special consideration because the evaluation and management of an infant with suspected glaucoma is an especially difficult task for all involved. Limited patient cooperation, a difficult office examination, parental apprehension, complex surgery, and the fear of a lifetime of blindness complicate the situation. The surgical skills of goniotomy, trabeculotomy, and examination under anesthesia (EUA) are difficult to master because the condition is uncommon, occurring in one of 10,000 to 15,000 live births. Even the most gifted surgeons may struggle with some aspect of pediatric glaucoma care.

Pediatric glaucomas encompass a challenging diverse group of ocular and systemic abnormalities ultimately requiring physician teamwork and perhaps

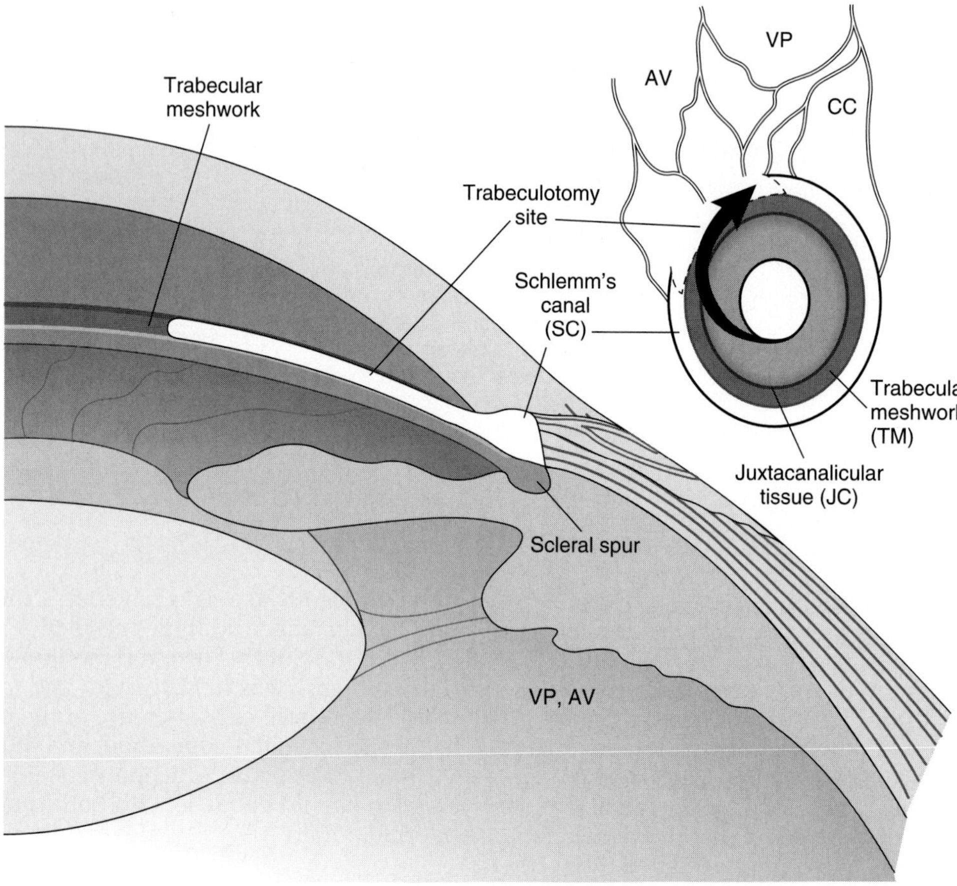

Figure 38–1. Outflow system and trabeculotomy site. Normal outflow resistance is approximately distributed in the following fashion: 60% in the trabecular meshwork (TM) and juxtacanalicular tissue (JC), 25% in Schlemm's canal (SC) and immediate collector systems, and 15% in the scleral collector system (CC). The trabecular meshwork is 750 microns in width, Schlemm's canal is 36 mm in circumference with an average width of 300 microns, and roughly 30 collector channels connect the canal to the venous plexus (VP). Approximately 6 to 8 aqueous veins (AV) exit Schlemm's canal and bypass the collector channels directly connecting to the venous plexus. Trabeculotomy is designed to decrease the area of greatest resistance to outflow by cleaving the TM, JC tissue and trabecular meshwork (black curved arrow). The major advantage over trabeculectomy is the lack of bleb formation. Successful trabeculotomy reestablishes drainage downstream into the episcleral collector system.

A

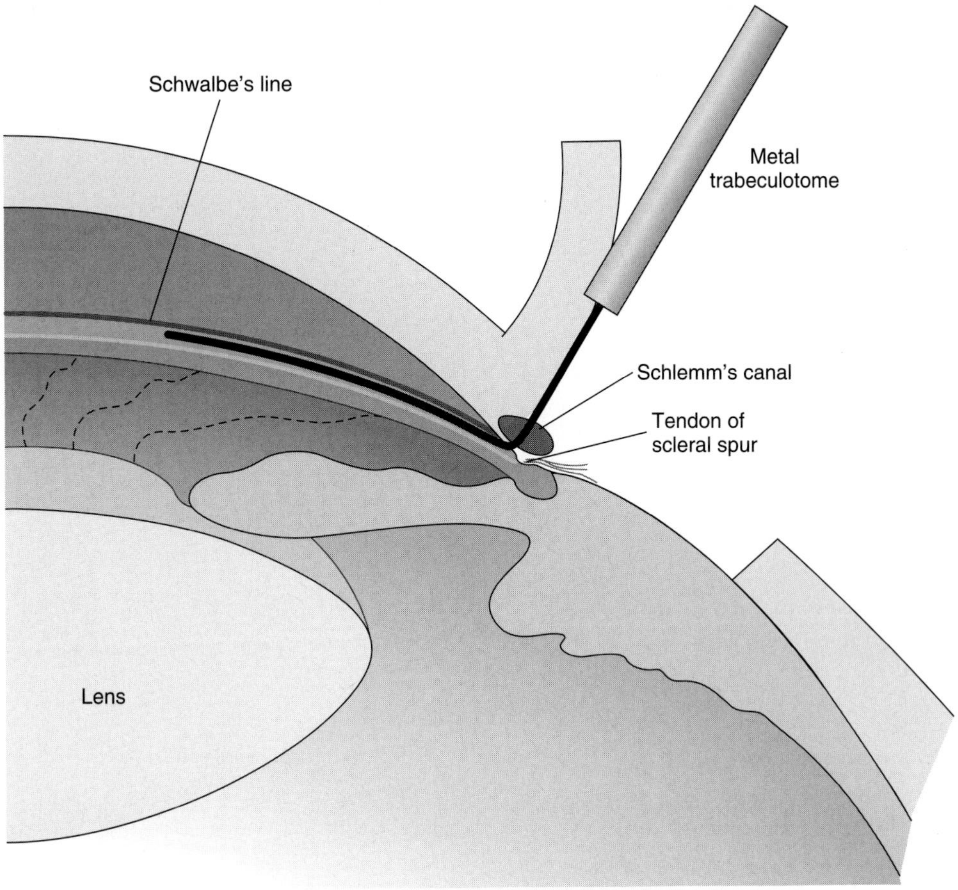

B

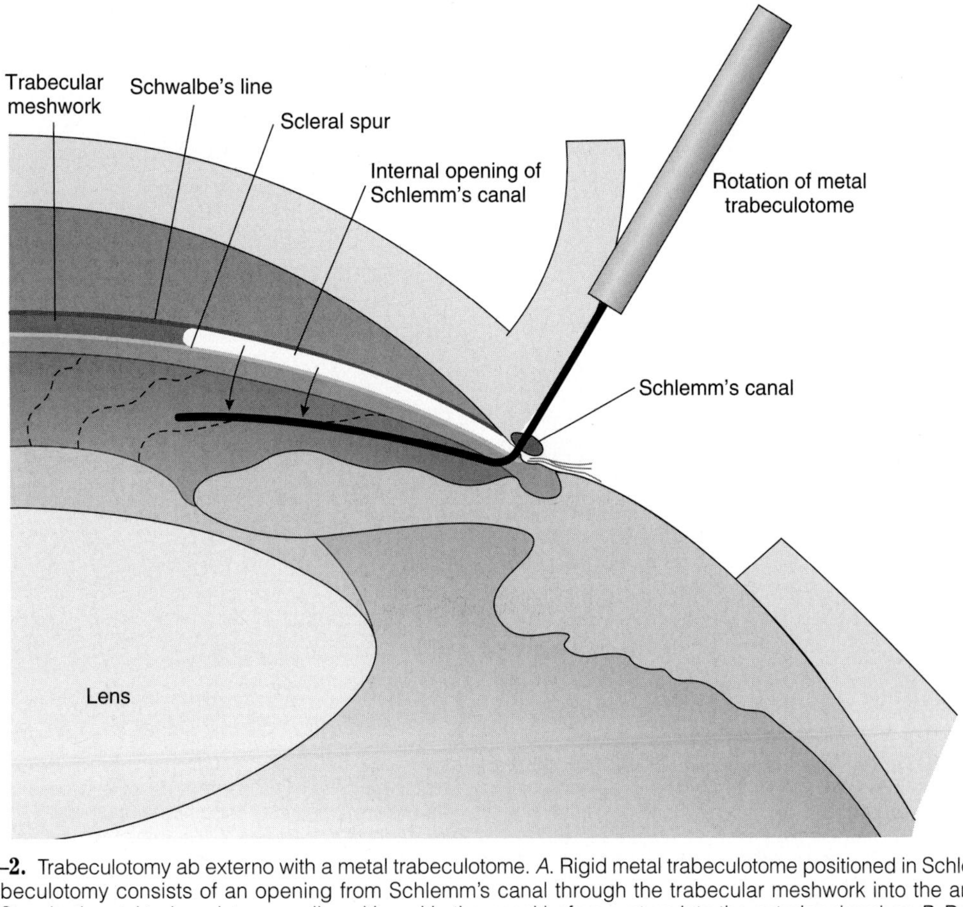

Figure 38–2. Trabeculotomy ab externo with a metal trabeculotome. *A*. Rigid metal trabeculotome positioned in Schlemm's canal. Trabeculotomy consists of an opening from Schlemm's canal through the trabecular meshwork into the anterior chamber. Standard metal trabeculotome well positioned in the canal before rupture into the anterior chamber. *B*. Rotation with rupture through the inner wall of Schlemm's canal and trabecular meshwork. Limitations of rigid trabeculotomes include creation of false passageways, premature angle entry, inability to accurately follow the curvature of the eye, and incapacity to open the entire angle at one sitting. The trabeculotome can be seen sweeping into the angle.

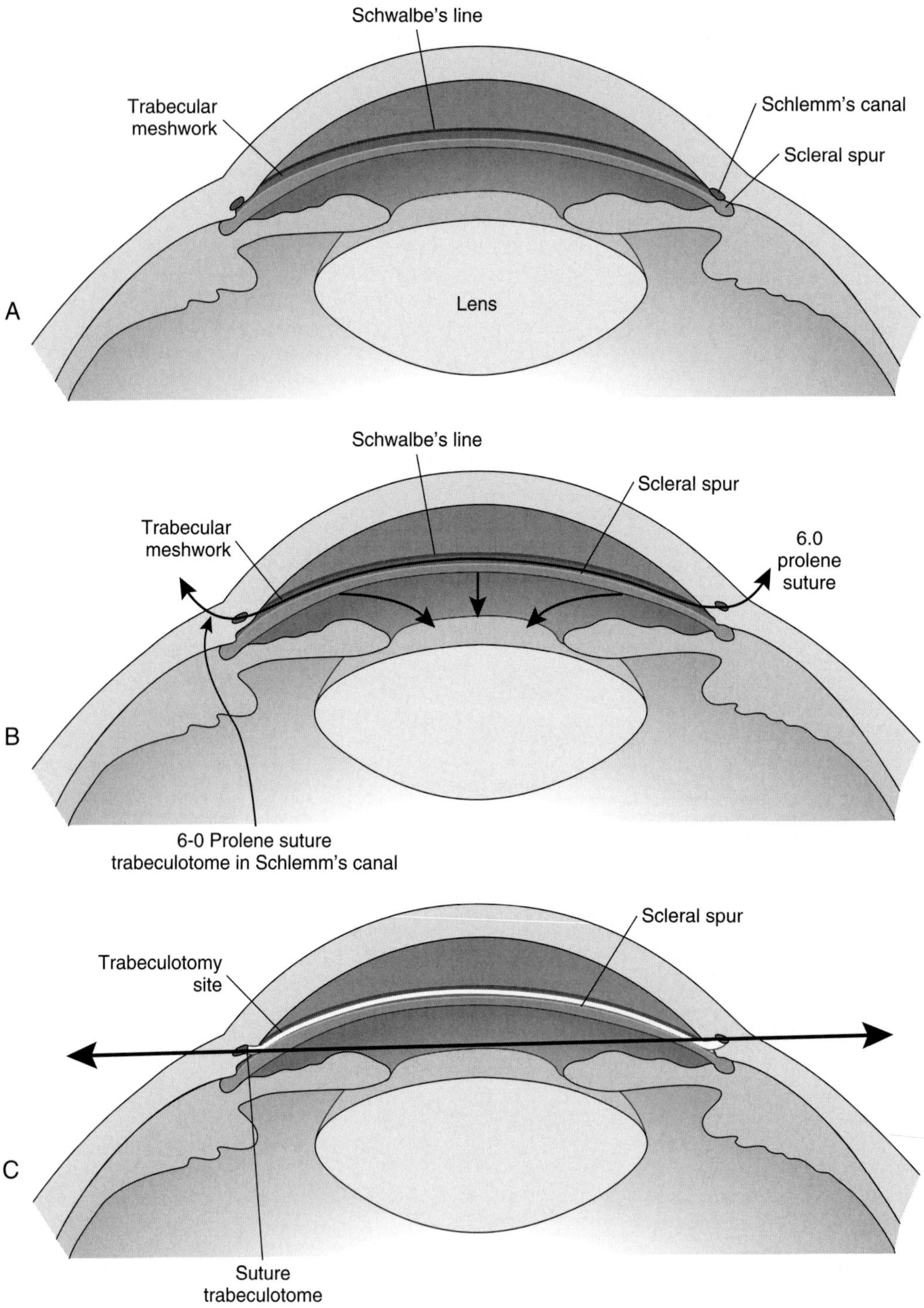

Figure 38–3. Filamentary trabeculotomy ab externo. *A.* Chamber angle before trabeculotomy. It is imperative to have a scholarly knowledge of angle anatomy with an appreciation of all the landmarks. Schlemm's canal is located between the scleral spur and Schwalbe's line. *B.* Chamber angle with filament (suture) in place prior to trabeculotomy. A 6-0 blue prolene suture is threaded into the canal for 360 degrees or, in this example, 180 degrees. *C.* Chamber angle after filamentary trabeculotomy. The ends of the suture are grasped and pulled apart, cleaving open the angle.

multiple microsurgical therapies. Approximately two-thirds of the glaucomas of childhood are primary developmental anomalies of the outflow system, and the remaining secondary glaucomas are more complex anterior segment dilemmas, yielding poorer prognoses.[9] The treatment of infantile (less than 3 years of age) and juvenile glaucoma is largely surgical. Microsurgical therapy revolves around trabeculotomy and goniotomy, two equally effective[10] anterior chamber angle procedures designed to improve outflow by incising and uncovering a maldeveloped anterior chamber outflow system. Visual prognosis depends on the surgeon's ability to accurately incise the iridocorneal angle, the age of onset, and the type of disease. When the glaucoma presents at birth or within the first month of life, the prognosis is significantly worsened because goniotomy and trabeculotomy are equally ineffective procedures in neonates, with success rates of 30% to 50%. Prognosis dramatically improves when the disease presents between 2 months of age and 3 years, yielding 70% up to 100% success for goniotomy or trabeculotomy, although several angle procedures may be included in overall success rates.

Goniotomy is a transcorneal ab interno method of incising the iridocorneal angle with a goniotomy blade. It is an effective method of pressure reduction,[11,12] yet limitations include difficulty incising the tissues when the cornea is cloudy, the necessity to repeat the procedure, and inability to open the entire chamber angle at one sitting. Some of these limitations are overcome with standard trabeculotomy. Trabeculotomy is an ab externo approach to angle surgery designed to uncover, cannulate, and open Schlemm's canal and adjacent trabecular tissue. However, even rigid metal trabeculotomes designed for standard trabeculotomy do not guarantee that the surgeon has correctly identified Schlemm's canal. An alternative to rigid trabeculotomes is filamentary full circumference trabeculotomy, upon which the entire procedure hinges on the surgeon's ability to accurately identify and fully cannulate the canal for 360 degrees. The recovery of the trabeculotome suture from the canal a considerable distance from the initial canal entry site unequivocally reassures the surgeon of the exact location of Schlemm's canal.

PATHOPHYSIOLOGY

Classification of anterior chamber angle anomalies is instrumental in determining surgical prognosis. Developmental defects of the chamber angle typically fall into three categories: (1) high insertion of anterior uvea, (2) incomplete development of outflow systems, and (3) iridocorneal adhesions. It is important to classify the glaucoma properly, for prognosis is inherently intertwined with diagnosis. The apparent abnormality in most developmental glaucomas is a cleavage problem between the trabecular meshwork and iris root–ciliary body. Anderson[13] states that the iris and ciliary body fail to recede posteriorly, causing the anterior uvea to overlap the trabecular meshwork. In addition, histologic abnormalities[14] include compressed and thickened trabecular beams with a narrowing of trabecular spaces. Schlemm's canal does not appear to be the site of obstruction to aqueous outflow in congenital glaucoma.[15] This is clinically demonstrated after successful goniotomy, where the site of incision varies and Schlemm's canal may not be incised at all.

DIAGNOSIS

Signs and Symptoms

Any one or a combination of the signs or symptoms of photophobia, epiphora, blepharospasm, globe enlargement, elevated intraocular pressure, cloudy cornea, or optic nerve head cupping should arouse suspicion of pediatric glaucoma. The disease is easier to detect in infants with unilateral glaucoma (Fig. 38-4) where anatomic asymmetry brings rapid attention to the problem. The pediatrician may be the first to notice asymmetry of ocular growth, a cloudy cornea, or a problem with tearing. Occasionally a parent will notice intermittent clouding of the eye. Later in life, as in juvenile glaucoma, the disease is silent and detectable only with examination.

Typically, the diagnosis hinges on a combination of signs and symptoms. Increased corneal diameter, corneal haze or edema, increased cup–disc ratios, gonioscopic evidence of chamber angle abnormalities, tears in Descemet's membrane, family history, and abnormal intraocular pressure are all involved in making the diagnosis.

EXAMINATION

Examination techniques for infants and children are far more difficult than for adults and may be a frustrating experience. Cooperative parents are essential in en-

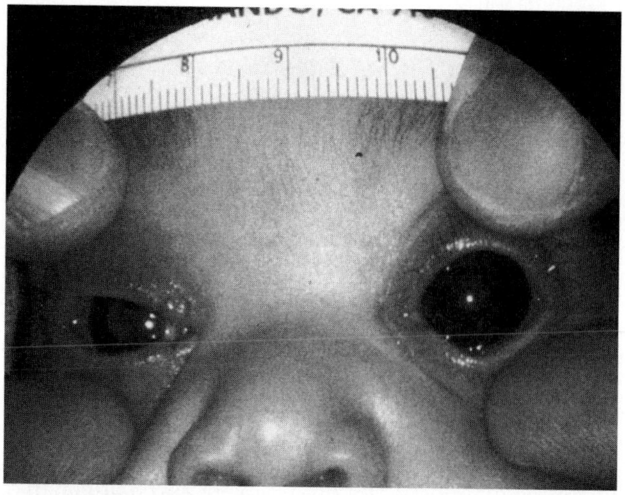

Figure 38–4. Unilateral buphthalmos. Globe enlargement secondary to elevated intraocular pressure is a hallmark of congenital glaucoma. When the disease is unilateral, the obvious asymmetry leads to an earlier diagnosis.

couraging their children to cooperate. A family history of developmental glaucoma or any of the above signs or symptoms are elicited. Occasionally, the diagnosis is obvious from across the room when the patient has unilateral buphthalmos with a cloudy cornea. In more subtle cases, the heart of the office examination is intraocular pressure, hand-held slit-lamp exam, and optic nerve analysis.

Office Examination

In infants younger than 6 months of age, a topical anesthetic is applied, and the eyelids are gently separated. With the infant cradled in a parent's arms and often asleep after a bottle-feeding, an accurate intraocular pressure measurement can be obtained with either a Perkins hand-held tonometer or Tonopen device. The ability to obtain an accurate intraocular pressure measurement in the office allows more definitive surgical planning. A hand-held portable slit-lamp device is especially useful in discovering anterior segment anomalies such as Haab's striae, corneal edema, iridocorneal adhesions, lenticular opacities, and iris abnormalities. A dilated pupil exam is essential to rule out other causes of glaucoma, especially rare pressure-producing tumors. Gross optic nerve head asymmetry may be detected even with low-illumination indirect ophthalmoscopy. The combination of an enlarged cornea, corneal edema, elevated intraocular pressure, and optic disc cupping are sufficient office evidence of the disease, and surgical planning may ensue. Traumatizing the infant will only make future examinations more difficult. An uncooperative patient may be more cooperative at a second visit, allowing additional data gathering for a more definitive diagnosis. However, the partial or incomplete office examination of a child with suspect glaucoma mandates an examination under anesthesia. Children may be coaxed into a slit-lamp exam by using different colored lights, distracting them by playing games with the slit-lamp handlebars (lawnmower, car driving, etc.), and having the patience to persist in the exam.

Examination Under Anesthesia

General anesthesia affords the physician the time and luxury of a thorough documented exam in the confines of the operating room. In a healthy child, there is little risk involved in the hands of an anesthesiologist experienced in dealing with infants. Children with multiple systemic abnormalities present more challenging risk-management problems and the consequences of an EUA may be more profound. Before this, consultation may be necessary before deciding on an appropriate course of action. A major problem with most general anesthetics is an unwanted reduction in intraocular pressure.

There are two types of EUA in infants and children, ketamine diagnostic/follow-up exam and halogenated anesthetics with diagnostic and planned surgery. For pure documentation purposes, ketamine is an excellent dissociative anesthetic administered intramuscularly or intravenously that allows general anesthesia without intubation or intraocular pressure reduction. Typically, anticholinergic agents are administered prior to the EUA to avoid excessive laryngeal secretions. In patients profoundly uncooperative in the office, in whom reliable intraocular pressure measurements have not been obtained, the diagnosis is in doubt, and a patient-physician-family bond has not been established, the situation may be best served by performing a straightforward ketamine diagnostic EUA without concomitant surgery. This type of exam is useful to establish a diagnosis or for follow-up evaluations after surgery. Some physicians prefer not to use ketamine in patients with seizure disorders. If the EUA indicates the need for surgery, the baseline clinical status is recorded and the procedure terminated. The appropriate amount of time can now be spent with family members. This is the best time to use diagrams to explain the type of glaucoma, the surgery to be performed, and the prognosis. Informed consent, risks, benefits, and alternatives of surgery are then reviewed. This is usually a lengthy discussion. Definitive surgery may be carried out within 24 to 72 hours and, if indicated, small doses of aqueous suppressants can be used to suppress the intraocular pressure. A cherry-flavored elixir of acetazolamide 10 mg/kg in 4 divided doses is useful to suppress aqueous production prior to surgery (10 kg infant = 100 mg, 25 mg per dose). If surgery is urgently indicated immediately following the EUA, some surgeons and anesthesiologists favor changing from ketamine to halogenated agents with endotracheal intubation and proceeding with the intraocular surgery.

Ketamine Diagnostic or Follow-up Examination Under Anesthesia

General anesthesia with halogenated gases may lower intraocular pressure rapidly.[16] Depending on the depth and time of anesthesia, intraocular pressures of 40 to 50 mm Hg may be reduced to normal levels. This problem is not encountered with ketamine, a dissociative anesthetic. In fact, intraocular pressure may be slightly elevated 3 to 5 mm Hg with this anesthetic. Airway obstruction at appropriate doses does not occur, atropine may be necessary to prevent excessive secretions, and oxygen is administered via mask. Following satisfactory ketamine general anesthesia with the patient in the supine position, the intraocular pressure measurement and the examination may be carried out safely. Premature infants under general anesthesia require even greater vigilance.

Measurement of Intraocular Pressure

Lid positioning is critical while obtaining an intraocular pressure measurement in infants. Improperly spreading the lids apart while checking the pressure may lead to falsely elevated levels because of the pressure transmitted to the globe by the physician's fingers and the lids. A pediatric or adult wire-lid speculum, depending on the relative dimensions, usually allows a more reliable method of pressure measurement. If anesthesia is not deep enough, the Bell's phenomenon occurs, and the eye is positioned underneath the lid preventing accurate measurement. Ample anesthesia should be administered to facilitate an accurate exam. With the globe in the straight-ahead position and a topical anesthetic applied, a Perkins hand-held tonometer is used to obtain a reliable intraocular pressure. Typically, three measurements are recorded and an average obtained. If the cornea is grossly edematous, a pneumotonometer reading may be useful. A Tonopen may be helpful in some circumstances when applanation is difficult. Intraocular pressure in infants is lower than in adults,[17] averaging 11.4 mm Hg. Asymmetric intraocular pressures coupled with clinical findings represent a significant finding.

Corneal Diameter Measurement

The collagen fibers of an infant's eye up to approximately age 3 years are soft and very elastic. This lesson is readily learned during congenital glaucoma or cataract surgery when the globe rapidly collapses with scleral infolding upon anterior chamber entrance. Conversely, when the intraocular pressure is markedly elevated as in congenital glaucoma, the collagen fibers stretch the globe, increasing axial length, corneal diameter, and producing myopia. Normal horizontal corneal diameter in a premature infant is 8.22 mm; in a full-term infant, 10 to 10.5 mm.[18] It typically increases to 11 or 12 mm at 1 year. Corneal diameter is measured with calipers from horizontal white to white limbus, and values greater than 12 mm prompt an evaluation for glaucoma. Subsequent evaluations should include corneal diameter measurements, which are helpful to follow disease progression.

Corneal Edema

Distension of the cornea may cause a tear in Descemet's membrane allowing the ingress of aqueous humor. These defects are best seen after endothelial overgrowth repair and normalization of intraocular pressure. Haab's striae or ruptures of Descemet's membrane, may be multiple and are easily seen as linear opacities with the operating microscope or during slit-lamp examination (Fig. 38–5). Such striae are commonly associated with congenital glaucoma but are not exclusively seen with this entity.

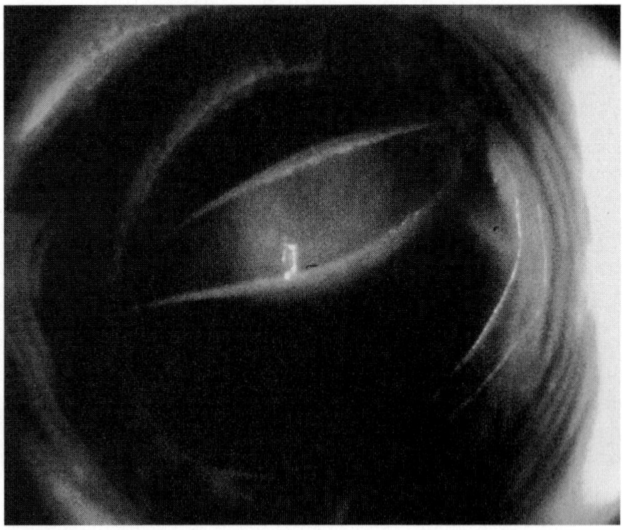

Figure 38–5. Haab striae. Corneal striae aid in the diagnosis of congenital glaucoma. These striae are almost always the telltale sign of a history of elevated intraocular pressure.

Gonioscopy

The appearance of the chamber angle may very well be the key to the diagnosis of congenital glaucoma. When an experienced gonioscopist identifies classic iridotrabecular dysgenesis, the diagnosis is complete. If the disease is unilateral, the gonioscopist may easily detect a striking difference between angle outflow anatomy. However, with bilateral disease and cloudy corneas, the diagnosis may be more difficult. Removing unhealthy central edematous epithelium with a cotton-tipped swab or Weck-cell sponge may enhance the angle view. Fine-tuned adult gonioscopy skills are essential to understand normal variation, for this can be extrapolated to infantile angles. Ophthalmologists who do not perform gonioscopy on a routine basis will quickly be lost trying to solve the mysteries of the infantile angle. In premature infants, the angle is even more complex. In the normal infant eye, the peripheral chamber is slightly shallow, for the angle recess has not fully formed. The collagenous white scleral spur is still an excellent infantile landmark. However, normal angle variety, even in healthy infants is diverse and variable. Details are confusing because the classic landmarks of trabecular pigment are nonexistent, and the meshwork has a smooth, uniform, ground glass appearance.

The gonioscopic hallmark of congenital glaucoma is a variable anterior insertion of the iris into the trabecular meshwork together with an ill-defined scleral spur. The iris may insert directly flat into the meshwork, but with a concave iris insertion, the uveal tissue then sweeps upward variably to insert into the meshwork (Fig. 38–6). Hoskins and coworkers have described this wraparound configuration, as well as an excellent developmental angle classification system.[19]

A variety of gonioprisms are used depending on the examiner's expertise, training, and preference. A Koeppe lens allows a panoramic angle view through a hand-held slit lamp. This diagnostic gonioprism may be used on both eyes simultaneously, allowing rapid viewing of both chamber angles and the posterior pole. This comparison facilitates the detection of such subtle differences in angle pathology as a higher iris insertion onto the inner wall of the eye. Expertise with this lens is difficult to acquire because the only time it is used is in the operating room. The angle view with the Koeppe lens is similar to a Barkan goniotomy lens, and both these lenses are excellent for angle photography. A Barkan goniotomy lens is useful to view the angle with the operating microscope tilted for the typical goniotomy position. Conversely, the angle may be viewed through the operating microscope using a four-mirror gonioprism. Posner or Zeiss prisms with a natural tear

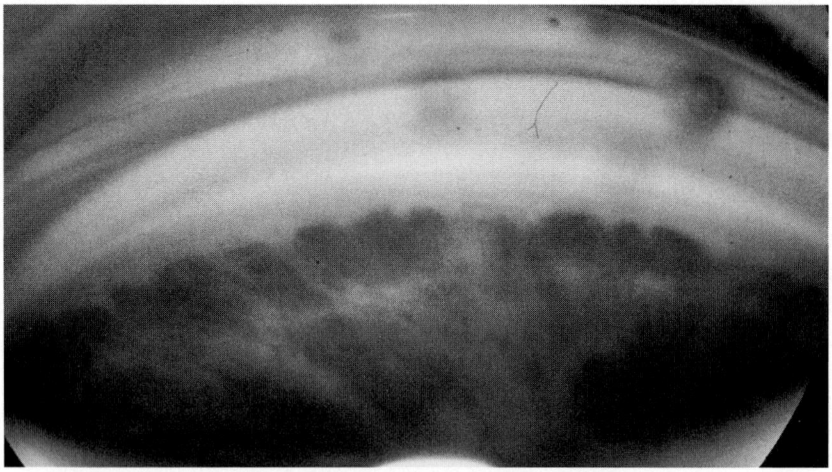

Figure 38–6. Goniophotograph of trabeculodysgenesis. Chamber angle of a 9-month-old with congenital glaucoma. The landmarks are poorly differentiated. The iris sweeps up into the angle and the scleral spur is difficult to locate. The best view of the chamber angle is obtained with the hand-held slit lamp and Koeppe goniolens.

fluid bridge allow a more familiar vista for most ophthalmologists, and magnification may be adjusted for improved viewing. Intraoperative gonioscopy with this technique is useful for chromatic suture identification inside Schlemm's canal during filamentary trabeculotomy. The angle findings are carefully documented.

The iris and lens are then evaluated before proceeding to the dilated fundus exam. An abnormality of these structures implies a more complicated secondary glaucoma with a poorer prognosis.

Fundus Examination

Following dilation of the pupil, the lens is reexamined for abnormalities and the optic disc and retina are evaluated. Baseline optic nerve head photography is critical to document disease progression, regression, or stability; disc drawings are also made in case of equipment failure. Notching of the disc and disc hemorrhages are infrequently detected in pediatric glaucomatous optic neuropathy. Classically, cupping occurs in the center of the disc, the rim remains relatively intact but thinned, and the scleral canal may enlarge before the age of 3 years. Disc pallor may occur and appears to be more common in premature infants, especially those with a history of intracranial demise. Pallor should always prompt neuroophthalmologic thinking. Cupping of the optic nerve is often reversible after normalization of the intraocular pressure, and it should be documented with serial photographs. Intracranial compressive lesions may cause nonglaucomatous cupping of the optic nerve.

Diagnostic Examination Under Anesthesia with Anticipated Surgery

Some physicians do not recommend changing from ketamine to intubation with inhalational anesthetics because of the risk of apnea or cardiac compromise. The safest approach is probably using ketamine for pure diagnosis and follow-up evaluations. If the physician anticipates a procedure, especially a lengthy one, it is probably better to use halogenated agents. After rapid induction by mask inhalation, an intraocular pressure measurement may be obtained. Intubation is then performed and the rest of the exam and potential procedure carried out. With this technique, it is not necessary to change anesthetics. The methodology that best befits the surgeon and clinical situation is typically used. Some physicians prefer not to use ketamine because of postoperative hallucinations, and they use halogenated agents for all examinations and surgery.

Trabeculotomy still has a role in management of the adult primary glaucomas[20] and is often combined with phacoemulsification.[21] Pressure reduction with trabeculotomy in adult glaucoma is less than with trabeculectomy, but postoperative complications are fewer.

Reasonable control of intraocular pressure is achieved in 75% of cases with the aid of medicines, even in steroid-induced glaucoma.[22] Patients who are poor candidates for standard trabeculectomy may be treated successfully with trabeculotomy. Patients with juvenile glaucoma at any age are candidates for trabeculotomy.

TRABECULOTOMY AB EXTERNO

LOCATION AND DISSECTION OF CONJUNCTIVAL AND SCLERAL FLAPS

After satisfactory anesthesia induction and routine preparation and draping, a lid speculum is inserted. If limbal exposure is inadequate, a lateral canthotomy is required.The location of the superior trabeculotomy site is between the 10 o'clock and 2 o'clock positions, depending on surgeon handedness and preference. If the expected success of the trabeculotomy is low because of altered limbal anatomy as in aniridia, the proposed trabeculotomy site can be made closer to 12 o'clock. In this case, if Schlemm's canal is absent, conversion to trabeculectomy with superior bleb formation is not a problem.

A corneal traction suture is used to rotate the globe in the appropriate direction. Depending on the above preference, a 5-mm fornix-based conjunctival flap is prepared. This creates a large enough conjunctival flap

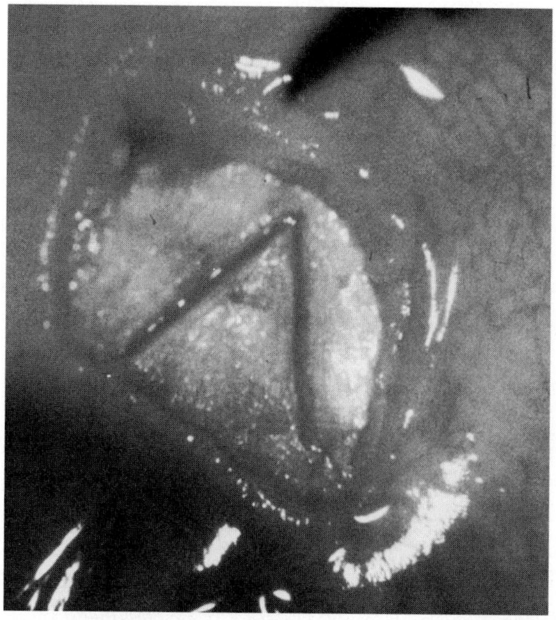

Figure 38–7. Fashioning the scleral flap. After making a fornix-based conjunctival flap, a 2/3-thickness scleral flap is dissected into clear cornea to gain access to the deeper limbal structures that contain Schlemm's canal.

for adequate wound closure, even if converting to a trabeculectomy. Apply light wet-field cautery for hemostasis avoiding excessive scleral shrinkage.

Construct a 2/3-thickness scleral flap, triangular in shape and limbal-based (Fig. 38–7), applying cautery judiciously to a barely moist flap bed. A triangular flap allows adequate anterior and posterior exposure of Schlemm's canal. A thin scleral flap is difficult to close and leaves excess tissue over the canal. The scleral flap dissection should proceed 1 mm into clear cornea, permitting appreciation of a relatively blue-white color zone within the bed of the flap. Schlemm's canal is located in this zone immediately anterior and external to the heavy white fiber band of the scleral spur. It is much more difficult to locate Schlemm's canal without the aid of a superficial scleral flap. Thus, a straight radial cutdown to seek Schlemm's canal without the benefit of a scleral flap is inadvisable.

LOCALIZATION OF SCHLEMM'S CANAL

Radial Incision Technique

With meticulous, cautious, purposeful, skillful movements and under high magnification, a radial incision is begun in the scleral bed equally overlapping the blue and white zones (Fig. 38–8). The scleral spur resembles a shining white circumferential tendon and is one of the best landmarks during trabeculotomy. Usually the canal is located just anterior to the scleral spur. The location of the scleral spur is highly variable, and in congenital glaucoma it may be more posteriorly located. A triangular scleral flap is more desirable than a rectangular one because there is a higher likelihood of unveiling a more posteriorly located canal.

Exteriorization of Schlemm's Canal

Once the suspected roof of Schlemm's canal is visualized through the radial incision site, incise the canal circumferentially across the radial incision for 2 mm, creating a T cut over the canal. The circumferential incision will open the roof of the canal enough to see down to its floor. Some pigment may be present in the canal creating a yellowish-brown color, and the roof of the canal is composed of epithelial cells finer than surrounding scleral fibers. This textural difference should be looked for during the procedure. Exercise extreme care at this stage to avoid premature entry into the anterior chamber. If the chamber is entered prematurely, create a paracentesis site and instill viscoelastic material to allow continued probing for the canal.

Identification of Schlemm's Canal

Once the suspected canal has been exteriorized, many surgeons will proceed with a rigid metal trabeculotomy. Unfortunately, limbal anatomy is confusing and highly variable, and without absolute canal verification, false passages are created. The surgeon will likely never

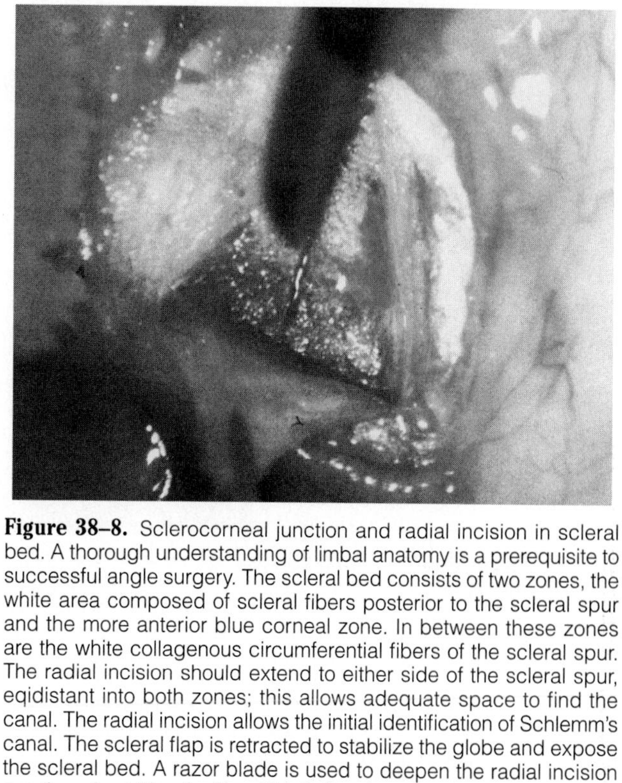

Figure 38–8. Sclerocorneal junction and radial incision in scleral bed. A thorough understanding of limbal anatomy is a prerequisite to successful angle surgery. The scleral bed consists of two zones, the white area composed of scleral fibers posterior to the scleral spur and the more anterior blue corneal zone. In between these zones are the white collagenous circumferential fibers of the scleral spur. The radial incision should extend to either side of the scleral spur, eqidistant into both zones; this allows adequate space to find the canal. The radial incision allows the initial identification of Schlemm's canal. The scleral flap is retracted to stabilize the globe and expose the scleral bed. A razor blade is used to deepen the radial incision evenly, scleral *fiber by fiber.* This is the slowest, most important, and most laborious part of the procedure. The lips of the radial incision are continually spread apart during dissection to create a viewing area. Schlemm's canal is usually located just anterior to the white circumferential fibers of the scleral spur, the best limbal landmark for angle surgeons. There may be light pigment in the canal, an important distinguishing feature.

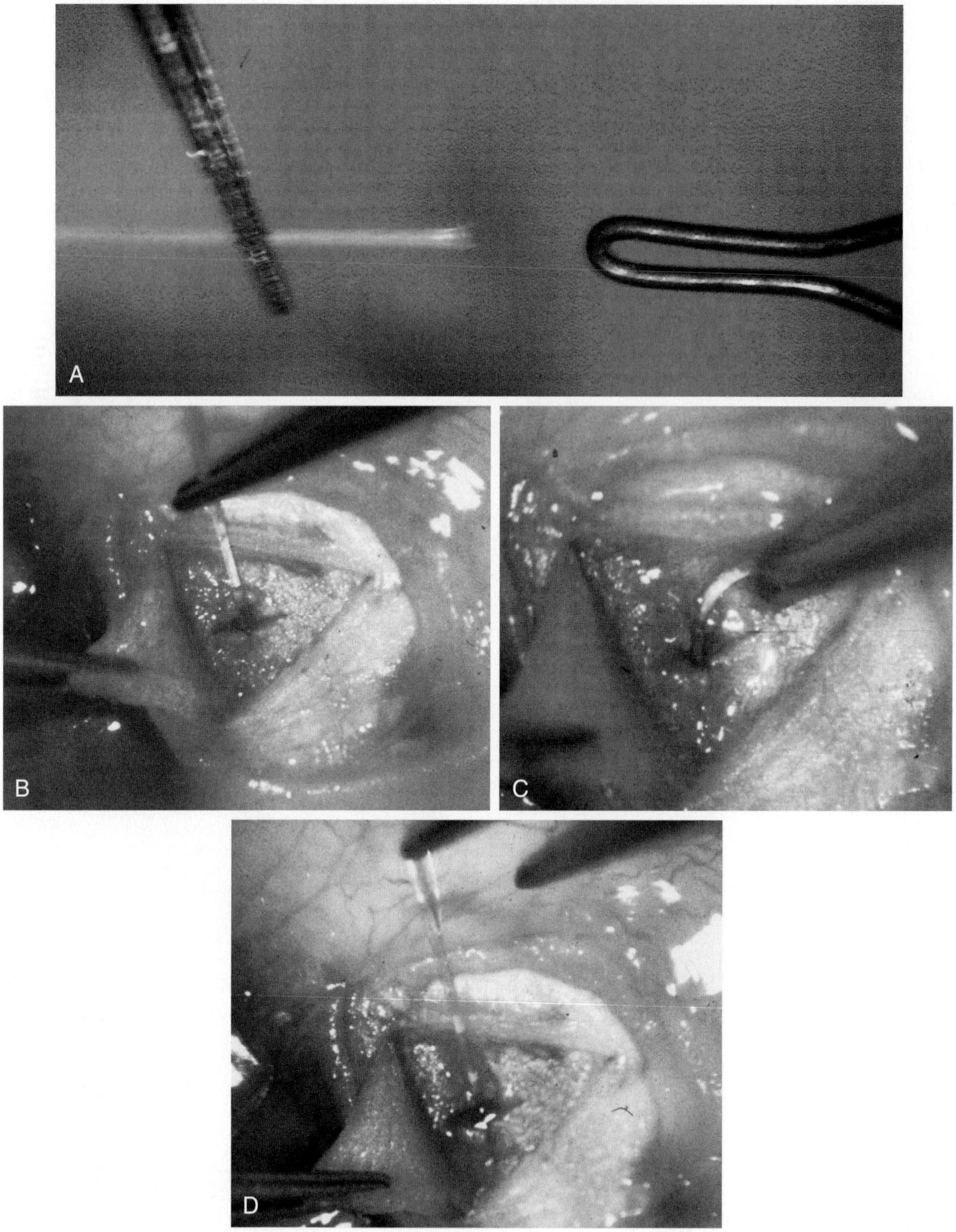

Figure 38–9. 5-0 nylon suture probe. *A.* A 5-0 clear nylon suture is thermally blunted into a bulb shape by slowly bringing the end of the suture adjacent to the tip of a thermal cautery during microscopic observation. *B.* Suture probe inserted into canal. The thermally blunted flexible 5-0 clear nylon suture probe is introduced into the suspected Schlemm's canal. The area of the T-cut incision is easily seen. If it is in the correct location, the suture will gently slide into the canal with minimal resistance. If resistance is met, continue dissection with the razor blade into a deeper plane and try probing the canal again. The 5-0 nylon suture probe will facilitate insertion of the smaller 6-0 prolene trabeculotome. In this example, the probe is inserted into the superotemporal flap site in a clockwise direction. *C.* Suture flexion. The next step is to prove the identity of Schlemm's canal by rotation of the flexible suture probe. The nylon probe should be approximately 20 mm in length with approximately 3 to 4 mm positioned inside the suspected canal. Grasp the proximal end of the suture with a forceps and flex posteriorly. *D.* Proper position upon release of probe. If the distal end of the probe is properly positioned in the canal, the proximal end will rapidly spring forward, back to its original position. If the distal end is malpositioned anterior to the canal, posterior flexion results in suture entry into the anterior chamber. The probe can easily be seen in the anterior chamber. When the proximal tip of the probe is flexed anteriorly and released, the probe promptly returns to a position tangential to the limbus if truly in contact with the posterior canal wall. If the probe is incorrectly positioned in the supraciliary space, following anterior flexion and release, the suture tip will not assume a position tangent to the limbus but will stop over the cornea.

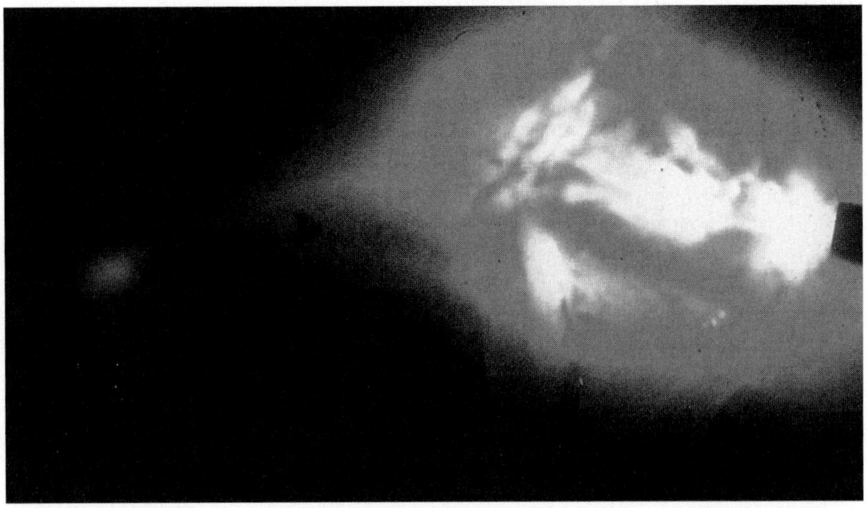

Figure 38–10. Fiberoptic illumination of suture probe. The suture probe is illuminated by contact with a light pipe. The distal end lights up and is in the expected position of the canal. Sometimes, the distal end will light up several millimeters posterior to the limbus, indicating improper intubation of the canal.

know of erroneous passageway and the procedure may fail. To avoid this problem, Lynn[23] described a method to evaluate and verify canal position before performing the trabeculotomy (Fig. 38–9). This consists of the insertion and flexion of a thermally blunted clear 5-0-nylon suture probe into the suspected canal. If insertion is difficult, further radial and/or circumferential incisions are necessary, for it is possible that the canal roof is located deeper or farther anterior in the tissues. Repeat the suture probing to find the actual canal; lateral insertion should be easy and not forceful. These flexion maneuvers help the physician find the true location of Schlemm's canal and are valuable learning tools for all interested in angle surgery. Another method of verifying the canal is by fiberoptic illumination (Fig. 38–10). With the clear 5-0-nylon suture in place, a light pipe is brought in contact with the proximal end. This is best viewed through the microscope with the coaxial light turned off. Upon contact with the suture, the blunted end of the suture will light up like a searchlight. If in the canal, the light will be seen at the limbus, if in the supraciliary space, the light will be seen a few millimeters from the limbus, under the sclera.

OPENING SCHLEMM'S CANAL

Rigid Metal Trabeculotomy

Once the canal has been located with the above technique, the canal on the other side of the radial incision is probed in a similar fashion. A paracentesis followed by intracameral acetylcholine and viscoelastic prepares the anterior segment for canal rupture. Do not overfill the chamber with viscoelastic material because this may cause pupillary sphincter rupture with permanent postoperative atonic pupil. A rigid metal trabeculotome is used to rupture the canal wall (Fig. 38–11 *A* and *B*). Before scleral flap closure, viscoelastic is irrigated from the anterior chamber and the scleral flap closed in a watertight fashion with a minimum of 3 9-0 nylon sutures. The conjunctival flap is reapproximated and the radial wing closed with an absorbable 9-0 Vicryl suture.

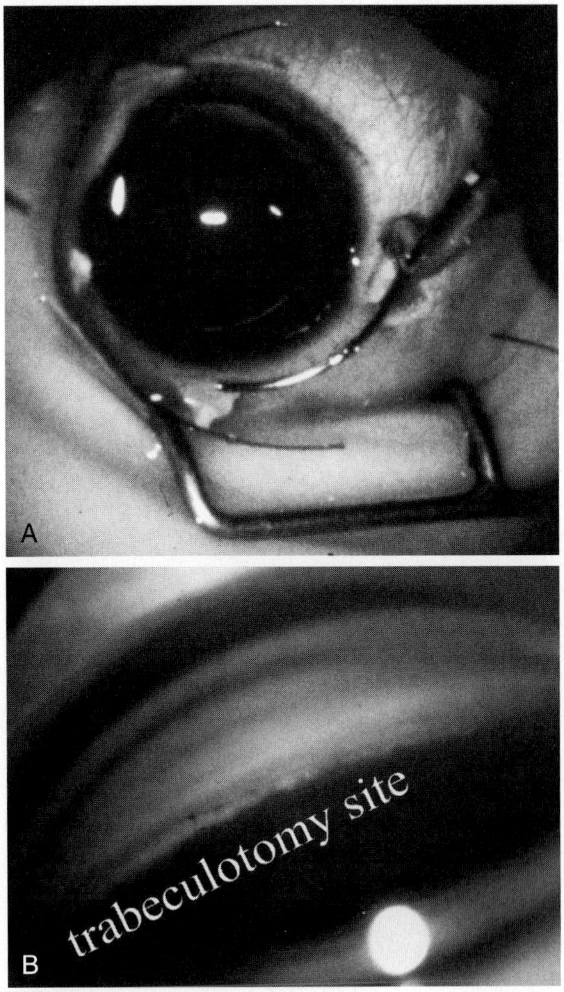

Figure 38–11. *A*. Trabeculotomy with metal trabeculotome. The metal trabeculotome is carefully inserted into the canal. Once fully inserted, the instrument is turned into the anterior chamber, cleaving the inner wall of the canal and trabecular meshwork. *B*. Chamber angle following trabeculotomy. The area over the lettering has the typical gonioscopic appearance of a white band-like structure best seen with a hand-held slit lamp through a Koeppe lens. Months postoperatively, iris processes may form, blood may be seen in the canal, and a fine gossamer filtering membrane forms anterior to the canal.

Filamentary Full Circumference Trabeculotomy (FFCT)

An alternative method of opening the canal is with a suture trabeculotome. There are three levels of assurance for finding Schlemm's canal. The least guarantee is simple pure visualization. Probing with a suture at the trabeculotomy site is the next level, and probing with distant suture retrieval from the canal provides the highest level of assurance. The suture may be retrieved from the canal after intubation for 180 degrees or 360 degrees. Distant suture retrieval from the canal proves Schlemm's location, for there is no other way to reach that destination.

One obstacle to FFCT is the presence of 3 o'clock and 9 o'clock septae, making it difficult to pass the suture a full 360 degrees. Threading a suture into the canal from a point closer to these obstructions provides a better vantage point and facilitates passage through these difficult areas. The initial scleral flap may be constructed closer to 10 o'clock or 2 o'clock, alleviating this problem. The exact same procedure for identifying the suspected Schlemm's canal is performed as outlined above. Once the suspected canal has been identified by the 5-0 clear nylon blunted suture probing technique, the canal is cannulated with a flexible suture. Smith[24] initially described this technique. Lynn and Fellman[7] revisited and improved upon the methodology 25 years later, and Lynch[8] further refined the surgery.

Suture Passage and Rupture of Canal

After identifying Schlemm's canal as instructed above, pass a thermally blunted 5-0 nylon probe counterclockwise beyond 3 o'clock, and then remove it. This facilitates probing with the blue prolene trabeculotome.

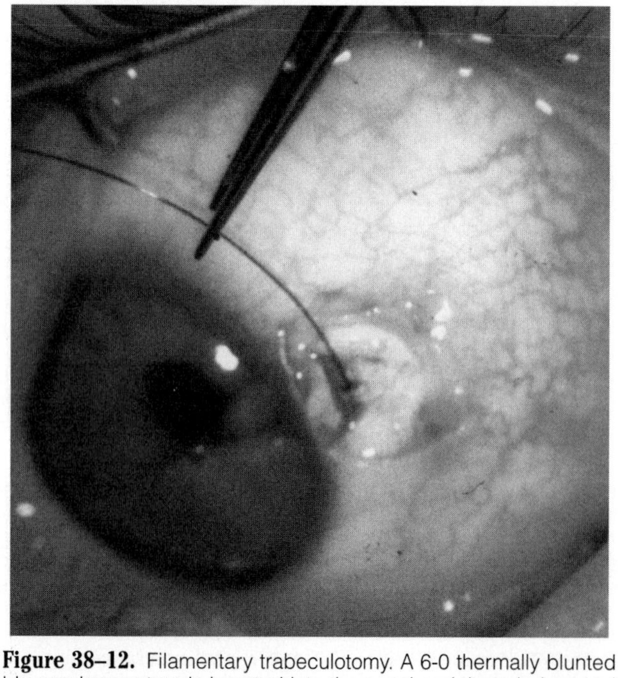

Figure 38–12. Filamentary trabeculotomy. A 6-0 thermally blunted blue prolene suture is inserted into the canal and threaded around for 360 degrees.

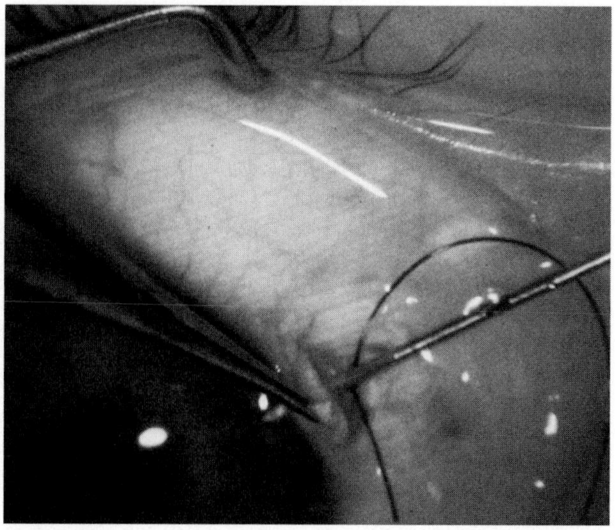

Figure 38–13. A 360-degree filamentary trabeculotomy. After threading the suture for 360 degrees, the end of the suture is retrieved from the cutdown site and exteriorized. The end of the prolene suture can be seen for 3 mm as it exits from the canal after going around for 360 degrees. Miochol is inserted through the base of the flap, followed by viscoelastic material to tamponade bleeding. The ends of the suture are grasped and pulled in opposite diretions to finish the filamentary trabeculotomy.

Select the curved portion of a thermally blunted 6-0 prolene suture, then insert it clockwise as far as it will go into Schlemm's canal without excessive force (Fig. 38–12). If possible, check the progress of the 6-0 prolene in Schlemm's canal with a gonioprism. After threading for 360 degrees, the blunted end of the blue suture will come into view at the adjacent end of the canal (Fig. 38–13). Retrieving the suture is an exhilarating experience for the surgeon, because he or she knows positively that the entire canal has been captured. After paracentesis and injection of intracameral acetylcholine and a viscoelastic agent, both ends of the crossed prolene suture are grasped with needle holders and pulled tangentially, opening the canal for 360 degrees in one fluid motion. The suture trabeculotome is then gently removed from the anterior chamber, approximately half of the viscoelastic material is irrigated out, and the flap closed in a watertight fashion.

Occasionally, septae in the canal will prevent 360-degree cannulation, and a second triangular flap site 180 degrees away is necessary. It usually is much easier and faster to create the second cut-down site because the blue prolene suture is easily seen in the scleral bed and rapidly identifies the true location of the canal. From the second flap site, it is possible to retrieve the previously hidden prolene suture and exteriorize it. It is then necessary to insert a second curved piece of thermally blunted 6-0 Prolene from the new site clockwise past 9 o'clock to the 2 o'clock entry point and retrieve its tip (Fig. 38–14*A*). Retrieve the suture from the second flap. Holding both ends of one Prolene arc with needle holders, tighten the suture until it bow strings abruptly into the anterior chamber (Fig. 38–14*B*). Release one end and remove the suture by gentle traction

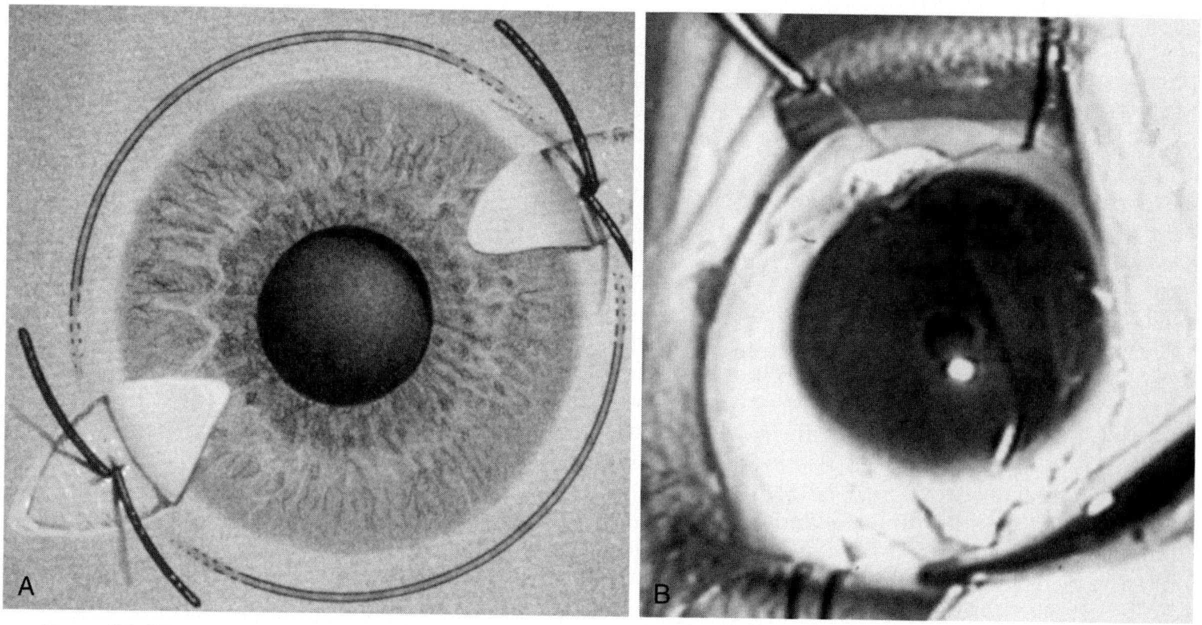

Figure 38–14. *A.* Two-site 360-degree filamentary trabeculotomy. Occasionally, the surgeon is unable to pass the suture all the way around to the original cutdown site. If this occurs, a second site is required to find the suture. Gonioscopy is helpful in determining the exact course of the blue suture to determine the cutdown site. *B.* Suture trabeculotomy. The opposite ends of the suture are grasped and the suture is bow stringed into the anterior chamber.

on the other end. Open the remaining 180 degrees of the angle in a similar fashion by tightening the other suture and removing it. Close the scleral flap "doors" securely with multiple interrupted nylon sutures. Close the conjunctiva with an 8-0 Vicryl taper point suture. Apply antibiotic-steroid ointment and an eye shield.

Alternative Deep Scleral Flap Approach to Isolating Schlemm's Canal

The surgical techniques for nonpenetrating filtration surgery involve the isolation of Schlemm's canal. These deep sclerectomy techniques reveal a completely different method of isolating the canal. During deep sclerectomy, Schlemm's canal is routinely unroofed. This is certainly not the case with the traditional method of finding Schlemm's canal with a radial cut-down. Nonpenetrating surgery requires the surgeon to create a second scleral flap that leaves only a few scleral fibers visible over the choroid. If in the proper plane, continued deep anterior dissection exposes the scleral spur. As the flap dissection continues, Schlemm's canal becomes exposed because its roof is contained in the flap. This is demonstrated by watching for the transition zone on the under side of the flap as the coarse scleral fibers give way to the smooth endothelial cells of the roof of the canal (Fig. 38–15). Simultaneously, the collagenous characteristics of the base of the flap bed change as the spur is reached, because the fibers of the spur become circumferential and the floor of the canal is translucent. If the surgeon desires to use this technique, the scleral flap is dissected as a single flap initially all the way down to choroid. This is an alternative method of localizing the canal.

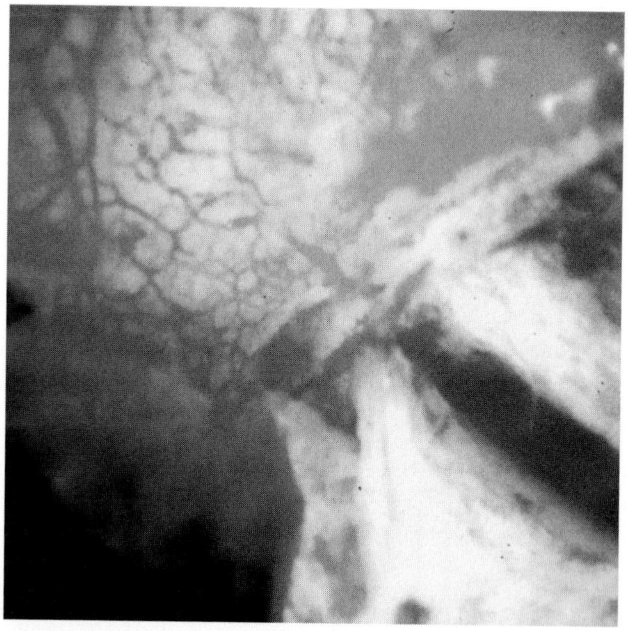

Figure 38–15. Deep scleral flap approach to Schlemm's canal. The coarse scleral fibers give way to the smooth endothelial cells that constitute the roof of Schlemm's canal. The canal is widely exposed with this dual flap technique.

POSTOPERATIVE MANAGEMENT

The patient is examined on the first postoperative day. Evaluation is hampered by periorbital swelling and the patient's inability to cooperate. If there are no overt signs of infection, the anterior chamber deep and the cornea relatively clear, a topical combination steroid-antibiotic drop is administered 4 times a day, with follow-up in 1 week. If stable, the infant is evaluated 2 weeks later in the office, and by EUA within 6 weeks, obtaining optic disc photographs, measuring corneal diameter, and performing a complete evaluation.

Postoperative hyphemas are a common result of bleeding from the incised iridocorneal angle, and they usually clear rapidly. Large hyphemas with significant pressure elevation are rare but should be observed closely for blood staining; if indicated, anterior chamber washout can be performed.[25] False passages created during trabeculotomy may result in a cyclodialysis or stripping of Descemet's membrane. This may be associated with increased bleeding, hypotony, or sudden closure of the cleft, with a marked rise in intraocular pressure. Peripheral anterior synechiae may form over a period of a few weeks but unless extensive, they do not significantly alter postoperative intraocular pressure. Filtering blebs may develop in approximately 10% of cases. Persistent corneal edema may be a sign of continued increased intraocular pressure.[26] Endophthalmitis is always a concern, especially with bilateral surgery. Bilateral surgery is typically avoided unless necessary.

Normalizing the intraocular pressure is just one part of the battle in caring for an infant with congenital glaucoma. If chamber angle procedures fail to control glaucoma, other procedures such as filtration, drainage implants, and cyclodestruction may be necessary. Associated systemic disorders require attention, amblyopia is a constant concern, and cornea and retinal problems are common. Teamwork with multiple sub-specialists is usually required to maintain optimal visual function.

REFERENCES

1. Burian HM: A case of Marfan's syndrome with bilateral glaucoma: With description of a new type of operation for developmental glaucoma (trabeculotomy ab externo). Am J Ophthalmol 1960;50:1187–92.
2. Smith R: A new technique for opening the canal of Schlemm. Br J Ophthalmol 1960;44:370–3.
3. Harms H: Glaukom-Operationen am Schlemm'schen Kanal. Sitzungsber. Der 114. Versammlung des Verens Rhein-Westf. Augenartze, 1966.
4. Harms H, Dannheim R: Trabeculotomy—Results and problems. Adv Ophthalmol 1970;22:121.
5. Lynn JR, Berry PB: A new trabeculotome. Am J Ophthalmol 1969; 68:430.
6. McPherson SD Jr: Results of external trabeculotomy. Am J Ophthalmol 1973;76:918.
7. Lynn JR, Fellman RL, Starita RJ: Full circumference trabeculotomy: An improved procedure for primary congenital glaucoma (Abstr). Ophthalmology 1988;95(suppl):168.
8. Beck AD, Lynch MG: 360° Trabeculotomy for Primary Congenital Glaucoma. Arch Ophthalmol 1994;113:1200-2.
9. Barsoum-Homsy M, Chevrette L: Incidence and prognosis of childhood glaucoma. A study of 63 cases. Ophthalmology 1986; 93:1323.
10. Anderson DR: Trabeculotomy compared to goniotomy for glaucoma in children. Ophthalmology 1983;90:805.
11. Barkan O: Technic of goniotomy. Arch Ophthalmol 1938;19:217.
12. Hodapp E, Heuer DK: A simple technique of goniotomy. Am J Ophthalmol 1986;102:537.
13. Anderson DR: The development of the trabecular meshwork and its abnormality in primary infantile glaucoma. Trans Am Ophthalmol Soc 1981;79:458.
14. Broughton WL, Fine BS, Zimmerman LE: A histologic study of congenital glaucoma associated with a chromosomal defect. Ophthalmology 1980;87:96.
15. Maumenee AE: The pathogenesis of congenital glaucoma. Am J Ophthalmol 1959;47:827.
16. Dominquez A, Banos MS, Alkvarez MG, et al: Intraocular pressure measurement in infants under general anesthesia. Am J Ophthalmol 1974;78:110.
17. Radtke ND, Cohen BF: Intraocular pressure measurement in the newborn. Am J Ophthalmol 1974;78:501.
18. Shaffer RN, Weiss DI: Congenital and Pediatric Glaucomas. St. Louis, CV Mosby, 1970; p 37.
19. Hoskins HD Jr, Shaffer RN, Hetherington J Jr: Anatomical classification of the developmental glaucomas. Arch Ophthalmol 1984; 102:1331.
20. Chihara E, Nishida A, Kodo M, et al.: Trabeculotomy ab externo: An Alternative treatment in adult patients with primary open-angle glaucoma. Ophthalmic Surg 1993; 24:735–9.
21. Tanihara H, Honjo M, Inatani M, et al.: Trabeculotomy combined with phacoemulsification and implantation of an intraocular lens for the treatment of primary open-angle glaucoma and coexisting cataract. Ophthalmic Surg Lasers 1997;28:810–7.
22. Honjo M, Tanihara H, Inatani M, Honda Y: External trabeculotomy for the treatment of steroid-induced glaucoma. J Glaucoma 2000;9:483–5.
23. Lynn JR: Trabeculotomy ab externo versus cyclotherapy. In Symposium on Glaucoma, Transactions of the New Orleans Academy of Ophthalmology, St. Louis, CV Mosby, 1975; pp 292–322.
24. Smith R: Nylon filament trabeculotomy in glaucoma. Trans Ophthalmol Soc UK 1962;82:439.
25. Tanihara H, Nakayama Y, Honda Y: Intraocular pressure elevation caused by massive and prolonged hemorrhage after trabeculotomy ab externo. Acta Ophthalmol Scand 1995;73:281–2.
26. Inatani M, Tanihara AH, Muto T, et al.: Transient intraocular pressure elevation after trabeculotomy and its occurrence with phacoemulsification and intraocular lens implantation. Jpn J Ophthalmol 2001;45:288–92.

CHAPTER 39

Shallow or Flat Anterior Chamber

LEON W. HERNDON, JR., M.D.

One feared complication after glaucoma filtering surgery is the flat, or shallow anterior chamber. The term "flat anterior chamber" may have different connotations under certain situations[1–5] with varied consequences. It is helpful, therefore, to classify shallow or flat anterior chambers into three groups. In type 1 there is contact between the peripheral iris and the corneal endothelium, with preservation of the anterior chamber over the pupillary portion of the iris (Fig. 39–1). In type 2 the iris touches the posterior surface of the cornea in all areas, but there is a space between the anterior surface of the lens (or vitreous) and the corneal endothelium. In type 3 the iris and cornea are in contact in all areas, and, in addition, the lens (or formed vitreous face) comes into contact with the central cornea. Types 1 and 2 might be thought of as shallow chambers, whereas type 3 represents a truly flat chamber.

In type 1 shallow chambers, the cornea is typically clear and the iris stroma has not been flattened by the gentle contact with the cornea. The anterior chamber in these eyes usually deepens spontaneously with time, requiring no special management. With a type 2 chamber, the cornea is also clear and the iris stroma has not been flattened. These eyes can also recover spontaneously or may progress to type 3 flat anterior chambers. Stewart and Shields[6] studied 36 consecutive phakic eyes with shallow or flat anterior chambers after filtering surgery and found that only those with type 3 chambers, as defined here, required surgical re-formation. All eyes with shallow chambers spontaneously re-formed within 1 to 3 weeks on conservative medical management, which consisted of topical atropine, antibiotic, and steroid. A type 3 flat anterior chamber is a surgical emergency. If not corrected promptly, there is significant risk of corneal endothelial cell loss[7,8] and irreversible decompensation, cataract formation, bleb failure, and formation of anterior[9] and posterior[10] synechiae. Depending on a variety of factors, the surgeon may choose among several different forms of management for the patient with a flat chamber: (1) applying a pressure patch; (2) re-forming the anterior chamber with air, viscoelastic material, expansile gas, or saline; or (3) draining the choroidal detachment and re-forming the anterior chamber. In addition, it may become necessary to intervene with a shallow anterior chamber if it is progressively shallowing or if it has persisted for more than 2 to 3 weeks. In all cases, treatment depends primarily on the mechanism of the flat or shallow chamber.

MECHANISMS OF SHALLOW OR FLAT ANTERIOR CHAMBERS

The major causes of shallow or flat anterior chambers are shown in Table 39–1. The determination of the responsible mechanism is based primarily on the nature of the filtering bleb, the intraocular pressure, and the depth of the anterior chamber (Table 39–2). It is helpful to categorize flat anterior chambers into those with hypotony and those with elevated intraocular pressure.

When a flat or shallow anterior chamber in the early postoperative period is associated with a low intraocular pressure, the most likely causes are excessive filtra-

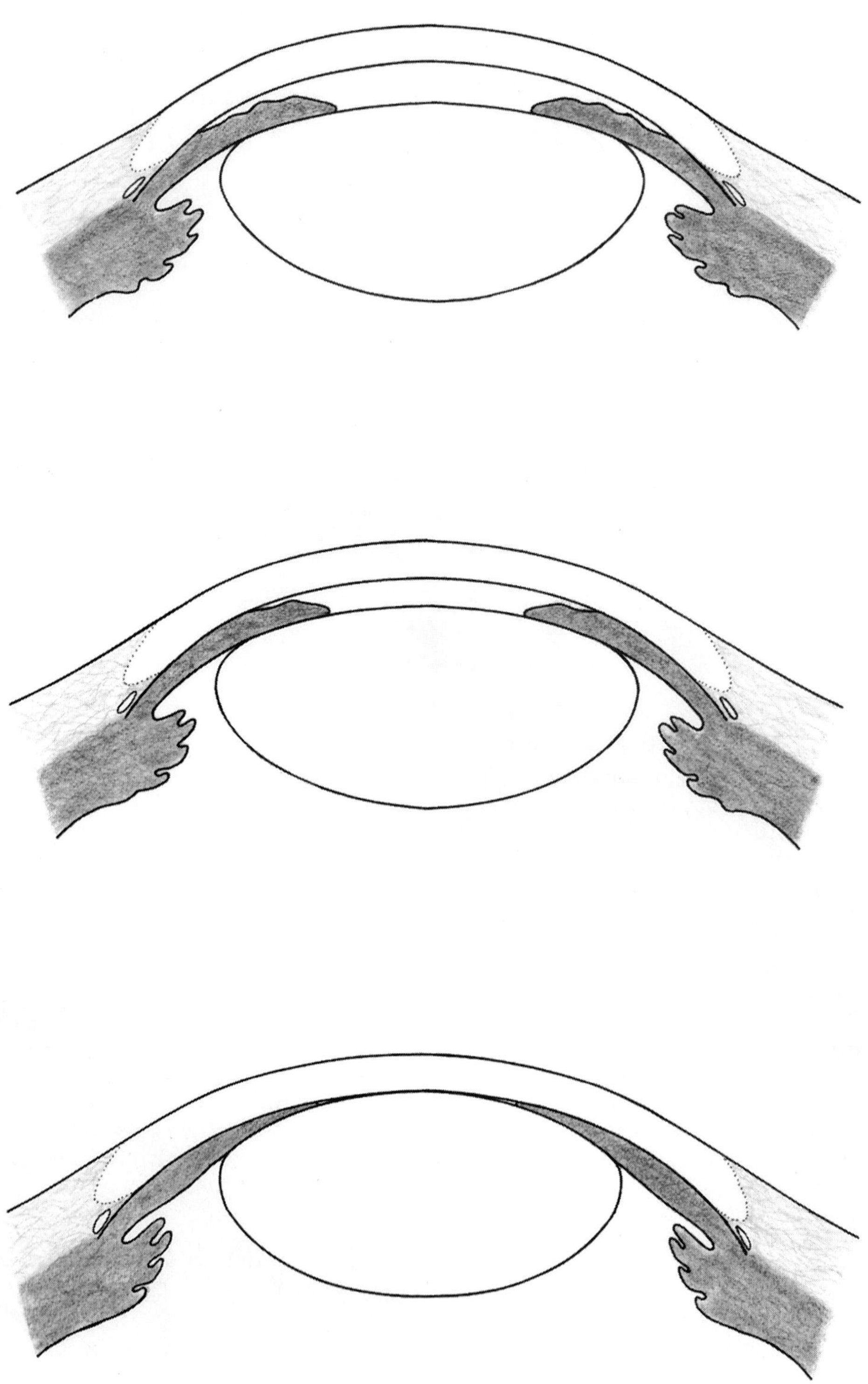

Figure 39–1. Classification of the different types of "flat anterior chambers." In type 1 *(top)* there is contact between the peripheral iris and the corneal endothelium, but the chamber is formed centrally over the iris. In type 2 *(middle)* the iris touches the posterior surface of the cornea in all areas, even centrally. In a type 3 flat anterior chamber *(bottom)* no chamber is present anywhere. (From Spaeth GL: Ophthalmic Surgery: Principles and Practice, 2nd Edition. Philadelphia: WB Saunders; 1990:336.)

TABLE 39–1. Causes for Shallow or Flat Anterior Chamber

Cause	Important Associated Findings
1. Inadequate resistance to aqueous outflow	High bleb or positive Seidel test
2. Fluid in the suprachoroidal space	Ophthalmoscopic or ultrasound evidence of choroidal or ciliary body detachment
3. Inadequate aqueous formation	Low bleb, low intraocular pressure, and inflamed eye
4. Interference with flow of aqueous humor from the posterior to the anterior chamber	Adherence of the iris to lens or vitreous: positive fluorescein appearance test
5. Anterior displacement of the lens–iris diaphragm	
a. Misdirection of aqueous flow into the vitreous	High intraocular pressure: positive intravenous fluorescein appearance test
b. Ciliary body swelling	Inflamed eye; tight scleral band
c. Constriction of the ciliary body sphincter	Use of strong miotic
d. Increase in size of lens	Slit-lamp evidence of increasing cataract
e. Partial or complete dislocation of lens	Phakodonesis
f. Swelling of vitreous contents	Intravitreal blood or gas (SF_6)

From Spaeth GL: Glaucoma surgery: In Spaeth GL (ed), Ophthalmic Surgery: Principles and Practice. Philadelphia: WB Saunders; 1990.

TABLE 39–2. Diagnosis of Postoperative Complications of Glaucoma Filtering Surgery

Condition	Intraocular Pressure	Bleb	Anterior Chamber	Other Findings
No filtration	High	None	Deep	—
Malignant glaucoma	Often high	None	Flat–II-III	Fluorescein pools behind vitreous face
Excessive filtration	Less than 10 mm Hg	High	Normal to flat	—
Inadequate aqueous humor production	Less than 5 mm Hg	Low and getting lower	Flat (I-III) until sclerostomy closes, then deep	Inflamed eye
Excessive filtration with developing inadequate aqueous production	Less than 5 mm Hg and falling	Low or none	Flattening	Increasingly inflamed eye
Pupillary block				
Early in association with excess filtration	5–15 mm Hg	Moderate	Flat with iris bombé	Posterior synechiae
In association with inadequate aqueous production	0–10 mm Hg	None	Flat	Posterior synechiae
After closure of sclerostomy	High	None	Flat	Posterior synechiae
Suprachoroidal hemorrhage	5–50 mm Hg	High	Flat	Severe pain
Ciliary body detachment	0–10 mm Hg	None–high	Flat	Detachment visible

From Spaeth GL: Glaucoma surgery: In Spaeth GL (ed), Ophthalmic Surgery: Principles and Practice. Philadelphia: WB Saunders; 1990.

tion, ciliochoroidal effusion, or a wound leak. A flat or shallow anterior chamber with a normal or high intraocular pressure is usually the result of malignant (ciliary block) glaucoma, suprachoroidal hemorrhage, or pupillary block. Because the appropriate management of a flat anterior chamber depends on the cause, it is crucial to know if the pressure is high or low. In the face of a flat anterior chamber, standard tonometric measurements may be unreliable, and tactile assessment of the intraocular pressure may provide an additional indication of the relative tension height.

Slit-lamp examination is also critical in determining the mechanism causing a shallow or flat anterior chamber. If the iris is in the bombé configuration and there is no patent iridectomy, pupillary block may be present. A flat or shallow central chamber with elevated pressure suggests malignant glaucoma or suprachoroidal hemorrhage. Ophthalmoscopy should also be performed to rule out choroidal effusion or hemorrhage. B-scan ultrasonography allows for accurate determination of these features in eyes with hazy or opaque media. High-frequency ultrasound biomicroscopy also provides imaging of the anterior segment anatomy not possible by other means.[12]

HYPOTONY AND FLAT ANTERIOR CHAMBER

A low, often unrecordable, intraocular pressure is common during the early postoperative period and is frequently associated with a shallow anterior chamber.

Kao and co-authors[13] evaluated anterior chamber depth in 20 consecutive phakic eyes undergoing glaucoma filtering procedures. The natural postoperative course showed maximum shallowing of the anterior chamber on the second and third postoperative days, with gradual deepening thereafter. Two eyes required surgical re-formation of the chamber.

PREVENTION

As with any procedure, the best way to avoid potential complications is to adhere to meticulous surgical detail. Careful wound closure is one means of avoiding a flat anterior chamber. Another measure that has been evaluated is injection of sodium hyaluronate into the anterior chamber perioperatively. Most studies have shown that this practice does not reduce the incidence of flat anterior chambers when injected at the end of the filtering operation.[14,15] Wand has suggested that deepening the anterior chamber with sodium hyaluronate at the beginning of the procedure and maintaining a deep chamber throughout the operative procedure may result in deeper chambers postoperatively.[16] However, Raitta and co-workers,[17] in a prospective study, found the incidence of shallow/flat anterior chamber after a guarded filtration procedure to be equal in a group of eyes that received sodium hyaluronate before fistulization compared to a group of eyes that did not receive an injection of sodium hyaluronate.

We will now consider different causes of hypotony and a flat anterior chamber and how they can be managed.

CONJUNCTIVAL DEFECT

At the end of the filtering surgery, watertight closure of the conjunctival wound should be confirmed by injecting balanced salt solution into the anterior chamber to check for leaks. Applying a fluorescein strip to the bleb is helpful in checking for leaks (Fig. 39–2). Postoperatively, if there is an obvious hole in the conjunctival flap or a leak at the wound edge, it may be possible to achieve spontaneous closure with a pressure patch (Fig. 39–3). A fusiform-shaped cotton ball can be placed over the lid in the area of the fistula and held in place with gauze pads to produce mechanical pressure. The patient should be kept awake, with the fellow eye open and looking straight ahead, because the Bell's phenomenon of sleep may place the tamponade over the central cornea. Examination of the eye 1 to 4 hours later often reveals deepening of the anterior chamber. If the chamber is significantly deeper after removal of the patch, the patch is placed back on the eye, and the patient is discharged home with instructions to remove the patch in the evening before going to sleep.

CILIOCHOROIDAL EFFUSION

With periods of hypotony, fluid often collects in the suprachoroidal space postoperatively. Additional factors, such as inflammation and venous congestion may also be important in the pathogenesis of choroidal detachments.[18] In most cases of hypotony and flat anterior chamber, a serous choroidal detachment is present, with the characteristic smooth, dome-shaped elevation of the peripheral fundus. Serous detachments are high in protein (67% of plasma concentration), suggesting that a pressure differential causes fluid with small and medium-sized protein molecules to pass from choroidal capillaries to extravascular spaces.[19,20] Less commonly, a hemorrhagic choroidal detachment can develop from rupture of the capillary membrane.[19] This condition is usually associated with pain, intraocular pressure elevation, and a flat anterior chamber.

Serous choroidal detachments usually resolve spontaneously with the normal rise in intraocular pressure that occurs during the first days to weeks postopera-

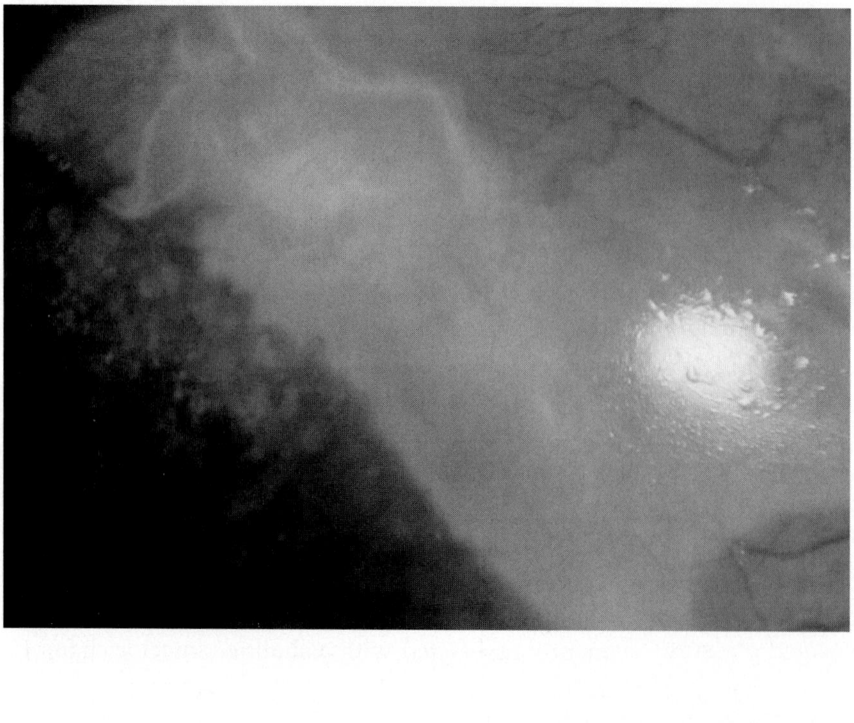

Figure 39–2. Bleb leak confirmed by 2% fluorescein solution.

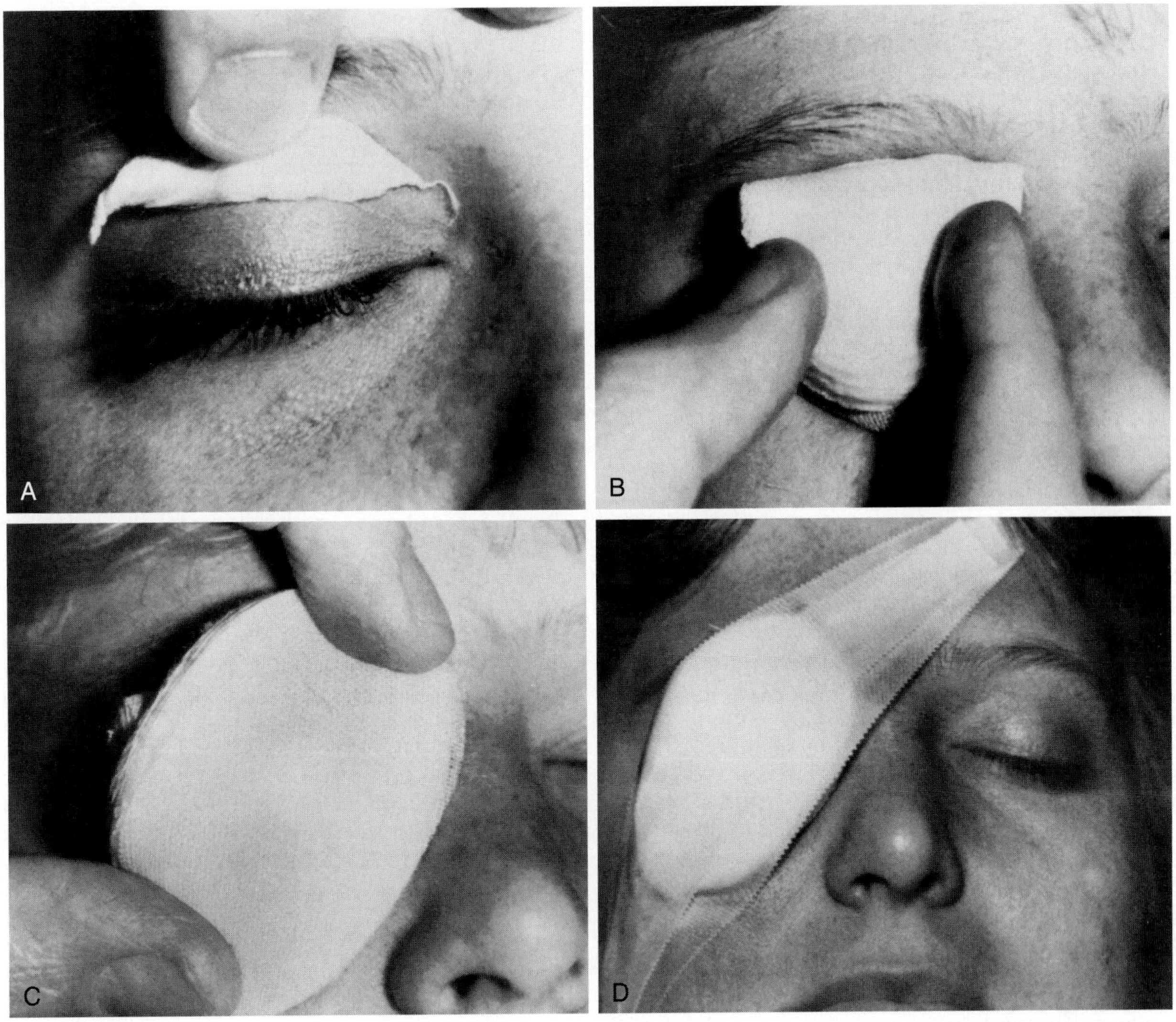

Figure 39–3. Pressure patching. A moistened torpedo-shaped cotton ball is placed over the upper lid *(A)* where it will exert pressure on the filtration site. A folded eye pad is placed over the cotton ball as shown *(B)*, followed by an additional open eye pad *(C)*. The eye pads and cotton ball are tightly opposed with tape *(D)*. The patient is reexamined 1 hour later, before being sent home. (From Shields MB: Textbook of Glaucoma, 3rd Edition. Baltimore: Williams & Wilkins; 1992. © Lippincott Williams & Wilkins, with permission.)

tively. It may be necessary to drain choroidal detachments when associated with a type 3 chamber, apposition or "kissing" contact of choroidals, prolonged hypotony, or a low bleb with a moderate to large choroidal effusion.

ANTERIOR CHAMBER RE-FORMATION

Re-formation of the anterior chamber can be performed by intraocular injection of balanced salt solution, air,[21,22] viscoelastic agents,[23,24] or expandable gases.[25,26] In most cases, the preferable method of management with flat anterior chambers is prompt re-formation of the anterior chamber with viscoelastic material.

At the time of the original surgery, it is good practice to place a paracentesis wound in the inferior temporal quadrant. If this was done, chamber re-formation can be performed with the patient's eye well anesthetized and the patient seated at a slit lamp, or under an operating microscope. Once the paracentesis track is identified, a 30-gauge blunt cannula is placed on the syringe containing the viscoelastic material. A variety of viscoelastic substances can be used. Sodium hyaluronate is less viscous than other materials, but more easily injected, and it is a suitable material for most eyes. A small amount of air may be left in the needle.

After the eye is appropriately prepped, the cannula tip is slowly introduced, on a plane absolutely parallel with the iris, into the anterior chamber through the paracentesis. As the plunger of the syringe is depressed, forcing air and viscoelastic material out of the needle, an air bubble rising spontaneously in the anterior chamber provides evidence that the cannula is in the chamber. The viscoelastic material is then slowly injected so that it does not push the iris in front of it, which could lead to iris plugging of the sclerostomy. The chamber should be deepened gradually until it has resumed normal depth. If a paracentesis was not made during the original surgery, it is usually possible to enter the anterior chamber with a 30-gauge needle and then inject the viscoelastic.

The use of intraocular gas offers the potential advantages of an expansile effect and longer persistence within the eye.[26] In aphakic, vitrectomized eyes, keeping the patient supine helps confine the gas in the anterior chamber, allowing effective tamponade of aqueous outflow.[27] The use of intraocular air or perfluoropropane in the phakic eye may be associated with an increased risk of postoperative anterior subcapsular cataract formation.

DRAINAGE OF A CHOROIDAL DETACHMENT

The most definitive treatment of the flat anterior chamber associated with hypotony and choroidal detachment is drainage of the fluid in the suprachoroidal space and re-formation of the anterior chamber with saline solution or viscoelastic material. If the eye is extremely soft, we prefer to use a subconjunctival block.

If the original paracentesis cannot be found, a new beveled paracentesis is made slowly, and with a very sharp, pointed blade. Care in making this incision prevents rapid entry into the anterior chamber, which could result in damage to the iris or lens. If fixation of the globe becomes difficult, it may be helpful to place a small, partial-thickness scratch incision into the cornea near the limbus with a very sharp blade. An incision approximately 2 mm long and one-third thickness is usually adequate. This groove can then be used for fixation, permitting development of a paracentesis. Once the paracentesis is made, the anterior chamber is re-formed with injection of balanced salt solution through a 27-gauge cannula.

A circumferential or radial conjunctival incision is made 3 to 6 mm from the limbus in the inferonasal and inferotemporal quadrants (away from the filtering site). Small blood vessels are gently cauterized before sclerotomy. Two 2- to 3-mm radial sclerotomies are centered in the inferior quadrants 3 to 4 mm from the limbus (Fig. 39–4). We prefer to use a No. 64 Beaver blade to make the sclerotomies because it is sharp enough to incise the sclera, but not sharp enough to cut through the choroid on contact. Xanthochromic fluid often drains spontaneously once the incision is carried into the suprachoroidal space. Once the fluid flow slows, the tip of a 0.5- to 1.0-mm cyclodialysis spatula can be carefully inserted into the suprachoroidal space in a circumferential direction (Fig. 39–5). This procedure is not usually necessary and is not recommended to be used routinely. The spatula is then removed and reinserted in the opposite direction. Periodically, the anterior chamber is re-formed with balanced salt solution when the eye softens. This cycle of fluid drainage and chamber re-formation is carried out until no further fluid drains from the suprachoroidal space. The cyclodialysis spatula is then withdrawn and the same procedure is carried out through the other sclerotomy. The anterior chamber is re-formed once again, with special emphasis on elevating the filtering bleb (Fig. 39–6).

Once the anterior chamber has been re-formed and the choroidal effusions drained, the edges of the sclerotomies are left unopposed to allow for continued drainage.[28] This can be accomplished by gaping the edges of the scleral wound with cautery or by excising a small piece of sclera with a punch or trephine.[29] The conjunctival wounds are closed with absorbable suture and atropine and antibiotic ointment applied to the eye, followed by a patch and eye shield. If cataract extraction needs to be performed, it may be combined with choroidal drainage.[30]

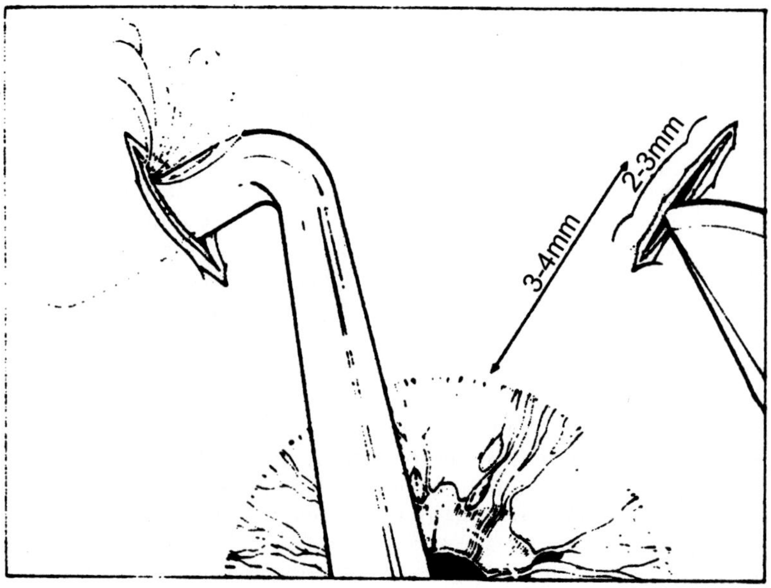

Figure 39–4. Sclerotomy sites in the inferior quadrants, 2- to 3-mm in length and centered 3 to 4 mm from the limbus. A No. 64 Beaver scalpel blade is used because it is not extremely sharp and thus there is less danger of inadvertently penetrating into the vitreous cavity. (From Epstein DL, Allingham RR, Schuman JS [eds]: Chandler and Grant's Glaucoma, 4th Edition. Baltimore: Williams & Wilkins; 1997. © Lippincott Williams & Wilkins, with permission.)

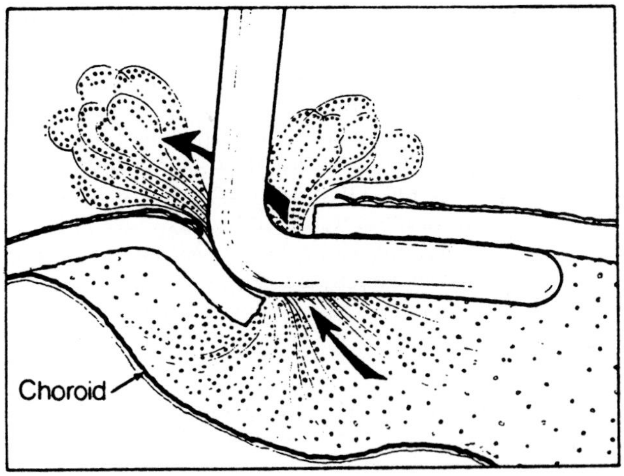

Figure 39–5. Side view of sclerotomy. The heel of the cyclodialysis spatula is used to depress the lip of the wound to aid the escape of suprachoroidal fluid. (From Epstein DL, Allingham RR, Schuman JS [eds]: Chandler and Grant's Glaucoma, 4th Edition. Baltimore: Williams & Wilkins; 1997. © Lippincott Williams & Wilkins, with permission.)

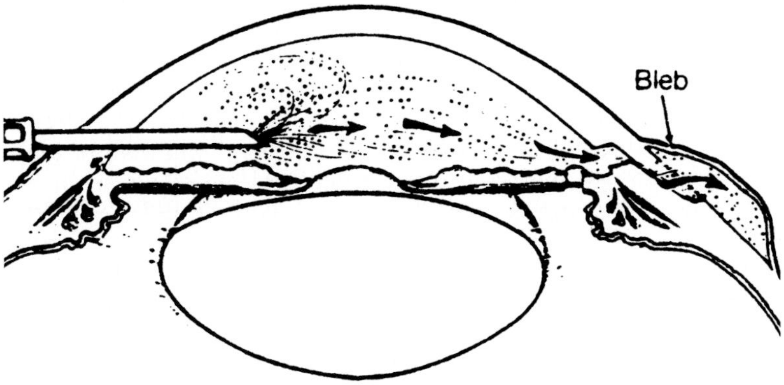

Figure 39–6. Injection of balanced salt solution deepens the anterior chamber and elevates the filtration bleb. (From Epstein DL, Allingham RR, Schuman JS [eds]: Chandler and Grant's Glaucoma, 4th Edition. Baltimore: Williams & Wilkins; 1997. © Lippincott Williams & Wilkins, with permission.)

ELEVATED INTRAOCULAR PRESSURE AND FLAT ANTERIOR CHAMBER

As previously noted, the differential diagnosis of a postoperative shallow anterior chamber in the face of an elevated intraocular pressure includes pupillary block, suprachoroidal hemorrhage, and malignant (ciliary block) glaucoma.

PUPILLARY BLOCK

Pupillary block may occur in the presence of normal intraocular pressure, although it is usually elevated. The inability of aqueous to pass from the posterior chamber to the anterior chamber results in the forward movement of the peripheral iris and closure of the anterior chamber angle. Pupillary block occurs when no patent peripheral iridectomy is present. It may be associated with adhesions of the iris to the lens (posterior synechiae) with resultant iris bombé or with an anterior chamber lens that prevents aqueous movement between the pupillary margin and the edges of the lens optic. A laser iridotomy is the treatment of choice, although laser pupilloplasty or peripheral iridoplasty may be helpful when an iridotomy is not effective or cannot be performed.

SUPRACHOROIDAL HEMORRHAGE

A suprachoroidal hemorrhage is one of the most serious complications of filtering surgery. It usually occurs within the first few postoperative days. The patient typically complains of the sudden onset of severe eye pain, which is virtually diagnostic when associated with choroidal detachment (often with central touch), a shallow anterior chamber, and a highly elevated intraocular pressure.[31,32] However, if the choroidal attachments are not large, the intraocular pressure is not always elevated by the time the patient seeks medical evaluation. After the acute event, the eye frequently becomes inflamed. This complication is not common (2% or less in most large series), but the incidence increases considerably with certain risk factors, especially aphakia and vitrectomy.[31–34] In one series of 305 filtering procedures, the overall incidence of delayed suprachoroidal hemorrhage was 1.6%, but rose to 13% in aphakic eyes and to 33% in aphakic, vitrectomized eyes.[32] In the Fluorouracil Filtering Surgery Study,[35] 6.2% of eyes that had undergone previous cataract extraction developed a suprachoroidal hemorrhage after filtering surgery. The risk of suprachoroidal hemorrhage was strongly associated with the level of the preoperative intraocular pressure, as none of the patients with a preoperative intraocular pressure less than 30 mm Hg developed a suprachoroidal hemorrhage.

A waiting period of 7 to 10 days after suprachoroidal hemorrhage is advised before surgical intervention to allow the fibrinolytic response to liquefy the clot, which permits more effective evacuation of the suprachoroidal space, with retinal and choroidal flattening.[36] At the time of suprachoroidal drainage, using vitrectomy techniques with the instillation of intraocular expandable gases can effectively decrease the incidence of rebleeding and can tamponade the choroid and the retina in their anatomic positions so that reoperation is less likely.

AQUEOUS MISDIRECTION SYNDROME (MALIGNANT OR CILIARY BLOCK GLAUCOMA)

This final differential diagnostic category of a shallow to flat anterior chamber postoperatively is characterized by an intraocular pressure elevated to moderate or high levels and is due to aqueous misdirection into the vitreous cavity.[37] This type of glaucoma was initially called malignant glaucoma, and later, ciliary block glaucoma. Because the basic problem is misdirection of the flow of aqueous humor posteriorly we here use this newer term. Classically, aqueous misdirection syndrome occurs after glaucoma filtration surgery, peripheral iridectomy, or combined cataract/filtration surgery. The diagnosis of aqueous misdirection syndrome typically includes (1) axial shallowing of the anterior chamber, (2) elevated intraocular pressure, (3) the presence of a patent iridectomy, and (4) the absence of suprachoroidal fluid or blood. However, in the presence of a functioning filtration bleb, the intraocular pressure may be only in the mid-to-low teens.

The anterior hyaloid, either because of inherent "permeability" or the amount of available hyaloid surface area for fluid transfer, is involved in the pathogenesis of aqueous misdirection syndrome. A maintained increase in total vitreous volume is responsible for the axial flattening of the anterior chamber.

The first major success in medical therapy for aqueous misdirection syndrome came in 1962 with the report of successful relief with mydriatic-cycloplegic drops, specifically, atropine 1% and phenylephrine 2.5%.[38] This treatment is thought to relieve the ciliary block by relaxation of the ciliary muscle. The intraocular pressure should be lowered with aqueous suppressants (beta-blockers, alpha-agonists, and carbonic anhydrase inhibitors) while simultaneously initiating mydriatic-cycloplegic drug therapy. Thought should also be given to administering osmotics[39] to lower the intraocular pressure and to temporarily dehydrate and thus decrease the vitreous volume. Medical therapy is successful in about 50% of cases of aqueous misdirection syndrome within 4 to 5 days. Patients who respond favorably to atropine treatment may need to continue the atropine for the rest of their lives. After this, surgical intervention is required.

When medical treatment is unsuccessful, laser therapy may be a useful option. Herschler[40] reported success with the technique of argon treatment of ciliary processes through the peripheral iridectomy in five of six cases of aqueous misdirection syndrome unresponsive to medical treatment. Epstein et al.[41] suggested neodymium: YAG laser hyaloidotomy to disrupt the anterior vitreous face in malignant glaucoma in aphakia and pseudophakia. Relief of the aqueous misdirection syndrome after laser treatment may be due to establishment of communication between the vitreous cavity and the posterior chamber.

Many surgical procedures have been employed for aqueous misdirection syndrome since its description in 1869. Posterior sclerotomies and lens extractions were used until 1954, when Shaffer[42] called attention to the importance of vitreous humor in phakic and aphakic eyes affected by malignant glaucoma. He noted that when lens extraction was performed without vitreous loss, the malignant course persisted, but that the glaucoma would respond to subsequent deep incision into the vitreous, which presumably disrupted the anterior and posterior hyaloid membranes. In 1964 Chandler[43] devised a surgical technique involving puncture and aspiration of the vitreous. This procedure was successful in relieving aqueous misdirection syndrome, but it was abandoned because of the high incidence of postoperative cataract formation. In an effort to prevent damage to the lens, Chandler devised a manual technique that came to be known as the *surgical confirmation procedure.*[37]

Vitrectomy has replaced many surgical procedures and has been shown to be effective in relieving ciliary block unresponsive to other treatment options.[44–46] Byrnes et al.[47] reviewed the medical records of 21 consecutive patients with refractory aqueous misdirection syndrome treated by pars plana vitrectomy and found that the initial vitrectomy was successful in alleviating ciliary block in 70% of eyes.

Management of the shallow or flat anterior chamber requires thorough evaluation and investigation of the many possible causes. Diligence on the part of the surgeon in seeking to make the correct diagnosis is crucial to offer the patient the greatest possibility of a successful outcome.

REFERENCES

1. Allen JC: Delayed anterior chamber formation after filtering operations. Am J Ophthalmol 1966;62:640.
2. Hoskins HD, Migliazzo C: Management of failing filtering blebs with the argon laser. Ophthalmol Surg 1984;15:731.
3. Traverso CE, Greenidge KC, Spaeth GL, et al.: Focal pressure: a new method to encourage filtration after trabeculectomy. Ophthalmol Surg 1984;15:62.
4. Chandler PA, Grant WM: Lectures on glaucoma. Philadelphia: Lea & Febiger; 1965:393–403.
5. Sampaolesi R: Postoperative flat anterior chamber after glaucoma surgery. Inst Barraquer 1972;10:124.

6. Stewart WC, Shields MB: Management of anterior chamber depth after trabeculectomy. Am J Ophthalmol 1988;106:41–4.
7. Fiore PM, Richter CU, Arzano G, et al.: The effect of anterior chamber depth on endothelial cell count after filtration surgery. Arch Ophthalmol 1989;107:1609.
8. Smith DL, Skuta GL, Lindenmuth KA, et al.: The effect of glaucoma filtering surgery on corneal endothelial cell density. Ophthalmic Surg 1991;22:251.
9. Kronfeld P: Delayed restoration of the anterior chamber. Am J Ophthalmol 1954:38:453.
10. Phillips CT, Clark CV, Levy AM: Posterior synechiae after glaucoma operations: aggravation by shallow anterior chamber and pilocarpine. Br J Ophthalmol 1987;71:428.
11. Wright MM, Grajewski AL: Measurement of intraocular pressure with a flat anterior chamber. Ophthalmology 1991;98:1854–7.
12. Pavlin CJ: Practical application of ultrasound biomicroscopy. Can J Ophthalmol 1995;30:225–9.
13. Kao SF, Lichter PR, Musch DC: Anterior chamber depth following filtration surgery. Ophthalmic Surg 1989;20:332–6.
14. Hung SO: Role of sodium hyaluronate (Healonid) in triangular flap trabeculectomy. Br J Ophthalmol 1985;69:46.
15. Teekhasaenee C, Ritch R: The use of PhEA 34c in trabeculectomy. Ophthalmology 1986;93:487.
16. Wand M: Viscoelastic agent and the prevention of post-filtration flat anterior chamber. Ophthalmic Surg 1988;19:523.
17. Raitta C, Lehto I, Puska P, et al.: A randomized, prospective study on the use of sodium hyaluronate (Healon) in trabeculectomy. Ophthalmic Surg 1994;25:536–9.
18. Brubaker RF, Pederson JE: Ciliochoroidal detachment. Surv Ophthalmol 1983;27:281.
19. Bellows AR, Chylack LT, Hutchinson BT: Choroidal detachment: clinical manifestation, therapy and mechanism of formation. Ophthalmology 1981;88:1107.
20. Chylack LT, Bellows AR: Molecular sieving in suprachoroidal fluid formation in man. Invest Ophthalmol Vis Sci 1978;17:420.
21. Asamoto A, Yablonski ME: Posttrabeculectomy anterior subcapsular cataract formation induced by anterior chamber air. Ophthalmic Surg 1993;24:314.
22. Stewart RH, Kimbrough RL: A method of managing flat anterior chamber following trabeculectomy. Ophthalmic Surg 1980;11:382.
23. Doro D, Mantovani E, Moro F: Sodium hyaluronate in the management of persistent flat anterior chamber after trabeculectomy. Glaucoma 1989;11:42.
24. Gerber SL, Cantor LB: Slit-lamp reformation of the anterior chamber following trabeculectomy. Ophthalmic Surg 1990;21:404.
25. Franks WA, Hitchings RA: Intraocular gas injection in the treatment of cornea-lens touch and choroidal effusion following fistulizing surgery. Ophthalmic Surg 1990;21:831.
26. Wilson MR, Yoshizumi MO, Lee DA, et al.: Use of intraocular gas in flat anterior chamber after filtration surgery (correspondence). Arch Ophthalmol 1988;106:1345.
27. Hykin PG, Hitchings RA: Alteration of patient posture to control immediate postoperative hypotony after fistulizing surgery (correspondence). Arch Ophthalmol 1991;109:920.
28. Abrams GW, Thomas MA, Williams GA, et al.: Management of postoperative suprachoroidal hemorrhage with continuous-infusion air pump. Arch Ophthalmol 1986;104:1455.
29. Dellaporta A: Scleral trephination for subchoroidal effusion. Arch Ophthalmol 1983;101:1917.
30. Berke SJ, Bellows AR, Shingleton BJ, et al.: Chronic and recurrent choroidal detachment after glaucoma filtering surgery. Ophthalmology 1987;94:154.
31. Gressel MG, Parrish RK, Heuer DK: Delayed non-expulsive suprachoroidal hemorrhage. Arch Ophthalmol 1984;102:1757.
32. Givens K, Shields MB: Suprachoroidal hemorrhage after glaucoma filtering surgery. Am J Ophthalmol 1987;103:689.
33. Ruderman JM, Harbin TS, Campbell DG: Postoperative suprachoroidal hemorrhage following filtration procedures. Arch Ophthalmol 1986;104:201.
34. Canning CR, Lavin M, McCartney ACE, et al.: Delayed suprachoroidal hemorrhage after glaucoma operations. Eye 1989;3:327.
35. The Fluorouracil Filtering Surgery Study Group: Risk factors for suprachoroidal hemorrhage after filtering surgery. Am J Ophthalmol 1992;113:501.
36. Lambrou FH, Meredith TA, Kaplan HG: Secondary surgical management of expulsive choroidal hemorrhage. Arch Ophthalmol 1987;105:1195.
37. Chandler PA, Simmons RJ, Grant WM: Malignant glaucoma: medical and surgical treatment. Am J Ophthalmol 1968;66:492.
38. Chandler PA,Grant WM: Mydriatic-cycloplegic treatment in malignant glaucoma. Arch Ophthalmol 1962;68:353.
39. Weiss DI, Shaffer RN: Treatment of malignant glaucoma with intravenous mannitol infusion. Arch Ophthalmol 1963;69:154.
40. Herschler J: Laser shrinkage of the ciliary processes—a treatment for malignant (ciliary block) glaucoma. Ophthalmology 1980; 87:1155.
41. Epstein DL, Steinert RF, Puliafito CA: Neodymium-YAG laser therapy to the anterior hyaloid in aphakic malignant glaucoma. Am J Ophthalmol 1984;98:137.
42. Shaffer RN: The role of vitreous detachment in aphakic and malignant glaucoma. Trans Am Acad Ophthalmol Otolaryngol 1954;58:217.
43. Chandler PA: A new operation for malignant glaucoma: a preliminary report. Trans Am Ophthalmol Soc 1964;62:408.
44. Duy TP, Wollensak J: Ciliary block (malignant) glaucoma following posterior chamber lens implantation. Ophthalmic Surg 1987; 18:741.
45. Lynch MG, Brown RH, Michels RG, et al.: Surgical vitrectomy for pseudophakic malignant glaucoma. Am J Ophthalmol 1986; 102:149.
46. Weiss H, Shin DH, Kollarits CR: Vitrectomy for malignant (ciliary block) glaucomas. Int Ophthalmol Clin 1981;21:113.
47. Byrnes GA, Leen MM, Wong TP, et al.: Vitrectomy for ciliary block (malignant) glaucoma. Ophthalmology 1995;102:1308.

CHAPTER 40

Low Postoperative Intraocular Pressure

MARTHA MOTUZ LEEN, M.D. and RICHARD P. MILLS, M.D., M.P.H.

Low intraocular pressure has traditionally been called *hypotony,* a term that usually implies an intraocular pressure less than 9 mm Hg, two standard deviations lower than for the mean population. It has long been recognized, however, that most eyes meeting the statistical definition of hypotony have no visual consequences of the "abnormally low" eye pressure. Such eyes are analogous to the ocular hypertensive eye that may suffer no visual consequences of "abnormally high" intraocular pressure. Some hypotonous eyes, however, have a variety of visually significant complications, including so-called hypotonous maculopathy, hypotonous choroidal effusion, and variable astigmatism of hypotony. Because of these visually disabling associations, the word "hypotony" carries the often unwarranted connotation of abnormal visual function. To obviate confusion in this chapter, we refer to *hypotony* in the statistical sense as intraocular pressure lower than 9 mm Hg, and the visual symptomatology associated with low intraocular pressure as the *low pressure syndrome.*

CAUSES OF POSTOPERATIVE HYPOTONY

Postoperative hypotony commonly occurs in association with a guarded filtration procedure, especially when adjunctive antimetabolites such as 5-fluorouracil or mitomycin are used. Hypotony may also develop after cataract extraction, cyclodestruction, goniotomy, trabeculotomy and cyclodialysis. A careful search for the mechanism of postoperative hypotony is essential to guide management (Table 40–1).

OVERFILTERING BLEB

In the early postoperative period after a guarded filtration procedure, overfiltration may occur as a result of a large bleb with little outflow resistance, conjunctival buttonhole, or conjunctival wound leak. Inadvertent filtration with or without a bleb may occur after cataract extraction, more commonly with larger wounds. However, unintended filtration may also occur with smaller cataract wounds in the setting of poor wound construction or faulty wound closure. In the later postoperative period, overfiltration may occur from a spontaneous pinpoint leak in the bleb or from slow transudation of aqueous humor in an excessively thin cystic bleb. Painting a bleb or incision site with a dry fluorescein strip and viewing the area with a cobalt blue light (Seidel test) will delineate an area of leak or transudation. Although a leak can be immediately identified, a bleb may need to be observed for several seconds to delineate an area of transudation. Blebs associated with excessive filtration are usually avascular and very thin, occuring more commonly with antimetabolite use.

TABLE 40–1. Differential Diagnosis of Hypotony after Glaucoma Surgery

- Overfiltering bleb
- Cyclodialysis cleft
- Choroidal effusion
- Retinal detachment
- Suppression of aqueous formation

CYCLODIALYSIS CLEFT

Disinsertion of the ciliary body from the scleral spur results in a cyclodialysis cleft (Fig. 40–1). This allows direct access of aqueous humor to the supraciliary space, with detachment of the anterior choroid over a much greater circumference than the cyclodialysis occupies, resulting in a low intraocular pressure. Cyclodialysis clefts are unusual after glaucoma filtering surgery, created when a block of scleral spur tissue is inadvertently excised. Clefts occur most often in the context of combined surgery with phacoemulsification, resulting from dissection of a scleral tunnel that is too deep. Diagnosis can be difficult because of a shallow anterior chamber, corneal distortion during gonioscopy, and peripheral anterior synechiae that can sometimes hide a cleft. In such cases, a viscoelastic agent injected intracamerally through a corneal paracentesis may aid in identification and localization of a cyclodialysis cleft by improving the gonioscopic view. High-frequency ultrasound biomicroscopy may be useful in identifying those clefts obscured by peripheral anterior synechiae.

CHOROIDAL EFFUSION

In almost all severely hypotonous eyes, some degree of choroidal effusion is present. This may be subtle, with a collection of fluid anteriorly, and difficult to detect with conventional b-scan ultrasonography. In such cases, use of high-frequency ultrasound biomicroscopy may demonstrate the effusion. When seen clinically, choroidal effusions appear smooth, dome-shaped, gray in color, and varying from one to four in number. Although the suprachoroidal space may be considered as one continuous entity, a lobulated appearance of choroidal effusions results from firm connections of the vortex veins and optic nerve head. Occasionally, the effusions may be extensive with "kissing" of convex choroidal detachments in the mid-vitreous. In any case, the presence of this fluid contributes to a vicious cycle of reduced aqueous humor production and, possibly, enhanced uveoscleral outflow, in turn aggravating hypotony and the tendency for more choroidal effusion (Fig. 40–2).

RETINAL DETACHMENT

A retinal detachment seen on fundus examination or ultrasonography can be associated with hypotony. More than one mechanism may contribute to the reduction in intraocular pressure. A retinal tear allows access of aqueous fluid to the subretinal space, probably enhancing choroidal absorption. There may also be a reduction in aqueous humor formation, perhaps related in part to an associated low-grade iridocyclitis.

AQUEOUS SUPPRESSION

When structural abnormalities have been ruled out after examination, suppression of aqueous humor formation by the ciliary body as a result of current or prolonged prior use of aqueous suppressants or active inflammation should be considered. After discontinuation of aqueous suppressants postoperatively, some degree of continued suppression may persist for 2 to 3 weeks. Alternatively, the possibilty of a chemical cyclodestructive effect resulting from transscleral mito-

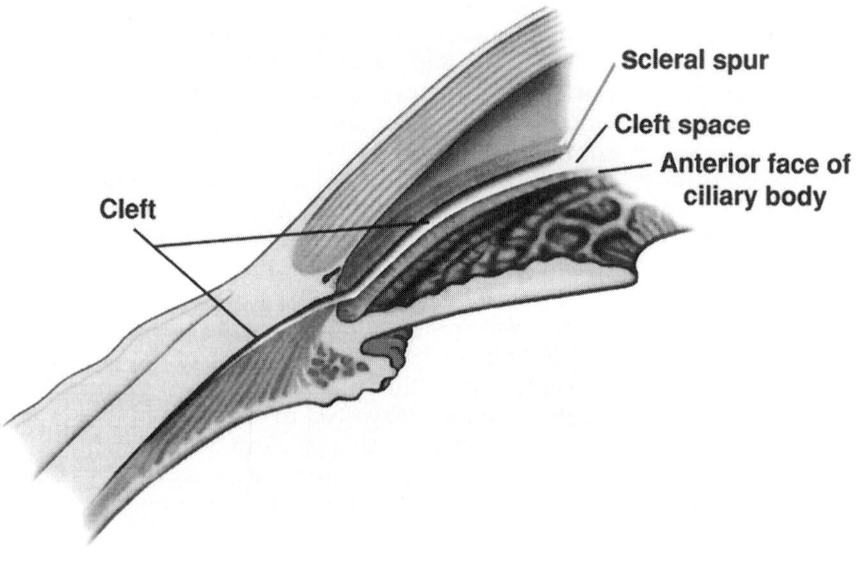

Figure 40–1. Cyclodialysis cleft. The ciliary body is detached from the scleral spur, allowing direct access of aqueous humor into the supraciliary space.

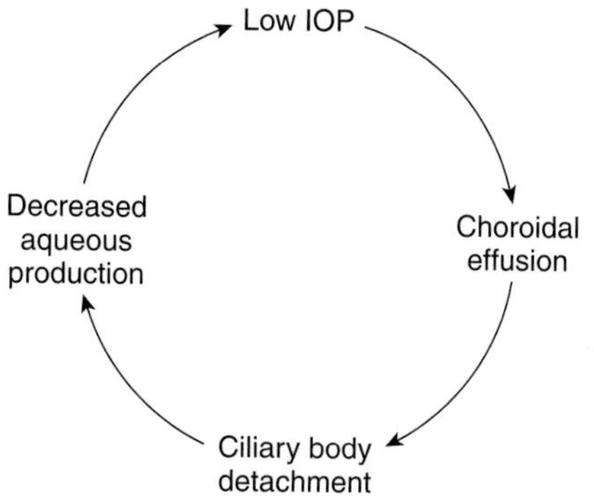

Figure 40–2. A vicious cycle. A low intraocular pressure can lead to a choroidal effusion resulting in decreased aqueous production, further lowering the intraocular pressure.

TABLE 40–2. Structural Characteristics of the Low Pressure Syndrome

- Corneal astigmatism
- Corneal edema
- Macular edema
- Disc edema
- Hypotonous maculopathy
- Breakdown of blood-aqueous barrier
- Shallow anterior chamber
- Choroidal effusion or hemorrhage
- Exudative retinal detachment

mycin diffusion has been suggested.[1] This possibility should be considered, especially if thin or friable sclera was noted intraoperatively.

THE LOW-PRESSURE SYNDROME

Hypotony, even extreme hypotony with intraocular pressure of 1 mm Hg, may be well tolerated, with no symptoms or secondary ocular signs. In that case, there is seldom an indication to intervene. In some hypotonous eyes, the low-pressure syndrome may occur when a low intraocular pressure is associated with structural and functional changes, sometimes requiring intervention. Although the presence of hypotony increases the risk of the low-pressure syndrome, the level of intraocular pressure required to produce this syndrome varies with individual eyes, and in some cases, it may occur at intraocular pressures that are higher than the hypotonous range (i.e., higher than 9 mm Hg).

STRUCTURAL CHANGES

The structural changes associated with the low-pressure syndrome may include corneal astigmatism, corneal edema, macular edema, disc edema, hypotonous maculopathy, corneal astigmatism, breakdown of the blood–aqueous barrier, shallow anterior chamber, choroidal effusion or hemorrhage, and exudative retinal detachment (Table 40–2).

Hypotonous maculopathy is diagnosed when the triad of macular choroidal folds, retinal vascular tortuosity, and optic disc edema are present in the setting of a low intraocular pressure (Fig. 40–3). In discs with advanced cupping and little or no remaining axonal tissue, disc edema, a collection of fluid within the axons, cannot develop. Choroidal folds are usually horizontally oriented, probably representing the resting tone of the inferior oblique muscle, which has a broad submacular insertion.[3] Although hypotonous maculopathy may occur more frequently following use of adjunctive antimetabolites, it can also occur after a standard guarded filtration procedure.[4] Risk factors include young patient age and high myopia.[5] It is likely that the thinner sclera of a young myopic eye is more easily deformed by contraction of the inferior oblique muscle. Permanent macular retinal pigment epithelial disturbances may occur if the period of hypotonous maculopathy is prolonged, limiting visual potential.

When a choroidal effusion is present in the setting of a low intraocular pressure, it is often difficult to establish which is the cause and which is the effect. The effusion is usually serous fluid, but it can occasionally contain blood. Low intraocular pressure, postoperative inflammation, and the acute decompression of the eye during surgery can contribute to the choroidal effusion. Nevertheless, persistence of the choroidal effusion leads to reduction in aqueous humor production and, possibly, enhanced uveoscleral outflow, further exacerbating the low intraocular pressure.

Exudative retinal detachment occurs infrequently and is generally accompanied by a large choroidal effusion. It is characterized by a smooth translucent appearance with shifting of subretinal fluid and usually resolves when the choroidal effusion resolves.

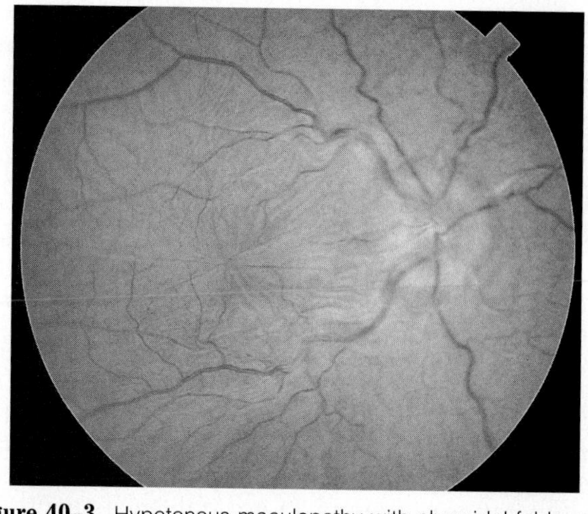

Figure 40–3. Hypotonous maculopathy with choroidal folds, vascular tortuosity, and disc edema.

FUNCTIONAL CHANGES

Each of these structural findings can be associated with functional symptoms, including reduced visual acuity and ocular discomfort. The most common cause of symptoms in the low-pressure syndrome is visual instability related to changing refractive error from variable amounts of astigmatism. Blurring of vision can be especially severe upon awakening due to pressure on the eye during sleep and may require an eye shield to mitigate. A hyperopic shift in refractive error may occur with edema or folds in the macula from anterior displacement of the sensory retina. A myopic shift in refractive error may occur with a shallow anterior chamber from anterior movement of the lens–irisdiaphragm. A choroidal effusion may result in reduced vision, not only from shallowing of the anterior chamber but also from blockage of peripheral and central vision by huge or "kissing" choroidals. Ocular pain and general discomfort is also quite common and may be related to defects in the blood–aqueous barrier with low-grade inflammation that can occur in eyes with low pressures, or it may have no identifiable cause other than the low intraocular pressure. Even a small amount of hemorrhage in the choroid can produce severe pain, often excruciating.

In many cases vision can be restored to normal with modest elevation of intraocular pressure, perhaps still remaining in the hypotonous range. However, in other cases, vision may remain permanently reduced after resolution of the low-pressure syndrome, especially if the duration of visual loss was prolonged. The duration of hypotony necessary to cause permanent damage varies from patient to patient. Macular edema lasting more than 1 month is of great concern, but complete visual recovery may occur even after edema has been present for as long as 6 months.

AVOIDANCE OF POSTOPERATIVE HYPOTONY

Because postoperative hypotony is often difficult to manage successfully, its avoidance is desirable. Preventive strategies include judicious use of antimetabolites, meticulous scleral flap closure, avoidance of premature flap suture release, and special attentiveness to patients with high-risk characteristics for hypotony.

RESTRICT USE OF ANTIFIBROTIC AGENTS

Antimetabolites enhance the success of filtration surgery and generally result in lower postoperative intraocular pressures. In general, mean postoperative pressures are lowest with mitomycin, a little higher after use of 5-fluorouracil, and higher yet when no antifibrotic agent has been used. The use of immunosuppressing agents is associated with a higher incidence of postoperative hypotony. In general, such agents are used most effectively and safely in eyes with poor surgical prognoses or eyes in need of a very low postoperative intraocular pressure. Unfortunately, badly damaged eyes may be those most liable to develop hypotony, because they make less aqueous humor and the sclera is likely to be less healthy.

ATTEND TO METICULOUS FLAP CLOSURE

Scleral flaps that are too thin may transude aqueous humor and become the source of excess leakage that cannot be easily controlled with suture. Sutures may also "cheese-wire" through thin flaps, further exacerbating the leakage. For these reasons, the scleral flap should be fashioned at least half thickness, especially if the sclera is noted to be thin or friable. Scleral sutures that are placed with a cutting needle vertically through the full thickness of the scleral flap can produce small defects in the flap that stretch open when the suture is tied, causing excess leakage. To avoid this, when possible, the suture should be placed only partially through the scleral flap, exiting horizontally at the edge of the flap (Fig. 40–4). This is easier to accomplish with thicker flaps.

PLACE EXTRA SCLERAL FLAP SUTURES

The amount of aqueous leakage can be controlled intraoperatively by adjusting the number and tightness of sutures reapposing the scleral flap to its bed. In general, postoperatively elevated intraocular pressures resulting from a scleral flap that is too tight are easier to manage than intraocular pressures too low resulting

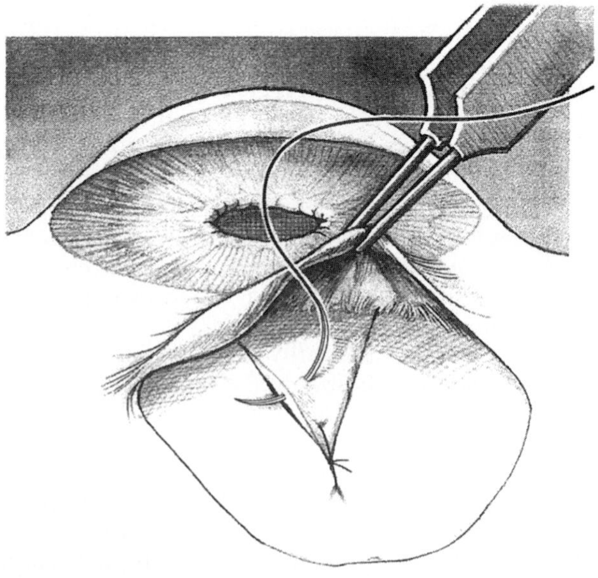

Figure 40–4. To avoid producing needle defects in the flap, the needle should exit the edge of the scleral flap.

from a loose scleral flap. Interrupted sutures securing the scleral flap can be cut with an argon laser postoperatively without violating the integrity of the conjunctiva. In cases where visibility of the sutures is expected to be difficult, such as with a thick Tenon's capsule or conjunctival hemorrhage, a releasable suture can be placed so it may easily be removed at the slit lamp (see Chapter 12, Surgery for Pediatric Cataracts).

AVOID RELEASING SUTURES TOO EARLY

Release of scleral flap sutures too early can increase the risk of postoperative hypotony, especially if antimetabolites have been used. In general, when 5-fluorouracil has been used either intraoperatively or by postoperative injection, initial suture lysis should be delayed at least 1 week. When mitomycin has been used, suture lysis should be delayed at least 2 weeks. Even with observance of these precautions, prolonged hypotony can occur after suture lysis performed as late as several months after a guarded filtration procedure with mitomycin.

TAKE EXTRA PRECAUTIONS IN EYES AT HIGH RISK OF HYPOTONY

Eyes of patients who are young, highly myopic or who have a lower aqueous production are at greater risk of developing hypotonous maculopathy. In these eyes, extra precautions should be taken to avoid this complication, such as tighter closure of the scleral flap and delayed suture lysis.

INDICATIONS FOR INTERVENTION

Not all hypotonous eyes require intervention. Some eyes with low pressures function well with good visual acuity, others do not, developing the low-pressure syndrome. The indications for intervening in an eye with prolonged hypotony must be individualized. The following indications should be considered: (1) low-pressure syndrome that is visually significant, (2) persistent bleb leak that places the eye at high risk of infection (i.e., history of prior blebitis or endophthalmitis, chronic blepharitis, or poor patient hygeine), (3) imminent risk of bleb failure (i.e., scarring of a shallow bleb to the underlying sclera or peripheral anterior synechia over the fistula from shallow anterior chamber), or (4) persistent ocular pain.

In many cases, simple observation will yield spontaneous resolution. This is more likely to occur in the early postoperative period than when prolonged hypotony exists in the late postoperative period. When time is not remedial, other measures can be considered. Management of overfiltering blebs is discussed in Chapter 41 by Lynch and Brown.

REPAIR OF A CYCLODIALYSIS CLEFT

OBSERVATION

Cyclodialysis clefts associated with the low-pressure syndrome may be observed for 6 to 8 weeks. Cycloplegia with atropine may enhance apposition of ciliary body to the sclera. Some degree of inflammation is beneficial, so steroids should be minimized or discontinued. Viscoelastic material injected to enhance gonioscopic view may also have a therapeutic effect by reversing the vicious cycle of hypotony. Clefts that do not resolve with medical treatment can be treated with laser, cryotherapy, or incisional surgery.

ARGON LASER SURGERY

Argon laser surgery should be attempted as the initial procedure for all clefts associated with the low-pressure syndrome. Pretreatment with pilocarpine and modest hyperinflation of the anterior chamber with viscoelastic material will enhance the view into the cleft, if needed. Laser parameters should be set at 50 to 100 μm spot size, 0.1 second duration, and 1000 to 3000 mW power. Using a Goldmann 3-mirror lens, rows of heavy confluent burns should be placed on the scleral aspect of the cleft first, from the scleral spur toward the depths of the cleft. Laser parameters are then changed to 100 to 200 μm spot size, 0.1 second duration, and 800 to 1200 mW power. The uveal aspect of the cleft should then be treated, starting in the depth of the cleft and working anteriorly to avoid an obscured view from uveal edema and pigment dispersion (Fig. 40–5). The viscoelastic agent should then be removed to blunt the intraocular pressure elevation that may occur immediately after the procedure. Postoperatively, atropine is instilled for 2 to 3 weeks. Steroids and miotics should be avoided.

CRYOTHERAPY

Cryotherapy over the cyclodialysis cleft can be attempted, but is best used as an adjunct to surgical repair. The applications should be of short duration to create an ice ball that is superficial, avoiding cyclodestruction. The goal of treatment is to induce inflammation in the iris/ciliary body root.

INCISIONAL SURGERY

If laser treatment is unsuccessful in closing the cleft, then incisional surgery can be attempted. Various surgical techniques have been described for repair of cyclodialysis clefts, and three methods will be described in detail:

1. The *direct cyclopexy technique* of Naumann[6,7] has the advantage of allowing a direct view of the disinserted ciliary body and scleral spur, resulting in the

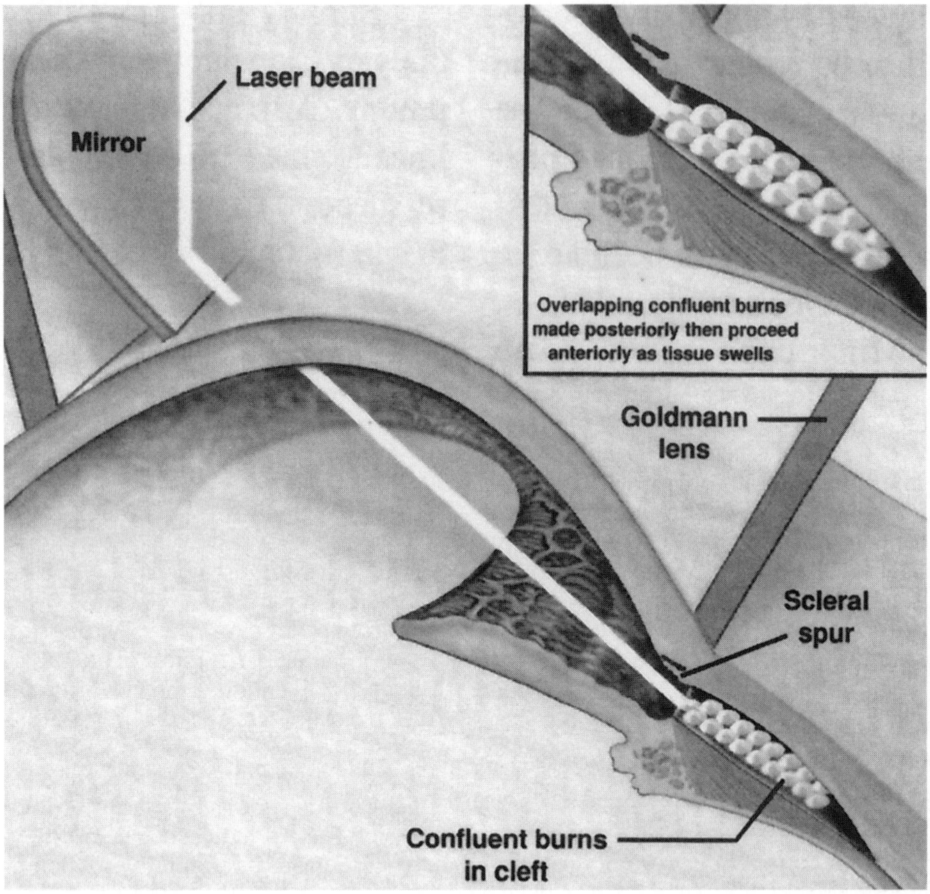

Figure 40–5. Argon laser cleft repair. Heavy confluent laser burns are delivered on the scleral aspect of the cleft first, followed by the uveal side.

most anatomically correct closure. This procedure is more difficult and requires intimate knowledge of limbal anatomy.

2. The *cross chamber cyclopexy technique* described by Metrikin[8] is an indirect method of closure using techniques derived from suturing posterior chamber intraocular lenses; it is less difficult than direct cyclopexy. However, it is applicable only in aphakic and pseudophakic eyes.
3. Finally, a method of *iris base fixation* described by Mills[9] is the easiest of the techniques and is generally appropriate for smaller clefts because it creates broad peripheral anterior synechiae along the length of the cleft.

Each of the procedures begins with injection of viscoelastic material into the anterior chamber to firm the globe and to allow better visualization of the cleft. The location of the cleft is confirmed by gonioscopy under the microscope. A disposable cautery can be used to mark the extent and location of the cleft by making small burns at the limbus. A limbal conjunctival peritomy is created adjacent to the cleft.

Direct Cyclopexy Technique

A two-thirds scleral thickness rectangular flap is created extending radially 4 mm from the limbus and 1-2 mm beyond the edge of the cleft in length. Then, within the remaining scleral bed, a full-thickness circumferential incision is made 1.5 mm posterior to the limbus, entering the cyclodialysis cleft and releasing aqueous. The cleft is directly visualized and light cautery is applied to the exposed surface of ciliary body. Ciliary body is directly sutured to the sclera using interrupted 10-0 nylon suture on a tapered vascular needle placed 1 mm apart. Each suture passes through the anterior lip of the scleral wound exiting in the region of scleral spur, then through ciliary muscle away from iris root vessels, then out through the posterior lip of the scleral flap. The sutures are tied after all have been inserted (Fig. 40–6). Light cryotherapy can then be applied at the base of the scleral bed to potentiate adhesion and the scleral flap is closed with interrupted 10-0 nylon sutures. The conjunctiva is closed and viscoelastic is removed from the anterior chamber.

Cross Chamber Cyclopexy Technique

The aphakic or pseudophakic eye is dilated preoperatively. A 1 to 2-mm corneal keratotomy is made 180 degrees opposite the cleft with a sharp blade. A 27-gauge needle is passed ab externa through the sclera 1.5 mm posterior to the limbus at one end of the cleft and exited

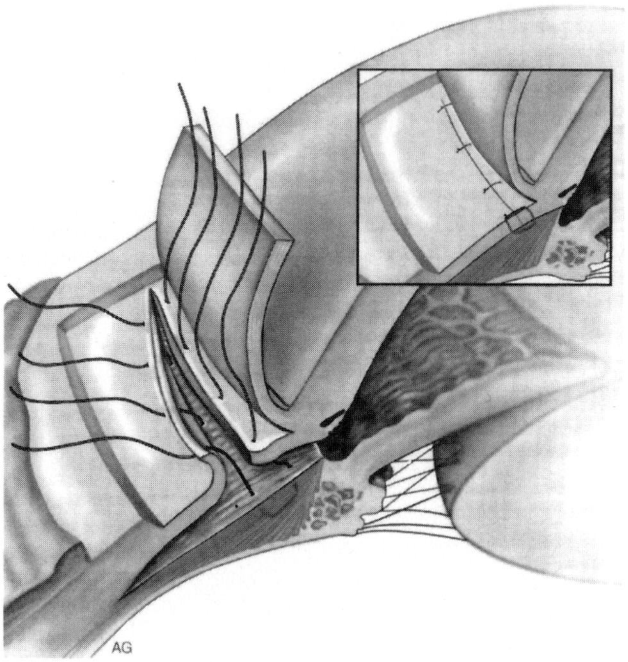

Figure 40–6. Direct cyclopexy. Each suture is passed through the anterior lip of the scleral wound, exiting the scleral spur region through ciliary muscle, and out through the posterior lip of the scleral wound. After all sutures have been placed, each is tied, closing the cleft.

through the ciliary sulcus between the iris and the posterior chamber lens. One arm of a 10-0 double-armed polypropylene suture on straight needles is simultaneously introduced into the anterior chamber through the keratotomy and threaded deep into the barrel of the 27-gauge needle (Fig. 40–7). The 27-gauge needle is pulled out of the eye, together with the straight needle, leaving the polypropylene suture passing through the keratotomy, across the anterior chamber, through the ciliary sulcus, across the cleft, and out through the sclera. The 27-gauge needle is reinserted in the same fashion 3 mm adjacent to the previous entry site. The second arm of the suture is then passed through the keratotomy, inserted into the barrel of the needle, and extracted out of the eye in the same fashion, pulling suture with it (Fig. 40–8). The two suture ends are then grasped where they exit the sclera, and a loop of suture is pulled into the anterior chamber toward the ciliary sulcus. When the suture is tightened, the ciliary body is pulled up against the scleral wall, closing the cleft. This maneuver is repeated as often as needed to close the length of the cleft (Fig. 40–9). The suture knots are buried. Light cryotherapy can be applied to the sclera posterior to the sutures to encourage adhesion. The viscoelastic material is removed and the keratotomy and conjunctiva are closed.

Iris Base Fixation Technique

A 1- to 2-mm keratotomy is made through peripheral clear cornea 1 mm anterior to the limbus adjacent to the cleft. A two-thirds-thickness rectangular scleral flap is dissected overlying the region of the cleft. For larger clefts, the keratotomy is enlarged to be 1 mm shorter than the extent of the cleft. Taking care not to snag corneal tissue with the needle, the surgeon passes one

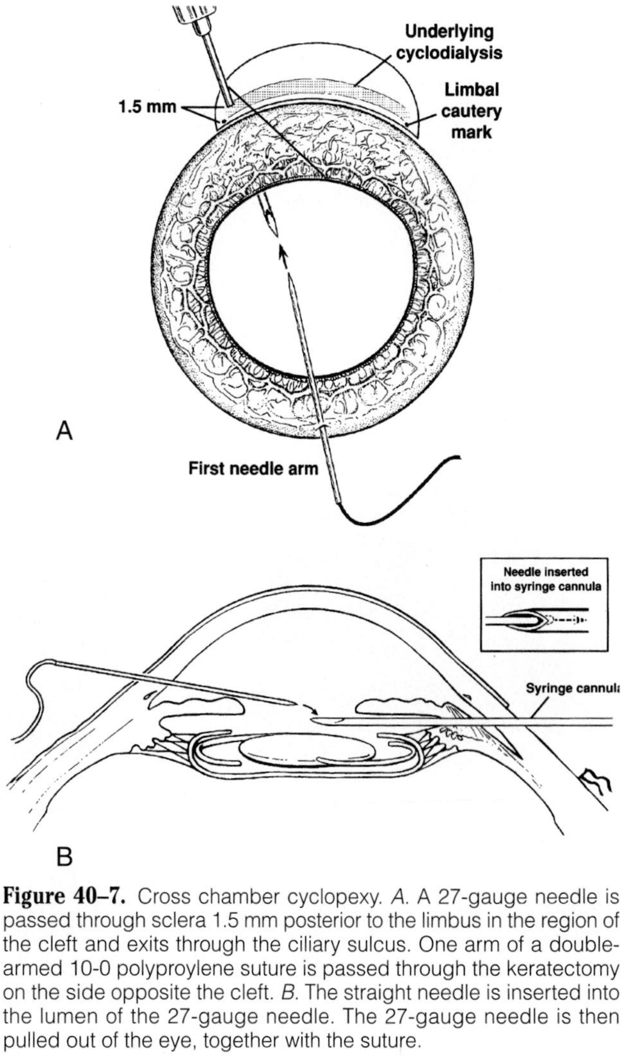

Figure 40–7. Cross chamber cyclopexy. *A.* A 27-gauge needle is passed through sclera 1.5 mm posterior to the limbus in the region of the cleft and exits through the ciliary sulcus. One arm of a double-armed 10-0 polyproylene suture is passed through the keratectomy on the side opposite the cleft. *B.* The straight needle is inserted into the lumen of the 27-gauge needle. The 27-gauge needle is then pulled out of the eye, together with the suture.

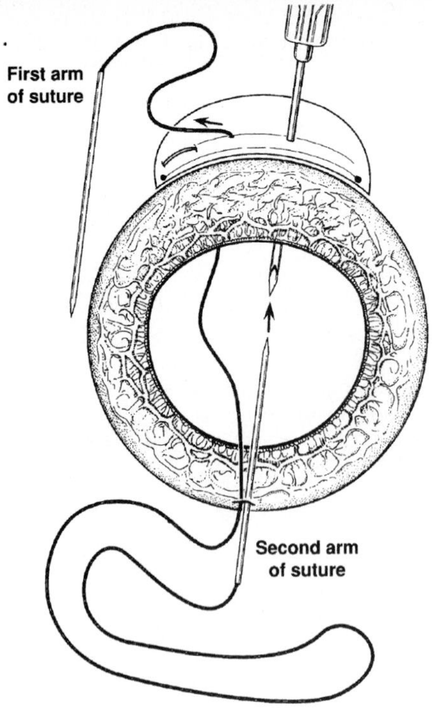

Figure 40–8. To continue the cross chamber cyclopexy, the suturing maneuver (Fig. 40–7) is repeated by reinserting the 27-gauge needle through the sclera 3 mm adjacent to the first pass. The second arm of the polypropylene suture is then passed through the keratectomy into the lumen of the 27-gauge needle and pulled out of the eye.

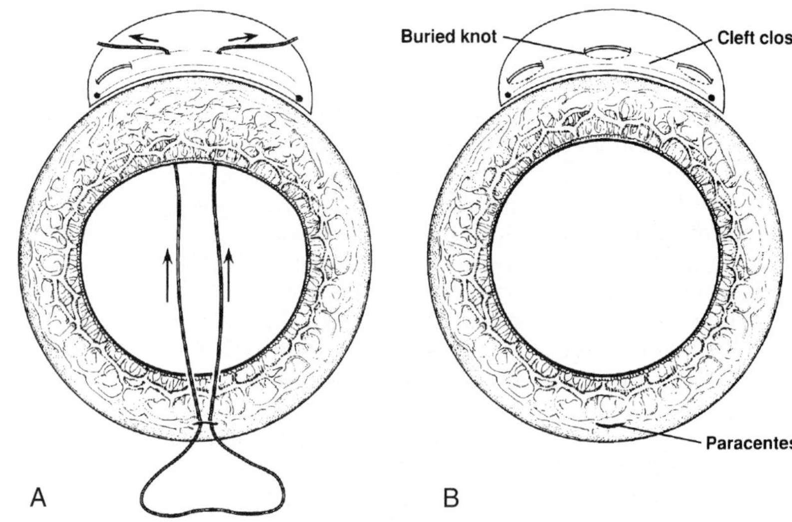

Figure 40–9. Completing the cross chamber cyclopexy. *A.* Both suture ends are grasped where they exit the sclera, pulling a loop of suture into the anterior chamber toward the cleft. *B.* The suture is tightened, pulling the cleft against the scleral wall. This technique is repeated as needed to close the length of the cleft.

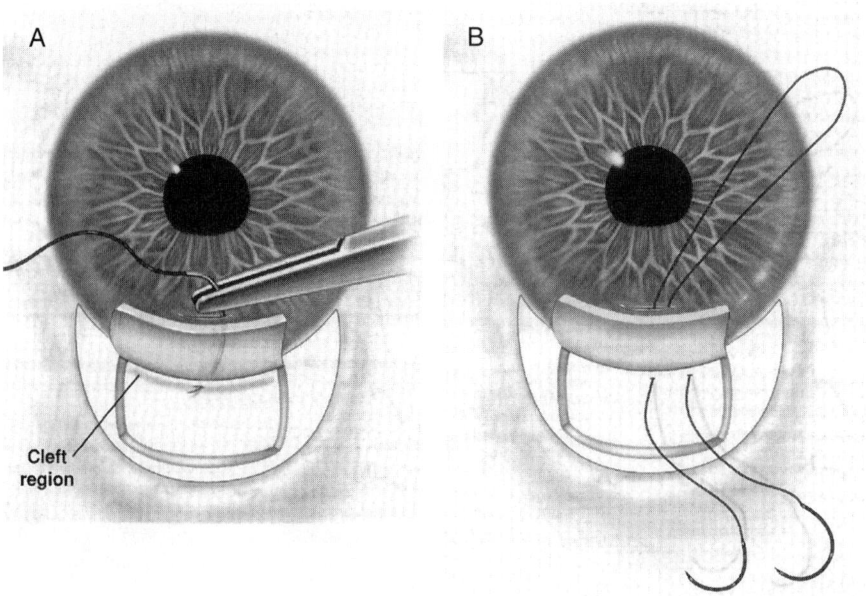

Figure 40–10. Iris base fixation. *A.* One arm of the needle is passed through the keratotomy, catches peripheral iris, and exits beneath the scleral flap. *B.* This maneuver is repeated with the second arm of the suture.

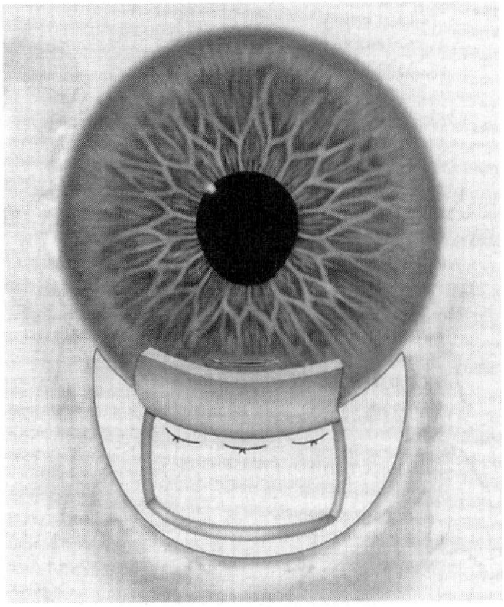

Figure 40–11. Completing the iris base fixation. Additional mattress sutures are placed as needed to close the length of the cleft.

arm of a double-armed 10-0 nylon suture on curved cutting needles through the keratotomy to catch peripheral iris at one end of the cleft, exiting through the scleral bed 0.5 to 1 mm behind the limbus. This maneuver is repeated with the second arm of the suture, catching iris 1 mm from the first iris pass (Fig. 40–10). As the suture is pulled taut, the nylon loop enters the anterior chamber and pulls peripheral iris against the scleral wall, often causing the pupil to peak a bit toward the cleft. The suture is tied. Additional mattress sutures are placed in a similar fashion as needed to span the width of the cleft (Fig. 40–11). Light cryotherapy may be applied to the base of the scleral flap to incite inflammation. Viscoelastic material is removed from the anterior chamber. The scleral flap and keratotomy are closed with interrupted 10-0 nylon sutures. The conjunctiva is closed.

Postoperatively for all three of the procedures described above, atropine is instilled for 2 to 4 weeks, and steroids are usually avoided. Sometimes the cleft does not immediately close, and a few weeks may elapse before the hypotony is reversed. When it does reverse, a pronounced intraocular pressure spike may ensue and is treated with aqueous suppressants. Prophylactic ocular hypotensive agents are not used.

SUMMARY

Postoperative hypotony is a common complication of glaucoma filtering surgery, particularly with adjunctive use of antifibrotic agents. Associated structural sequelae and reduced visual function may occur in some eyes, resulting in the low-pressure syndrome. Precautions may be taken intraoperatively and postoperatively to decrease the likelihood of hypotony. Sometimes, despite these measures, low-pressure syndrome can still occur and be difficult to manage. When simple observation over time does not result in spontaneous resolution, several noninvasive and invasive techniques are available, targeted at the cause of low intraocular pressure. If a cyclodialysis cleft is identified, laser and incisional surgical techniques are available to reverse the hypotony. When other causes of hypotony are identified, such as overfiltration or choroidal effusion, appropriate management options are available, as discussed in Chapter 41.

REFERENCES

1. Gandolfi SA, Vecchi M, Braccio L: Decrease of intraocular pressure after subconjunctival injection of mitomycin in human glaucoma. Arch Ophthalmol 1995:113;582–585.
2. Dellaporta A: Fundus changes in postoperative hypotony. Am J Ophthalmol 1955;40;781–785.
3. Greene P: Mechanical considerations in myopia: relative effects of accommodation, convergence, intraocular pressure, and the extraocular muscles. Am J Optometry Physiol Optics 1980;57:902–914.
4. Costa V, Smith M, Spaeth G, et al: Loss of visual acuity after trabeculectomy. Ophthalmology 1993;100:599–612.
5. Stamper RL, Mcmenemy MG, Lieberman MF: Hypotonous maculopathy after trabeculectomy with subconjunctival 5-fluorouracil. Am J Ophthalmol 1992;114:544–553.
6. Kuchle M, Naumann GOH: Direct cyclopexy for traumatic cyclodialysis with persisting hypotony. Report in 29 consecutive patients. Ophthalmology 1995;102:322–333.
7. Naumann GOH, Volcker HE: Direct cyclopexy for persisting hypotony syndrome due to traumatic cyclodialysis. In Koch DD, Parke DW, Paton D (eds.), Current management in ophthalmology. New York: Churchill Livingstone, 1983:143–150.
8. Metrikin DC, Allinson RW, Snyder RW: Transscleral repair of recalcitrant, inadvertent, postoperative cyclodialysis cleft. Ophthalmic Surg 1994;25:406–408.
9. Stewart JFG, Leen MM, Mills RP. Identification and management of cyclodialysis clefts. In Lindquist TD, Lindstrom RL (eds.), Ophthalmic surgery, 5th edition, Section I. Chicago: Mosby-Year Book Medical Publishers, 1996.

CHAPTER 41

Treatment of Excessive or Overfiltering Blebs

MARY G. LYNCH, M.D. and REAY H. BROWN, M.D.

OVERFILTRATION

Blebs can function excessively from overfiltration or from leaks (Tables 41-1 and 41-2. Some blebs overfilter immediately after surgery[1]; others develop overfiltration at a later time in the postoperative course.[2-4] This phenomenon occurs because the structure and function of filtering blebs can change over time.[5] The avascular, acellular blebs that often develop after antimetabolite therapy are particularly likely to change, not only in the early postoperative period but also years after the surgical procedure. A "stable," well-functioning bleb can slowly become a large, overfiltering bleb and can render an eye hypotonous after years of good pressure control. For the most part, the changes in bleb structure and function are due to the dynamic instability and weakness of the conjunctival tissue and the continued internal "barotrauma" of aqueous outflow. However, external trauma also can cause a bleb to grow in size, to become thinner, and to become multilobulated. Trauma can be incidental and isolated, such as with a sports injury, or it can be repetitive such as with chronic rubbing by the patient or inadvertent pressure during sleep. In a situation of excessive filtration it is important to look for a history of trauma or of ocular irritation that could lead to continued rubbing or scratching.

BLEB LEAKS

Leaks or holes in the bleb itself are not infrequent causes of overfiltration. Bleb leaks generally fall into two categories. "Traumatic" tears usually occur from a single event such as patient rubbing or a blunt injury. They are often accompanied by an acute change in bleb function (i.e., a sudden decrease in intraocular pressure) and symptoms (i.e., blurred vision) (Fig. 41-1). Such tears can be slit-like or flap-like in configuration, and because their edges are relatively "raw," they often can be treated with aqueous suppression and patching.

A second type of leak appears more like a "hole" and occurs in "threadbare" conjunctiva (Fig. 41-2). These atrophic holes usually follow a more chronic course and develop in very thin blebs that are unstable and expanding. Often, the hole is round, with a raised cuff around the opening; however, some occur at the edge of a lobulated area. With the more "threadbare" holes, changes in bleb function and the patient's symptoms may be slow and progressive. The treatment of threadbare holes is more challenging than the treatment of acute tears because the edges of the opening are lined with conjunctival epithelium. These tears often require more aggressive surgical intervention.

GENERAL CONSIDERATIONS FOR INTERVENTION

When and how to intervene with a troublesome bleb depends on the cause of the problem, its duration, and the individual circumstances of the patient. For example, a simple, acute bleb tear caused by inadvertent rubbing is a surface problem and might be treated conservatively with aqueous suppression and patching. In contrast, an intact but excessively filtering bleb that has caused

TABLE 41–1. Elements of Overfiltration

Avascular, acellular conjunctiva
Antimetabolite use
Internal aqueous barotrauma
External trauma
Incidental
Repetitive (rubbing)

TABLE 41–2. Elements of a Bleb Leak

Tear
Generally traumatic
Often slit-like or flap-like
Acute change in bleb function
Suddenly symptomatic
Hole
"Threadbare" in thin conjunctiva
Often round with raised cuff
Slow change in bleb function
Insidiously symptomatic

profound hypotony, visual loss, and maculopathy may require an aggressive approach that attacks the internal portion of the bleb (area of sclerectomy and flap) as well as the thin, avascular conjunctiva. The circumstances of the individual patient also must be kept in mind. For instance, an elderly, monocular patient with an overfiltering bleb, mild maculopathy, but good visual acuity might be followed without surgical intervention.

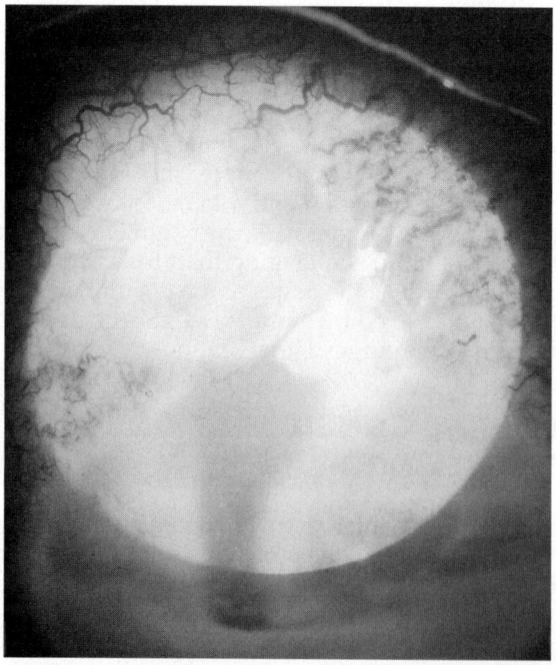

Figure 41–1. A 66-year-old woman with a well-functioning bleb bumped her eye on the corner of a shelf. The trauma caused a slit tear at the edge of the bleb and a sudden decrease in vision.

The following parameters usually dictate a more conservative approach: (1) acute tear, (2) monocular patient, (3) good central acuity, (4) reliable patient (will notify physician of any change in symptoms), (5) hypotony with no change in vision or macular function. In the following situations, a more aggressive course may be followed: (1) expanding, unstable, and overfiltering bleb; (2) overhanging, irritating bleb; (3) chronic threadbare hole in bleb; (4) history of bleb-related infection; (5) unreliable patient or one with poor hygiene for whom repeated trauma is a concern; (6) change in vision from maculopathy, hyperopic shift, or astigmatism.

MEDICAL INTERVENTION

There are several methods of stenting excessive blebs with minimally invasive techniques (Table 41-3). Surgery may also become appropriate (Table 41-4).

AQUEOUS SUPPRESSION

Reducing the rate of aqueous formation can limit the impact of internal barotrauma on the bleb. By simply "turning down the faucet," some intact but thin blebs will remodel on their own, especially in the early postoperative period. Acute bleb tears also respond to aqueous suppression, especially when combined with torpedo patching. When the eye is patched, oral carbonic anhydrase inhibitors (CAIs) should be considered. If the eye is not patched, topical beta-blockers and CAIs can be used.

TOPICAL ANTIBIOTICS

Some surgeons anecdotally recommend the use of topical antibiotic drops with bleb leaks as a means of irritating the ocular surface and perhaps stimulating a fibrotic response. According to these authors, acute bleb tears can seal on their own without antibiotics, but chronic, threadbare holes do not respond to any conservative therapy. These holes usually require some type of surgical repair. Therefore, because chronic antibiotic therapy could theoretically select-out resistant organisms, we do not recommend their use.

BLEB COMPRESSION

Bleb compression can be effective in changing the appearance and function of a troublesome bleb. Torpedo

TABLE 41–3. Medical Intervention

Aqueous suppression
Oral agent
Topical agents
Torpedo patch
Trichloroacetic acid

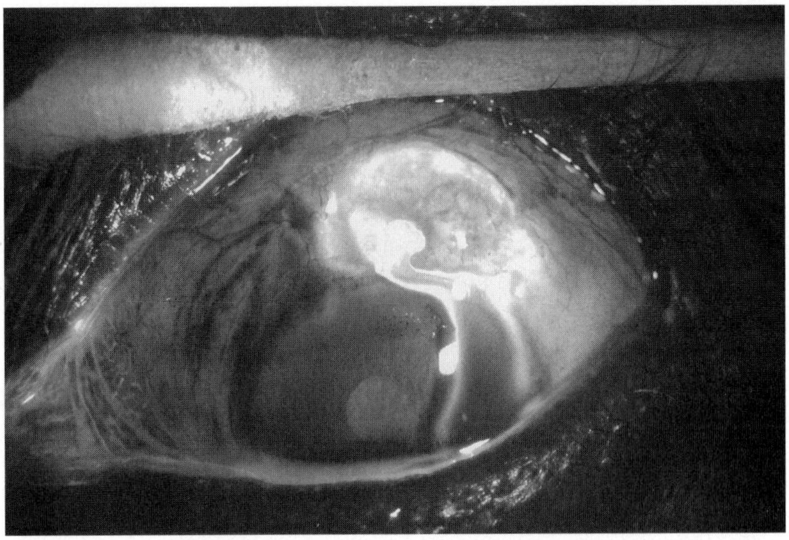

Figure 41–2. A patient with an avascular bleb presented with a round, well-defined hole in the dome of the bleb. A cuff of tissue surrounded the opening.

patching and aqueous suppression alone often suffice for an acute bleb tear or a bleb leak that occurs in the early postoperative period.[6] An effective torpedo patch should put direct pressure over the bleb, and can be created with cotton pads. Approximately one third of the inner cotton material is removed from a standard cotton pad, rolled into a torpedo shape, and then folded in half. With the patient's eyelid closed, the "pea patch" is placed over and depresses the bleb. Accurate placement of the patch is essential and can be ensured by having the patient look down with the fellow eye. Two additional cotton pads are placed over the "pea patch" and fixed in position with transpore tape.

An over-sized bandage contact lens[7–9] and a Simmons shell[10] also can be effective methods of bleb compression.

TRICHLOROACETIC ACID

Topical application of trichloroacetic acid (TCA) has been advocated as a means of shrinking thin conjunctiva.[11] The acid is applied topically to the bleb with a small stick. This intervention theoretically should work in cases of acute bleb tears because the therapy is directed to surface tissue only. However, the general experience with this therapy has been disappointing. For cases of overfiltration caused by both deep problems (i.e., large sclerectomy) and surface problems (i.e., large avascular bleb), TCA application is not indicated.

SURGICAL INTERVENTION

There are a majority of different surgical approaches to the excessive bleb (Table 41-4).

TABLE 41–4. Surgical Intervention

Cryotherapy
Suturing
Cataract extraction
Autologous blood injection
Without cryotherapy
With cryotherapy
Laser revision
Surgical revision

CRYOTHERAPY

For many years, cryotherapy to the bleb surface was the mainstay of therapy for overfiltering and leaking blebs.[12–14] However, the efficacy of this maneuver compared to other, more recently developed approaches is poor. Nevertheless, cryotherapy is a relatively low-risk procedure and may be indicated for large overfiltering blebs, overhanging and irritating blebs, and blebs that develop spontaneously after cataract surgery. Cryotherapy is not effective in cases with more deep-seated problems, as might occur after excessive antimetabolite use or early, aggressive suturolysis.

Usually, peribulbar anesthesia is required for a comfortable treatment. The 3-mm flat glaucoma probe is used to treat the surface of the bleb with four to six applications. With each application, the iceball penetrates the bleb and reaches the episclera after 6 to 10 seconds. The probe tip does not reach the low temperature levels ($-60°$ to $-80°$ Celsius).

After cryotherapy, a torpedo patch is placed (see above) and if possible, oral CAIs are begun to reduce aqueous production. After 24 to 48 hours the patch may be removed and the eye treated with topical aqueous suppressants. If possible, topical steroids are avoided because local inflammation may help in the remodeling process.

SUTURING

Two types of suturing techniques have been used for troublesome blebs: "closure" sutures and "compression" sutures. Large, acute bleb tears and bleb leaks that occur in the early postoperative period may require a suture for closure. Suturing often can be done under topical anesthesia. A fine monofilament material (10-0 nylon or 9-0 Vicryl) is used on a fine vascular needle. Care must be taken not to create additional holes in adjacent conjunctiva by unnecessarily passing and repassing the needle.

A compression suturing technique has also been advocated for leaking or overfiltering blebs.[15] Compression sutures consist of 9-0 nylon placed in a mattress fashion directly over the bleb. The suture is initially passed through peripheral cornea just anterior to the bleb and parallel to the limbus. It is then draped over the bleb and a second parallel bite is taken through Tenon's capsule and conjunctiva just posterior to the bleb. The suture is tied tightly and the knot is buried in the peripheral cornea. After several weeks, the suture can be removed. One complication of this procedure is the inadvertent creation of a bleb leak.

Another suturing technique, described by Murray Johnstone, M.D. (personal communication), is a "shoelace" method, forming a continuous running suture around the bleb.

LENS EXTRACTION

When an eye with an overfiltering or leaking bleb also has a cataract, both problems can be addressed with cataract extraction.[16] Often the inflammation associated with cataract surgery alone can stimulate fibrosis of the bleb, which changes its structure and function. The surgeon must keep in mind that additional glaucoma surgery may be necessary in the future so the cataract incision should be either clear cornea or temporal in position. Minimal steroids should be used in the postoperative period.

AUTOLOGOUS BLOOD INJECTION

The injection of autologous blood directly into the bleb has been advocated for overfiltering and leaking blebs.[17–19] Theoretically, this procedure places plasma proteins and other factors to stimulate fibroblast ingrowth within the bleb to induce fibroblast migration and proliferation. Success rates of up to 60% have been reported with this technique. Complications include hyphema, a transient rise in intraocular pressure, bleb failure, corneal graft rejection, corneal blood staining, and endophthalmitis.[20,21]

Autologous blood injection can be performed with topical anesthesia at either the slit lamp or with the patient supine. The eye is pretreated with a topical broad-spectrum antibiotic and the area around the eye is swabbed with povidone-iodine. A proparacaine hydrochloride drop is administered and a lid speculum is placed. A cotton-tipped applicator soaked in tetracaine or a 4% solution of lidocaine is held over the injection site to achieve maximal anesthesia. Approximately 1 mm of venous blood is withdrawn from the patient's arm. The needle is exchanged for a sterile 30-gauge needle that is bent to an angle. Blood is advanced through the needle. With the patient looking down, the needle is inserted into the conjunctiva posterior to the bleb and advanced into the bleb. From 0.2 to 0.5 ml of blood is injected into the bleb. With lobulated blebs it may be necessary to partially withdraw the needle and reinsert it into a different portion of the bleb. An attempt should be made to fill the bleb with blood, but it should be injected slowly to avoid creating or extending a bleb leak. After the procedure, an additional antibiotic drop is administered.

A torpedo patch is placed over the bleb for 24 to 48 hours and if possible, CAIs are begun. The success rate with this procedure is low in eyes with large, avascular, multilobulated blebs.[8,22,23] In such cases, autologous blood injection is followed by cryotherapy to shrink the bleb surface (Fig. 41–3). Again, a torpedo patch is placed postoperatively.

LASER TREATMENT TO THE BLEB

Two laser procedures have been described for troublesome blebs. In one procedure, the argon laser is used with a tissue-staining dye to treat overhanging or cystic blebs.[24] It is recommended that this technique not be used for blebs that are transparent without underlying connective tissue because it may create a bleb leak. The procedure is performed under topical anesthesia. A proparacaine drop is instilled, and a lid speculum is put in place. The epithelium over the bleb is abraded with a cotton-tipped applicator that has been soaked in additional anesthetic. A solution of either methylene blue or rose bengal is "painted" over the surface of the bleb. The bleb surface then is treated with a grid pattern of argon laser burns with the following laser parameters: 500 to 800 micron spot size, 0.1 to 0.5 second, 300 to 500 mW. With each application, the bleb should show visible shrinkage. Up to 200 applications may be necessary. At the end of the procedure, a broad-spectrum antibiotic drop is administered, and a torpedo patch is placed over the bleb for 24 to 48 hours; oral CAIs may be prescribed. Complications with this procedure include inadvertent bleb leaks. Theoretically, the technique alters the bleb surface rather than the episcleral or internal bleb structure; it is less effective for the troublesome blebs that develop after excessive antimetabolite use or aggressive suturolysis.

A second procedure employed the Microrupter II or III Nd:YAG laser, a multifunctional laser that was used during the 1980s and 1990s.[25] The continuous-wave multimode could be used to achieve a thermal reaction rather than mechanical tissue reaction. The point of laser impact also could be "offset" up to 3 mm distal to the aiming beam. The offset option was available in nine increments of 0.3 mm each. Thus, the bleb could be treated internally with this laser, with thermal spread to the overlying conjunctival epithelium (Fig. 41–4). For maximum comfort, the procedure was performed after peribulbar anesthesia. A lid speculum was placed. With the laser in the continuous-wave, multimode, the bleb was treated with a grid pattern of approximately 30 to 40 applications. The following laser parameters were

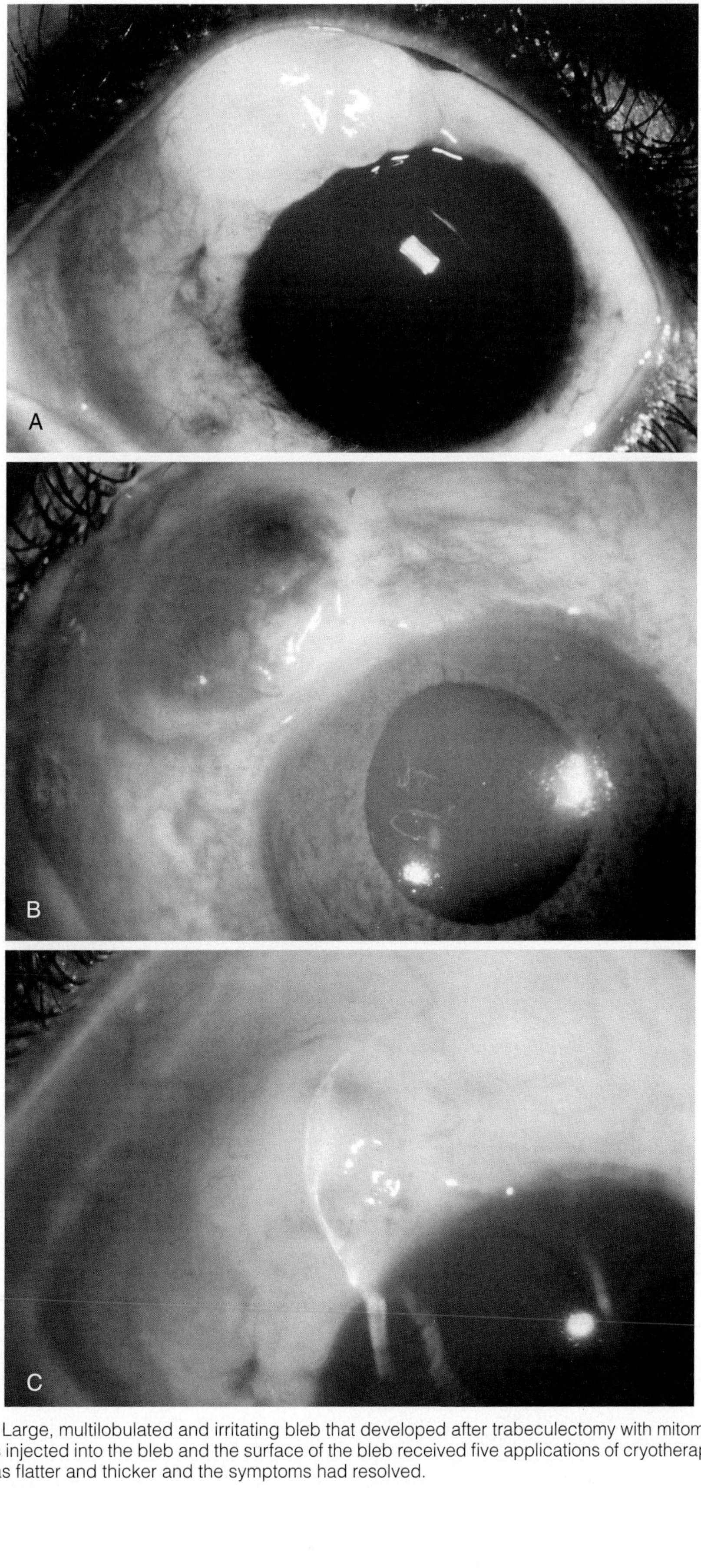

Figure 41–3. *A.* Large, multilobulated and irritating bleb that developed after trabeculectomy with mitomycin C. *B.* Autologous blood was injected into the bleb and the surface of the bleb received five applications of cryotherapy. *C.* Two weeks later, the bleb was flatter and thicker and the symptoms had resolved.

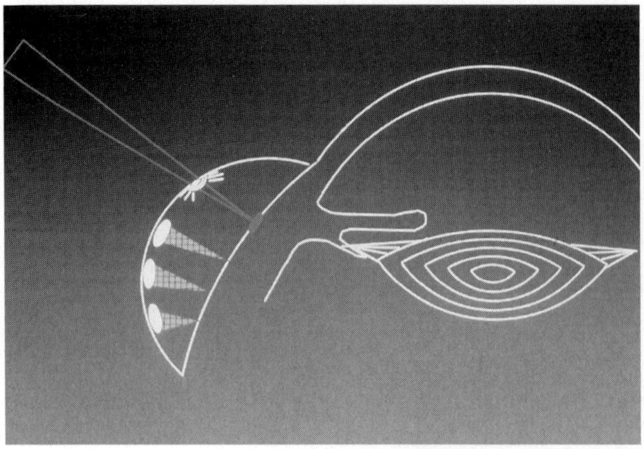

Figure 41–4. With the continuous-wave Nd:YAG laser, the laser–tissue interaction can be offset to occur within the bleb. A thermal effect from the laser is spread to overlying conjunctiva. Thus, the bleb is treated both at the surface and internally.

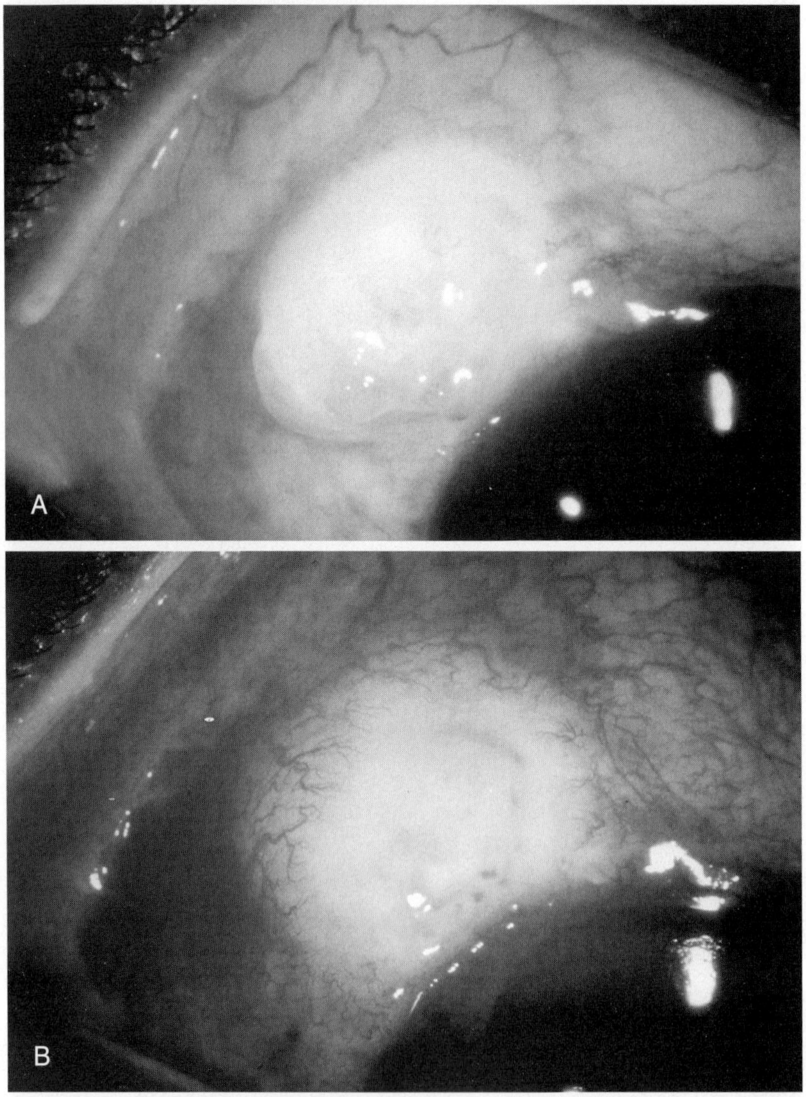

Figure 41–5. *A.* Large, overhanging bleb that developed following a guarded filtration procedure with mitomycin C for traumatic glaucoma. The eye also had a scleral buckle, which limited the posterior spread of the bleb and directed it anteriorly. *B.* One week after laser treatment of the bleb, the surrounding conjunctiva showed moderate injection. The bleb was lower and thicker and had mild pigmentation along the inner wall. *Illustration continued on opposite page*

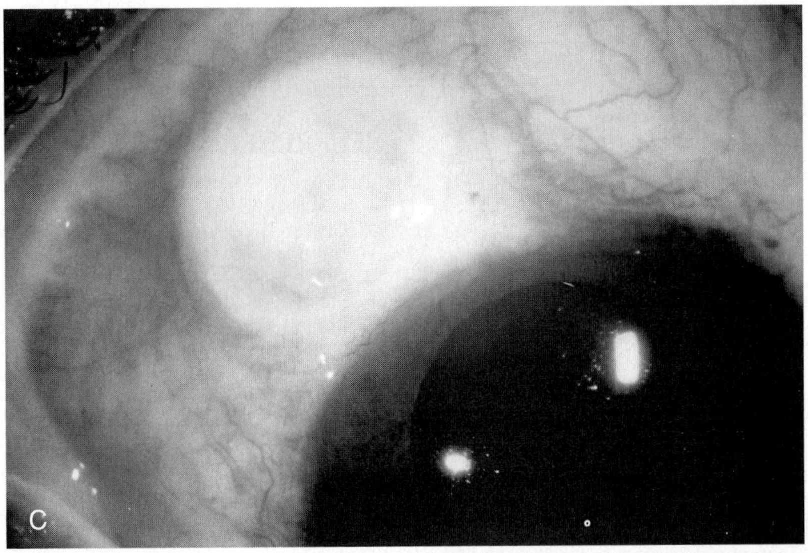

Figure 41–5 *Continued.* *C.* One month later, the bleb was lower and thicker and the symptoms had resolved.

used: 3 to 4 joules and an offset of 3 to 4 mm. The aiming beam was focused on the conjunctival epithelium and the energy and depth of focus were adjusted to achieve a whitening and wrinkling of the conjunctival epithelium. The periphery of the bleb was treated until these parameters were determined, and then the entire bleb surface is treated. At the end of the procedure, a topical antibiotic and aqueous suppressants were instilled. A torpedo patch was placed for 24 to 48 hours and if tolerated, oral CAIs are given. Once the patch was removed, topical aqueous suppressants were continued for several weeks and steroids were avoided.

In the early postoperative period, the eye ached, requiring cycloplegia and analgesia. As the bleb remodeled, pigmentation spots often appeared along its inner surface. Complications included discomfort, a transient rise in intraocular pressure, and uveitis. Bleb leaks were occasionally created during retreatments in areas of bleb pigmentation. Because this technique treats both the surface and internal portions of the bleb, it can be used for overfiltering, overhanging, and leaking blebs (Fig. 41–5).

Initial success rates with the Nd:YAG Microrupter II were very encouraging. One year after treatment, 9 of 14 eyes (64%) with overfiltration and hypotony had an increase in the pressure.[25] In 4 of 5 eyes (80%) with a leaking bleb, the leak was sealed. However, longer follow-up yielded more disappointing results.[35] At 4 years, only 5 of the 14 parents (36%) in the overfiltering group had maintained a good pressure and only 1 of 5 eyes (20%) in the bleb leak group was free of a leak. Ongoing barotrauma to the blebs reversed the laser effects for many of the patients.

A diode laser has been used to shrink filtering blebs in rabbit eyes.[26] The laser surgery involves 22 to 34 applications at a power of 3000 mW. A G-probe is used and held 3 mm above the ocular surface. A THC:YAG (Holmium) laser also has been used to treat overfiltering blebs.[36]

SURGICAL REVISION

When more conservative interventions are unsuccessful, surgical revision of the bleb may be necessary. This can take the form of (1) resuturing the scleral flap and reclosing the conjunctival flap,[27] (2) bleb excision with autologous conjunctival transplantation,[40,41] (3) conjunctival advancement with or without bleb excision[37,39] or (4) amniotic membrane graft.[34] With extremely thin or leaking blebs and excessive outflow, a combination of flap resuturing and bleb excision[28] or conjunctival advancement[29] may be necessary. These procedures should be performed in the operating room under a microscope. The surgeon should be prepared with donor scleral tissue,[30–32] preserved pericardium, or another reinforcing material[33] in case the area of the scleral flap is necrotic and impossible to suture.

In the case of an overfiltering bleb, the conjunctiva should be opened along the same incision and the area of the scleral flap carefully examined. If the tissue has good integrity, then additional sutures may be placed to close the flap. These should be 10-0 nylon and the knots should be buried. The ability of the eye to maintain a firm pressure should be tested by infusing balanced salt solution intracamerally. If a good pressure is achieved, the conjunctiva is reclosed with a monofilament suture on a vascular needle (10-0 nylon or 9-0 Vicryl).

If a good pressure cannot be achieved, then a scleral patch graft or other reinforcing material should be used to cover the scleral flap. The graft should be slightly bigger than the involved area and should be sutured in place with 10-0 nylon. The knots should be buried within the graft.

If the bleb problem is a leak or a terribly avascular conjunctiva following antimetabolite use, then the conjunctiva must be reinforced. The bleb may be excised or left in place but abraded with a surgical blade. If

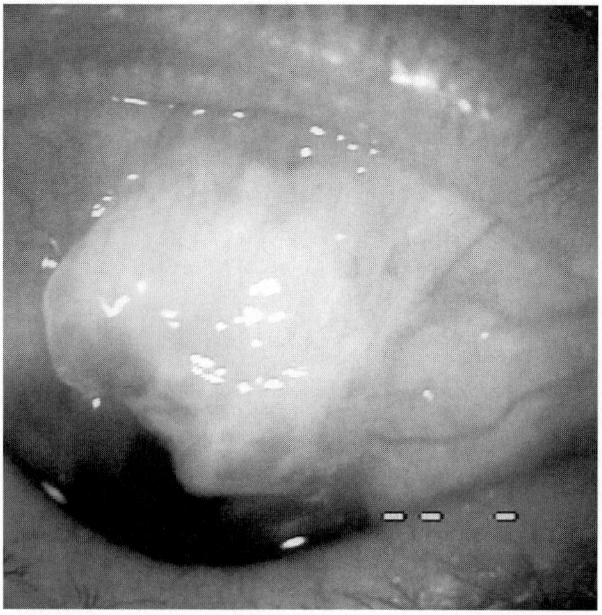

Figure 41–6. A 62-year-old man underwent excision of an overfiltering bleb with conjunctival autograft. Two years later, a large, multilobulated filtering bleb has developed over the surgical site.

sufficient Tenon's capsule and conjunctiva remain, these tissues can be advanced directly over the leaking area. The posterior conjunctiva and Tenon's should be undermined and sutured to the peripheral cornea with 10-0 nylon. If the tissue is tight, a relaxing incision can be made in the conjunctiva deep in the fornix. The anterior edge of the relaxing incision is then sutured to the sclera with 9-0 Vicryl.

If conjunctiva cannot be safely advanced, then a conjunctival autograft is made. First the bleb is excised and the widest diameter of the defect is measured. If possible, the autograft should be obtained from the same eye, inferotemporally. The size of the graft should be 50% larger than the defect because the grafted tissue will contract. The graft is sutured to the host bed with interrupted sutures of either 10-0 nylon or 9-0 monofilament Vicryl. The knots may be buried or left with long tails to minimize discomfort. The donor site is left unsutured and heals within weeks with granulation tissue.

Postoperatively, it is not unusual for a bleb to reform in the area of revision and for pressure control to be maintained (Fig. 41-6).

Amniotic membrane transplantation to cover a bleb leak has been reported but with mixed results.[34,38]

SUMMARY

The incidence of overfiltering, overhanging, and leaking blebs has increased dramatically in recent years. Appropriate preoperative precautions and postoperative patient education can help to minimize the problem. However, troublesome blebs will develop despite the best intentions because of the intrinsic weakness of the conjunctival tissues. When a bleb goes awry, it is important to determine the primary etiologic factors before embarking on what is often a difficult and frustrating therapeutic journey.

REFERENCES

{ED: Note style for pa ranges changed ir this chapte ok?}

1. Popovic V: Early hypotony after trabeculectomy. Acta Ophthalmol Scand 1995;73:255–260.
2. Costa VP, Wilson RP, Moster MR, et al.: Hypotony maculopathy following the use of topical mitomycin C in glaucoma filtration surgery. Ophthal Surg 1993;24:389–394.
3. Stamper RL, McMenemy MG, Lieberman MF: Hypotonous maculopathy after trabeculectomy with subconjunctival 5 FU. Am J Ophthalmol 1992;114:544–553.
4. Zacharia PT, Depperman SR, Schuman JS: Ocular hypotony following trabeculectomy with mitomycin C. Am J Ophthalmol 1993;116:314–326.
5. Augusto AB, Katz LJ: Dysfunctional filtering blebs. Surv Ophthalmol 1998;43:93–126.
6. Liebmann JM, Sokol J, Ritch R: Management of chronic hypotony after glaucoma filtration surgery. J Glaucoma 1996;5:210.
7. Blok MDW, Kok JHC, Mil C, et al.: Use of the megasoft bandage lens for treatment of complications after trabeculectomy. Am J Ophthalmol 1990;110:264.
8. Nuyts RMMA, Greve EL, Geijssen HC, Langerhorst CT: Treatment of hypotonous maculopathy after trabeculectomy with mitomycin C. Am J Ophthalmol 1994;118:322–331.
9. Smith MF, Doyle JW: Use of oversized bandage soft contact lenses in the management of early hypotony following filtration surgery. Ophthal Surg Lasers 1996;27:417–421.
10. Simmons RJ, Kimbrough RL: Shell tamponade in filtering surgery for glaucoma. Ophthal Surg 1979;10:17–34.
11. Gehring JR, Ciccarelli EC: Trichloroacetic acid treatment of filtering blebs following cataract extraction. Am J Ophthalmol 1972;74:662–665.
12. Cleasby GW, Fung WE, Webster RG: Cryosurgical closure of filtering blebs. Arch Ophthalmol 1972;87:319.
13. Douvas NG: Cystoid bleb cryotherapy. Am J Ophthalmol 1972;69:1972.
14. Yanuzzi LA, Theodore FH: Cryotherapy of post-cataract blebs. Am J Ophthalmol 1973;76:217.
15. Palmberg P: Late complications after filtering surgery. In Leader B, Calkwood J (eds), Proceedings of the 45th Annual Symposium of the New Orleans Academy of Ophthalmology. Kulger Publications, The Hague, 1998:183–193.
16. Sibayan SAB, Igarashi S, Kasahara N, et al.: Cataract extraction as a means of treating postfiltration hypotony maculopathy. Ophthal Surg Lasers 1997;28:241–243.
17. Wise JB: Treatment of chronic postfiltration hypotony by intrableb injection of autologous blood. Arch Ophthalmol 1993;111: 827–830.
18. Chen PP, Palmberg PF, Culbertson WW, Davis JL: Management of overfiltering and leaking blebs with autologous blood injection. Arch Ophthalmol 1996;114:633–634.
19. Leen MM, Moster MR, Katz LJ, et al.: Management of overfiltering and leaking blebs with autologous blood injection. Arch Ophthalmol 1995;113:1050–1055.
20. Ayyala RS, Urban RC, Krishnamurthy MS, Mendelblatt DJ: Corneal blood staining following autologous blood injection for hypotony maculopathy. Ophthal Surg Lasers 1997;28:866–868.
21. Zaltas MM, Schuman JS: A serious complication of intrableb injection of autologous blood for the treatment of postfiltration hypotony. Am J Ophthalmol 1994;118:251–253.
22. Hyung SM, Choi MY, Kang SW: Management of chronic hypotony following trabeculectomy with mitomycin C. Korean J Ophthalmol 1997;11:15–24.
23. Vela MA, Long T, Ozment RR: Filtering bleb autologous blood injection. Invest Ophthalmol Vis Sci 1994;35(Suppl):1421.
24. Fink AJ, Boys-Smith JW, Brear R: Management of large filtering blebs with the argon laser. Am J Ophthalmol 1986;101:695–699.
25. Roesch M, Lynch MG, Brown RH: Remodeling filtering blebs with the YAG laser. Ophthalmology 1996;103:1700–1705.
26. Leen MM, Takahashi Y, Li Y, et al.: Mitotic effect of autologous blood injection and diode laser bleb revision on rabbit filtration blebs. Arch Ophthalmol 1999;117:77–83.

27. Cohen SM, Flynn HW, Palmberg PF, et al.: Treatment of hypotony maculopathy after trabeculectomy. Ophthal Surg Lasers 1995;26: 435–441.
28. Buxton JN, Lavery KT, Liebmann JM, et al.: Reconstruction of filtering blebs with free conjunctival autografts. Ophthalmology 1994;101:635–639.
29. Galin MA, Hung PT: Surgical repair of leaking blebs. Am J Ophthalmol 1977;83:328–333.
30. Haynes WL, Alward WLM: Rapid visual recovery and long-term intraocular pressure control after donor scleral patch grafting for trabeculectomy-induced hypotony maculopathy. J Glaucoma 1995;4:200–201.
31. Melamed S, Ashkenazi I, Belcher DL, Blumenthal M: Donor scleral graft patching for persistent filtering bleb leak. Ophthal Surg 1991;22:164–165.
32. Shingleton BJ: Management of the failing glaucoma filter. Ophthalmic Surg Lasers 1996;27:445–451.
33. Rumelt S, Rehany U: A donor corneal patch graft for an incompetent scleral flap following trabeculectomy. Ophthal Surg Lasers 1996;27:878–880.
34. Kee C, Hwang JM: Amniotic membrane graft for late-onset glaucoma filtering leaks. Am J Ophthalmol 2002;133:834-835.
35. Lynch MG: Surgical repair of leaking filtering blebs. Ophthalmology 2000;107:1687.
36. Iwach AG, Degando ME, Adachi M, et al.: Filtering bleb modification with a THC-YAG (Holmium) laser. Ophthalmic Surg Lasers 2002;33:181-187.
37. Burnstein AL, WuDunn D, Knotts SL, et al.: Conjunctival advancement versus nonincisional treatment for late-onset glaucoma filtering bleb leaks. Ophthalmology 2002;109:71-75.
38. Budenz DL, Barton K, Tseng SC: Amniotic membrane transplantation for repair of leaking glaucoma filtering blebs. Am J Ophthalmol 2000;130:580-588.
39. Wadhwani RA, Bellows AR, Hutchinson BT: Surical repair of leaking filtering blebs. Ophthalmology 2000;107:1681-1687.
40. Myers JS, Yang CB, Herndon LW, et al.: Excisional bleb revision to correct overfiltration or leakage. J Glaucoma 2000;9:169-173.
41. Harris LD, Yang G, Feldman RM, et al.: Autologous conjunctival resurfacing of leaking filtering blebs. Ophthalmology 2000; 107:1675-1680.

CHAPTER 42

The Underfiltering Bleb

ROBERT RITCH, M.D. and JEFFREY M. LIEBMANN, M.D.

Glaucoma filtering surgery is unusual in that its goal is the creation and maintenance of a nonhealing fistula between two anatomic spaces that are not normally connected. The desired result is a functional filtering bleb. The bleb and its surrounding tissues, from the internal ostium to the subconjunctival space, form the filtration pathway, which is not a static system but a dynamic one, subject to the effects of biological processes on its functionality throughout the life of the patient. Fibroblasts, connective tissue elements, cytokines, aqueous humor, and the surrounding vascular supply all influence what happens to a bleb over a long period of time. Because of the need to maintain this nonphysiological condition indefinitely, greater attention than heretofore afforded needs to be paid to the recognition of structural changes and potential signs of failure in all stages of the life of the bleb, from formation to maturity, in order to achieve long-term control of intraocular pressure.

Preoperative identification of features that can contribute to bleb failure permit earlier intervention to prevent it. Risk factors that predispose to filtration failure include neovascular glaucoma,[1–3] black race,[4–14] aphakia,[15-19] prior failed filtering procedures,[19,20] uveitis,[2,21–23] prior cataract surgery,[24,25] and young or relatively young age.[10,11,19,26–32,34–40] Coincident multiple risk factors further decrease the likelihood of success, and prolonged preoperative medical therapy may also increase the risk of filtration failure.[41,42] For all of the above reasons, earlier guarded filtration procedure has been advocated by some surgeons.[43–47] Identification of risk factors for surgical failure should prompt the surgeon to consider alternative forms of intervention. This includes the use of agents that inhibit fibroblast cell division and scarring. Both 5-fluorouracil[22,48–64] and mitomycin-C[65–92] improve the pressure-lowering effect of guarded filtration surgery, particularly in difficult cases. Newer methods of inhibition of wound healing are continually being investigated at the level of tissue culture, animal models, and glaucoma patients.[93–104]

Identification of risk factors after surgery has lagged. Very little has been done in terms of classification, understanding long-term structural and functional changes, methods of preventive manipulation to prevent sudden or gradual filtration failure, active means of bleb maintenance, and features that would enable prediction of whether the eye alone can manage the formation, establishment, and maintenance of a functional bleb or whether intervention is necessary at any particular time. The goal of this chapter is to describe those factors that are known to lead to filtration failure and to outline methods of approach to maintenance or restoration of function of the underfiltering bleb. For other reviews of this topic, see references 105 through 107.

The best way to treat filtration failure is to prevent it from developing. Antiglaucoma medications, particularly miotics and sympathomimetics, have been reported to have an adverse effect on the success of filtration surgery.[108] Discontinuation of sympathomimetic agents and initiation of topical steroid treatment 1 month prior to a guarded filtration procedure produced a decrease in the number of fibroblasts and inflammatory cells in the conjunctiva.[109] Vital data from examination, such as the presence of conjunctival adhesions or scarring from previous surgery, should influence the type of and approach to surgery. For example, scarring may preclude the safe creation of a limbus-based conjunctival flap, but may still permit development of an adequate fornix-based flap or may mandate moving the surgery site to a less scarred quadrant. Failure to note the presence of scarring might lead to inadvertent "buttonhole" formation and an inability to form a bleb in the early postoperative period. However, because relatively little attention has been paid to the dynamic aspects of primary bleb formation and maintenance, and because bleb failure after previous intraocular surgery must be tailored to the individual case, the focus of this chapter will be our approach to the "standard" filtration bleb after primary filtration surgery.

At the time of surgery, the scleral flap sutures should be visible through conjunctiva and Tenon's capsule, either spontaneously or with light pressure. Our rule of thumb to ensure this placement is to make sure that the sutures are visible through the conjunctiva at the end of surgery while the patient is on the table. We rarely perform a tenonectomy when using antifibrotic agents but do so if the Tenon's capsule is thick enough to prevent suture visualization for postoperative laser suture lysis. The injection of a perfluoropropane (C_3F_8) gas bubble into the bleb may be useful in augmenting or salvaging blebs at risk of failure[110] and has been reported to increase the success rate of the guarded filtration procedure in young patients.[111]

PHASES IN THE LIFE OF A BLEB

FORMATION PHASE

The life of a bleb can be divided into three phases, formation, establishment, and maturation. The formation stage comprises roughly the first 2 weeks after surgery. In this phase, lack of establishment of critical criteria for bleb function will lead to immediate postsurgical failure. Until now, the initial formation of a bleb has been regarded largely as an act of Divine Providence, its survival or demise to be passively witnessed at the slit lamp by the surgeon. However, it is actually a critical time during which interventive measures may need be taken to ensure the formation of an adequate bleb if it does not occur spontaneously.

Early Appearance of the Bleb

Successful blebs share certain common characteristics, including elevation and avascularity. Initial bleb survival is aided when the flow of aqueous humor maintains sufficient tissue turgor pressure to collapse the conjunctival and Tenon's capsule blood vessels.[112] Blebs have a wide range of appearance in terms of height, size, and wall thickness. They may be diffuse or localized, thin-walled or spongy, and they differ in height, pallor, and extent of conjunctival microcystic edema. Conjunctival microcysts indicate the presence of subconjunctival aqueous humor flow and can be easily seen using high magnification either with a very thin slit-beam or under cobalt blue illumination after application of fluorescein (Fig. 42–1). Thin, cystic blebs develop more frequently after the guarded filtration procedure with antifibrosis therapy or full-thickness surgery, and are associated with greater transconjunctival flow of aqueous across the bleb.[113]

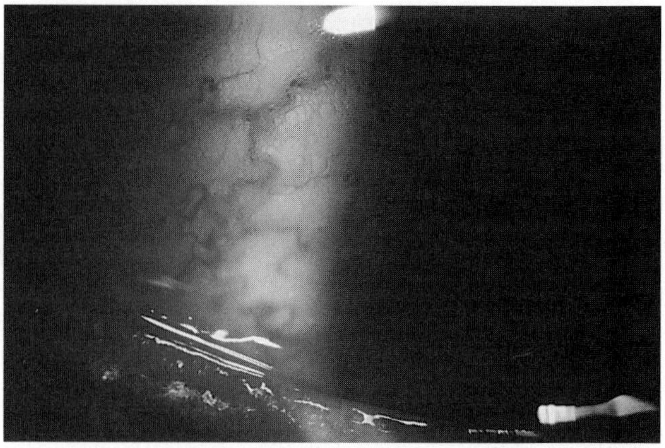

Figure 42–1. Conjunctival microcysts in a functioning bleb.

Early recognition of signs of failure to establish an initial bleb is particularly important during the first 2 weeks following surgery when the healing process is most active. Careful attention to the depth of the anterior chamber, appearance of the bleb, gonioscopic appearance of the internal ostium, and the response to digital pressure to the globe facilitate recognition of filtration failure, which may be classified by anatomic location (internal or external) and temporally (early or late in the postoperative period).

In the first 1 or 2 postoperative days, the bleb should be elevated and relatively ischemic (Fig. 42–2). A broad, diffuse bleb with microcysts is the most desirable type, irrespective of whether a fornix-based or limbus-based flap was created. It is during this period that the bleb appearance is likely to undergo its greatest changes in configuration. Postoperative injection of the bleb may be present and inflammation of the anterior chamber is

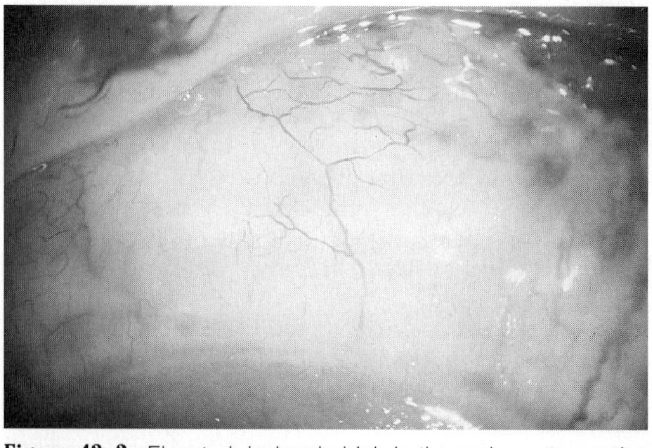

Figure 42–2. Elevated, ischemic bleb in the early postoperative period.

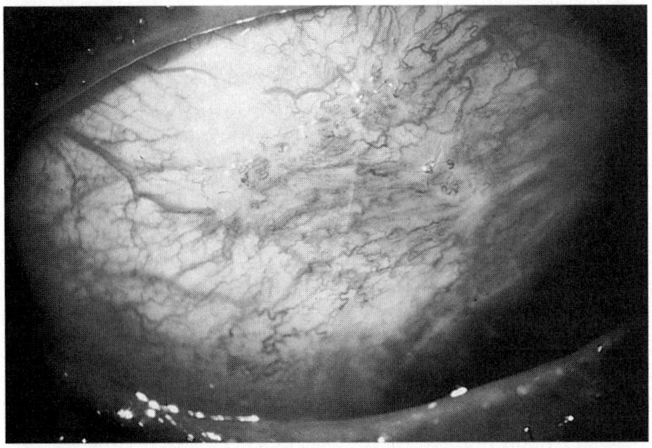

Figure 42–3. Large, ropy blood vessels carry a particularly bad prognosis for successful filtration.

always present. Large, ropy vessels crossing the bleb surface are particularly ominous (Fig. 42–3).

The absence of a bleb should be dealt with expeditiously. Continued absence of a bleb leads to bogginess, increased injection, and finally scarring together of conjunctiva, Tenon's capsule, and episclera, leading in turn to conjunctival immobility and poor chances of reviving the site into a functioning bleb. We regard it as highly desirable to achieve diffuse bleb elevation as early as possible postoperatively, and we now attempt to create a bleb if the conjunctiva is flat.

Management of the Flat Bleb

If the anterior chamber is shallow or flat, a wound leak or "buttonhole" must be suspected, particularly if hypotony is present. A Seidel test may be negative merely because there is insufficient aqueous flow to detect. We always create a paracentesis at the time of surgery in case the anterior chamber needs to be tapped or refilled postoperatively. It is useful to mark the site of the paracentesis at the time of surgery with a 10-0 nylon suture so that it can be easily identified later. Sodium hyaluronate or balanced salt solution can be injected at the slit lamp to fill the chamber. These problems are covered in Chapter 39.

If no wound leak is present, the anterior chamber is deep, and the intraocular pressure is normal or high, we attempt to initiate bleb formation, particularly if there are prominent conjunctival surface vessels, as is common in this situation. Gonioscopy should be performed to visualize the ostium and to rule out blockage by fibrin, blood, or, rarely, iris or lens. Events at surgery or complications in the perioperative period can lead to incarceration of iris, vitreous, ciliary body, ciliary processes, or lens into the internal ostium. Very often, the appearance of iris blocking the ostium is misleading, as on ultrasound biomicroscopy (UBM), the iris is usually adherent to the anterior edge of the ostium and the ostium remains patent behind it (Fig. 42–4). A 4-mirror gonioscopy lens should be used as this causes minimal trauma to the cornea and avoids contact with the filtering bleb. If blood or fibrin is blocking the ostium, waiting 2 or 3 days for it to clear will not interfere with successful creation of a bleb unless the conjunctiva over the area of the scleral flap is injected. In the latter case, we will persist in attempting to elevate the bleb rather than wait. Only rarely is intervention, in the form of intraocular tissue plasminogen activator, needed to dissolve plugs of fibrin or blood clots.

If no internal blockage is present and the anterior chamber is deep, the simplest step is to use digital massage gently.[114] We do this even if the intraocular pressure is in the low teens, just to elevate the conjunctiva slightly off the episclera. If direct massage does not work, then gentle pressure behind the scleral flap, whether with an applicator,[115] blunt instrument tip, or Ritch laser suture lysis lens[116] will often result in elevation. The procedure is not entirely benign.[114] Parenthetically, with the advent of newer techniques for the resurrection of bleb function, we no longer routinely place patients on digital massage two or three times daily. It is uncomfortable for many patients and may be damaging to thin-walled cystic blebs obtained with antifibrotic agents. We do use it in selected cases.

In a failing bleb, compression may result in either elevation of the bleb (focal or diffuse) or a resistance to elevation. If compression fails to elevate the bleb and the internal ostium is free of obstruction, the obstruction may be due to excessive inflammation with adherence of the conjunctiva, Tenon's capsule, and scleral flap together. This is often the case if very little Tenon's is present over the scleral flap itself. In other cases, fibrosis of the episclera around the scleral flap may be present. This can be suspected when the edges of the scleral flap are easily visible through the conjunctiva yet digital massage or pressure posterior to the scleral flap does not elevate the conjunctiva, especially when

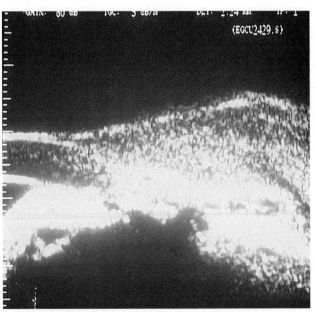

Figure 42–4. Ultrasound biomicrograph showing an open ostium posterior to iris adherent to the anterior edge of the ostium.

there appears to be a small space between the margins of the scleral flap and the surrounding sclera. This space often appears slightly darker than the sclera itself and gives the appearance of a space that should be there and that will open easily, but does not. In this case, elevation of the bleb with balanced salt solution or lidocaine 2% with nicking upward of the scleral flap with the needle tip opens the flap easily.

Transient bleb formation with massage resulting in lowering of the intraocular pressure suggests tight scleral flap sutures. Once further bleb treatment has been decided upon, either laser suture lysis or direct formation of a bleb with fluid injection is indicated. For early laser suture lysis, we use a Ritch suture lysis lens,[116] with 0.05 second duration, 100 microns spot size, and about 400 mW power. Injection of the conjunctiva or subconjunctival hemorrhage can result in damage to the conjunctiva and bleb leak or predisposition to a future bleb leak, and the krypton laser may be used in this situation.[117] For bleb elevation, using a tuberculin syringe with about 0.3 cc 1% lidocaine or balanced salt solution and a 30-gauge needle, we elevate the conjunctiva over the scleral flap after passing a needle from several millimeters away to avoid perforating the conjunctiva at the site of the bleb. If the Tenon's capsule is thick, we try to inject both intra-Tenon's and sub-Tenon's to "spongify" the bleb. Five or 10 mg of 5-fluorouracil is also injected above the newly created bleb. We like to compare the procedure to making puff pastry out of a wad of dough.

ESTABLISHMENT PHASE

Elevated intraocular pressure can occur transiently several weeks after surgery.[118,119] The bleb wall is elevated and the wall appears tense and cystic, even though it may be ischemic at this stage. This rise in intraocular pressure needs to be differentiated from an elevation in pressure caused by blockage of the internal ostium, tight scleral flap sutures, or external scarring. This situation responds poorly to bleb needling (see below), and medical treatment is indicated until the bleb can establish itself.[120] In a randomized trial, medication for cyst formation at this stage proved more successful than needling.[120] If medication does not work, then needling should be attempted. The needle should be passed through the cyst wall several times. We often needle from both the nasal and the temporal directions to try to improve the chance of success. More than one attempt may be needed before needling is successful. We generally supplement needling procedures at this stage with 5-fluorouracil injections.

Prolonged or excessive inflammation can also result in failure of the bleb to become established. At present, continued vascularization of the bleb surface is treatable only with high-dose steroids. Nonsteroidal anti-inflammatory agents contribute to bleb injection and are not recommended.[121] Treatment with tissue plasminogen activator may be of some use when obstruction is due to a blood or fibrin clot.[122,123] Intracameral urokinase may also be successful.[124] It is anticipated that use of new agents, perhaps growth factors or cytokines or their antagonists, will ameliorate this problem. External blockage to aqueous outflow may also result in failure of the bleb to establish itself. This may be due to a combination of inadequate aqueous flow through the fistula, inflammation, and scarring. Inadequate flow and inflammation may result from a flat anterior chamber, ciliochoroidal detachment, or prolonged secretory hypotony, and they lead to injection, vascularization, leukocytic infiltration, and connective tissue proliferation.

In cases in which the anterior chamber is deep and the internal ostium remains free of obstruction, efforts to reduce the external resistance to aqueous outflow should be attempted. Laser suture lysis is especially useful when scleral flap sutures have been tied tightly during surgery. It is important to lyse only one suture, and then to determine the effect of that single suture lysis. Only rarely will one lyse all the flap sutures at one time. Hypotony may be the unfortunate result of cutting too many sutures.

The procedure is readily performed with topical anesthesia and the overlying conjunctiva remains intact. We use a Ritch laser suture lysis lens, which simultaneously compresses the conjunctiva and holds up the upper lid. Gentle pressure on the conjunctiva blanches the overlying conjunctival vessels and allows visualization of the scleral flap sutures. After the sutures are found, they can be released with the argon laser using applications of 50 micron spot size, 0.05 second duration, and about 400 mW power. We release (one suture at a time) to prevent sudden decompression of the eye and flattening of the anterior chamber or hypotony. Digital massage often helps to elevate the scleral flap from its bed. The procedure should be performed within the first few postoperative weeks, as episcleral scarring later limits the amount of aqueous outflow and the effect of releasing the scleral flap sutures. Occasionally, subconjunctival hemorrhage or thickened, opaque connective tissue prevents successful lysis of the sutures.

MATURE PHASE

Filtration blebs vary widely in their clinical appearance. After a successful guarded filtration procedure, blebs characteristically have a diffuse, spongy appearance (Fig. 42-1), whereas after full-thickness surgery or adjunctive antifibrosis chemotherapy blebs are typically more thin-walled and cystic (Fig. 42-2).[19,59,80,95,125–129] Encapsulated blebs tend to be elevated and localized, with or without prominent surface vessels.[130–132] Failed blebs are often totally flat and vascularized (Fig. 42-3).[133,134] The clinical appearance of a bleb is not always an accurate predictor of functional status (Fig. 42-4).[130,135]

Rather than being static structures, blebs are dynamic, and remodeling takes place over time.[136] This was more apparent when second procedures were performed from below, the effect of repeated contact with the lower lid margin serving to reshape the bleb over time. Broadly speaking, functional blebs can be divided into three general categories (Fig. 42–5): broad, diffuse,

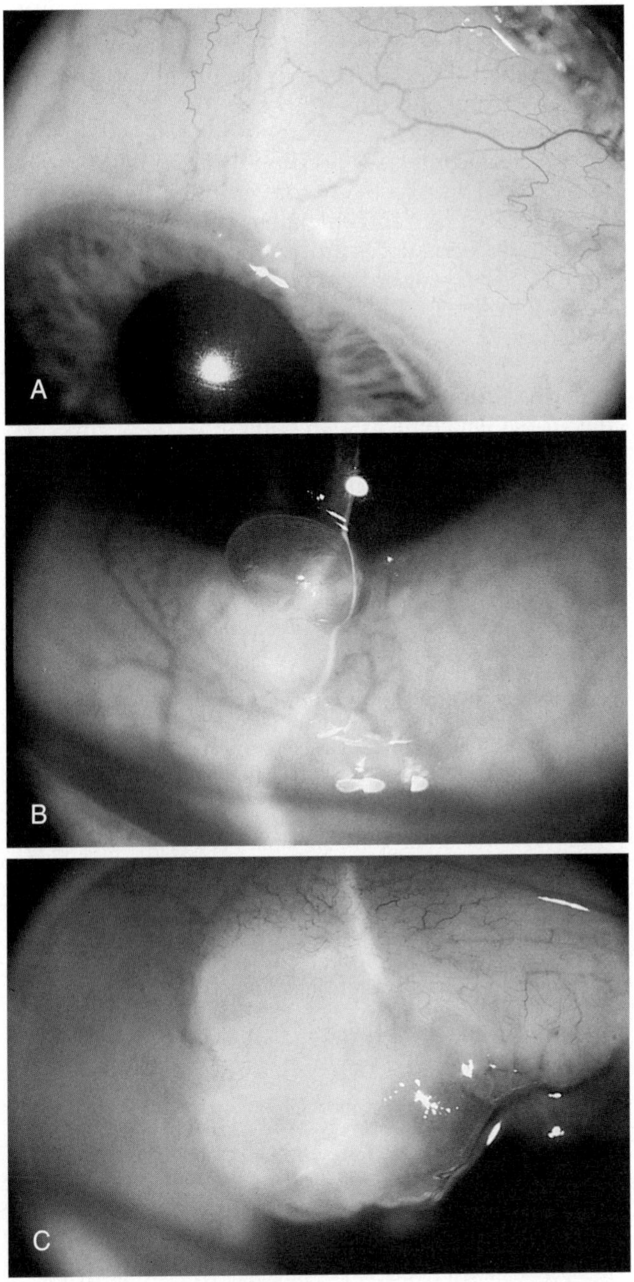

Figure 42–5. *A.* Broad, diffuse, ischemic bleb. *B.* Localized, thin-walled bleb. *C.* Multiloculated bleb.

ischemic blebs; localized, thin-walled blebs; and multi-loculated blebs.

Bleb failure can occur at five structural levels from peripheral to central, which can be grouped into three categories: (1) blockage at the level of the bleb wall (the conjunctival–Tenon's–episcleral interface or a cystic bleb), (2) scleral level (episcleral overgrowth over the scleral flap or sealing down of the scleral flap), and (3) the internal ostium.

Ultrasound biomicroscopy (UBM) can be useful in identifying the site of filtration failure and in suggesting an approach to needling. We classify failure into four categories based on the ultrasound appearance of the bleb. These are the level of the internal ostium, beneath the scleral flap, at the episclera, and within the subconjunctival space.

The UBM appearance of filtering blebs following a guarded filtration procedure with adjunctive mitomycin C was described by Yamamoto and colleagues, who created a bleb classification system.[137] Blebs with low internal reflectivity tended to have better intraocular pressure control and required fewer antiglaucoma medications. In addition, the route under the scleral flap could be clearly visualized in 81/82 eyes with good pressure control, compared with only 21/35 eyes with fair or poor control (Fig. 42-4).[137] We have used a classification system based on slit-lamp appearance (Fig. 42-5). Type 1 blebs are cystic, ischemic blebs with thin walls and multiple fluid-filled spaces separated by septa (Fig. 42-5*A*). Type 2 blebs are diffusely elevated, more opacified, pale and deeper in the epibulbar tissues (Fig. 42-5*B* and *C*). Type 3 blebs are flat, failed blebs with subconjunctival scarring. Type 4 blebs are those that were encapsulated (Tenon cyst) and in which intraocular pressure normalizes after needling.

Blockage at the Level of the Bleb Wall

Bleb encapsulation (Tenon cyst) develops in approximately 10% to 13% of eyes following a guarded filtration procedure.[118,119,131] A histopathological study of tenon cyst walls revealed fibroblastic proliferation of a Tenon's capsule that was acellular.[138] Risk factors for development of bleb encapsulation have been thought to include postoperative hypotony, flat anterior chamber, postoperative hyphema, age less than 35 years, and previous intraocular surgery.[131] Ultrasound biomicroscopy shows a discrete cystic encapsulation with an echolucent area between the conjunctiva and the outer cyst wall, possibly representing an area of subconjunctival aqueous flow.

In the vast majority of cases, external blockage is the cause of bleb failure.[128,139–142] In UBM images of failed blebs, the internal ostia are often patent with a filtration space beneath the scleral flap (Fig. 42–4), but without a filtration track at the external entrance of the scleral flap, suggesting that the blockage of aqueous outflow appears to be at the level of the episclera.

Late encapsulation consists of fibroblastic overgrowth that results in a tense, opalescent bleb with a thick wall in direct communication with the anterior chamber.[131,138] Histopathology reveals dense subconjunctival connective tissue, few cells, and no cellular lining.[138,139] Bleb encapsulation may be accompanied by progressive conjunctival hyperemia. One typically finds loculation, thickening of the subconjunctival connective tissue, and elevated intraocular pressure. The appearance ranges from incomplete loculation and mild hyperemia to complete encapsulation. The dome-like region is firm, although the overlying conjunctiva may be mobile, and is in direct communication with the anterior chamber.

Revision of guarded filtration procedure through a small conjunctival incision for filtration failure was described in 1941.[143] Discission with a needle-knife was first described in 1962.[144] Bleb needling, as currently performed, was described by Pederson and Smith,[131] and is capable of restoring function to clinically failed blebs that would otherwise require reoperation.[145–154] This procedure allows the surgeon to create an opening(s) in the wall of an encapsulated bleb or raise a flattened bleb at the slit lamp or in the operating room via subconjunctival manipulation with a small-gauge needle. The technique involves elevation of the conjunctiva off the surface of the globe with balanced salt solution or anesthetic with a small-gauge needle. The underlying episcleral/Tenon's capsule scarring is then incised with the needle. If this does not succeed in restoring filtration, the edge of the scleral flap may be elevated. Using this technique, Pederson and Smith[131] achieved successful control of intraocular pressure in 96% of cases with or without more complete surgical revision. Shin et al.[154] reported restoration of bleb function in 80% of eyes with flat, failed blebs undergoing needle revision with supplemental 5-fluorouracil. Ewing and Stamper[155] reported successful outcome in 11/12 patients without significant surgical complications. Common complications include conjunctival hemorrhage and transient wound leak. Ocular hypotony may occur, and although rare, choroidal effusion has been reported.[156] Aqueous humor may occasionally leak from the needle entry site for several days but does not usually require any intervention. The main advantages of the procedure include its ease, minimal anesthesia, and few complications.[154] Reoperation, however, is often required.[131,157] Our current regimen employs a course of 5-fluorouracil to decrease the tendency toward recurrent scarring.

Blockage at the Scleral Flap Level

Blockage at the scleral flap level is often amenable to needling but requires that the needle tip be inserted under the scleral flap, and preferably into the anterior chamber so that perforation can be verified. Caution should obviously be used in phakic patients.

The use of lasers, including argon laser internally[158] and externally,[159] or Nd:YAG laser internally[160–164] and externally,[165,166] are less safe and more complicated and we rarely use these techniques any more.

Blocked Internal Ostium

Late internal blockage may result from anterior chamber membrane proliferation over the internal ostium such as a fibrovascular membrane in neovascular glaucoma, fibrous tissue in fibrous ingrowth, epithelium in epithelial downgrowth, or corneal endothelium and Descemet's membrane in the iridocorneal-endothelial syndrome. Iris pigment epithelium may occasionally proliferate and block the internal ostium.

The argon and Nd:YAG lasers have been used successfully to open internally blocked sclerostomy sites. In addition, a transcorneal approach with a curved needle and a transanterior chamber approach with a goniotomy-type blade have also been successful in cases where aqueous outflow is blocked through the internal sclerostomy. These techniques, however, are more easily described than performed; we have had few successes with any of them.

Internal blockage or blockage at the scleral flap level may be treated by laser revision or automated trephination.[167,168] This effectively converts a partial-thickness operation to a late full-thickness procedure. This approach has been successful in our hands when a mature bleb is present but aqueous flow is blocked at the scleral flap level and needling procedures have been unsuccessful.

Acknowledgment This work was supported by the New York Glaucoma Research Institute, New York, NY.

REFERENCES

1. Allen RC, Bellows AR, Hutchinson BT, et al.: Filtration surgery in the treatment of neovascular glaucoma. Ophthalmology 1982;89:1181–7.
2. Mietz H, Raschka B, Krieglstein GK: Risk factors for failures of trabeculectomies performed without antimetabolites. Br J Ophthalmol 1999;83:814–21.
3. Parrish RK II, Herschler J: Eyes with end-stage neovascular glaucoma; natural history following successful modified filtering operation. Arch Ophthalmol 1983;101:745–6.
4. Ben Sira I, Ticho U: Excision of Tenon's capsule in fistulizing operations on Africans. Am J Ophthalmol 1969;68:336–40.
5. Broadway D, Grierson I, Hitchings R: Racial differences in the results of glaucoma filtration surgery; are racial differences in the conjunctival cell profile important? Br J Ophthalmol 1994;78: 466–75.
6. David R, Freedman J, Luntz MH: Comparative study of Watson's and Cairns trabeculectomy in a black population with open-angle glaucoma. Br J Ophthalmol 1977;61:117–19.
7. Ferguson JG Jr, MacDonald R Jr: Trabeculectomy in blacks: a two-year follow-up. Ophthalmic Surg 1977;8:41–43.
8. Freedman J, Shen E, Ahrens M: Trabeculectomy in a black American glaucoma population. Br J Ophthalmol 1976;60:573–4.
9. Kietzman B: Glaucoma surgery in Nigerian eyes: a five-year study. Ophthalmic Surg 1976;7:52–8.
10. Merritt JC: Filtering procedures in American blacks. Ophthalmic Surg 1980;11:91–4.
11. Miller RD, Barber JC: Trabeculectomy in black patients. Ophthalmic Surg 1981;12:46–50.
12. Sandford-Smith JH: The surgical treatment of open-angle glaucoma in Nigerians. Br J Ophthalmol 1978;62:283–6.
13. Thommy CP, Bhar IS: Trabeculectomy in Nigerian patients with open-angle glaucoma. Br J Ophthalmol 1979;63:636–42.
14. Welsh NH: Failure of filtration operations in Africans. Br J Ophthalmol 1970;54:594–8.
15. Bellows AR, Johnstone MA: Surgical management of chronic glaucoma in aphakia. Ophthalmology 1983;90:807–13.
16. Herschler J: The effect of total vitrectomy on filtration surgery in the aphakic eye. Ophthalmology 1981;88:229–32.
17. Herschler J, Litinsky SM, Shaffer RN, et al.: Surgical treatment of glaucoma in the aphakic patient. In Emery JM (ed.), Current concepts in cataract surgery: selected proceedings of the Fifth Biennial Cataract Surgical Congress. St. Louis: CV Mosby; 1978; 426-8.
18. Heuer DK, Gressel MG, Parrish RK II, et al.: Trabeculectomy in aphakic eyes. Ophthalmology 1984;91:1045–51.
19. Schwartz AL, Anderson DR: Trabecular surgery. Arch Ophthalmol 1974;92:134–8.
20. Shirato S, Kitazawa Y, Mishima S: A critical analysis of the trabeculectomy results by a prospective follow-up design. Jpn J Ophthalmol 1982;26:468–80.
21. Hoskins HD Jr, Hetherington J Jr, Shaffer RN: Surgical management of the inflammatory glaucomas. Perspect Ophthalmol 1977;1:173–81.

22. Jampel HD, Jabs DA, Quigley HA: Trabeculectomy with 5-fluorouracil for adult inflammatory glaucoma. Am J Ophthalmol 1990;109:168–73.
23. Liesegang TJ: Clinical features and prognosis in Fuchs' uveitis syndrome. Arch Ophthalmol 1982;100:1622–6.
24. Broadway DC, Grierson I, Hitchings RA: Local effects of previous conjunctival incisional surgery and the subsequent outcome of filtration surgery. Am J Ophthalmol 1998;125:805–18.
25. Gross RL, Feldman RM, Spaeth GL, et al.: Surgical therapy of chronic glaucoma in aphakia and pseudophakia. Ophthalmology 1988;95:1195–1201.
26. Cadera W, Pachtman MA, Cantor LB, et al.: Filtering surgery in childhood glaucoma. Ophthalmic Surg 1984;15:319–22.
27. D'Ermo F, Bonomi L, Doro D: A critical analysis of the long-term results of trabeculectomy. Am J Ophthalmol 1979;88:829–35.
28. Gressel MG, Heuer DK, Parrish RK II: Trabeculectomy in young patients. Ophthalmology 1984;91:1242–6.
29. Inaba A: Long-term results of trabeculectomy in the Japanese: an analysis by life-table method. Jpn J Ophthalmol 1982;26:361.
30. Kwitko ML: Glaucoma in Infants and Children. New York: Appleton-Century-Crofts; 1973
31. Lamping KA, Bellows AR, Hutchinson BT, et al.: Long-term evaluation of initial filtration surgery. Ophthalmology 1986;93: 91–101.
32. Levene RZ: Glaucoma filtering surgery: factors that determine pressure control. Trans Am Ophthalmol Soc 1984;82:282.
33. Mills K: Trabeculectomy: a retrospective long-term follow-up of 444 cases. Br J Ophthalmol 1981;65:790–5.
34. Shaffer RN, Weiss DI: Congenital and Pediatric Glaucomas. St. Louis: CV Mosby; 1970.
35. Shields MB: Trabeculectomy vs. full-thickness filtering operation for control of glaucoma. Ophthalmic Surg 1980;11:498–505.
36. Spaeth GL, Poryzees E: A comparison between peripheral iridectomy with thermal sclerostomy and trabeculectomy: a controlled study. Br J Ophthalmol 1981;65:783.
37. Stewart RH, Kimbrough RL, Bach H, et al.: Trabeculectomy and modifications of trabeculectomy. Ophthalmic Surg 1979;10: 76–80.
38. Stürmer J, Broadway DC, Hitchings RA: Young patient trabeculectomy. Assessment of risk factors for failure. Ophthalmology 1993;100:928–39.
39. Sugar HS: Limboscleral trepanation: eleven years' experience. Arch Ophthalmol 1971;85:703–8.
40. Sugar HS: Limbal trepanation: four years' experience. Ann Ophthalmol 1975;7:1399–404.
41. Batterbury M, Wishart PK: Is high initial aqueous outflow of benefit in trabeculectomy? Eye 1993;7:109–12.
42. Lavin MJ, Wormald RPL, Migdal CS, et al.: The influence of prior therapy on the success of trabeculectomy. Arch Ophthalmol 1990;108:1543–8.
43. Jay JL: Earlier trabeculectomy. Trans Ophthalmol Soc UK 1983;103:35.
44. Jay JL, Allan D: The benefit of early trabeculectomy versus conventional management in primary open-angle glaucoma relative to severity of disease. Eye 1989;3:528–35.
45. Jay JL, Murray SB: Early trabeculectomy versus conventional management in primary open-angle glaucoma. Br J Ophthalmol 1988;72:881–9.
46. Migdal C, Hitchings R: The role of early surgery for open angle glaucoma. Ophthalmol Clin N Amer 1991;4:853–61.
47. Wax MB, Adelson A: Indications for early glaucoma surgery. Ophthalmol Clin North Am 1988;1:175–80.
48. Bansal RK, Gupta A: 5-fluorouracil in trabeculectomy for patients under the age of 40 years. Ophthalmic Surg 1992;23: 278–80.
49. Fluorouracil Filtering Surgery Study Group T: Five-year follow-up of the Fluorouracil Filtering Surgery Study. Am J Ophthalmol 1996;121:349–66.
50. Goldenfeld M, Krupin T, Ruderman JM, et al.: 5-Fluorouracil in initial trabeculectomy, a prospective, randomized, multicenter study. Ophthalmology 1994;117:149–54.
51. Gressel MG, Parrish RK 2nd, Folberg R, et al.: 5-Fluorouracil and glaucoma filtering surgery. I. An animal model. Ophthalmology 1984;91:1242.
52. Heuer DK, Parrish RK II, Gressel MG, et al.: 5-Fluorouracil and glaucoma filtering surgery. II. A pilot study. Ophthalmology 1984;91:384–94.
53. Heuer DK, Parrish RK II, Gressel MG, et al.: 5-Fluorouracil and glaucoma filtering surgery. III. Intermediate follow-up of a pilot study. Ophthalmology 1986;93:1537–46.
54. Hugkulstone CE, Vernon SA: Low-dose perioperative 5-fluorouracil in trabeculectomy. Ophthalmic Surg Lasers 1996;27: 910–16.
55. Kitazawa Y, Taniguchi T, Nakano Y, et al.: 5-Fluorouracil for trabeculectomy in glaucoma. Graefe's Arch Clin Exp Ophthalmol 1987;225:403.
56. Liebmann JM, Ritch R: 5-Fluorouracil in glaucoma filtration surgery. Ophthalmol Clin North Am 1988;1:125–31.
57. Liebmann JM, Ritch R, Marmor M, et al.: Initial 5-fluorouracil trabeculectomy in uncomplicated glaucoma. Ophthalmology 1991;98:1036–41.
58. Mora JS, Nguyen N, Iwach AG, et al.: Trabeculectomy with intraoperative sponge 5-fluorouracil. Ophthalmology 1996;103: 963–70.
59. Ruderman JM, Welch DB, Smith MF, et al.: A randomized study of 5-fluorouracil and filtration surgery. Am J Ophthalmol 1987;104:218–24.
60. Sidoti PA, Choi JC, Morinelli EN, et al.: Trabeculectomy with intraoperative 5-fluorouracil. Ophthalmic Surg Lasers 1998;29:552–61.
61. Singh CK, Egbert PR, Byrd S, et al.: Trabeculectomy with intraoperative 5-fluorouracil vs mytomycin C. Am J Ophthalmol 1997;123:48–53.
62. Taniguchi T, Kitazawa Y, Shimizu U: Long-term results of 5-fluorouracil trabeculectomy for primary open-angle glaucoma. Int Ophthalmol 1989;13:145–9.
63. Weinreb RN: Adjusting the dose of 5-fluorouracil after filtration surgery to minimize side effects. Ophthalmology 1987;94: 564–70.
64. Whiteside-Michel J, Liebmann JM, Ritch R: Initial 5-fluorouracil trabeculectomy in young patients. Ophthalmology 1992;99:7–13.
65. Al-Hazmi A, Zwaan J, Awad A, et al.: Effectiveness and complications of mitomycin C use during pediatric glaucoma surgery. Ophthalmology 1998;105:1915–20.
66. Azuara-Blanco A, Wilson RP, Spaeth GL, et al.: Filtration procedures supplemented with mitomycin C in the management of childhood glaucoma. Br J Ophthalmol 1999;83:151–6.
67. Beatty S, Potamitis T, Kheterpal S, et al.: Trabeculectomy augmented with mitomycin C application under the scleral flap. Br J Ophthalmol 1998;82:397–403.
68. Beeson C, Skuta GL, Higginbotham EJ, et al.: Randomized clinical trial of intraoperative subconjunctival mitomycin-C versus postoperative 5-fluorouracil. Invest Ophthalmol Vis Sci 1991;32 (Suppl):1122.
69. Cheung JC, Wright MM, Urali S, et al.: Intermediate-term outcome of variable dose mitomycin C filtering surgery. Ophthalmology 1997;104:143–49.
70. Cohen JS, Novack GD, Li ZL: The role of mitomycin treatment duration and previous intraocular surgery on the success of trabeculectomy surgery. J Glaucoma 1997;6:3–9.
71. Costa VP, Comegno PE, Malta RF, et al.: Low dose mitomycin C trabeculectomy in patients with advanced glaucoma. J Glaucoma 1996;5:193–9.
72. Honjo M, Tanihara H, Inatani M, et al.: Mitomycin C trabeculectomy in eyes with cicatricial conjunctivitis. Am J Ophthalmol 1998;126:823–5.
73. Hung PT, Lin LLK, Hsieh JW, et al.: Preoperative mitomycin-C subconjunctival injection and glaucoma filtering surgery. J Ocul Pharmacol Ther 1995;11:233–41.
74. Jacobi PC, Dietlein TS, Krieglstein GK: Adjunctive mitomycin C in primary trabeculectomy in young adults: a long-term study of case-matched young patients. Graefes Arch Clin Exp Ophthalmol 1998;236:652–7.
75. Katz GJ, Higginbotham EJ, Lichter PR, et al.: Mitomycin C versus 5-fluorouracil in high-risk glaucoma filtering surgery. Extended follow-up. Ophthalmology 1995;102:1263–9.
76. Kim YY, Sexton RM, Shin DH, et al.: Outcomes of primary phakic trabeculectomies without versus with 0.5- to 1-minute versus 3- to 5-minute mitomycin. C. Am J Ophthalmol 1998;126:755–62.

77. Kitazawa Y, Kawase K, Matsushita H, et al.: Trabeculectomy with mitomycin: a comparative study with fluorouracil. Arch Ophthalmol 1991;109:1693–8.
78. Kitazawa Y, Suemori-Matsushita H, Yamamoto T, et al.: Low-dose and high-dose mitomycin trabeculectomy as an initial surgery in primary open-angle glaucoma. Ophthalmology 1993;100:1624–8.
79. Kupin TH, Juzych MS, Shin DH, et al.: Adjunctive mitomycin C in primary trabeculectomy in phakic eyes. Am J Ophthalmol 1995;119:30–9.
80. Lamping KA, Belkin JK: 5-Fluorouracil and mitomycin C in pseudophakic patients. Ophthalmology 1995;102:70–5.
81. Levkovitch-Verbin H, Goldenfeld M, Melamed S: Fornix-based trabeculectomy with mitomycin-C. Ophthalmic Surg Lasers 1997;28:818–22.
82. Matsuda T, Tanihara H, Hangai M, et al.: Surgical results and complications of trabeculectomy with intraoperative application of mitomycin C. Jpn J Ophthalmol 1996;40:526–32.
83. Mietz H, Krieglstein GK: Three-year follow-up of trabeculectomies performed with different concentrations of mitomycin-C. Ophthalmic Surg Lasers 1998;29:628–34.
84. Palmer SS: Mitomycin as adjunct chemotherapy with trabeculectomy. Ophthalmology 1987;98:317–21.
85. Bindlish R, Condon GP, Schlosser, et al.: Efficacy and safety of mitomycin-C in primary trabeculectomy: five-year follow-up. Ophthalmology 2002;109:1336–41.
86. Perkins TW, Gangnon R, Ladd W, et al.: Trabeculectomy with mitomycin C: Intermediate-term results. J Glaucoma 1998;7:230–6.
87. Robin AL, Ramakrishnan R, Krishnadas R, et al.: A long-term dose-response study of mitomycin in glaucoma filtration surgery. Arch Ophthalmol 1997;115:969–74.
88. Sanders SP, Cantor LB, Dobler AA, et al.: Mitomycin C in higher risk trabeculectomy: a prospective comparison of 0.2- to 0.4-mg/cc doses. J Glaucoma 1999;8:193–8.
89. Scott IU, Greenfield DS, Schiffman J, et al.: Outcomes of primary trabeculectomy with the use of adjunctive mitomycin. Arch Ophthalmol 1998;116:286–91.
90. Skuta GL, Beeson CC, Higginbotham EJ: Intraoperative mitomycin versus postoperative 5-fluorouracil in high-risk glaucoma filtering surgery. Ophthalmology 1992;99:438–44.
91. Stone RT, Herndon LW, Allingham RR, et al.: Results of trabeculectomy with 0.3 mg/ml mitomycin C titrating exposure times based on risk factors for failure. J Glaucoma 1998;7:39–44.
92. Ustundag C, Diestelhorst M: Effect of mitomycin C on aqueous humor flow, flare and intraocular pressure in eyes with glaucoma 2 years after trabeculectomy. Graefes Arch Clin Exp Ophthalmol 1998;236:734–8.
93. Akimoto M, Hangai M, Okazaki K, et al.: Growth inhibition of cultured human Tenon's fibroblastic cells by targeting the E2F transcription factor. Exp Eye Res 1998;67:395–402.
94. Al-Aswad LA, Huang M, Netland PA: Inhibition of Tenon's fibroblast proliferation and enhancement of filtration surgery in rabbits with cytosine arabinoside. J Ocular Pharmacol Ther 1999;15:41–49.
95. Avila M, Ortiz G, Lozano JM, et al.: The effects of RGD (arg-gly-asp) peptides on glaucoma filtration surgery in rabbits. Ophthalmic Surg Lasers 1998;29:309–17.
96. Constable PH, Crowston JG, Occleston NL, et al.: Long term growth arrest of human Tenon's fibroblasts following single applications of β radiation. Br J Ophthalmol 1998;82:448–52.
97. Cordeiro MF, Gay JA, Khaw PT: Human anti-transforming growth factor-β2 antibody: a new glaucoma anti-scarring agent. Invest Ophthalmol Vis Sci 1999;40:2225–34.
98. Cunliffe IA, Richardson PS, Rees RC, et al.: Effect of TNF, IL-1, and IL-6 on the proliferation of human Tenon's capsule fibroblasts in tissue culture. Br J Ophthalmol 1995;79:590–5.
99. Gillies MC, Brooks AMV, Young S, et al.: A randomized phase II trial of interferon-alpha 2b versus 5-fluorouracil after trabeculectomy. Aust NZ J Ophthalmol 1999;27:37–44.
100. Haas AL, Boscoboinik D, Mojon DS, et al.: Vitamin E inhibits proliferation of human Tenon's capsule fibroblasts in vitro. Ophthalmic Res 1996;28:171–5.
101. Heilmann C, Schönfeld P, Schlüter T, et al.: Effect of the cytostatic agent idarubicin on fibroblasts of the human Tenon's capsule compared with mitomycin C. Br J Ophthalmol 1999;83:961–6.
102. Mietz H, Chevez-Barrios P, Feldman RM, et al.: Suramin inhibits wound healing following filtering procedures for glaucoma. Br J Ophthalmol 1998;82:816–20.
103. Saika S, Yamanaka O, Okada Y, et al.: Pentoxifylline and pentifylline inhibit proliferation of human Tenon's capsule fibroblasts and production of type-1 collagen and laminin in vitro. Ophthalmic Res 1996;28:165–70.
104. Salas-Prato M, Assalian A, Mehdi AZ, et al.: Inhibition by rapamycin of PDGF- and bFGF-induced human Tenon fibroblast proliferation in vitro. J Glaucoma 1996;5:54–9.
105. Azuara-Blanco A, Katz LJ: Dysfunctional filtering blebs. Surv Ophthalmol 1998;43:93–126.
106. Haynes WL, Alward WLM: Control of intraocular pressure after trabeculectomy. Surv Ophthalmol 1999;43:345–55.
107. Shingleton BJ: Management of the failing glaucoma filter. Ophthalmic Surg Lasers 1996;27:445–51.
108. Broadway DC, Grierson I, O'Brien C, et al.: Adverse effects of topical antiglaucoma medication. II. The outcome of filtration surgery. Arch Ophthalmol 1994;112:1446–54.
109. Broadway DC, Grierson I, Stürmer J, et al.: Reversal of topical antiglaucoma medication effects on the conjunctiva. Arch Ophthalmol 1996;114:262–7.
110. Tym WH, Seah SKL: Augmentation of filtering blebs with perfluoropropane gas bubble. An experimental and pilot clinical study. Ophthalmology 1999;106:545–9.
111. Lu DW, Tai MC, Chiang CH: Subconjunctival retention of perfluoropropane (C3F8) gas increases the success rate of trabeculectomy in young people. Asian J Ophthalmol 1999;1:8–9.
112. Palmberg P: The failing filtering bleb. Ophthalmol Clin N Amer in press, 2000.
113. Franks WA, Hitchings RA: Complications of 5-fluorouracil after trabeculectomy. Eye 1991;5:385–9.
114. Segrest DR, Ellis PP: Iris incarceration associated with digital ocular massage. Ophthalmic Surg 98;12:349–51.
115. Traverso CE, Greenidge KC, Spaeth GL, et al.: Focal pressure: a new method to encourage filtration after trabeculectomy. Ophthalmic Surg 1984;15:62.
116. Ritch R, Potash SD, Liebmann JM: A new lens for argon laser suture lysis. Ophthalmic Surg 1994;25:126–7.
117. Aktan SG, Mandelkorn RM: Krypton laser suture lysis. Ophthalmic Surg Lasers 1998;29:635–8.
118. Scott DR, Quigley HA: Medical management of a high bleb phase after trabeculectomies. Ophthalmology 1988;95:1169.
119. Sherwood MB, Spaeth GL, Simmons ST, et al.: Cysts of Tenon's capsule following filtration surgery. Medical management. Arch Ophthalmol 1987;105: 1517–21.
120. Costa VP, Correa MM, Kara-Jose N: Needling versus medical treatment in encapsulated blebs: a randomized, prospective study. Ophthalmology 1997;104:1215–20.
121. Migdal C, Hitchings R: Effect of antiprostaglandins on glaucoma filtration surgery. Trans Ophthalmol Soc UK 1982;102:129.
122. Lee PF, Myers KS, Hsieh MM, et al.: Treatment of failing glaucoma filtering cystic blebs with tissue plasminogen activator (tPA). J Ocul Pharmacol Ther 1995;11:227–32.
123. Lundy DC, Sidoti P, Winarko T, et al.: Intracameral tissue plasminogen activator after glaucoma surgery. Ophthalmology 1996;103:274–82.
124. WuDunn D: Intracameral urokinase for dissolution of fibrin or blood clots after glaucoma surgery. Am J Ophthalmol 1997; 124:693–5.
125. Blondeau P, Phelps CD: Trabeculectomy vs thermosclerostomy. A randomized prospective clinical trial. Arch Ophthalmol 1981;99:810–16.
126. Cairns JE: Trabeculectomy. Trans Am Acad Ophthalmol Otol 1972;76:384.
127. Lewis RA, Phelps CD: Trabeculectomy vs thermosclerostomy—a five year follow-up. Arch Ophthalmol 1984;102:533–6.
128. Skuta GL, Parrish RK II: Wound healing in glaucoma filtering surgery. Surv Ophthalmol 1987;32:149–70.
129. Wilson MR: Posterior lip sclerostomy vs trabeculectomy in West Indian blacks. Arch Ophthalmol 1989;107:1604–8.
130. Cohen JS, Shaffer RN, Hetherington J Jr, et al.: Revision of filtration surgery. Arch Ophthalmol 1977;95:1612–5.
131. Pederson JE, Smith SG: Surgical management of encapsulated filtering blebs. Ophthalmology 1985;92:955–8.

132. Richter CU, Shingleton BJ, Bellows AR, et al.: The development of encapsulated filtering blebs. Ophthalmology 1988;95:1163–8.
133. Galin MA, Baras I, McLean JM: How does a filtering bleb work? Trans Am Acad Ophthalmol Otol 1965;69:1082–91.
134. Maumenee AE: External filtering operations for glaucoma: the mechanism of function and failure. Tr Am Ophthalmol Soc 1960;58:319–28.
135. Migdal C, Hitchings R: The developing bleb: effect of topical antiprostaglandins on the outcome of glaucoma fistulizing surgery. Br J Ophthalmol 1983;67:655–60.
136. Sugar HS: The course of change in size of successful filtering cicatrices. Am J Ophthalmol 1960;49:795–800.
137. Yamamoto T, Sakuma T, Kitazawa Y: An ultrasound biomicroscopic study of filtering blebs after mitomycin C trabeculectomy. Ophthalmology 1995;102:1770–6.
138. Van Buskirk EM: Cysts of Tenon's capsule following filtration surgery. Am J Ophthalmol 1982;94:522–7.
139. Addicks EM, Quigley HA, Green WR, Robin AL: Histologic characteristics of filtering blebs in glaucomatous eyes. Arch Ophthalmol 1983;101:795.
140. Desjardins DC, Parrish RK, Folberg R, et al.: Wound healing after filtering surgery in owl monkeys. Arch Ophthalmol 1986; 104:1835–9.
141. Durcan FJ, Cioffi GA, van Buskirk EM: Same-site revision of failed filtering blebs. J Glaucoma 1992;1:2–6.
142. Teng CC, Chi HH, Katzin HM: Histology and mechanism of filtering operations. Am J Ophthalmol 1960;47:16–34.
143. Ferrer H: Conjunctival dialysis in the treatment of glaucoma recurrent after sclerectomy. Am J Ophthalmol 1941;24:788–90.
144. Fitzgerald JR, McCarthy JL: Surgery of the filtering bleb. Arch Ophthalmol 1962;68:453–67.
145. Azuara-Blanco A, Bond JB, Wilson RP, et al.: Encapsulated filtering blebs after tbcy with mitomycin-C. Ophthalmic Surg Lasers 1997;28:805–9.
146. Chen PP, Palmberg PF: Needling revision of glaucoma drainage device filtering blebs. Ophthalmology 1997;104:1004–10.
147. Gillies WE, Brooks AMV: Restoring the function of the failed bleb. Aust NZ J Ophthalmol 1991;19:49–51.
148. Greenfield DS, Miller MP, Suner IJ, et al.: Needle elevation of the scleral flap for failing filtration blebs after trabeculectomy with mitomycin C. Am J Ophthalmol 1996;122:195–204.
149. Hayashi M: Use of the Hoskins lens in needle revision of a failed bleb after filtration surgery. Am J Ophthalmol 1995;119:232–3.
150. Hodge W, Saheb N, Balazsi G, et al.: Treatment of encapsulated blebs with 30-gauge needling and injection of low-dose 5-fluorouracil. Can J Ophthalmol 1992;27:233–6.
151. Liebmann J, Ritch R: Management of the failing filtering bleb. Semin Ophthalmol 1991;6:1–6.
152. Mardelli PG, Lederer CM Jr, Murray PL, et al.: Slit-lamp needle revision of failed filtering blebs using mitomycin C. Ophthalmology 1996;103:1946–55.
153. Morales J, Ritch R: Treatment of failing filtering blebs. Clin Decisions Ophthalmol 1987;11:4–11.
154. Shin DH, Juzych MS, Khatana AK, et al.: Needling revision of failed filtering blebs with adjunctive 5-fluorouracil. Ophthalmic Surg 1993;24:242–8.
155. Ewing RH, Stamper RL: Needle revision with and without 5-fluorouracil for the treatment of failed filtering blebs. Am J Ophthalmol 1990;110:254–9.
156. Potash SD, Ritch R, Liebmann J: Ocular hypotony and choroidal effusion following bleb needling. Ophthalmic Surg 1993;24:279.
157. Shingleton BJ, Richter CU, Bellows AR, et al.: Management of encapsulated filtration blebs. Ophthalmology 1990;97:63–8.
158. Ticho U, Ivry M: Reopening of occluded filtering blebs by argon laser photocoagulation. Am J Ophthalmol 1977;84:413.
159. Kurata F, Krupin T, Kolker AE: Reopening filtration fistulas with transconjunctival argon laser photocoagulation. Am J Ophthalmol 1984;98:340.
160. Budenz DL, Brown SVL, Thomas JV, et al.: Laser therapy for internally failing glaucoma filtration surgery. Ophthalmic Laser Ther 1986;1:169.
161. Cohn HC, Whalen WR, Aron-Rosa D: YAG laser treatment in a series of failed trabeculectomy. Am J Ophthalmol 1989;108:395.
162. Cohn JH, Aron-Rosa D: Reopening blocked trabeculectomy sites with the YAG laser. Am J Ophthalmol 1984;102:1024.
163. Dailey RA, Samples JR, Van Buskirk EM: Reopening filtration fistulas with neodymium-YAG laser. Am J Ophthalmol 1986;102:491.
164. Oh Y, Katz LJ: Indications and technique for reopening closed filtering blebs using the Nd:YAG laser - A review and case series. Ophthalmic Surg 1993;24:617.
165. Van Rens GH: Transconjunctival reopening of an occluded filtration fistula with the Q-switched neodymium-YAG laser. Doc Ophthalmol 1988;70:205.
166. Weber PA, Jones JH, Kapetansky F: Neodymium:YAG transconjunctival laser revision of late-failing filtering blebs. Ophthalmology 1999;106:2023–6.
167. Brown RH, Lynch MG, Denham DB, et al.: Internal sclerectomy with an automated trephine for advanced glaucoma. Ophthalmology 1988;95:728.
168. Brown RM, Denham DB, Bruner WE, et al.: Internal sclerectomy for glaucoma filtering surgery with automated trephine. Arch Ophthalmol 1987;105: 133–6.

CHAPTER 43

Suprachoroidal Hemorrhage

LOUIS B. CANTOR, M.D.

Suprachoroidal hemorrhage is among the most feared complications of ophthalmic surgery. The occurrence of this complications may leave the patient with an eye that becomes immediately blind, and painful, and could lead to eventual enucleation. However, with appropriate patient assessment, identification and management of risk factors, and prompt recognition and appropriate treatment of a hemorrhage when it does occur, severe complications of a suprachoroidal hemorrhage can be reduced.

RISK FACTORS

Suprachoroidal hemorrhage, both intraoperative and delayed postoperative, is nearly ten times more common in patients undergoing intraocular surgery who have glaucoma than in those without glaucoma. There is also a much higher risk of suprachoroidal hemorrhage associated with glaucoma surgery than with other ophthalmic procedures. The incidence of suprachoroidal hemorrhage following modern cataract surgery is reported to be between 0.03% and 0.06%. The incidence of this complication following glaucoma surgery is reported to be 1.6% to 2.0%. The risk of delayed suprachoroidal hemorrhage is particularly high after glaucoma procedures because of prolonged hypotony, development of serous choroidal effusions, and inflammation.

Most evidence suggests that the source of the hemorrhage is from one of the short or long posterior ciliary arteries at the point where they enter the suprachoroidal space from their intrascleral canals. In an acute intraoperative expulsive hemorrhage there is most likely a rupture of a necrotic or weakened vessel wall associated with hypotony during the procedure. Delayed postoperative suprachoroidal hemorrhage is usually preceded by hypotony and the development of serous ciliochoroidal effusions, which stretch and rupture one of the vessels where it bridges the suprachoroidal space (Fig. 43-1).

Conditions that predispose to vascular fragility or forward displacement of the retina and choroid may predispose to suprachoroidal hemorrhage. Advanced age, hypertension, arteriosclerosis, blood dyscrasias, anticoagulation, or other conditions that may affect the vascular system increase the risk of a hemorrhage. Ocular conditions that have been associated with an increased risk of suprachoroidal hemorrhage include glaucoma, high myopia, aphakia or pseudophakia, hypotony, trauma, uveitis, intraocular surgery, and a history of a suprachoroidal hemorrhage in the fellow eye. Perioperatively, sudden decompression of the globe (especially if the preoperative intraocular pressure was markedly elevated), Valsalva, general anesthesia, vitreous loss, inadequate local anesthesia, patient agitation from IV sedation, or intraoperative elevations of the blood pressure increase the risk of hemorrhage. Postoperatively, Valsalva, prolonged hypotony, hypertension, ocular trauma, and inflammation increase the risk of bleeding. The use of antifibrosis agents (5-fluorouracil or mitomycin C) also significantly increases the risk of a suprachoroidal hemorrhage. These agents predispose to prolonged postoperative hypotony and a shallow anterior chamber, either by delayed would healing with excessive filtration or secondary to conjunctival wound leaks.

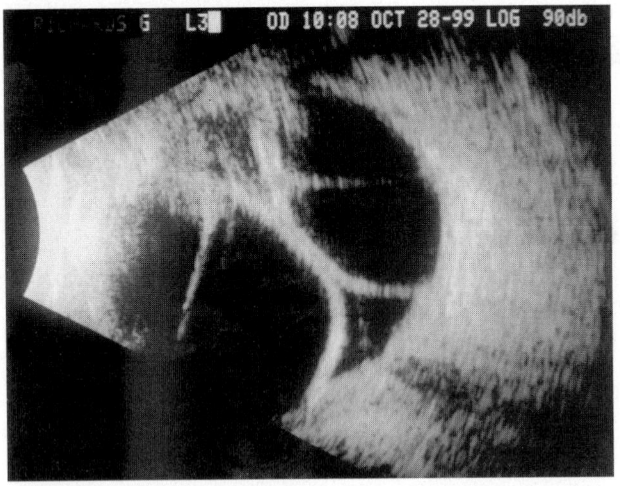

Figure 43–1. B-scan ultrasound demonstrating ciliochoroidal effusion with a vessel bridging the suprachoroidal space. When such a vessel is placed under traction, it is prone to rupture.

PREVENTION

When possible, the intraocular pressure should be lowered as much as possible before decompressing the globe. Sudden decompression of the globe from a high intraocular pressure is perhaps the most important single risk factor for acute intraoperative suprachoroidal hemorrhage. Unfortunately, it is not always possible to reduce the intraocular pressure. If the patient has systemic hypertension, controlling the blood pressure prior to and especially during surgery is recommended. Minimizing increases in central venous pressure by avoiding general anesthesia, administering adequate preoperative sedation and analgesia, and assuring optimal management of any pulmonary or cardiovascular disease will decrease the risk of coughing or Valsalva. If possible, discontinuation of aspirin or warfarin will reduce the risk of bleeding.

INTRAOPERATIVE SUPRACHOROIDAL HEMORRHAGE

Several signs may alert the surgeon to an intraoperative suprachoroidal hemorrhage. Iris prolapse, shallowing of the anterior chamber, vitreous prolapse, gaping of the incision, firmness of the globe, striae in the cornea, or a change in the red reflex may be the earliest sign of a hemorrhage. The hallmark of a suprachoroidal hemorrhage is often severe, sudden pain that often is noted by the patient despite an apparently adequate retrobulbar or peribulbar local anesthetic nerve block. Prompt recognition is vital to minimizing the complications of an acute intraoperative hemorrhage.

The first priority following recognition of a possible intraoperative suprachoroidal hemorrhage is secure closure of the incision. If the surgery was planned to involve a large incision, as in extracapsular cataract surgery, preplaced sutures are recommended in eyes that are at risk for a hemorrhage. These sutures can then be pulled tight and tied quickly. The sutures must be of sufficient tensile strength to withstand a very high intraocular pressure and sutures of less than 8-0 are generally not sufficient.

Once the globe is secured and any prolapsed uvea reposited, the eye can be evaluated. It is generally recommended that the remainder of the planned surgery be aborted unless the eye appears well stabilized and additional surgery is absolutely necessary. If the intraocular pressure remains significantly elevated hyperosmotic agents can be administered along with topical or oral intraocular pressure-lowering medications. The anterior chamber can be re-formed, if necessary, with a viscoelastic agent. Unless there are specific indications to do so, immediate drainage of the suprachoroidal hemorrhage is not necessary and may precipitate further bleeding. However, if the eye cannot be closed, the anterior chamber reformed, the intraocular pressure controlled, or if there is intractable pain it may be necessary to consider drainage intraoperatively.

DELAYED SUPRACHOROIDAL HEMORRHAGE

Delayed or postoperative suprachoroidal hemorrhage generally behaves differently from an acute intraoperative hemorrhage. This type of hemorrhage usually occurs between the third to fifth postoperative day and in most cases is preceded by hypotony and the development of ciliochoroidal serous effusions. The patient will generally have a history of sudden onset of eye pain, often with nausea, vomiting, decreased vision, headache, tearing, and possible lid swelling or chemosis. At times the patient may be awakened from sleep with these symptoms.

On examination there will often be shallowing of the anterior chamber, vitreous prolapse, and loss of the red reflex. The intraocular pressure may be elevated, though in eyes with a filtering sclerostomy the aqueous may decompress into the subconjunctival space causing a large filtering bleb and chemosis. If the suprachoroidal hemorrhage is large, the choroidal detachments may be visible on slit-lamp examination behind the lens. The presence of blood in the vitreous or the anterior chamber should be noted. If there has been "breakthrough" bleeding to beneath or through the retina, the prognosis for recovery of vision is diminished.

Initial treatment is directed at the relief of pain and control of the intraocular pressure if necessary. Oral or topical ocular hypotensive agents such as topical beta-adrenergic antagonists, topical and oral carbonic anhydrase inhibitors, and alpha-2-adrenergic agonists can usually manage the intraocular pressure. Intravenous or oral hyperosmotic agents may also be considered. Pain can be relieved in most cases with cycloplegic agents such as atropine and analgesics. If necessary, potent analgesics containing codeine or other medications may be useful for immediate or short-term relief. The use of topical and oral corticosteroids will help decrease the inflammatory response, which often accompanies a severe hemorrhage.

ULTRASONOGRAPHY

The diagnosis of a suprachoroidal hemorrhage is usually made based on the clinical presentation and ophthalmic examination. However, the use of ultrasonography may aid in the diagnosis, especially when there is media opacification or blood present. Ultrasonography may help detect if a retinal detachment is present in addition to the hemorrhagic choroidal effusion. The use of serial ultrasound can aid in following the hemorrhage for clot lysis, which is essential if drainage of the blood is being contemplated. In the early period following a hemorrhage, ultrasound will reveal high reflective, solid, irregular masses within the suprachoroidal space (Fig. 43-2*A* and *B*). With eye movement these masses can be seen to actually move in the suprachoroidal space. As the clot lyses, more regular and lower internal reflectivity is seen (Fig. 43-3). Complete clot lysis will generally require 5 to 14 days, although this time may be variable in different individuals. With ultrasound, the timing of the drainage, if needed, can be optimized to the time when all or most of the blood is amenable to drainage (Fig. 43-4).

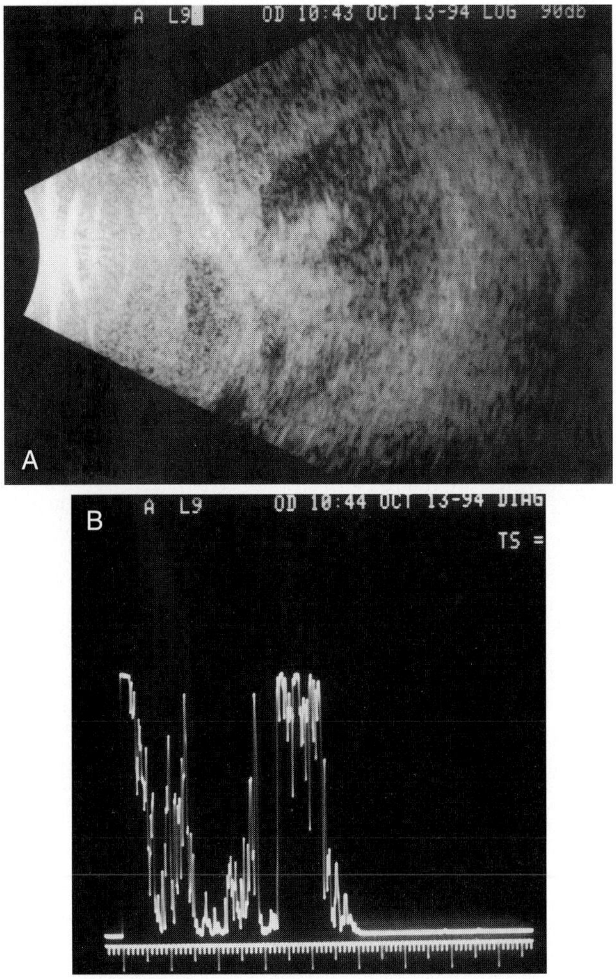

Figure 43–2. *A.* B-scan ultrasound demonstrating suprachoroidal hemorrhage with clotted blood filling the suprachoroidal space. *B.* Corresponding A-scan ultrasound demonstrating characteristic internal reflectivity.

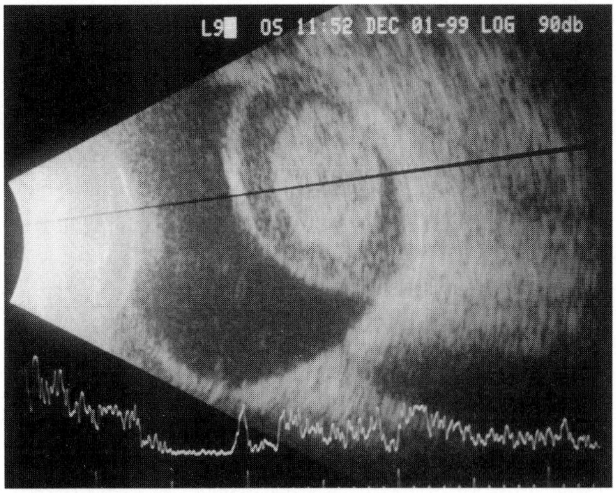

Figure 43–3. B-scan ultrasound with partial resolution and liquefaction of the suprachoroidal hemorrhage. A blood clot is visible within the suprachoroidal space surrounded by liquefied blood.

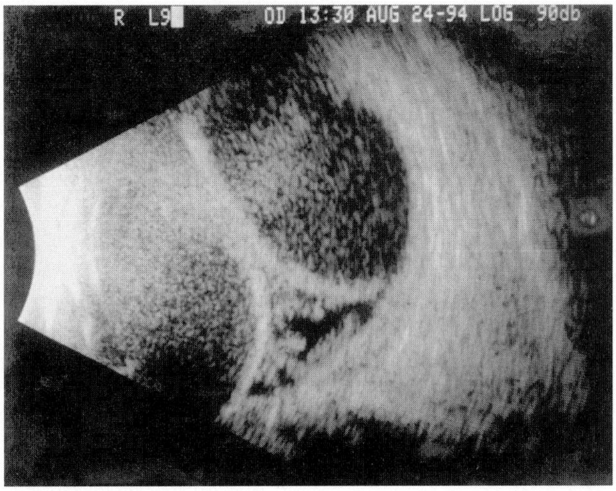

Figure 43–4. B-scan ultrasound revealing complete liquefaction of the suprachoroidal hemorrhage. At this stage, the hemorrhage is amenable to drainage if deemed necessary.

DRAINAGE APPROACHES

Several factors may influence the decision to consider drainage of a suprachoroidal effusion. It is well established that most suprachoroidal hemorrhages will eventually clear spontaneously. It also appears that the final visual outcome may be similar whether early drainage is performed or the hemorrhage is allowed to resolve on its own. However, the presence of massive "kissing" effusions, intractable pain, persistent or recurrent flat anterior chamber, prolapse of intraocular contents, suspicion of a retinal detachment, vitreous hemorrhage, retained lens fragments, or the need for more rapid visual rehabilitation are among the indications for drainage. When drainage is undertaken, depending on the circumstances, drainage alone may be performed through a posterior sclerostomy with injection of fluid into the anterior chamber of the eye, or more involved vitreoretinal or anterior chamber manipulation may be required. In general, it is probably best to be conservative and do only as much surgery as is necessary until the eye has had time to stabilize.

Current techniques for drainage involve placement of one or more posterior sclerotomies and injection into the eye of a vitreous substitute consisting of fluid, viscoelastic material, or air. Expansile gasses and silicone oil may be used when vitreoretinal approaches are required. A sclerostomy placed in the inferior temporal quadrant is usually sufficient for drainage if there has been clot lysis. The sclerostomy need not be placed directly under the hemorrhage, even if it is a more localized hemorrhage, as the suprachoroidal space is one large communicating space. By means of either repeated injections of fluid or viscoelastic material or a continuous infusion cannula by gravity, the blood can be drained from the sclerostomy site. If the drainage appears incomplete, either through the operating microscope or via intraoperative indirect ophthalmoscopy, a second sclerostomy site can be attempted. It is not required that all blood be drained to be successful. If most of the blood can be removed, the remainder will be reabsorbed spontaneously. Any vitreous that has prolapsed can be removed by vitrectomy. It is prudent to inspect the glaucoma filtration site and to remove any vitreous, blood, iris, lens capsule, or fibrin that may be obstructing the internal sclerostomy.

Whenever drainage of a suprachoroidal hemorrhage is undertaken, one must be aware that retinal complications may be uncovered that were not evident previously. The presence of vitreous hemorrhage should alert the surgeon to the possibility of a retinal detachment. Retinal incarceration into the wound, retinal detachment, and other complications requiring vitreoretinal surgery carry a much poorer prognosis. If the blood has remained confined in the suprachoroidal space with no loss of ocular contents or other complication, the prognosis for visual recovery is good.

SECTION V

Robert Alan Goldberg, M.D.

Oculoplastic Surgery

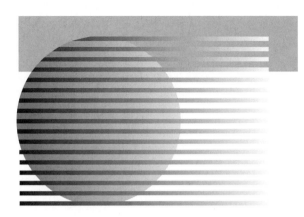

CHAPTER 44

Orbitotomy: Surgical Approaches

JONATHAN W. KIM, M.D., ROBERT ALAN GOLDBERG, M.D., and NORMAN SHORR, M.D.

INTRODUCTION

Orbitotomy techniques and surgical approaches continue to evolve. There has been a recent paradigm shift away from traditional cutaneous approaches involving time-consuming dissections toward direct, rapid approaches that offer equal or superior exposure through hidden incisions. Because no two cases are alike, individualization of approach and technique is of paramount importance if the optimal surgical result is to be achieved. An ideal orbitotomy approach should not only offer maximal exposure to the site of pathology, it should also allow for flexibility and customization of the technique to the patient and to the orbital disease process. The modern surgeon who is willing to embrace the latest surgical techniques and has the flexibility to customize the procedure is optimally prepared to patients. Stressing these concepts, we will review our favorite surgical approaches for performing orbital biopsy, exploration, tumor extirpation, and orbital reconstruction.

An extensive range of the orbital space can be safely accessed through orbitotomy approaches that use cosmetically hidden incisions. In particular, the medial (transcaruncular) and inferior (forniceal) conjunctival approaches provide outstanding, unencumbered access to the obit without creating any visible cutaneous scar. The upper eyelid crease incision is also versatile in providing exposure to the lacrimal gland fossa, deep lateral orbit, and orbital apex. These three approaches fulfill the criteria of providing wide exposure through cosmetically hidden incisions and, alone or in combination, these can be used to access the vast majority of orbital tumors encountered in clinical practice. These approaches are also quite versatile, and if required, can be combined with removal of the superior, lateral, or inferior orbital rim for additional exposure. Finally, the coronal approach also results in a hidden scar as long as the patient has an adequate hairline, and provides enormous wide-open exposure to the entire orbit, at the expense of a somewhat longer opening and closing procedure.

TRANSCARUNCULAR (BAYLIS) APPROACH

The transcaruncular (Baylis) approach was developed at UCLA in the mid-1980s. The transcaruncular incision has become our preferred approach for performing a medial orbitotomy because it provides rapid and wide exposure of the entire medial wall through a cosmetically hidden incision. Advantages over the classic Lynch transcutaneous incision include more rapid orbital entry and avoidance of a noticeable cutaneous scar. The transcaruncular approach is also quite versatile, providing wide exposure and safe access to the medial extraperiosteal space, ethmoid and sphenoid sinuses, orbital apex, and optic canal. A transcaruncular incision can also be combined with a fornix approach to gain 270 degrees of continuous exposure to the entire medial and inferior orbit.

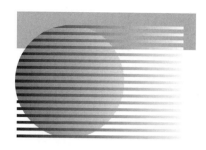

One of the keys to performing the transcaruncular approach is to create a wide enough opening in both the conjunctival incision and the periosteal incision to provide exposure of the entire medial orbit. Another critical point is to create the proper surgical plane to the posterior lacrimal crest, which will avoid damage to the anterior nasolacrimal system while simultaneously avoiding entry into the posterior orbital fat, which would prolapse into the field and diminish exposure. If the subperiosteal dissection is extended into the inferomedial orbit, care should be taken to avoid damaging the nasolacrimal duct and the insertion of the inferior oblique muscle. Finally, careful edge-to-edge closure of the conjunctiva is critical to avoid cicatricial changes in the medial conjunctiva.

SURGICAL TECHNIQUE

The procedure can be performed under local or general anesthesia, although general anesthesia is usually indicated.

Step 1. Infiltration with lidocaine containing 1:100,000 epinephrine is performed into the caruncle and along the medial orbit to facilitate hemostasis. If indicated, the infiltration is extended into the inferior conjunctival fornix.

Step 2. The assistant uses two 0.5 Castroviejo forceps to grasp the eyelid near the puncta and expose the caruncle for the surgeon (two lacrimal rakes can also be used) (Fig. 44–1). The transcaruncular incision is made at the junction of the medial ¾ and lateral ¼ of the caruncle with Wescott scissors. The conjunctival incision is extended superiorly and inferiorly to both puncta (12 mm in each direction), with care to create one continuous incision and avoiding macerating the delicate conjunctiva (Fig. 44–2).

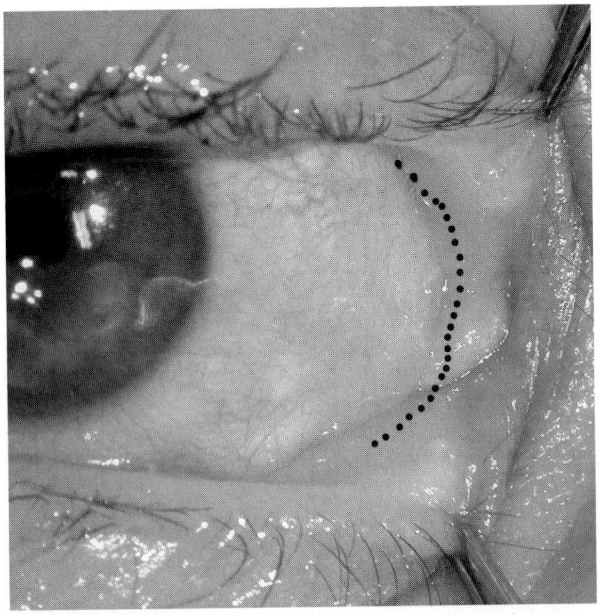

Figure 44–1. The medial eyelid is grasped with a fine-toothed forceps adjacent to the upper and lower puncta, and a conjunctival incision is made from the superior to the inferior fornix, cutting across the lateral 1/4 junction of the caruncle. (© copyright 2001, Regents of the University of California; reprinted with permission.)

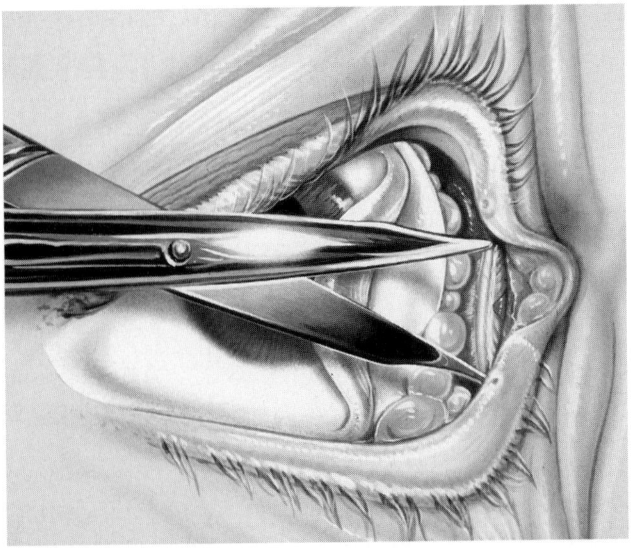

Figure 44–2. The surgeon strums the scissors tips in order to feel the posterior lacrimal crest, and the blades of the scissors are opened while the scissors is pressed against the posterior lacrimal crest. (© copyright 2001, Regents of the University of California; reprinted with permission.)

Step 3. A curved Stevens scissors is then inserted into the incision and blunt and sharp scissors dissection is performed until the posterior lacrimal crest can be palpated with the scissors tips. The surgeon gently strums the scissors tips in an anteroposterior direction until the proper location of the posterior lacrimal crest is verified (Figs. 44–3, 44–4).

Step 4. Maintaining the position on the posterior lacrimal crest, the surgeon opens the tips of the scissors to expose the whitish line of the arcus marginalis.

Step 5. The surgeon continues to maintain the position of the scissors tips and places a malleable retractor over the scissors. Once the malleable retractor is properly positioned, the scissors are removed. The assistant switches to a lacrimal rake and retracts the medial edge of conjunctiva. Blunt dissection with cotton-tipped applicators can be useful to visualize the arcus marginalis and the anterior red fibers of Horner's muscle where it inserts onto the posterior lacrimal crest. This plane of dissection is posterior to the lacrimal drainage apparatus and anterior to the orbital fat (Fig. 44–5).

Step 6. A No.15 Bard-Parker blade or the monopolar cautery can be used to incise the periosteum, following the arcus marginalis at the posterior lacrimal crest. This incision should extend inferiorly behind the nasolacrimal duct and superiorly to the orbital roof for wide exposure of the entire medial orbit (Fig. 44–6).

Step 7. Periosteal elevators are used to dissect posteriorly along the medial orbital wall, achieving the

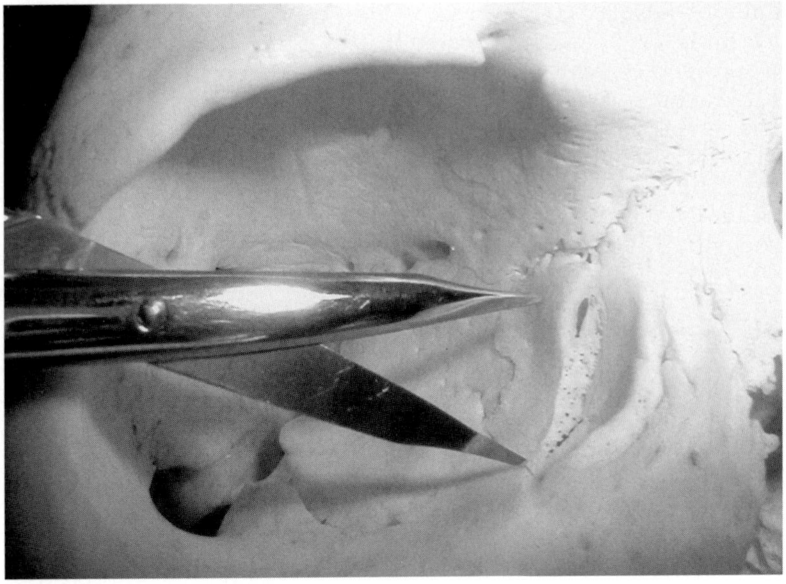

Figure 44–3. The proper position of the scissors tips relative to the poster lacrimal crest is demonstrated on a skull. (© copyright 2001, Regents of the University of California; reprinted with permission.)

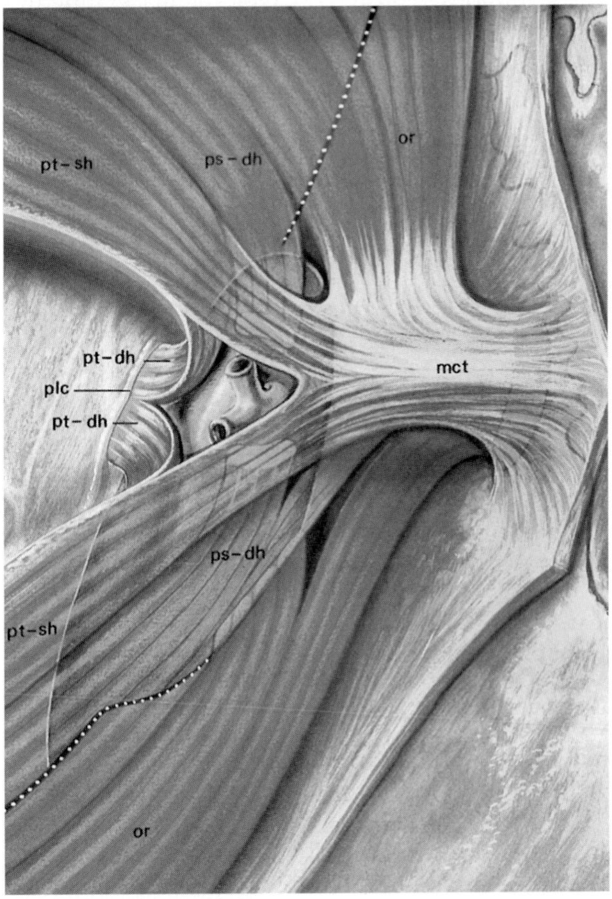

Figure 44–4. Horner's muscle (pt-dh, pretarsal muscle deep head) is a slip of orbicularis that inserts on the posterior lacrimal crest, brushing against the posterior wall of the lacrimal sac. The anterior limb of the medial canthal tendon (mct) brushes along the anterior wall of the lacrimal sac. (pt-sh: pretarsal superficial head; ps-dh: preseptal deep head; or: orbit; plc: posterior lacrimal crest). (From Rootman J, Stewart B, Goldberg RA: Orbital Surgery: A conceptual approach. Philadelphia: Lippincott, Williams & Wilkins, 1995, p 140. © copyright 1995, Bruce Stewart; used with permission.)

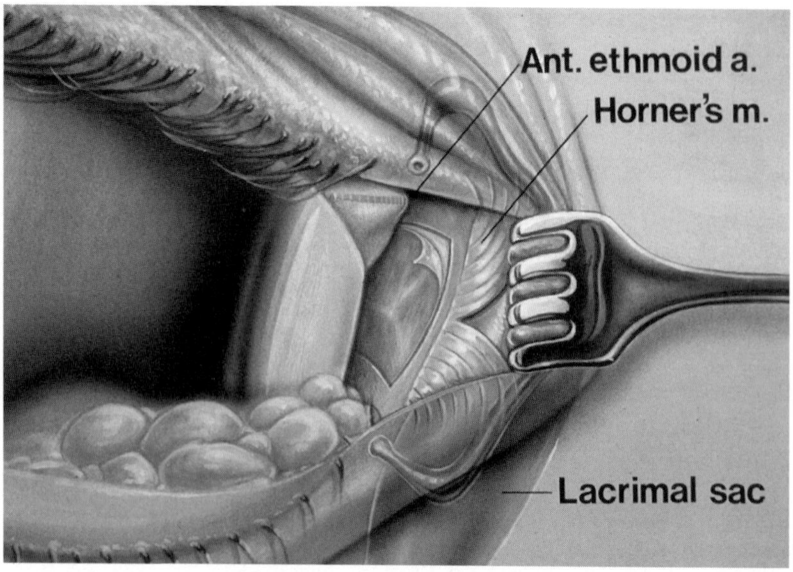

Figure 44–5. By blunt dissection, the periosteum overlying the posterior lacrimal crest and the junction of Horner's muscle with the lacrimal crest is exposed. Illustrated here is the creation of a periosteal flap for use in strabismus surgery, an example of one of the many uses of the caruncular approach. (© copyright 2001, Regents of the University of California; reprinted with permission.)

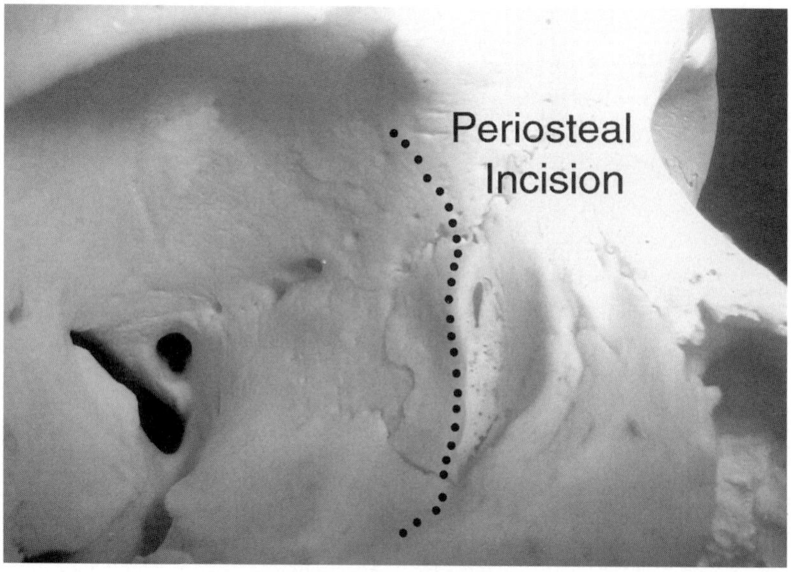

Figure 44–6. To access the deep orbit, a wide periosteal incision is made. A beginner's mistake is to make a periosteal incision that is too small, limiting the deep exposure. (© copyright 2001, Regents of the University of California; reprinted with permission.)

desired extraperiosteal plane (Fig. 44–7). Superiorly, the subperiosteal dissection is extended onto the roof of the orbit. The trochlea lies anterior to the plane of dissection and is relatively easy to avoid.

Step 8. Identification of the anterior ethmoidal artery can be facilitated by carrying the subperiosteal dissection from the orbital roof down onto the medial wall. The anterior ethmoidal foramina is 24 mm posterior to the medial orbital rim, and the posterior ethmoidal foramina is 12 mm posterior to the anterior ethmoidal foramina. These arteries are at the level of the roof of the ethmoid sinus (fovea ethmoidalis). These vessels are cauterized with the bipolar cautery to obtain better exposure to the medial wall. Surgical exposure during the subperiosteal dissection is facilitated by maintaining an intact periosteum and, whenever possible, avoiding orbital fat prolapse into the field.

Step 9. Inferiorly, the subperiosteal dissection is carried over the maxilloethmoid strut onto the medial floor of the orbit. As the surgeon approaches the insertion of the inferior oblique, a strong periosteal adhesion will be noted just superior to the insertion of the muscle (Fig. 44–8). This most likely represents fascial extensions of Lockwood's ligament to the medial orbit, and these attachments should be dissected off to provide wider exposure.

Step 10. The surgeon can either extend the subperiosteal incision posteriorly behind the insertion of the inferior oblique muscle, or alternatively, the subperiosteal incision can be

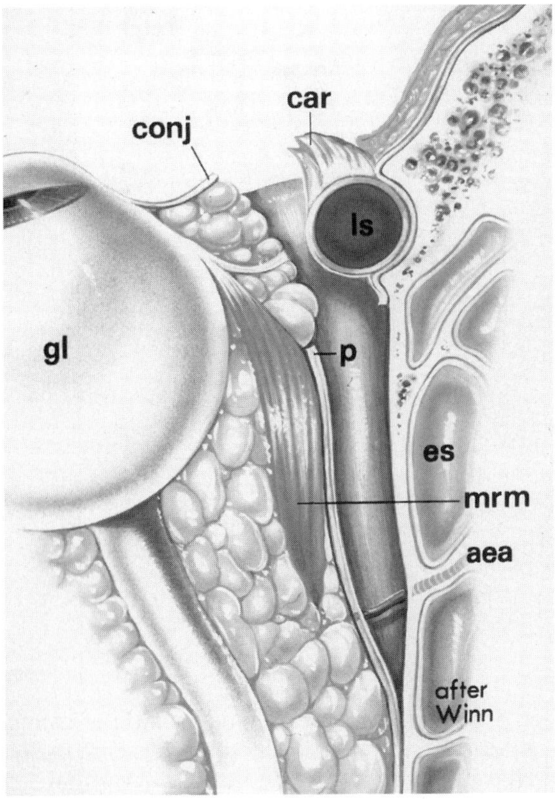

Figure 44–7. Axial view of the subperiosteal dissection plane created with the caruncular approach; the anterior ethmoid artery (aea) bridges across the subperiosteal dissection. (conj: conjunctiva; car: caruncle; gl: globe; p: periosteum; es: ethmoid sinus; mrm: medial rectus muscle; ls: lacrimal sac). (© copyright 2001, Regents of the University of California; reprinted with permission.)

extended anterior to the insertion of the muscle, with care not to damage the nasolacrimal duct. The muscle can also be cut at its insertion, usually with impunity, if it is resutured at the end of the case.

Step 11. Closure is accomplished with 1 to 3 interrupted 6-0 absorbing sutures. Identifying the cut edges of conjunctiva and performing careful edge-to-edge closure will avoid symblepharon formation as well as possible globe restriction.

MEDIAL CUTANEOUS (LYNCH) APPROACH

A curvilinear incision over the superomedial orbital rim (Lynch incision) has classically been used to begin a subperiosteal dissection plane into the medial and superomedial orbit. The Lynch approach also provides good access to the ethmoid and sphenoid sinuses and the orbital apex. Because this approach enters immediately into the subperiosteal, extraorbital plane, one avoids the problem of orbital fat prolapsing into the surgical field. The main disadvantage of this procedure is that a cutaneous incision is created and the resulting scar may be visible and prominent. Other potential complications include medial canthal webbing and damage to the nasolacrimal outflow system. If wider surgical access is required to gain access to the lateral wall or orbital floor, a new and discontinuous incision becomes necessary. Because the transcaruncular approach offers all of the advantages of the Lynch approach, without producing a cutaneous scar, we now use a transcaruncular incision exclusively when approaching the medial orbit. However, in keeping with the theme of an individualized approach to the management of orbital disease, it is important for orbital surgeons to be aware of this approach.

SURGICAL TECHNIQUE

Step 1. The proposed incision is marked. There are several variations on the Lynch incision to help minimize scarring (Fig. 44–9 *A,B*).

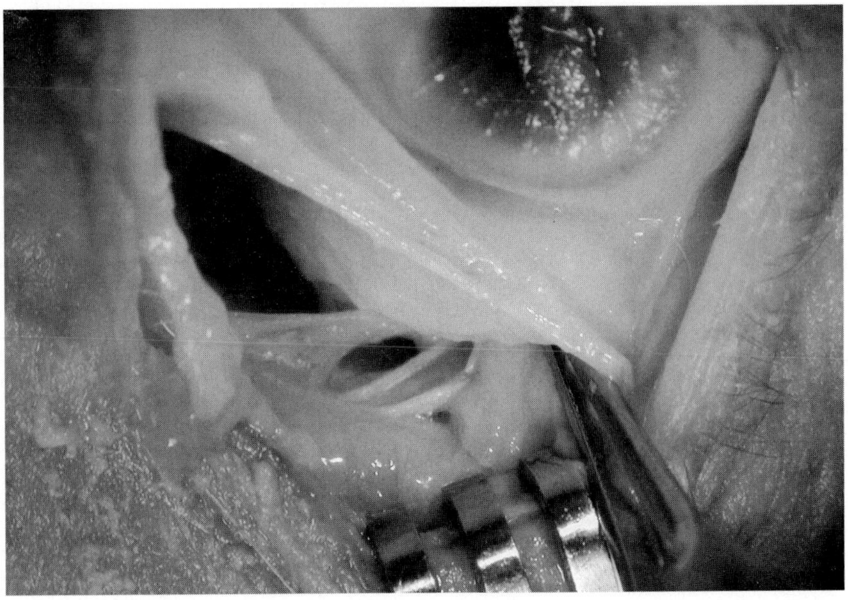

Figure 44–8. Strong fibrous attachments of Lockwood's ligament are noted along the inferior aspect of the posterior lacrimal crest, near the junction of the lacrimal duct. These should be dissected off of the bone to provide wider exposure. (© copyright 2001, Regents of the University of California; reprinted with permission.)

Step 2. A lidocaine solution with 1:100,000 epinephrine is injected subcutaneously to aid in hemostasis, regardless of whether the patient is under local or general anesthesia.
Step 3. A No. 15 Bard-Parker blade is used to make the incision through the skin to the level of the periosteum.
Step 4. The angular vessels are identified with blunt dissection and then cauterized.

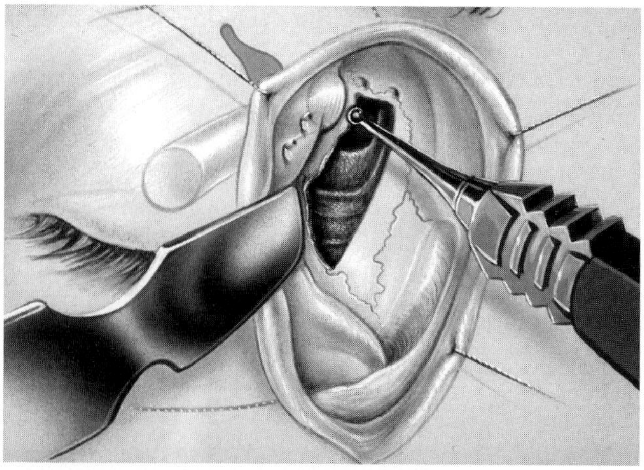

Figure 44–10. Wide exposure of the medial orbit and apex can be achieved through the Lynch incision, and orbital fat is typically not spilled, improving visualization of the apical structures, for example, in optic nerve canal decompression, pictured here. (From Rootman J, Stewart B, Goldberg RA: Orbital Surgery: A Conceptual Approach. Philadelphia: Lippincott, Williams & Wilkins, 1995, p. 286. © copyright 1995, Bruce Stewart and Lippincott, Williams & Wilkins.)

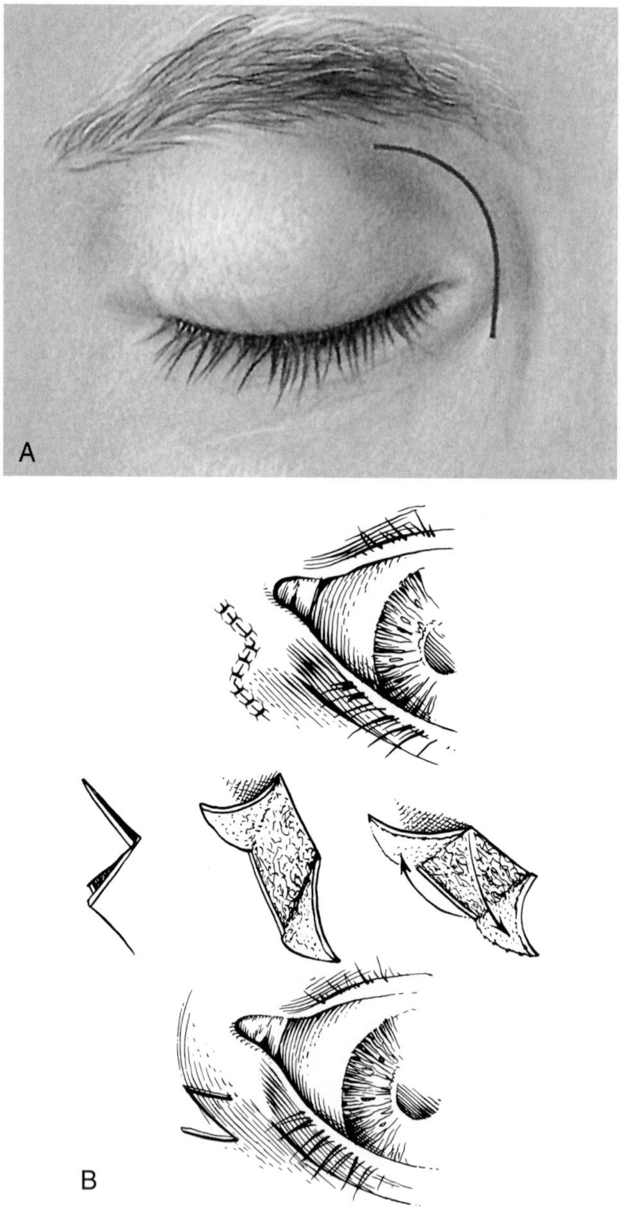

Figure 44–9. *A.* The standard curved Lynch incision is constructed overlying the nasal bone; it provides wide subperiosteal exposure at the expense of a visible scar and the need to dissect through highly vascular tissue planes. (From Rootman J, Stewart B, Goldberg RA: Orbital Surgery: A Conceptual Approach. Philadelphia: Lippincott, Williams & Wilkins, 1995, p 219. © copyright 1995, Bruce Stewart and Lippincott Williams & Wilkins.) *B.* The incision can be broken up as a Z-plasty in order to decrease scarring and web formation. (From Leone CR Jr: Plastic Surgery. In Spaeth GA [ed]: Ophthalmic Surgery: Principles and Practice, 2nd ed. Philadelphia: WB Saunders, 1990, p. 538.)

Step 5. The medial canthal tendon and periosteum anterior to the anterior lacrimal crest are incised. This allows reflection of the medial canthal tendon and lacrimal drainage apparatus.
Step 6. The periorbita is carefully elevated off the lamina papyracea with a periosteal elevator to obtain access to the subperiosteal plane.
Step 7. The anterior and posterior ethmoidal arteries are identified and cauterized with the bipolar cautery to obtain exposure of the entire medial wall (Fig. 44–10).
Step 8. After the goals of the procedure have been achieved, the medial canthal tendon and periosteum are approximated with absorbable sutures. The skin incision is carefully closed with a two-layered closure.

INFERIOR FORNIX (SWINGING EYELID) APPROACH TO THE ORBITAL FLOOR

The transconjunctival inferior fornix approach provides direct entry and wide exposure of the orbital floor, zygoma, and midface through a cosmetically hidden incision while minimizing the risk of postoperative lower eyelid retraction and ectropion. We believe that septal scarring, which is unavoidably created through any of the cutaneous approaches to the inferior orbit, is the primary cause of lower eyelid retraction and lateral canthal rounding. Therefore, we strongly discourage the use of the subciliary or transcutaneous approach to the orbital floor. We also do not recommend a transconjunctival, preseptal approach, which has similar disadvantages of inducing middle lamellar scarring and contracture. Ideally, the transconjunctival approach completely avoids the plane of the orbital septum and follows a direct route through the fat pockets to the inferior orbital rim.

As with the other approaches that we describe, the transconjunctival fornix incision is a versatile approach for performing an inferior orbitotomy. For most patients, the fornix approach should be combined with a lateral canthotomy and cantholysis (swinging eyelid) for adequate exposure. The fornix approach can also be combined with a transcaruncular incision to obtain continuous 270 degrees of access to the inferior and medial orbit. For some patients with lower eyelid laxity, it is possible to obtain enough exposure to the orbital floor through an isolated fornix approach alone. Again, we stress that the approach should be individualized to the patient. For tumors that involve the posterior aspect of the inferior orbital fissure or the pterygopalatine fossa, the swinging eyelid technique can be combined with removal of the entire zygoma to obtain panoramic exposure of the inferolateral orbit. When using the swinging eyelid fornix approach, it is imperative that the surgeon re-form the lateral canthus in its proper anatomic location at the end of the case, as lateral canthal dystopia is a potential complication of this technique.

SURGICAL TECHNIQUE

Step 1. The lateral canthotomy incision is marked with a 10-mm horizontal line placed in a lateral canthal crease.

Step 2. To facilitate hemostasis, local infiltration into the lateral canthal region and inferior fornix is performed with a solution of lidocaine containing 1:100,000 epinephrine.

Step 3. A No. 15 Bard-Parker blade is used to make the lateral canthotomy incision (Fig. 44–11). The incision is carried down to the level of the periosteum. Exposing the lateral canthal periosteum becomes important when reattaching the tarsotendinous strap.

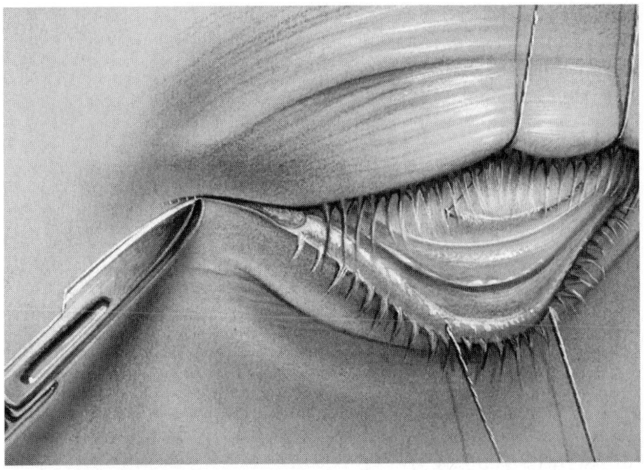

Figure 44–11. A canthal incision is carried out between the upper and lower eyelid margin, down to the level of periosteum. (From Rootman J, Stewart B, Goldberg RA: Orbital Surgery: A Conceptual Approach. Philadelphia: Lippincott, Williams & Wilkins, 1995, p. 371. © copyright 1995, Bruce Stewart and Lippincott, Williams & Wilkins.)

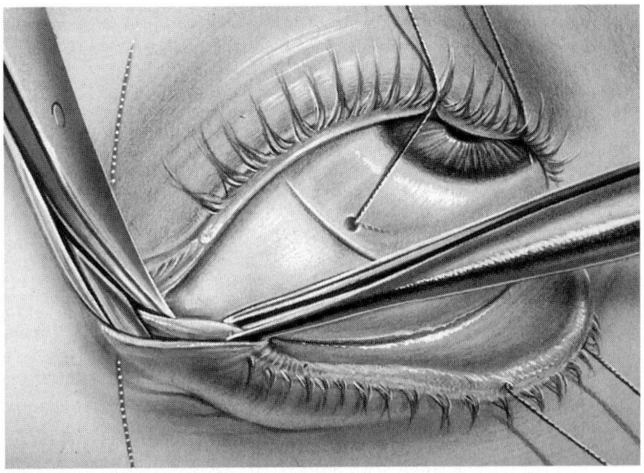

Figure 44–12. Stevens scissors are used to perform the lateral cantholysis, detaching the inferior crus of the lateral canthal tendon. (From Rootman J, Stewart B, Goldberg RA: Orbital Surgery: A Conceptual Approach. Philadelphia: Lippincott, Williams & Wilkins, 1995, p. 193. © copyright 1995, Bruce Stewart and Lippincott, Williams & Wilkins.)

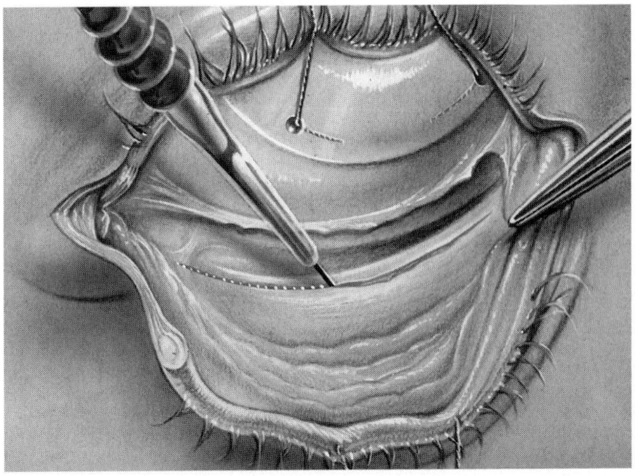

Figure 44–13. With the globe protected by use of a nonconducting retractor, and the eyelid pulled forward over the rim with a Desmarres retractor, cutting cautery is used to cut through the lower eyelid retractors and anterior rim of orbital fat, to expose the periosteum of the inferior orbital rim at the arcus marginalis. (From Rootman J, Stewart B, Goldberg RA: Orbital Surgery: A Conceptual Approach. Philadelphia: Lippincott, Williams & Wilkins, 1995, p. 373. © copyright 1995, Bruce Stewart and Lippincott, Williams & Wilkins.)

Step 4. Stevens scissors are used to perform the lateral cantholysis, detaching the inferior crus of the lateral canthal tendon from the lateral orbital rim (Fig. 44–12).

Step 5. The lower eyelid is retracted anteriorly with a Desmarres retractor, and the transconjunctival incision is extended across the horizontal length of the eyelid to the caruncle, approximately 4 mm below the inferior border of tarsus (Fig. 44–13). This will avoid the plane of the orbital septum. The incision can extend through the caruncle if additional exposure is needed.

Step 6. Blunt and sharp scissors dissection is performed through the fat pads until the inferior orbital rim is visualized. To protect the globe, an assistant can grasp the lower lid retractors, or a 4-0 silk traction suture can be placed through the cut edge of the lower lid retractors. The assistant should also retract the anterior lamella against the inferior orbital rim with the Desmarres retractor to protect it from inadvertent injury. The optimal plane of dissection is immediately posterior to the plane of the orbital septum. In the proper plane, septi within the orbital fat will allow the surgeon to keep the fat posterior to the surgical field.

Step 7. The arcus marginalis at the inferior orbital rim is identified and serves as an important landmark. The dissection can now proceed in a subperiosteal plane, or in the supraperiosteal plane for an extraconal tumor. For dissection in a subperiosteal plane, the periosteum is incised with a No. 15 Bard-Parker blade or the monopolar cautery along the arcus marginalis.

Step 8. The subperiosteal dissection is initiated with the periosteal elevator (Fig. 44–14). The thicker edge of periosteum at the arcus marginalis can be grasped with forceps to aid in the dissection.

Step 9. Once a subperiosteal pocket has been formed, a malleable retractor is inserted to gently retract the orbital contents superiorly (Fig. 44–15). Keeping the periorbita intact during the dissection will facilitate maintaining wide exposure of the entire orbital floor.

Step 10. The closure of the periorbita is usually not indicated. If an orbital floor implant has been placed, the periorbita can be reapproximated to the arcus marginalis over the implant to prevent implant migration, with care not to incorporate the orbital septum in the closure. If there is concern about lower lid retraction (i.e., in a case of multiple previous surgeries), injection of triamcinolone acetonide (Kenalog 40 mg/cc) into the plane of the lower lid retractors and orbital septum can be performed before closure.

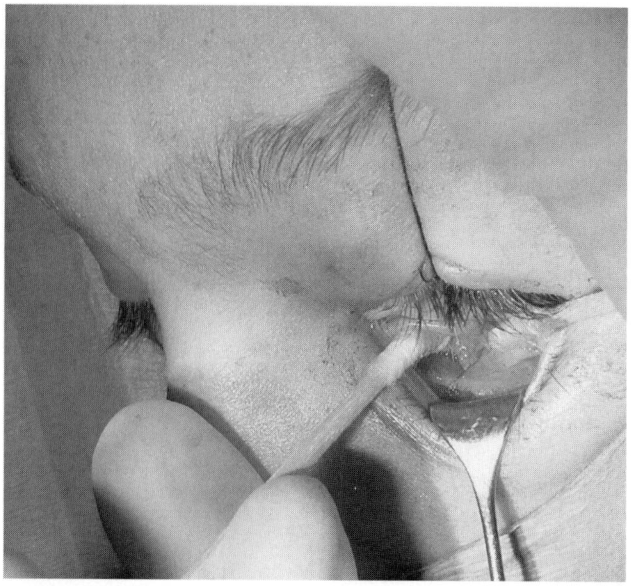

Figure 44–15. The orbital contents are elevated with a malleable retractor or, as pictured here, cotton-tipped applicators, in order to visualize the bony orbital floor. (© copyright 2001, Regents of the University of California; reprinted with permission.)

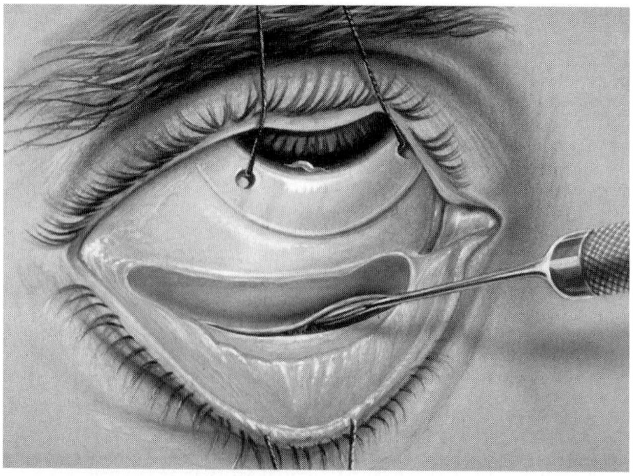

Figure 44–14. The subperiosteal dissection is initiated with a periosteal elevator. (From Rootman J, Stewart B, Goldberg RA: Orbital Surgery: A Conceptual Approach. Philadelphia: Lippincott, Williams & Wilkins, 1995, p. 203. © copyright 1995, Bruce Stewart and Lippincott, Williams & Wilkins.)

Step 11. The conjunctiva and lower lid retractors are closed with several interrupted absorbable sutures. The lateral canthal tendon is reattached to the periosteum at the lateral orbital rim with an absorbable suture.

Step 12. The lateral canthotomy skin incision is closed with interrupted sutures. It is helpful to carefully approximate the eyelid margins at the lateral canthus with a horizontal mattress suture (Fig. 44–16).

UPPER EYELID CREASE APPROACH

Traditionally, lateral orbitotomies were performed through noticeble brow incisions, as described by Berke, Stallard, and Wright. We now use a cosmetically hidden eyelid crease incision for performing a lateral and superomedial orbitotomy, obtaining wide access to the lacrimal fossa, lateral intraconal or extraconal space, and deep lateral orbit, often without the need for bone flap. This incision is particularly useful for accessing the lacrimal gland for biopsy and/or removal, although complete extirpation of the gland is probably more safely performed by removing the lateral wall of the orbit. Fortunately, the eyelid crease incision affords the opportunity to create various lateral bone flaps that can be individualized to the patient if additional access is required. An important concept in obtaining adequate exposure of the deep orbit through an eyelid crease incision is to create a wide opening through the periosteum and soft tissues at the lateral canthus. Accordingly, we recommend extending the subperiosteal

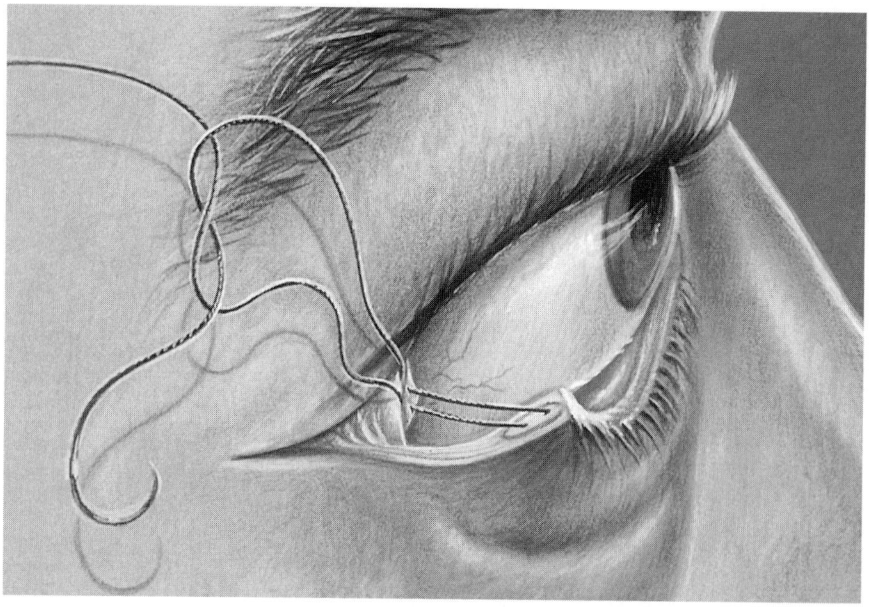

Figure 44–16. The lateral canthal tendon is reattached to the periosteum at the lateral orbital rim using a nonabsorbable suture. (From Rootman J, Stewart B, Goldberg RA: Orbital Surgery: A Conceptual Approach. Philadelphia: Lippincott, Williams & Wilkins, 1995, p. 195. © copyright 1995, Bruce Stewart and Lippincott, Williams & Wilkins.)

dissection onto the malar region, which will help "open" up the exposure to the deep lateral orbit and the lateral orbital floor.

SURGICAL TECHNIQUE

Step 1. Mark the skin incision along the lateral two thirds of the upper eyelid crease. Typically, this incision extends laterallyto the lateral orbital rim, approximately 3 to 5 mm past the lateral canthus (Fig. 44–17).

Step 2. With a No. 15 Bard-Parker blade, make the incision through skin and orbicularis, avoiding entry into the orbital septum.

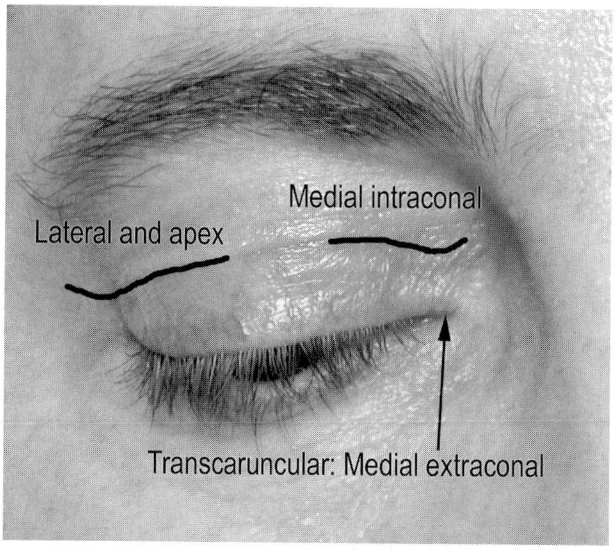

Figure 44–17. The canthal angle is carefully re-formed, and the skin is closed with interrupted sutures. (From Rootman J, Stewart B, Goldberg RA: Orbital Surgery: A Conceptual Approach. Philadelphia: Lippincott, Williams & Wilkins, 1995, p. 195. © copyright 1995, Bruce Stewart and Lippincott, Williams & Wilkins.)

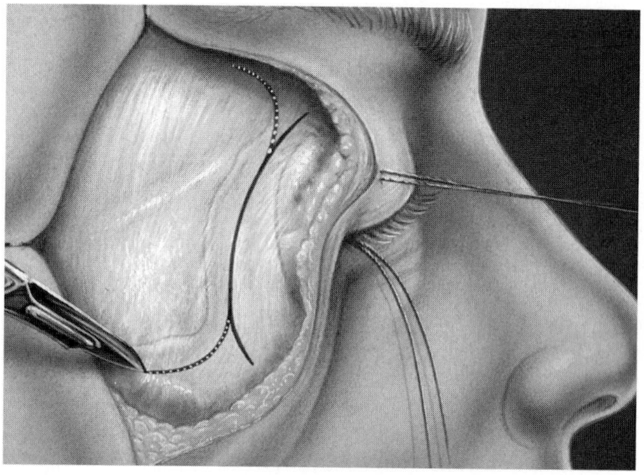

Figure 44–18. The eyelid crease incision begins in the eyelid crease, as in a blepharoplasty, and extends in "lazy S" fashion to the level of the lateral orbital rim. (Modified From Rootman J, Stewart B, Goldberg RA: Orbital Surgery: A Conceptual Approach. Philadelphia: Lippincott, Williams & Wilkins, 1995, p. 230. © copyright 1995, Bruce Stewart and Lippincott, Williams & Wilkins.)

Step 3. The monopolar cautery or the Stevens scissors is used to dissect in the suborbicularis plane to the superolateral orbital rim. Maintaining an intact orbital septum during this dissection will avoid prolapse of fat into the field.

Step 4. The superolateral orbital rim is marked by placement of a cotton-tipped applicator just inside the orbital rim. The surgeon then dissects through the brow fat pad and identifies the arcus marginalis. The periosteum at the rim of the orbit is incised with the monopolar cautery or a No. 15 Bard-Parker blade, carefully following the normal curvature of the orbit (Fig. 44–18). This will leave a 5-mm cuff of periosteum at the arcus marginalis to assist in the intraorbital, subperiosteal dissection.

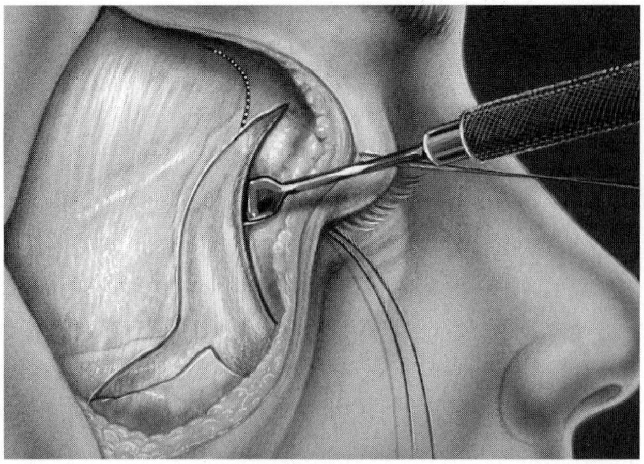

Figure 44–19. The periosteum at the rim of the orbit is incised with monopolar cautery, carefully following the normal curvature of the orbit. (From Rootman J, Stewart B, Goldberg RA: Orbital Surgery: A Conceptual Approach. Philadelphia: Lippincott, Williams & Wilkins, 1995, p. 230. © copyright 1995, Bruce Stewart and Lippincott, Williams & Wilkins.)

Step 5. Subperiosteal dissection is extended medially along the superior orbital rim, where it is limited medially by the supraorbital neurovascular bundle. Inferiorly, the subperiosteal dissection is continued onto the face of the zygoma, where it is limited by the zygomaticofacial nerve formaina. It is often necessary to dissect the temporalis fascia off the lateral orbital rim during this dissection. This superior and inferior extension of the subperiosteal dissection is critical to open up exposure to the deep orbit.

Step 6. The subperiosteal, intraorbital dissection is initiated with a periosteal elevator and a 0.5 Cassie forceps, which is used to grasp the cuff of periosteum (Fig. 44–19).

Step 7. As the subperiosteal dissection proceeds into the inferior orbit, the surgeon will encounter the zytomaticotemporal nerve and artery. This neurovasular bundle is cauterized with the bipolar cautery and cut with the periosteal elevator.

Step 8. The anterior half of the inferior orbital fissure is now visualized at the junction of the lateral wall and the floor of the orbit. Because no critical structures are contained in this portion of the fissure, the anterior 1 cm is cauterized with the bipolar cautery to "open" up the inferior orbital exposure and to serve as a landmark during the surgery.

Step 9. The subperiosteal, intraorbital dissection is then extended superiorly toward the orbital roof. It is critical to identify the junction between the thicker bone of the lateral wall and the thin roof of the orbit. There is a distinct color difference at this junction, with the thinner bone of the roof appearing purplish from the underlying dura, while the thicker greater wing of the sphenoid appears whitish. Another useful landmark for this junction is the meningolacrimal artery, which is located 6 mm lateral to the tip of the superior orbital fissure. This artery can be cauterized with the bipolar cautery if additional deep exposure is required.

Step 10. The next landmark to identify is the anterior tip of the superior orbital fissure, which marks the medial limit of the dissection from this approach. The entire lateral orbit should now be exposed, from the inferior orbital fissure to the superior orbital fissure.

Step 11. If a bony orbitotomy will be performed for additional exposure, a customized bone flap can be fashioned (Fig. 44–20 *A,B,C*). Typically, the bony incisions are made just above the zygomaticofrontal suture line and inferiorly along the line of the superior margin of the body of the zygoma. The bone flap is removed with an oscillating saw and rongeurs.

Step 12. After the goals of the procedure have been achieved, the periosteum and fascia overlying the lateral orbital rim are closed with interrupted, absorbable sutures to prevent unsightly adhesions between the skin and orbital rim. The upper eyelid crease incision is closed with either an interrupted suture or a running suture.

CORONAL APPROACH FOR ORBITAL RECONSTRUCTION

The coronal incision is a versatile approach for orbitotomy because it provides maximal surgical exposure to all four orbital walls, facilitates the harvesting of cranial bone grafts and regional soft-tissue flaps, and produces good cosmesis in patients with an adequate hairline. Because it requires a large incision and time-consuming dissection of the forehead and scalp, the bicoronal flap should be reserved for patients who cannot be treated by direct orbital approaches. The patient's hair "density" is an important factor to consider. Because of the high incidence of male-pattern baldness in men, the coronal approach is primarily employed in women. Possible complications specifically related to the coronal approach include numbness in the supraorbital nerve distribution, alopecia at the incision site, flap hematoma, temporalis muscle atrophy with late depressed contour abnormality, and most important, facial nerve damage. Despite these possible limitations, it behooves the modern orbital surgeon to become familiar with the versatile coronal approach, because many multidisciplinary orbital cases involve a bicoronal incision and flap. We describe our surgical technique for performing a bicoronal approach to the orbits and discuss methods of avoiding complications.

SURGICAL TECHNIQUE

Preoperatively, evaluation of the patient's forehead, hairline, and hair density are all factored into the deci-

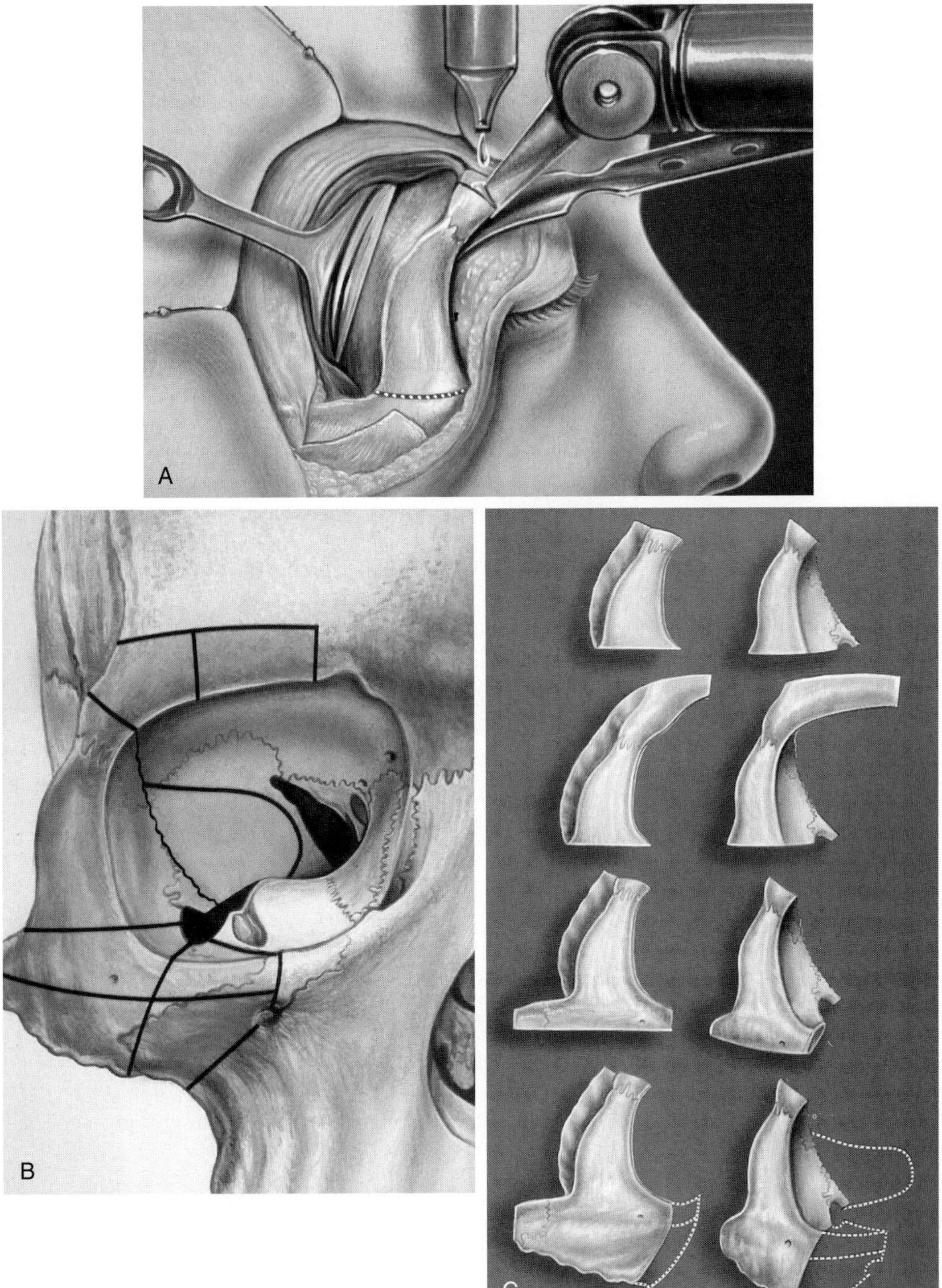

Figure 44–20. *A.* The subperiosteal dissection into the orbit is carefully created to avoid spilling orbital fat into the field; relaxing incisions are needed only rarely, and with practice, the surgery can be performed through a much smaller exposure than the one pictured here. *B.* The bony incisions are carried out with the sagittal saw; typically, bony incisions are made in the area of the frontozygomatic suture and at the takeoff of the zygomatic arch. *C.* The bony incisions can be customized to the exposure needed for each individual case. Some options are pictured here. (From Rootman J, Stewart B, Goldberg RA: Orbital Surgery: A Conceptual Approach. Philadelphia: Lippincott, Williams & Wilkins, 1995, pp. 231, 232 & 229. © copyright 1995, Bruce Stewart and Lippincott, Williams & Wilkins.)

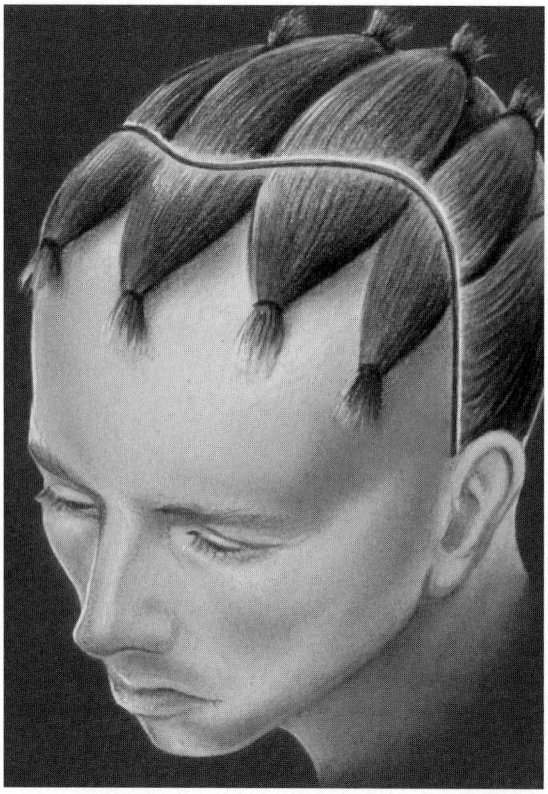

Figure 44–21. The coronal incision is made at least 2 cm posterior to the hairline, and should be carried inferiorly into the postauricular sulcus. (Modified From Rootman J, Stewart B, Goldberg RA: Orbital Surgery: A Conceptual Approach. Philadelphia: Lippincott, Williams & Wilkins, 1995, p. 228. © copyright 1995, Bruce Stewart and Lippincott, Williams & Wilkins.)

sion of whether to employ a pretrichial (hairline) or posthairline scalp incision. The posthairline incision will usually move the hairline posteriorly and increase the vertical height of the forehead, while a pretrichial incision can reduce the size of the forehead by allowing resection of forehead tissue anterior to the incision (Fig. 44–21). The posthairline coronal incision and approach will be described here.

Step 1. With the patient under general anesthesia, the hair is parted and braided along the proposed posthairline coronal incision line (a lubricating jelly like K-Y jelly can be useful in separating the hair and keeping it out of the surgical field). The incision line extends from the superior aspect of one ear along the scalp to the superior aspect of the other ear. If indicated, continuing the incision anterior to the ear can "relax" the flap and allow it to be retracted further inferiorly for better exposure of the inferior orbit.

Step 2. Local anesthetic solution containing 0.5% lidocaine with 1:200,000 epinephrine and hyaluronidase is injected subcutaneously along the coronal incision line and in the temporal regions bilaterally. Additional local anesthetic is injected into the area of interest in the orbit. Supraorbital nerve blocks with 0.75% bupivacaine may be administered for postoperative analgesia.

Step 3. After a full betadine prep of the face and hair, the coronal scalp incision is made with a No. 15 Bard-Parker blade and carried down to the level of the periosteum, entering the subgaleal (preperiosteal) plane. Bleeding from the wound edge is controlled with Raney clips and careful cautery to prevent the significant blood loss that can result from this scalp wound. Excessive cautery should be avoided to prevent hair loss, although a segment of scalp along the anterior edge of the incision may be excised at the end of surgery to prevent alopecia along the incision site.

Step 4. The scalp and forehead flap is elevated in the subgaleal plane with blunt (the surgeon's fingers) or sharp (scissors) dissection inferiorly to the lower forehead, approximately 1.5 cm above the brow (Fig. 44–22). At this point, the periosteum is incised, and the dissection is continued down to the superior orbital rims in the subperiosteal plane with a periosteal elevator. This maneuver will avoid injury to the supraorbital neurovascular bundle.

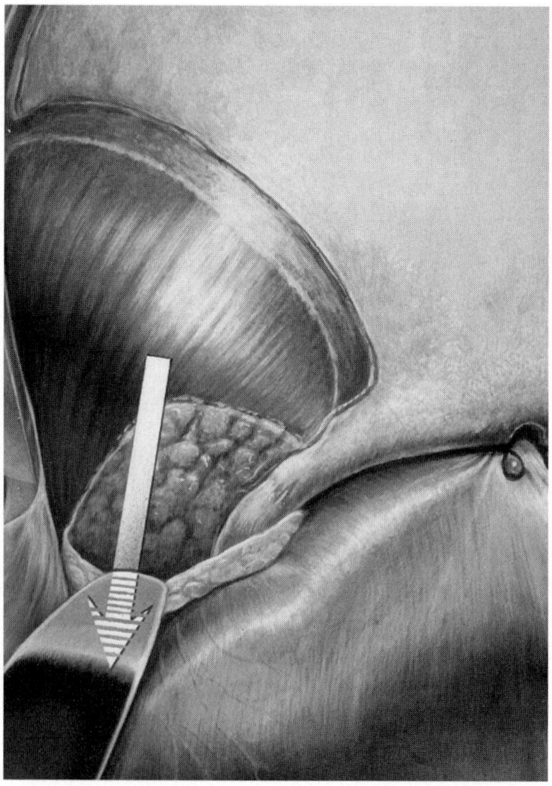

Figure 44–22. The flap is carried down in the subperiosteal plane; over the temporalis muscle, the flap is carefully dissected at the level of the deep and temporalis fascia and within the intermediate temporal fat pad, so that the surgeon is in the plane deep to the branches of the facial nerve, which travel through the superficial temporal fascia. (Modified From Rootman J, Stewart B, Goldberg RA: Orbital Surgery: A Conceptual Approach. Philadelphia: Lippincott, Williams & Wilkins, 1995, p. 169. © copyright 1995, Bruce Stewart and Lippincott, Williams & Wilkins.)

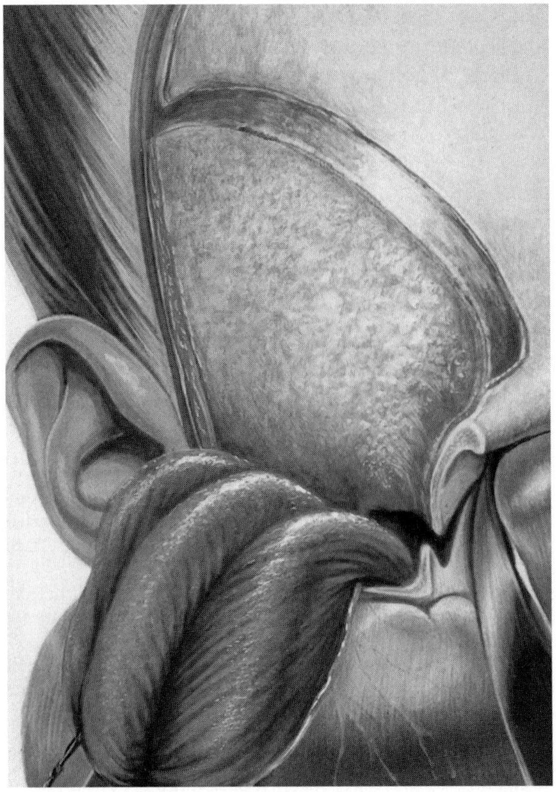

Figure 44–23. To provide wide exposure to the deep orbit, the temporalis muscle can be elevated out of its fossa; to decrease temporalis atrophy, a cuff of muscle is left attached to bone, and the muscle can be rotated anteriorly at the end of the case as it is closed to the remaining cuff. (From Rootman J, Stewart B, Goldberg RA: Orbital Surgery: A Conceptual Approach. Philadelphia: Lippincott, Williams & Wilkins, 1995, p. 169. © copyright 1995, Bruce Stewart and Lippincott, Williams & Wilkins.)

Step 5. Dissection over the temporalis fossa carries the risk of facial nerve injury, and careful attention to the plane of surgical dissection is essential in this region. The frontal (temporal) branches of the facial nerve lie within the deeper layers of the superficial temporal fascia (temporoparietal fascia), just superficial to the deep temporalis fascia. While dissection along the surface of the deep temporal fascia is generally safe, a surgical plane within or beneath the temporalis fascia assures additional safety in avoiding the temporal branches of the facial nerve.

Step 6. Below the superior orbital rim and above the zygomatic arch, the deep temporalis fascia divides into two layers and forms the intermediate temporal fat pad (Fig. 44–23). Inferior dissection within this fat pad avoids damage to the branches of the facial nerve, but the dissection should be as atraumatic as possible to minimize postoperative atrophy of this region.

Step 7. If additional exposure of the deep lateral orbit and orbital apex is required, the temporalis muscle can be disinserted from its fossa for maximal exposure of this region; however, some degree of temporalis muscle atrophy can result whenever the muscle is disinserted from its fossa. Relaxing incisions are made in the temporalis fascia superolaterally, and the temporalis muscle is dissected off the anterior temporalis fossa with cutting cautery and a periosteal elevator to expose the external aspect of the lateral orbital wall. A 1-cm cuff of muscle is left at its insertion to allow re-attachment at the conclusion of the case (Fig. 44–24 *A*).

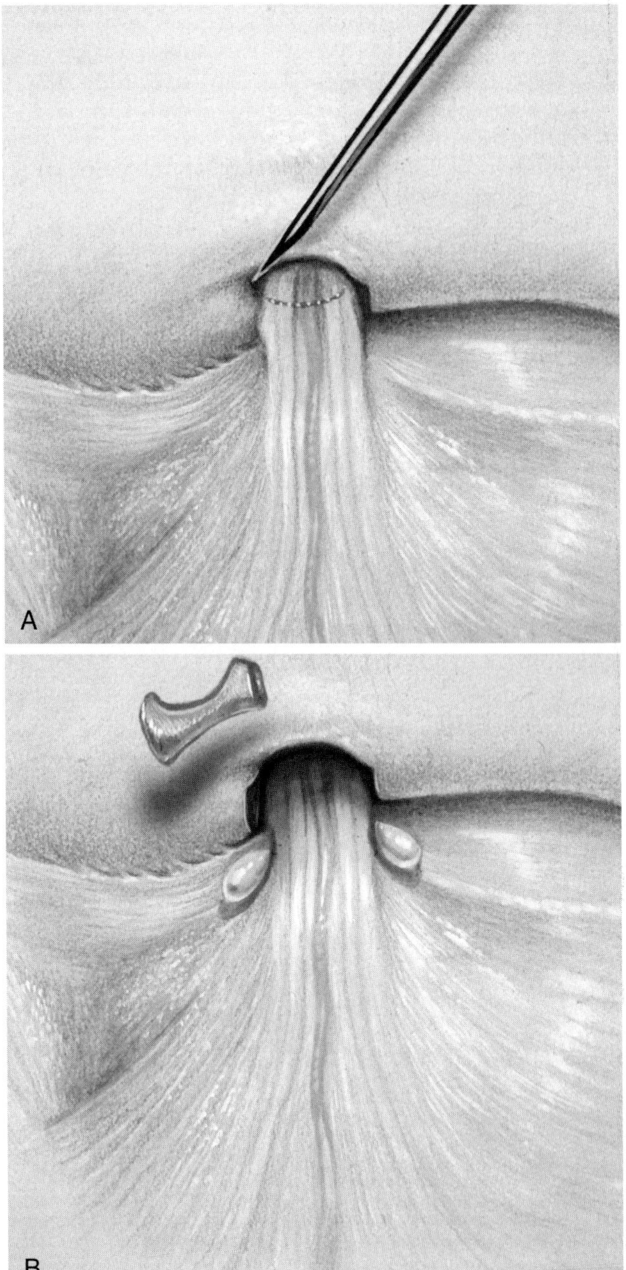

Figure 44–24. *A.* A sharp osteotome can be used to chip out to the bar of bone that forms the canal of the supraorbital nerve. *B.* Once the canal is chipped out, the nerve can be safely lifted out of the canal so that the orbit can be widely exposed in the subperiosteal plane. (From Rootman J, Stewart B, Goldberg RA: Orbital Surgery: A Conceptual Approach. Philadelphia: Lippincott, Williams & Wilkins, 1995, p. 170. © copyright 1995, Bruce Stewart and Lippincott, Williams & Wilkins.)

Step 8. When a coronal flap is being employed, a subperiosteal dissection into the orbit is usually appropriate. The subperiosteal plane can be either continued or initiated along the superior, medial, and lateral orbital rims and into the orbit along the corresponding orbital walls with a periosteal elevator. If the supraorbital neurovascular bundle emerges from a canal rather than a notch, the canal may be carefully opened with an osteotome to free the nerve and allow better surgical exposure of the orbit (Fig. 44–24 *B*). For exposure of the medial orbit, the trochlea is disinserted superonasally with the periosteum, and the medial canthal tendon may also be disinserted for additional exposure, although this is generally unnecessary. The medial orbital floor may be accessed by elevating the lacrimal sac out of its fossa.

Step 9. If the temporalis muscle was disinserted, it is resutured to its anterior muscle stump. Anterior temporal wasting may be minimized by either rotating the temporalis muscle anteriorly when reattaching it, or placing an autogenous graft or flap in the anterior temporalis fossa (such as a free dermis-fat-galeal graft from the anterior edge of the coronal incision or a periosteal-galeal flap transposed laterally from the forehead).

Step 10. The scalp flap is replaced in the normal anatomic position, and the scalp incision is closed with surgical staples. No drains are required. The hair is rinsed with baby shampoo to remove residual blood. A compressive head dressing is placed at the end of the procedure to prevent hematoma formation beneath the scalp flap. The staples are removed 10 days postoperatively.

SUGGESTED READINGS

Cartwright MJ, Elner VM, Polley JW, et al.: A modification of the transcoronal flap that enhances orbital exposure and cosmesis. Ophthal Plast Reconstr Surg 1993;9:139–142.

Goldberg RA, Weinberg DA, Shorr N, Wirta D: Maximal, three-wall, orbital decompression through a coronal approach. Ophthal Surg Lasers 1997;28:832–843.

Goldberg RA, Lessner AM, Shorr N, Baylis HI: The transconjunctival approach to the orbital floor and orbital fat. A prospective study. Ophthal Plast Reconstr Surg 1990;6:241–246.

Holtman B, Wray RC, Little AG: A randomized comparison of four incisions for orbital fractures. Plast Reconstr Surg 1981;67:731–737.

Lacey M, Antonyshyn O, MacGregor JH: Temporal contour deformity after coronal flap elevation: an anatomical study. J Craniofac Surg 1994;5:223–227.

Magnus WW, Castner DV, Schonder AA, Salz JJ: A conjunctival approach to repair of medial wall of orbit: report of case. J Oral Surg 1971;29:664–667.

McCord CD: Orbital decompression for Graves' disease. Exposure through lateral canthal and inferior fornix incision. Ophthalmology 1981;88:533–541.

Mourits M, Kornneef L, Wiersinga WM, et al.: Orbital decompression for Graves' ophthalmopathy by inferomedial, by inferomedial plus lateral, and by coronal approach. Ophthalmology 1990;97:636–641.

Rootman J, Stewart B, Goldberg RA: Orbital Surgery: A Conceptual Approach. New York, Raven Press, 1995.

CHAPTER 45

Entropion and Ectropion

MICHAEL J. GROTH, M.D.

ENTROPION

Entropion is the inward turning or rotation of the eyelid margin, which may cause the lashes or the skin of the lid margin to rub against the eye. Symptoms include scratching, foreign body sensation, photophobia, and tearing. Mechanical trauma from an entropion may result in conjunctivitis, keratitis, corneal scarring, corneal ulceration, or loss of the globe. Surgery is indicated when an entropion poses a threat to comfort or vision.

Entropion should be differentiated from other conditions in which there may be irritation from lashes but where there is no true inward turning of the lid margin. These conditions include epiblepharon, a congenital condition in which an abnormal fold of pretarsal skin and muscle turns the lashes inward; trichiasis, a misdirection of the eyelashes; and distichiasis, a congenital condition in which there is an accessory row of lashes emanating from the meibomian gland orifices.

Entropion can be classified as congenital, spastic, involutional, or cicatricial. Congenital entropion may result from developmental defects in the posterior lamella. Spastic entropions are usually transient and related to swelling of the eyelid associated with spasm of the orbicularis muscle. Involutional entropion results from an attenuation of the structures that maintain a normal eyelid position. Cicatricial entropion results from an acquired shrinkage of the posterior lamellae of the eyelid. Trichiasis may accompany an entropion, especially the cicatricial form.

CONGENITAL ENTROPION AND EPIBLEPHARON

Congenital entropion is a rare condition related to developmental defects in the eyelid that result in marginal rotation. These defects may include lower eyelid retractor dysgenesis, structural abnormalities of the tarsal plate, hypertrophy of the pretarsal orbicularis muscle, or a relative vertical deficiency of the tarsal plate. Repair of a congenital entropion is directed at the underlying anatomic defect and may include repair of the lower lid retractor detachment as discussed later, under Involutional Entropion.[1]

In contrast, epiblepharon is a more common congenital condition related to a developmentally weak attachment of the tarsus to the pretarsal muscle and skin causing a fold of pretarsal skin and muscle to rise above the lid margin, forcing the cilia into a vertical position. In epiblepharon there is no true rotation of the lid margin; however, the lashes may touch the eye, particularly in down gaze. Epiblepharon usually resolves with maturation of the facial structures. Occasionally a significant keratitis necessitates surgical intervention. Orbicularis muscle resection with skin tarsal fixation is frequently successful.

ORBICULARIS RESECTION WITH SKIN TARSAL FIXATION

Technique

A line is drawn 2 mm below the lash line, beginning lateral to the punctum and continuing to the lateral canthus, or 5 mm beyond where the lashes are affected (Fig. 45–1*A*). An incision is then made along this infraciliary line through the skin and orbicularis muscle to the inferior border of the tarsus. The orbicularis muscle over the tarsus is resected up to the margin (Fig. 45–1*B*). The incision is closed with 6-0 plain gut suture. With each bite of the suture, the needle is first passed through the superior skin edge, then through the inferior border of the tarsus, and finally through the inferior skin edge (Fig. 45–1C). This attachment of the skin to the inferior border of the tarsus rotates the lid margin outward. Adjustment of this suture may be necessary to achieve the desired eversion. More severe cases may necessitate the excision of a 2-mm strip of skin in order to effectively evert the lid margin (Fig. 45–1D).

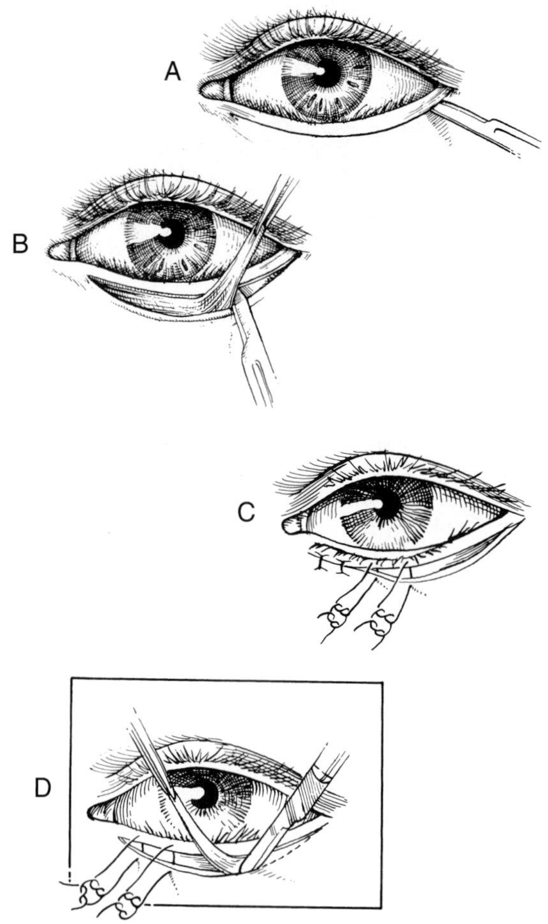

Figure 45–1. Orbicularis resection with skin tarsal fixation.

SPASTIC ENTROPION

Spastic entropion is often associated with acute swelling of the eyelid and reactive spasm of the orbicularis muscle. Often there is a history of ocular or eyelid inflammation, prolonged patching, or recent intraocular surgery that initiates the edema and the spasm. Once the entropion develops the ocular irritation increases, aggravating the spasm. Spastic entropion is usually a transient condition that may resolve with the breaking of this cycle. Treating the underlying cause of the inflammation along with lid taping is usually successful. Rarely, full-thickness rotational sutures (discussed later, under Involutional Entropion) are necessary. Some patients who develop a spastic entropion have an underlying laxity of the eyelid and are predisposed to develop involutional entropion and should be followed with this in mind.

INVOLUTIONAL ENTROPION

Involutional entropion is the most common type of entropion and most commonly affects the elderly. The etiology is thought to include varying degrees of three anatomic abnormalities: attenuation or disinsertion of the lower eyelid retractors creating vertical instability, attenuation of the canthal tendons creating horizontal lid laxity, and superior displacement or overriding of the preseptal orbicularis muscle over the pretarsal space, creating inward rotation of the lid margin (Fig. 45–2).[2,3] Additionally, in cases of enophthalmos, the lack of posterior globe support may contribute to entropion formation. Although involutional entropion primarily affects the elderly it can occur whenever the supporting ligaments and tendons that stabilize the lid margin are attenuated or disinserted.

Over 100 procedures have been described to repair involutional entropion. Most of them address one or more of the three anatomic defects described above. The most successful procedures address all three anatomic defects and permit individual adjustment based on the relative contributions of each etiologic factor.[4] The following description of involutional entropion repair illustrates this concept. The horizontal lid laxity is corrected at the lateral canthus via a mod-

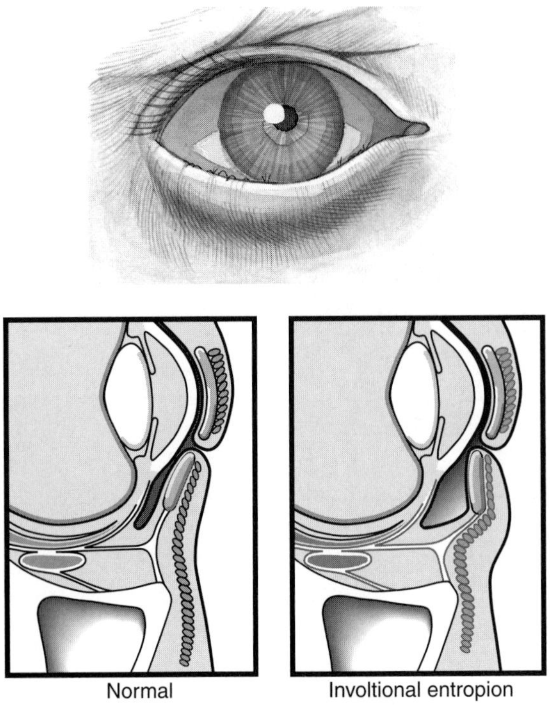

Figure 45–2. Involutional entropion.

ified lateral tarsal strip procedure.[5–7] The lower lid retractor defect is corrected by attaching the lower lid retractors to the inferior border of the tarsus. The override of the preseptal orbicularis is minimized by excising a strip of orbicularis and creating a barrier to superior migration.

INVOLUTIONAL ENTROPION REPAIR

Technique

The proposed incision site is outlined. The incision begins medially, inferior to the lacrimal punctum, and extends along the lower eyelid, paralleling the lid margin at a distance 4 mm from the lid margin to a point inferior to the lateral canthal angle. The incision is then directed upward toward the lateral canthal angle and extended lateral to the lateral canthal angle for a distance of 12 mm (Fig. 45–3*A*).

The incision is made with a No. 15 Bard Parker blade. The incision extends through the skin and subcutaneous muscle to the orbital septum along the infraciliary region and to the lateral canthal tendon in the region lateral to the lateral canthal angle.

A lateral canthotomy is performed with Steven's tenotomy scissors (Fig. 45–3*B*). This separates the superior from the inferior limb of the lateral canthal tendon. In making this incision the scissors are directed from the lateral canthal angle toward the lateral orbital tubercle. This incision extends to the orbital rim.

The Steven's tenotomy scissors are then turned 90 degrees to the canthotomy incision and the inferior limb of the lateral canthal tendon is cut near its insertion onto the lateral orbital rim (Fig. 45–3*C*). The inferior limb of the lateral canthal tendon is dissected free from the adjacent structures with sharp dissection. The mucocutaneous border is dissected off the superior border of the tendon with Wescott scissors for a distance of approximately 4 mm. The conjunctiva and lower lid retractors are dissected off the inferior border of the tendon with Wescott scissors for a distance of 4 mm. The skin and subcutaneous muscle are dissected off the anterior surface of the tendon for a distance of 6 mm, medially and inferiorly. This dissection isolates the inferior limb of the lateral canthal tendon prior to shortening and reattaching it. Next, attention is directed toward the lateral orbital rim. The periosteum of the lateral orbital rim is incised vertically, creating a medial and lateral flap of periosteum (Fig. 45–3*D*).

The inferior limb of the lateral canthal tendon is draped over the orbital rim and the excess tendon is excised with Steven's tenotomy scissors. The amount the tendon to be shortened depends on the degree of the laxity of the lower eyelid as well as the proximity of the cantholysis incision to the orbital rim. The amount to be resected ranges from 0 to 8 mm, and the average is approximately 3 mm.

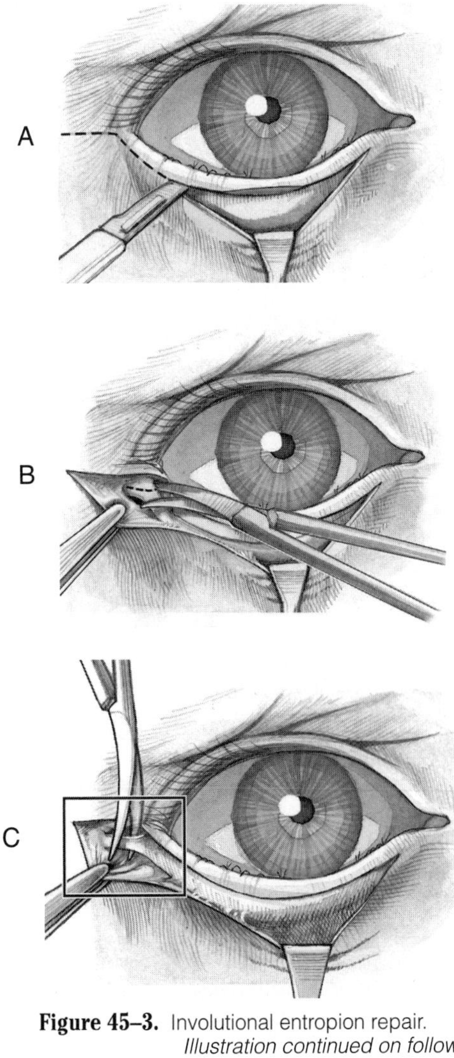

Figure 45–3. Involutional entropion repair.
Illustration continued on following page

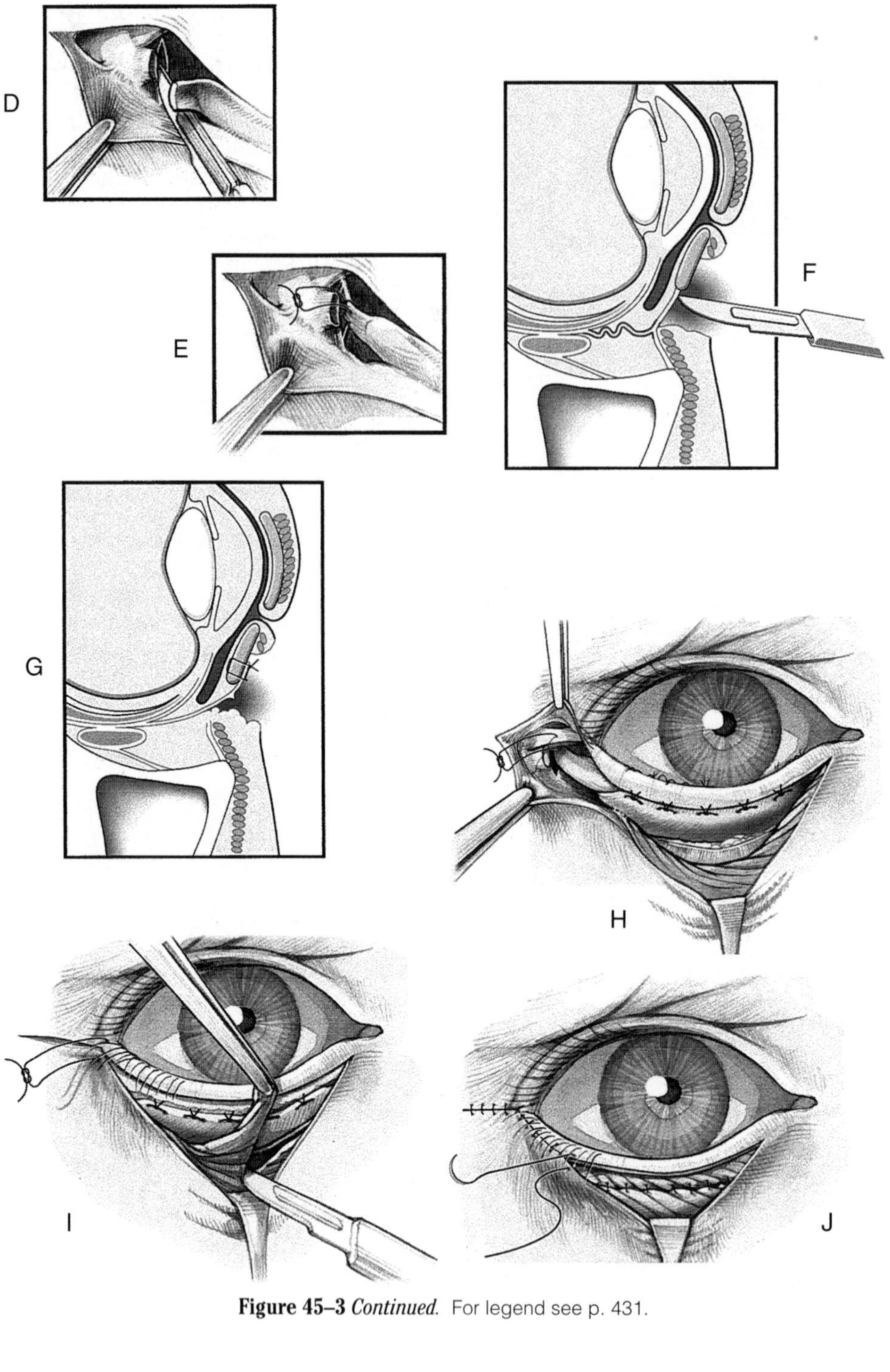

Figure 45–3 *Continued.* For legend see p. 431.

The tendon is then reattached to the medial flap of periosteum at the lateral orbital rim with interrupted 5-0 or 6-0 Prolene sutures (Fig. 45–3*E*). One suture is placed near the superior aspect of the tendon and the other suture is placed near the inferior aspect of the tendon. The tendon is directed along the medial aspect of the orbital rim to permit the eyelid to follow the curvature of the globe.

The orbital septum is incised along the infraciliary portion of the wound with Steven's tenotomy scissors, exposing the inferior orbital fat (Fig. 45–3*F*). The inferior orbital fat is bluntly dissected off the lower eyelid retractors with a moistened cotton-tipped applicator. Attenuation or disinsertion of the lower eyelid retractors is identified. The lower eyelid retractors are advanced and reattached to the inferior aspect of the lower eyelid tarsus with four interrupted 6-0 Dexon sutures tied in a horizontal mattress fashion (Fig. 45–3*G*). This maneuver stabilizes the position of the eyelid and prevents rotation of the lid margin. Advancing the retractors too far onto the anterior surface of the tarsus can result in ectropion formation, and should be avoided. Prominent orbital fat may be excised if desired. The gray lines of the upper and lower eyelids are then approximated with a single interrupted 6-0 mild chromic gut suture at the lateral canthal angle (Fig. 45–3*H*). The knot of this suture is buried within the substance of the lateral canthus. This re-forms the lateral canthal angle.

The skin and subcutaneous muscle are redraped over the lower eyelid and the lateral canthus and any excess is excised. A strip of preseptal orbicularis muscle can be excised along the inferior aspect of the infraciliary region of the wound (Fig. 45–3*I*). This weakens the preseptal orbicularis and prevents preseptal orbicularis override. The cicatrix formed by this excision forms a barrier to superior migration of the remaining preseptal orbicularis. The skin and subcutaneous muscle are then approximated with 7-0 Prolene suture (Fig. 45–3*J*).

FULL-THICKNESS ROTATIONAL SUTURES

In some patients with involutional entropion a full surgical correction may not be advisable or possible, because of health concerns, an inability to be transported to an appropriate surgical facility, or patient refusal of surgery. In such cases, full-thickness rotational (Quickert-Rathbun) sutures may be a suitable temporizing measure.[8]

Technique

In this procedure rotational sutures are places in the eyelid without incising the eyelid. Typically, three double-armed 5-0 chromic gut sutures are placed through the eyelid from a posterior inferior to anterior superior location (Fig. 45–4). Each arm is passed first through the conjunctiva and lower lid retractors in the inferior fornix; then the needle is directed superiorly through the pretarsal orbicularis muscle and exits the eyelid in the infraciliary region. When the sutures are tied and tightened the suture creates an outward rotation of the lid margin. The cicatrix along the suture tract may help maintain the lid position even after the suture is removed. Unfortunately recurrence of the entropion is common, making this a temporary solution in many cases.

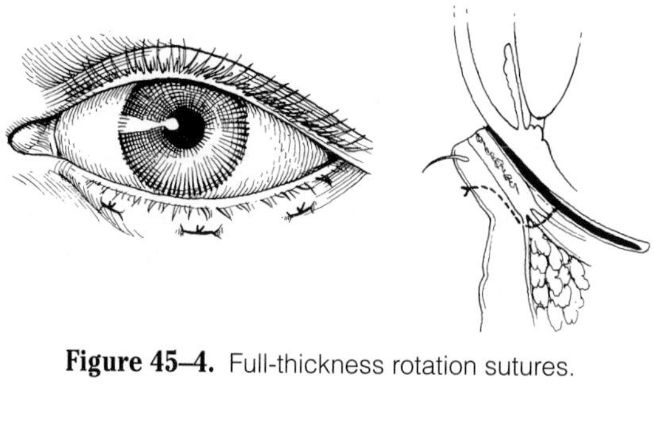

Figure 45–4. Full-thickness rotation sutures.

CICATRICIAL ENTROPION

Cicatricial entropion arises from an acquired shrinkage of the posterior lamellae (tarsus and conjunctiva) of the eyelid that results in the inward turning of the lid margin. Common causes of cicatricial entropion include inflammation (ocular cicatricial pemphigoid, atopic keratoconjunctivitis, erythema multiforme, Stevens-Johnson syndrome, pseudopemphigoid secondary to certain eye drops such as miotic and idoxuridine), infection (trachoma, herpes zoster), and trauma (chemical burns, thermal burns, and surgery). The diagnosis of cicatricial entropion is made by noting the inward turning of the eyelid margin in conjunction with a shortened and often scarred posterior lamella. It is important to distinguish involutional from cicatricial entropion because the surgical repair of the two conditions is quite different. Unlike involutional entropion, the margin malposition cannot be corrected by digital pressure on the inferior border of tarsus in cicatricial entropion.

Cicatricial entropion is one of the more difficult forms to repair. The surgical correction may involve incisions and sutures that permit the rotation of the lid margin outward, grafting techniques to lengthen the vertical height of the posterior lamellae, or both. Because the underlying cause of cicatricial entropion is a shortened posterior lamella the most anatomical solution is to replace the deficient tissue with a graft. In moderate to severe cases a graft is often necessary. In mild cases, several techniques involving blepharotomy or tarsotomy without grafting may be useful.

FULL-THICKNESS TRANSVERSE BLEPHAROTOMY WITH MARGINAL ROTATION

This technique first described by Wies,[9] involves a full-thickness eyelid incision with the creation of a bipedicle flap. This flap is then rotated outward and sutured in place in a more everted position.

Technique

A horizontal incision is made through the skin and subcutaneous muscle to the tarsal plate at a distance 3 mm from the lash line (Fig. 45–5*A*). The incision extends both medially and laterally at least 5 mm beyond the affected area, or if the entire lid is involved, from the lateral canthus to a point 2 mm lateral to the punctum. Care is taken to preserve the marginal artery. To prevent an irregular cut, the eyelid is everted and a separate incision is made in the conjunctiva and tarsus 3 to 4 mm from the lid margin (Fig. 45–5*B*).

The two incisions are connected with scissors (Fig. 45–5C). and the lid margin is then separated from the rest of the eyelid, forming a bipedicle flap.

Four 6-0 polyglactin double-armed sutures are passed through the cut edge of the attached tarsus through the pretarsal orbicularis of the detached portion of the lid margin, exiting the skin at a variable dis-

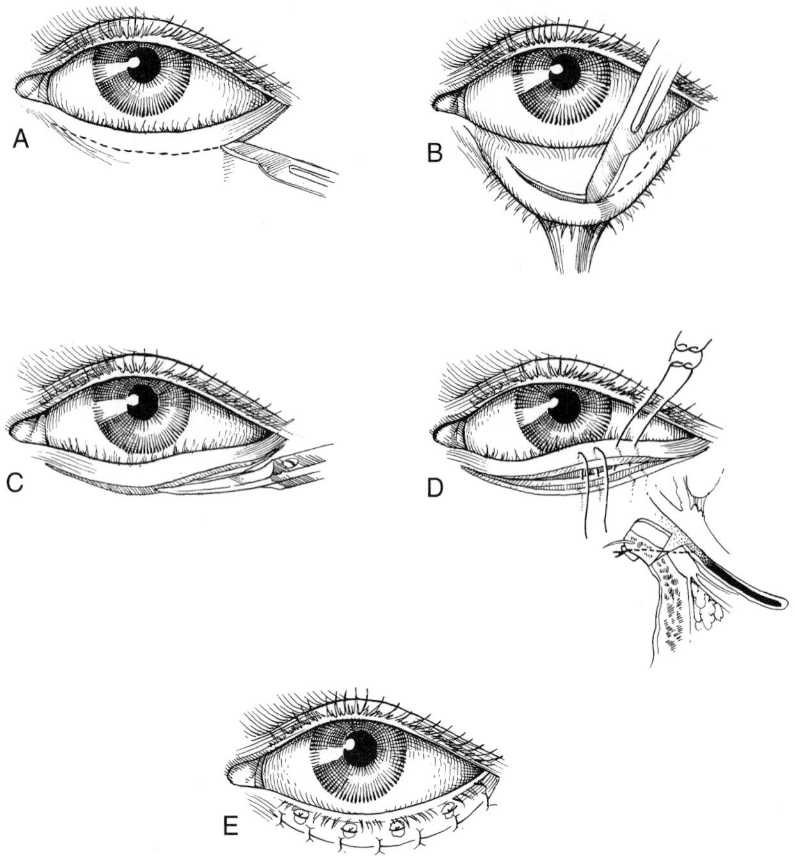

Figure 45–5. Full-thickness transverse blepharotomy with marginal rotation.

tance below the cilia (Fig. 45–5*D*). The amount of eversion can be adjusted through the placement of this suture. The closer to the cilia the suture exits the skin, the greater the eversion.

The sutures are tied over cotton bolsters (rolled-up cotton wool measuring 2 × 4 mm) to avoid excessive pressure on the lid margin. The cutaneous incision is closed with a running 7-0 Prolene suture (Fig. 45–5*E*). The marginal sutures are removed in 10 days, or sooner if a gross overcorrection is noted.

Although used for many years, the Wies procedure has been associated with complications. It creates ischemic stress and can result in ischemic sloughing of the lid margin. Other complications include overcorrection, with resultant ectropion and lid retraction.

TRANSVERSE TARSOTOMY WITH MARGINAL ROTATION

Another procedure that may be effective is the partial-thickness transverse tarsotomy with marginal rotation. This procedure reduces distortion and ischemic stress on the lid margin when compared to the Wies procedure.

Technique

The eyelid is everted over a Desmarres retractor and a horizontal incision is made in the conjunctiva and tarsus at a distance 3 mm from the margin (Fig. 45–6*A*). The incision extends medially and laterally to a point 5 mm beyond the affected area. To permit eversion of the lid margin, sharp dissection may be necessary to release attachments anterior to the tarsus.

The eyelid margin is then rotated outward through the placement of 6-0 polyglactin double-armed sutures (Fig. 45–6*B*). Each suture is placed first through the proximal tarsus and then through the pretarsal orbicularis, and exiting the skin near the cilia. The closer to the cilia the suture exits the greater the degree of eversion. A moderate overcorrection is desired, as wound contracture will reverse this effect.

The sutures are left to dissolve in 4 to 6 weeks (Fig. 45–6*C*).

ANTERIOR LAMELLA RECESSION WITH OR WITHOUT MUCOUS MEMBRANE GRAFTING

Moderate to severe degrees of cicatricial entropion may require more extensive surgery. One such procedure is eyelid splitting with rotation of the lid margin and recession of the anterior lamella. This may be combined with an oral mucous membrane graft for even greater effect.

This procedure is used most often on the upper eyelid, but it can be used on the lower eyelid as well. One advantage of this procedure is that it avoids a graft on the posterior lamella and thus reduces postoperative

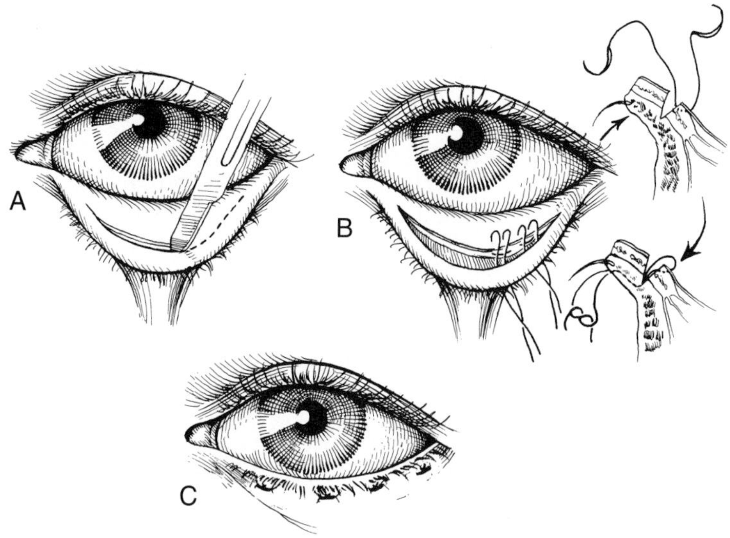

Figure 45–6. Transverse tarsotomy with marginal rotation.

corneal irritation. The one that follows is widely used, though many variations have been described.

Technique

The eyelid is everted on a Desmarres retractor. A horizontal incision is made just posterior to the lid margin at a point where all cilia are anterior to the incision (Fig. 45–7*A*). Sharp dissection is carried superiorly in the plane between the tarsus and the orbicularis for a variable distance separating the anterior from the posterior lamella. The greater the dissection the greater the amount the anterior lamella can be recessed.

The anterior lamella is recessed with respect to the posterior lamella leaving 3 to 4 mm of bare tarsus exposed along the anterior aspect of the posterior lamella. The two lamellae are sutured in this position with four or five 6-0 polyglactin sutures on a spatulated needle passed in a horizontal mattress fashion through the anterior lamella and partial-thickness tarsus (Fig. 45–7*B*). The tarsus can be left bare to heal by secondary intention, or a mucous membrane graft can be used to cover the bare tarsus.

A full-thickness mucous membrane graft can be harvested from the lower lip. The lip is infiltrated with lidocaine and epinephrine. The lip is everted and an oversized graft is outlined to allow for postoperative

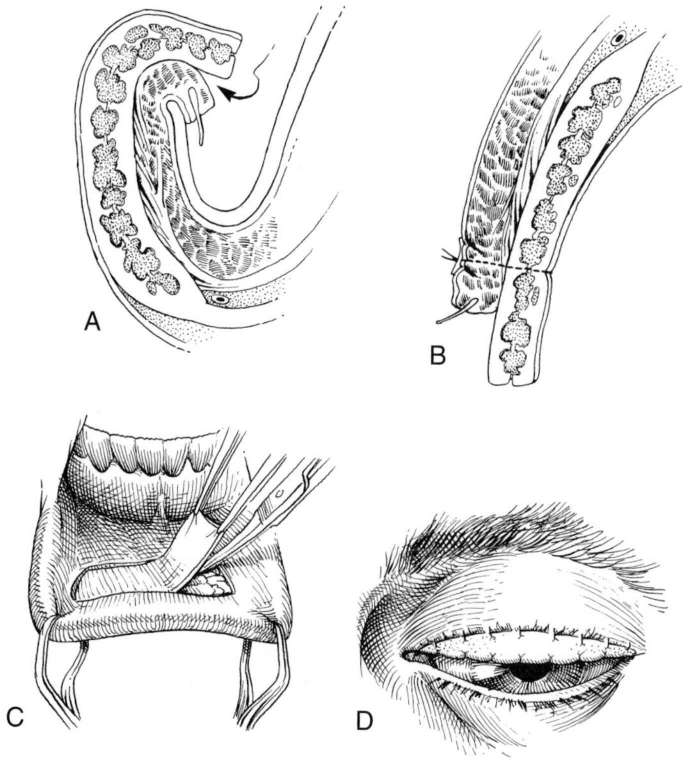

Figure 45–7. Anterior lamellar recession with mucous membrane graft.

shrinkage. The mucosa is incised with a scalpel blade and excised with scissors (Fig. 45–7*C*). A full-thickness graft is preferred because it will shrink less than a partial-thickness graft. The lip is allowed to heal by secondary intention.

The graft is thinned of submucosal tissue and laid in the dried recipient bed. The graft is sutured in place with 6-0 plain gut suture and the knots are kept away from the cornea (Fig. 45–7*D*). An overcorrection is desired because the graft will shrink 30% to 60% postoperatively. If the graft remains redundant beyond 3 months it can be trimmed. It is important for the surgeon to keep in mind that cicatricial entropion may be an ongoing process.

FREE TARSAL–CONJUNCTIVAL GRAFT

Severe cases of cicatricial entropion or recurrent cases in which there is significant loss of tarsus may require a grafting procedure to lengthen the posterior lamella. A free tarsal–conjunctival graft is a logical choice to replace a deficiency in tarsus causing the eyelid margin to turn in.[10] The ideal circumstance for finding tarsal–conjunctival tissue for grafting would be ptosis of one of the upper eyelids where a tarsal–conjunctival tissue specimen will be generated as part of the ptosis repair. Nevertheless, a tarsal–conjunctival graft can be taken from a non-ptotic lid if the donor site is left unsutured. This frequently results in minimal effect on lid height. In lower lid entropion this graft can come from the ipsilateral upper lid. In upper lid entropion the graft can come from the contralateral upper lid.

Although tarsal–conjunctival tissue is the best match, an adequate source of excess tarsal–conjunctival tissue is frequently not present. Many times the underlying disease process that resulted in the cicatricial entropion affects the other eyelids, resulting in inadequate tarsal–conjunctival tissue on all eyelids. Other tissues that are suitable grafts for the posterior lamella of the eyelid include oral mucous membrane, hard palate mucosa, nasal chondromucosa, dermal allografts, and scleral allografts. The hard palate has the advantage that it is rigid and resists shrinkage and is an excellent choice for lower lid reconstruction. Unfortunately, hard palate mucosal grafts have been associated with chronic keratitis when used in the posterior lamella of the upper eyelid and thus are best reserved for the lower eyelid. Donor tissue has the advantage that it obviates the necessity for harvesting of the graft; however donor tissue may be more prone to absorption and shrinkage than autogenous grafts. The choice of grafting material depends on availability of tissue, site to be grafted, and patient and surgeon preference.

POSTERIOR LAMELLAR GRAFTING PROCEDURE

Technique

The eyelid is everted on a Desmarres retractor. A horizontal incision is made through the conjunctiva and tarsus 2 mm from the lid margin along the full length of the tarsus (Fig. 45–8*A*). Sharp dissection is used to separate attachments anterior to the tarsus. The cut edges

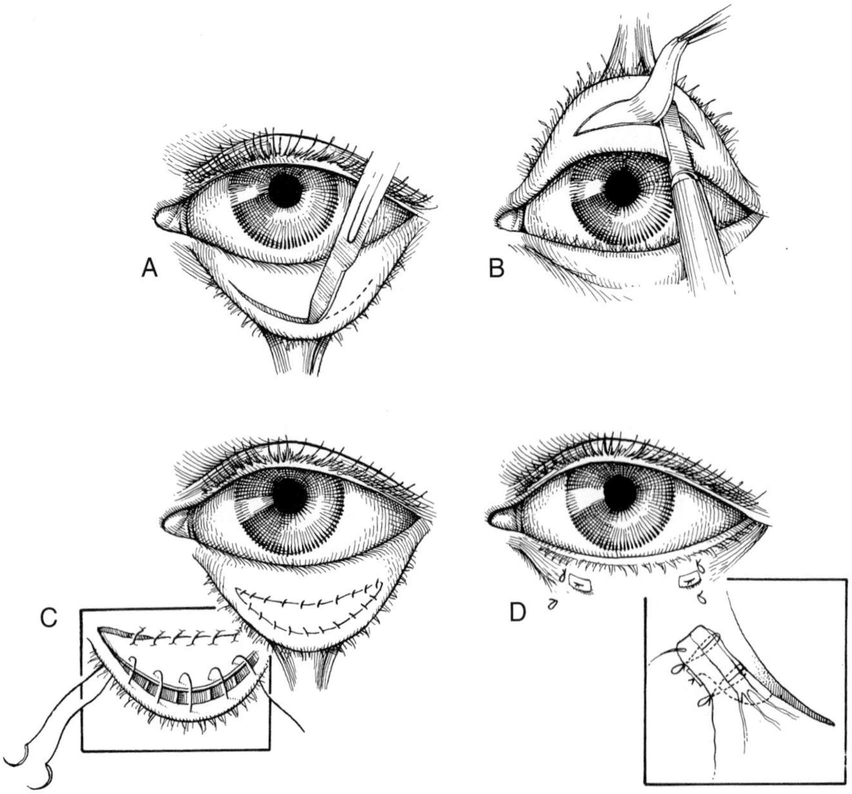

Figure 45–8. Posterior lamellar grafting procedure.

of the tarsus are separated, and the lid margin is rotated outward, opening up a bed for the graft.

The upper eyelid is everted on a Desmarres retractor, and the graft is taken from the mid-tarsal area (Fig. 45–8*B*). The graft is usually 2 to 3 mm wide. A slightly oversized graft is planned to permit for postoperative shrinkage. The tarsal defect is left to heal unsutured. Alternatively, one of the grafts mentioned previously may be used.

The graft is placed in the recipient bed and sutured in place with running 6-0 Prolene sutures (Fig. 45–8*C*). The suture knots are externalized to prevent corneal irritation and to facilitate removal. A bandage contact lens may be used further to protect the cornea.

Sutures of 6-0 double-armed silk are placed from the inferior cul de sac through the orbicularis and out through the skin beneath the cilia and are tied over silicone pegs (No. 40 silicone band) (Fig. 45–8*D*). These sutures brace the lid in an everted position during the healing process. Alternatively, traction sutures may be used to place the eyelid on traction and immobilize the lid in the postoperative period. The Prolene sutures are removed in 1 week and the silk sutures in 2 weeks.

ECTROPION

Ectropion is the outward turning or rotation of the lid margin which leads to poor eyelid apposition to the globe. This may result in exposure of the eye and eversion of the punctum. Symptoms may include a red eye, dryness, foreign body sensation, and tearing. Exposure and drying of the eye may produce conjunctivitis and keratitis. Eversion of the punctum may produce epiphora. Surgery is indicated when exposure of the eye impairs comfort or vision, or when epiphora impairs function.

Ectropion may be classified as congenital, involutional, paralytic, and cicatricial. Congenital ectropion is a rare condition that is usually caused by congenital deficiency of anterior lamellar tissue. Involutional ectropion is due to laxity or attenuation of the supporting structures of the lower eyelid. Paralytic ectropion is due to paralysis of the facial nerve or one of its branches with resultant weakness of the orbicularis oculi muscle. Cicatricial ectropion results from an acquired deficiency or shrinkage of anterior lamellar tissue. Other forms of ectropion are inflammatory and mechanical.[11]

CONGENITAL ECTROPION

Congenital ectropion is a rare condition that is most frequently seen in Down syndrome. There is usually a congenital vertical shortage of anterior lamellar tissue. It may also be seen as part of the autosomal dominant condition known as the "congenital eyelid" (blepharophimosis) syndrome. This syndrome may include blepharophimosis, blepharoptosis, epicanthus inversus, telecanthus, and congenital ectropion. Many of these patients require several surgical procedures to address each of these problems. Often there is a deficiency of the eyelid skin. In mild cases of congenital ectropion where corneal exposure is mild, no treatment is necessary. In more severe cases where the exposure keratitis threatens vision, skin grafts may be necessary.

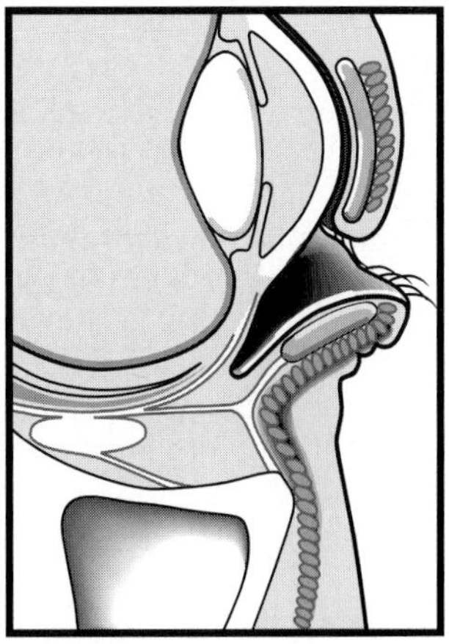

Figure 45–9. Involutional ectropion.

INVOLUTIONAL ECTROPION

The most common type of ectropion, involutional ectropion results from laxity of the structures that maintain the normal eyelid position (Fig. 45–9). These structures include the tarsal ligamentous sling and to a lesser degree the lower eyelid retractors. Although this condition primarily affects the elderly, it may occur whenever sufficient laxity develops in the structures that support the eyelid position. Typically, involutional ectropion begins in the medial eyelid and may be manifest as punctal eversion or medial ectropion. As the condition worsens the entire eyelid can become involved. In severe cases, particularly when the lower eyelid retractors are disinserted, there can be complete eversion of the tarsus. Longstanding involutional ectropion may lead to shrinkage of the anterior lamella of the eyelid, and thus develop a cicatricial component.

The surgical correction of involutional ectropion is directed at the underlying anatomic abnormalities. The horizontal laxity of the eyelid is corrected by horizontal tightening procedures. Laxity of the tarsal ligamentous sling is usually secondary to a stretching and attenuation of the canthal tendons and not the tarsus. Tightening the eyelid by shortening the lateral canthal tendons may address the underlying anatomic problem better than the tarsal resection of a full-thickness eyelid resection. The advantages of tightening the eyelid at the lateral canthus include reduced likelihood of causing corneal irritation, lid margin irregularities, and a horizontally shortened palpebral fissure. Shortening the lateral canthal tendon is technically easier than shortening the medial canthal tendon, because of the absence of the lacrimal drainage ducts laterally. Medial canthal tendon plication should be avoided whenever practical. The procedure selected for repair of the involutional ectropion is selected based on the location and severity of the ectropion as well as the degree of laxity of the supporting structures of the eyelid.

EVERSION OF THE LACRIMAL PUNCTUM

Excessive tearing may be one of the most bothersome symptoms of ectropion. The epiphora seen in some patients with ectropion is due to eversion of the lacrimal punctum out of the lacrimal lake. In patients with reduced tear production, epiphora may not be present despite eversion of the punctum. This is occasionally the case in the elderly. When symptoms of tearing are bothersome to the patient, a tarsal–conjunctival resection may be indicated.[12]

TARSAL–CONJUNCTIVAL RESECTION

Technique

The lower eyelid is everted on a retractor, exposing the inferior conjunctival fornix. The globe is protected with a Jaeger lid plate. A Bowman probe is placed in the inferior canaliculus to identify it. The incision is kept at least 3 mm inferior to the lid margin to prevent damage to the lacrimal canaliculus (Fig. 45–10). A spindle-shaped block of tissue consisting of conjunctiva and lower lid retractors is excised from the medial conjunctival fornix inferior to the punctum. The size of this resection varies depending on the degree of punctal eversion. Typically, the spindle measures 3 to 4 mm vertically and 6 to 8 mm horizontally. One-third of this resection is medial to the punctum and two-thirds is lateral. The conjunctiva and lower lid retractors are reapproximated with interrupted 6-0 plain gut sutures (Fig. 45–10 Inset).

MEDIAL ECTROPION

Correction of a medial ectropion is accomplished by combining a tarsal–conjunctival resection with a horizontal tightening procedure. Commonly, this includes combining a tarsal–conjunctival resection with a lateral tarsal strip procedure. Another popular yet less desirable combination procedure is the "lazy T" operation.[13] This procedure combines a tarsal–conjunctival resection with a full-thickness eyelid resection. The tarsal strip procedure may be technically easier and more successful than the full-thickness eyelid resection for the reasons mentioned previously.

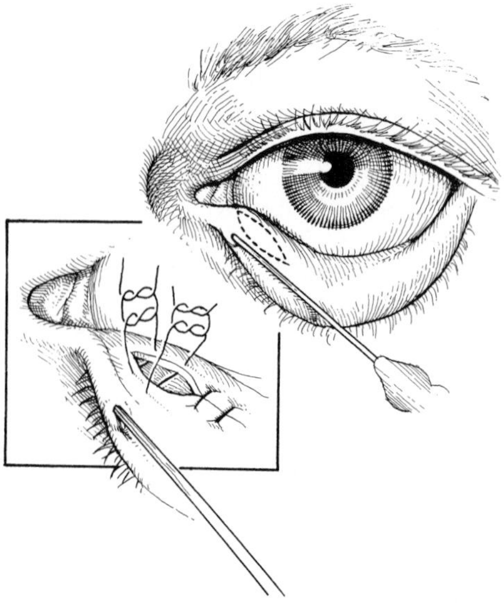

Figure 45–10. Tarsal–conjunctival resection.

"LAZY T" PROCEDURE

Technique

A full-thickness vertical lower eyelid incision is made 5 mm lateral to the punctum. The incision is then extended from the lid margin to the cul-de-sac (Fig. 45–11*A*). A Bowman probe is placed in the inferior canaliculus to identify it (Fig. 45–11*B*).

The conjunctiva and tarsus are incised horizontally 2 mm below the lid margin. Care must be taken to avoid the canaliculus (Fig. 45–11*C*). The incision extends from a point 4 mm medial to the punctum to the edge of the full-thickness incision. The conjunctiva and lower lid retractors are undermined inferiorly for a distance of 5 to 6 mm (Fig. 45–11*D*). The tarsal–conjunctival flap is then advanced superiorly (Fig. 45–11*E*), and triangle-shaped block of tarsus, conjunctiva, and lower lid retractors is resected from this flap (Fig. 45–11*F*). The horizontal incision is closed by approximating the tarsus to the conjunctiva and lower lid retractors with interrupted 6-0 plain catgut sutures (Fig. 45–11*G*).

The cut edges of the vertical incision are overlapped, and a block of redundant full-thickness eyelid is excised by making a second full-thickness vertical incision lateral to first (Fig. 45–11*H*). The two incisions are connected inferiorly in the cul-de-sac. The full-thickness vertical eyelid incision is then approximated in the standard fashion (Fig. 45–11*I*).

HORIZONTAL TIGHTENING AT THE LATERAL CANTHUS

This procedure is perhaps the most useful procedure for involutional ectropion. It also may be used to repair a longstanding paralytic entropion and as a component of the repair of cicatricial ectropion. Many variations of this procedure have been described. The following is a modified form of the popular tarsal strip procedure.[5–7]

Technique

The skin is incised, extending from the lateral canthal angle laterally for a distance of 12 mm (Fig. 45–12*A*). The incision is then extended through the skin and subcutaneous muscle exposing the lateral canthal tendon. A lateral canthotomy is performed with Steven's tenotomy scissors (Fig. 45–12*B*). This separates the superior limb from the inferior limb of the lateral canthal tendon. To make this incision, the scissors are directed from the lateral canthal angle toward the lateral orbital

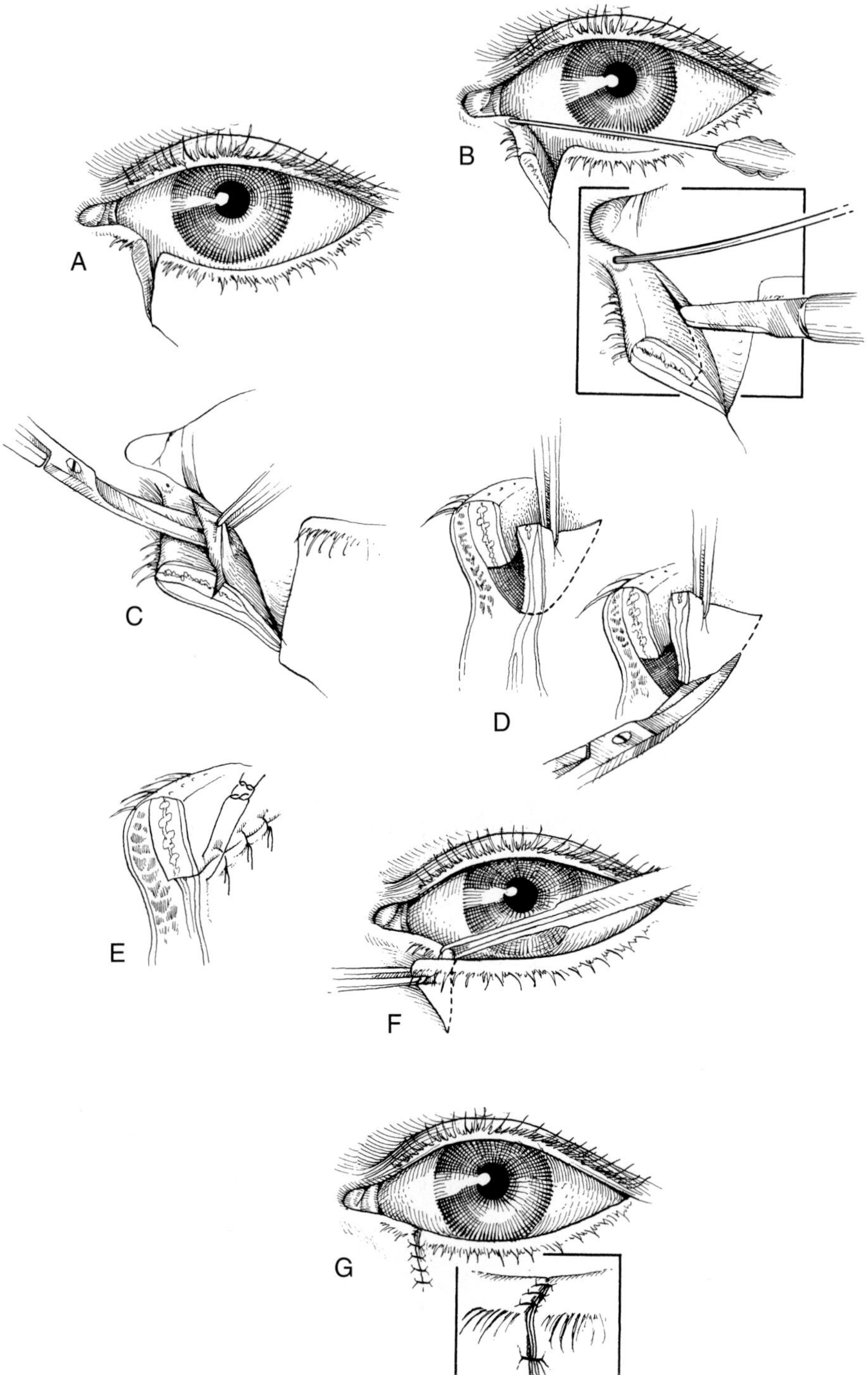

Figure 45–11. Lazy "T" procedure.

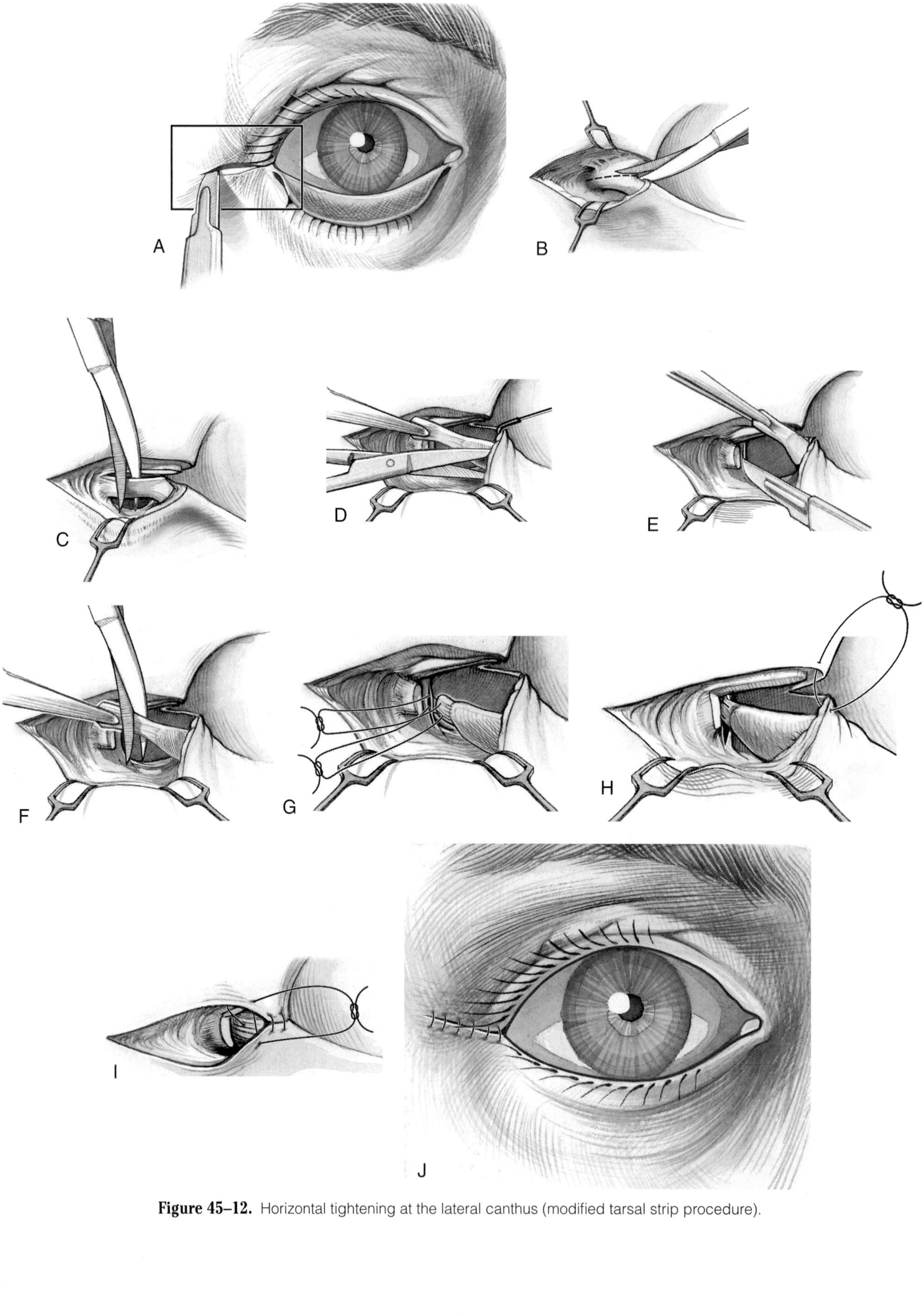

Figure 45–12. Horizontal tightening at the lateral canthus (modified tarsal strip procedure).

tubercle, and the incision is extended to the orbital rim. The Steven's tenotomy scissors are then turned 90 degrees to the canthotomy incision and the inferior limb of the lateral canthal tendon is cut near its insertion into the lateral orbital rim (Fig. 45–12*C*).

The inferior limb of the lateral canthal tendon is dissected free from the adjacent structures with sharp dissection (Fig. 45–12*D*). The mucocutaneous border is dissected off the superior border of the tendon with Wescott scissors for a distance of approximately 4 mm. The conjunctiva and lower lid retractors are dissected off the inferior border of the tendon with Wescott scissors for a distance of 4 mm. The skin and subcutaneous muscle are dissected off the anterior surface of the tendon for a distance of 6 mm, medially and inferiorly. This dissection isolates the inferior limb of the lateral canthal tendon prior to shortening and reattaching it. Next, attention is directed toward the lateral orbital rim. The periosteum of the lateral orbital rim is incised, creating a medial and lateral flap of periosteum (Fig. 45–12*E*). The inferior limb of the lateral canthal tendon is draped over the orbital rim and the excess tendon is excised with Steven's tenotomy scissors (Fig. 45–12*F*). The amount the tendon is shortened depends on the degree of laxity of the lower eyelid as well as the proximity of the cantholysis incision to the orbital rim. The amount resected ranges from 0 to 8 mm, and the average is 3 mm.

The tendon is then reattached to the medial flap of periosteum at the lateral orbital rim with interrupted 5-0 or 6-0 Prolene sutures (Fig. 45–12*G*). One suture is placed near the superior aspect of the tendon and the other is placed near the inferior aspect of the tendon. The tendon is directed along the medial aspect of the orbital rim to permit the eyelid to follow the curvature of the globe. Attaching the tendon to the lateral aspect of the orbital rim can result in formation of an unnatural-appearing space between the globe and the eyelids at the lateral canthal angle.

The gray lines of the upper and lower eyelids are then approximated with a single interrupted 6-0 mild chromic gut suture at the lateral canthal angle (Fig. 45–12*H*). The knot of this suture is buried within the substance of the lateral canthus. This re-forms the lateral canthal angle.

The skin and subcutaneous muscle are redraped over the lateral canthus and any excess is excised. The skin and subcutaneous muscle are then approximated with 7-0 Prolene suture (Fig. 45–12 *I* and *J*).

MEDIAL CANTHAL TENDON PLICATION

In some patients with involutional lower lid laxity there is significant laxity of the inferior limb of the medial canthal tendon as well as the lateral canthal tendon. Plication of the inferior limb of the medial canthal tendon is best avoided whenever practical because it may interfere with the outflow of tears through the lacrimal drainage apparatus. Nevertheless, when the lid is distracted laterally and the punctum is displaced beyond the pupil in primary gaze, there is significant medial canthal tendon laxity that warrants consideration of medial canthal tendon plication.

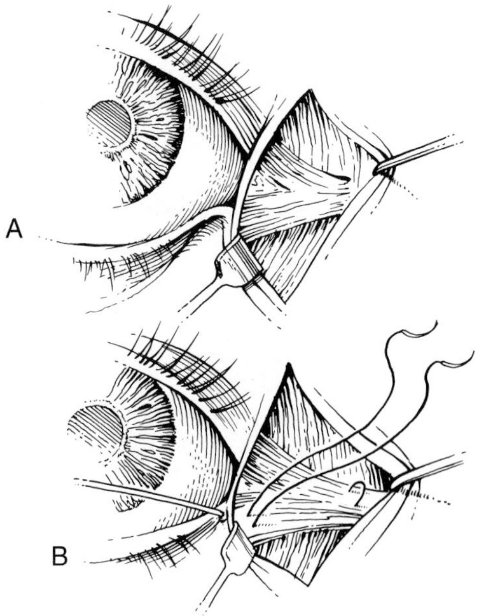

Figure 45–13. Medial canthal tendon plication.

Technique

The skin is incised just medial to the medial canthal angle, exposing the medial canthal tendon (Fig. 45–13*A*). The inferior canaliculus is identified by placing a Bowman probe along its course. A double-armed 5-0 Prolene suture is passed in a horizontal mattress fashion from the main canthal tendon to the stretched inferior limb of the medial canthal tendon and is tied, plicating and tightening the tendon (Fig. 45–13*B*). Care is taken to avoid over-tightening of the tendon and obstructing the lumen of the canaliculus. A horizontal shortening at the lateral canthus is then performed as previously described.

TARSAL ECTROPION REPAIR

Tarsal ectropion occurs when the entire eyelid rotates outward and creates complete eversion of the tarsus. This may occur in involutional ectropion when there is significant attenuation or disinsertion of the attachment of the capsulopalpebral fascia (lower eyelid retractors) into the inferior border of the lower eyelid tarsus.[14–17] Usually, there is some component of horizontal lid laxity; however, a simple horizontal lid tightening procedure may not be enough to correct this ectropion. Combining a horizontal tightening procedure with reattachment of the lower eyelid retractors is frequently successful.

Technique

An ellipse of conjunctiva and attenuated lower lid retractors measuring approximately 2 to 3 mm in verti-

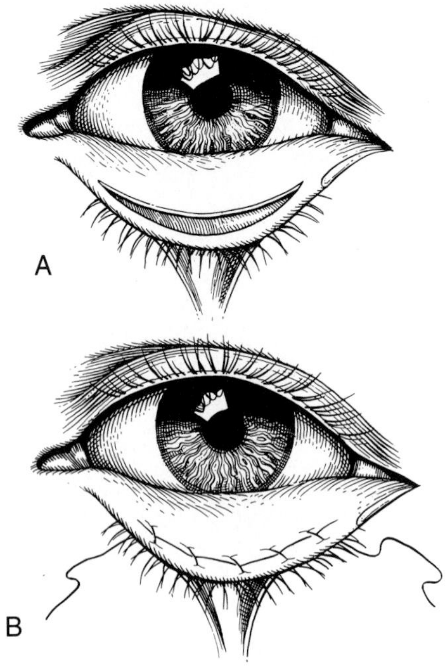

Figure 45–14. Tarsal ectropion repair.

cal height is excised along the inferior border of the lower eyelid tarsus (Fig. 45–14*A*). The conjunctiva and lower lid retractors are then reattached to the inferior border of tarsus with a running 6-0 plain gut suture, with the suture knots buried or directed away from the cornea (Fig. 45–14*B*). A horizontal tightening procedure is then performed as described previously.

PARALYTIC ECTROPION

Paralytic ectropion results from paralysis of the facial nerve in conjunction with an underlying laxity of the tarsal ligamentous sling. In the young patient, a facial nerve paralysis seldom results in ectropion because of the support of the tarsal ligamentous sling. In the elderly patient, however, a facial nerve palsy frequently results in an ectropion because there is usually some degree of laxity of the tarsal ligamentous sling. If the facial nerve paralysis is expected to be temporary, the patient may be managed with ocular lubricants, lid taping, moisture chambers, or if necessary a temporary tarsorrhaphy. If the facial nerve palsy is expected to be longstanding or permanent, then a horizontal tightening procedure as described for involution ectropion repair may be indicated. In cases of facial nerve paralysis the necessary degree of lid tightening is greater than in cases of involutional ectropion because there is no support from the paralytic orbicularis muscle.

CICATRICIAL ECTROPION

Cicatricial ectropion results from a shortening of the anterior lamella of the eyelid. This shortening may involve skin alone or both skin and orbicularis muscle. Causes of cicatricial ectropion include actinic skin damage, inflammations, infections, trauma, surgery, chemical or thermal burns, and sclerosing tumors.

The repair of cicatricial ectropion frequently involves three steps. First, the anterior lamella is incised, releasing tension on the lid and permitting superior displacement of the lid margin. Next, the eyelid is horizontally tightened to reduce lid laxity and to gain support for a normal eyelid position. Finally, the anterior lamella is vertically lengthened with a skin graft or flap to prevent further cicatricial contracture. Skin grafts are preferred over flaps for vertically augmenting the anterior lamella of the eyelid, because the necessary flaps would be exceedingly long and the available skin grafts take exceptionally well on the lower eyelid. However, flaps may be useful in select cases such as, an ectropion isolated to the region of the lateral or medial canthus, where grafting tissue is scarce (burn patients), or where skin graft take may be limited (prior irradiation).[18] The most desirable donor site for lower eyelid defects is the postauricular region. Upper eyelid skin is also excellent when available. Other less desirable sites include supraclavicular, medial upper arm, and preauricular skin.

TRANSPOSITIONAL FLAP FOR REPAIR OF CICATRICIAL ECTROPION

Technique

The proposed incision sites on the eyelids are outlined with a marking pen (Fig. 45–15*A*). The incisions must be hinged beyond the lateral canthus and straddle the canthal angle to permit transposition. The flap is kept as wide at the base and as short in length as practical to maximize blood supply to the flap, while providing enough tissue to vertically augment the lower eyelid. A mark is made 3 mm below the lid margin throughout the interval of the ectropion.

A lateral canthotomy and inferior cantholysis is performed. The lower lid incision is made through the skin and subcutaneous tissue, releasing attachments in this plane and permitting superior displacement of the lid margin (Fig. 45–15*B*). The lower eyelid is horizontally tightened at the lateral canthus as described previously. The previously marked incision sites on the flap are incised. The skin and subcutaneous muscle are undermined with scissors and the flap is elevated. The subcutaneous muscle is included to reduce shrinkage of the flap and to improve blood supply. The flap is transposed across the canthal angle and laid in the recipient bed in the lower eyelid (Fig. 45–15*C*).

The flap is sutured in place and the upper lid and canthal incisions are closed with 6-0 plain gut sutures (Fig. 45–15*D*). The lower eyelid can be placed on traction by placing three 5-0 Prolene sutures in a horizontal mattress fashion through the gray line of the lower lid margin (Fig. 45–15*E*) and taping them to the forehead with benzoin and steri-strips (Fig. 45–15*F*). A pressure

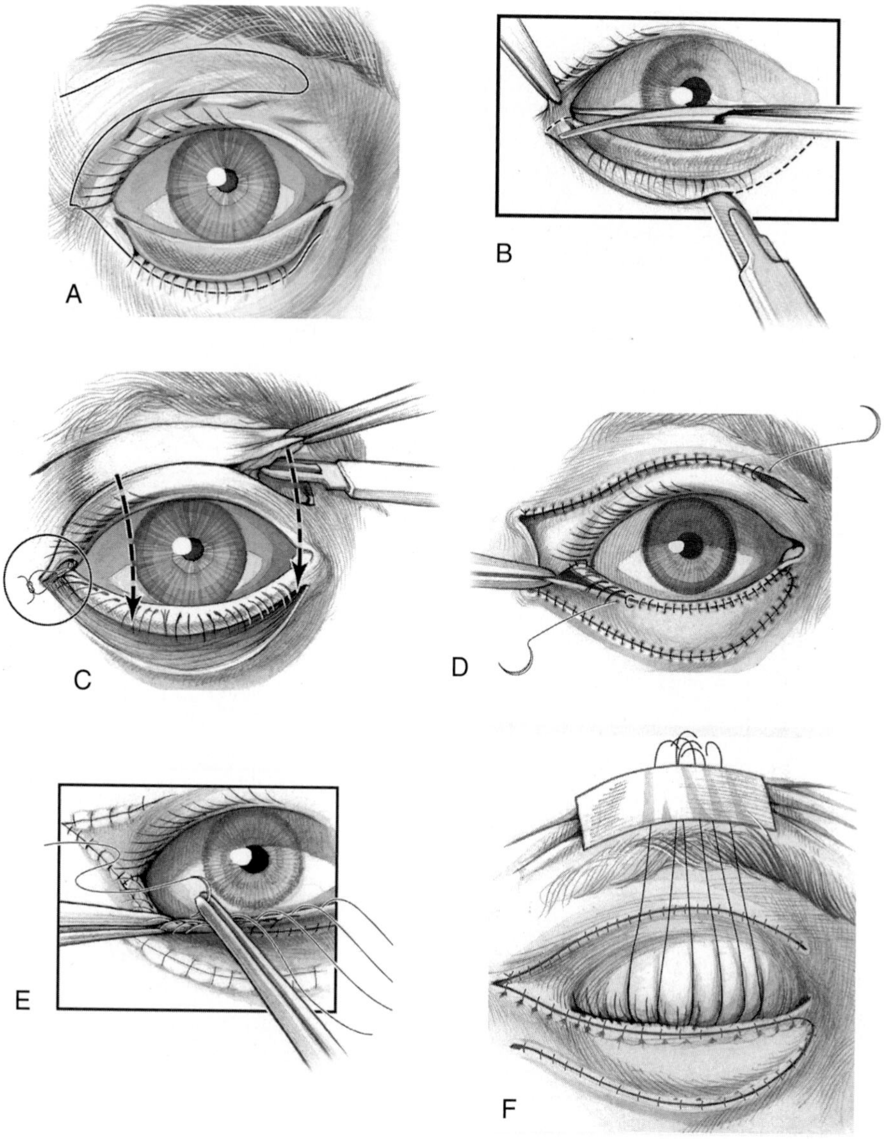

Figure 45–15. Transposition flap for repair of cicatricial ectropion.

patch is then applied. (Alternatively, a cotton bolster can be tied over the flap.) The sutures are removed in 1 week.

FULL-THICKNESS SKIN GRAFT FOR REPAIR OF CICATRICIAL ECTROPION

Technique

An incision is made 3 mm below the lid margin along the involved portion of the eyelid (Fig. 45–16*A*). This may include the full length of the eyelid from canthus to canthus or, in severe cases, the incision may be extended beyond the canthi for 3 to 5 mm. Sharp dissection is used to release superficial attachments in the anterior lamella of the eyelid, allowing superior displacement of the lid margin to the superior limbus in primary position. The orbicularis is left intact when possible to provide a vascularized bed for the graft. A horizontal tightening is performed at the lateral canthus as described previously to support the tarsal ligamentous sling. Traction sutures of 5-0 Prolene are placed in a horizontal mattress fashion from the lower eyelid margin through the upper eyelid margin and to the eyebrow, medially, centrally, and laterally (Fig. 45–16*B*). These sutures will hold the eyelid in position and immobilize the skin graft in the immediate postoperative period.

A suitably sized skin graft is then harvested from the postauricular region (Fig. 45–16*C*). The graft is thinned of subcutaneous tissue and laid in the dried recipient

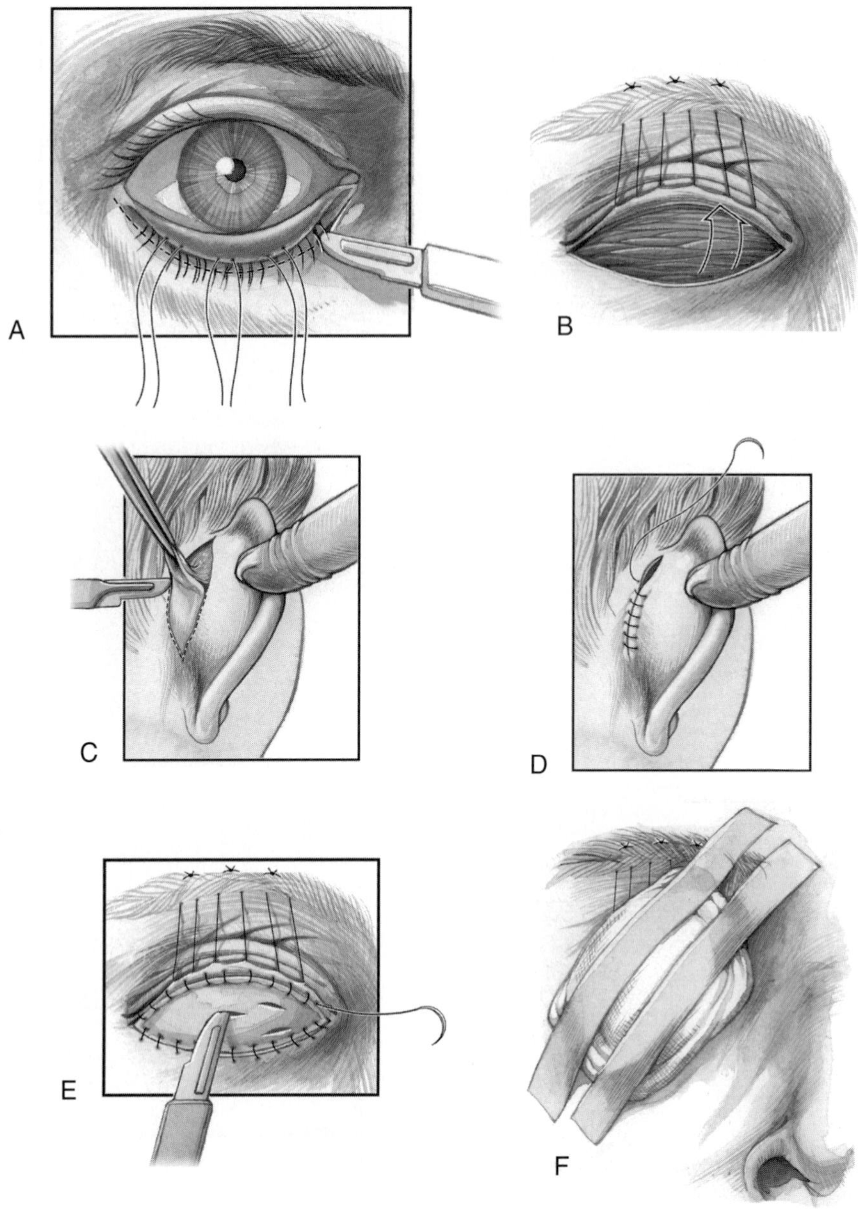

Figure 45–16. Full-thickness skin graft for repair of cicatricial ectropion.

bed. The graft is sutured in place with 6-0 plain gut suture. The postauricular wound is closed with 5-0 Prolene suture (Fig. 45–16*D*). Several 3-mm incisions are made in the skin graft to permit the egress of subgraft fluid in the postoperative period (Fig. 45–16*E*). A telfa pad and a pressure patch are applied over the graft (Fig. 45–16*F*). Alternatively, a bolster of cotton can be placed over the graft and tied in place by leaving the graft sutures long. The pressure patch and the traction sutures can be removed in 7 to 10 days.

The repair of entropion and ectropion must be individualized. The procedure selected is based on the underlying etiologic mechanism and the severity of the condition.

REFERENCES

1. Tse DT, Anderson RL, Fratkin JD: Aponeurosis disinsertion in congenital entropion. Arch Ophthalmol 1983;101:436–440.
2. Dortzbach RK, McGertrick JJ: Involutional entropion of the lower eyelid. In Advances in Ophthalmic Plastic and Reconstructive Surgery. New York: Pergamon Press; 1983:257–267.
3. Jones LT, Reeh MJ, Wobig JL: Senile entropion. A new concept for correction. Am J Ophthalmol 1972;74:327–329.
4. Wesley RE, Collins JW: Combined procedure for senile entropion. Ophthalmic Surg 1983;14:401–405.
5. Anderson RL, Gordy DD: The tarsal strip procedure. Arch Ophthalmol 1979;97:2192–2196.
6. Jordan DR, Anderson RL: The lateral tarsal strip revisited: the enhanced tarsal strip. Arch Ophthalmol 1989;107:604–606.
7. Weber PJ, Popp JC, Wulc AE: Refinements of the tarsal strip procedure. Ophthalmic Surg 1991;22:687–691.

8. Quickert MH, Rathbun E: Suture repair of entropion. Arch Ophthalmol 1971;85:304–305.
9. Wies FA: Spastic entropion. Trans Am Acad Ophthalmol Otolaryngol 1955;59:503–505.
10. Leone CR: Mucous membrane grafting for cicatricial entropion. Ophthalmic Surg 1974;5:24.
11. Frueh BR, Schoengarth LD: Evaluation and treatment of the patient with ectropion. Ophthalmology 1982;89:1049–1054.
12. Nowinski TS, Anderson R: The medial spindle procedure for involutional medial ectropion. Arch Ophthalmol 1985;103:1750.
13. Smith B: The lazy "T" correction of ectropion of the lower punctum. Arch Ophthalmol 1976;94:1149.
14. Hawes MJ, Dortzbach RK: The microscopic anatomy of the lower eyelid retractors. Arch Ophthalmol 1982;100:1313–1318.
15. Putterman AM: Ectropion of the lower eyelid secondary to Muller's muscle-capsulopalpebral fascia detachment. Am J Ophthalmol 1978;85:814–817.
16. Tse D, Kronish JW, Buus D: Surgical correction of lower eyelid tarsal ectropion by reinsertion of the retractors. Arch Ophthalmol 1991;109:427–432.
17. Wesely RE: Tarsal ectropion from detachment of the lower eyelid retractors. Am J Ophthalmol 1982;93:491–495.
18. Leone CR: Repair of cicatricial ectropion by horizontal shortening and pedicle flap. Ophthalmic Surg 1976;606:47.

CHAPTER 46

Eyelid Reconstruction

GEORGE C. CHARONIS, M.D.

Eyelid reconstructive surgery can test the ingenuity of every surgeon. The surgeon must not only address the obvious tissue deficit but also restore the structure, function, and cosmesis in the best possible physiologic way. It is very important to be able to analyze the eyelid defects in a systemic way and chose the procedure that will provide the best result. In the repair of the more complex eyelid and periorbital defects, the surgeon combines several surgical techniques and modifies them to get the structurally normal, functionally sound, and aesthetically pleasing eyelid.

The major indication for eyelid reconstructive surgery is after the removal of malignant lesions that involve the eyelid and periorbital area. The created defects can vary in size and location and are often much larger than anticipated preoperatively. Basal cell carcinoma is the most common eyelid malignancy and occurs on the lower lid in 90% of the cases, followed in order of frequency by the medial canthus, the lateral canthus, and the upper eyelid.[1] Squamous cell carcinoma, meibomian gland carcinoma, and melanoma are less frequent malignant eyelid lesions, but must be carefully looked for and aggressively treated because they can metastasize.

Eyelid and periorbital trauma constitutes another indication for reconstructive surgery in the area. The sequelae of trauma can be devastating for the visual function as well as the function and aesthetics of the patient. Adherence to reconstructive principles and techniques is crucial, as secondary defects can be very difficult or even impossible to correct in repeat surgical attempts.

The last important indication for reconstructive surgery involves a variety of congenital and acquired blepharocanthal abnormalities that require reconstructive techniques that vary in complexity and severity.

There are certain aspects of the reconstructive process that must be understood before such surgery is attempted. The first involves the eyelid tissues, which do not have the same tissue properties in all individuals. Usually the eyelid stretches more with age, which allows tissue defects to be reduced to a substantially smaller size by simple stretching alone. In general, the defect can be reduced 10% to 15% more in older patients with tissue laxity than in younger patients with tighter eyelids.[2] Certain patients have particularly rigid eyelids: previously irradiated lids, actinic skin changes, previous surgery, scars, burns, and cicatrizing processes that produce eyelids that are stiff and difficult to reconstruct. Keeping these tissue characteristics in mind, the surgeon can group defects in three categories. Small defects comprise loss of tissue of up to 20% to 30%. Moderate defects involve tissue loss between 30% and 50%, and large defects have tissue loss greater than 50%. This categorization, although somewhat arbitrary, can be helpful, because it allows grouping of different procedures and understanding the anatomic elements of every such procedure.

Canthal fixation is a very important reconstructive element that must not be overlooked. Good apposition of the eyelid to the globe, normal eyelid movement, and lacrimal outflow depend on this critical anatomic relationship and can only be accomplished with proper canthal fixation. In the medial canthus, this involves direct suturing of the eyelid to the periosteum of the posterior lacrimal crest or to a periosteal flap in that area and transnasal wiring or miniplate fixation if increasing amounts of bone and soft tissue have been removed. In the lateral canthus, fixation is accomplished by direct suturing of the lateral tarsus or lateral canthal tendon to the periosteum overlying Whitnall's tubercle inside the lateral orbital rim, creation of periosteal flaps, and placement of wires through drill holes in the bone of the lateral orbital rim or insertion of miniplates if the bone has been removed.

Restoration of the lacrimal drainage system should be accomplished primarily by silicone intubation and canaliculoplasty when the resection involves part of the proximal canaliculus. In cases with extensive damage or removal of the lacrimal drainage apparatus, the timing of the lacrimal reconstruction depends on the nature of the initial injury (trauma vs. malignancy) and the condition of the canthal angle. In most cases it is usually best to wait until the canthus has assumed a more normal configuration and the patient is tumor free for several months before performing more complicated lacrimal procedures such as placement of Jones tubes.

FULL-THICKNESS DEFECTS OF THE LOWER EYELID

SMALL DEFECT

In small lower eyelid defects (tissue loss up to 20% to 30%) the reconstruction can be accomplished by direct closure (Fig. 46–1). The resected margins are "freshened up" prior to reconstruction, and the repair is the same as that described for the upper eyelid.

MODERATE DEFECT

Direct Closure with Canthotomy and Cantholysis

In lower eyelid defects that fall into the lower range of moderate (tissue loss between 30% and 50%), canthotomy and cantholysis of the inferior crus of the lateral canthal tendon can provide sufficient release of lower eyelid tissues to allow reconstruction of the defect by direct closure. The technique is the same as that described for the upper eyelid.

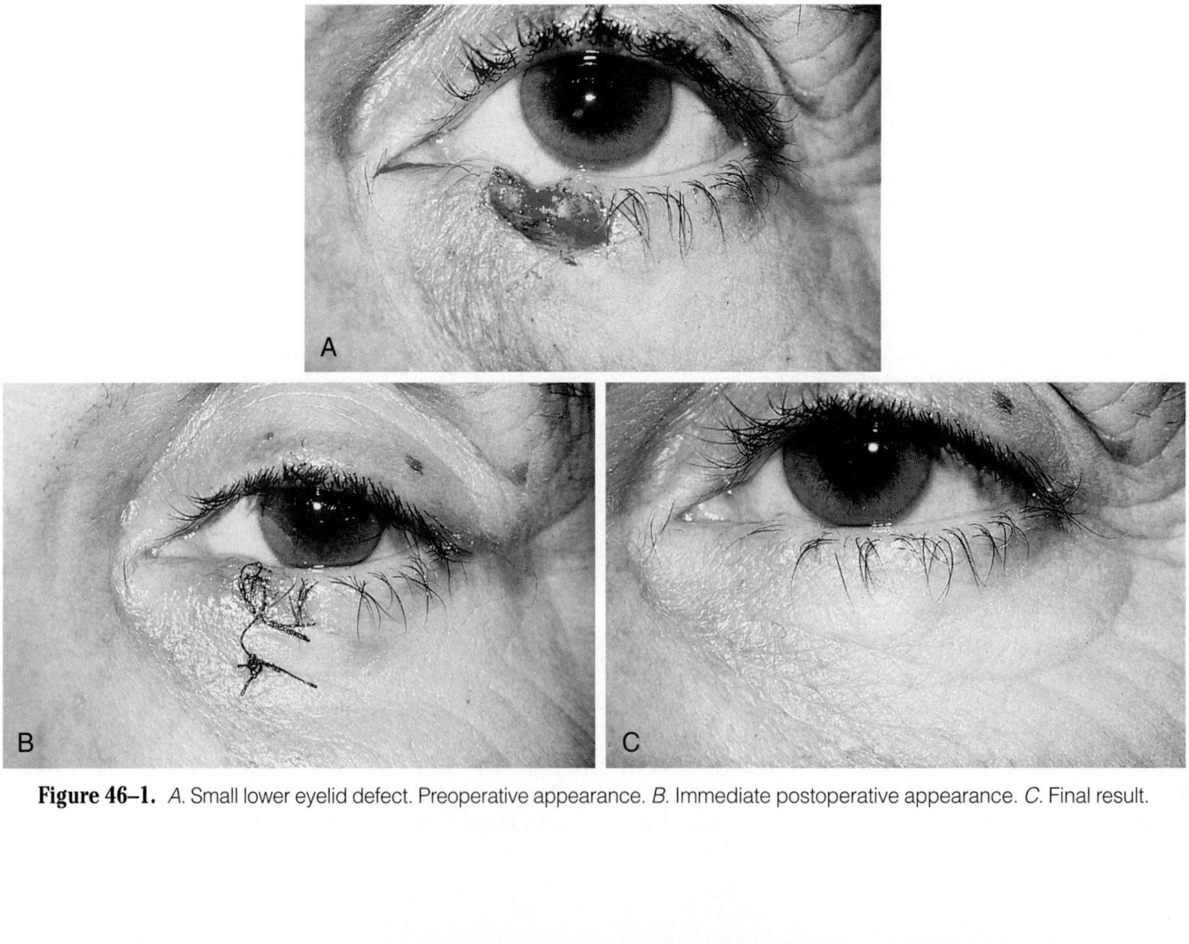

Figure 46–1. *A.* Small lower eyelid defect. Preoperative appearance. *B.* Immediate postoperative appearance. *C.* Final result.

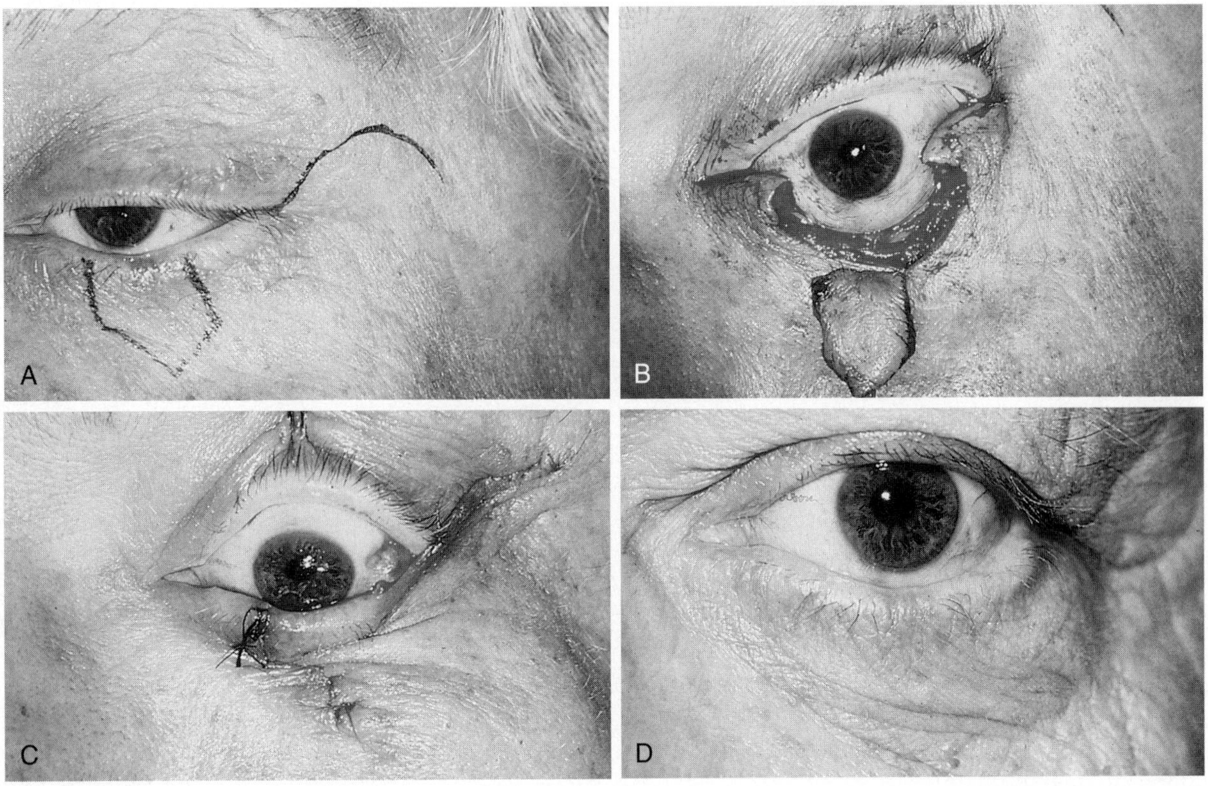

Figure 46–2. *A.* A pentagonal wedge is outlined around a lower eyelid malignant lesion. The semicircular flap is marked in the lateral canthal area. *B.* The lesion has been removed. *C.* Immediate postoperative appearance. The reconstructed eyelid will appear tight initially. *D.* Final result.

Tenzel Rotational Flap

In larger lower eyelid defects, the Tenzel rotational flap technique[4] can give excellent results. A detailed description of the technique can be found in the section of upper eyelid moderate defects (Fig. 46–2). Meticulous attention to the surgical details, especially in the lateral canthal fixation will give a highly desirable structural, functional, and aesthetic result. When the defect is getting progressively larger, further advancement of the myocutaneous flap in the lower eyelid away from the lateral orbital rim, and gravity will cause lower eyelid retraction and scleral show. In such situations, the use of a periosteal flap, hard palate mucoperichondrium, ear cartilage graft, or nasal chondromucosal graft will provide adequate posterior lamella support and is highly recommended.

LARGE DEFECT

Repair of large tissue defects (tissue loss greater than 50%) of the lower eyelid require supplemental tissue from adjacent regions. Reconstruction should be thoughtful and include separately the posterior and anterior lamella of the lower eyelid in order to achieve the best possible structure, function, and cosmesis of the reconstructed eyelid.

Modified Hughes Tarsoconjunctival Flap

For large lower eyelid defects (that can involve almost the total lower eyelid), the modified Hughes technique[9–11] can be the procedure of choice. This is particularly true for large, centrally located lower eyelid defects with sparing of the eyelid margins medially and laterally. This method produces a dynamic, movable lower eyelid, it has withstood the test of time, and it is one of the most favored procedures by eyelid reconstructive surgeons.[2] This two-staged procedure involves the advancement of a tarsal–conjunctival flap from the upper eyelid to reconstruct the posterior lamella of a large lower eyelid defect. A full-thickness skin graft can provide the anterior lamella of the reconstructed lower eyelid segment. The disadvantage of this procedure is that the eye is kept closed for several weeks until viability of the flap is ensured. This can be a significant problem in monocular patients or in young children, where amblyopia is a serious consideration.

Technique (Fig. 46–3)

After the tumor has been removed, a large, central defect in the lower eyelid is created. The upper eyelid is everted over a Desmarres retractor. A horizontal incision is made 4 mm from the upper eyelid margin. The length is approximately the same as the size of the

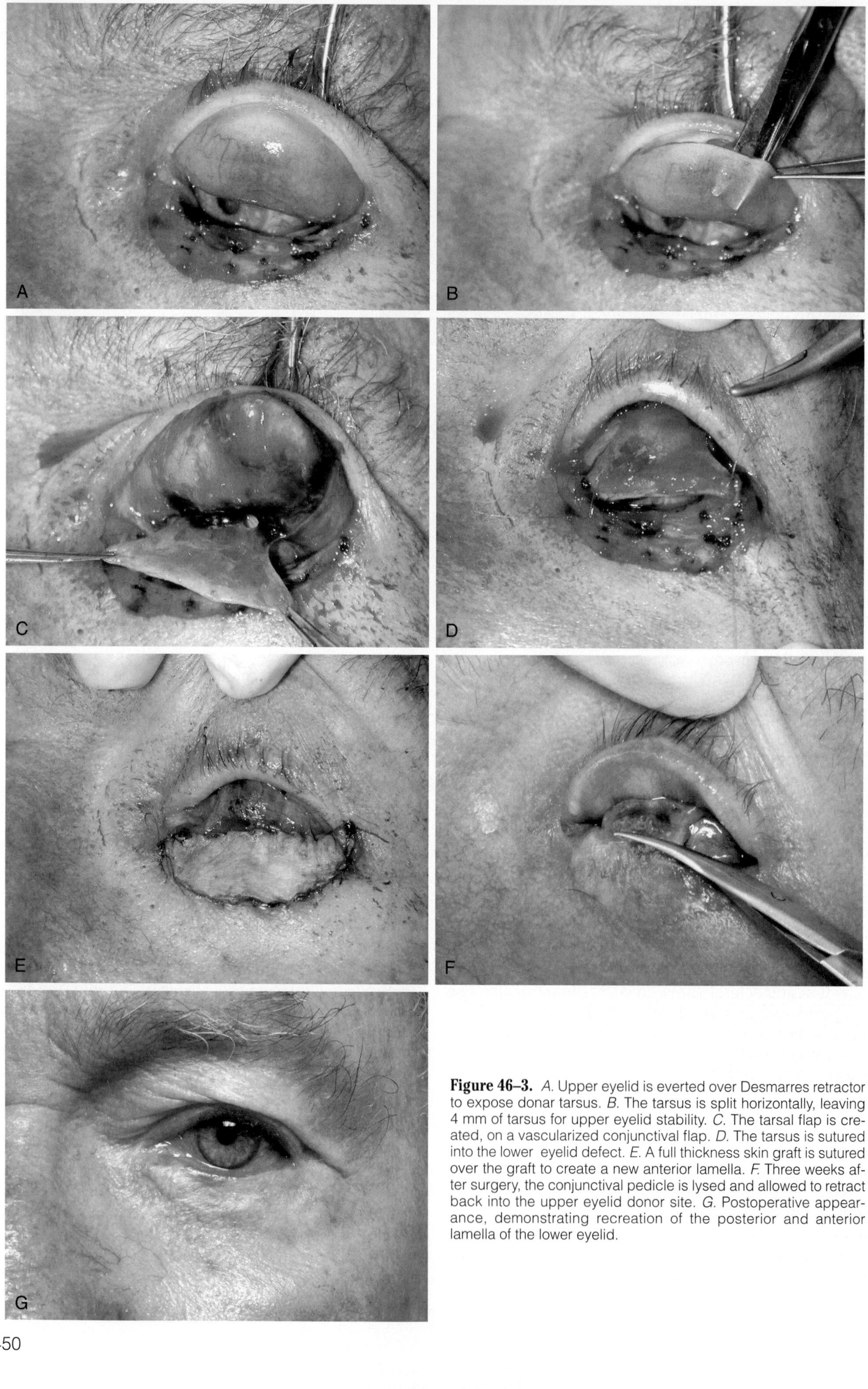

Figure 46–3. *A.* Upper eyelid is everted over Desmarres retractor to expose donar tarsus. *B.* The tarsus is split horizontally, leaving 4 mm of tarsus for upper eyelid stability. *C.* The tarsal flap is created, on a vascularized conjunctival flap. *D.* The tarsus is sutured into the lower eyelid defect. *E.* A full thickness skin graft is sutured over the graft to create a new anterior lamella. *F.* Three weeks after surgery, the conjunctival pedicle is lysed and allowed to retract back into the upper eyelid donor site. *G.* Postoperative appearance, demonstrating recreation of the posterior and anterior lamella of the lower eyelid.

lower eyelid defect when it is kept under stretch. It is important to leave at least 4 mm of tarsus in the upper eyelid to prevent the occurrence of postoperative upper eyelid deformities from the creation of an unstable upper eyelid.

The dissection is then continued in the pretarsal plane until the superior tarsal border is reached and then between Müller's muscle and conjunctiva. Some surgeons prefer to include Müller's muscle in the flap to allow greater vascularization of the flap in marginal cases. However, postoperative eyelid contour and height problems may be encountered if Müller's muscle is included in the flap. Each surgeon should exercise judgment on this. The dissection can be continued all the way to the superior fornix until the tarsoconjunctival flap can be rotated into the lower eyelid defect without any tension. Meticulous dissection is needed to achieve this and to prevent postoperative complications of the upper eyelid contour.

In the lower eyelid the conjunctiva is separated from the lower eyelid retractors to avoid placing vertical traction on the graft. The flap is then sutured to the edge of the lower eyelid tarsus with partial-thickness tarsal bites. If no lower eyelid tarsus is available at the margins of the defect, then the tarsoconjunctival flap is attached to the medial canthal remnants or to the periosteum of the posterior lacrimal crest medially and to the periosteum overlying Whitnall's tubercle inside the lateral orbital rim laterally. The inferior margin of the flap is sutured to the remaining conjunctiva below with a 6-0 absorbable suture (such as plain gut or mild chromic).

Next, the anterior lamella is reconstructed with a full-thickness skin graft taken from the contralateral eyelid or from the postauricular area. A light pressure dressing is placed over the graft for 5 days until the time for suture removal. The eye must remain closed for 4 to 8 weeks to allow the development of adequate blood supply from the graft margin and to provide an upward pull that counteracts the natural process of eyelid retraction that occurs in the early postoperative period.[2]

In the second stage, the flap is severed close to the upper eyelid margin to prevent lower eyelid margin distortion. A grooved director is useful and provides adequate corneal protection during this step. If Müller's muscle has been advanced with the tarsus, it should be separated from its attachment to the superior tarsal border and from the advancing conjunctiva. This will prevent upper eyelid retraction from Müller's muscle advancement. Finally, the conjunctiva is draped over the lower eyelid margin and sutured to the anterior mucocutaneous junction with a 6-0 to 7-0 absorbable suture to avoid corneal irritation.

Hewes Transposition Tarsoconjunctival Flap

This is a one-stage procedure[12] that is particularly helpful in addressing large but shallow lateral lower eyelid defects. It uses the superolateral portion of the upper eyelid tarsus as an axial-based flap. The flap is brought down and sutured to the tarsus and conjunctiva in the lower eyelid defect. The transposed tarsoconjunctival flap is covered with a full-thickness skin graft from a suitable donor site, or with a myocutaneous flap that is based in the lateral canthus.

The tumor is resected from the lower eyelid and the skin–muscle transposition flap is drawn in the upper eyelid. The inferior line follows the upper lid crease. The width of the flap is determined by the extent of the defect and the amount that can be removed without causing vertical eyelid inadequacy. This flap is based at the lateral canthal area. Next, the upper eyelid is everted over a Desmarres retractor and the flap is outlined. The flap involves a 4-mm-wide strip that includes the superior tarsal border and its conjunctiva and is hinged in the lateral fornix and canthal angle. Its length corresponds to the length of the lower eyelid defect when it is kept under moderate stretch. It is a true axial flap in that the peripheral arcade at the superior tarsal edge is included. Care must be taken during the dissection to spare the arcade as it enters the base of the flap. The flap is then rotated and transposed into the lower eyelid defect. If there is too much laxity in the graft, a tuck can be taken between the lateral canthal tendon and the flap.

The flap is then lined with the remaining lower eyelid tarsal segment and sutured to it with partial-thickness lamellar bites of a 6-0 absorbable suture (such as plain or chromic). The flap is also sutured to the inferior conjunctiva with similar sutures. Finally, the flap is covered with a musculocutaneous transposition flap from the upper eyelid that is based at the lateral canthal angle or with a full-thickness skin graft from a suitable donor site.

Mustardé Rotational Cheek Flap

The Mustardé flap[13] is a large rotational musculocutaneous cheek flap that can, if necessary, be relied on to cover virtually any lower eyelid defect. It may be considered a progression in size from the smaller Tenzel semicircular rotational flap. It is most useful for large, deep, medial, full-thickness lower eyelid defects and is performed in one stage. It should be considered in individuals where the lid should not be closed for any period of time (such as in monocular patients, patients with severe glaucoma, or amblyopia risk in a child) or in patients that are poor candidates for repeated staged reconstructions. Posterior lamellar support is provided by a graft of hard palate mucoperichondrium, ear cartilage, or nasal chondromucosa. This procedure has significant drawbacks, which should be carefully thought through before making a decision to proceed. The reconstructed lower eyelid is adynamic, and the facial scars created are long and visible. A triangle of normal tissue in the eyelid and cheek is sacrificed. Furthermore, there is always a risk of facial palsy from inadvertent injury to the facial nerve during dissection of the flap. Cheek skin is not good replacement for eyelid skin, and it may cause significant anterior ocular surface irritation and discomfort.[14]

The semicircular flap that begins at the lateral canthal angle and extends to the tragus of the ear is outlined with a marking pen. Its superior limit should extend to the level of the eyebrow or above. This arching of the incision high above the lateral canthal tendon is helpful in preventing lower eyelid sag. A large isosceles triangle with its base along the lower eyelid margin and its medial edge along the nasolabial fold is outlined also. It measures twice the length of the lower eyelid defect.

The semicircular flap is then dissected and undermined, with care to avoid the branches of the facial nerve. Hemostasis is achieved with cautery. The posterior lamella spacer graft is then trimmed to the appropriate size and placed with the mucosal surface over the cornea. It is sutured inferiorly to the conjunctiva of the inferior fornix. The cheek flap is then rotated medially to fill the triangular defect. A suture is placed between the dermis of the cheek flap and the remnant of the medial canthal tendon or the periosteum of the posterior lacrimal crest. The posterior lamella spacer graft is then sutured to the posterior surface to the cheek flap and tied externally to prevent corneal irritation. The lateral margin of the graft is anchored to the inner surface of the periosteum of the lateral orbital rim and kept high to prevent lower eyelid sagging. Additional sutures are placed between the posterior surface of the cheek flap and the anterior surface of the lateral orbital rim to further support the lower eyelid. Finally, the skin is closed in two layers in a standard fashion. The lateral edge of the cheek flap may need excision of a triangle or a V to Y closure to avoid dog-ears.

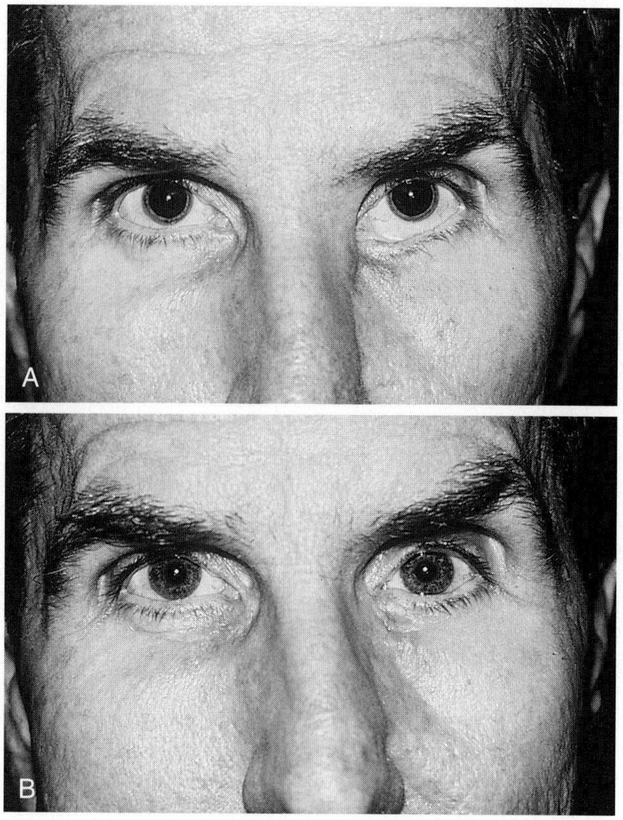

Figure 46–4. *A.* Posttraumatic medial canthal dystopia. The primary reconstruction did not address the proper fixation and reconstruction of the medial canthal tendon unit. *B.* The same patient after medial canthal reconstruction.

MEDIAL CANTHAL RECONSTRUCTION

Reconstruction involving the medial canthal area is a common procedure because this is an area that is frequently involved by eyelid malignancies. It can also be very challenging because this is an anatomically complex multicontoured area. The thick skin of the nose meets with the thin skin of the eyelid, and any reconstruction has the potential to violate this fine balance of tissues. Furthermore, from a physiologic standpoint, the complex relationships between the medial canthal tendon unit and the lacrimal sac, and between the orbicularis oculi muscle and the lacrimal crests form the basis for the proper function of the lacrimal pump and the lacrimal apparatus. These fine anatomic relationships must be preserved when reconstructing the medial canthal area (Fig. 46–4). Proper medial canthal fixation and, therefore, apposition of the eyelid to the globe is crucial for a functioning lacrimal apparatus. The four main ways to reconstruct defects that involve the medial canthal area are described in the paragraphs that follow.

"OPEN TECHNIQUE" OF HEALING: NATURAL GRANULATION

Small medial canthal defects can be left to heal by natural granulation. This can be a useful alternative for patients who are poor surgical candidates who would not be able to withstand surgery. Sometimes, a very aesthetic and functionally pleasing result may be accomplished with this method, as it tends to leave a normal concavity and contour to the medial canthal area. Moreover, tumor recurrences in this area are identified more readily as myocutaneous flaps and skin grafts can hide the early tissue changes that signify malignancy. The disadvantage is the obvious lengthy healing phase that requires meticulous wound care with daily dressing changes until granulation tissue develops.

FREE FULL-THICKNESS SKIN GRAFT

A full-thickness skin graft taken from a suitable donor site (commonly from the postauricular area) can be used to repair medial canthal area defects (Fig. 46–5). It is important to emphasize that before such a skin graft is used, all margins of the excised tissues must be free of residual tumor because unsuspected residual tumor covered with a skin graft can extend insidiously into the orbit.

Technique (Fig. 46–5)

A full-thickness skin graft is harvested in the standard fashion from a suitable donor site. The graft is placed

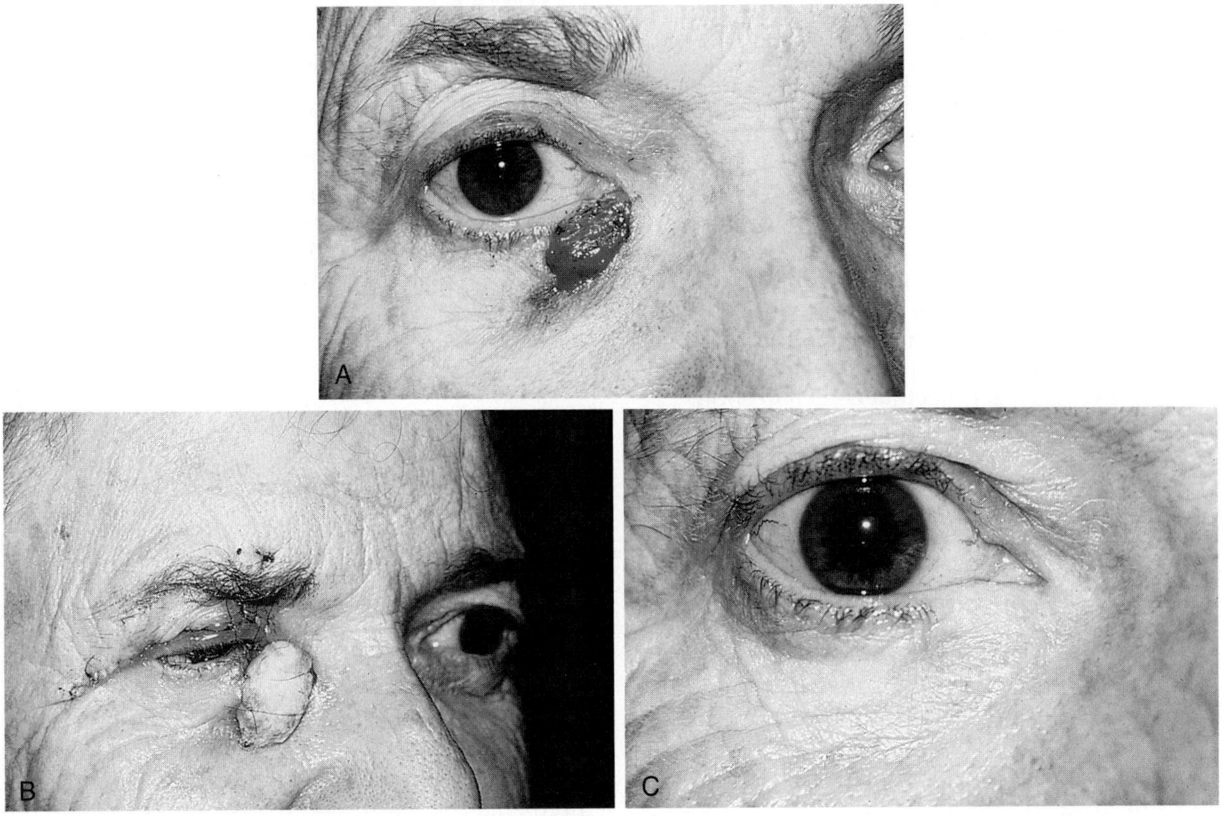

Figure 46–5. *A.* Shallow lower eyelid and a medial canthal defect that is ideal for reconstruction with a full-thickness skin graft. *B.* Immediate postoperative appearance. A pressure bolster has been applied over the graft. *C.* Final result.

over the defect and trimmed to the appropriate size. It is then sutured meticulously with several interrupted 6-0 sutures with the ends left long. It is important to achieve hemostasis in the bed of the graft because a hematoma may cause graft necrosis and sloughing.

A pressure bolster made from a cotton roll and soaked in antibiotic ointment is placed and tied over the graft with the long 6-0 silk sutures. The patient is asked to avoid any manipulation of the grafted area. The bolster and all the sutures are removed in 5 to 7 days. It is important to realize that if the resulting defect in the medial canthal area involves the medial canthal tendon, proper medial canthal fixation to the periosteum of the posterior lacrimal crest should be done prior to the coverage of the defect with a skin graft to prevent medial canthal dystopia and ectropion.

GLABELLAR FOREHEAD FLAP

This is a rotational myocutaneous flap that incorporates a V to Y advancement in the glabellar region.[15,16] It is the time-honored method of reconstruction in this area but unfortunately it can have significant disadvantages. The reconstructed area appears thickened, and the lines of incision are placed in a rather obvious place. Furthermore, some distortion in the medial end of the eyebrows and of the interbrow distance can develop from the closure of the donor defect.

The lesion is resected and the flap is designed with a marking pen. From the point of excision, an oblique line is drawn through the medial canthus to a point 2 to 3 cm above the eyebrows in the midline. Another line is drawn from this point toward the opposite medial canthus and stops just below the opposite eyebrow. The incisions are done next, and the flap is raised at the level just above the glabellar musculature. The movement of the flap is part rotational and part transpositional. It is sutured with 5-0 silk into the medial canthal defect. The donor defect is closed in a standard two-layer fashion with 5-0 Vicryl and 5-0 silk or Prolene sutures.

FINGER FLAP

This is a midline transposition flap that can be very helpful in reconstructing medial canthal defects. It has a simple design and allows transfer of non-hair-bearing thin skin to the medial canthal area.[16]

After excision of the medial canthal lesion, the flap is outlined with a marking pen. Its width should correspond to the size of the defect. The flap is then lifted from the deep tissues and transposed to the defect. If it has any skin excess it will be exhibited in the inferior rotation area and trimmed without difficulty. Finally, the flap is sutured in a standard two-layer fashion.

LATERAL CANTHAL RECONSTRUCTION

Isolated lateral canthal defects do not occur frequently. When they do occur, however, they pose a challenging reconstructive problem because of the lack of a suitable local flap donor site that shares the same skin quality characteristics with the lateral canthus and the eyelids.[17] If the created defect does not expose bare bone, a proper lateral canthal fixation to reestablish the lateral canthal position vertically and horizontally and a full-thickness skin graft is probably the best reconstructive option. If, however, bare bone is exposed, a local myocutaneous flap should be utilized. The latter option has inherent disadvantages. The local anatomy can be distorted as tension is placed to the eyebrow and the eyelid. Furthermore, as mentioned, the skin quality and texture of the flap donor site is different and also the additional incision lines characteristic of flap reconstruction are rather obvious.

PERIOSTEAL FLAP WITH LATERAL FOREHEAD TRANSPOSITION FLAP

In this technique,[1] periosteal flaps are used as posterior lamella substitutes at the lateral upper and lower eyelid. They are covered with a lateral forehead transposition flap. Unfortunately, the thick quality of the forehead skin produces a very obvious and bulky reconstruction. If the donor site is closed directly, eyebrow position and shape is distorted.[17] If it is grafted, the skin graft, placed in an obvious place, will cause a definite cosmetic defect.

The tumor is removed and the created defect involves both of the lateral aspects of the upper and lower eyelids. A vertical flap is drawn, starting in the lateral aspect of the defect and carried upward, just lateral to and above the eyebrow. The periosteum overlying the lateral orbital rim and the adjacent deep temporal fascia are exposed. Two parallel incisions 1.5 cm apart are made, starting at the medial aspect of the lateral orbital rim and extending into the deep temporal fascia. The two incisions are joined with a vertical connecting incision laterally over the temporalis fascia. The flap is raised and is hinged medially.

The rotated flap is then divided horizontally. The two resulting flaps are crossed and sutured to the posterior lamella of the remaining upper and lower eyelids with a 6-0 Vicryl suture, establishing the normal tension of the eyelids and a good lid-to-globe apposition.

The lateral forehead flap, which includes subcutaneous tissue, is raised and transposed into the defect. The flap is split at the end to allow formation of the lateral canthal angle and to cover the periosteal flaps. The donor area can be closed primarily, or a full-thickness skin graft can be used to cover the area. Either alternative has potential pitfalls, as primary closure will result in eyebrow distortion, whereas grafting will create a cosmetic defect in a rather obvious area of the face.

CONGENITAL EPICANTHAL FOLDS

Traditionally, congenital epicanthal folds have been classified as four entities: epicanthus inversus, tarsalis, palpebralis, and supracilliaris.[18] Epicanthus inversus is the commonest form and involves a fold that arises in the lower eyelid and extends upward, partially covering the medial canthus. These folds can range in severity and can also be accompanied by other congenital periorbital abnormalities, such as ptosis, phimosis, and telecanthus.

A Y TO V OPERATION

A Y to V advancement flap can be effective in correcting epicanthus.[1]

A horizontally oriented Y is drawn over the medial canthal angle area. Each arm is approximately 10 mm long and runs parallel to the eyelid margin. The point of intersection is 5 mm from the canthal angle. The base of the stem should be at the desired new position of the canthus, which is determined by pinching the skin together over the nasal dorsum.

The skin is undermined adjacent to the horizontal incision to allow movement of the canthal angle in a nasal direction. The medial canthal tendon can be exposed and tucked with a suture, if necessary. A purchase of periosteum will augment this tuck and advance the canthus farther toward the midline. The incision is closed as a "V" in a standard two-layer fashion.

MUSTARDÉ TECHNIQUE

The Mustardé technique[19] is effective and has withstood the test of time, but it is more complicated to perform than the Y to V operation. It eradicates epicanthal folds by breaking up the right vertical line in the fold. The excess skin on either side of the fold is thus utilized to make up for the shortness in the vertical line. If telecanthus is present it can be corrected with a medial canthal tendon tuck or with transnasal wiring, depending on its magnitude.

The site of the desired canthus (point X) is marked. Point Y represents the current location of the canthus, and the two points are joined. This line is measured, giving the basis for the other lines, which are all drawn 1 to 2 mm smaller. Another line is drawn from the midpoint of the X-Y line, angled 60 degrees inferiorly toward the eye. At the end of these two lines, additional lines are drawn at a 45 degree angle back toward the nose. From point Y, two additional lines are drawn parallel and 2 mm away from the eyelid margins. The incisions are made and the flaps are raised and separated from one another. The medial canthal tendon is exposed and can be tucked, if necessary. In severe forms of telecanthus, transnasal wiring can be performed. The flaps are then transposed and trimmed appropriately to fit into place. Finally, the flaps are sutured with 6-0 sutures. The obvious postoperative scarring fades within a year.

FULL-THICKNESS DEFECTS OF THE UPPER EYELID

SMALL DEFECT

Direct Closure

If the loss of tissue in the upper eyelid is small (up to 20% to 30%), the repair can generally be closed primarily. However, it is often necessary to "freshen-up" the resected margins prior to reconstruction. Excision should extend in a perpendicular fashion from the eyelid margin to the tarsal border to allow even wound closure and to avoid buckling of the eyelid or a lid notch.[3] This type of repair by direct closure requires meticulous eyelid approximation.

The repair begins with the placement of a 6-0 suture in the plane of the meibomian glands at the eyelid margin approximately 2 mm from the wound edges, and 2 mm deep. Historically, these margin sutures are nonabsorbable. However, we have routinely used absorbable sutures (such as 6-0 Dexon; Davis Geck) without experiencing complications from premature suture absorption. This option can be particularly useful in children.

The initial traction suture is pulled to determine whether satisfactory approximation of the margin edges has been accomplished. A good margin eversion should be the goal. This suture is left long and untied to facilitate repair of the tarsal segments.

The tarsus is then closed with fine interrupted partial-thickness sutures such as 6-0 or 7-0 Dexon or silk. The knots are tied on the anterior tarsal surface to avoid corneal irritation. Additional margin sutures are then placed, usually in the posterior eyelash line and in the gray line. These sutures are tied and left long. The anterior lamella of the eyelid is next closed with fine interrupted sutures, and the margin sutures are tied through these sutures to prevent the suture ends from abrading the cornea. When nonabsorbable sutures are used, they are removed in approximately 2 weeks.

MODERATE DEFECT

Direct Closure with Canthotomy and Cantholysis

In situations when tissue loss is in the low moderate range (between 30% and 50%), canthotomy and cantholysis of the inferior crus of the lateral canthal tendon can provide additional tissue in the lower eyelid to allow adequate closure. This technique can be important in situations where eyelid laxity and lateral canthal laxity is present. When the eyelid is rigid, the contribution of the cantholysis, may not be clinically significant.

A horizontal incision is made through the lateral canthus for 1 to 1.5 cm to the lateral orbital rim. The lower arm of the lateral canthal tendon is then identified, and the structures that lie anterior (skin) and posterior (conjunctiva) are dissected away from the tendon before the tendon is cut. An immediate release of the lower eyelid can be felt and when all attachments of the lateral retinaculum are cut; maximum relaxation of the lower eyelid is noted.

The closure is done as described for direct closure (see Fig. 46–1 for details). The canthal incision is closed in two layers.

Tenzel Rotational Flap

A very useful technique,[4] the Tenzel rotational flap can be very effective for the reconstruction of moderate upper eyelid defects of approximately 30% to 40% (Fig. 46–1). It is usually the first option when the defect is felt to be too large to be addressed with canthotomy and cantholysis.

An inferior arching semicircular line is drawn with a diameter of approximately 20 mm that follows the natural downward curve of the upper eyelid laterally. The semicircular musculocutaneous flap is then elevated and undermined. The superior crus of the lateral canthal tendon is cut and the upper eyelid is advanced medially. The semicircular flap is also advanced medially. The medial edge of the flap is approximated to the edge of the defect and closed in the standard fashion (see Fig. 46–1).

Lateral canthal fixation is accomplished by suturing the flap to the periosteum inside the lateral orbital rim over Whitnall's tubercle. This step allows the upper eyelid to curve inward and follow the contour of the globe. Conjunctiva can be dissected and advanced to cover the posterior surface of the flap to complete the reconstruction and prevent symblepharon formation. Final closure is done in a standard two-layer fashion.

Tenzel Rotational Flap with Periosteal Flap

When the upper eyelid defect is in the upper range of moderate (approximately 40% to 50%) the Tenzel flap can be supplemented with a periosteal flap that is elevated from the lateral orbital rim and is based medially.[2,3] This periosteal flap is rotated and sutured to the lateral tarsal edge and remains hinged at the lateral orbital rim. Conjunctiva can sometimes be advanced to cover the posterior surface of the flap. The myocutaneous flap is rotated medially and covers the anterior surface of the periosteal flap.

Tenzel Rotational Flap Combined with a Posterior Lamella Spacer

When the defects are even larger (around 50%), tend to involve the lower eyelid, or if the remaining eyelid tissue is attenuated, a posterior lamella substitute needs to be provided to ensure proper structure and stability of the eyelid. Available materials include hard palate mucoperichondrium, nasal chondromucosal grafts, and ear cartilage grafts.[3] Alloplastic materials have also been used with variable success. Initially the eyelid may appear tense, but it will gradually relax over time.

Horizontal Sliding Tarsoconjunctival Flap Combined with a Full-Thickness Skin Graft or Cutaneous Flap

This is another useful technique to address moderate to large (30% to 50%) upper eyelid defects when the previously described procedures are not considered appropriate.[2] A tarsoconjunctival flap is harvested in the upper eyelid and rotated to provide adequate posterior lamellar support in the newly reconstructed portion of the upper eyelid. The anterior lamella is reconstructed with a full-thickness skin graft from the opposite eyelid, from the retroauricular area, or from an advancement cutaneous flap if excess skin is present in the periorbital area.

For repair of a lateral upper eyelid defect, the upper eyelid is everted over a Desmarres retractor and a tarsoconjunctival graft is prepared to fill the defect. A horizontal incision is made in the tarsus approximately 4 mm above the eyelid margin. This is done to maintain the stability of the donor site in the upper eyelid and to prevent postoperative entropion or ectropion. The horizontal width of the flap is determined by the size of the defect when the lid is placed under moderate stretch. This will allow appropriate tension in the final closure to prevent excessive postoperative lid laxity and dystopia. The vertical portions of the flap are constructed up to the superior tarsal border. It is important to dissect the tarsoconjunctival graft free from the underlying Müller's muscle to avoid postoperative retraction or tethering of the upper eyelid from Müller's muscle contraction.

The graft is then rotated and sutured in place. One edge is attached to the lateral canthal tendon remnants or to the periosteum inside the lateral orbital rim. The outer edge is attached to the levator aponeurosis in the upper eyelid, with sutures placed partial-thickness through the tarsus and the tarsoconjunctival graft to avoid postoperative corneal irritation and keratopathy. A full-thickness skin graft can be placed over the graft and sutured carefully to the newly created upper eyelid margin. If an adequate amount of skin is present, an advancement cutaneous flap can provide efficient anterior lamella support in the defect.

LARGE DEFECT

When reconstructing large upper eyelid defects, the surgeon must appreciate the effects of both horizontal and vertical tension on the final result. Excessive horizontal tension on the upper eyelid will cause tether ptosis. Excessive vertical tension will cause lagophthalmos. Care must be taken to avoid these postoperative complications. There are multiple surgical modalities available to address full-thickness tissue loss greater than 50% of the upper eyelid, all of them sharing the principles of replacing both the posterior and the anterior lamella structures.

Cutler-Beard Bridge Flap

A Cutler-Beard bridge flap reconstruction[5,6] is useful for large full-thickness upper eyelid defects covering up to 100% of the eyelid margin. This technique borrows tissues from the lower eyelid to reconstruct the upper eyelid. In the original procedure[5] a full-thickness segment of the lower eyelid is advanced under a bridge of lower eyelid margin into the upper eyelid defect. Because this flap contains little or no tarsus, however, the flap can be modified from the original Cutler-Beard procedure by inserting a posterior lamella spacer (such as hard palate mucoperichondrium or ear cartilage graft) under the skin muscle flap. This creates a more stable upper eyelid. It is a two-step procedure and the eye is, unfortunately, occluded for 6 to 12 weeks. It does not replace lost eyelashes of the upper eyelid and is also fraught with the need for secondary corrective procedures.

The tumor is removed from the upper eyelid and a large defect is created. In the lower eyelid a horizontal line is drawn 4 to 5 mm below the eyelid margin with a length equal to the stretched upper eyelid defect. Keeping this distance from the margin helps preserve the vascular supply to prevent necrosis of the remaining bridge of the lower eyelid margin. Unfortunately, very little (if any) tarsus is present in the lower lid at such a distance below the lid margin. Vertical lines are drawn from each end of the horizontal line to the inferior orbital rim and are angled outward to achieve greater flap length.

A full-thickness incision is carried in this lower lid flap. This can be done by making a separate incision on the skin and tarsal surfaces and connecting them, to avoid a miscut and compromise of the marginal artery of the lower lid. The flap is then advanced under the lower lid margin to the rectangular-shaped upper lid defect. If more advancement is necessary, the outward angulated incisions are extended to achieve further release of the flap. The tarsoconjunctival portion of the flap is sutured to the remaining tarsus and conjunctiva with a 6-0 absorbable suture.

When further stability of the reconstructed portion of the upper lid is necessary, hard palate, ear cartilage, or alloplastic material (Gortex) can be trimmed to the appropriate size and sutured to the tarsal remnant medially and laterally with 7-0 suture.

The musculocutaneous portion of the flap is sutured in the defect with 7-0 sutures, and the raw inferior lower lid surface is left open.

Postoperatively, when the adequate time has elapsed—usually takes 6 to 12 weeks—and there is not a great deal of vertical tension on the flap, it may be released. During this time the raw surface of the lower lid margin epithelializes. At this stage, the flap is separated, with a bit more conjunctiva left inferiorly, in order to rotate it and cover the raw upper lid margin, thereby keeping the keratinized skin from irritating the anterior ocular surface. Final closure is then accomplished.

Mustardé Lid-Switch Technique

Another very useful technique[7] for the reconstruction of large upper lid defects is Mustardé's lid-switch. It can be especially helpful in patients with broad shallow defects of the upper lid that resist reconstruction by conventional methods. It is a two-staged procedure

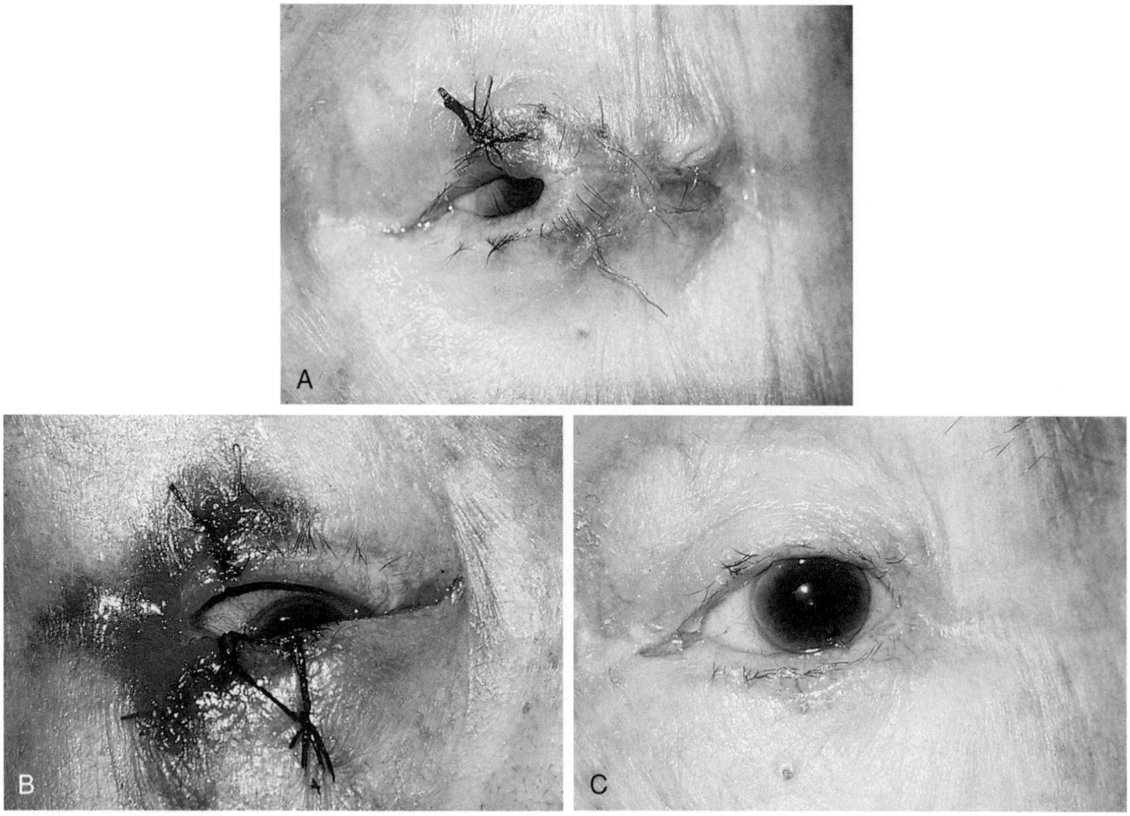

Figure 46–6. *A.* A Mustardé pedicle from the lower eyelid has been rotated to reconstruct a broad, shallow upper eyelid defect. *B.* Immediate appearance following the second stage. The flap has been separated and the lower eyelid has been reconstructed. *C.* Final result.

performed by transferring a pedicle flap from the lower lid to the upper lid (Fig. 46–2). The advantage of this flap is that eyelashes are transferred to the upper lid. As the middle portion of the lower lid has the longest eyelashes and is away from the canthal region, this is often the best donor site. This second stage, where the pedicle is separated, should be performed 4 to 6 weeks after the first stage.

Technique (Fig. 46–6)

The lower lid pedicle, which has the necessary size to close the upper lid defect, is marked. The amount of tissue that can be transferred without having to reconstruct the lower lid is 6 mm. The width of the pedicle should be at least 6 to 7 mm in height to include the marginal artery and thus ensure viability of the pedicle.[3]

Full-thickness incisions are then carried, the lower lid pedicle flap is elevated and rotated in the upper lid defect, and sutured by first placing partial-thickness tarsal sutures between the upper eyelid tarsus and the lower eyelid tarsus. Some kinking may be encountered, but good vascular supply will ensue if the marginal vascular arcade from the lower eyelid is intact. The entire pedicle flap cannot be sutured in position in the upper eyelid, but multiple interrupted sutures are used to approximate the flap to the edge, and so establish adequate blood supply to the upper eyelid. This concludes the first stage of the reconstruction. Excessive pressure patching is avoided in order to maximize the vascular supply of the flap.

In 4 to 6 weeks the second stage can be performed, which includes separation of the base of the flap from the lower eyelid, its rotation into the upper eyelid defect and, finally, reconstruction of the lower eyelid defect.

REFERENCES

1. Spaeth GL: Ophthalmic Surgery: Principles and Practice, 2nd Edition. Philadelphia: WB Saunders, 1990, pp 606–613.
2. McCord CD Jr: System of repair of full thickness lid defects. In McCord CD Jr, Tanenbaum M, Nunery WR (eds.), Oculoplastic surgery, 3rd Edition. New York: Raven, 1995:85–97.
3. Green JP, Charonis GC, Goldberg RA: Eyelid trauma and reconstruction techniques, Chapter 7.13. In Yanoff M, Duker JS (eds.), Ophthalmology. St. Lous: CV Mosby, 1998, pp 13.1-8.
4. Tenzel RR: Reconstruction of the central one half of an eyelid. Arch Ophthalmol 1975;93:125–126.
5. Cutler N, Beard C: A method for partial and total upper lid reconstruction. Am J Ophthalmol 1955;39:1–7.
6. Smith B, Obear MF: Bridge flap technique for reconstruction of large upper eyelid defects. Plast Reconstr Surg 1966;38:45–48.
7. Mustardé JC: Eyelid reconstruction. Orbit 1982;1:33–43.
8. Shorr N, Goldberg RA, Green JP: The SOOF lift in aesthetic and reconstructive surgery. Paper presented at the ASOPRS Fall Symposium, Chicago, 1996.
9. Hughes WH: Reconstruction of the lids. Am J Ophthalmol 1945;28:1203–1211.
10. Hughes WH: Total lower lid reconstruction: Technical details. Trans Am Ophthalmol Soc 1976;74:321–329.
11. Cies WA, Bowlett RE: Modification of the Mustarde and Hughes methods of reconstruction of the lower lid. Ann Ophthalmol 1967;7:1497–1501.

12. Hewes EH, Sullivan JH, Beard C: Lower eyelid reconstruction by tarsal transpositions. Am J Ophthalmol 1976;81:512–514.
13. Mustardé JC: Repair and reconstruction in the orbital region, Ch. 7 and 8. Edinburgh, Churchill Livingstone.
14. Dryden RM, Wulc AE: Reconstruction of the lower eyelid: Major defects. In Hornblass A (ed.), Oculoplastic, Orbital and Reconstructive Surgery, Vol. 1. Ch. 69. Baltimore: Williams & Wilkins, 1988:630–642.
15. Kazanjjan VH, Roopenian A: Median forehead flaps in the repair of defects of the nose and surrounding area. Trans Am Acad Ophthalmol Otolaryngol 1956;60:557–566.
16. In Jackson IT, editor, Local flaps in head and neck reconstruction. Ch 4. St. Louis; CV Mosby, 1985:91–95.
17. In Jackson IT (ed.), Local flaps in head and neck reconstruction. Ch 7. St. Louis: CV Mosby, 1985:323–325.
18. Liu D: Oriental eyelids: anatomic difference and surgical consideration. In Hornblass A (ed.), Oculoplastic, orbital and reconstructive surgery, Vol. 1, Ch. 57. Baltimore: Williams & Wilkins, 1988:513–524.
19. Mustardé JC: In Tessier P, et al.: Symposium on plastic surgery in the orbital region, Vol. 12. Ch. 12. St. Louis: CV Mosby, 1976.

CHAPTER 47

Comprehensive Ptosis Management

NICOLAS UZCATEGUI, M.D. and STEVEN C. DRESNER, M.D.

Ptosis of the upper eyelid is a condition in which the upper eyelid margin is in an abnormal inferiorly displaced position. With ptosis, the eyelid may cover a significant portion of the cornea and pupillary aperture, sometimes enough to cause visual impairment. The treatment of ptosis requires accurate evaluation, consistent measurement of the eyelid position and function, and careful documentation of the functional deficit, as well as skillful use of surgical techniques to implement a functional and aesthetic correction. This chapter describes the evaluation and measurement of ptosis, the corrections for minimal ptosis (Muellerectomy, Fasanella-Servat procedure) and levator aponeurotic repair for patients with involutional changes. Frontalis suspension and Whitnall's sling are also described for those cases of ptosis with myogenic, neurogenic, or paralytic etiology. A clinical pathway summary for management of ptosis is included (Fig. 47–1).

EVALUATION OF THE PTOSIS PATIENT

History taking is one of the most important elements in evaluating the ptosis patient. If the ptosis is congenital, the physician should question the patient or family about the absence or presence of jaw winking and family history of ptosis. With acquired ptosis, the timing of onset is of extreme importance (acute vs. progressive or chronic). A history of fatigability or variable ptosis with exercise or through the day should warrant a work-up for myasthenia gravis, especially if there is noticeable improvement with rest. Associated neurologic symptoms, if any, should also be investigated. History of orbital or ocular trauma, previous ocular histories of inflammatory disorders, or contact lens wear may also be germane.

Although there are numerous classifications for ptosis; such as congenital versus acquired; neurogenic, myogenic, traumatic and mechanical,[1] none of those classifications provides a complete approach to the ptosis patient, nor do any of them guide the clinician to the development of a system for adequate repair. Classifying ptosis as *minimal, moderate, or severe* provides a practical framework for a logical system of repair. The appropriate choice of surgical strategy can then be applied to each of these three categories.

OCULAR EXAM

In addition to documenting the patient's visual acuity and ocular motility, the importance of the pupillary function exam should not be underestimated. Anisocoria suggestive of Horner's syndrome should be fully evaluated. The presence or absence of Bell's phenomenon should be documented, as well as quantitative and qualitative properties of the tear film both by Schirmer's testing and study of tear break-up time. Slit-lamp examination should be used to assess the integrity of the cornea and the conjunctiva and to detect any inflammatory disease or subclinical pathology.

Children with ptosis should have full-dilated exams, retinoscopy, and assessment of occular motility and sensory function with either fixation preference, the 10Δ base down prism test, or a formal stereopsis test to rule out amblyopia. Careful motility examination in pediatric patients may uncover a double elevator palsy

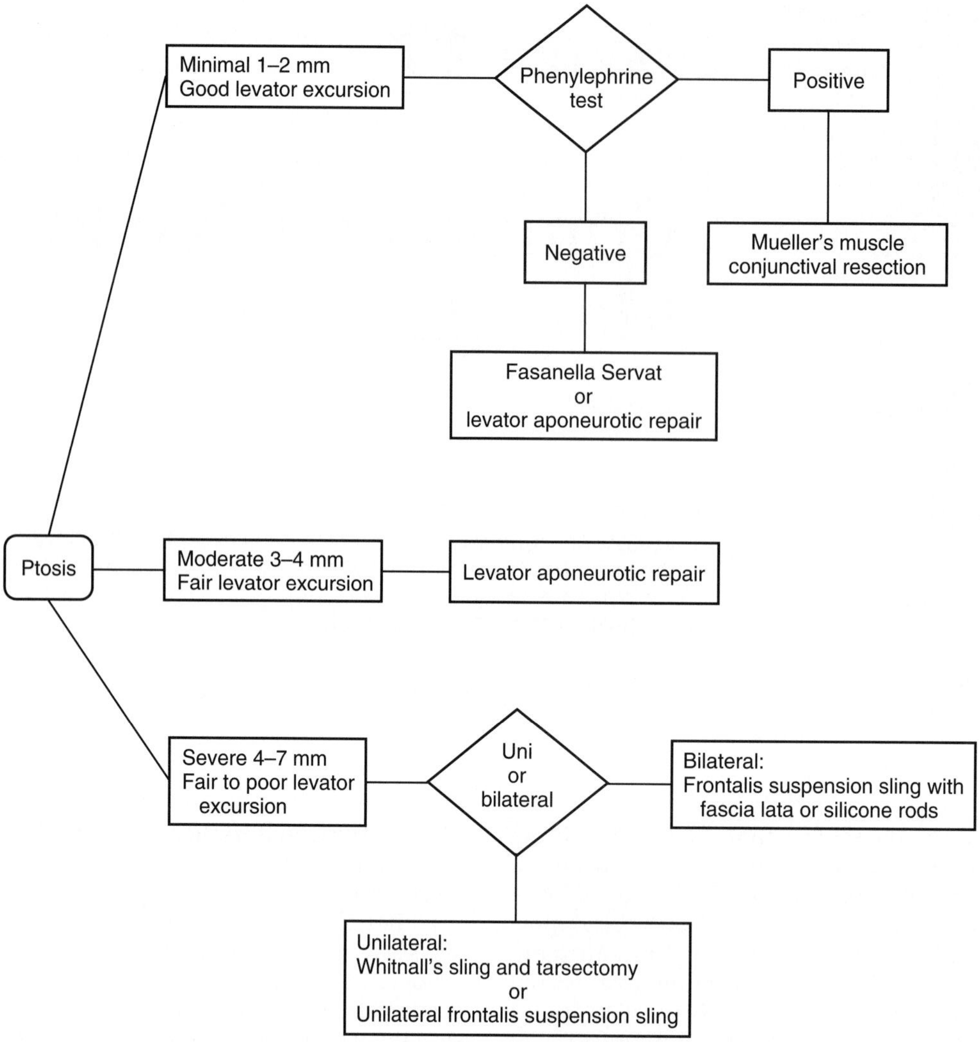

Figure 47–1. The clinical pathway in the following algorithm summarizes the surgical management of ptosis.

associated with the ptosis or partial third cranial nerve involvement causing the ptosis.

PTOSIS ASSESSMENT AND DOCUMENTATION

Ptosis is documented by the margin to reflex distance 1 (MRD_1),[2] which is the distance from the central pupillary light reflex to the upper eyelid margin, measured in millimeters. It is important to document the amount of ptosis to the nearest 0.5 mm, if possible. The margin to reflex distance 2 (MRD_2) is the distance from the central pupillary light reflex to the lower eyelid margin. The MRD_1 plus the MRD_2 should equal the palpebral fissure.

The levator excursion test is the best clinical means for assessing levator function. The levator excursion is documented in millimeters, measuring the distance from extreme upgaze to downgaze with the brow immobilized by the examiner's thumb to eliminate any contribution of the brow to lid elevation. A millimeter ruler is used vertically in the pupillary axis to assess the full excursion. Levator excursion of 10 mm or greater is considered good function; 5 to 9 mm of excursion is fair function; and 4 mm or less is poor function.

Patients with minimal ptosis (2 mm or less) should have a phenylephrine test performed in the involved eye or eyes after appropriate ptosis measurements have been documented. Either 2.5% or 10% phenylephrine is instilled in the affected eye or eyes. Usually two drops are instilled and the patient is reexamined 5 minutes later. The MRD_1 is rechecked in the affected and unaffected eyes (Fig. 47–2). A rise in the MRD_1 of 1.5 mm or greater is considered a positive phenylephrine test. This indicates that Mueller's muscle is viable, and the Mueller's muscle conjunctival resection procedure can be performed, also giving the patient a reasonable prediction of the desired result.

The contralateral eye must also be rechecked in patients with unilateral ptosis. When the ptotic eye is occluded, if the MRD_1 decreases appreciably in the opposite eye, this usually indicates that bilateral ptosis is present; this finding is consistent with Herring's law.[3] The patient may require bilateral surgery. A negative phenylephrine test precludes the use of the Mueller's muscle conjunctival resection procedure, because the outcome of the procedure is unpredictable in this setting. Callahan and Beard[1] have stated that minimal or mild ptosis is 2 mm or less, moderate ptosis is 3 to 4 mm, and severe ptosis is 4 mm or greater. Usually patients with minimal ptosis will have good levator excursion. The moderate ptosis patients usually have good to fair excursion, and typically patients with severe ptosis have poor levator excursion.

SURGICAL OPTIONS BASED ON LEVATOR FUNCTION

For patients with minimal ptosis (2 mm or less) there are three surgical options: (1) Mueller's muscle conjunctival resection, (2) the Fasanella-Servat procedure, or (3) levator aponeurotic surgery. If the phenylephrine test is positive, the Mueller's muscle conjunctival resection procedure is the most precise and predictable surgical option.[2] For many ptosis surgeons, this is the preferred approach for minimal ptosis because of its ease, predictability, and the ability to grade or titrate the correction according to the preestablished nomograms. The surgeon can also calculate, with time and personal experience, his or her own nomogram.[19] If, however, the phenylephrine test is negative, one must consider other procedures because of the unpredictability of Mueller's muscle conjunctival resection in this subset of patients. The Fasanella-Servat procedure is the next option for minimal ptosis and a negative phenylephrine test. The Fasanella-Servat procedure is nearly as predictable as Mueller's muscle conjunctival resection and equally easy to perform.[4] Because it is in a sense a tarsectomy with little Mueller's muscle resected, it is viable in the absence of a positive phenylephrine test.

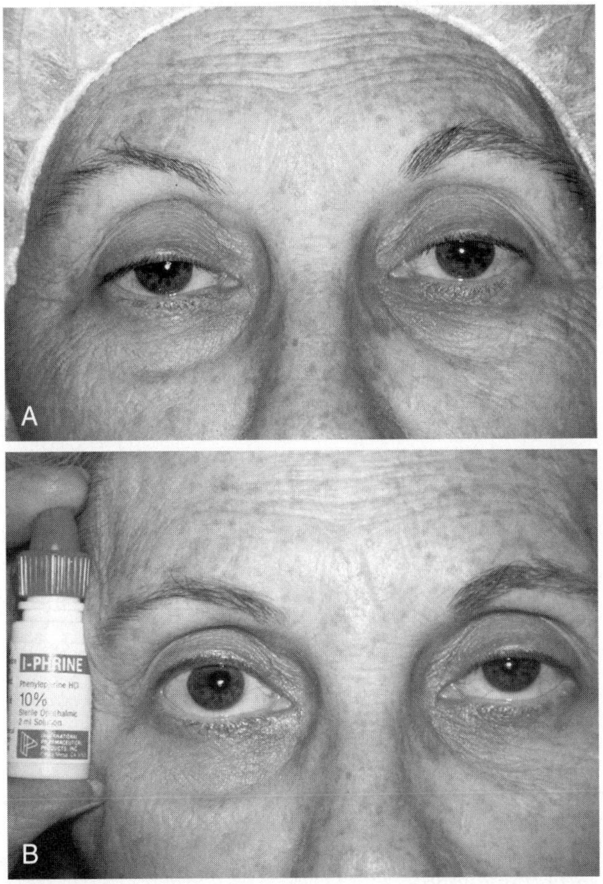

Figure 47–2. The phenylephrine test. *A.* The margin-to-reflex distance (MRD_1) is measured on both upper eyelids and repeated 5 minutes after instillation of 2.5% to 10% phenylephrine eye drops in the ptotic eye. *B.* The right upper eyelid responds to the stimulating effects of the phenylephrine and shows a reduction of the ptosis (an increase in the MRD_1).

Levator aponeurosis repair is the third option for minimal ptosis. Many surgeons prefer this technique because it allows them to set the eyelid height while the patient is on the operating table. It is particularly useful for patients who have contour abnormalities and who have ptosis that requires concomitant blepharoplasty.[3] There are, however, many variables that may affect the results, including the need for patient cooperation, the effects of sedation or local anesthetic infiltration, and the need to overcorrect the affected side or sides. It is also difficult to grade the degree of correction under general anesthesia. Indeed, many reports have suggested that predictability and success with this procedure may vary as much as 2 mm between the two affected eyelids.[6,7,20] In the setting of minimal ptosis, however, success ought to be judged to within 0.5 mm. Nonetheless, levator aponeurotic repair is useful for many minimal ptosis patients.

Levator aponeurosis repair is the treatment of choice for nearly all patients with moderate ptosis. These patients usually have good to fair levator excursion, and they usually have negative phenylephrine tests.

Patients with severe ptosis typically have poor levator excursion and require some type of frontalis suspension. Patients with unilateral congenital ptosis and levator excursion of only 4 to 5 mm are often helped with Whitnall slings or maximal levator aponeurotic advancement. This treatment can be augmented by simultaneous tarsectomy as well.

Bilateral severe ptosis patients, or patients with very poor levator excursion, need some type of frontalis suspension. Congenital severe ptosis with little levator excursion is best served with autogenous fascia lata sling grafts. Nonautogenous materials are available and can be used, if necessary; however, the long-term results are poorer than with autogenous materials.[8] Acquired severe ptosis, as seen with third nerve palsy, progressive external ophthalmoplegia, or oculopharyngeal dystrophy, is best treated by frontalis suspension sling with a silicone (Silastic) rod because of its adjustability and the possibility for subsequent removal if the cornea becomes compromised.[9]

SURGICAL METHODS

Mueller's Muscle Conjunctival Resection

Mueller's muscle conjunctival resection is reserved for patients with minimal ptosis (2 mm or less) with normal levator excursion and a positive phenylephrine test. Putterman and Urist[10] originally described this technique in 1975. Various modifications have since been described.[2,11]

Mueller's muscle is a smooth muscle that originates from the undersurface of the levator and inserts with a 0.5- to 1-mm tendon into the superior tarsal plate.[12] When denervated in Horner's syndrome, this muscle relaxes, causing 2 to 3 mm of clinical blepharoptosis. The levator aponeurosis has been shown to insert on the anterior surface of the tarsus within 7 to 8 mm of the upper tarsal border. Additional interdigitations with the intermuscular septum of the orbicularis oculi form the eyelid crease.[13] Whitnall, however, recognized Mueller's muscle as another important primary attachment or insertion of the levator. When Mueller's muscle is advanced it strengthens the posterior lamella and appears to plicate the levator aponeurosis, with healing and subsequent scarring in the posterior lamella. This plication is successful in maintaining constant elevation of the upper eyelid in the open eyelid positioning primary gaze.[2]

Surgical Technique

A frontal nerve block is unnecessary for the procedure; 1% or 2% Xylocaine is used as a regional block for the upper eyelid. Epinephrine is omitted to avoid stimulation of Mueller's muscle. Approximately 5 cc of the solution, mixed with hyaluronidase (10 cc of anesthetic is mixed with 150 units of hyaluronidase), is injected just below the superior orbital rim. Tetracaine topical anesthetic eye drops are then placed on the conjunctival surface. A 4-0 silk suture is placed through the tarsus at the eyelid margin in the pupillary axis. The eyelid is reflected over a Desmarres retractor. Marks are made at one half the distance of the total resection amount medially, centrally, and laterally, measured with a caliper, and beginning 0.5 mm above the tarsal plate. Another mark is made centrally to measure the total extent of resection desired[4] (Fig. 47–3).

Three 4-0 silk traction sutures are placed through the conjunctiva and Mueller's muscle centrally, medially, and laterally at the halfway marks. Each bite is approximately 3 mm long and deep to the underlying Mueller's muscle but should not penetrate to the levator aponeurosis or orbicularis muscle. The sutures are separated into two bundles and tied on themselves, to be used as traction sutures to elevate the required amount of conjunctiva and Mueller's muscle to be resected (Fig. 47–4).[5]

The Desmarres retractor is removed and the lid marginal suture is clamped superiorly to the head drape. The bundles of sutures are elevated, with one bundle held by the surgeon and the other by an assistant. The Mueller's muscle conjunctival resection clamp (Karl ILG Instruments, 6N601 Route 31 Saint Charles, IL 60174) is placed over the elevated tissues. The clamp is placed so that the most superior central mark is adjacent to the resection clamp.

A 6-0 plain horizontal mattress suture is placed under the clamp approximately 0.5 to 1 mm below the clamp (Fig. 47–5). The clamped tissues are excised with a no. 15 blade metal on metal (Fig. 47–6). The conjunctiva is closed with a running baseball stitch in the reverse direction of the original pass. The suture is tied on itself (Fig. 47–7). Exteriorizing the suture is not required. The eyelid is returned to its anatomic position, and the eyelid margin suture is removed. Antibiotic ointment is placed in the eye and no patch is necessary. Excellent results can be seen, with minimal ptosis ranging between 1 and 2 mm (Fig. 47–8). The advantages of this technique are that it is quick, predictable, and quantifiable. Late failures are rare. Complications include a rare superior corneal abrasion, undercorrection, or overcorrection. Usually an abrasion heals spontaneously if it is small. A bandage contact lens can also be placed if desired. Overcorrection is rare with this technique. If it occurs, the plain suture can be cut under topical anesthetic in the office, and the wound can be separated gently with a cotton swab. Undercorrection requires another procedure at a later date.

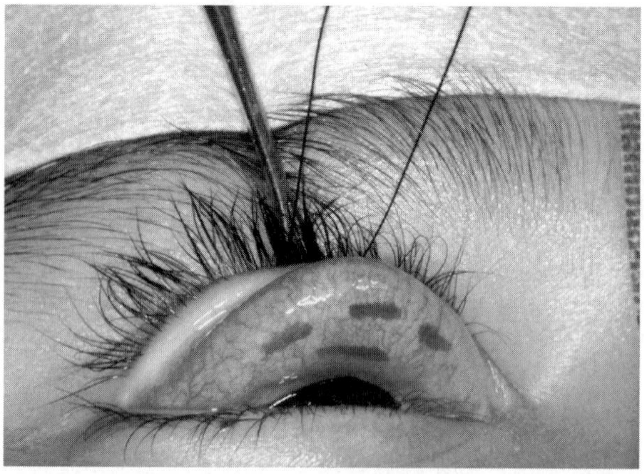

Figure 47–3. Mueller's muscle conjunctival resection. A 4-0 silk traction suture is placed through the tarsus and the eyelid is reflected over a Desmarres eyelid retractor. Marks are made medially, centrally, and laterally at one-half the distance of the total vertical amount of resection desired. A separate mark is made centrally to indicate the height of the total resection desired.

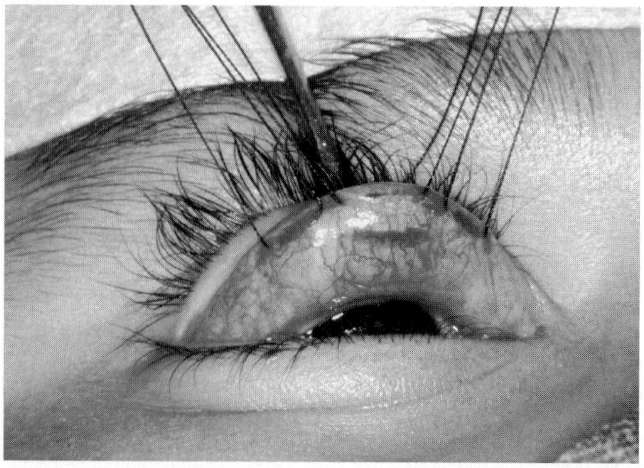

Figure 47–4. Mueller's muscle conjunctival resection. Three 4-0 silk traction sutures are placed through Mueller's muscle and conjunctiva.

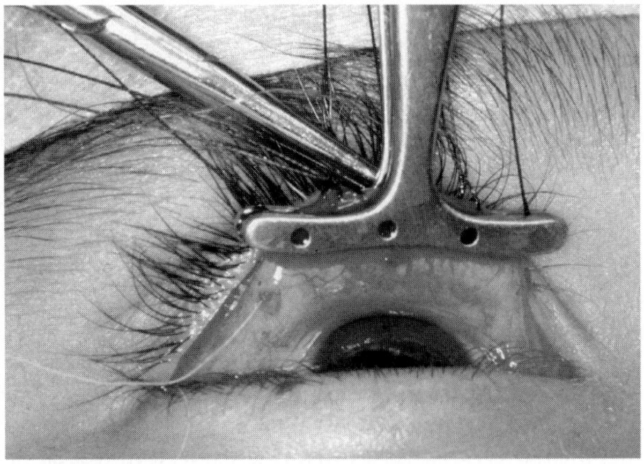

Figure 47–5. Mueller's muscle conjunctival resection. The sutures are elevated in two bundles and the clamp is placed over the tissues. A 6-0 plain catgut suture is placed underneath the clamp.

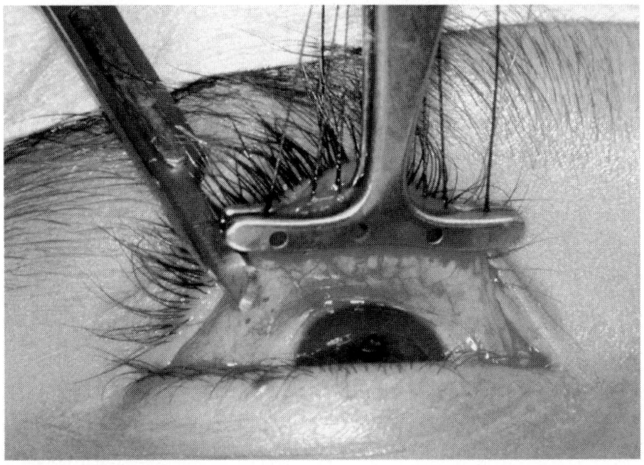

Figure 47–6. Mueller's muscle conjunctival resection. The clamped tissues are incised with a no. 15 Bard-Parker blade, along the lower edge of the clamp.

FASANELLA-SERVAT PROCEDURE

In 1961 Fasanella and Servat[13] described their tarsectomy operation for correcting small amounts of ptosis in patients with normal levator function. In 1972 Putterman developed a clamp to supplant the use of curved hemostats for the Fasanella-Servat procedure. This clamp is best known today for its use in the Mueller's muscle conjunctival resection procedure. The Fasanella-Servat procedure is well suited for minimal ptosis because patients with a positive phenylephrine test are treated with a Mueller's muscle conjunctival resection procedure, the Fasanella-Servat is reserved for patients with minimal ptosis and a negative phenylephrine test who, in general, do not require blepharoplasty.

Surgical Technique

Fasanella and Servat described performing their procedure with two curved hemostats. Placing these hemostats can be cumbersome, and misplacement can lead to postoperative contour abnormalities or central peaking. A modified Putterman clamp (Karl ILG Instruments) can be used in place of the two hemostats (Fig. 47–9). This clamp is modified with a screw closure, which assists in crushing the tarsus.

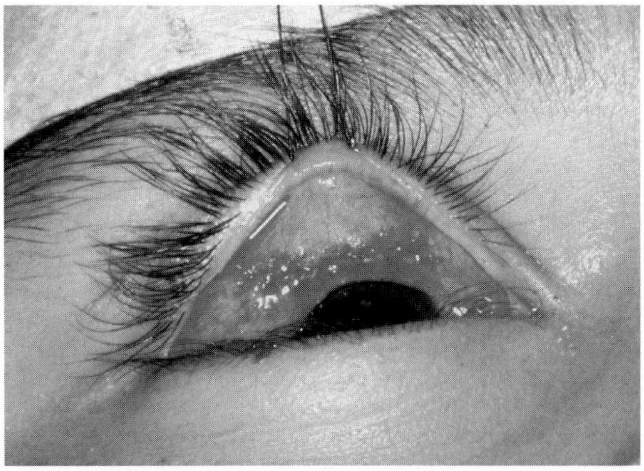

Figure 47–7. Mueller's muscle conjunctival resection. The conjunctiva is closed with the 6-0 fast absorbing plain gut suture.

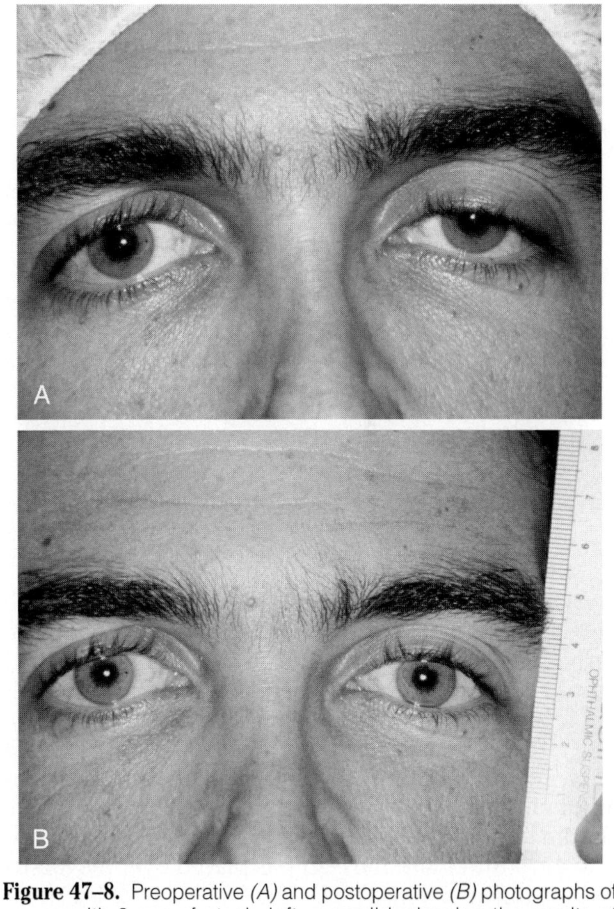

Figure 47–8. Preoperative *(A)* and postoperative *(B)* photographs of a man with 2 mm of ptosis left upper lid, showing the results of Muellerectomy.

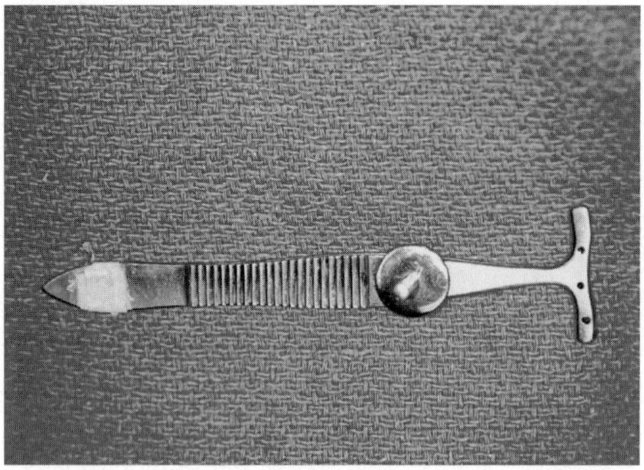

Figure 47–9. The modified Putterman clamp can be used in place of two hemostats in performing the Fasanella-Servat procedure.

Although the outcome of this procedure is not as predictable as the Mueller's muscle conjunctival resection procedure, it is nearly so, and can yield excellent results in patients who have 1 to 2 mm of ptosis (Fig. 47–13). Correction of 3 mm of ptosis is not recommended with this procedure because of the need to excise large amounts of tarsus. Complications include undercorrection, overcorrection, and the rare corneal epithelial defect. Overcorrection can usually be treated by early removal of the suture and by digital message; undercorrection will need either a full-thickness eyelid resection or a levator aponeurotic repair.

This procedure can be performed on patients with or without positive phenylephrine tests; however, patients with a positive phenylephrine test are usually better served with Mueller's muscle conjunctival resection. The advantages of this modified Fasanella-Servat technique include avoiding the need for two hemostats, the

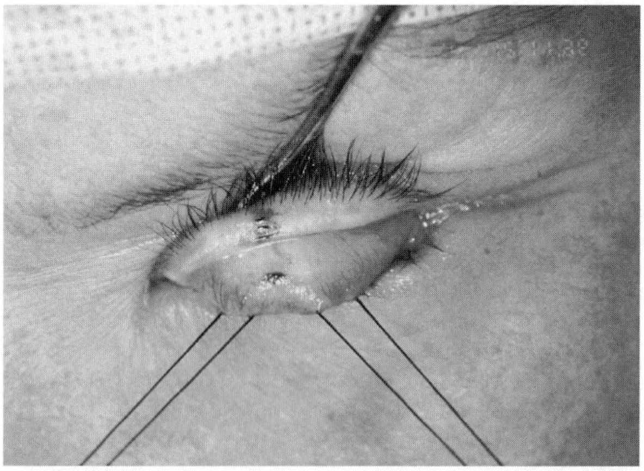

Figure 47–10. The Fasanella-Servat procedure. Two 4-0 silk traction sutures are placed through the conjunctiva toward a subcutaneous plane along the superior tarsal border medially and laterally.

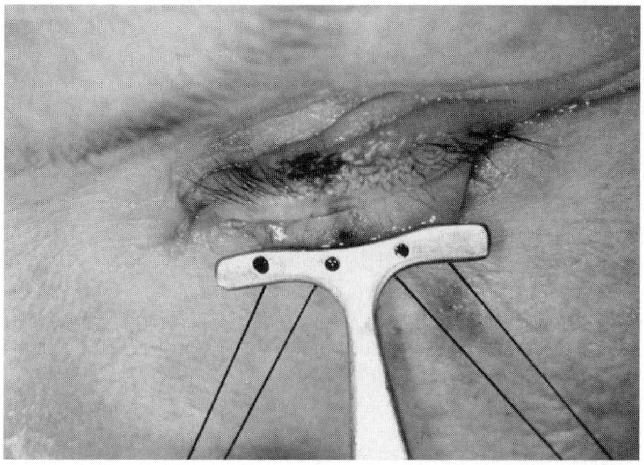

Figure 47–11. The Fasanella-Servat procedure. The tarsal resection is marked and the clamp is placed over the tissues. A 6-0 Prolene suture is placed under the damped tissues, originating externally in the pretarsal skin areas and terminating externally as well.

Anesthesia is obtained by injecting 1% Xylocaine with 1:100,000 dilution epinephrine and hyaluronidase through the superior cul-de-sac. The eyelid is everted and two 4.0 silk sutures placed through the conjunctival tarsal border medially and laterally (Fig. 47–10). The tarsus is marked centrally along the pupillary axis after the surgeon has measured the proposed resection amount. For each millimeter of ptosis, 2 mm of tarsus should be resected. The tissues are elevated via the two traction sutures and the clamp is placed over the tarsus and conjunctiva (Fig. 47–11). The screw device is turned until the tissues are firmly crushed. A 6-0 Prolene suture is placed through the anterior lamella under the clamp, then passed back and forth in horizontal mattress fashion and exteriorized through the anterior skin lamella at the other end of the clamp.[14] The clamped tissues are excised with a no. 15 Bard Parker blade (Fig. 47–12). The eyelid is reflected back in its anatomic position, and the suture is tied to itself in the pretarsal area. The suture is removed in 5 to 7 days.

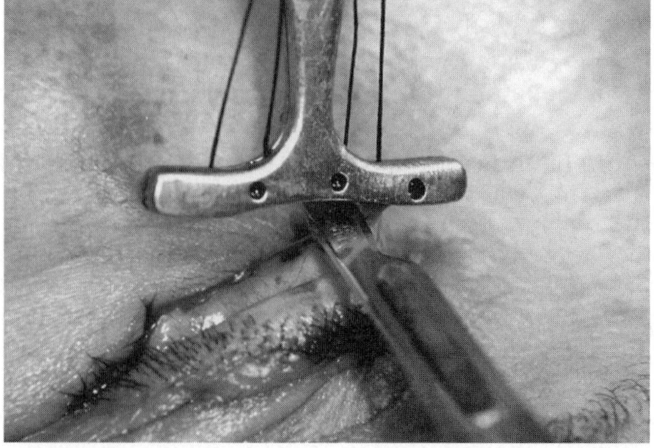

Figure 47–12. The Fasanella-Servat procedure. The clamped tarsus levator aponeurosis Mueller's muscle, and conjunctiva are excised with a no. 15 Bard-Parker blade, cutting along the lower border of the clamp. At both ends, the externalized suture is tied to itself in the pretarsal area.

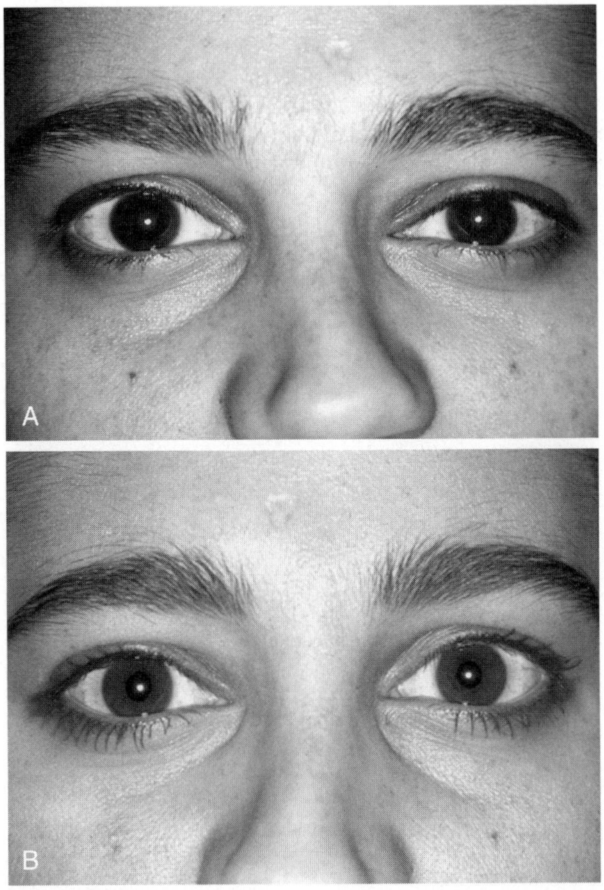

Figure 47–13. Preoperative *(A)* and postoperative *(B)* photographs of a woman with 1.5-mm ptosis, right upper lid show the result of the Fasanella-Servat procedure.

absence of contour abnormalities, and the ability to quantitate the procedure well.

LEVATOR APONEUROSIS REPAIR

Levator aponeurosis repair is useful for minimal to moderate ptosis and can be employed when Mueller's muscle conjunctival resection or Fasanella-Servat are not indicated, as in the patient with a large conjunctival filtering bleb or when concomitant blepharoplasty it desired. For moderate ptosis (3 to 4 mm), it is the procedure of choice. A maximal levator aponeurotic advancement or Whitnall sling can be employed for patients with severe unilateral ptosis; excising additional amounts of tarsus to elevate the eyelid margin can further augment it.

The levator palpebrae superioris extends from the annulus of Zinn traveling anteriorly through the superior orbit to Whitnall's ligament, which serves as a suspensory ligament for the upper eyelid (Fig. 47–14). At this point the muscle appears aponeurotic and has a whitish color. The levator aponeurosis courses downward to insert on the inferior two thirds of the anterior surface of the tarsal plate, the fibrous septi of the orbicularis and the subcutaneous tissues.[15] Anterior to the levator aponeurosis is the pre-aponeurotic fat pad and the orbital septum.

Surgical Technique

The procedure is best performed under local anesthesia with minimal intravenous sedation; small amounts of local anesthetic are used to avoid paralyzing the levator muscle. Epinephrine is recommended for adequate hemostasis. Approximately 1 to 2 cc of 1% Xylocaine with epinephrine is usually sufficient. The eyelid crease should be marked prior to local infiltration. If unilateral ptosis is to be performed, the incision is marked approximately 1 mm below the crease on the opposite eyelid. Postoperatively the crease will rise slightly. If bilateral surgery is planned, the incision can be symmetrically placed at the desired location, but placing the incision too high beyond the superior tarsal border of the upper tarsus should be avoided.

After the local anesthetic is injected into the eyelid, topical tetracaine eye drops are placed on the conjunctival surface. The patient is prepped, and protective corneal shields can be placed over the globes. The incision can be made with a no. 15 Bard-Parker blade, a Colorado needle tip (Colorado Biomedical, 6851 Highway 73 Evergreen, CO 80439) in cut mode, or a CO_2 laser set to incisional mode. A skin muscle flap is developed to expose the orbital septum. The septum is incised over the upper one third to avoid

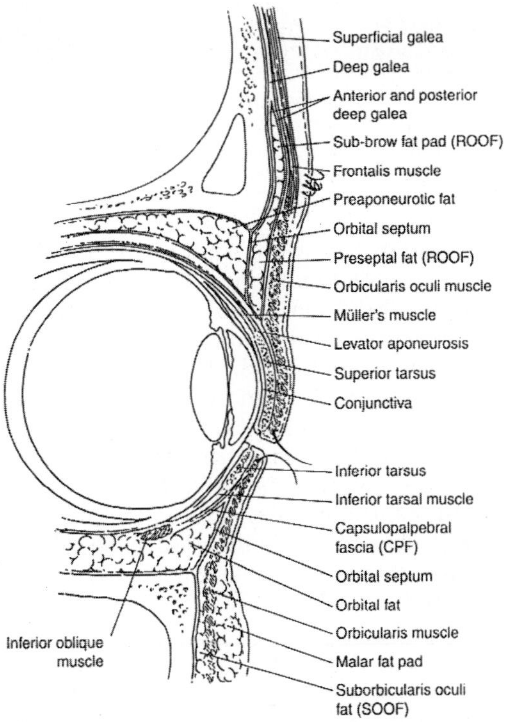

Figure 47–14. Levator aponeurosis repair. Schematic line drawing of upper lid. The levator muscle extends from the annulus of Zinn anteriorly to Whitnall's ligament, where it transitions into the levator aponeurosis. It courses downward to insert into the anterior two thirds of the tarsal plate.

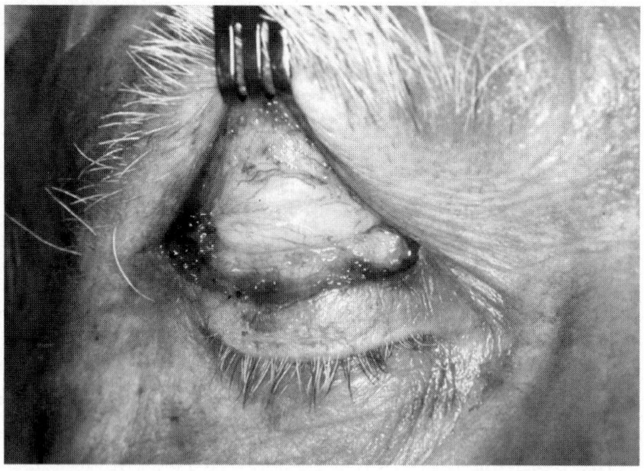

Figure 47–15. Levator aponeurosis repair. The orbital septum is transected in the upper one third.

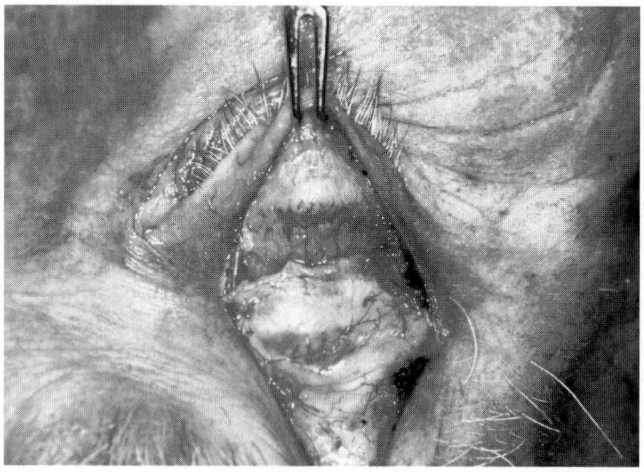

Figure 47–16. Levator aponeurosis repair. The levator is dissected off of the tarsus with a hand-held cautery.

incising or damaging the underlying levator (Fig. 47–15).[18] The preaponeurotic fat pad is reflected upward to reveal the whitish aponeurosis beneath. A high-temperature hand-held cautery is used to disinsert the aponeurosis from the tarsal plate, which separates the aponeurosis from the underlying Mueller's muscle (Fig. 47–16). Dissection is carried upward, as high as Whitnall's ligament if necessary. A double-arm 5-0 Vicryl suture is placed partial thickness through the central portion of the upper tarsus in two 3 mm bites. This suture is then taken up through the aponeurosis at the desired height (Fig. 47–17). This is temporarily tied and the level is examined. Usually sitting the patient up on the table gives a more accurate assessment. A 1-mm to 1.5-mm overcorrection is desirable because the protractors (orbicularis) are paralyzed by local anesthetic and there can be some stimulation of Mueller's muscle by the epinephrine. Additional sutures can be placed medially and laterally for contour adjustment; often, however, they are unnecessary. The excess levator aponeurosis is trimmed. A strip of skin-orbicularis flap superiorly can be excised if necessary, or bilateral blepharoplasties can be performed. The wound is then closed with a 6-0 suture of choice with supratarsal fixation on every other bite of the suture. Excellent results can be obtained with this approach (Fig. 47–18).

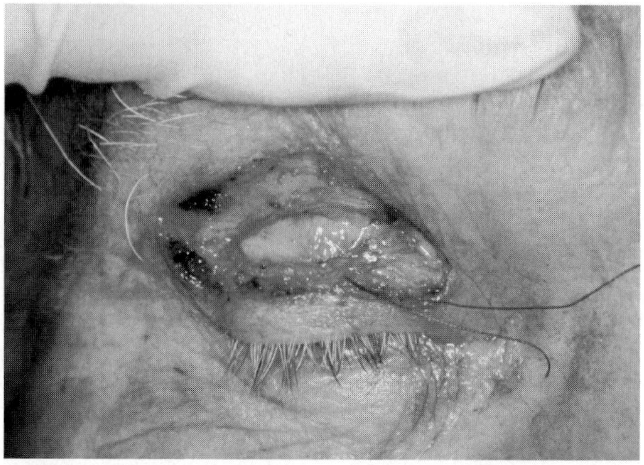

Figure 47–17. Levator aponeurosis repair. Double-armed 6-0 Vicryl sutures are placed through the central superior tarsus in two broad bites and then up through the aponeurosis and tied.

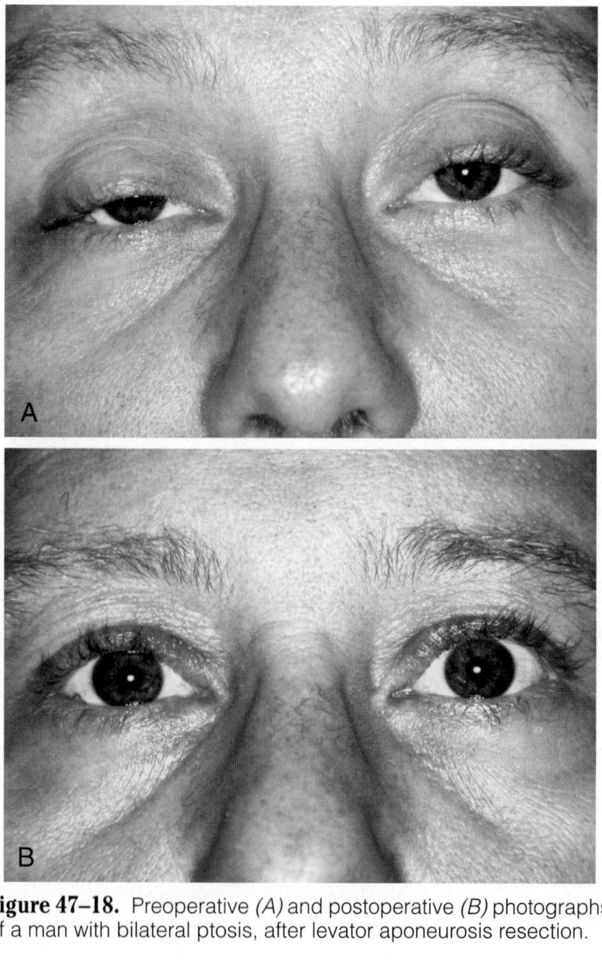

Figure 47–18. Preoperative *(A)* and postoperative *(B)* photographs of a man with bilateral ptosis, after levator aponeurosis resection.

WHITNALL SLING PROCEDURE

The Whitnall sling procedure is a *maximal levator aponeurosis advancement.* In actuality, the levator muscle's Whitnall's ligament is sewn to the superior tarsal plate, with no cutting of the medial and lateral horns of the levator and aponeurosis. This is usually employed in unilateral congenital ptosis with levator function in the 5-mm range.

Surgical Technique

Because this technique is often performed under general anesthesia, an empiric formula needs to be used to set the height of the lid margin. The gaping technique described by McCord[16] suggests that in congenital ptosis, 3 mm should be added to the amount of ptosis present; this numeric value equals the amount of gaping or lagophthalmos that will be established on the operating room table. For instance, if there is 3 mm of ptosis present, the eyes should be left open or "gaped" 6 mm on the operating table. Another formula that can be used is to subtract the levator excursion in the affected eyelid from the levator excursion on the normal side; this number is then multiplied by 1.2 to calculate the amount of levator aponeurotic advancement. For example, if one ptotic side has a levator excursion of 6 mm and the unaffected side has a levator excursion of 14 mm; the difference in levator function is 8 mm. This value of 8 mm is then multiplied by 1.2, for a total of 9.6 mm of levator advancement.

If additional elevation is required, a tarsectomy can be performed at the same time that the Whitnall's sling is being performed; up to 2 to 4 mm of tarsus can be excised at the time of surgery.[17] With this method, each millimeter of tarsus is equivalent to 2 mm of aponeurosis advancement.

Complications with aponeurosis surgery include contour abnormalities, overcorrection, undercorrection, and conjunctival prolapse, which is rare. Complications are usually best addressed 1 week into the postsurgical period.[7] With overcorrection, the wound can be opened and the aponeurosis sutures cut. The aponeurosis is then recessed slightly with cotton swabs and the eyelid level is reassessed. Undercorrections are opened and the aponeurosis advanced appropriately to the desired position, and contour abnormalities are handled in a similar fashion.

FRONTALIS SUSPENSION USING FASCIA LATA

Patients with severe ptosis and poor levator function are candidates for frontalis suspension with auto-genous fascia lata. Patients with synkinetic ptosis (Marcus-Gunn jaw-winking ptosis) may also be candidates for this procedure with or without levator extirpation. Generally, autogenous fascia lata gives more predictable and long-lasting results.[8] Eye bank preserved tissues can be utilized when the patient is younger than 3 years of age or at the family's request.

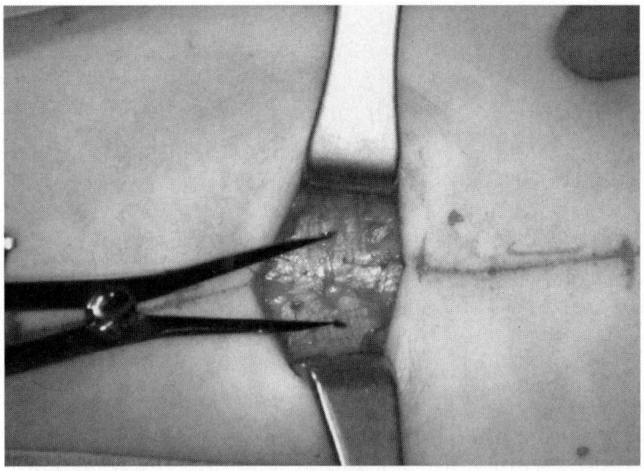

Figure 47–19. Frontalis suspension. A 3- to 4-cm incision is made at the lateral surface of the mid-thigh to obtain autogenous fascia lata.

Autogenous fascia lata is easily harvested "freehand," obviating the need for any kind of fascial strippers. An incision of approximately 3 to 4 cm is marked in the mid-thigh longitudinally, halfway between the head of the fibula and the anterior superior iliac spine (Fig. 47–19). Although this procedure is usually performed under general anesthesia, 0.5% Marcaine with 1:100,000 epinephrine is injected subcutaneously for hemostasis and postoperative analgesia. The foot is pronated slightly by a nonscrubbed assistant, or it can be taped to immobilize the leg and place the fascia lata on stretch. The incision is begun with a no. 15 Bard-Parker blade, and dissection is carried down through the subcutaneous fat to the fascia. For bilateral surgery, the harvested strip of fascia needs to be at least 6 mm in width and 8 to 10 cm in length. Two incisions are made 8 to 10 cm apart into the fascia with a no. 15 Bard-Parker blade. The fascia is exposed superiorly and inferiorly by dissecting bluntly with small "peanuts" (small gauze-wrapped cotton balls). A surgical assistant moves along the incisions with army–navy retractors to expose the field. Using long Metzenbaum scissors, the fascial strips are incised lengthwise. Each strip is transected at both ends with curved scissors or Jorgenson's scissors, and pulled out of the wound. The fascia lata is not repaired primarily. The subcutaneous tissues are closed with 4-0 or 5-0 Vicryl sutures, and the skin can be closed with a 5-0 plain gut suture.

Surgical Technique

A number of patterns for frontalis suspensions have been described. A simple pentagonal pattern is useful for both fascia lata and silicone rod and requires less graft material, which is advantageous for two reasons: less foreign material is implanted and, in the cases of small children, the available length of autologous material will not be a limiting factor.

Local anesthetic with epinephrine is injected pretarsally and to the suprabrow region. Two marks are drawn adjacent to the medial and lateral corneal limbus over the midtarsus, and 3-mm-long incisions are made over the previously placed marks down to the tarsal plate with a no. 15 Bard-Parker blade. A fascial strip 2 to 3 mm in width is then pulled through the incisions with a Wright fascia lata needle. The fascial strips can be pulled upward to the medial and lateral eyebrow to mark the two brow incisions, ensuring a proper vector and eyelid contour. The medial and lateral suprabrow incisions are incised down to the periosteum with a no. 15 Bard-Parker blade. While the globe is protected by a lid plate or a corneal protector, a Wright needle is passed downward from the medial and lateral brow incisions through the pre-aponeurotic fat pads to the lid incisions. The fascial strip is then pulled through the medial and lateral brow incisions and crossed centrally over the pupil to mark the central incision at a point 5 to 7 mm above the two incisions. The central incision is made down to the periosteum, and the two ends of the fascial strip are tunneled into the central incision with the Wright needle. This approach helps ensure the proper vectors of pull and respects the normal eyelid contour. The fascia is pulled up until the lid margin approximates the upper limbus and is then tied with one half of a surgeon's knot. A 6-0 Prolene suture or braided nylon suture is sewn through the knotted strips and tied, securing the knot. It is then sewn into the frontalis muscles superiorly. Excess fascia is trimmed, and 4 to 5 mm of remnant fascia is tucked under the central skin incision, into frontalis muscle. The eyelid and brow incisions are then closed with 6-0 plain gut suture.

Variations

A variation of this technique involves making a lid crease incision and sewing the fascia directly to the tarsal plate. This is helpful when it is useful to excise excess skin or to provide a more defined lid crease. The pretarsal incision technique described previously, however, is faster and creates an appropriate upper eyelid crease in most instances, obviating the need for eyelid crease reformation sutures.

FRONTALIS SUSPENSION USING A SILICONE (SILASTIC) ROD

Silicone (Silastic) rod suspension is useful in myogenic ptosis conditions such as progressive external ophthalmoplegia, oculopharyngeal dystrophy, and myasthenia gravis, or in third nerve palsy patients. Rarely, an adult with severe bilateral congenital ptosis with no previous surgical correction or with undercorrection from previous surgeries may present with absent or poor Bell's protective eye phenomenon. These patients are usually better served with silicone rod frontalis suspension.

Silicone rod frontalis suspension is recommended in patients with progressive neuromuscular disorders and third nerve palsy because of the possibility of recovery from illness, possible favorable response to therapeutics, and allowance for postoperative adjustment. The 1 mm solid silicone (Silastic) rods are available commercially (Fig. 47–20). Some of the available silicone rod packages come with passing needles and a silicone sleeve, which eliminate the need for the Wright fascia lata needle (BD Visitec Frontalis suspension set (Seiff, 1 Becton Drive, Franklin Lakes, NJ 07417)

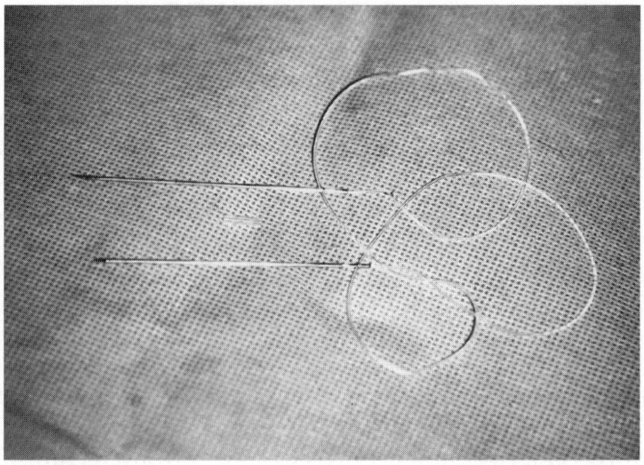

Figure 47–20. Frontalis suspension. Commercially available Silastic rod set from Visitec (no. 5192; 7575 Commerce Court, Sarasota, FL 34243-3212). The set comes with 0.9-mm stainless-steel threading needles, a 40-cm length of Silastic rod, diameter 0.8 mm, and a 10-mm segment of Silastic sleeve that has an external diameter of 2 mm and an internal diameter of 1 mm.

Surgical Technique

The surgery can be performed under general anesthesia or local anesthesia; however local anesthesia is preferred because it allows the surgeon to fine-tune the eyelid level and contour intraoperatively. A simple pentagonal design similar to that used for the fascial frontalis suspension works well for this procedure. A lid crease incision, however, is more appropriate in this situation because it permits attachment of the silicone rod directly to the tarsal plate.

One percent Xylocaine with epinephrine and hyaluronidase is injected under the lid crease incision and just above the eyebrow centrally, medially, and laterally. The lid crease incision is made and the tarsal plate is exposed by dissection through the orbicularis. The silicone rod is sewn onto the tarsal plate with three to five interrupted 6-0 braided nylon or polypropylene sutures (Fig. 47–21). The rod is then pulled up to the eyebrow to mark the medial and lateral brow incisions. This will help to optimize the contour of the upper eyelid margin. Incisions are made down to the periosteum. With the globe protected, in a similar fashion as described above, the rods are passed through the preaponeurotic space to the medial and lateral brow incisions with the passing needles (Fig. 47–22) or the Wright fascia needle. The medial and lateral ends of the silicone rod are then pulled up and crossed centrally to mark the central incision above the pupillary optic axis, which is usually above the pupil or just slightly medial to it. The two ends of the rod are passed through a small silicone sleeve to secure them at optimum length and tension. This maneuver can be performed using either a Watzke or a Lambert silicone sleeve spreader. The lid level is set between 1 and 3 mm above the pupil, depending on the condition being treated. (When dealing with adult myogenic or neurogenic ptosis, the surgeon should not elevate the margin of the superior eyelid to the limbus, as for correction of congenital ptosis.) The rods are trimmed and left with 5 to 8 mm at either end for possible future adjustment. The ends of these rods are then tucked into the wound. A 6-0 braided nylon or polypropylene suture is sewn around the sleeve, with cutting into the silicone sleeve, which is then sewn superiorly to the deeper frontalis muscle (Fig. 47–23). The brow incisions are closed and the lid crease incision is closed, usually with supratarsal fixation every other bite to create a defined lid crease. One can adjust the lid level and contour postoperatively in the office by exposing the silicone sleeve under the central suprabrow incision. This is best done within the first few weeks after surgery, because, once a pseudocapsule forms around the rods, adjustment may prove to be more difficult. If indicated, the rod can be entirely removed at any time postoperatively. The silicone rod offers the extra advantage and flexibility of adjustability, and results comparable to those obtained with fascia lata techniques can be achieved (Fig. 47–24).

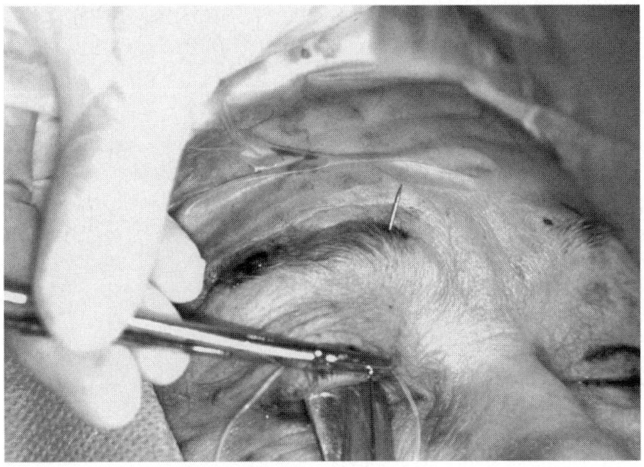

Figure 47–21. Frontalis suspension. The Silastic rod is sewn to the tarsal plate.

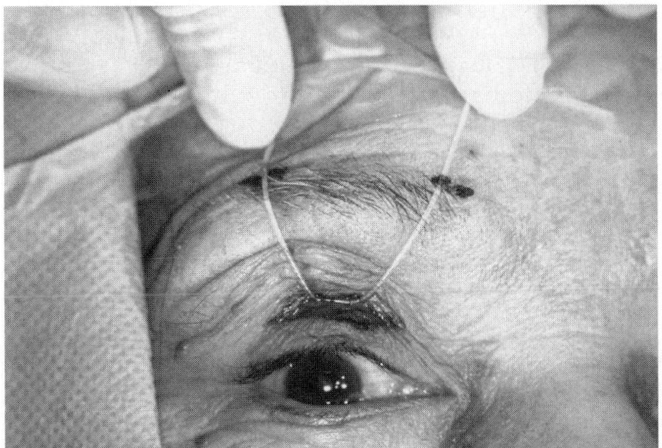

Figure 47–22. Frontalis suspension. The rods are passed through the preaponeurotic space to the medial and lateral suprabrow incisions.

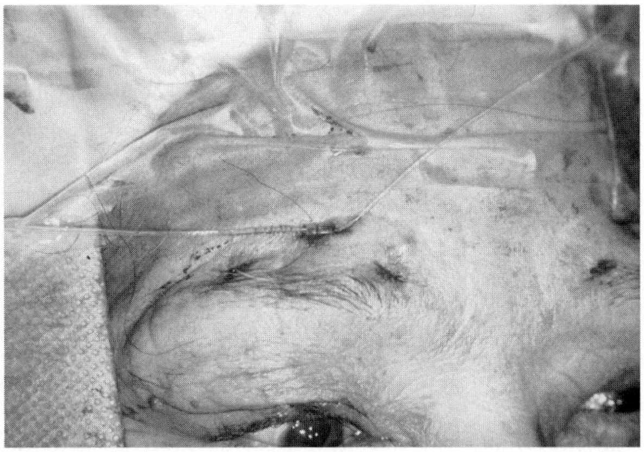

Figure 47–23. Frontalis suspension. The medial and lateral ends are crossed centrally to mark the exact central incision. The ends are passed through the central brow incision and then through the Silastic sleeve. The appropriate tension adjustment is made so that the lid is at the desired level and the contour is judged optimal. A 6-0 permanent suture is sewn around the sleeve and then stitched into the frontalis muscle under the superior edge of the incision.

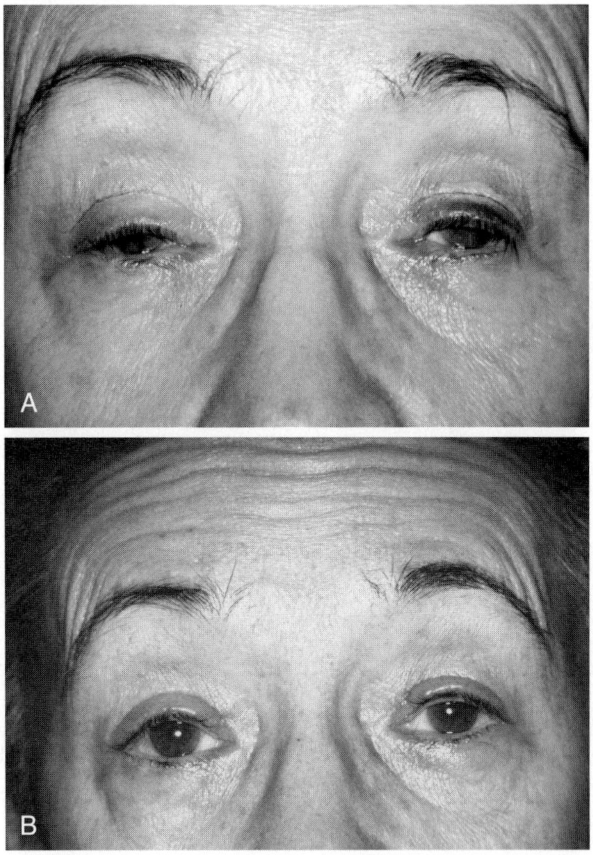

Figure 47–24. Preoperative *(A)* and postoperative *(B)* photographs of a woman with chronic progressive external ophthalmoplegia after frontalis suspension using Silastic rods.

REFERENCES

1. Callahan M, Beard C: Ptosis, 4th ed. Birmingham: Aesculapius, 1990.
2. Dresner SC: Further modifications of the Miller's muscle conjunctival resection procedure. Ophthalmic Plast Reconstr Surg 1991;7:114–122.

3. Meyer DR, Wobig JL: Detection of contralateral eyelid retraction associated with blepharoptosis. Ophthalmology 1992;99:366–369.
4. Dresner SC: Minimal ptosis management. In Kikkawa DO (ed), Aesthetic Ophthalmic Plastic Surgery. Philadelphia: Lippincott-Raven, 1997:151–162.
5. Older JJ: Ptosis repair and blepharoplasty in the adult. Ophthalmic Surg 1995;4:304–308.
6. Shore JW, Berlnin DJ, Garrett SN: Results of blepharoptosis surgery with early postoperative adjustment. Ophthalmology 1990;97:1502.
7. Berlin AJ, Vestal KP: Levator aponeurosis surgery. Ophthalmology 1989;96:1033–1037.
8. Crawford JS: Repair of ptosis using frontalis muscle and fascia lata: a 20 year review. Ophthalmic Surg 1977;8:31–40.
9. Older JJ, Dunne PB: Silicone slings for the correction of ptosis associated with progressive external ophthalmoplegia. Ophthalmic Surg. 1984;15:379–381.
10. Putterman AM, Urist MJ: Muller muscle-conjunctival resection. Arch Ophthalmol 1975;93:619–623.
11. Weinstein GW, Buerger GF: Modifications of the Mueller's muscle-conjunctival resection operation for blepharoptosis. Am J Ophthalmol 1982;93:647.
12. Beard C: Mueller's superior tarsal muscle: anatomy, physiology and clinical significance. Ann Plast Surg 1985;14:324–333.
13. Fasanella RM, Servat J: Levator resection for minimal ptosis: another simplified operation. Arch Ophthalmol 1961;65:493–496.
14. Putterman AM: A clamp for strengthening Mueller's muscle and the treatment of ptosis: modification, theory and a clamp for Fasanella-Servat operation. Arch Ophthalmol 1972;87:665–667.
15. Collin JRO, Beard C, Wood L: Experimental and clinical data on the insertion of the levator palpebral superioris muscle. Am J Ophthalmol 1978;85:792–801.
16. McCord CD, Tannenbaum M: Oculoplastic Surgery. New York: Raven Press; 1987.
17. McCord CD: An external tarso-aponeurectomy. Trans Am Acd Ophthalmolo Otol 1975;79:683.
18. Anderson RL, Dixon RS: Aponeurotic ptosis surgery. Arch Ophthalmol 1979;79:1123–1128.
19. Mercandetti M, Putterman AM, Cohen ME, et al.: Internal levator advancement by Müller's muscle-conjunctival resection: technique and review. Arch Facial Plast Surg 2001;3:104–110.
20. Linberg JV, Vasquez RJ, Chao GM: Aponeurotic ptosis repair under local anesthesia. Prediction of results from operative lid height. Ophthalmology 1988;95:1046–1052.

CHAPTER 48

Blepharoplasty

ROBERT ALAN GOLDBERG, M.D., KYLE C. BALCH, M.D.,
CHAIM EDELSTEIN, M.D., NORMAN SHORR, M.D., and
TINA G. LI, M.D.

INTRODUCTION

Upper blepharoplasty deals with the contours of the upper eyelid space, mainly the region between the eyebrow and the eyelashes. It is not about skin, although removal of skin is typically part of the operation. Rather, it is about sculpture and contouring of this aesthetic unit. The eyebrow, orbital fat, and skin, as well as the underlying structures including the tarsal plate, levator muscle, and bony orbital rim, all play a role in determining the contours of the upper eyelid aesthetic unit. Each of these components must be considered in evaluation and surgical planning for upper blepharoplasty, and often, each of these components may need to be addressed surgically to achieve the results desired by the patient. Eyelid sculpture is an art, not a science. Blepharoplasty planning and execution is quite obviously an individualized process; the surgeon must determine (with variable amounts of suggestion, depending on the sophistication of the patient) the desired aesthetic result, and then work with the patient to determine which techniques and surgeries might be used in that case to achieve some or all of the desired aesthetic changes. This intermingling of art and technique, of patient desires and technical realities, in addition to the physician–patient relationship makes aesthetic eyelid surgery both gratifying and challenging.

Mid-face rejuvenation, also the responsibility of the ophthalmologist, includes midface lifting and suborbicularis oculi fat (SOOF) repositioning. An in-depth discussion of midface rejuvenation is beyond the scope of this chapter, but the midface structures must be considered by the physician evaluating any patient for lower blepharoplasty. Having said that, within the eyelid complex proper, lower blepharoplasty is primarily about removing or repositioning orbital fat; this is almost always done through a conjunctival approach.

ANATOMY

Thorough knowledge of the surgical anatomy of the eyelids and eyebrows is essential for the successful performance of blepharoplasty. For a detailed description of this anatomy, the reader is referred to chapter 46 of this volume. An important, and very often overlooked point, is the need for the understanding of the surface anatomy of the eyelid and eyebrow aesthetic unit. Such knowledge will facilitate the preoperative evaluation, which is the most important aspect of blepharoplasty surgery.

It is important to develop the ability to "see through" the skin and subcutaneous tissues that drape over the deep anatomic substrates of the periorbital area. The surgeon should get a sense of the contribution of these various substrates to the existing surface anatomy, and therefore a sense of which substrates are available for surgical modification. Figure 48–1 demonstrates the important characteristics of surface anatomy. Skin and subcutaneous tissues can be excised to reduce redundancy, and fat can be removed to expose the deeper structures, such as the levator aponeurosis and bony orbital rim.

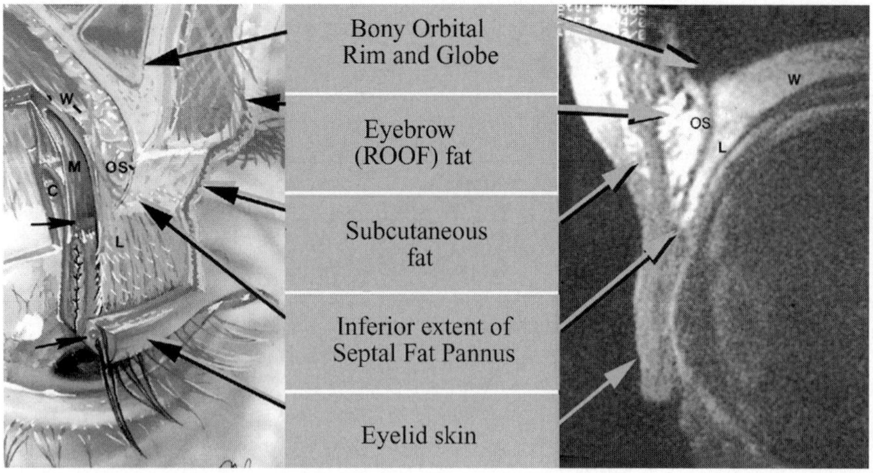

Figure 48–1. Sagittal section of upper eyelid anatomy. (From Goldberg RA, Wu JC, Jesmanowicz A, Hyde JS: Eyelid anatomy revisited. Dynamic high-resolution magnetic resonance images of Whitnall's ligament and upper eyelid structures with the use of a surface coil. Arch Ophthalmol 1992;110:1598–1600, with permission.)

The vertical proportions of the midface should be well appreciated. The area between the eyebrows and the upper eyelid margin can be divided into thirds. The distance between the eyebrows and the upper eyelid crease occupies two thirds while that between the upper eyelid crease and the upper eyelid margin is one third (Fig. 48–2). The eyebrow fat is usually located above the superior orbital rim. Hereditary factors and involutional changes can cause a descent of this eyebrow fat, which thus encroaches on the upper eyelid space and gives a "full" appearance. A beginning surgeon might erroneously attribute this fullness to preaponeurotic fat prolapse and formulate an inaccurate operative plan.

The upper eyelid crease is formed by the farthest superior attachments of the levator aponeurosis to the skin. The actual crease is not typically visible in occidental eyelids because a variable flap of skin, the eyelid fold, hangs down over the crease. The exact positions, extents, and definitions of both the crease and the fold, as well as any subtle asymmetries, should be noted preoperatively and incorporated into the operative plan.

The contour of the tightly attached skin over the levator aponeurosis and tarsus forms the eyelid "platform," the area upon which, for example, eye shadow would be applied. The septal fat pannus overlies the levator and upper tarsal plate. Racial variations exist, and are important here. At one extreme lies the Asian patient, with an abundant septal fat pannus consisting of eyelid and eyebrow fat that covers the entire tarsal plate, and essentially obliterates any visible platform. At the other extreme lies the aged Caucasian patient with superior sulcus fat atrophy, in which case the entire levator can often be followed up into the orbit, sometimes even with Whitnall's ligament exposed as a horizontal band just below the orbital rim (Fig. 48–3*A* and *B*).

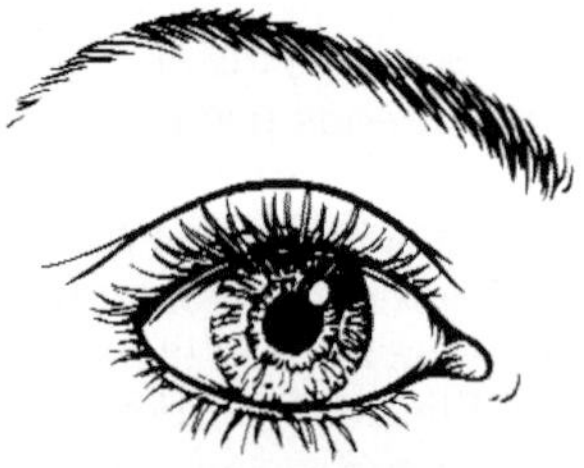

Figure 48–2. The distance between the eyebrows and the upper eyelid crease occupies two thirds, while that between the upper eyelid crease and the upper eyelid margin is one third. (Figure copyright 1996, UC Regents, University of California, Los Angeles reprinted with permission.)

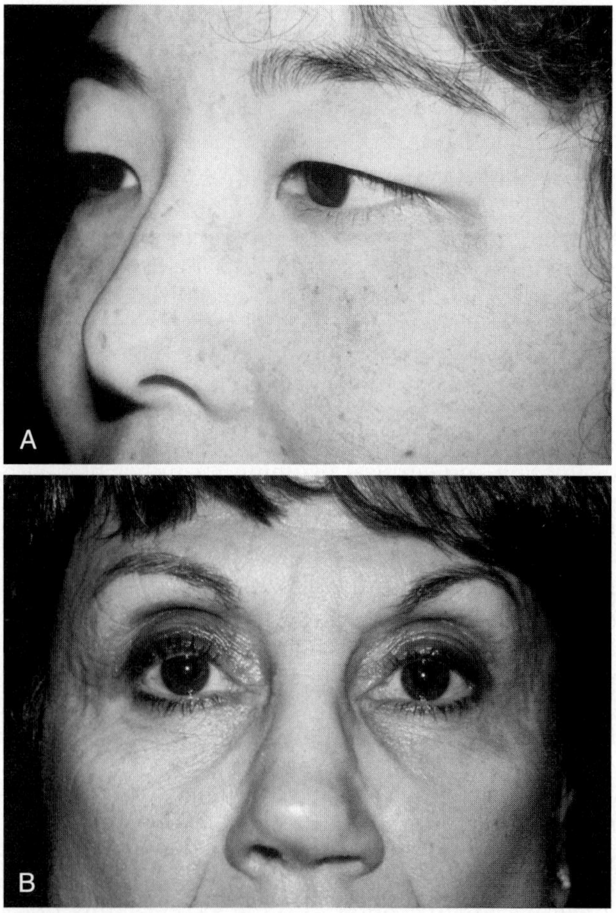

Figure 48–3. *A.* Typical upper eyelid appearance and contour of Asian patient demonstrating full upper eyelid and lack of noticable crease. *B.* Typical upper eyelid appearance and contour of elderly Caucasian patient demonstrating superior sulcus atrophy and visible underlying structures.

The most medial portion of the upper eyelid, combined with the lateral surface of the nose and the medial canthus, constitutes an area that deserves particular attention. Redundancy in this area is often related to eyebrow ptosis, with tissues encroaching from the glabella to form a diamond-shaped deformity (Fig. 48–4). This anatomically complex area has different tissue characteristics from the interdigitation of different skin textures. Incisions should not extend into this area because of the high likelihood of producing postoperative webs or other irregularities that give an aesthetically unpleasant outcome. Elevation of the redundant eyebrow tissues out of the multicontoured space is often more effective in restoring the normal width of the radix, by reducing the redundancy in the multicontoured area.

The lower eyelid is composed of skin and underlying orbicularis muscle, which continues past the lower orbital rim onto the face. Behind the orbicularis, near the lid margin, is the tarsal plate. The orbital septum fuses with the inferior border of the tarsus and continues caudally to attach to the crest of the lower orbital rim at the arcus marginalis. Just behind the orbital septum are the lower eyelid orbital fat compartments. The orbital fat is bordered posteriorly and superiorly by the lower eyelid retractors, which arise from the inferior rectus muscle and tendon. The lower lid retractors fuse with the orbital septum approximately 5 mm inferior to the inferior tarsal border before inserting onto the tarsal plate. Posteriorly, the lower eyelid retractors are closely adherent to the palpebral conjunctiva of the lower lid (Fig. 48–5).

The orbital fat is surrounded by many fine connective tissue septae (septae of Koorneef). A fascial extension of the sheath of the inferior oblique muscle and Lockwood's ligament called the *arcuate expansion* inserts on the inferolateral orbital rim and separates the central from the lateral fat compartments. The inferior oblique muscle originates from the anterior medial orbital floor and separates the medial fat compartment from the central fat compartment as it passes posteriorly and laterally beneath the equator of the globe. As shown in Figure 48–5, the orbital fat can be easily accessed by incising the conjunctiva and lower lid retractors in the fornix while the orbital septum remains well anterior to these structures.

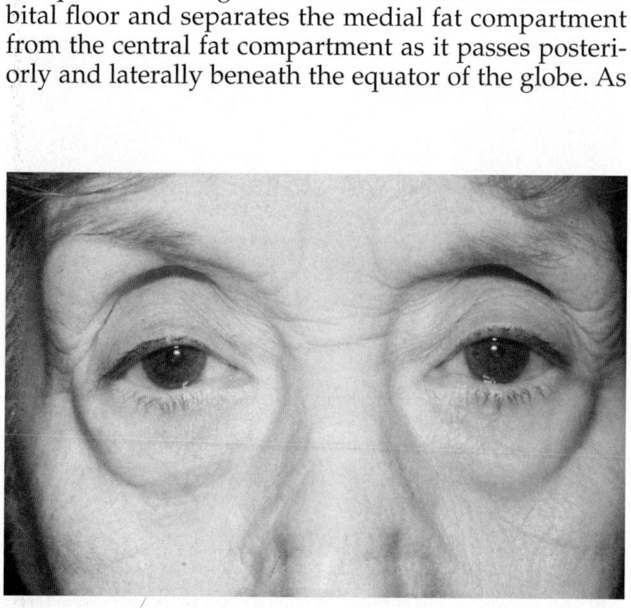

Figure 48–4. Eyelid changes with aging include loss of superior orbital fat and deepening of the superior sulcus, lower orbital fat prolapse, as well as skin changes and eyebrow descent. (© Figure copyright 1996: Regents UC, University of California, Los Angeles, reprinted with permission.)

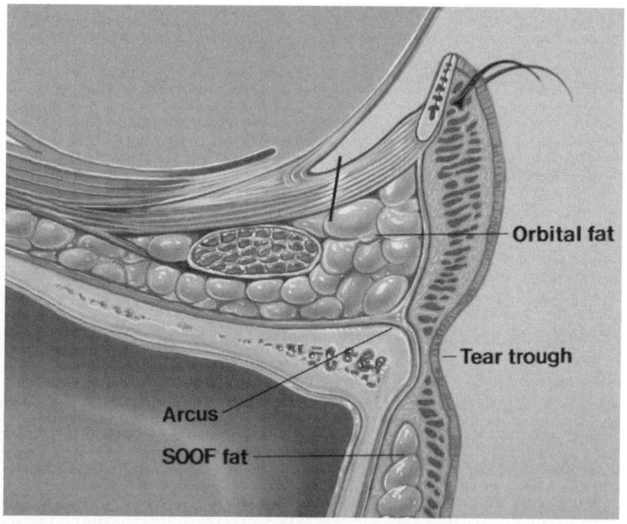

Figure 48–5. Sagittal section of the lower eyelid demonstrating the relationship of the conjunctiva, lower eyelid retractors, and orbital septum to the orbital fat. (From Baylis HI, Long JA, Groth MJ: Transconjunctival lower eyelid blepharoplasty: Technique and complications. Ophthalmology 1989;96:1027-1032, with permission.)

EYELID ASSESSMENT AND SURGICAL PLANNING

UPPER BLEPHAROPLASTY

Because blepharoplasty surgery is concerned with anatomy, understanding the surface anatomy of the eyelid complex and its deep underpinnings leads to an accurate assessment of the individual patient, as well as to a sound surgical plan. The best way to learn what blepharoplasty accomplishes is by examining preoperative and postoperative photographs of blepharoplasty patients. This discipline of photograph review should extend to the individual surgeon's own patients, so that one can learn from one's own experience.

Aging changes are important. Although some young patients come in for blepharoplasty because of congenital characteristics that displease them, most patients seek blepharoplasty surgery because of age-related changes in the eyelid complex, which are characterized by skin texture changes (with loss of elasticity and formation of wrinkles), enophthalmos (with loss of fat), and inferior displacement of fat (with lower eyelid fat prolapse) (Fig. 48–4). It is important to avoid excessive fat removal from the upper eyelid, and attention to eyebrow position is critical for successful rejuvenation of the aging eyelid complex.

Upper eyelid fullness is generally a congenital condition (Fig. 48–6*A*). It can be addressed by removal of fat from the upper eyelid, exposing the underlying levator aponeurosis and tarsus (Fig. 48–6*B* and *D*). The

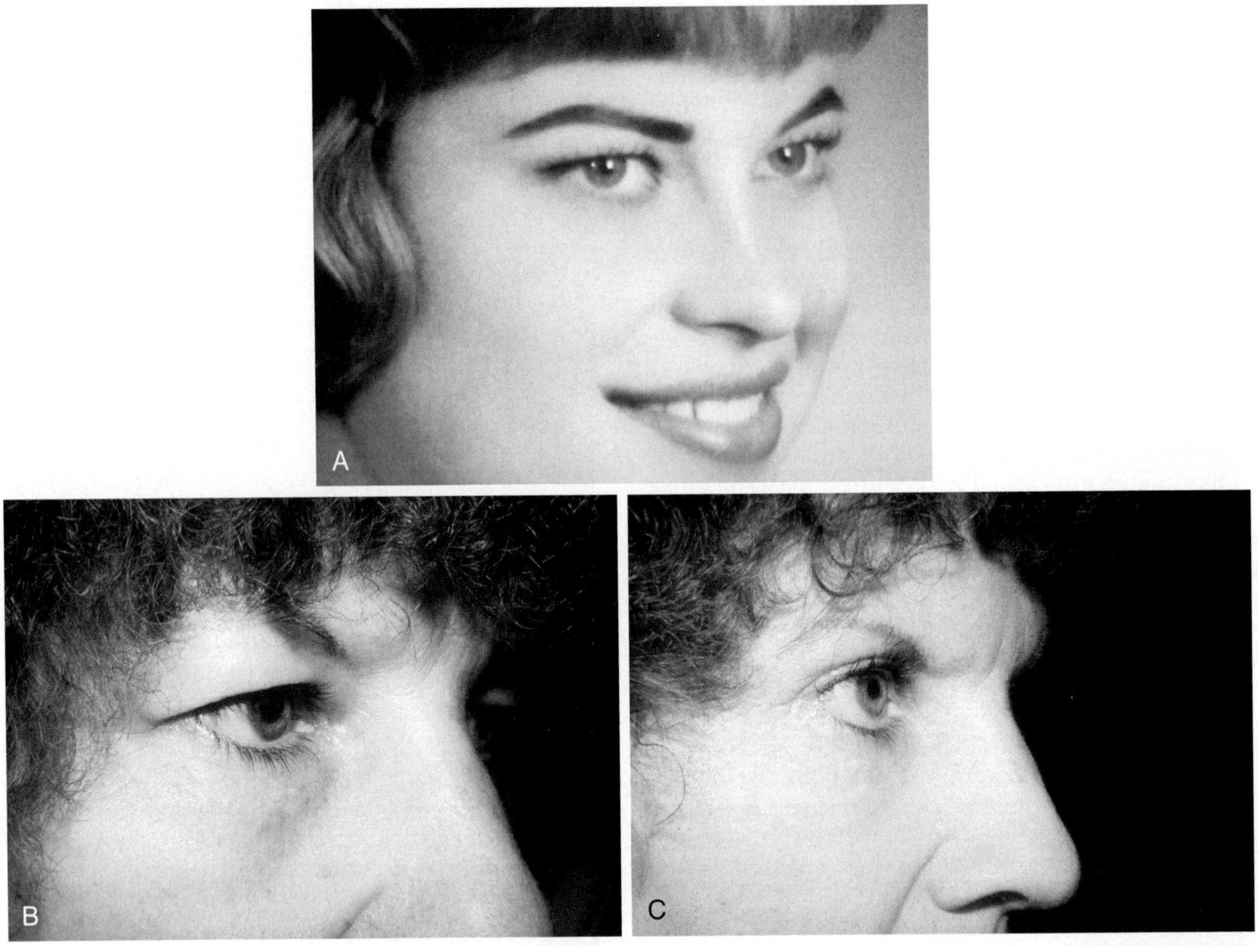

Figure 48–6. *A.* Upper eyelid fullness is generally a congenital condition as demonstrated in photographs of this patient at a young age (upper left) *(B)* in middle life (upper right). *C.* The same patient with good structure and good eyebrow position demonstrating effective conservative removal of redundant tissue to display the underlying structure of the septal fat pannus in the upper eyelid to reveal the underlying platform of tightly apposed skin, levator, and tarsal plate. (© Figure copyright 1996: Regents UC, University of California, Los Angeles reprinted with permission.)

surgeon must recognize when the fullness in the eyelid complex is caused by eyebrow descent. The eyebrows are held at a certain position by the tone of the frontalis muscle, which maintains comfortable vision. If heavy tissues are removed from below the brow, it will descend to its resting position (Figs. 48–7 and 48–8).

If too much of the septal fat pannus and ROOF (retro orbicularis oculi fat or eyebrow fat pad) is removed, the underlying structures will be exposed to an undesirable degree (Fig. 48–9 *A* and *B*). As already mentioned, excessive hollowness of the superior sulcus gives an aged appearance to the eyelid complex. Blepharoplasty in the thin aged upper eyelid must be conservative, with minimal removal of fat. Because there will not be much of a septal fat pannus or eyelid fold to cover the incision, the crease is often made high in the eyelid where it will fall into the shadow of the superior sulcus and be relatively hidden.

If the globe is relatively prominent, the tarsus and levator platform will be more readily exposed by removing orbital fat (Fig. 48–10 *A* and *B*). The orbital fat and full eyelid tissues actually benefit the patient by masking underlying proptosis. In this situation the admonition "big eye, big trouble" should be heeded, and fat removal should be conservative or even avoided altogether in favor of orbital decompression for proptosis reduction.

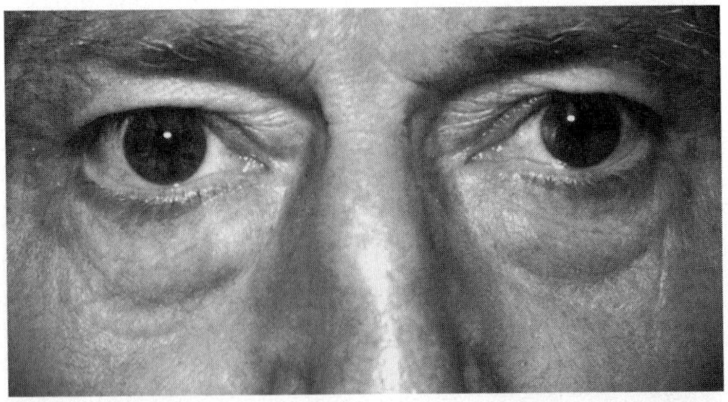

Figure 48–7. Eyebrows maintained in comfortable position for vision by frontalis tone. (© Figure copyright 1996: Regents UC, University of California, Los Angeles reprinted with permission.)

Among Caucasian patients, the most obvious structural variations are those between men and women.

Women should have a high, arched brow with a relatively deep superior sulcus, and a well-defined upper eyelid crease. Men should have a straight brow, perpendiculear to the nose, with a minimal sulcus and a low, subtle upper eyelid crease. Clearly, with different goals in mind, different approaches must be employed for men and women. There are, however, a few consistencies. Of note, the lateral canthus generally lies 2 mm superior to the medial canthus; the upper eyelid generally crosses the cornea 1 to 2 mm below the superior limbus; and the lower eyelid generally crosses the cornea tangential to the inferior limbus.

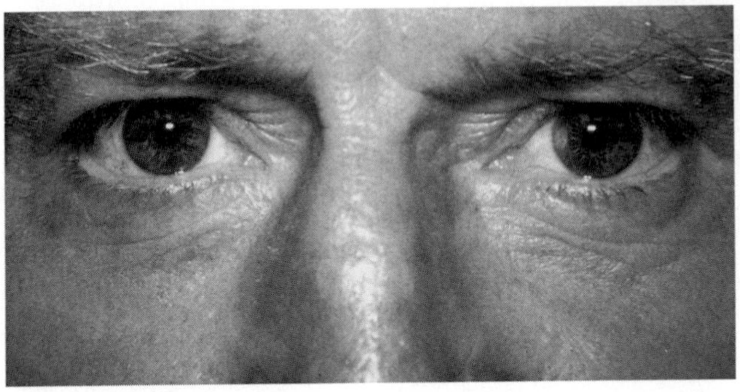

Figure 48–8. Eyebrow descent cause by release of frontalis tone following blepharoplasty. (Figure copyright © 1996: Regents UC, University of California, Los Angeles reprinted with permission.)

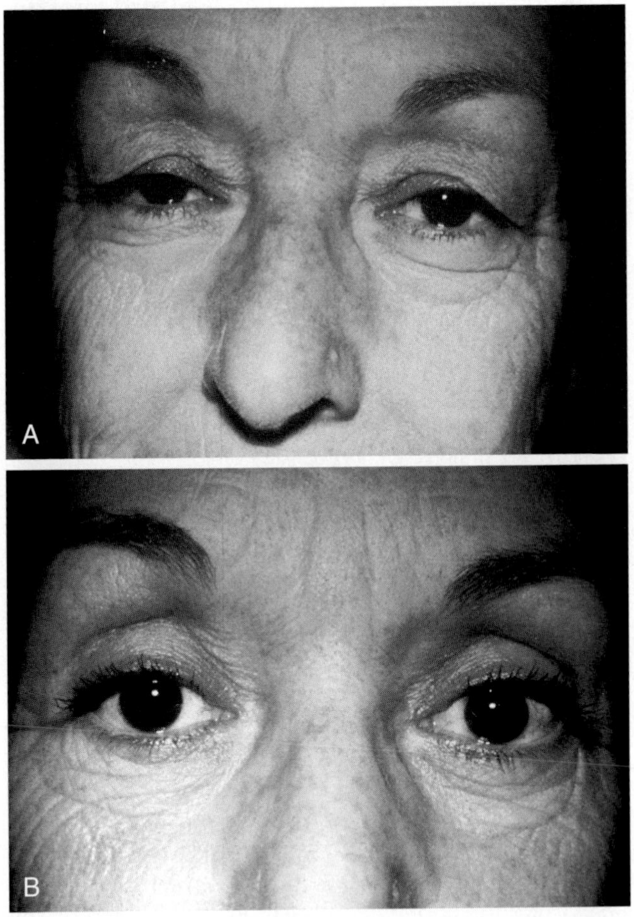

Figure 48–9. *A.* Removal of too much of the orbital fat and associated soft tissue reveals the deep structures of the levator and orbital rim *(B)* (including the inverted "V" of the superior orbital notch and valley of the superior oblique tendon). (Figure copyright © 1996: Regents UC, University of California, Los Angeles reprinted with permission.)

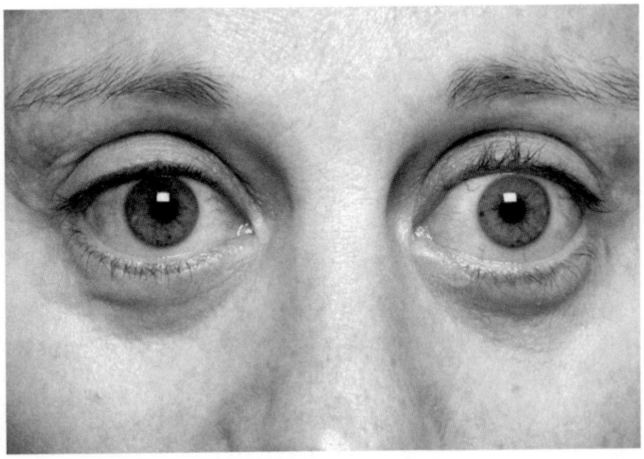

Figure 48–10. The orbital fat and full eyelid tissues actually benefit the patient by masking underling proptosis. Prominent globe is revealed by orbital fat removal. In the circumstance of a prominent globe, fat removal should be conservative or avoided altogether. (© Figure copyright 1996: Regents UC, University of California, Los Angeles reprinted with permission.)

Racial variations are also significant in planning and executing upper blepharoplasty. For example, the Asian eyelid is characterized by a full, sometimes bulging superior sulcus and a low crease with narrow or absent tarsal platform. The crease narrows medially to form an epicanthal fold. The fullness is based anatomically on abundant and somewhat fibrotic fat in the suborbicularis, orbital, and postaponeurotic spaces. This abundant fat can be carefully sculpted because it is fibrotic, but it is unforgiving, so it is easy to create a contour abnormality, a visible dent, or an undesired second crease if the fat is not evenly, or conservatively, sculpted. The goal of Asian blepharoplasty is usually to retain the characteristic of the eyelid while better defining the thin tarsal platform and low crease. To accomplish this, conservative debulking of the inferior edge of the septal fat pannus (with sparing and avoidance of the remainder) is performed. And fixation of the orbicularis or skin edge to the exposed tarsus is performed to create a firm, low, and meticulously symmetric crease (Fig. 48–11 *A* and *B*).

Skin removal is one of the least important parts of upper blepharoplasty. Removal of more skin and associated orbicularis muscle than is necessary is not only the mark of the inexperienced or unsophisticated blepharoplasty surgeon, it is also the cause of most of the functional problems associated with the surgery. The significant effect of minimal skin removal can be appreciated in "touch-up," or reconstructive, upper eyelid surgeries.

LOWER BLEPHAROPLASTY

Lower blepharoplasty addresses the contours of the lower eyelid and cheek. When evaluating patients for

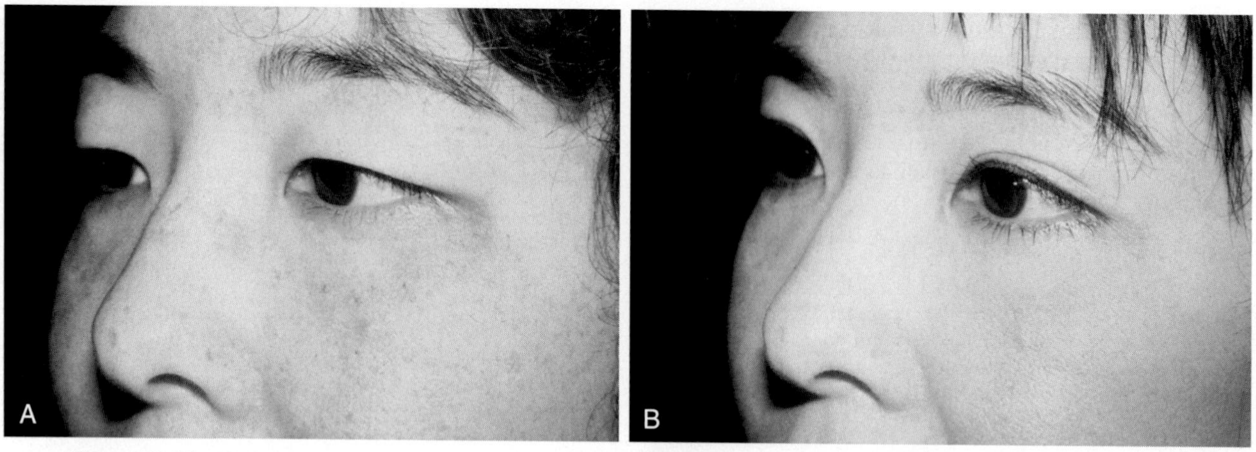

Figure 48–11. Blepharoplasty in the Asian eyelid must respect the fullness of the orbital, preseptal and eyebrow fat pads: to preserve the racial characteristic, a low tarsal platform is maintained by designing a low crease incision that follows the medial epicanthal fold and by excising fat conservatively at the inferior edge of the septal fat pannus allowing the crease to form onto the tarsal plate. In this Asian patient with full septal fat pannus and preorbicularis fat, *(A)* conservative tissue removal preserves the full Asian eyelid and low eyelid crease *(B)*. (© Figures copyright 1996: Regents UC, University of California, Los Angeles reprinted with permission.)

possible lower eyelid surgery, the contours of the orbital fat should be observed. Often the medial, central, and lateral fat pads can be identified and individually graded (Fig. 48–12 *A* and *B*). This type of analysis helps with surgical planning. Inferior to the fat pads, the orbital rim can be seen as a groove marking the arcus marginalis, or orbital septal insertion. There exists an orbitomalar ligament that folds the skin. Medially, the groove can be quite prominent and is often referred to as the "tear trough deformity." Inferior to the groove of the orbital rim the cheek fat forms various contours over the face of the maxilla and malar prominence. Descent of the SOOF fat pad gives rise to a hollow region below the orbital rim, that is bordered inferiorly by a visible trailing edge of the descended SOOF fat pad. Young patients may have a congenitally prominent tear trough deformity.

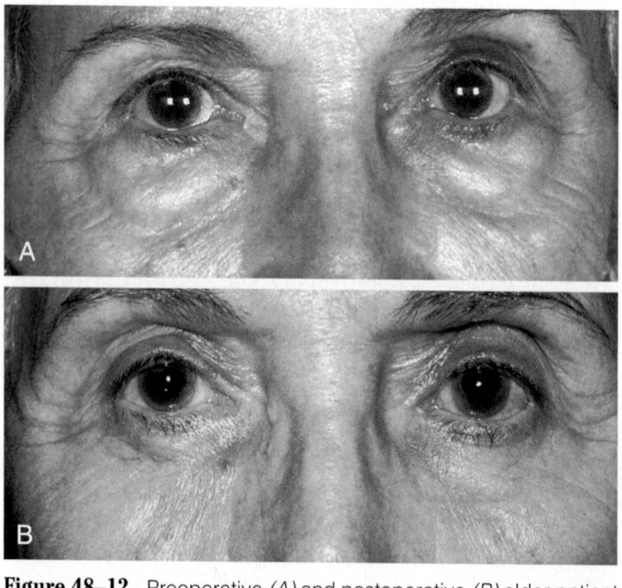

Figure 48–12. Preoperative *(A)* and postoperative *(B)* older patient with fat atrophy and hollow superior sulcus. (© Figures copyright 1996: Regents UC, University of California, Los Angeles reprinted with permission.)

The lower eyelid skin should be evaluated for wrinkles and folds of skin and orbicularis muscle. Discrete folds of skin and orbicularis can be removed by a skin pinch technique. Fine wrinkles are best removed with CO_2 laser resurfacing, which can be performed at the time of blepharoplasty. In general, we advise patients that lower lid wrinkles cannot be improved with surgery. Additional preoperative evaluation includes assessment of the lower eyelid position and tension. In patients with extreme lower eyelid laxity, retraction, ectropion, or entropion, consideration may be given to performing a lateral canthal tightening procedure, or even a transconjunctival entropion surgery, at the time of transconjunctival fat excision.

PROCEDURES: UPPER BLEPHAROPLASTY

ANESTHESIA

Blepharoplasty surgery is most often performed under local anesthesia. In our experience, 2% lidocaine is necessary, to achieve adequate anesthesia of the eyelid and deep periorbital structures. Epinephrine is important for hemostasis; we use a concentration of 1:100,000. Addition of Wydase (hyaluronidase) to the anesthetic mixture allows more rapid, and more even, spreading of the anesthesia through the tissues. One vial (75 units) is added to a 25 cc bottle of 2% lidocaine with epinephrine (this bottle is then used for all of the morning cases). We inject 3–5 cc of anesthetic into each of the four eyelids. In the upper eyelid, the injection is performed just subcutaneously by making a single puncture and "milking" the fluid across the eyelid. It is often possible to anesthetize the entire lid through one puncture, thus reducing the risk of hematoma formation with the needlestick. If the injection is then given slowly, through a 30-gauge needle, successful eyelid anesthesia can be achieved comfortably with little, or no sedation. Removal of orbital fat is usually the most uncomfortable part of the surgery for the patient, especially when unipolar electrocautery is used. Therefore, in both the upper and lower eyelids, we make a point of injecting behind the orbital septum so that a deep orbital block is achieved.

We almost always use intravenous sedation. The surgery can be performed under straight local anesthesia in appropriately selected patients with careful slow injections, but deep fat removal usually necessitates intravenous sedation. In this regard, use of the CO_2 laser may be advantageous in minimizing the need for electrocautery. Intravenous sedation also affords the availability of the anesthesiologist, or nurse anesthetist, who can provide additional psychological support to the patient with continuous communication, reassurance, hand-holding, and other physical contact.

The incisions are typically marked prior to anesthesia administration. They are made best with the patient in the sitting position, with patient cooperation, and with the tissues in their normal gravitational relationships (significant change in eyebrow, cheek, and orbital fat position occurs when patients relax into a supine position). Injection anesthesia is then performed. Even in the rare case performed under general anesthesia we use regional injections of lidocaine and epinephrine to provide hemostasis and decrease the requirement for general anesthesia.

For eyelid work alone, it is unlikely that the toxic dose of lidocaine (7 mg/kg) will be reached. In the average-sized adult, a full 25-cc bottle of 2% lidocaine with epinephrine would be required to reach the toxic level. The same is true of epinephrine (toxic level 7 mcg/kg). In patients who are sensitive to epinephrine, more dilute solutions such as 1:200,000 or even 1:400,000 can be used to achieve similar degrees of hemostasis.

One of the most important aspects of local anesthesia surgery is "staying ahead of the curve" with regard to the anesthetic wearing off. Even with epinephrine, the effect of lidocaine begins to wear off 45 minutes after the injection. Many cases take longer than this, so it is important to pay attention to the clock and to re-inject before the anesthetic wears off. Otherwise, negative consequences may ensue, including a rise in blood pressure in response to pain and increased bleeding in the field, requiring the surgeon to use more cautery—and more time—all of this creating a cycle that can double the case time. It is far better to stay ahead of the curve by reinjecting the lidocaine/epinephrine mixture every 30 to 45 minutes.

DESIGNING AND MARKING THE EYELID CREASE

There can be no standard formula for measuring and marking the upper blepharoplasty incisions. The primary decisions involve the location of the inferior crease incision, and how much skin to remove vertically. Secondary decisions involve deciding how much tissue to excise medially and laterally.

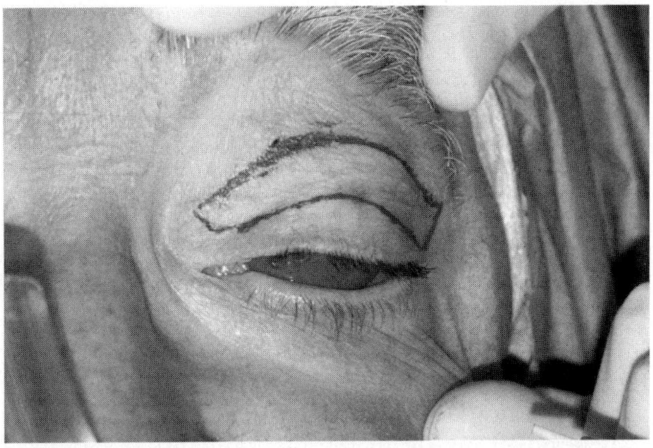

Figure 48–13. Skin markings in upper blepharoplasty: skin excision should be conservative, and the position of the lower incision is designed to be hidden in the eventual eyelid fold. (© Figure copyright 1996: Regents UC, University of California, Los Angeles reprinted with permission.)

The inferior incision, to a certain extent, determines the height of the "platform" of the tarsal plate. However, it is incorrect to assume that the incision will form the eyelid crease and determine its height. If we remember the sagittal anatomy of the eyelid, it is clear that the redundant eyelid and eyebrow complexes will cover the surgical crease in most cases unless aggressive brow and lid surgery is performed.

In a very thin eyelid, for example in a very aged Caucasian patient, there will be little fat and skin to drape over the crease incision, and the incision itself may be visible. In this situation, it may be advantageous to make a high incision that will fall into the shadow of the superior sulcus. In such thin lids, minimal fat will be taken, with the goal of surgery being to remove some redundant skin in the superior sulcus, while smoothing out the long tarsal platform. In this setting a more inferiorly placed eyelid crease incision might not only be visible but might also predispose to a second crease forming higher up on the levator aponeurosis.

In a more typical patient, a certain amount of the septal fat pannus will hang over the surgical incision, and therefore the inferior incision is drawn slightly higher than the height of the desired tarsal platform. In a woman, this will typically result in a lower incision, approximately 7 to 10 mm above the eyelash line centrally (Fig. 48–13). And in a man, an incision typically 5 to 8 mm above the lash line is indicated. In an Asian patient, the range might be 3 to 6 mm above the eyelash line centrally. Laterally, the incision dips down to pick up some of the temporal hooding. It is best to address this temporal hooding through eyebrow elevation (see appropriate chapter), but if eyebrow surgery cannot be performed, or if redundant tissue persists after eyebrow elevation, temporal hooding can be excised directly at the expense of a scar in the thicker skin of the temple and at the expense of decreasing the distance between the tail of the brow and the lateral eyelid. Medially, it is also best to elevate redundant tissue out of the multicontoured area (the medial one fifth of the upper eyelid) through appropriate eyebrow elevation. However, if the surgeon elects to compromise and remove redundant skin in this area directly, a "lazy S" incision helps to decrease webbing in this susceptible region by converting the vector of skin tension (upon closure) to a more horizontal direction. This incision is accomplished by dipping down the medialmost component of the incision to pick up the medial redundancy. The proliferation of creative flaps such as W-plasties and T-shaped incisions is indicative of the difficulty encountered by surgeons working in the medial canthal region. It is not uncommon to see early web formation even preoperatively, and any surgery that removes tissue in the medial canthal region is prone to web formation. Web formation is caused primarily by the tendency for the scar to contract, and to "clothesline" the tissues from the nasal bridge across the hollowed concave region of the medial canthal multicontoured surface. The more the surgeon can lift these tissues out of the multicontoured area through eyebrow surgery, and avoid the temptation to draw the medial canthal incision line far into the multicontoured area, the less chance there is of web formation and other contour problems in this region.

In upper blepharoplasty, the vertical excision of skin should always be conservative. Flowers has suggested that at least one inch (25 mm) of skin between the eyebrow and eyelashes is necessary for proper eyelid closure. Certainly, older techniques, such as the "skin pinch," in which the surgeon tries to maximize skin removal while narrowly avoiding lagophthalmos, are philosophically and technically inappropriate. Rather, the goal should be just the opposite: How little skin can we remove from the lid and still accomplish our surgical goal of creating an eyelid platform while sculpting the eyelid tissues to reveal more of the underlying deep structures? In the presence of uncorrected eyebrow ptosis, the surgeon has to be especially careful to avoid the temptation to address heavy eyebrow tissues by excising them from below, in the eyelid space. This can create a situation in which the "eyebrows are sutured to the eyelids," so that the patient is functionally and aesthetically crippled with persistence of heavy eyebrow tissues in the eyelid space and an inability to elevate the eyebrows without creating lagophthalmos (Figs. 48–7 and 48–8). Very rarely is it necessary to excise more than 10 mm of skin in the vertical direction. Typically, a 5- to 7-mm excision is appropriate, and an excision of 3 to 5 mm of skin is not uncommon, especially in younger patients.

UPPER EYELID BLEPHAROPLASTY TECHNIQUE

After the surgeon marks the incision, either the steel blade or the CO_2 laser can be used to accomplish the actual cutting. More surgical precision, easier tissue dissection, a relatively bloodless field, and more rapid postoperative recovery are generally seen with the laser unit. At the same time, the need for an instrument that costs between $40 thousand and $140 thousand demands tighter safety principles and necessitates additional training is debated by some eyelid surgeons. But in times where publicity and patient demand can be the governing factors, other eyelid surgeons would argue that laser blepharoplasty is the way to a thriving cosmetic surgery practice.

In most instances the musculocutaneous flap is removed in one piece (Fig. 48–14). In rare instances, where pronounced attenuation and involutional upper eyelid thinning is noted, some or most of the orbicularis oculi muscle can be left intact and the dissection can be done in a subcutaneous plane.

After removal of the musculocutaneous flap, the orbital septum can be visualized. In some patients a pronounced preseptal fat pannus can be noticed. This should not be confused with the preaponeurotic fat pads of the upper eyelid. This preseptal fat may represent a gravitational descent of the ROOF, which is the sub-brow fat that has descended to encroach on the upper eyelid aesthetic unit, giving a full appearance. This fat can be sculpted or repositioned to its anatomic area with sutures.

Excessive "fullness" or "bulging" of the lateral aspect of the upper eyelid may be due to a prominent orbital rim. Osteoplastic techniques utilizing bone burrs and chisels can smooth these projections, to give a satisfactory result. A bit more dissection into the subperiosteal plane is all that is necessary to address this problem. Alternatively, and perhaps preferably, the rim can be contoured via a coronal approach.

The orbital septum is incised horizontally (Fig. 48–15), usually across the full extent of the upper eyelid to provide an "open-sky" approach to the underlying structures. The septum is not a single layer as is usually described, but rather, a multilaminar structure with varying thickness in different areas of the upper eyelid. As Flowers has suggested, the orbital septum should be opened just above its insertion into the aponeurosis, with particular attention to avoiding accidental sectioning of the underlying aponeurosis. The preaponeurotic

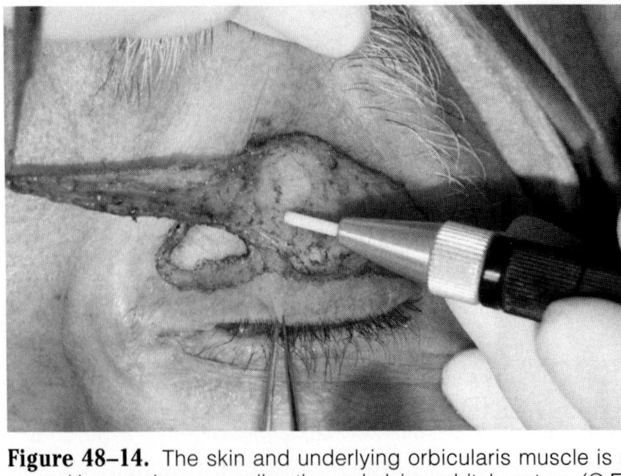

Figure 48–14. The skin and underlying orbicularis muscle is removed in one piece, revealing the underlying orbital septum. (© Figure copyright 1996: Regents UC, University of California, Los Angeles reprinted with permission.)

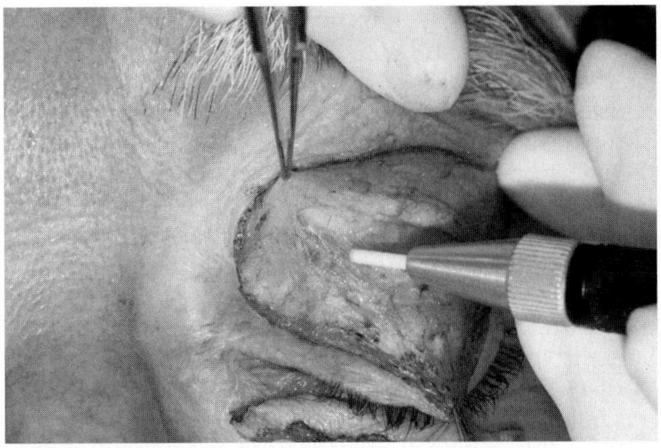

Figure 48–15. The orbital septum is opened just superior to its attachment onto the levator aponeurosis. This leaves the septal fat pannus intact above the incision and allows graded sculpting of the septal fat pannus; it also sets the stage for sculpture of the pretarsal septal remnant and orbicularis. (© Figure copyright 1996: Regents UC, University of California, Los Angeles reprinted with permission.)

fat pads will be viewed next. Most of the fullness of the upper eyelid is the result of herniation of the larger central fat pad, but occasionally the smaller nasal fat pad can contribute to significant and localized bulging. The fat that was preoperatively planned for reduction is removed (Fig. 48–16). This can be accomplished in a piecemeal fashion when using electrocautery by alternating the cautery and coagulation. Alternatively, fat vaporization can be accomplished with the CO_2 laser. Excessive pulling on the fat pads must be avoided to prevent avulsion of the orbital vessels that usually run within these fat compartments. In some individuals there is excessive fullness at the lateral aspect of the upper lid as a result of involutional stretching and descent of the lacrimal gland into the preaponeurotic tissue plane. Obviously, it is important to identify the more orange-looking friable lacrimal gland tissue, and to avoid its amputation. The lacrimal gland can be repositioned inside the lacrimal gland fossa and sutured to the overlying periosteum.

To reiterate, it is important to avoid excessive reduction of the preaponeurotic fat pads. Its ease of removal with the "open-sky" approach should never lead to excessive removal. Enough fat should be left to serve as a physiologic sliding tissue for upper eyelid excursion. Sometimes, fat repositioning is all that it is required. The "valley" of the superior oblique tendon separates the central fat pads from the nasal fat pads, and it is usually a hollow area (Fig. 48–17). Fat repositioning into this area can reduce the inverted "V" deformity that characterizes the aged eyelid.

After the judicious removal of preaponeurotic fat, the septal edge can be trimmed to provide a flatter, smoother, and tighter upper eyelid platform (Fig. 48–18). This step can be supplemented with excision of a strip of pretarsal orbicularis oculi muscle along the inferior edge of the incision for further debulking of the pretarsal area. The CO_2 laser is an excellent instrument

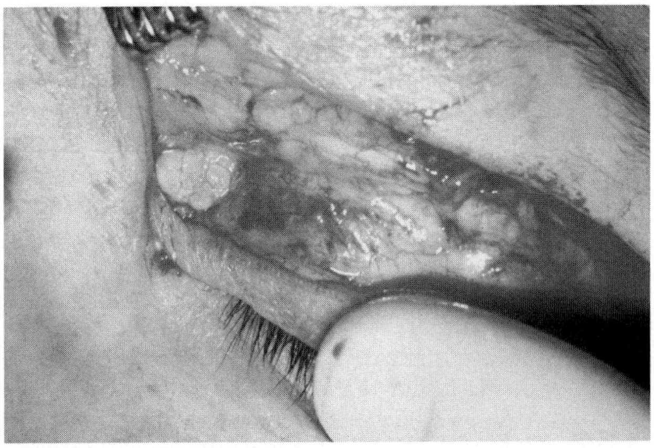

Figure 48–17. The medial fat pad is white in color. It lies medial to the valley of the superior oblique muscle. (© Figure copyright 1996: Regents UC, University of California, Los Angeles reprinted with permission.)

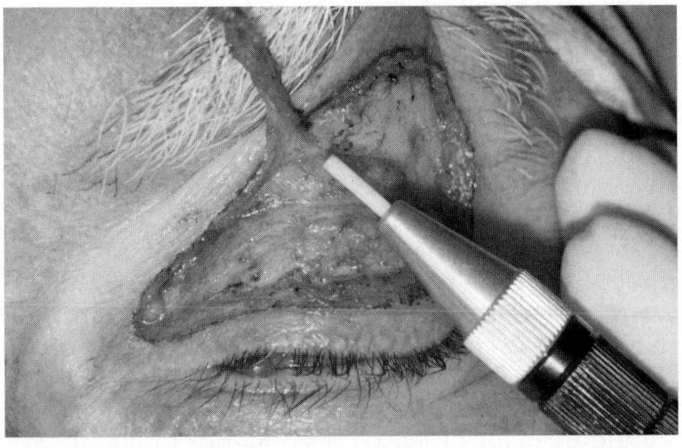

Figure 48–16. The orbital fat (septal fat pannus) is excised in graded fashion, with care taken to minimize excess excision over the superior orbital notch/valley of the superior oblique. (© Figure copyright 1996: Regents UC, University of California, Los Angeles reprinted with permission.)

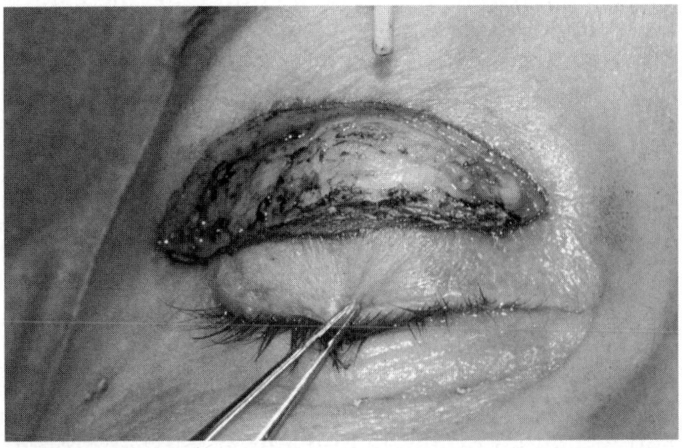

Figure 48–18. The CO_2 laser is an excellent instrument to vaporize and tighten these preaponeurotic tissues to create a tight platform and well-defined eyelid crease. (© Figure copyright 1996: Regents UC, University of California, Los Angeles reprinted with permission.)

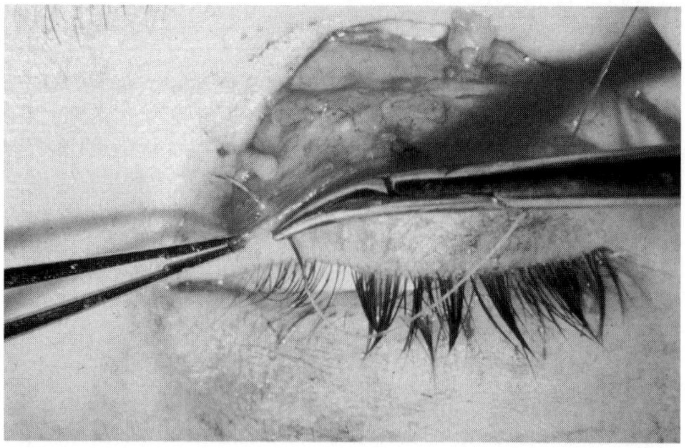

Figure 48–19. For supratarsal fixation, a bite of levator is included in each of the running suture bites. (© Figure copyright 1996: Regents UC, University of California, Los Angeles reprinted with permission.)

that can vaporize and tighten these preaponeurotic tissues to create a tight platform and a well-defined eyelid crease.

The last step of the procedure, wound closure, includes the consideration of supratarsal fixation. The preoperative planning will determine whether a well-defined "hard" crease or a more conspicuous "soft" crease is desirable. Generally, a "hard" crease is optimal for women to provide a well-demarcated upper eyelid platform for the application of eye shadow, whereas most men do not benefit from such an abrupt definition of the upper eyelid crease. When supratarsal fixation is performed, the skin and orbicularis oculi muscle of the pretarsal flap along the inferior edge of the incision are anchored together to the "leathery" preaponeurotic fascia at the level of the superior portion of the tarsus. The exact anchoring level varies with each patient and is another manifestation of the individualization that is required in blepharoplasty surgery. Several interrupted sutures can be placed for supratarsal fixation, or a running suture that is used for skin closure can include a purchase of the preaponeurotic fascia (Fig. 48–19). A 6-0 or 7-0 running absorbable or nonabsorbable suture on a cutting needle can be used to close the cutaneous incision; some surgeons insist on a subcuticular running closure, but we have not noticed any difference in wound healing or postoperative appearance.

PROCEDURES: LOWER BLEPHAROPLASTY

Local anesthesia for transconjunctival blepharoplasty is somewhat different from that for other lower eyelid surgeries. The injection must be made through the conjunctiva because the sensory nerves of the conjunctiva and orbital fat originate in the orbit. First, a drop of proparacaine HCL 0.5% is placed on the conjunctiva. Then, a cotton-tipped applicator soaked in 4% lidocaine is held on the conjunctival surface for 1 to 2 minutes without touching the cornea. This step may be omitted if the patient has deep intravenous sedation. Two percent lidocaine with 1:100,000 epinephrine and Wydase (one vial of Wydase per 50 cc bottle of lidocaine) is then injected with a 27- or 30-gauge needle. The surgeon sits at the head of the table and tents up the eyelid so that the injection can be delivered through the conjunctival fornix under direct visualization. The needle is directed slightly posteriorly to the inferior orbital rim behind the orbital septum and then walked posteriorly until the needle literally touches the floor of the orbit. Injections of 1 cc are made in this fashion medially, centrally, and laterally to anesthetize each individual fat pocket. The Wydase in the injection allows for posterior spread, and it is not uncommon to see pupillary dilation and weakness of the extraocular muscles causing temporary diplopia after the injection. Gentle intermittent pressure is applied to the lids, and 15 minutes is allowed to elapse for the hemostatic properties of epinephrine to become effective.

SURGICAL TECHNIQUE

After sterile preparation with betadine solution and open-face draping of awake patients, the surgery begins with the transconjunctival incision. An assistant retracts the medial third of the lower eyelid downward with a medium or small Desmarres retractor to expose the cul-de-sac. A nonconductive eyelid plate (a Pyrex plate is available from Weiss Scientific Glass Blowing, Portland, OR, which also makes Jones tubes) is placed over the globe into the inferior fornix and is used to balotte the globe posteriorly. This action with the lid plate prolapses the orbital fat over the orbital rim. If the lower eyelid is too tight to allow adequate exposure, a lateral canthotomy and inferior cantholysis can be performed. This is rarely necessary, however. A needle-tip monopolar cutting cautery unit on a low setting is then used to palpate the medial, inferior orbital rim. We prefer the Valley Labs cautery unit set on 1.5 to 2.0 watts, and an insulated Colorado MicroDissection needle tip (available from Colorado Biomedical, Inc., Evergreen, CO). If the insulated cutting cautery needle tip is not available, a 19-gauge intracath can be placed over any cautery needle tip to avoid inadvertent cauterization of adjacent structures. An alternative cutting instrument that is very effective in lower blepharoplasty is the CO_2 laser, which can be used in the continuous or ultrapulse mode at a power of 7 to 10 watts to incise the conjunctiva. This setting may also be used to incise and vaporize the orbital fat.

The conjunctiva and lower lid retractors are incised directly over the fat with the needle tip directed 1 to 2 mm posterior to the inferior orbital rim. The incision may be made from medial to lateral beginning at the apex of the caruncle and extending to the lateral canthus, if necessary, to expose the lateral fat. The incision should be made at least 4 mm inferior to the inferior punctum to avoid damage to the canaliculus. An alternative technique is to make several small (5–7 mm) incisions over the individual fat pockets and connect them as necessary for full exposure. After incising the conjunctiva and lower lid retractors, yellow orbital fat can be seen bulging into the field (Fig. 48–20). Once the fat is noted, the connective tissue septae can be dissected away with the needle tip or toothed forceps until a tuft of fluffy yellow fat is exposed. At this point, the glass lid plate is removed, and the assistant grasps the posterior edge of the wound (lower lid retractors) with a 0.5-mm toothed forceps and lifts it up and over the globe. This maneuver protects the globe and further prolapses the fat into the surgical field. The Desmarres retractor can now be repositioned so that the blade is itself in the wound, providing wider exposure. With the connective tissue septae on stretch, the cutting cautery can then be used to open the fat compartments widely. The closer the fat compartment is opened to the orbital rim, the easier the exposure and the less chance of encountering bleeding or damage to the inferior oblique muscle.

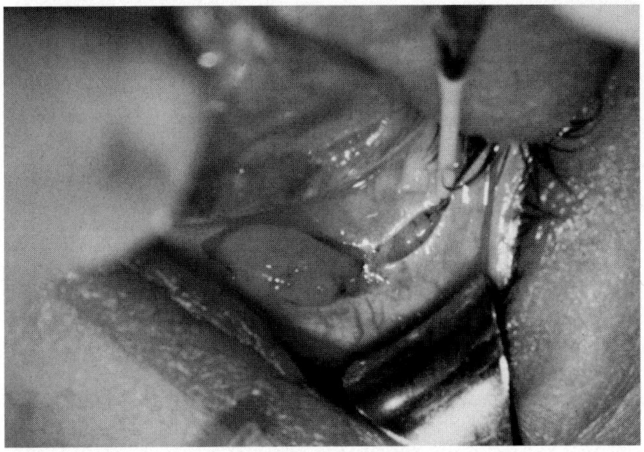

Figure 48–20. The conjunctiva is exposed, using a plastic eyelid plate over the cornea and a Desmarres retractor on the lower eyelid, and incised using cutting cautery or laser. (© Figure copyright 1996: Regents UC, University of California, Los Angeles reprinted with permission.)

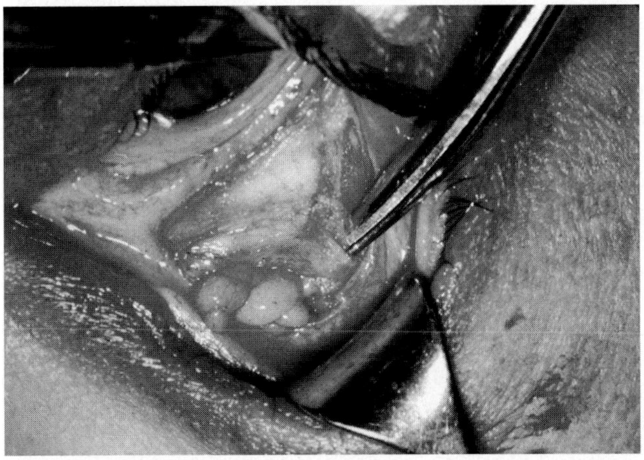

Figure 48–21. The arcuate expanse of the inferior oblique muscle separates the central and lateral fat pockets: here it is cut with a scissors. (© Figure copyright 1996: Regents UC, University of California, Los Angeles reprinted with permission.)

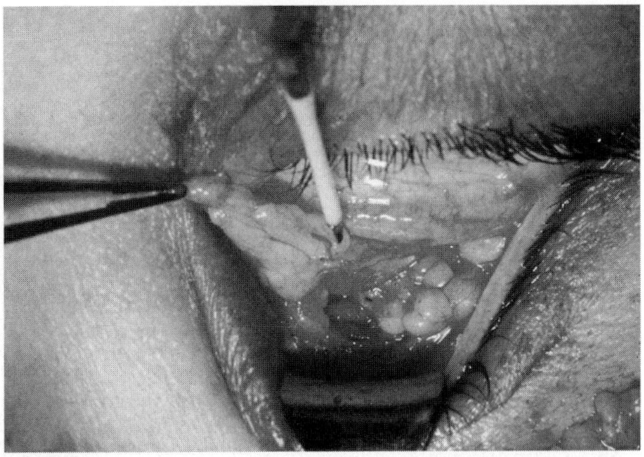

Figure 48–22. Medially, the valley of the inferior oblique muscle separates the central and medial fat compartments. Note the white appearance of the medial fat pad. (© Figure copyright 1996: Regents UC, University of California, Los Angeles reprinted with permission.)

Laterally, the arcuate expansion of the inferior oblique muscle separates the central fat pocket from the lateral fat pocket (Fig. 48–21). Incision of this fascial band at its attachment to the orbital rim, with scissors or cutting cautery, makes the central fat pocket continuous with the lateral fat pocket. This permits identification and exposure of the lateral fat pocket. The lateral fat pad is covered with more septae than the central pad and may not spring forward as easily. With excision of the superficial portion of the lateral pad, the fat posterior to this point comes forward more freely.

The medial fat compartment is the most difficult to locate, and partial resection of the central fat may be necessary to allow identification of the medial fat. Of note medially, the inferior oblique muscle separates the central and medial fat compartments. It is important to identify this "valley," especially for the surgeon who is learning this technique. Early identification will ensure that both the medial and central fat compartments are excised, and will avoid injury to the inferior oblique muscle. After identification and exposure of the central fat, the medial fat may be totally obscured, or may present as a slight bulge in the superior medial aspect of the wound. The glass lid plate can be replaced at this point and pressure placed on the globe to ballotte the fat forward. The needle tip can be used to sharply dissect the overlying septae. The medial fat is different from the central and lateral fat in that it appears white and membranous (Fig. 48–22). Additionally, it may not be postseptal at all; rather, it may come from the muscle cone, bulging around the edge of the lower eyelid retractors. The only difference between tthe lower eyelid medial fat pad and the medial fat pad in the upper lid is that the palpebral vessels go directly through the medial fat pad, as opposed to the upper eyelid where the medial vessels lie on the surface of the fat pad. Once the central and medial fat pads are excised, the inferior oblique muscle will be in plain view.

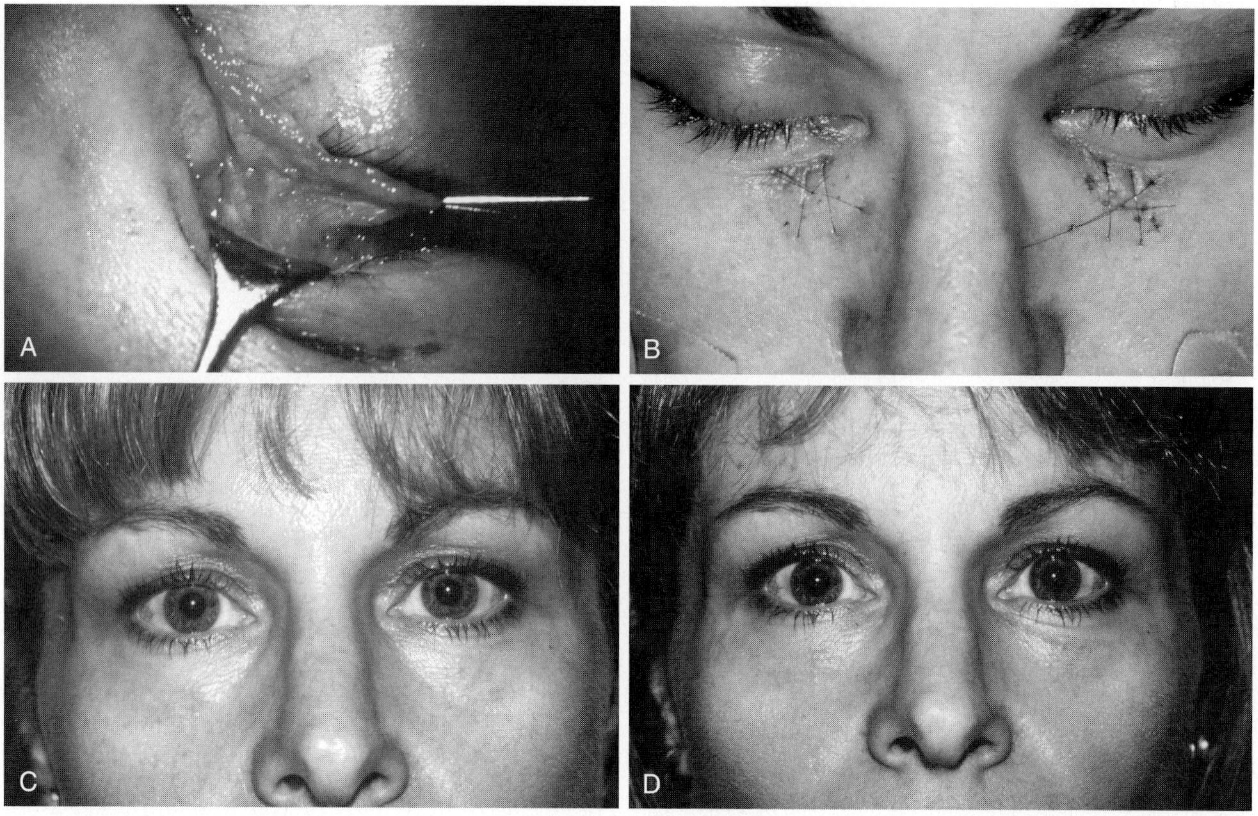

Figure 48–23. *A.* Surgical photo of medial fat pedicle prepared for placement outside the orbit, through the orbital septum. *B.* Photograph demonstrating construction of a 6-0 Prolene "cage." *C.* Preoperative photograph of young patient with prominent tear trough deformity. *D.* Postoperative photograph demonstrating improvement in lower eyelid contour of the patient in *C.* (© Figure copyright 1996: Regents UC, University of California, Los Angeles reprinted with permission.)

With advanced techniques, the medial fat pad can be sculpted into a pedicle that can then be transposed outside the orbit along the inferior orbital rim to fill in the tear trough deformity. The orbital septum is opened along the arcus marginalis, and the fat pedicle is arranged in a supraperiosteal, suborbicularis pocket (Fig. 48–23 *A–D*)

With the standard techniques, once all the fat is exposed as described above, the fat is excised in a careful graded fashion with a cutting monopolar cautery or a scissors. A small hemostat or clamp can be used to help define the line of excision when the exposure is tight. Before any excision of fat, it is useful to expose the fat of both lower eyelids, especially for the beginning surgeon, to allow for more symmetric fat excision. The end point of fat excision is reached when the anterior border of the fat is seen to be flush with the orbital rim while light pressure is applied to the globe, simulating upright posture. This results in a slight concavity of the lower lid when the patient lies supine. Meticulous hemostasis is necessary during the procedure. The blood vessels associated with each fat compartment should be directly visualized via blunt dissection with applicator tips, followed by cauterization with the monopolar cautery unit (Valley Labs cautery unit on Coag set at 2.0–2.5 Ws). Even when the CO_2 laser is used, it is best to have electrocautery available for the occasional vessel that is refractory to coagulation with the laser. There are some large vessels in the orbital fat pockets medially and, to a lesser extent, laterally. These can often be identified and cauterized before they are violated.

After excising the fat, the lower lid margin is pulled superiorly to release any adhesions that might result in lid retraction, as well as to realign the tissue planes. With the lid on stretch, gentle pressure on the globe reveals any residual fat bulges. If necessary, further fat can be excised at this point. In our experience, it is not necessary to close the conjunctiva and lower lid retractors; however, a single interrupted suture of 6-0 mild chromic gut is used to close the conjunctiva centrally if the tissues do not appear well opposed.

POSTOPERATIVE CARE AND COMPLICATIONS

UPPER BLEPHAROPLASTY

Upon completion of the procedure, antibiotic ophthalmic ointment is applied to the suture line and to the cornea. This ointment can be applied daily for approximately 1 week postoperatively. Because of the rich vascularity of the eyelids, eyelid infections after blepharoplasty are exceedingly rare, and so we do not use systemic antibiotic prophylaxis.

Ice "burritos" made with gauze or clean washcloths wrapped around crushed ice are applied continuously over the operated area for 24 to 48 hours to achieve local vasoconstriction and to minimize postoperative ecchymosis and edema. A mild, non-aspirin-containing, analgesic is used to control postoperative discomfort.

Blepharoplasty surgery should not result in significant discomfort. It is imperative that the patient be examined immediately if any pain is noted that is not relieved by analgesics. In patients with excessive pain, acute postoperative hemorrhage is present until proven otherwise. Blindness after blepharoplasty is the most dreaded complication, with an incidence of approximately 1/40,000. Early recognition and prompt intervention is the only way to minimize progression to blindness. The patient should be examined immediately and have a visual acuity and pupillary examination. Should any evidence of optic nerve compromise be present, the wound should be opened without hesitation, and all blood should be evacuated. Medical decompression of the orbit with systemic osmotic agents and corticosteroids should also be initiated. If no response is noted, radical cantholysis and surgical decompression of the orbit should be considered.

It is good practice for the surgeon to contact the patient on the evening of the surgery. A simple telephone call can alleviate the patient's anxiety and also identify potential warning signs that need immediate attention. The patient is usually examined 5 days after the surgery, as long as earlier problems do not arise. At that time, any nonabsorbable sutures are removed. We have noticed that absorbable sutures are more reactive, especially in the younger patients.

The postoperative ecchymosis and edema is expected to gradually improve over the following 2 to 3 weeks. When all the edema has subsided, the surgeon should critically examine the eyelid contour and shape, identifying suboptimal results such as noticeable asymmetry, irregularity, or webbing. In these circumstances, additional touch up or "enhancement" surgery may be required. The optimal timing for this surgery should be individualized, realizing that healing changes may continue for as long as 3 months, or even 6 months, after surgery. Therefore, there is often an advantage to waiting out subtle asymmetries or undercorrections.

LOWER BLEPHAROPLASTY

Antibiotic ophthalmic ointment is applied to the conjunctiva and ice compresses are immediately applied to the lower lids and, as much as tolerated, for the first 48 hours postoperatively. After the first 48 hours, warm compresses are used four times per day for an additional 7 to 10 days. The conjunctival incision makes soft contact lens wear difficult for the first week or two, but generally soft contacts can be successfully resumed within 10 days. Hard contact lenses can be resumed after 3 to 4 days. Postoperative bruising lasts 10 to 14 days, in general, and patients should be warned that postoperative ecchymosis may increase, or may first appear on the third postoperative day (with the switchover to warm compresses).

The most common complication of transconjunctival blepharoplasty, as reported in five published series, is inadequate fat excision, ranging from 0% to 20% of cases. As previously stated, we do not consider this a complication at all, rather an expected sequela given our conservative philosophy of graded fat excision. No cases of overexcision of fat have been reported; however, we have recently had one case of an overcorrection severe enough to warrant a postoperative fat graft. Lower eyelid malpositions have not previously been reported, but, again, we have recently seen several cases of lower eyelid retraction and malposition. Increased skin wrinkling and redundant lower eyelid skin were reported as complications in 1.6% to 3.3% of patients, while one small series of seven patients reported redundant skin in two (28.6%) cases. Again, this is easily remedied with careful preoperative evaluation and patient counseling, along with a skin-pinch excision or laser resurfacing at the time of transconjunctival fat excision.

No cases of permanent inferior oblique palsy have been reported after this procedure, but transient inferior oblique weakness has been noted. We have seen two cases of restrictive strabismus, with diplopia in the extremes of gaze associated with conjunctival symblepharon, neither of which completely resolved despite reoperation. Additionally, we consulted on a bizarre case of inadvertent disinsertion of the inferior rectus muscle from the globe during transconjunctival blepharoplasty. Fortunately the muscle was retrieved via an anterior orbitotomy 3 months later; it was reattached, and the diplopia resolved. We have reported one postoperative wound hemorrhage that resolved spontaneously without permanent ocular sequelae. Additionally, we have seen several cases of persistent conjunctival chemosis after transconjunctival blepharoplasty, all of which resolved over several months. Persistent chemosis was thought to be a direct result of incision placement too close to the globe. The potential complications of ocular infections, or periocular infections, and blindness have not been reported to date, nor have we observed these serious complications in any of our patients.

SUMMARY

Most blepharoplasty patients seek eyelid surgery because of age-related changes in the eyelid complex, while a minority are young, with "undesirable" congenital characteristics. The aging process in the eyelid complex is characterized by skin texture changes (with loss of elasticity and formation of wrinkles), enophthalmos (due to loss of fat), and lower eyelid fat prolapse (with inferior displacement of fat). Upper eyelid blepharoplasty is not a matter of skin removal; rather, it involves sculpturing and contouring of the asthetic init. Transconjunctival lower eyelid blepharoplasty is extremely effective at reducing lower eyelid "bags" caused by prolapsed orbital fat. The anterior-posterior blepharoplasty, consisting of transconjunctival lower blepharoplasty (or repositioning), and laser resurfacing is, in our hands, one of the most successful surgical procedures in facial aesthetic surgery. The blepharoplasty surgeon should avoid excessive fat removal. Instead, the focus should be on conservative fat removal, with or without fat repositioning. Total awareness will lead to successful rejuvenation of the aging eyelid complex.

SUGGESTED READINGS

Aiache AE, Ramirez OH: The suborbicularis oculi fat pads: An anatomic and clinical study. Plast Reconstr Surg 1995;95:37–42.

Baylis HI, Sutcliffe T, Fett DR: Levator injury during blepharoplasty. Arch Ophthalmol 1984;102:570–571.

Baylis HI, Long JA, Groth MJ: Transconjunctival lower eyelid blepharoplasty: Technique and complications. Ophthalmology 1989;96: 1027–1032.

Baylis HI, Wilson MC, Groth MJ: Complications of lower blepharoplasty. In Putterman AM (ed): Cosmetic Oculoplastic Surgery, 2nd Edition. Philadelphia, WB Saunders, 1993; pp. 356–388.

Dresner SC, Karesh JW: Transconjunctival entropion repair. Arch Ophthalmol 1993;111:1144–1148.

Edgerton MT Jr: Causes and prevention of lower eyelid ectropion following blepharoplasy. Plast Reconstr Surg 1972;49:367–373.

Flowers RS: Periorbital aesthetic surgery for men. Eyelids and related structures. Clin Plast Surg 1991;18:689–729.

Flowers RS: Optimal procedure in secondary blepharoplasty. Clin Plast Surg 1993;20:225–237.

Flowers RS: Canthopexy as a routine blepharoplasty component. Clin Plast Surg 1993;20:351–365.

Flowers RS, Caputy GG, Flowers SS: The biomechanics of brow and frontalis function and its effect on blepharoplasty. Clin Plast Surg 1993;20:255–268.

Flowers RS: Upper blepharoplasty by eyelid invagination. Anchor blepharoplasty. Clin Plast Surg 1993;20:193–207.

Flowers RS, Flowers SS: Precision planning in blepharoplasty. The importance of preoperative mapping. Clin Plast Surg 1993;20: 303–310.

Flowers RS, Flowers SS: Diagnosing photographic distortion. Decoding true postoperative contour after eyelid surgery. Clin Plast Surg 1993;20:387–392.

Goldberg RA, Edelstein C, Balch K, Shorr N: Fat repositioning in lower eyelid blepharoplasty. Semin Ophthalmol 1998;13:103–106.

Goldberg RA, Shorr N, Marmor MF, Christenbury JD, et al.: Blindness following blepharoplasty: Two case reports, and a discussion of management. Ophthal Surg 1990;21:85–89.

Hamako C, Baylis HI: Lower eyelid retraction after blepharoplasty. Am J Ophthalmol 1980;9:517–521.

Jelks GW, Jelks EB: Preoperative evaluation of the blepharoplasty patient. Bypassing the pitfalls. Clin Plast Surg 1993;20:213–223.

Koorneef L: Spatial Aspects of Orbital Musculo-fibrous Tissue in Man, Amsterdam, Swets and Zeitlinger, 1977; pp. 1–168.

Levine MR, Boyton J, Tenzell RR, Miller GR: Complications of blepharoplasty. Ophthal Surgery 1975;6:53–57.

May JW Jr, Fearon J, Zingarelli P: Retro-orbicularis oculus fat (ROOF) resection in aesthetic blepharoplasty: A 6-year study in 63 patients. Plast Reconstr Surg 1990;86:682–689.

McKinney P, Zukowski ML, Mossie RD: The fourth option: A novel approach to lower lid blepharoplasty. Aesth Plast Surg 1991;15: 293–296.

Neuhaus RW: Lower eyelid blepharoplasty. J Dermatol Surg Oncol 1992;18:1100–1109.

Palmer FR, Rice DH, Churukian MM: Transconjunctival blepharoplasty complications and their avoidance: A retrospective analysis and review of the literature. Arch Head Neck Surg 1993; 119:993–999.

Parkes M, Fein W, Brennan HG: Pinch technique for repair of cosmetic eyelid deformities. Arch Ophthalmol 1973;89:324–328.

Perman KI: Upper eyelid blepharoplasty. J Dermatol Surg Oncol 1992;18:1096-1099.

Sheen JH: Supratarsal fixation in upper blepharoplasty. Plast Reconstr Surg 1974;54:424–431.

Suh CD: Laser double eyelid operation. Aesth. Plast. Surg. 1999;23:343–348.

Sutcliffe T, Baylis HI, Fett DR: Bleeding in cosmetic blepharoplasty: An anatomical approach. Ophthal Plast Reconstr Surg 1985;1: 107–113.

Tomlinson FB, Hovey LM: Transconjunctival lower blepharoplasty for removal of fat. Plast Reconstr Surg 1975;56:314–318.

Warwick R: Eugene Wolff's Anatomy of the Eye and Orbit: Including the Central Connections, Development and Comparative Anatomy of the visual Apparatus, 7th Edition. Philadelphia, WB Saunders, 1976; p. 273.

CHAPTER 49

Enucleation and Evisceration

WILLIAM R. NUNERY, M.D., JOHN D. NG, M.D.,
and KATHY J. HETZLER, B.C.O., F.A.S.O.

Enucleation is the removal of the globe from the orbit. Evisceration is the removal of the intraocular contents, including the uvea but leaving the sclera, the optic nerve, and the extraocular muscles intact. To achieve maximum cosmetic outcome, both enucleation and evisceration are usually accompanied by surgical placement of an orbital implant within the orbit or the remaining scleral shell.

In this chapter, we present the indications for enucleation and evisceration, the importance of a sound patient-physician relationship, our surgical techniques for enucleation and evisceration along with their complications and the prosthetic rehabilitation of the enucleated or eviscerated socket.

Tables are included to facilitate quick reference to the indications for these procedures and to provide step-by-step references to the procedure described.

INDICATIONS FOR ENUCLEATION AND EVISCERATION

The first indication for enucleation is a blind eye that causes chronic pain from elevated pressure, chronic inflammation, or ciliary sensitivity (Table 49–1). Topical medications to alleviate pain include cycloplegics, nonsteroidal anti-inflammatory agents, steroids, and ocular antihypertensives. Topical medications are usually only temporarily effective and occasionally produce chronic irritation or allergic reaction. Long-term use of systemic pain control such as narcotics is unjustifiable because of addictive or abuse potential. Retrobulbar alcohol blocks may provide temporary relief, but they induce a prominent acute inflammatory response and may produce cosmetically objectionable results by inducing an orbital apex syndrome. Enucleation is permanent, effective, and safer than most alternatives when chronic pain occurs in a blind eye.

In general, no eye with nonmalignant disease should be enucleated or eviscerated while light perception exists, because even bare light perception is preferable to no light perception, which might occur in the event of unforeseen loss of the better eye. Exceptional indications for enucleation in an eye with vision include the presence of intraocular malignancy and following severe penetrating globe trauma with a poor visual prognosis, to prevent sympathetic ophthalmia. Also, patients with severe pain in an eye with minimal vision must evaluate the merits of enucleation for pain relief versus the risk of some future injury to the better eye. Table 49–1 lists the indications for both enucleation and evisceration.

TABLE 49–1. Indications for Enucleation and Evisceration

Enucleation
- In a blind eye:
  1. Chronic pain
  2. Objectionable appearance
  3. Atrophy bulbi
  4. Unilateral uncontrollable glaucoma
  5. Unilateral uncontrollable iritis
  6. Hypoplasia in childhood
  7. Prevention of sympathetic ophthalmia
- In a seeing eye:
  1. Treatment of intraocular malignancy
  2. Prevention of sympathetic ophthalmia
  3. Severely painful eye with very poor vision

Evisceration
- In a blind eye:
  1. Active endophthalmitis
  2. In a severely ill patient who cannot tolerate general anesthesia and would benefit from a shorter procedure under local anesthesia
  3. In a patient with a bleeding disorder

A cosmetically disfiguring blind eye is the second indication for enucleation. In view of the importance of the eyes to the patient's overall appearance and self-image, a cosmetically objectionable blind eye is ample reason for enucleation, even when no other indication is present.

The third indication for enucleation in a blind eye is atrophy bulbi. Because phthisis is a histologic term and not a clinical term, the presence of phthisis bulbi must be inferred from the clinical findings of a hypotonic, atrophic, and opaque globe.[1] In atrophy bulbi, the cornea may be opaque and shrunken. The normally spherical eye may become squared, and the detached retina may be replaced with a dense cyclitic membrane. Hyaline degeneration occurs in the choroid and connective tissue. Calcification may also occur in the retina and choroid.[1]

Phthisical eyes have an increased incidence of choroidal malignant melanoma. This incidence has been estimated at 4% to 15%.[1,2] Melanomas have been found in 21% of enucleated eyes that had opaque media,[1] and 12% of these melanomas had been unsuspected prior to enucleation.[3] Because eyes with opaque media are difficult to examine clinically for choroidal melanoma, enucleation can be prophylactic for the development of malignant disease in the degenerating eye.

Eyes with unilateral glaucoma or uveitis may also harbor melanoma. This is particularly true when opaque media are present. Ten percent of eyes enucleated for end-stage uncontrollable glaucoma and opaque media harbor unsuspected choroidal melanoma.[2] Enucleation may therefore be preferable to filtering procedures or cyclodestructive procedures for relief of pain caused by elevated intraocular pressure in a blind eye. If an atrophic eye is not enucleated, it should be examined on a yearly basis with A-scan and B-scan ultrasonography to rule out the development of melanoma.

A fourth indication for enucleation in a blind or seeing eye is the presence of suspected intraocular malignancy, such as retinoblastoma or melanoma. Unnecessarily traumatic enucleation for malignant disease, however, may actually hasten metastatic spread.[4,5] When enucleation is undertaken for malignant disease, careful attention should be paid to technique. Technique modifications for malignant disease will be discussed below.

A fifth indication for enucleation—with placement of an orbital implant—is aplasia or severe hypoplasia of a globe in childhood. Full orbital volume is essential for the development of the bony structure of the orbit.[6] Experimental anophthalmos in kittens demonstrates reduction of orbital volume by 30% or more following removal of a normal volume eye. Observation on human skulls with congenital anophthalmos demonstrates reduction in skull size up to 60%.[6,7] Loss of orbital volume following enucleation in childhood without an implant may be 30%. This bony asymmetry can be minimized by early placement of a large orbital implant. The implant may be progressively enlarged as the child grows if asymmetry is observed. Alternatively, an expandable implant may be used until the orbit and skull have reached mature size, when a permanent implant should be substituted.[8,9] The child remains at risk for bony asymmetry until after age 13 years.[7]

A sixth indication for enucleation is prophylaxis against the development of sympathetic ophthalmia after penetrating ocular trauma. Sympathetic ophthalmia is an autoimmune, lymphocytic attack on the uveal tract of both eyes following sensitization of lymphocytes to uveal tissue after penetrating trauma in one eye.[10] It may also occur rarely after intraocular surgery or in the presence of choroidal melanoma. Histologically, nodular aggregates of lymphocytes are seen within the uvea, particularly the choroid.[1] This ultimately leads to choroidal atrophy with secondary retinal atrophy.

Sympathetic ophthalmia occurs most commonly after penetrating ocular trauma. Rare cases have been reported as early as 5 days following injury, and as late as 50 years later.[10] Ninety percent, however, occur between 2 weeks and 1 year after penetrating ocular injury.[10] The incidence of sympathetic ophthalmia after penetrating ocular injury is not completely agreed upon. It has been estimated to be as high as 3% to 5% of cases in one series.[1] While this figure may seem high, it is clear that sympathetic ophthalmia does occasionally occur and compounds the tragedy of a penetrating ocular injury.[11]

Enucleation of the injured eye prior to the development of sympathetic ophthalmia may prevent its occurrence. Enucleation to prevent sympathetic ophthalmia is usually performed in either a blind eye or a poorly seeing eye with very poor visual prognosis. Enucleation after the development of sympathetic ophthalmia, however, has no beneficial effect. Evisceration does not protect against sympathetic ophthalmia and may actually encourage its development.

The actual presence of sympathetic ophthalmia is clearly not an indication for enucleation. The presence of sympathetic ophthalmia may be a relative contraindication to enucleation, since enucleation will not be therapeutic once the sympathetic ophthalmia has been initiated. Because sympathetic ophthalmia is a bilateral disease, the originally injured eye may, at some point in the course of the disease, become the better eye, and should therefore, be preserved.

After penetrating ocular injury, a discussion with the patient should outline the likelihood of visual recovery in the individual case, as well as the possibility of development of sympathetic ophthalmia. The decision to enucleate or not to enucleate the injured eye should be made within the first 7 to 10 days after injury and should be based on the relative severity of the injury as well as the patient's informed knowledge of the risks of sympathetic ophthalmia.

Treatment of sympathetic ophthalmia, after the diagnosis is made, is with topical and systemic steroids and immunosuppressive agents, depending on the severity of the inflammation.[10,11]

Evisceration is performed for many of the same reasons as enucleation, with the exception of a few circumstances discussed below. The first indication for evisceration is in a blind eye with active, uncontrolled endophthalmitis. Evisceration may be less likely to lead to spread of infection to cerebral spinal fluid than would enucleation, in which severing of the optic nerve sheath is required.[12] If infection has already spread through the sclera, however, enucleation may be necessary to remove all the infected tissue. Oftentimes, a secondary enucleation is performed after the infection has cleared.

The second relative indication for evisceration occurs in a severely ill patient who cannot tolerate general anesthesia. Evisceration of a blind eye is technically easier and quicker to perform under local anesthesia than enucleation and therefore may be of benefit to the severely ill or elderly patient.

A third indication for evisceration is a blind eye in a patient with a severe bleeding disorder or in anticoagulated patients. Fewer orbital blood vessels are severed in an evisceration, thereby reducing the risk of greater blood loss or orbital hemorrhage.

Evisceration is contraindicated in the presence of intraocular malignancy, because it may contribute to dissemination of the disease. Similarly, evisceration should not be used in atrophi bulbi and hypoplasia in childhood because an adequate sized implant cannot be placed inside the scleral shell, if one is even present in the latter entity. As stated earlier, an eye with atrophy bulbi may also harbor an unsuspected malignancy, which may be disseminated by an evisceration. Evisceration should not be performed for prophylaxis against sympathetic ophthalmia, because choroidal tissue may not be completely removed even with the best of techniques. Figure 49–1 is a decision flow chart demonstrating a useful method of choosing between performing an enucleation and an evisceration.

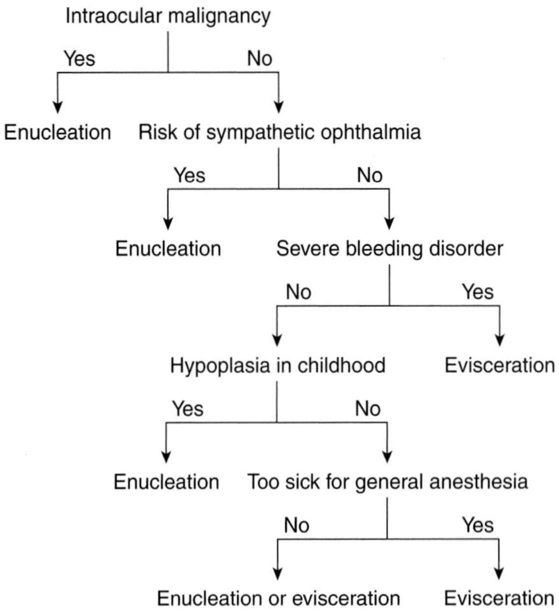

Figure 49–1. Flow chart for enucleation vs. evisceration.

PSYCHOLOGICAL CONSIDERATIONS

Once a recommendation for enucleation or evisceration is determined, the surgeon must be prepared to recognize and deal with the psychological sequelae the patient will experience. This requires a sound physician–patient relationship from the outset. Regardless of the clinical situation, the enucleation/evisceration patient will experience predictable phases of psychiatric adjustment. The first stage after the procedure is usually a period of denial, followed by depression or anger, and finally, the patient reaches a stage of acceptance and rehabilitation.

These responses occur in any loss of a significant body part, but the loss of an eye is particularly traumatic. In addition to the sensory deprivation associated with loss of vision, the patient must adjust to altered body image for the most cosmetically crucial part of the body. Also, because direct eye-to-eye contact is the basis for communication and self-expression, and plays a role in social-interpersonal relationships, anophthalmic patients may have to adjust their entire method of communication and social interaction, as well as their self-image.

Because the loss of an eye often occurs suddenly due to trauma, infection, or unsuspected malignancy, the patient is poorly prepared to deal with these crises. Even when the patient has many years to contemplate enucleation, as in progressive glaucoma or diabetes, we can expect the same reactions.

We have found that the best method of promoting psychiatric rehabilitation following enucleation is to expect these reactions, and allow time to deal with them. Patients are given the opportunity to express anger or depression. They should be reassured that these feelings are normal, healthy, and typical of any anophthalmic patient's reaction. Patients should be encouraged to allow themselves a period of grief.

Many patients are comforted to learn that the condition of anophthalmos is common in the population. The likelihood is that they know other anophthalmic patients, perhaps without being aware of their anophthalmic condition.

When patients express cosmetic concerns or insist on wearing a patch to cover the socket, they should be encouraged to accept the new body image without shame or apology. When patients accept this, they will also accept the way they imagine that others see them. We encourage all our patients to discard patches or cover shields within 4 weeks of enucleation.

Finally, patients should be encouraged by the physician's or ocularist's experience of seeing many other patients pass through these cycles of grief and depression and emerge again into a productive, self-confident life. When the physician observes unusually severe or prolonged grief responses to enucleation, or believes depression may be suicidal in severity, the patient should be referred to a psychiatrist for further treatment.

TECHNIQUES FOR ENUCLEATION

Various techniques for enucleation have been available since the 16th century, although the lack of anesthesia and the brutality of the procedure made enucleation an operation that was performed only under the most dire circumstances. Bartisch, in 1583,[13] first recorded a technique that involved engaging the eye with a hook or other retraction instrument and making random slashes with a variety of blunt or sharp instruments until adequate tissue was removed from the socket.

It was not until 1841 that O'Farrell described an enucleation technique similar to current techniques.[14] Spivey described elevating the conjunctiva, separating the rectus muscles from the globe, and transecting the optic nerve.[14]

Modifications and improvements have been introduced since that time. In 1885, Mules described the use of a spherical orbital implant to reduce the volume loss after enucleation.[14,15]

Most enucleation techniques are derived from similar principles and vary only in the subtleties of location of the implant and technique of reattaching disinserted extraocular muscles. The author's preferred modification of the enucleation technique will be presented.

Enucleation can be performed under either general or local anesthesia, although general anesthesia is preferable. Under local anesthesia, stimulation of the optic nerve at the time of transection may lead to sudden, intense visual perception known as the Augenblick phenomenon. This may be distressing to the patient and lead him or her to question whether the enucleated eye was truly blind. Also, retrobulbar anesthesia may not lead to complete loss of sensation in the extraocular muscle tissue. This may result in a procedure that is uncomfortable for the patient and technically difficult for the surgeon.

AUTHORS' TECHNIQUE

After administration of general anesthesia, 10 cc of 1% lidocaine with 1:100,000 dilution epinephrine in a 50:50 mixture with 0.5% plain bupivacaine are injected subconjunctivally around the limbus and into the retrobulbar space. The injection of local anesthesia assists in the separation of the conjunctiva from the sclera, aids in the hemostasis of the orbit, and provides temporary postoperative pain control.

Sutures of 4-0 silk are then placed through the center of the lid margin in the upper and lower eyelids. These sutures are attached to hemostats and used for retraction of the eyelids during the procedures. An eyelid speculum may be used as a substitute for the eyelid retraction sutures (Fig. 49–2). A 360 degree limbal peritomy is performed with Wescott scissors, simultaneously dissecting off Tenon's fascia down to

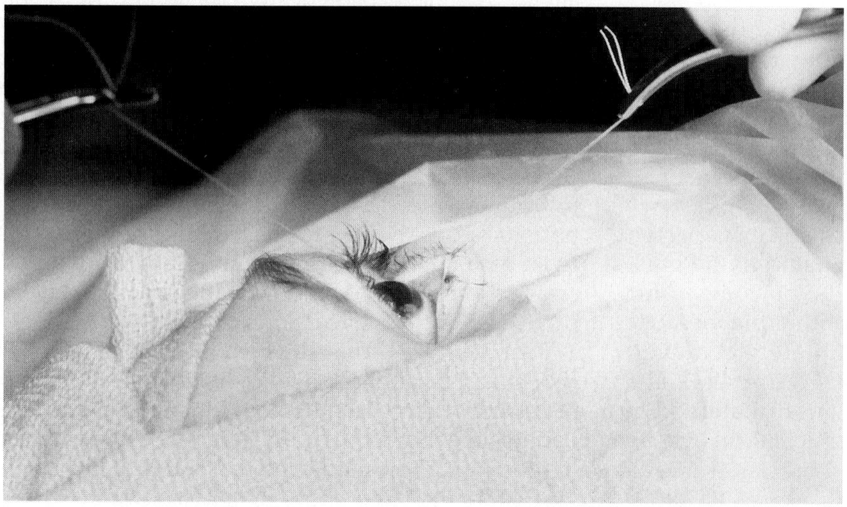

Figure 49–2. Lid retraction sutures.

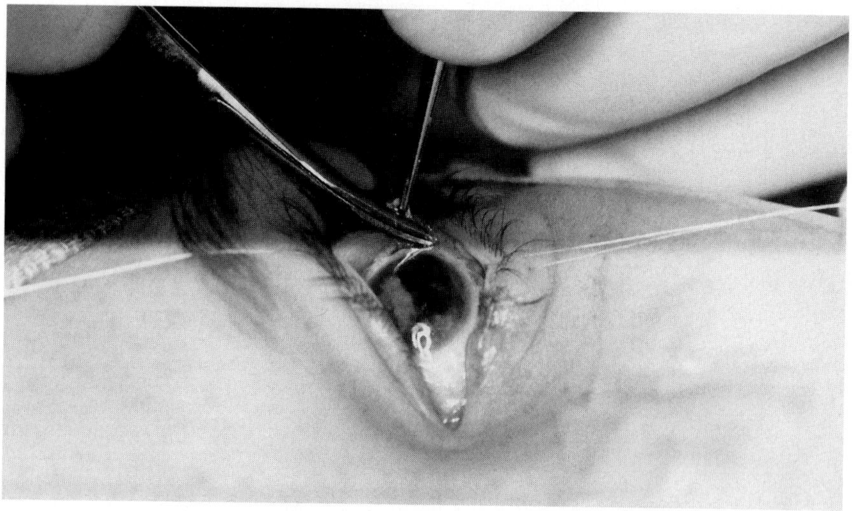

Figure 49–3. Conjunctival peritomy.

bare sclera and taking care to preserve all conjunctival tissue (Fig. 49–3).

Once the conjunctiva and Tenon's fascia are elevated off the sclera, a curved hemostat is used to bluntly dissect the posterior Tenon's fascia off the globe in all four quadrants between the four rectus muscles. The tips of the hemostat should be kept on the surface of the sclera while they are spread. This provides an accessible plane from which to isolate the extraocular muscles (Fig. 49–4).

A muscle hook is inserted behind the medial rectus muscle to engage it. Keeping the tip of the muscle hook against the sclera while passing it behind the muscle insertion will keep it from snagging Tenon's fascia. A second muscle hook passed from the opposite edge of the muscle will help ensure that the entire muscle is isolated. A small amount of Tenon's fascia may be carefully dissected from the muscle insertion site for better visualization. The integrity of Tenon's fascia should otherwise be maintained to facilitate placement of the orbital implant later in the procedure.

A doubled-armed 5-0 Vicryl suture is passed through the substance of the muscle near its insertion site. Locking bites at each edge of the muscle will provide added security. The muscle tendon is then transected from the globe using Wescott scissors (Fig. 49–5). A small stump of tendon may be left on the sclera to assist in manipulation and retraction of the globe. In a similar manner, the remaining three rectus muscles are isolated, ligated with 5-0 Vicryl sutures, and disinserted from the globe. All needles are left on the sutures for later use in the procedure. Small bulldog clamps may be applied to the sutures of each muscle to reduce tangling of the sutures.

The superior oblique muscle tendon is then engaged with the muscle hook by passing it from the superonasal quadrant out laterally. Once isolated, the tendon is transected with Wescott scissors. The superior oblique muscle may be secured to the superior rectus muscle by passing the sutures already attached to the superior rectus through the superior surface of the superior oblique tendon and securing it with several knots. Once again, the sutures are left intact.

In a similar manner, the inferior oblique muscle is isolated by passing a muscle hook from the inferonasal quadrant, sweeping it posterolaterally toward the area of the macula. The inferior oblique tendon is transected and secured to the lateral rectus muscle just as the superior oblique muscle was to the superior rectus.

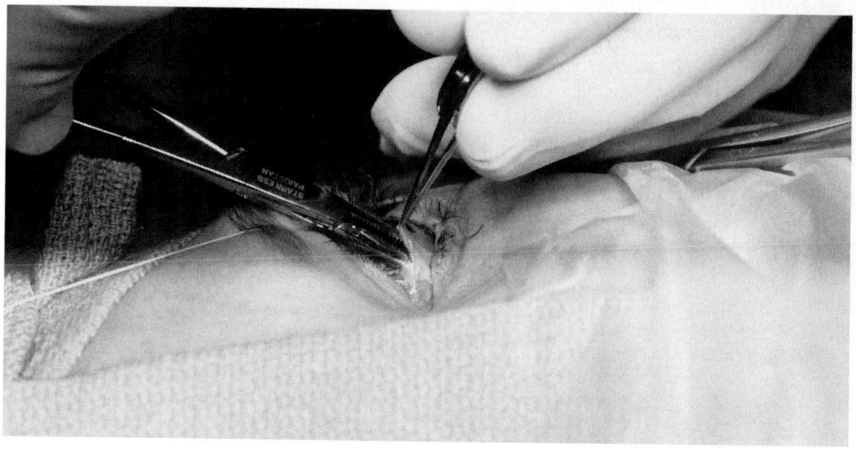

Figure 49–4. Clearing of Tenon's fascia from quadrants with hemostat.

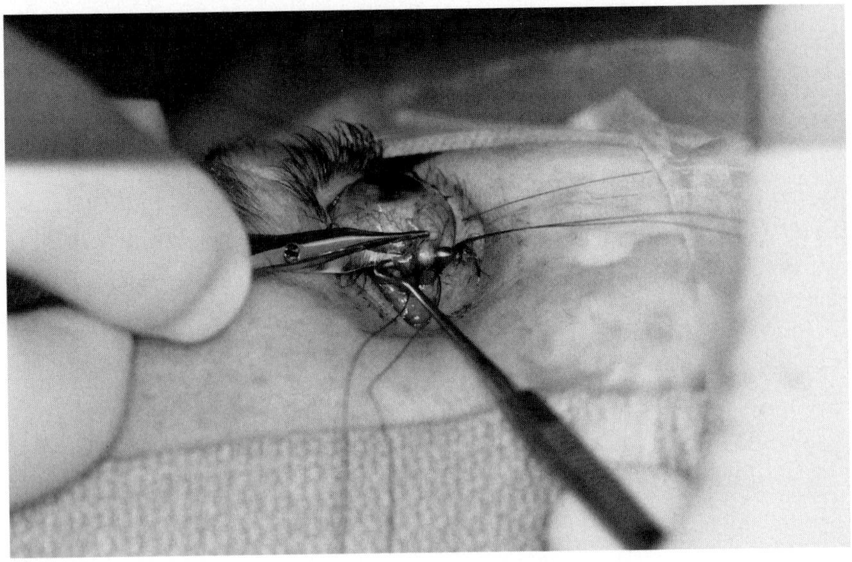

Figure 49–5. Hooked muscle with sutures attached, being cut with Wescott scissors.

This maneuver provides an inferior hammock that may help support the weight of the orbital implant (Fig. 49–6).

After disinsertion of all extraocular muscle attachments, a careful inspection of the globe is made to be certain that all Tenon's fascia attachments have been bluntly dissected away from the globe. The vortex veins can be identified and cauterized to reduce bleeding. Blunt dissection and inspection are carried back to the optic nerve sheath.

The nerve is transected with either a pair of enucleation scissors or an enucleation snare (Fig. 49–7*A* and *B*). If scissors are used, it may be helpful to crush the optic nerve with a hemostat prior to transection. In this technique, a curved hemostat is inserted behind the globe from a medial approach with the concave angle facing anteriorly and the tip toward the optic nerve. The hemostat is used to feel the optic nerve with the tips closed. Once the nerve is located the tips of the hemostat are separated and the instrument is slipped around the nerve. The hemostat is then slid posteriorly along the nerve toward the apex of the orbit while the tips are angled toward the medial wall. Once the hemostat is as far posterior along the nerve as possible, the nerve is clamped for hemostasis. A curved enucleation scissors is placed just above the hemostat using the same maneuver. Next, transect the nerve just above the hemostat. Bipolar cautery may be used to coagulate the transected nerve end to seal off the central retinal artery.

If an enucleation snare is used, clamping of the nerve is not necessary as the snare will crush the nerve

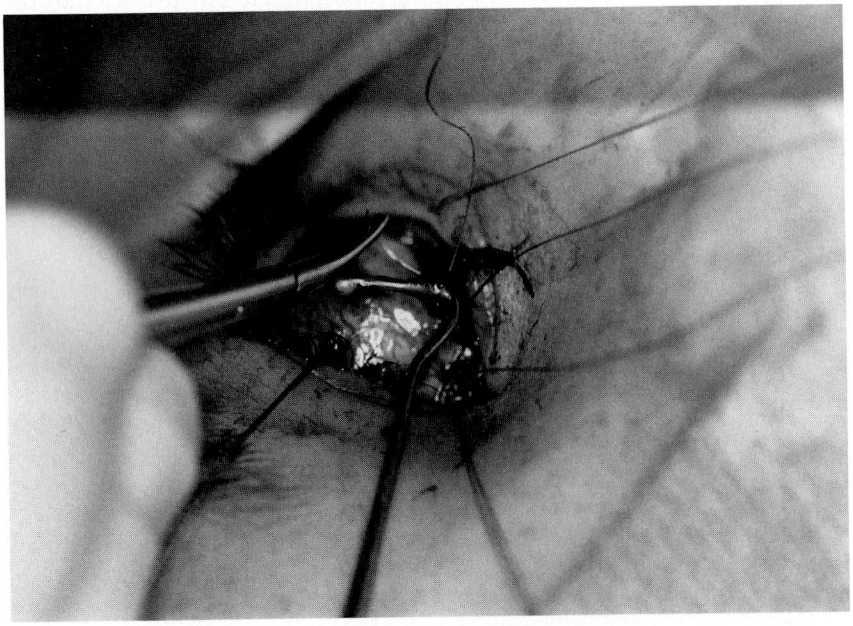

Figure 49–6. Attaching inferior oblique to lateral rectus muscle.

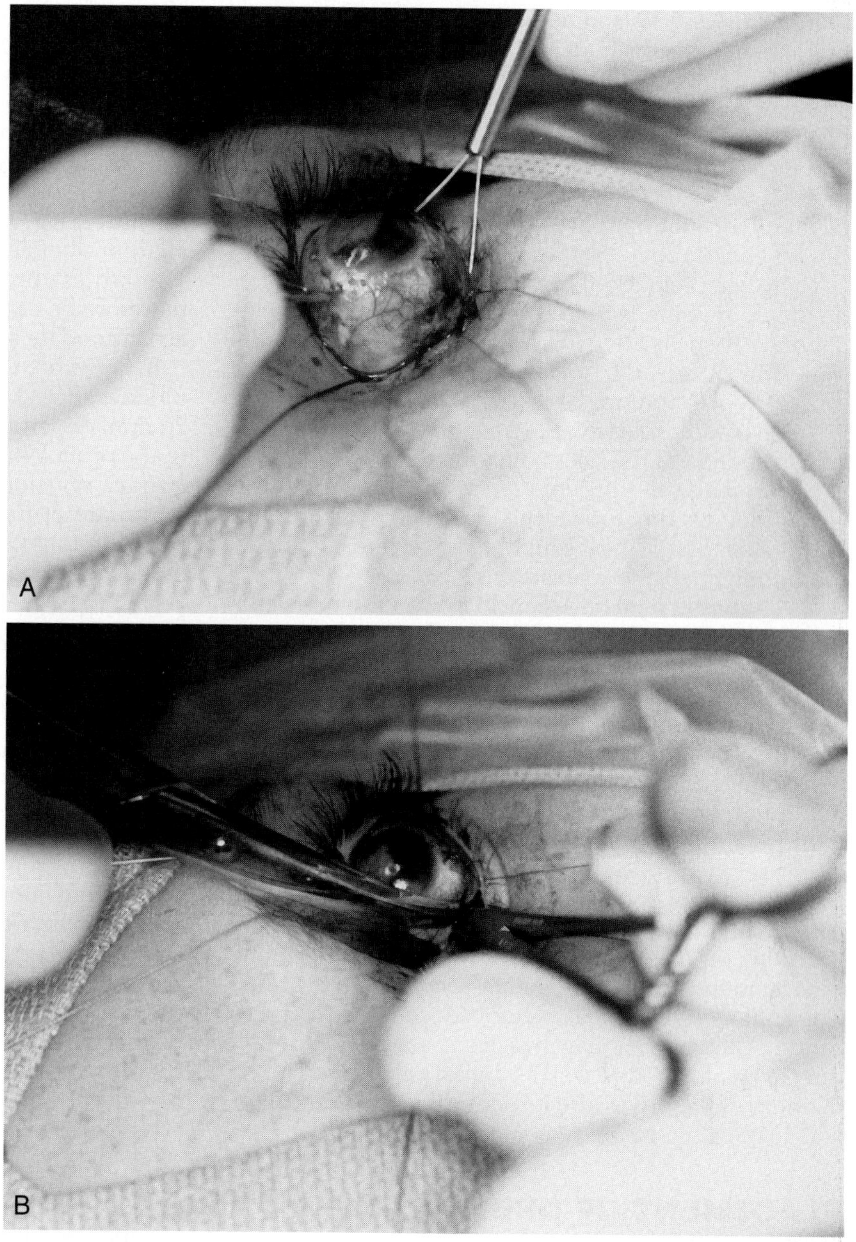

Figure 49–7. *A.* Enucleation snare in place. *B.* Clamp and enucleation scissors in place.

during transection. The snare loop is placed around the globe, being sure the extraocular muscles and other orbital tissue are not engaged. This can be done from either a lateral or a medial approach. Once around the globe, the wire loop is tightened so it is just slightly larger than the diameter of the nerve. The snare is then slid posteriorly along the nerve to the apex before it is used to sever the nerve. This maneuver minimizes the risk of transecting other orbital contents. The severed nerve end may be located and cauterized if desired. When done properly, there should be at least a 5 mm segment of optic nerve attached to the globe. In cases of intraocular malignancy, a longer segment of 10 mm is desired.

Bleeding is usually minimal, especially when the snare is used. When bleeding does occur one can pack the orbit with thrombin soaked gelfoam and apply direct pressure. Random and excessive cautery must be avoided as damage to apical structures or chiasmal injury from transmission along the optic nerve toward the chiasm may result. Likewise, excessive traction on the optic nerve should be avoided.

THE "NO TOUCH" TECHNIQUE

The "no touch" technique was advocated by Fraunfelder and Wilson[4] for enucleation of eyes that harbor intraocular malignancy such as choroidal melanoma. Zimmerman, McLean, and Foster[5] have suggested that enucleation may precipitate metastatic spread of melanoma through the dissemination of tumor emboli.

Fraunfelder and Wilson demonstrated that intraocular pressure may rise as high as 370 mm during scleral depression, rapid injection of retrobulbar medication, or pressure on the eye during enucleation.[4] They further demonstrated that hamsters with intraocular melanoma survived longer when an atraumatic enucleation technique was used than did hamsters in which the melanoma-containing eye was deliberately massaged during enucleation.

They then proposed the no touch technique, in which no direct pressure is placed on the eye during enucleation. All tissue is lifted away from the eye prior to cutting. The extraocular muscles are cut without using muscle hooks, and no blepharostat is used to hold the lids open. After release of extraocular muscles, a cryo ring is applied to the sclera over the tumor. The tumor is frozen with intermittent cryo treatment during the remainder of the procedure. With this technique, Fraunfelder and Wilson sought to lessen the likelihood of tumor emboli and metastatic spread.

No studies to date have conclusively shown the efficacy of the no touch technique in reducing the mortality associated with enucleation for intraocular melanoma. Prudence, however, would dictate the most delicate enucleation possible when dealing with an intraocular malignancy. In eyes with tumors, we modify our technique by keeping the traction on the eye to a minimum when hooking the extraocular muscles. The muscles are transected from the globe with a slightly larger segment of tendon left on the globe. Minimal traction on the globe is used when severing the optic nerve with the snare or scissors. Attention to leaving a very long segment of optic nerve attached to the globe is paramount. Sutures are not passed through the muscles until after the globe is removed from the orbit. Location of the extraocular muscles is achieved through direct visualization as well as digital palpation. The remainder of the procedure is identical to the non-tumor enucleations.

PLACEMENT OF ORBITAL IMPLANT

Placement of an orbital prosthesis is almost universally performed in tandem with an enucleation. Patients with psychiatric disorders involving ritualistic rubbing of the eye would be one reason to avoid placement of an implant as it would assuredly extrude. We will describe our technique for placement of both the silicone sphere and the hydroxyapatite implant. Dermal-fat grafting will also be described because it is a valuable technique for replenishing surface area and orbital volume.

SILICONE SPHERE

Once the enucleation has been performed as described above, a silicone sphere of appropriate size is selected. A 22.4-mm spherical implant coupled with an average-sized ocular prosthesis will adequately fill orbital volume in an enucleated socket.[16] If the implant is less than 20 mm, orbital volume loss with secondary orbital deformities will result.

Fox has stated that implants larger than 18 mm may contribute to high extrusion rates.[17] Secondary extrusion of the orbital implant, however, is related more to the integrity of the Tenon's fascia closure and the anatomic barriers to extrusion than to the implant size. The largest implant possible, up to 20 mm, should therefore be employed. Most anophthalmic orbits can accommodate a 20-mm sphere.

In children, the largest implant the orbit can accommodate should be placed. This may be between 14 and 20 mm, depending on the age of the child and the size of the orbit. When smaller implants are employed, secondary revisions of the implant may be necessary to stimulate optimal growth of the orbit during childhood. In infants, the largest implant the orbit will tolerate should be used.

Authors' Technique

Once the silicone sphere is selected, it may be placed into the orbit unwrapped. Alternatively, it may be wrapped in banked or autogenous sclera or fascia lata or a 1 mm thickness piece of Gortex sheet. The wrapping material is placed around the implant and trimmed to minimize excess material, which will form dog ears when sewn. Once trimmed, 5-0 Vicryl or a permanent suture such as silk or prolene may be used to approximate the edges of the wrap (Fig. 49–8). If sclera is used, the implant will be exposed at the corneal opening, which will be placed facing the apex of the orbit. If donor tissue is used, the patient must be made aware of the risks of viral transmission. If autogenous sclera from the enucleated eye is used, residual fascia, extraocular muscle, and optic nerve should be trimmed off. The uvea must be meticu-

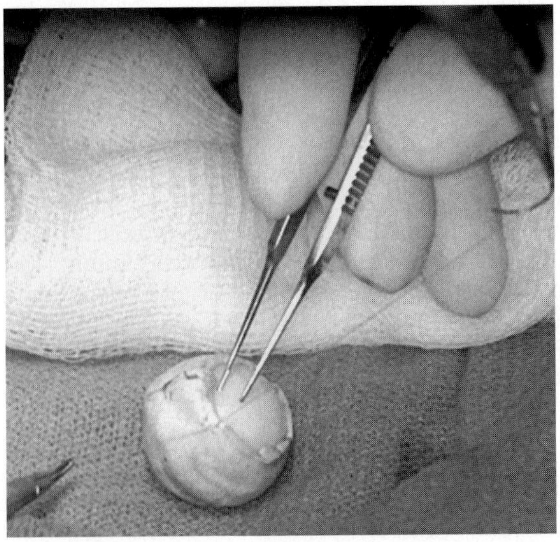

Figure 49–8. Wrapping of implant sphere.

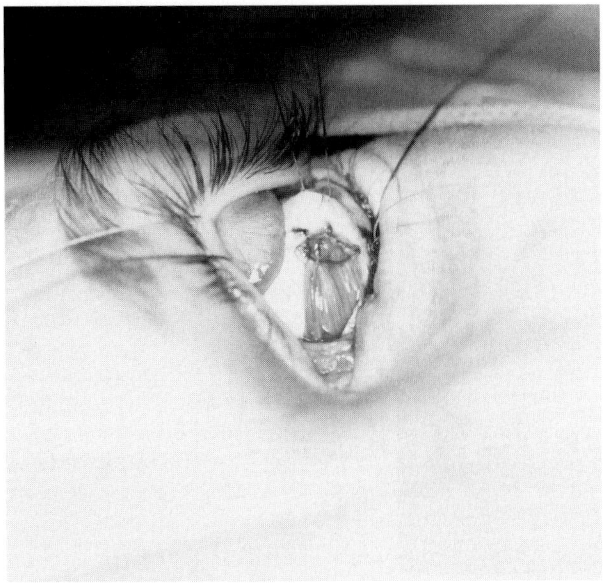

Figure 49–9. Muscles sewn onto implant.

lously scrubbed off the sclera. To ensure complete removal and denaturing of uveal antigens, the sclera may be scrubbed with 100% ethanol or 10% phenol and then rinsed thoroughly with normal saline or antibiotic solution. Autogenous sclera should never be used in a case involving intraocular infection or suspected malignancy.

The prepared implant is then placed deep within the muscle cone. The extraocular muscles are sewn to the implant in their approximate normal anatomical positions. The muscles are sewn to the wrapping material or directly to the silicone sphere, using the previously placed sutures. The needles are left on the sutures after the muscles are attached to the implant (Fig. 49–9). The muscles should not be imbricated over the anterior surface of the implant because this will not provide a barrier for extrusion, as the implant may easily extrude through the area between the rectus muscles. Furthermore, the imbricating technique encourages migration of the implant, usually in the superior temporal direction.[17,18] Problems associated with the migrated implant include a socket difficult to fit prosthetically, ptosis of the upper eyelid, and compromise of the fornices.

Tenon's fascia and the conjunctiva are then draped over the implant. Next, all four double-armed sutures still attached to the muscles and implant are passed full thickness through the overlying fascia and conjunctiva from the deep to anterior surface, without shortening the fornices or retracting the tissue edges. The sutures are then tied and trimmed (Fig. 49–10). This maneuver pulls the tissue layers posteriorly onto the implant. When this is done properly, the conjunctival edges should be nearly approximated. Tenon's fascia is then closed in two layers with interrupted, 5-0 Vicryl sutures with buried knots (Fig. 49–11). The conjunctiva should be easily closed with a running 5-0 Vicryl suture without any tension on the wound (Fig. 49–12).

Once the wound is closed, antibiotic ointment is placed into the fornices and a plastic conformer is placed behind the lids. The conformer should be as large as possible but not so large that it places tension on the wound when the lids are closed over it. A 6-0 mild chromic suture tarsorrhaphy is then performed to keep the conformer in place during the first postoperative week (Fig. 49–13). No dressing is required, although a light dressing may be applied.

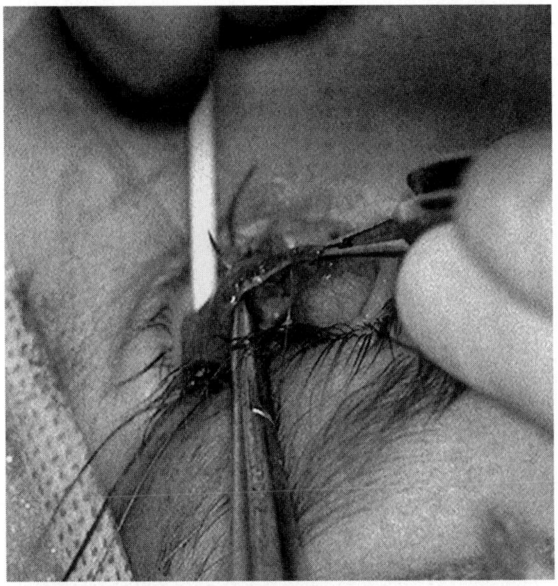

Figure 49–10. Sutures passed through Tenon's fascia and conjunctiva.

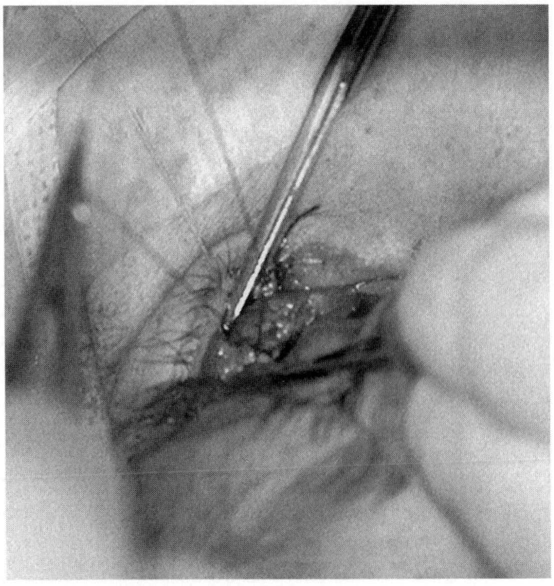

Figure 49–11. Suturing Tenon's fascia.

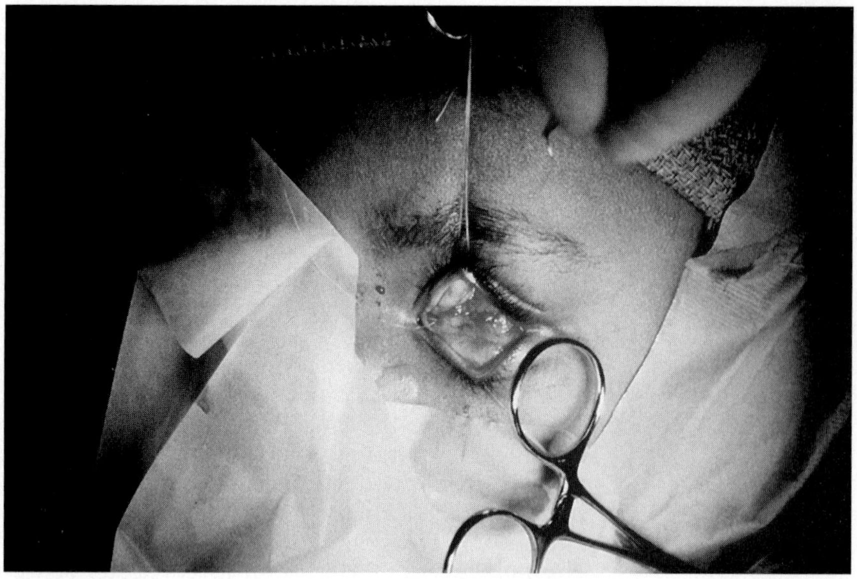

Figure 49–12. Suturing conjunctiva.

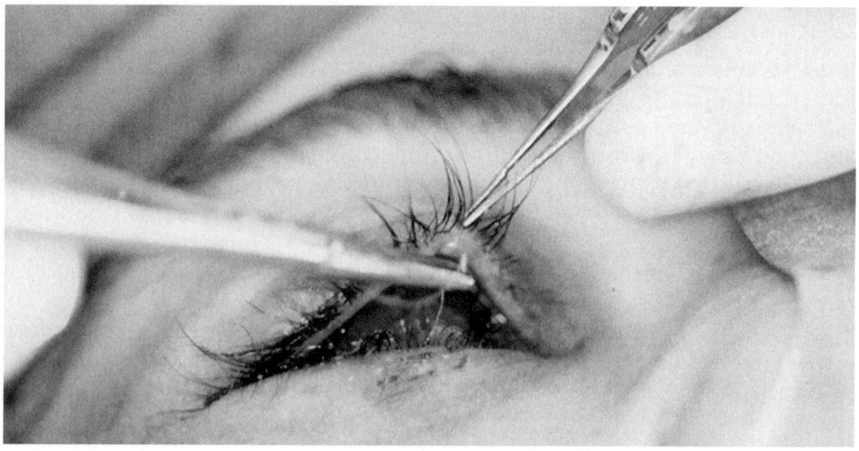

Figure 49–13. Conformer in place and 6-0 mild tarsorrhaphy suture placement.

HYDROXYAPATITE

An alternative to the silicone sphere is the hydroxyapatite implant. We use hydroxyapatite implants usually in young, motivated individuals with healthy sockets who desire the possibility of improved prosthetic mobility achieved by coupling it to the implant via a motility peg placed as a secondary procedure. The implant size is usually 18 to 19 mm in diameter so the socket can accommodate a thicker prosthesis with a peg receptacle. The implant should be soaked in antibiotic solution. Additionally, it should be placed in a syringe filled with antibiotic solution. Apply negative pressure by occluding the tip of the syringe and pulling on the plunger to extract air bubbles from the implant. The implant can be shaved down with a scalpel or a burr to flatten the surface that will face anteriorly. This will also help with later peg placement and prosthesis fitting. The hydroxyapatite implant is then wrapped in sclera or fascia lata as described for the silicone sphere, with the corneal opening facing posteriorly, away from the flattened surface of the implant. Four-millimeter-diameter openings

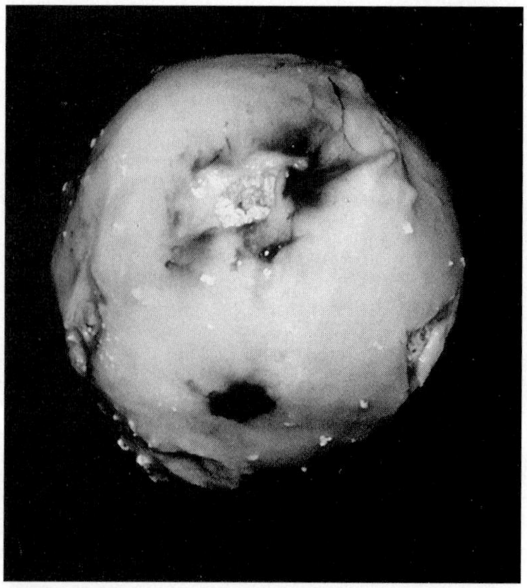

Figure 49–14. Fenestrating hydroxyapatite wrapping.

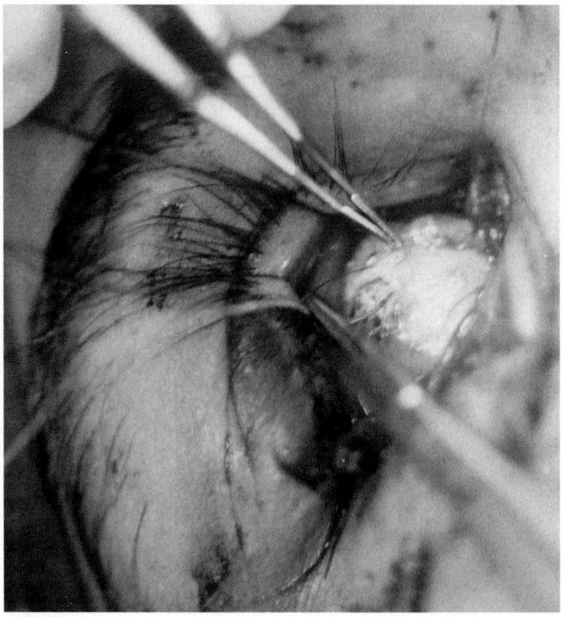

Figure 49–15. Suturing muscles to anterior lip of hydroxyapatite wrapping.

are made in the sclera or fascial wrap in the areas approximating the normal location of the extraocular muscle insertion sites (Fig. 49–14). Vascular access channels are created through these windows and into the center of the implant with an 18-gauge needle. The implant is then placed into the orbit with the corneal opening toward the apex. The extraocular muscles are sewed to the wrap over the 4-mm openings. The sutures are passed through the openings and secured to the anterior scleral lip of the fenestration (Fig. 49–15).[19–22] Synthetic materials are not used with hydroxyapatite because they would hinder fibrovascular ingrowth into the implant. Once all the muscles are attached, the procedure is performed in the same manner as was described for the silicone sphere. Once complete vascularization of the implant occurs, it can be drilled for peg placement. Complete vascularization usually takes 9 months to a year and can be confirmed with bone scan or MRI.

The silicone sphere and the hydroxyapatite implant are probably the most common synthetic implants in current use. Other surgeons are using materials such as the Universal Implant in an attempt to improve mobility.[23] As stated earlier, because of its low rate of complications and extrusions, our preference is the silicone implant. Alternatively, the hydroxyapatite implant may be used in selected cases where there is no microvascular disease, radiation exposure, or multiple surgeries that might hinder adequate fibrovascular ingrowth, resulting in an increased extrusion or exposure rate.[24,25] Reference to other texts regarding other implants is recommended.

Dermis-Fat Grafting

The dermis-fat grafting technique employs a composite graft of dermis and subdermal fat taken from the buttocks or abdominal area. The donor site is marked in an elliptical fashion (Fig. 49–16). The dermis and fat are incised with a No. 15 Bard-Parker blade to the gluteus muscle. The epidermis is excised with the blade, and the base is transected with a straight scissors. Hemostasis is managed with electrocautery. The donor site is then closed with 4-0 Vicryl interrupted deep sutures and a running 6-0 prolene suture for the skin.

After removal of the eye as described earlier, posterior Tenon's fascia is opened in all four quadrants of the intermuscular membrane. This allows orbital fat to come into contact with the grafted fat tissue. The dermal-fat graft is placed directly into the anophthalmic socket with the fat facing posteriorly. The rectus muscles are sutured to the margins of the dermis. Tenon's fascia and the con-

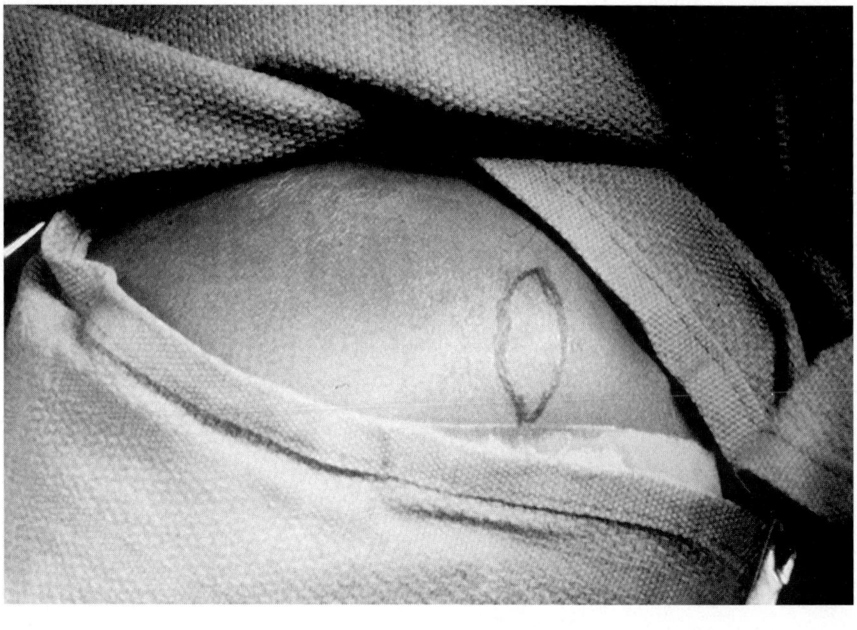

Figure 49–16. Dermal fat graft harvesting.

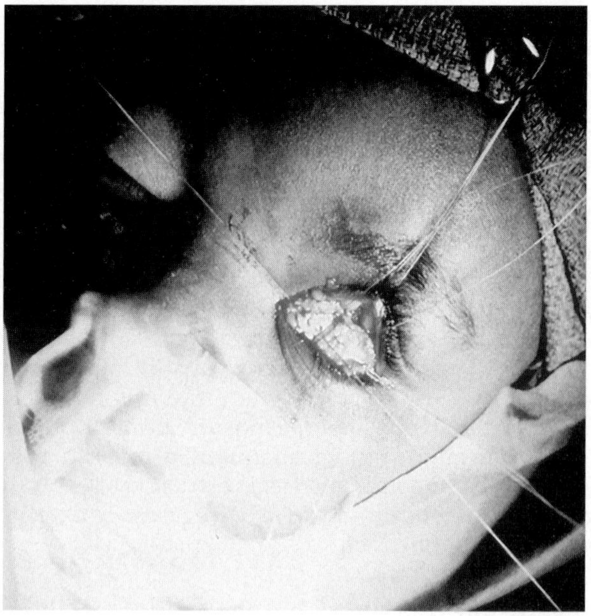

Figure 49–17. Suturing in of dermal fat graft (muscles, Tenon's, conjunctiva).

junctiva are then sutured directly to the margin of the dermal fat graft with 5-0 Vicryl sutures (Fig. 49–17). The desired orbital volume is overcorrected by approximately 20% to allow for reabsorption of the fatty graft.

Autogenous composite dermal fat grafting provides the advantage of no likelihood of implant extrusion, and no possibility of migration of implanted material. Dermal-fat grafted sockets frequently have good motility and are usually comfortable after prosthetic fitting.[26,27] Unfortunately, the rate of reabsorption of transplanted fatty tissue is unpredictable. If fat reabsoprtion is excessive, superior sulcus deformity may result. Another consequence of fat reabsorption is eyelid retraction. This occurs when rectus muscles become adherent to the fat graft. As the fat graft shrinks, the rectus muscles are also contracted. This posterior pull on the rectus muscles is transmitted secondarily to the levator aponeurosis and inferior retractor muscle layers. Clinically significant retraction may occur (Fig. 49–18).

In the authors' experience, reoperations within the first 3 years of dermal fat grafting are necessary in approximately 60% of cases.[28] Also, two of every three patients require major refabrication of the ocular prosthesis within 1 year of surgery, to compensate for changes in socket anatomy from fat reabsorption.

On at least one occasion, we encountered the complication of excessive fat deposition in the dermal fat grafted socket 20 years after fatty implantation after enucleation. This occurred after systemic weight gain in the patient. Because the volume of autogenously transplanted fat from the hip or abdominal area with systemic weight changes may fluctuate, deposition of increased fatty tissue in the orbit may result. This may require further revision of the anophthalmic socket (Fig. 49–19).

We have found the dermal-fat graft implant to be especially helpful in patients who have significant orbital tissue loss, patients with cicatricial shortening of the fornices, and patients who have had multiple implant extrusions. We have found this technique less suitable for routine postenucleation implants because of the high incidence of surgical and prosthetic revisions. (See Table 49–2 for summary of the procedure.)

ORBITAL IMPLANTATION IN PEDIATRIC PATIENTS

Pediatric anophthalmic and microphthalmic sockets pose an additional challenge. A normally growing eye stimulates expansion and development of the orbit until bony growth is complete. The orbit makes up most of the midface. Orbits without normal-sized eyes are hypoplastic and therefore cause ipsilateral facial hypoplasia.[6,7,29] Without treatment a 60% orbital volume deficit may occur. Significant facial deformity follows with its accompanying psychological sequelae. Treatment of the anophthalmic socket should begin as early as possible. Cepela, Nunery, and Martin demonstrated that bony stimulation was proportional to the volume of the implant placed into the orbit. Therefore, the

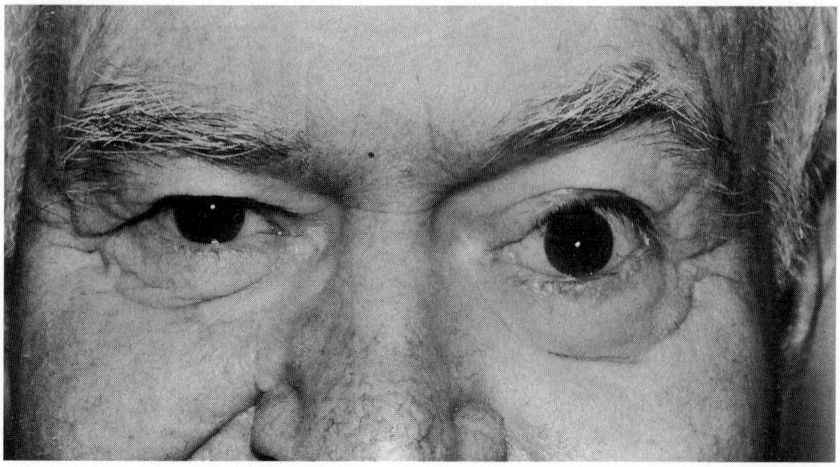

Figure 49–18. Fat-induced lid retraction.

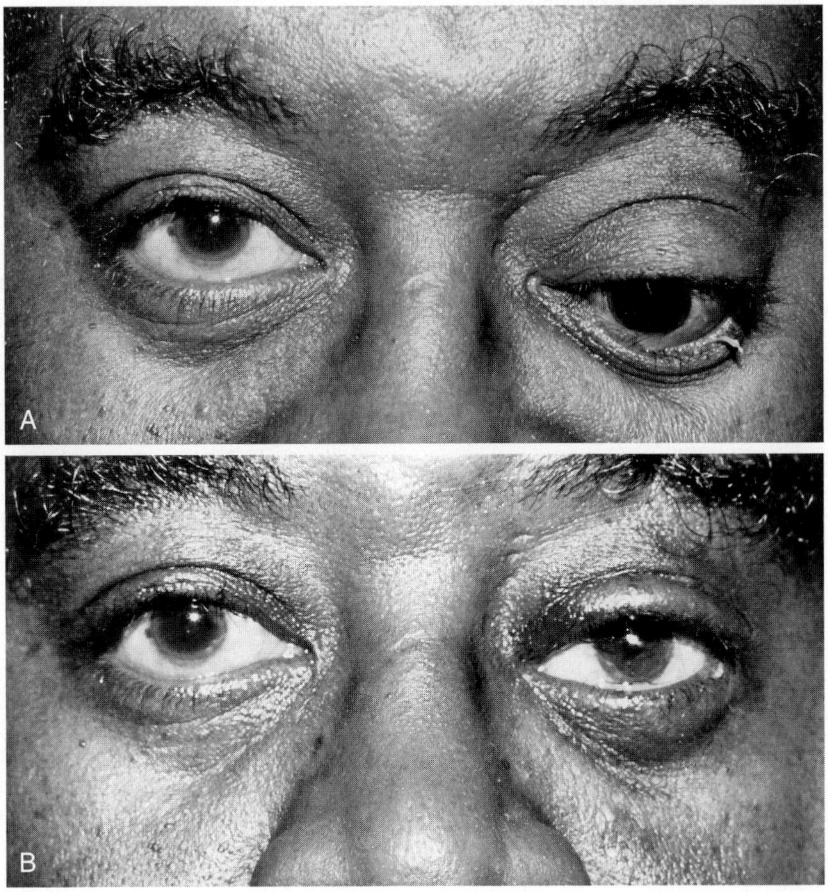

Figure 49–19. Proptosis from a dermal fat graft with weight gain.

TABLE 49–2. Enucleation Steps

1. Retrobulbar injection with anesthetic and epinephrine
2. Apply 4-0 silk lid retraction sutures or lid speculum
3. 360 degree limbal peritomy with Wescott scissors
4. Clear Tenon's fascia away from the globe in all four quadrants using a curved tip hemostat.
5. Sequentially isolate each rectus muscle with a muscle hook, secure each with a double-armed 5-0 Vicryl suture and disinsert each muscle from the globe with Wescott scissors.
6. Isolate and disinsert the superior oblique muscle and secure it to the superior rectus.
7. Isolate and disinsert the inferior oblique muscle and secure it to the lateral rectus.
8. Transect the optic nerve with a snare or a clamp and enucleation scissors.
9. Ensure hemostasis
10. Choose the largest implant up to 20-mm sphere to place into the socket.
11. Soak implant in antibiotics. (For hydroxyapatite, use antibiotic filled 30-gauge syringe to apply negative pressure to implant. See text.)
12. Wrap the implant with sclera, Gortex or fascia. Make fenestrations in wrap for hydroxyapatite implants.
13. For hydroxyapatite implants, use 18-gauge needle to create access channels into the implant.
14. Place the implant into the socket with the opening of the wrap facing posteriorly.
15. Reattach the extraocular muscles to the implant in the approximate anatomical positions and secure the sutures leaving the needles attached.
16. Pass the sutures full thickness through Tenon's fascia and conjunctiva without shortening the fornices or creating wound tension.
17. Close Tenon's layer in multiple layers with interrupted 5-0 Vicryl sutures.
18. Close conjunctiva with a running 5-0 Vicryl suture.
19. Apply antibiotic ointment and insert an appropriate sized conformer.
20. Apply a suture tarsorrhaphy with a single central 6-0 mild chromic suture.

largest implant possible (up to 20 mm in diameter) should be placed into the orbit. Heinz, Nunery, and Cepela also showed that the amount of achievable orbital expansion was inversely proportional to the age at which expansion begins. Treatment may consist of placing sequential orbital expanders, delaying placement of an orbital implant until maximum orbital size is reached.[9] We prefer to place sequentially larger implants into the orbit via a lateral orbital approach without disturbing the conjunctiva. Working in conjunction with the ocularist, who enlarges the fornices with conformers, is crucial. An expandable orbital implant that enlarges with saline injections is an alternative to sequential replacement of orbital sphere implants.

TECHNIQUE FOR EVISCERATION

Indications for evisceration were discussed in the Indications for Enucleation and Evisceration section. Historically, evisceration has been considered to be a technique that provides better motility of the prosthesis and a better cosmetic result than does enucleation.[30] This may be true if enucleation techniques such as release of the rectus muscles or imbrication over the anterior surface of the implant are employed.

With current enucleation techniques, however, the final cosmetic appearance of the enucleated socket is as good as or better than the eviscerated socket. The enucleated socket is more likely to achieve full volume. Prosthesis motility following enucleation in our experience compares favorably with prosthesis motility in the eviscerated socket. A cosmetic advantage, therefore, should not be considered an indication for evisceration vs. enucleation.

Evisceration may also have a higher incidence of implant extrusion than does enucleation. One series showed a 1.4% incidence of extrusion following enucleation. The incidence of extrusion following evisceration was 6% during the same time period. This demonstrates that the incidence of extrusion was four times greater with evisceration than with enucleation.[31]

In the authors' experience, enucleation provides the most satisfactory long-term result when any of the previously mentioned indications are present. When careful enucleation technique is employed, the result is a stable socket with good volume, good motility, and only a small chance of further surgical revision.

AUTHORS' TECHNIQUE

The patient is administered general or local anesthesia with monitored sedation as described for enucleation. Once the patient is prepped and draped according to sterile procedure, Wescott scissors are used to create a 360 degree limbal conjunctival peritomy. A No. 11 or No. 15 Bard-Parker blade is used to enter the eye at the limbus. The corneal edge is grasped with a forceps and the full-thickness incision around the entire limbus is completed either with the scalpel blade or the Wescott scissors (Fig. 49–20). Once the entire cornea is removed, the intraocular contents are removed from the eye. The lens, vitreous, retina, and uveal tissue may be removed with an evisceration spoon or similar instruments such as a periosteal elevator or flat spatula (Fig. 49–21). Once the contents are removed, the intraocular surface of the sclera is vigorously scrubbed free of uveal tissue with a moistened cotton-tipped applicator or small piece of gauze on a hemostat. The gauze may be soaked with 100% ethanol or 10% phenol to denature any remaining uveal protein and to possibly induce sclerosis of the ciliary nerves (Fig. 49– 22). The effect on decreasing ciliary pain is highly variable in the authors' experience. Extreme care must be used to avoid spilling ethanol or phenol on the conjunctival surface because both substances are quite irritating to the periocular tissue. Likewise, once the sclera is scrubbed, it should be irrigated with a copious amount of normal saline solution.

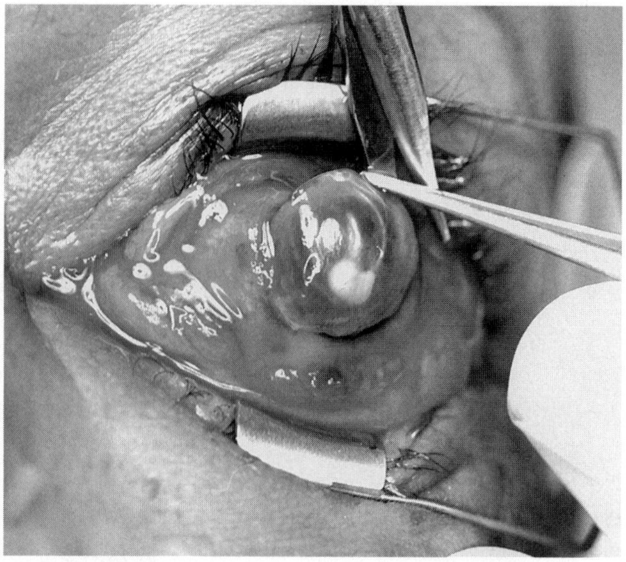

Figure 49–20. Removal of cornea from sclera.

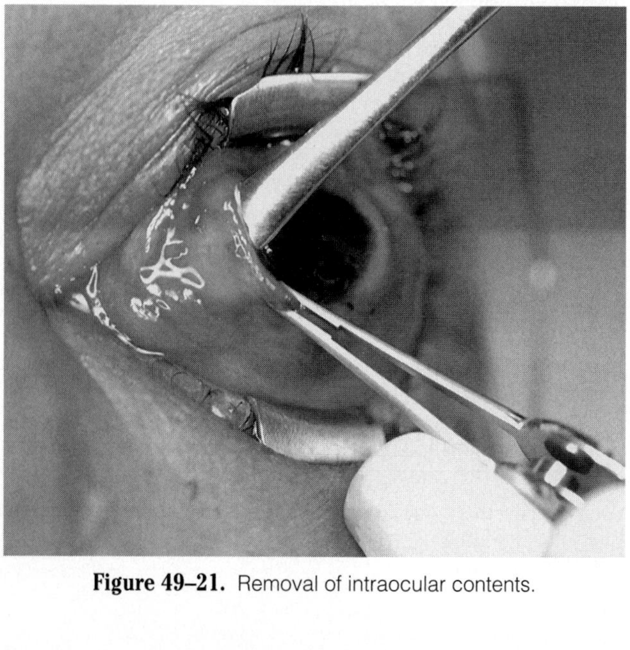

Figure 49–21. Removal of intraocular contents.

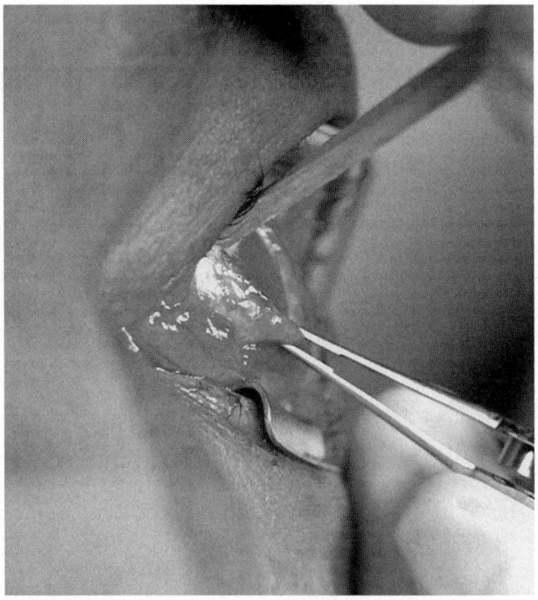

Figure 49–22. Scrubbing inside of scleral shell.

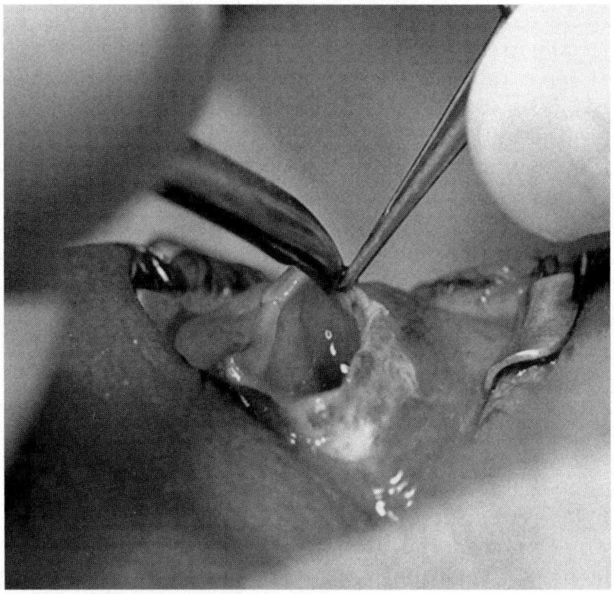

Figure 49–23. Limbal scleral relaxing incisions.

If evisceration is performed for intraocular infection, the sclera should be irrigated with antibiotic solution and packed with antibiotic gauze until the socket quiets down. The packing is usually removed after 24 to 48 hours. Once the infection is cleared, the rest of the sclera may be enucleated in preparation for placement of an orbital implant. Alternatively, an orbital implant such as a silicone sphere may be placed into the eviscerated scleral shell. Placement may be facilitated by incising the limbal scleral edge in an anterior–posterior direction to create a larger anterior opening through which to position the implant (Fig. 49–23). Once the implant is in the sclera, the relaxing incision should be sewn together with a 5-0 Vicryl suture. Next, Tenon's fascia is closed over the sclera in multiple layers with 5-0 Vicryl sutures as described for enucleation. The conjunctiva is closed with a running 5-0 Vicryl suture. Other surgeons advocate sewing the scleral edges over the implant prior to closing Tenon's fascia and conjunctiva. However, this requires the use of a much smaller implant, with a resulting decrease in orbital volume, mandating the use of a larger prosthesis, usually with less effective mobility. We avoid using hydroxyapatite implants in evisceration patients because we believe a higher exposure rate occurs as a consequence of the inability to place the implant far enough posterior in the orbit. Once the implantation is completed, a conformer is placed behind the lids and temporary 6-0 mild chromic suture tarsorrhaphy is placed. (See Table 49–3 for a summary of the procedure.)

COSMETIC COVER SHELL

When the sole indication for enucleation or evisceration is cosmesis, the cosmetic cover shell alternative may be considered. A cosmetic cover shell is similar to an ocular prosthesis fabricated following enucleation, except that the anterior-to-posterior thickness is less, and the radius of anterior curvature is greater. The greatest advantage of the cosmetic cover shell is that it does not require surgical intervention. This may be a particular advantage in patients who are medically unable to withstand surgery or who psychologically are not prepared for enucleation or evisceration.

Cosmetic cover shells, however, do have several dis-

TABLE 49–3. Evisceration Steps

1. Retrobulbar anesthesia with epinephrine.
2. Apply 4-0 silk lid retraction sutures or lid speculum.
3. 360 degree limbal peritomy with Wescott scissors.
4. Remove cornea at limbus with scalpel blade and Wescott scissors.
5. Remove all intraocular contents with evisceration spoon, periosteal elevator, or spatula.
6. Vigorously scrub the inner scleral surface with 100% ethanol or 10% phenol without spilling it on the ocular surface.
7. Rinse thoroughly with normal saline.
8. Create relaxing incisions at the scleral limbal edge with Wescott scissors.
9. Insert a silicone sphere implant.
10. Suture the scleral edges with 5-0 Vicryl to secure the implant.
11. Close Tenon's fascia over the globe and implant in several layers using interrupted 5-0 Vicryl sutures.
12. Close conjunctiva with a running 5-0 Vicryl suture.
13. Apply antibiotic ointment.
14. Insert an appropriately sized conformer.
15. Apply a suture tarsorrhaphy with a single central 6-0 mild chromic suture

advantages. Unless the eye is atrophic, the cover shell must be thin in the anterior-to-posterior diameter to avoid a proptotic appearance. Because of this thinning, the iris artwork has a flat appearance and is generally less cosmetically acceptable than a postenucleation prosthesis.

Second, a cosmetic cover shell may be irritating to the cornea. Some patients are unable to tolerate a cover shell due to corneal sensitivity. This is especially true if the patient has had ocular pain prior to the fitting of the cover shell. Mechanical abrasion of the cornea may pose concerns for corneal ulceration and possible perforation of the globe.

Another disadvantage is the tendency for atrophic globes to continue undergoing degeneration. The size and shape of the socket change continually, and this leads to frequent revisions of the cover shell to provide an adequate fit.

The final objection to a cosmetic cover shell, in the presence of atrophy bulbi, is the potential for development of an occult choroidal melanoma. The patient should understand this risk of leaving the degenerating eye in the socket and should be prepared to accept that risk in deciding to select the cosmetic cover shell alternative.

COMPLICATIONS OF ENUCLEATION AND EVISCERATION

EARLY ENUCLEATION COMPLICATIONS

Early complications after enucleation surgery include hemorrhage, infection, spread of infection to intracranial tissue, and injury to orbital apex structures.

Hemorrhage

Hemorrhage associated with enucleation may, in rare cases, be severe. Intraoperative hemorrhage can usually be minimized through the use of retrobulbar injection of epinephrine and careful enucleation technique. Crushing of the optic nerve prior to transection also helps to prevent hemorrhage. Direct electrocautery of the central retinal artery within the optic nerve stump is a useful technique for preventing later postoperative hemorrhage.

Patients most prone to develop excessive hemorrhage during enucleation are patients who use aspirin, patients with liver disease, and patients with endogenous abnormalities of the clotting mechanisms. The effect of salicylates on the inhibition of platelet aggregation may persist as long as 2 weeks after administration of only one aspirin tablet. Elective enucleation, therefore, should be postponed until the patient has been off all aspirin-containing products for a minimum of 2 weeks.

Patients who abuse alcohol or have liver abnormalities should have intramuscular or intravenous vitamin K replacement therapy until protime testing is within the normal range. Patients with other specific bleeding disorders such as hemophilia or absence of other clotting factors should be given specific clotting factors preoperatively to minimize the risk of excessive hemorrhage. Because it is associated with much less bleeding, evisceration rather than enucleation should be elected if bleeding time or clotting factors cannot be corrected preoperatively.

The use of pressure dressings over the enucleated socket is not warranted for routine enucleation, in our experience. Pressure dressings may, however, be a useful adjunct to tamponade hemorrhage postoperatively should excessive bleeding develop in the unusual case.

Infection

As with any surgical procedure, the risk of postoperative wound infection exists. Wound infection is uncommon, however, due to the excellent blood supply of the orbit. Patients with diabetes are at a higher risk than other patients for the development of postoperative wound infection. The use of prophylactic antibiotics may be considered postoperatively in diabetic patients.

The possibility of infectious organisms traveling from the orbit into the central nervous system by way of the transected optic nerve after enucleation is of concern, especially in cases of endophthalmitis or panophthalmitis. At least one case of meningoencephalitis occurred 9 months after enucleation for proven cryptococcal endophthalmitis.[3,12] The presumed, but unproved, portal of entry was the transected optic nerve at the time of enucleation. Although intracranial spread of infection is rare following contaminated enucleation, this theoretic concern provides a relative indication for evisceration rather than enucleation in the presence of endophthalmitis or panophthalmitis.

Orbital Apex Injury

Dysfunction of orbital apex structures, including complete loss of cranial nerves III, IV, V, and VI may occur following indelicate dissection of the orbital apex at the time of enucleation. This may occur if random electrocautery is undertaken in an effort to control operative hemorrhage. Orbital apex syndrome may also occur if enucleation scissors are indelicately placed in the orbital apex. Postoperative acute orbital hemorrhage, especially in an orbit with a pressure bandage on, may result in apex damage as well. Theoretically, excessive traction on the optic nerve may produce injury to the chiasm.

EARLY EVISCERATION COMPLICATIONS

Because of the nature of the procedure, evisceration is usually not associated with complications of orbital apex injury or intracranial spread of infection through the optic nerve. As with any surgical procedure, evisceration may be associated with infection and bleeding. Bleeding from evisceration is usually much less severe than in enucleation because fewer vessels are cut and bleeding should only occur from the retinal vessels and vortex veins, which can be directly visualized end cauterized intraoperatively.

LATE ENUCLEATION COMPLICATIONS

Late complications of enucleation include migration or extrusion of orbital implants, volume loss with superior sulcus deformity, loss of inferior fornix tissue with or without mucous membrane shrinkage, formation of orbital cysts, and eyelid malposition such as ectropion or ptosis.[32–39] The problems of persistent discharge and pain in the anophthalmic socket may also be considered a late complication.

Implant Migration and Extrusion

Implant migration and extrusion have been addressed previously.[39] A superior-temporal migration may cause ptosis by advancing and impeding the superior rectus and levator (Fig. 49–24). To minimize this ptosis, the prosthesis may be custom designed with minimal superior volume to eliminate further downward pull on the levator. Ptosis buckles on the prosthesis are ineffective when ptosis is caused by a migrated implant.

If ptosis persists, a minimal levator tightening procedure may be done. Care should be taken to avoid overcorrection of the ptosis, because anophthalmic ptosis responds well to minimal levator tightening. Revision of the implant may be considered prior to ptosis surgery in severely migrated implants.

Careful technique and proper choice of implant will minimize the incidence of late implant extrusion. When the orbital implant does become visible through a small external opening, this should be considered an indication to revise the implant immediately (Fig. 49–25). If the implant is allowed to extrude spontaneously and the socket is allowed to heal prior to socket revision, tissue contracture will occur and an optimal cosmetic result will be difficult to achieve. If the implant can be revised prior to complete extrusion, however, less tissue loss and contracture will be encountered and a more acceptable postrevision socket will be the result.

Patching the early implant extrusion defect with eyebank sclera may prevent complete extrusion in some cases.[34,38] This may, however, only delay the final extrusion and thus may not represent a long-term solu-

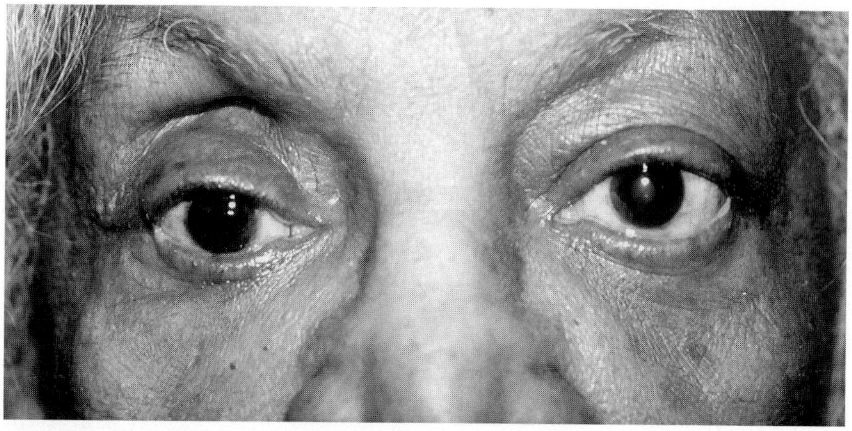

Figure 49–24. Ptosis secondary to implant migration.

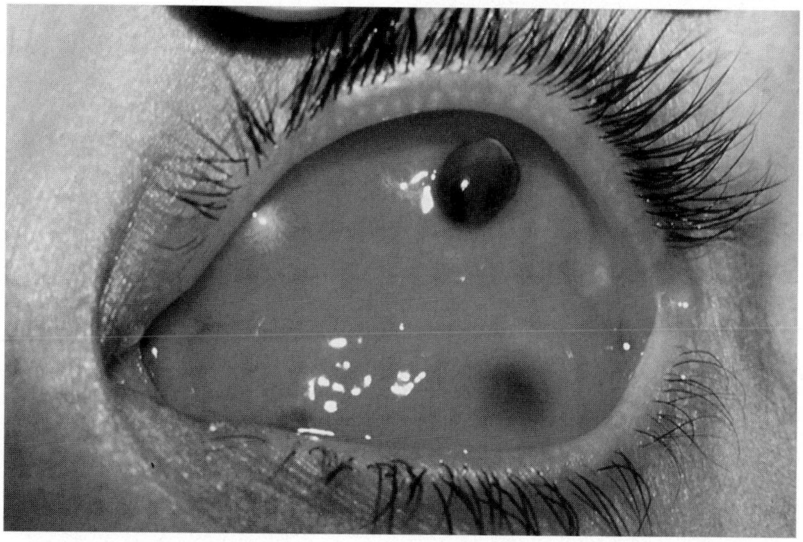

Figure 49–25. Exposed orbital implant.

tion to the problem. Autogenous composite dermal fat grafting may be a useful technique to add orbital volume where contracture of the socket has occurred after implant extrusion.

Volume Deficit

Volume deficit and superior sulcus deformity seem to be an almost inevitable part of anophthalmic socket reconstruction (Fig. 49–26). Volume loss should preferably be prevented through the use of a 20-mm sphere implant at the time of enucleation. The use of the 18-mm diameter (or smaller) sphere is more common, but most anophthalmic sockets can tolerate a 20-mm sphere without overstretching Tenon's capsule over the sphere implant or creating an additional risk of extrusion.

When enucleation is undertaken in small children, the largest implant possible should be placed. Otherwise, frequent revision with larger implants may be necessary to encourage growth of bony tissue until adolescence.

Prosthetically, superior sulcus deformity can be reduced by reshaping the prosthesis into a more vertically elongated design. Volume is then added anteriorly and superiorly to push more lid tissue into the superior sulcus. A posterior–superior flange will prevent the prosthesis from tipping posteriorly (Fig. 49–27). If excess volume is added, the additional weight may contribute to ectropion or inferior fornix instability. This can be minimized through the inferior fornix, ectropion prosthetic design (see below).

A marked superior sulcus deformity can be corrected surgically by placement of a larger sphere implant, or by placement of a subperiosteal volume implant along the floor of the orbit (Fig. 49–28).

If subperiosteal volume implants are undertaken to correct the superior sulcus deformity, we prefer the use of silicone precut into wedges of differing sizes and thickness, which can be cut and adjusted to the appropriate replacement volume intraoperatively.

Contracted Socket

The integrity of the inferior fornix is perhaps the most important aspect of secure fitting of the ocular prosthesis. Inadequate inferior fornix will result in frequent extrusion of the prosthesis and malposition of the lower eyelid. Loss of the inferior fornix may be due to upward traction on the conjunctiva and fornix tissue at the time of enucleation, migration of the implant postoperatively, or shrinkage of the mucosa. Laxity and ectropion of the lower eyelid also contribute to an inadequate lower fornix. This may be aggravated by an

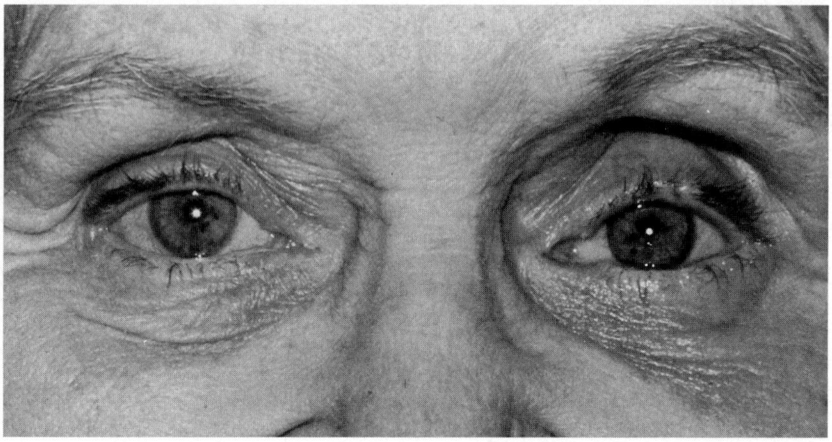

Figure 49–26. Superior sulcus deformity.

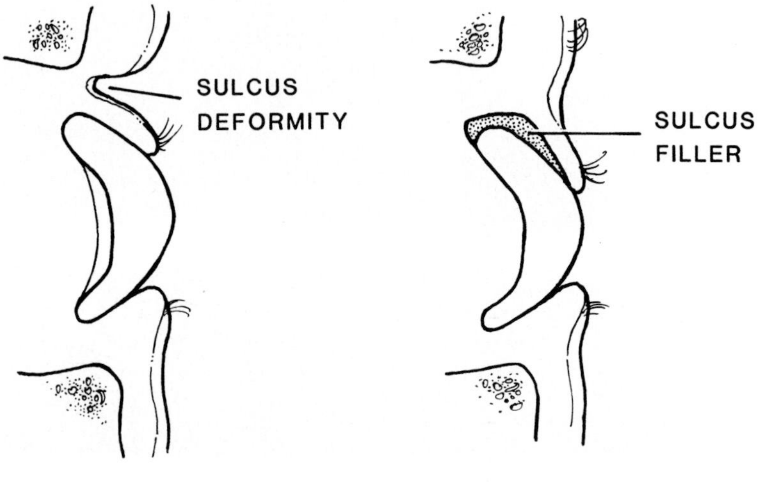

Figure 49–27. Superior sulcus flange on prosthesis.

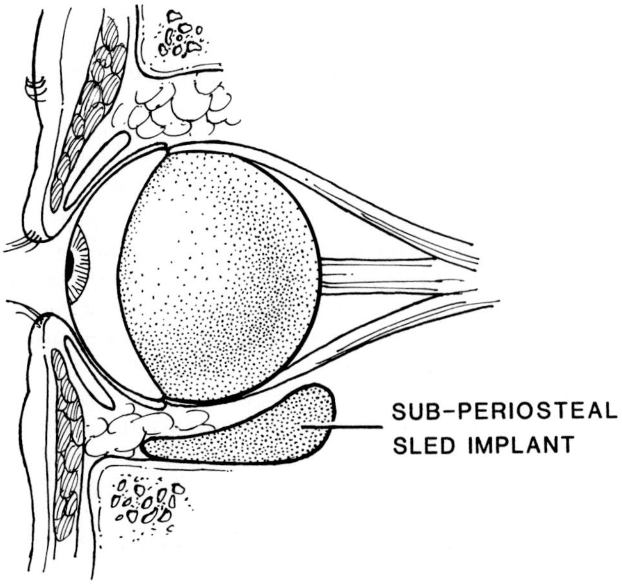

Figure 49–28. Subperiosteal volume implant.

oversized prosthesis that has been fabricated to compensate for volume loss in the orbit.

Instability of the prosthesis caused by a shallow inferior fornix can be minimized by making the inferior aspects of the prosthesis thin and vertically elongated (Fig. 49–29). The posterior aspect of the superior margin of the prosthesis is built up to prevent the superior prosthesis from tipping posteriorly. At the same time, the inferior aspect is engaged more securely in the shallow inferior fornix.

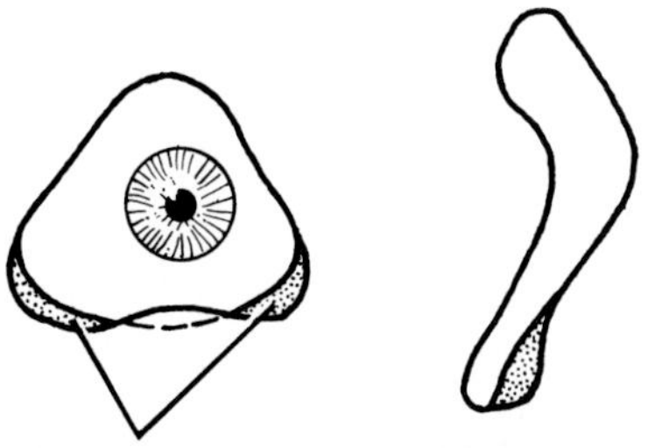

Figure 49–29. Inferior fornix modification of prosthesis.

Should the prosthetic manipulation be unsatisfactory in stabilizing the inferior fornix, the fornix conjunctiva may be redirected surgically when sufficient conjunctival tissue exists. In cases of inadequate conjunctival tissue, full-thickness buccal mucous membrane grafting may augment inferior fornix tissue and allow the placement of a secure prosthesis.

Conjunctival atrophy has also been noted following enucleation. Tissue factors leading to contracture of the mucosa have not been well defined. We have observed cases of pseudo-pemphigoid reaction in the enucleated eye only.

In the progressively contracting anophthalmic socket, buccal mucous membrane grafting may not survive or may undergo secondary shrinkage. In these cases, split-thickness skin grafting may be placed in the inferior fornix to ensure adequate fornix tissue. Although associated desquamation of keratin material and hygiene difficulties make split-thickness skin grafting less desirable than mucous membrane grafting, the split-thickness skin is a hearty tissue that can survive when mucous membrane tissue will not.

Eyelid Malpositions

Eyelid malposition is common following enucleation. Ptosis may be due to superior temporal implant migration, as previously described; to stretching of the levator aponeurosis at the time of surgery; or to direct trauma to the levator aponeurosis. Upper lid ptosis can sometimes be improved prosthetically. Unfortunately, some ocularists may fit an oversized prosthesis in an effort to lift the upper lid. The increased weight and volume often will put additional pressure on the lower lid and fornix. In addition to not correcting ptosis, these large prostheses may frequently extrude or cause a noticeable ectropion of the lower lid.

A more desirable way to elevate the upper lid is to add volume to the superior aspect of the cornea, which tends to open the fissure. Volume is then reduced superiorly to the upper limbus to create a more horizontal curvature in the area of the tarsal plate. Finally, a superior flange is added to the superior aspect of the prosthesis to elevate or buckle Mueller's muscle and levator aponeurosis (Fig. 49–30).

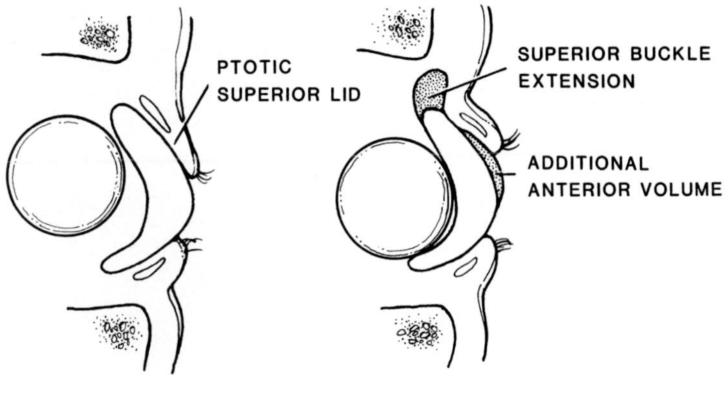

Figure 49–30. Superior prosthesis flange for ptosis.

If surgical repair of the anophthalmic socket ptosis is needed, the repair should be conservative, because these cases are usually accompanied by normal levator strength, and overcorrection of ptosis may occur if levator strength is underestimated.

Ectropion or malposition of the lower eyelid occurs as a result of prosthetic weight on the lower eyelid, upward traction or shortening of the inferior fornix conjunctiva, or dehiscence of the inferior retractor muscle. To improve ectropion, volume should be removed from the area immediately below the lower limbus, and volume should be added on the anterior aspect of the inferior edge of the prosthesis. The contour of the lower edge is then shortened in the area of greatest lid shortage to eliminate further downward pressure. Finally, volume is added anteriorly, in the area of the medial and lateral canthal tendons to better support the weight of the prosthesis (Fig. 49–31).

If these changes do not correct the ectropion, horizontal tightening procedures or advancement of the inferior retractor muscles is usually successful. Horizontal tightening procedures, particularly at the lateral canthus, are usually effective in maintaining a tight, well-placed lower lid margin. Advancement of the inferior retractor muscle may be done in severe cases of ectropion.

Painful Socket

Coexisting pain and excessive discharge in the anophthalmic socket can be difficult problems for the patient, the ophthalmologist, and the ocularist. Pain may be the result of tissue being pinched between the implant and the overlying ocular prosthesis. This may be more common with irregularly shaped motility implants.

A painful socket may signal the earliest phase of implant extrusion. Refitting of the anophthalmic socket with a custom-fit prosthesis technique may relieve pressure against inflamed conjunctival tissue and may delay implant extrusion.

Persistent discharge in the anophthalmic socket is generally due to (1) contaminants absorbed in the ocular prosthesis, (2) pooling of secretions behind an ill-fitting or stock prosthesis, (3) painful pressure points between

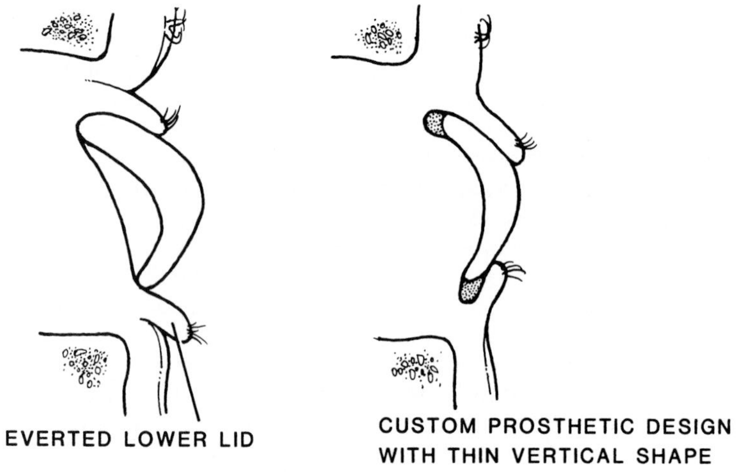

Figure 49–31. Ectropion modification of prosthesis.

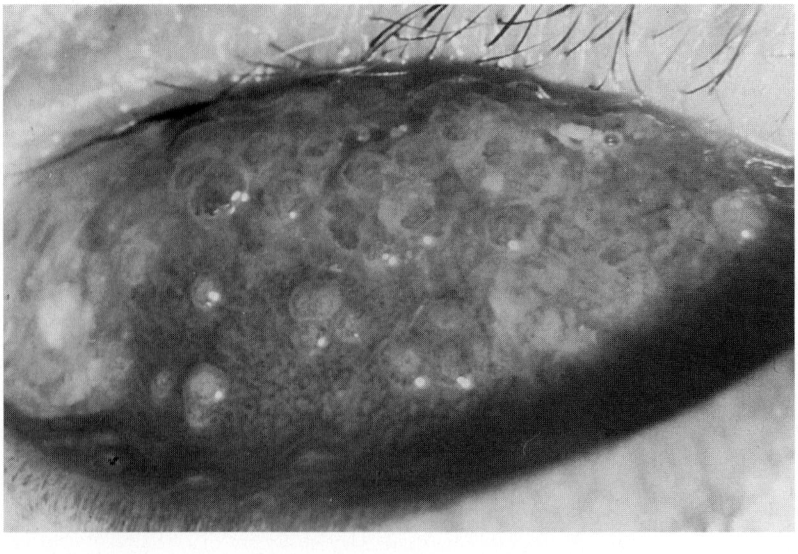

Figure 49–32. Giant papillary conjunctivitis.

prosthesis and implant, or (4) mucoid discharge secondary to keratitis sicca or giant papillary conjunctivitis.

The tarsal conjunctiva should be examined for evidence of acute socket infection or giant papillary response on the conjunctiva (Fig. 49–32).[40] Giant papillary conjunctivitis results from type IV (cell-mediated) hypersensitivity to polymers used in prosthesis fabrication, or to environmental allergens absorbed in the prosthesis.

Possible pressure points or tender areas in the socket tissue may indicate potential extrusion sites of the implant. Migration of the implant or evidence of a poorly fitting prosthesis should be noted.

If the implant is poorly fitting, excessive discharge will not resolve prior to eliminating areas of pooling through the use of the modified-impression custom-fitting technique. If socket hygiene is inadequate, cleaning and polishing of the prosthesis, along with hygiene instructions to the patient, lessen the discharge.

Prolonged indiscriminate use of antibiotic ointments is not advised in cases of excessive socket discharge because this may lead to the development of resistant organisms, and the conjunctival lining of the socket may react to the benzalkonium chloride, thimerosal, or chlorbutanol preservatives contained in most antibiotic preparations. The prosthesis may also absorb these preservatives and prolong the irritation and discharge.

Another cause for mucoid discharge in the anophthalmic socket is inadequate aqueous production, or sicca syndrome. This can be minimized by use of topical lubricants.

LATE EVISCERATION COMPLICATIONS

Late complications of evisceration include extrusion of implants, loss of inferior fornix tissue, eyelid malpositions such as ectropion or ptosis, and persistent discharge. Mechanisms of these complications are similar to those discussed for late enucleation complications.

PROTECTIVE EYEWEAR AFTER ENUCLEATION OR EVISCERATION

The ophthalmologist and ocularist have an obligation to educate the patient in ways of protecting the remaining eye following enucleation. Frequent routine examinations of the remaining eye should be undertaken on a schedule to be dictated by the health of the eye. Patients should be reminded of the hazards of activities such as hammering metal on metal, participating in racket sports, and using machinery such as lawn mowers, weed trimmers, or other machines capable of throwing foreign objects.

For daily wear, impact-resistant glasses, either piano or prescription, should be worn as protection against injury. For industrial wear, athletics, home workshop, or lawn care use, glasses meeting the American National Standard Practice for Occupational and Educational Eye and Face Protection (ANSI Z87.1-1979) standards should be used. This generally requires 2.2- to 3.2-mm polycarbonate lenses in impact-resistant frames. These glasses are monogrammed with "Z87 " on the frame front and temple.

The National Society to Prevent Blindness estimates that 35,000 eye injuries in the home workshop, and 5,000 eye injuries in the lawn and garden occur each year. Patients with one anophthalmic socket should be reminded of these dangers to the other eye.

PROSTHESIS FITTING

Successful prosthesis fitting and optimal postenucleation rehabilitation require a close association between the ocularist and the ophthalmic surgeon. Consultation with the ocularist prior to enucleation may allay the patient's anxieties and make postoperative expectations more realistic.

Following enucleation, a clear acrylic conformer is placed. It may be custom contoured by the ocularist. A slight vaulting over the conjunctival suture line is desirable to prevent pressure on the healing tissue. Excess vaulting, however, is undesirable, because it provides an area where pooling of secretions may promote infection. The fornices should be completely filled by the conformer to provide gentle deepening pressure on the fornices. The conformer should be worn continuously until the prosthesis is fabricated at 6 to 8 weeks post-enucleation, to prevent shortening of the fornices or socket contracture.

Fabrication of an optimum prosthesis requires custom fitting to design one that precisely fits the socket anatomy. This is best achieved through the modified impression technique of custom eye fitting.[41,42] The use of premade "stock" prostheses creates air pockets between the prosthesis and socket, which may provide a breeding ground for bacteria. A predesigned shape may also distort lid or socket anatomy and ultimately create the need for further surgical revision of the tissue. Unless the design of the prosthesis and the artwork of the iris and sclera precisely match the patient's socket and the other eye, optimal cosmesis cannot be achieved.

An impression of the anophthalmic socket is made by injecting a soft alginate impression material through a stemmed impression tray into the socket (Fig. 49–33). The correct consistency is necessary to avoid distortion of the soft socket tissue. Overfilling can also distort the tissue. The proper impression allows the ocularist to identify anatomic features such as conjunctival folds, the trochlear notch, tarsal plate height, migration of the implant, and anterior contour of the implant.

A semihard wax model is then molded using the alginate impression for the design. The wax model is placed in the socket and then carefully sculpted or modified to achieve the optimum function of the socket and cosmesis. The ocularist may reduce volume in one area to minimize tissue pressure, or add volume in another area to shape the lids, develop the fornices, or improve tissue dynamics.

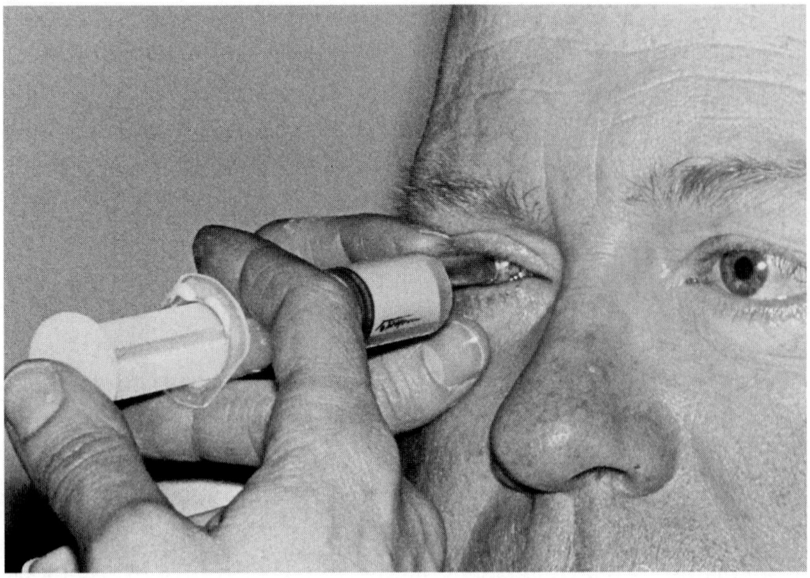

Figure 49–33. Impression molding for prosthesis.

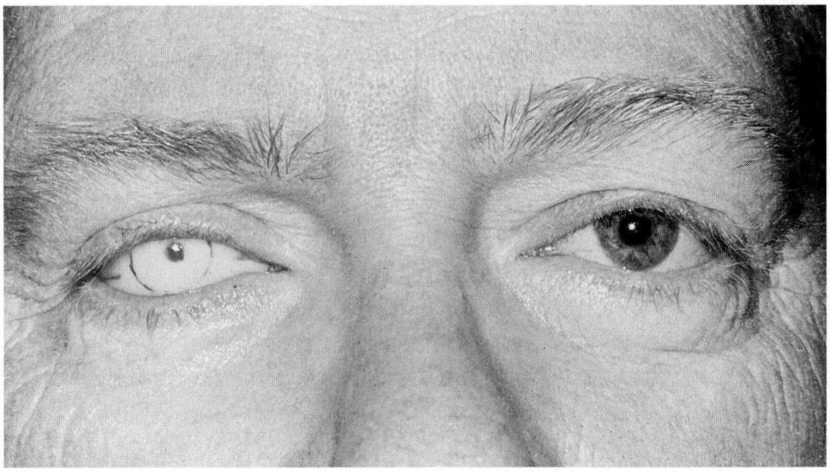

Figure 49–34. Button wax model for prosthesis fitting.

To maximize palpebral fissure dimensions, volume can be added anteriorly to both the horizontal and vertical axes as necessary. To reduce the palpebral fissure opening, anterior volume can be removed, or alteration in the anterior curvature can change the tarsal angulation, resulting in a more open or closed fissure.

The iris plane augmentation is accomplished by precise placement of the corneal-iris button in the wax model to achieve symmetry in the palpebral opening and parallel gaze with the companion eye (Fig. 49–34). Measurements should be made of the distance between the facial midline and pupillary reflex in the normal eye.

After detailed sculpting of the wax model, a glass-stone mold of the model is cast to be used in the fabrication of the initial white, acrylic shape. After the acrylic shape has been cured, the anterior surface is reduced for the scleral tinting, vesseling, and iris overpainting. Approximately 1 mm of the overall scleral surface is removed. The corneal-iris button should be meticu-

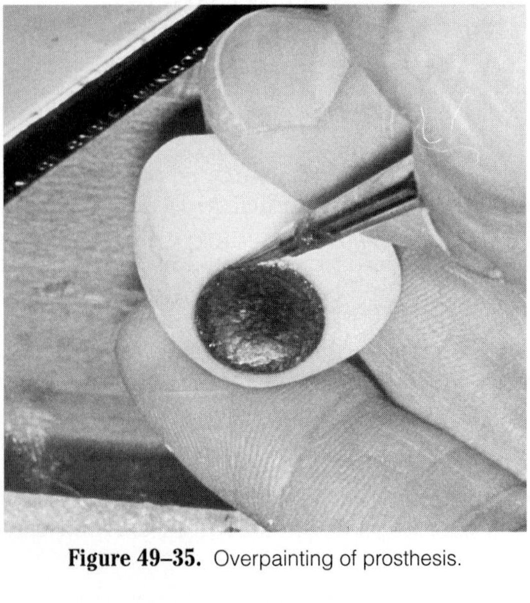

Figure 49–35. Overpainting of prosthesis.

lously exposed for desired limbal effect. Intricate iris overpainting can be accomplished at this stage, creating a third dimension in color and stroma (Fig. 49–35).

The painted white acrylic is thoroughly dried prior to the final casting in clear resin. The clear acrylic is cured under heat and pressure. It is then cooled in a cold water bath. Once cooled, the prosthesis is removed for the final pumice and polishing process. The prosthesis is then tested in the socket to be certain that the optimum fit and cosmesis have been achieved.

SUMMARY

The enucleated patient presents a special challenge to the ophthalmologist and the ocularist. The more thought applied to the enucleation technique and prosthetic fitting, and the more care exercised, the more favorable will be the cosmetic appearance. The ophthalmologist should be prepared to deal with the psychological aspects of enucleation, advise the patient on prophylactic protection of the uninjured eye, and redouble efforts to diagnose and treat any condition that may be a threat to the remaining eye.

REFERENCES

1. Hogan MJ, Zimmerman LE: Ophthalmic Pathology: An Atlas and Textbook, Philadelphia: WB Saunders; 1962.
2. Duke-Elder S (ed.): Cysts and tumors of the uveal tract: diagnosis of malignant melanoma. In System of Ophthalmology, Vol 9, Chap 6, St. Louis: CV Mosby; 1966:896.
3. Yanoff M, Fine B: Ocular Pathology, Hagerstown, MD: Harper & Row; 1975.
4. Fraunfelder FT, Wilson RS: A new approach for intraocular malignancy: the "no touch" technique. In Jakobiec FA (ed.), Ocular and Adnexal Tumors, Birmingham, UK: Aesculapius; 1978.
5. Zimmerman LE, McLean IW, Foster WD: Does enucleation of the eye containing malignant melanoma prevent or accelerate the dissemination of tumor cells? An unanswered question! In Jakobiec FA (ed.), Ocular and Adnexal Tumors, Birmingham, UK: Aesculapius; 1978.
6. Kennedy RE: Effects of early enucleation on the orbit in animals and humans. Trans Am Ophthalmol Soc 1964;62:459.
7. Osborne D, Hadden OB, Deeming LW: Orbital growth after childhood enucleation. Am J Ophthalmol 1974;77:756–9.
8. Cepela MA, Nunery WR, Martin RT: Stimulation of orbital growth by the use of expandable implants in the anophthalmic cat orbit. Ophthalmic Plast Reconstr Surg 1992;8:157–67.
9. Heinz GW, Nunery WR, Cepela MA: The effect of maturation on the ability to stimulate orbital growth using tissue expanders in the anophthalmic cat orbit. Ophthalmic Plast Reconstruct Surg 1997;13:115–28.
10. Duke-Elder S (ed.): Uveitis of unknown origin: sympathetic ophthalmitis—aetiological theories. In Systems of Ophthalmology, Vol 9, Chap 5, St. Louis: CV Mosby; 1966:566.
11. Chan C, Roberge FG, Witcup SM, Nussenblatt RB: 32 Cases of sympathetic ophthalmia: a retrospective study at the National Eye Institute, Bethesda, MD. Arch Ophthalmol 1995;113:597–600.
12. Berkmann LW, Bennett DR: Meningoencephalitis following enucleation for cryptococcal endophthalmitis. Ann Neurol 1978;4:476–7.
13. Youngs CW: Lack of motility in ocular prosthetics. Today's Ocularist 1977;3:10–14.
14. Spivey BE: Enucleation: a remaining challenge. Aust J Ophthalmol 1980;8:69–74.
15. Mules PH: Enucleation of the eye and its substitutes. Am Encyc Ophthalmol 1915;6.
16. Perry A: Volume of anophthalmic implants. Address to American Society of Ocularists, San Francisco, 1983.
17. Fox SA: Ophthalmic Plastic Surgery, New York: Grune & Stratton; 1976:543.
18. Allen L: The argument against imbricating the rectus muscles over spherical orbital implants after enucleation. Trans Am Acad Ophthalmol 1983;90:1116–20.
19. Dutton JJ: Coralline hydroxyapatite as an ocular implant. Ophthalmology 1991;98:370–7.
20. Ferone PJ, Dutton JJ: Rate of vascularization of coralline hydroxyapatite ocular implants. Ophthalmology 1992;99:376–9.
21. Perry AC: Advances in enucleation. Ophthalmol Clin North Am 1991;4:173–82.
22. Shields CL, Shields JA, De Potter P: Hydroxyapatite orbital implant after enucleation: experience with initial 100 consecutive cases. Arch Ophthalmol 1992;110:333–8.
23. Jordan DR, Anderson RL, Nerad JA: A preliminary report on the universal implant. Arch Ophthalmol 1987;105:1726.
24. Nunery WR, Cepela MA, Heinz GW, et al.: Extrusion rate of silicone spherical anophthalmic socket implants. Ophthalmic Plast Reconstr Surg 1993;9:90–5.
25. Nunery WR, Heinz GW, Bonnin JM, et al.: Exposure rate of hydroxyapatite spheres in the anophthalmic socket: histopathologic correlation and comparison with silicon sphere implants. Ophthalmic Plast Reconstr Surg 1993;9:96–104.
26. Guberina C, Hornblass A, Meltzer MA, et al.: Autogenous dermis-fat implantations. Arch Ophthalmol 1983;101: 1587–90.
27. Smith B, Petrelli R: Dermis-fat graft on a moveable implant within the muscle cone. Am J Ophthalmol 1978;85:62–6.
28. Nunery WR, Hetzler KJ: Dermal-fat graft as a primary enucleation technique. Ophthalmology 1985;92:1256–61.
29. Schaffer DP: Evaluation and management of the anophthalmic socket and socket reconstruction. In Nesi FA, RD Lisman, MR Levine (eds.), Smith's Ophthalmic Plastic and Reconstructive Surgery. St. Louis: CV Mosby; 1988:1079–1124.
30. Ruedemann AD Jr: Modified Burch-type evisceration with scleral implant. Am J Ophthalmol 1960;49:41.
31. Zolli CL: Implant extrusion in eviscerations. Paper presented at American Society of Ocularist Meeting, 1984, San Francisco.
32. Bayliss H, Shorr N: Evisceration, enucleation and correction of problems of anophthalmic sockets. In McCord CD Jr (ed.), Ophthalmic Surgery, New York: Raven Press; 1981:313–47.
33. Clodius L, Martin O: Problems of the anophthalmic orbit. In Hornblass AS, Meltzer A, Rees TD (eds.), Third International Symposium of Plastic and Reconstructive Surgery of the Eye and Adnexa, Baltimore: Williams & Wilkins; 1980:244–7.
34. Helveston EM: Human bank scleral patch for repair of exposed or extruded orbital implants. Arch Ophthalmol 1969;82:83.
35. Hornblass A, Bosniak S: Orbital cysts following enucleation: the use of absolute alcohol. Ophthalmic Surg 1981;12:123.
36. Mustarde JC: Repair and Reconstruction in the Orbital Region, 2nd Edition. Edinburgh and London: Churchill Livingstone; 1980:230–244.
37. Soll DB: Management of Complications in Ophthalmic Plastic Surgery, Birmingham, UK: Aesculapius; 1976:296–324.
38. Zolli C, Shannon GM: Experience with donor sclera for extruding orbital implants. Ophthalmic Surg 1977;8:63–70.
39. Zolli CL: Implant extrusion in enucleation. Ann Ophthalmol 1988;20:127.
40. Srinivasan BD, Jakobiec FA, Iwamoto T, DeVoe AG: Giant papillary conjunctivitis with ocular prostheses. Arch Ophthalmol 1979;97:892–5.
41. Allen L, Webster HE: Modified impression method of artificial eye fitting. Am J Ophthalmol 1969;67:189–218.
42. Bartlett SO, Moore DJ: Ocular prosthesis: a physiologic system. J Prosthet Dent 1973:29:450–9.

CHAPTER 50

Surgery of the Lacrimal System

ROGER A. DAILEY, M.D., SCOTT C. SIGLER, M.D.,
and STANLEY M. SAULNY, M.D.

ANATOMY

The lacrimal system is made up of a secretory portion and an excretory apparatus. The secretory part consists of the two lobes of the major lacrimal gland and its ducts and the accessory glands of Krause and Wolfring. The excretory apparatus contains the orbicularis muscle of the eyelids, lacrimal puncti and canaliculi, lacrimal sac, and nasolacrimal duct.

SECRETORY APPARATUS

The lacrimal gland is divided into two discrete lobes by the lateral horn of the aponeurosis of the levator palpebrae (Fig. 50–1). The palpebral lobe lies inferior to the lateral horn of the aponeurosis and the orbital lobe lies superior to that structure. The two lobes are connected posteriorly by shared parenchyma. The orbital lobe of the lacrimal gland lies in a shallow fossa of the frontal bone, the *lacrimal gland fossa.* The major lacrimal ducts open into the superior cul-de-sac 4 to 5 mm above the superior lateral tarsal border. There are approximately 12 excretory ductules of the lacrimal gland. Damage to the palpebral lobe can result in significant decrease in reflex tearing because the orbital lobe ducts must run through the palpebral lobe to empty onto the conjunctival surface.

Efferent innervation of the orbital and palpebral lobes is through the seventh cranial nerve. The innervation to the palpebral lobe travels through the orbital lobe; injury or removal of the orbital lobe can result in efferent denervation of the palpebral lobe. The glands of Wolfring, located just at the edge of the tarsus, and the glands of Krause, located near the fornix, do not require efferent innervation and are the basic lacrimal secretors. There are approximately 20 accessory glands in the upper lid and 10 in the lower lid. The afferent pathway is along the fifth cranial nerve via the lacrimal nerve. Sympathetic innervation is present, but the exact route is not clear. The lacrimal artery, which is a branch of the ophthalmic artery, and the lacrimal vein, which drains into the superior ophthalmic vein, represent the vascular support of the gland.

EXCRETORY APPARATUS

The pumping mechanism of the eyelids is a vital part of the excretion of tears. Tears from the lacrimal gland are secreted from the superior cul-de-sac and travel across the eye medially. The eyelids close during blinking secondary to the contraction of the orbicularis oculi muscle. The pretarsal portion of the muscle has a deep and superficial head. When these heads contract, they close the ampulla of the puncti, squeeze the canaliculi closed,

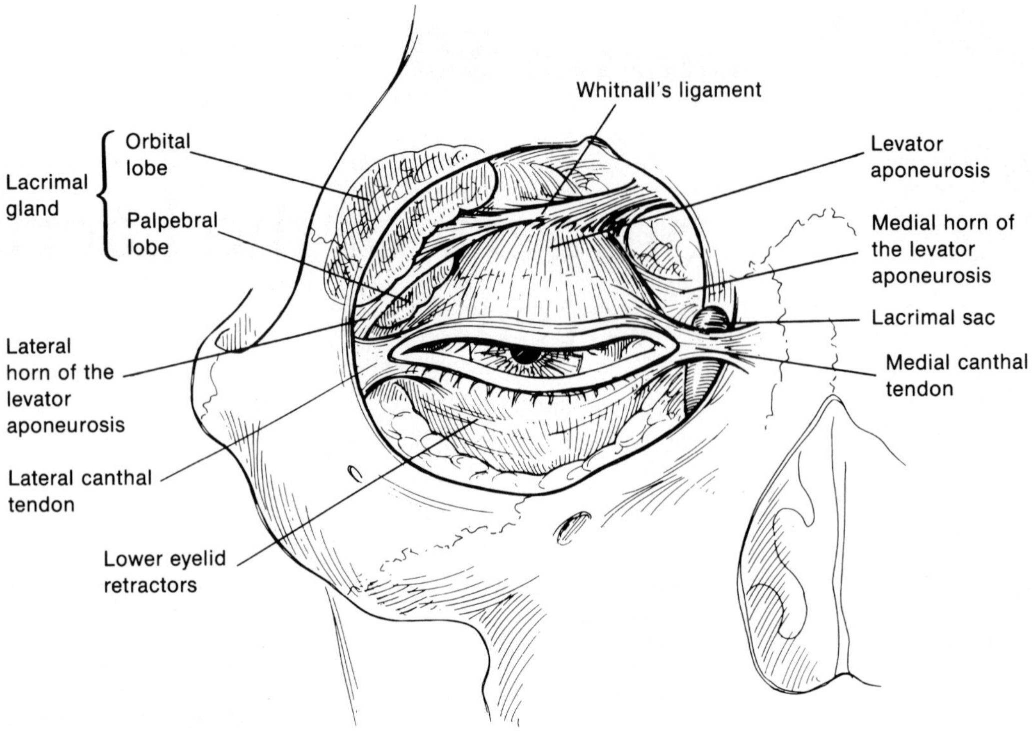

Figure 50–1. A frontal view of Whitnall's ligament and anterior orbital structures. As the levator muscle extends below the superior orbital.

and pull the puncti medially. The deep heads of the preseptal portion of the orbicularis oculi muscle simultaneously pull on the periosteum and the lateral wall of the lacrimal sac and cause the sac to expand laterally, creating negative pressure in the sac. Tears are pushed into the sac by the positive pressure formed by closure of the puncti and shortening of the canaliculi and they are pulled into the sac by the negative pressure formed by the deep heads of the preseptal orbicularis. On release of the blink and relaxation of the orbicularis muscle, the sac gains positive pressure as the lateral wall resumes its prior position more medially and the canaliculi lengthen and the puncti open, allowing tears to drain in again. This change from negative to positive pressure within the sac pumps the tears into the sac and down the nasolacrimal duct.[1] Gravity also assists in this drainage.

The lacrimal outflow tract starts with the punctum, which is slightly inverted on the lid margin. The punctum course is vertical in the lid for 2 mm. The canaliculus then courses slightly superiorly toward the medial canthal tendon for 8 to 10 mm. The upper and lower puncti join together to form a common canaliculus in 90% of individuals. This structure immediately opens into the lacrimal sac just posterior and superior to the center of the sac. The lacrimal sac is positioned in the lacrimal sac fossa, behind the medial canthal tendon. The fundus of the sac extends above the tendon 3 to 5 mm. The medial canthal tendon has two portions, the deep portion attaches to the posterior lacrimal crest behind the sac and the anterior portion attaches to the frontal process of the maxillary bone. The body of the sac is approximately 9 to 10 mm in height and drains into the nasolacrimal duct, which is 12 to 13 mm in length within the canal and extends another 2 to 3 mm into the inferior meatus (Fig. 50–2).[1]

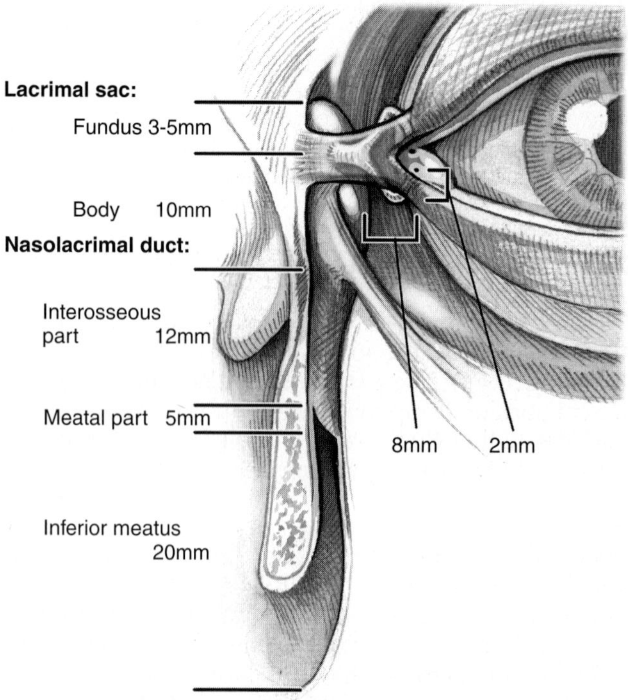

Figure 50–2. Lacrimal excretory anatomy.

EVALUATION OF LACRIMAL FUNCTION

SECRETION

Schirmers I

The Schirmers I test measures both reflex and basic secretions. Without topical anesthetic, a strip of filter paper is placed in the cul-de-sac and left there for 5 minutes. The normal amount is equal or greater than 15 mm of wetting.[2]

Basal Tear Secretion

With the conjunctiva anesthetized and any excess tears or anesthetic in the inferior fornix blotted up, a strip of filter paper is draped over the lower lid extending from the fornix for 5 minutes. This measures the basic secretion. The normal result is 10 mm of wetting or more. This test can be performed by the busy comprehensive ophthalmologist by taking the measurement obtained after 1 minute and multiplying it $\times$ 3 for an equivalent number to the straight 5-minute test.[3]

Schirmers II

With the conjunctiva anesthetized, the tears are blotted and the filter paper is placed. The middle turbinate on the ipsilateral side is then stimulated with a cotton tip or instrument. An increase in the measured amount of wetting as compared to the basal tear secretion test confirms activity of the reflex secretors and shows that the neurologic reflex arc is intact.[2]

EXCRETION

Dye Disappearance Test

A drop of 2% fluoroscein is placed in the conjunctival fornices in each eye and the tear film is observed. Asymmetric clearance of the dye after 5 minutes or retention of the dye in both lacrimal lakes indicates stasis of flow. This can be due to lid malposition, abnormal pumping mechanism of the lids, or abnormalities of the lacrimal outflow tract.

Primary Dye Test (Jones I)

This test evaluates the lacrimal outflow under physiological conditions. A drop of 2% flourescein is instilled in the inferior cul-de-sac. After 5 to 10 minutes, the inferior meatus is swabbed with a cotton applicator, dacroswab, or cotton-tipped nasal wire. If dye is retrieved from the meatus, the test is positive: open and functioning excretory system. If no dye is retrieved (negative), then the secondary dye test is performed. In children, examination of the oropharynx for dye after 10 minutes with a cobalt blue light indicates a positive test if dye is seen.[4]

Secondary Dye Test (Jones II)

When the Jones I test is negative, the residual dye and tears are wiped from the inferior cul-de-sac. Lacrimal irrigation is then attempted. The punctum is dilated and then, with a blunt 23-gauge cannula, saline or tap water is irrigated into the system. If irrigation of fluid is successful into the nose and the fluid has dye in it, the test is positive. A positive test means that tears are reaching the lacrimal sac and that the nasolacrimal duct is patent. A negative Jones I and a positive Jones II indicates a functional nasolacrimal duct block. If the irrigated fluid does not have dye in it, then this indicates that the dye/tears are not gaining entry to the lacrimal excretory system. This can be due to an abnormal lid position, a poor pumping mechanism, or stenosis of the puncti or canaliculi. The nasolacrimal duct, however, is patent. Dilatation of the puncti or canalicular system may have allowed the irrigation of fluid, while Jones I testing was negative because there was punctal or canalicular stenosis.[4]

Dacryocystogram

Although seldom used, a dacryocystogram uses radiopaque dye to image the excretory system. It is useful in identifying masses, diverticuli, or fistulas of the lacrimal canaliculi, sac, or nasolacrimal duct. In the angiography suite, x-rays are taken as dye is injected into the canaliculum via a sialogram angiocatheter. A baseline Caldwell and lateral view are taken. Additional imaging is performed immediately after injection, and again 30 minutes later. The failure of dye to leave the sac indicates a functional nasolacrimal duct obstruction.[5]

Microscintigraphy

The microscintigram is similar to the dacryocystogram, except that technetium is used instead of radiopaque dye.

Imaging studies in general are rarely needed in the evaluation of the lacrimal drainage system. Computed tomography (CT) scanning can assist in the evaluation of lacrimal obstruction caused by facial trauma, congenital craniofacial deformities, or when lacrimal neoplasms are suspected. Magnetic resonance imaging (MRI) can be used with larger tumors of the head when they are associated with the lacrimal system.

PUNCTAL DISORDERS

AGENESIS/DYSGENESIS/STENOSIS OF THE PUNCTUM

A transparent membrane may be present at birth in congenital atresia of the punctum. Usually the underlying system is normal. A punctal dilator with a sharp tip can usually "pop" through this membrane. Local infiltrative anesthesia or even topical anesthetic (cocaine 5% or lidocaine 4%) on the area prior to the procedure makes the procedure much more comfortable.[6]

Aging as well as ocular surface infections and chronic use of certain topical ophthalmic drops can result in stenosis of the punctum. Repeated dilation may be successful in relieving epiphora, however occasionally a one or two snip procedure is indicated to permanently open the punctum.

One Snip Procedure *(Fig. 50–3)*

A. Topical or infiltrative anesthetic is administered.
B. The punctum is dilated. One blade of a sharp scissors is placed in the punctum with the remaining blade on the palpebral conjunctival surface perpendicular to the lid margin. The tissue is cut.
C. The incision is left open. Laterally directed tension applied multiple times per day by the patient for 2 to 3 days after the procedure may facilitate patency.

Two-Step Procedure *(Fig. 50–4)*

A. Identical to the one-snip procedure through completion of part B above.
B. An additional incision is made through the proximal part of the punctum, and a small triangle of conjunctiva, with the apex pointing toward the inferior fornix, is cut away.

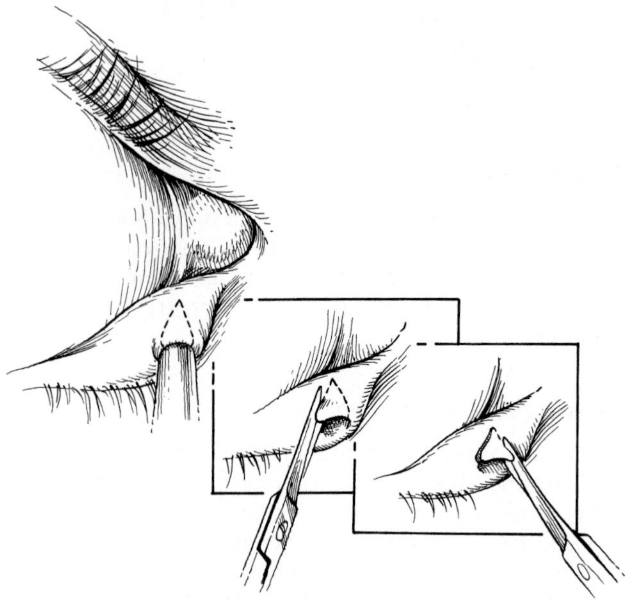

Figure 50–4. Two-snip punctalplasty.

Eversion of the Punctum *(Fig. 50–5)*

Occasionally the punctum may become everted away from the globe, often in association with ectropion. A diamond wedge procedure rotates the punctum posteriorly toward the globe secondary to vertical shortening of the posterior lamella. Reattachment of the retractors in the slightly more complicated medial spindle procedure will correct more severe lid eversion.[7]

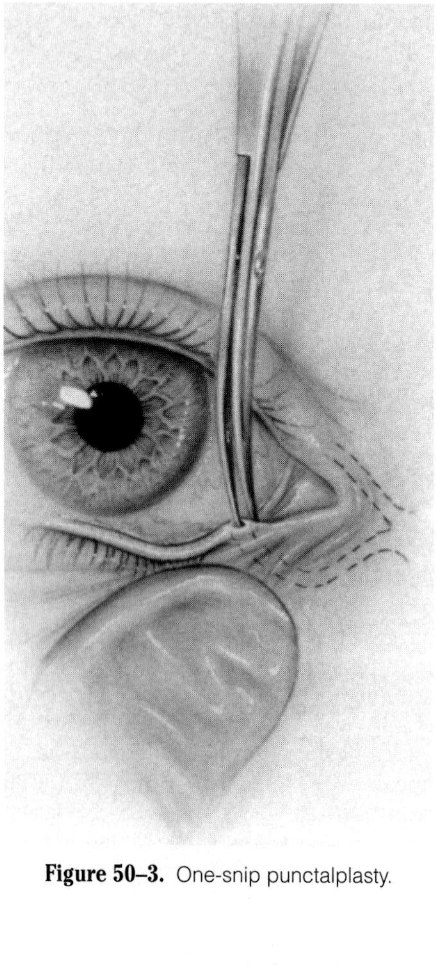

Figure 50–3. One-snip punctalplasty.

A. A horizontal diamond or ellipse of conjunctiva and underlying connective tissue is resected just inferior to the punctum.
B. The subconjunctival tissue is brought together with a buried interrupted absorbable suture like 5-0 polyglactin 910 suture.

CANALICULAR DISORDERS

Obstruction can occur in the inferior or superior canaliculi as well as in the common canaliculus. Probing will usually identify the obstruction. Irrigation is not successful through the canaliculus with obstruction. If the common canaliculus is closed, fluid irrigated into the upper or lower canaliculi results in flow out the uncannulated punctum. Acquired cases of canalicular obstruction include trauma, canaliculitis, chemotherapy (i.e., 5-fluorouracil), toxic topical medications, viral infections, and autoimmune disorders such as pemphigoid.

SILICONE INTUBATION

Attempts to open the obstruction should be performed first. Often there is a small stricture or obstruction that can be eliminated with probing alone. To prevent the tissues from growing together again, intubation with a silicone tube should be performed to allow re-epithelialization of the previously obstructed area.

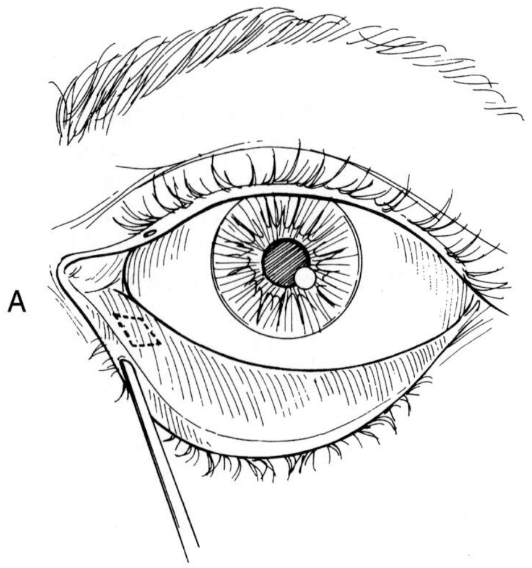

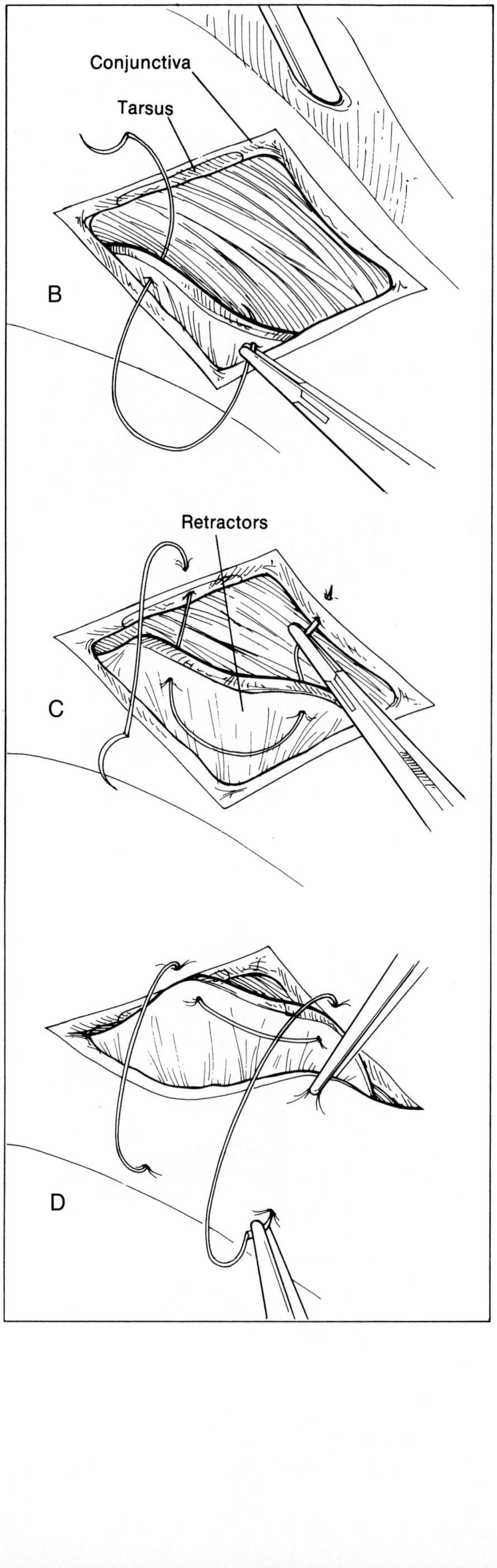

Figure 50–5. *A.* Surgeon's view from the head of the operating table. The medial eyelid is severed, a Bowman probe is inserted into the inferior canaliculus, and a diamond-shaped fusiform wedge of conjunctiva and lower lid retractors are excised inferior to the lower margin of the tarsal plate. The conjunctiva and underlying retractors are removed, with the vertical height being about 4 to 6 mm and the horizontal dimension approximately 6 to 8 mm. The vertical height of the fusiform excision depends on the amount of punctal ectropion. Its greatest vertical dimension should lie beneath the punctum. The inferior edge of this diamond-shaped incision points toward the inferior fornix and exposes the superior margin of the lower lid retractors. The surgeon should avoid cutting into the horizontal preseptal oribicularis muscle fibers. *B.* The defect is closed with a double-armed 5-0 chromic suture in a horizontal mattress fashion. The suture is initially passed through the retractors at the lower edge of the incision in a backhanded pass. *C.* The needle passes through the upper edge of the ellipse, uniting the tarsal plate and conjunctiva on the upper edge. After passing both arms of the suture, the suture is pulled superiorly, joining the edge of the retractors to the inferior tarsal border. *D.* With forceps grasping the conjunctival edge of the lower border of the incision, the suture is passed full-thickness through the eyelid. The needle should be brought through the skin 12 to 15 mm inferior to the lid margin. The other arm of the suture is passed in the same fashion. The sutures are tied on the skin surface. The suture tension should be adjusted as needed to invert the punctum to the proper position. Care should be taken not to tie too tightly as to overcorrect the medial eyelid margin and produce entropion. It may be helpful to have the patient sit up while tying the sutures. The suture is left in place until it is absorbed.

A. This procedure can be performed under general anesthesia or monitored anesthesia care with intravenous sedation. 0.5% to 0.75% bupivicaine (Marcaine) with 1:100,000 epinephrine is sprayed into the ipsilateral nares. Cotton strips soaked in cocaine 5% are placed into the nose, under the inferior turbinate in the meatus. Local injection of 2% lidocaine with 1:100,000 epinephrine is given in the upper and lower lids around the puncti and in the medial canthal area.
B. Once satisfactory anesthesia is obtained, the puncti are dilated with a 1-2 Jones punctal dilator. If significant resistance is encountered, a one-snip procedure can be administered as described earlier. A No. 0-00 probe is then used in either canaliculus to enter the lacrimal sac. The examiner must keep lateral tension on the lid to avoid an accordian effect of the canaliculus which increases the risk of creating a false passage if the epithelium is perforated (Fig. 50–6). Once inside the sac, the probe is advanced to hit the bony wall. Lateral tension on the lower lid should be released at this time.
C. The probe is then rotated superiorly about 90 degrees following the bony contour. If directed slightly temporally and posteriorly (aligned with the supraorbital notch or slightly medial to it), the probe should easily drop through the nasolacrimal duct into the inferior meatus (Fig. 50–7). This is

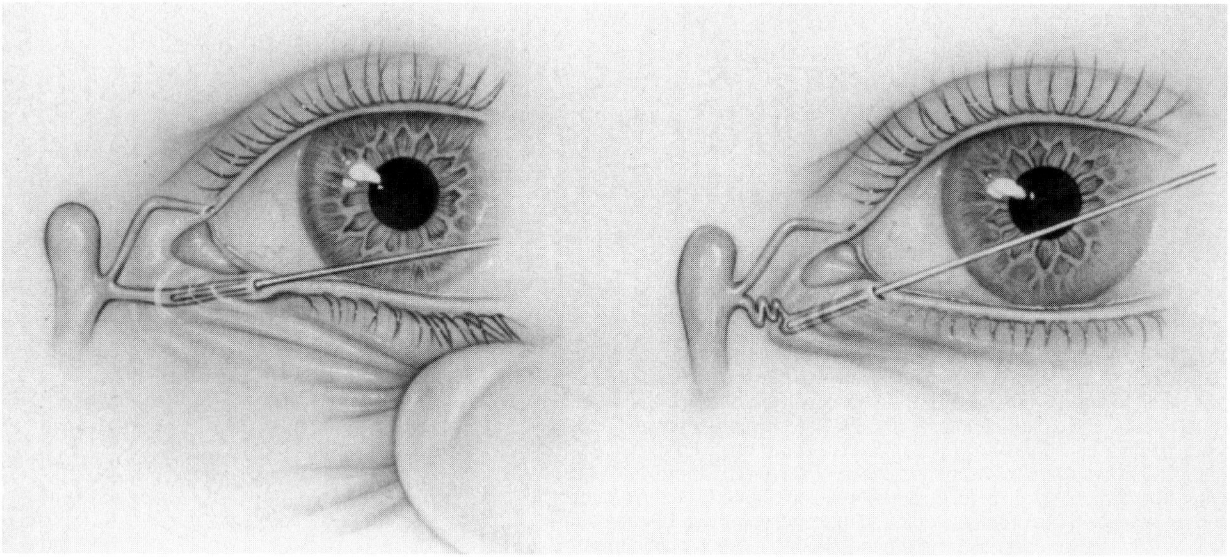

Figure 50–6. Lateral tension on the lower lid reduces the risk of creating a "false passage" during probing of the canaliculus.

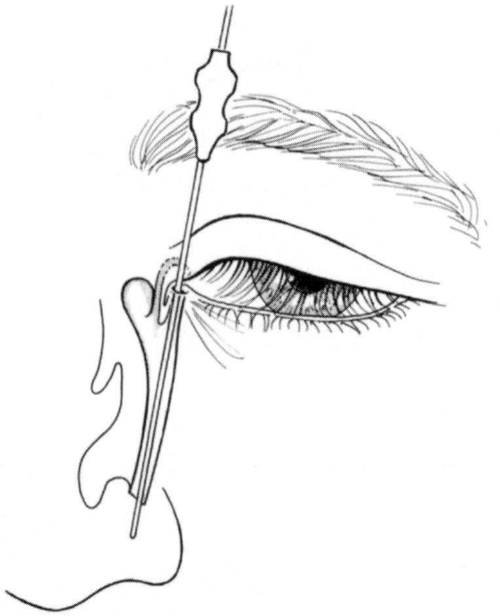

Figure 50–7. Nasolacrimal duct probing with Bowman probe.

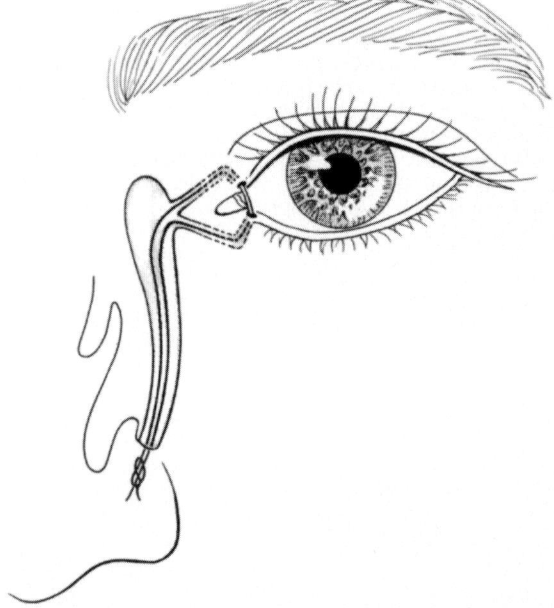

Figure 50–8. Silicone stent in place in lacrimal excretory system.

confirmed by direct visualization in the nose using a nasal speculum, headlight, and Freer elevator if necessary. Occasionally the inferior turbinate needs to be fractured medially with a caudal or Freer elevator to allow more room in the inferior meatus and better exposure.

D. Silicone tubing, 0.025 inch in diameter in infants and 0.037 inch in adults, is used to intubate the excretory system. Quickert-Dryden probes are attached to each end of the tubing with medical grade silicone adhesive. Crawford or Cline-Guibor probes with tubing can also be used. Once the end of the probe is seen in the inferior meatus, it is retrieved out the nares with a forcep. The other canaliculus is then probed and the opposite end of the silicone tubing is brought out through the nares. The probes are pulled off the tubing and the tubing is tied into a square knot. The tubing is then cut 1 cm away from the knot and is allowed to retract into the inferior meatus (Fig. 50–8). Any epistaxis encountered will usually stop with external tamponade; however, an anterior pack Vaseline gauze can be placed if necessary.

E. We have not found it necessary or desirable to suture the silicone to the nasal wall. Removal of the tube can then be easily performed in the office using only topical anesthetic. In children, topical anesthetic is placed in the eye. The tube is cut between the upper and lower puncti. A cut end is grasped and quickly pulled laterally, allowing the tube and knot to be brought out through the canaliculus and punctum. Children tolerate this well and it avoids general anesthesia, which is often required if the tubing is sutured to the nose. In adults, the knot is identified in the nose with the help of a nasal speculum and headlight. The tube is cut between the upper and lower puncti and the knot grasped in the nose with a bayonet forcep. The tube is then brought out through the nares.

CANALICULITIS

Canaliculitis is an inflammation of the canaliculus, most commonly caused by *Actinomyces israelii,* a filamentous gram-negative rod. This disorder can also be due to other bacterial, viral, mycotic, and chlamydial infections. Patients have an erythematous, dilated and "pouting" punctum, often with dilatation of the canaliculus. Usually, the involved area is edematous and has marked discharge and pain if acute. Probing and curettage often reveals yellow granules consistent with Actinomyces. Treatment includes curettage through the pouting punctum whch may be followed by penicillin irrigation along with warm compresses. Occasionally, the concretions must be removed directly.

CANALICULOTOMY (Fig. 50-9)

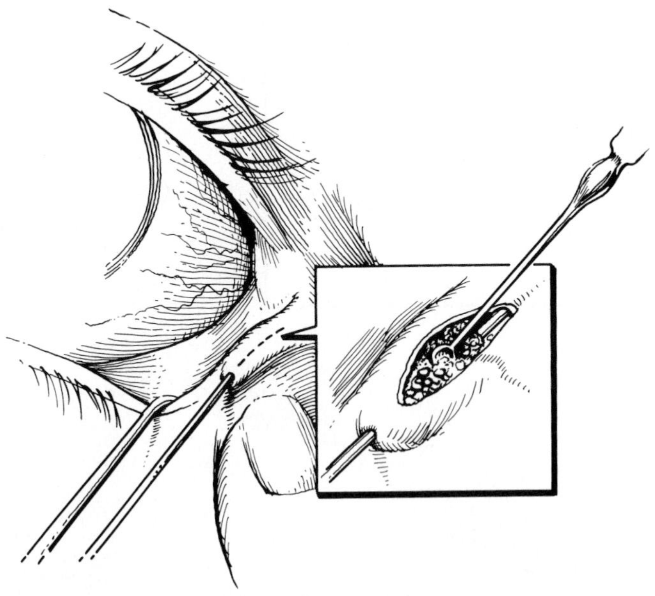

Figure 50–9. Canaliculotomy.

A. The canaliculus is probed and a full-thickness skin incision is made into the canaliculus down to the probe. Leave the fibroelastic ring around the punctum intact if possible, which will help prevent "cheesewiring" of the canaliculus.

B. Under direct visualization, a curette is used to remove the concretions.

C. The area is irrigated with antibiotic aqueous solution.

D. The incision can be left opened or repaired over a silicone tube.

LACERATIONS OF THE CANALICULAR SYSTEM

Lacerations of the medial eyelids and medial canthal area require careful inspection to rule out canalicular injury. Often the edema and distortion of normal anatomy will hide a canalicular laceration unless manipulation of the tissue in the injured area is performed. If a canalicular laceration is suspected, gentle probing of the area is recommended. This is usually not possible in children without sedation or general anesthesia. Bicanalicular silicone intubation is suggested to repair the canalicular laceration.[8,9]

Repair of Canalicular Lacerations (Fig. 50–10)

A. The puncti are dilated with a Jones punctal dilator or other dilating instrument and probed through the involved punctum with a No. 0-00 probe to identify the lateral cut end of the canaliculus.

B. The medial cut end needs to be identified. Magnification with either loupes or an operating microscope may be needed. Irrigation of the area with saline often will cause the cut end of the canaliculus to appear white, with the surrounding muscle appearing red. A No. 0-00 probe is passed into the medial cut end and into the nasolacrimal duct as

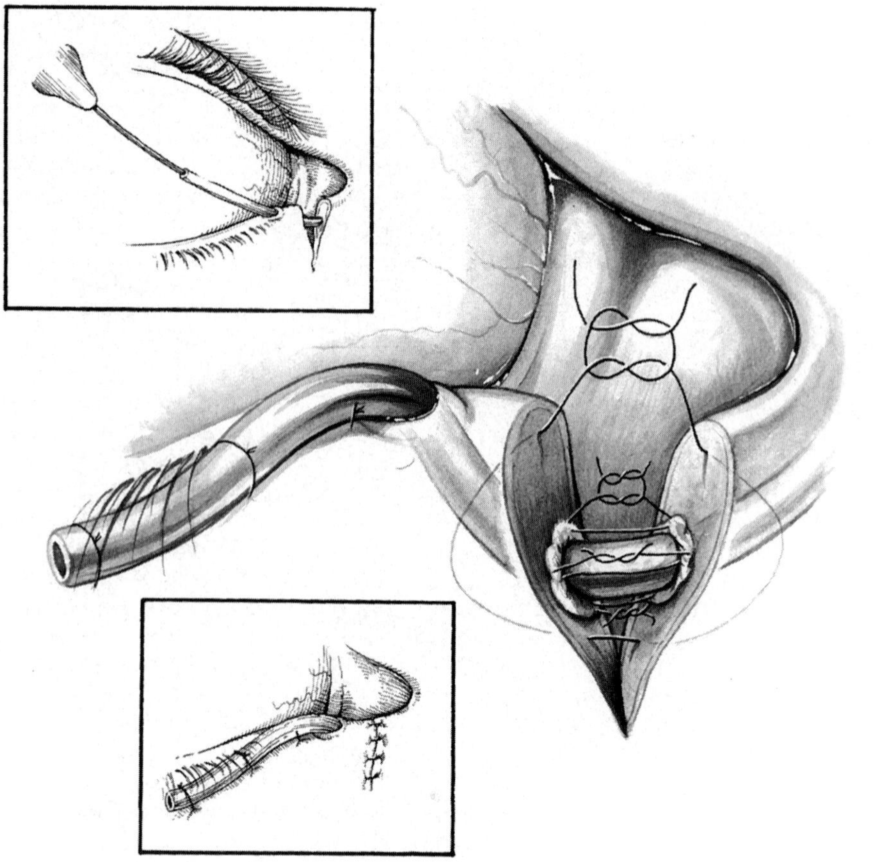

Figure 50–10. Repair of lacerated canaliculus.

described previously. If the medial end is difficult to find, the "bubble test" can be used.[10] Irrigation of air thru the intact uninvolved canaliculus can demonstrate the location of the cut end of the proximal involved canaliculus. Place a small pool of saline in the tear lake area prior to air irrigation and then look for where the bubbles are eminating.

C. The silicone tube with probe is placed in the medial cut end of the canaliculus and passed into the duct and out the nares.
D. The probe at the other end of the tube is placed into the lateral cut end of the canaliculus and brought out the punctum.
E. The second probe, after it is brought out of the involved canaliculus and punctum, is then placed in the uninvolved punctum and intubation occurs into the nares through the nasolacrimal system as previously described.
F. The probes are removed from the tubing and the tube is tied with a surgeon's knot and the excess tubing cut.
G. The laceration is then repaired with absorbable suture for deep tissue around the tubing with 5-0 polyglactin 910. 5-0 plain fast-absorbing gut is used to close the skin. These sutures will not need to be removed.
H. The tube should remain in place at least 6 weeks.

OBSTRUCTION OF THE NASOLACRIMAL DUCT

Congenital nasolacrimal duct obstruction is usually due to a membrane or obstruction of the valve of Hasner at the distal end of the nasolacrimal duct. The obstruction generally becomes apparent by 1 to 2 weeks of age in 2% to 4% of full-term infants, with one-third being bilateral. Most resolve within 4 to 6 weeks. Symptoms consist of epiphora, crusting, and discharge. Rarely, patients will have an acute dacryocystitis. Conservative treatment for congenital nasolacrimal obstruction consists of daily massaging of the tear sac. Massage should be performed in such a manner that positive pressure is created in the nasolacrimal sac and duct to force open the membranous obstruction. Topical antibiotic ointments or drops are occasionally used to clear up discharge. Rarely at birth, an infant may present with a bluish medial canthal mass which represents an underlying dilated lacrimal sac. The sac is filled with amniotic fluid as well as mucus secreted from the goblet cells of the conjunctiva. These are referred to as amniotoceles or dacryoceles and may be associated with nasal obstruction. In bilateral cases, the infants may not be able to feed as they are normally obligated to breath through the nose during feeding. This may create a failure to thrive. Occasionally, the nasal portion of the mass requires surgical marsupialization.

The nasolacrimal duct is obstructed, preventing drainage of the fluid. If there is no evidence of infection or airway obstruction, this condition can be first treated conservatively as described above.

If the nasolacrimal duct obstruction is not relieved by conservative measures or time, probing is indicated. Opinions vary as to the optimal timing of probing. It is clear that a delay in probing past 13 months of age is associated with a decreased success rate of initial probing.[11,12] Some physicians advocate office probing using topical anesthesia in a child 5 to 9 months old. This is arguably the safer, less expensive route and avoids general anesthesia, chronic conservative treatment by the parents, and epiphora-related pediatrician visits. In experienced hands, the immediate success rate is high, with virtually no morbidity, and the cost is low. However, in a number of these patients the obstruction will resolve without intervention. If probing is delayed too long, the patient may need silicone intubation for several months, or even a dacryocystorhinostomy, to maintain patency.

NASOLACRIMAL DUCT PROBING FOR CONGENITAL OBSTRUCTION

Probing of the nasolacrimal system can be accomplished either case in the operating room or in the office setting, depending on the age of the patient and the comfort level of the surgeon and family. General anesthesia is indicated if in the operating room. In either case, topical anesthetic is placed in the involved eye. If the child is awake, topical 5% cocaine on a cotton-tipped applicator can be placed on the punctum. If in the operating room, a cocaine-soaked cotton-tipped applicator may be placed in the inferior meatus after anesthesia induction.

A. The inferior punctum is dialted with a Jones punctal dilator.
B. A No. 00 probe is then inserted into the punctum and canalicular system until it hits the medial bony wall against the lacrimal sac. The probe is then rotated superiorly and angled slightly posteriorly and advanced into the nasolacrimal duct and into the inferior meatus. A popping sound or feeling often occurs as the membranous obstruction is elevated.
C. The probe is left in place for a minute to help dilate the opening. If the patient is under general anesthesia, the probe should be visualized within the nose with the aid of a nasal speculum and headlight. Fracturing of the inferior turbinate inward or medially with a Freer elevator or caudal elevator is performed. This has been demonstrated to be successful in reducing nasolacrimal duct obstruction.[13]

SILICONE INTUBATION FOR CONGENITAL NASOLACRIMAL DUCT OBSTRUCTION

Silicone intubation of the lacrimal excretory system is typically performed on children for nasolacrimal duct obstruction that fails to respond to conservative treatment or probing or in children too old to undergo probing in the office. It is occasionally performed on adults with partial obstruction of the nasolacrimal duct. The procedure is usually performed with the patient under general anesthesia but can be done using a local infiltrative anesthesia, topical nasal anesthetic, as well as intravenous sedation. The procedure has been described previously.

LACRIMAL ANLAGE

A lacrimal anlage is a congenital abnormality that occurs as a result of malformation of the lacrimal drainage apparatus. Multiple variations can occur but in general, this is an epithelium-lined passage somewhere in the medial canthal area that may be continuous with the lacrimal drainage system or be a "blind" cul-de-sac without connection. Those which are connected often will manifest by tears draining from the fistulous tract. If there is no connection to the drainage system, the anlage can be removed in the office (Fig. 50–11). If a connection is present, simultaneous canalicular intubation should be performed:

A. An appropriate Bowman probe is placed in the anlage tract.
B. Sharp dissection is used to cut around the probe, including all of the tract epithelium in the resection.
C. Once the deepest aspect of the tract is identified, the tissue surrounding the probe is removed entirely.
D. The deep subcutaneous tissues are closed with interrupted absorbable suture, and the skin is then closed to complete a two-layer closure.

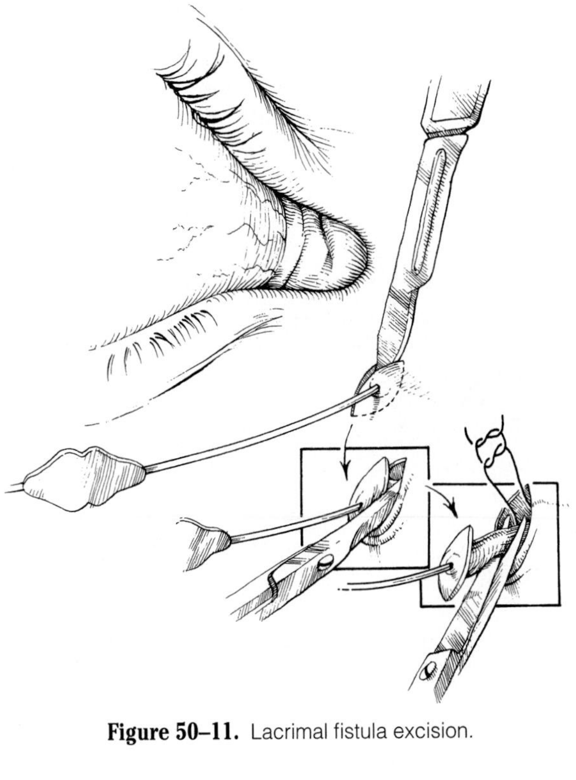

Figure 50–11. Lacrimal fistula excision.

ACQUIRED NASOLACRIMAL DUCT OBSTRUCTION

Acquired nasolacrimal obstruction can occur for various reasons. Trauma to the naso-orbital complex can result in a fracture of the lacrimal or maxillary bone, injuring the duct; chronic sinusitis, nasal or lacrimal sac inflammation, or infection can predisposition to obstruction. In addition, chronic ocular medications can accumulate in the lacrimal excretory system and cause blockage, as can lacrimal sac stones. In most cases, no clear cause is identified. Tumors are rare.

Although most patients present with epiphora, occasionally acute or chronic dacryocystitis is observed. Acute dacryocystitis treatment differs depending on the severity of the symptoms. For mild infections, a warm compress with topical antibiotics may be appropriate. More severe infections require oral antibiotics and, occasionally, decompression of the sac with massage, probing, or lancing with an 18-gauge needle or stab incision with a No. 11 blade. Probing is performed carefully in a severely infected sac with cellulitis to avoid spreading infection through false tracts.

DACRYOCYSTORHINOSTOMY (DCR)

External dacryocystorhinostomy (DCR) remains the "gold standard" for treating epiphora caused by nasal lacrimal duct obstruction.[14] As a general rule, dacryocystectomy is performed only when lacrimal sac masses are present. In an older or medically debilitated person or one with dry eyes who also has an incurable dacryocystitis, dacryocystectomy is probably a reasonable choice.[15] Lacrimal sac tumors are not common, but the malignancy rate is approximately 55% for those that do occur.[16] This problem may require management with a head and neck surgeon and an oncology team.

Endonasal DCR procedures were used for a long time prior to the introduction of endoscopy, but their best success rate was generally thought to be about 80%. A renewed interest in endonasal DCRs was sparked by the introduction of endonasal laser-assisted dacryocystorhinostomy.[17] The endoscope was added to this procedure shortly afterwards.[18] For the next few years, the success rates reported were generally poor. More recently, our experience and that of some others with endoscopic DCR has been equivalent to our success rates with external DCR. We now offer endoscopic DCR to patients who are concerned about the cosmetic blemish that a facial scar might produce.

Because good hemostasis is an important factor in dacryocystorhinostomy, every adult patient is urged to have a local anesthetic with monitored anesthesia care (MAC). The local anesthetic consists of an infiltrative anesthetic, a vasoconstrictor, and hyaluronidase. The maximum effect of the intravenous sedation administered by the anesthesiologist or certified registered nurse anesthetist should coincide with the administration of the local anesthetic.

After the eye on the operative side is topically anesthetized with proparacaine hydrochloride, infiltrate subcutaneously with lidocaine 2% with epinephrine (1:100,000) and hyaluronidase in the operative area below the medial canthus and in the region of the infratrochlear nerve above the medial canthus (Fig. 5–12). Packing gauze, 0.5 inch wide and 6 to 8 inches long, or 0.5 mm by 1.5 mm cottonoids, saturated with 5% cocaine and a trace of epinephrine hydrochloride (1:1000) or phenylephrine 2% is packed into the nose in the region of the attachment of the anterior tip of the middle turbinate (Fig. 50–13). When general anesthesia is used, the same infiltration and nasal packing are employed.

A. The skin is incised 11 mm nasal to the medial canthus, starting just superior to the medial canthal tendon insertion and extending inferiorly and slightly laterally for 20 mm (Fig. 50–14). The knife should not cut deeper than the subcutaneous tissue. The remaining subcutaneous tissue is cut with sharp Stevens scissors.

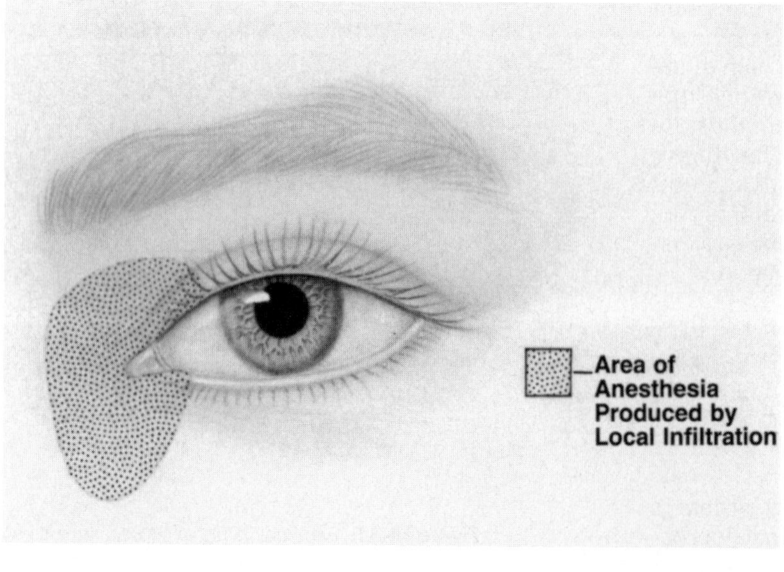

Figure 50–12. Local infiltrative anesthetic area.

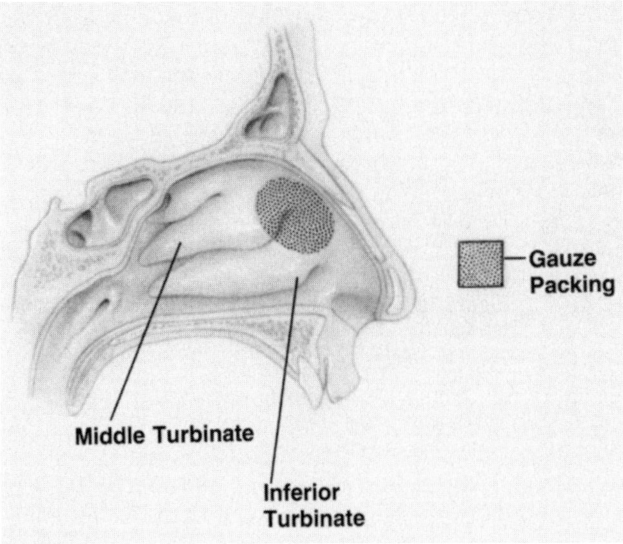

Figure 50–13. Intranasal location of infiltrative anesthetic and gauze packaging.

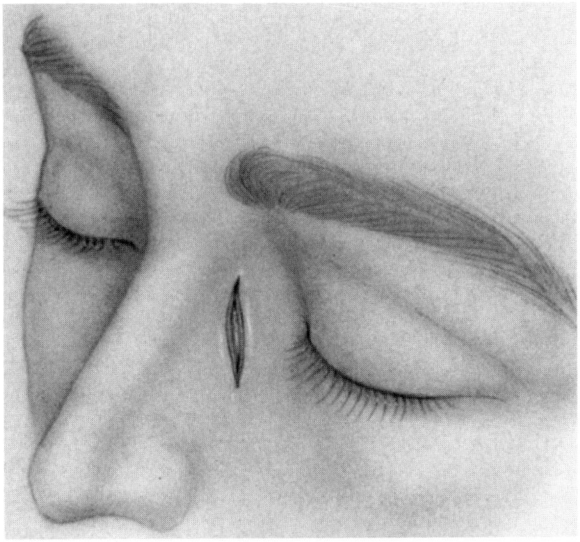

Figure 50–14. DCR incision.

B. A self-retaining, spring-type retractor like the Agricola is then inserted (Fig. 50–15). Separation of the initial orbicularis muscle fibers and hemostasis is performed with a hand-held battery high-temperature cautery unit (2200° F).

C. With two Freer elevators, locate the angular vein as it crosses the medial canthal tendon (Fig. 50–16). Press the vein to the medial or lateral side with an elevator to avoid injury to it and bleeding during the procedure. Dissect down using the elevators in the area just below the attachment of the medial canthal tendon to periosteum. Incise the periosteum with the sharp end of the elevator, parallel to the rim edge, and 2 to 3 mm medial to the anterior lacrimal crest. The periosteal incision on both sides is then raised and lightly elevated with the Freer elevator, and the periosteum is lifted off the bone. The lateral incision elevation will curve down into the orbit as it crosses the anterior lacrimal crest and continues to the posterior lacrimal crest. The periosteum is also elevated into the nasolacrimal canal as far as possible.

D. The lacrimal sac is then infiltrated with the same local anesthesia mixture used previously (Fig. 50–17), and a small square cottonoid that has been soaked in cocaine 5% is placed between the periosteum of the lacrimal sac and the bony wall of the medial orbit. This serves to help in hemostasis, anesthesia, and to protect the sac during bone removal.

E. At this time, exchange the spring-type retractor for one with longer teeth, such as a Goldstein retractor, which will reach the periosteum and give deeper exposure.

F. The nasal packing is removed prior to bone removal. Using a Hall drill or similar substitute with a 4-mm dental burr, an oblong area of bone anterior to the lacrimal crest is removed, taking care not to injure the nasal mucoperiosteum (Fig. 50–18). Use irrigation to prevent excessive heat build-up and to facilitate visualization.

G. Once a small opening has been made with the burr, elevate the nasal mucoperiosteum away from the bone with a dental burnisher or a Clev-dent No. 1 (Fig. 50–19).

H. Remove the cottonoid next to the periosteum and lacrimal sac, and inject the mucoperiosteum with local anesthetic.

I. A 45-degree Kerrison punch is then used to enlarge the vertical dimensions of the bony opening (Fig. 50–20). The most important area to remove lies just in front of the posterior lacrimal crest and under the medial canthal tendon.

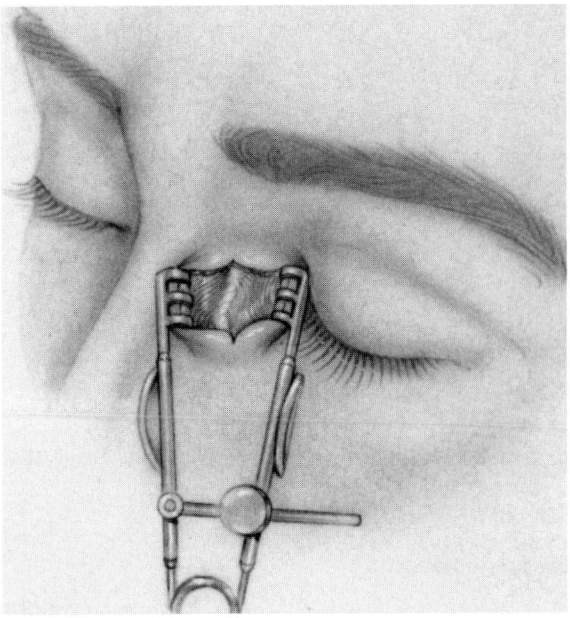

Figure 50–15. DCR dissection through orbicularis.

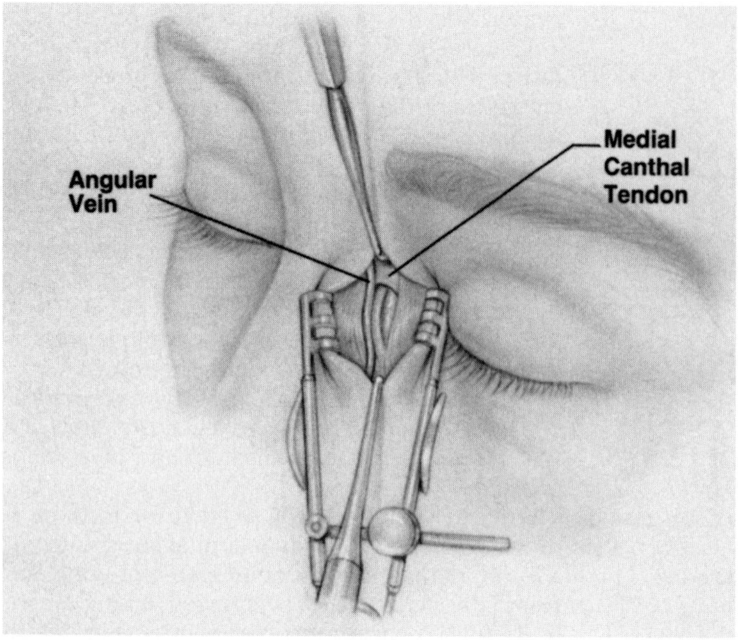

Figure 50–16. DCR dissection below medical canthal tendon.

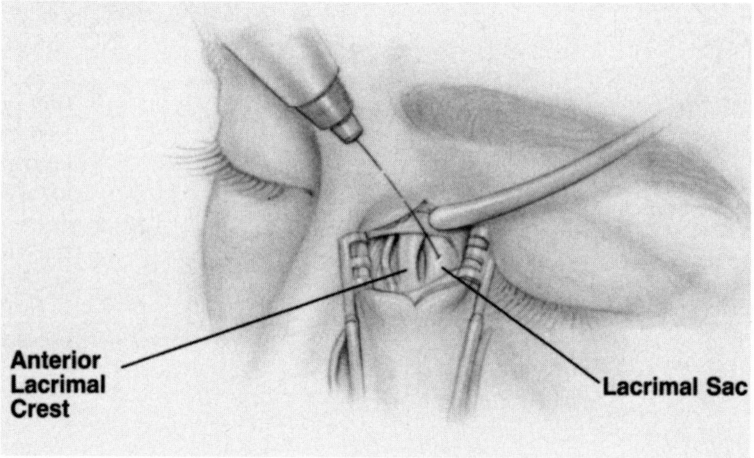

Figure 50–17. Local infiltration of lacrimal sac.

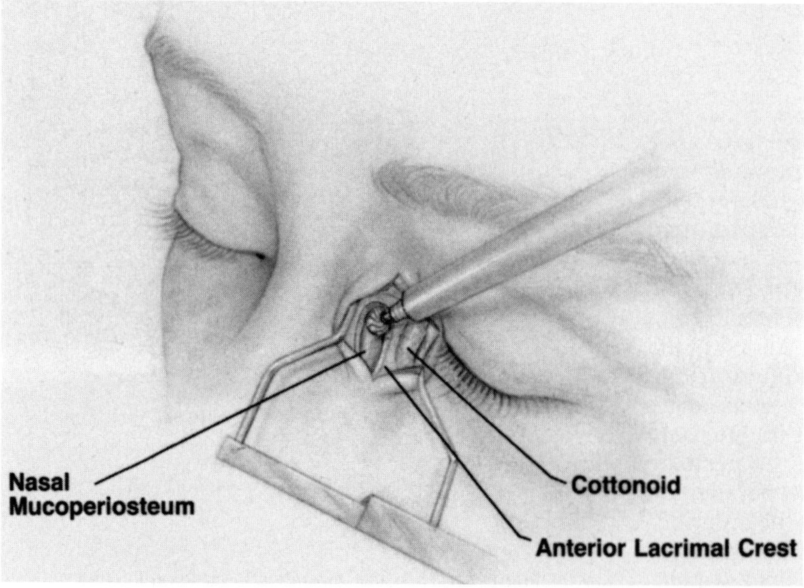

Figure 50–18. Creation of bony ostium with dental burr.

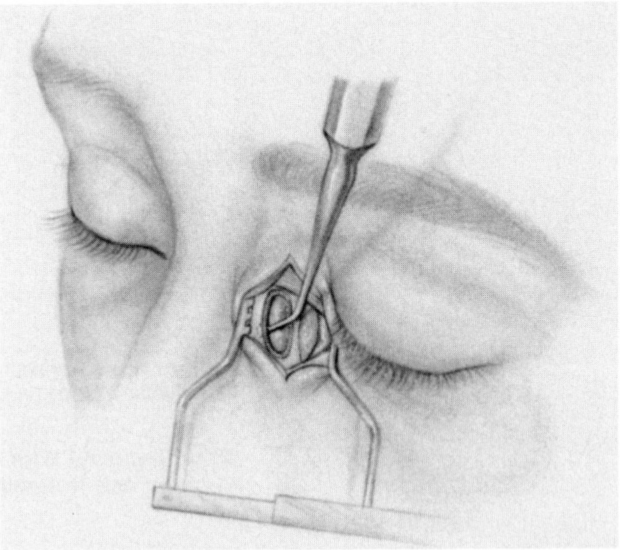

Figure 50–19. Separation of nasal mucoperiosteum from bone with dental burnisher.

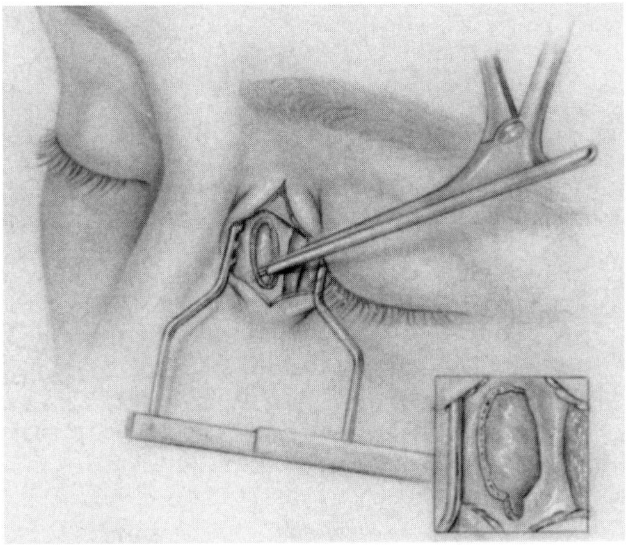

Figure 50–20. Enlarging bony ostium with rongeurs.

J. The bony bridge of the anterior lacrimal crest that remains is then removed with a rongeur (Fig. 50–21). The surgeon may encounter ethmoid air cells. We suggest a conservative "deskeletonization" of these cells.
K. The last portion of bone to be removed is the medial half of the bony nasolacrimal duct. First separate the nasal mucoperiosteum from the canal down to the inferior turbinate. A rongeur can be used to remove this bone.
L. Kerrison punches are used to smooth the rough edges of the hannulus, where the anterior and posterior lacrimal crests meet inferiorly. A good rule for all tear sac surgery is never to have a bony margin closer than 5 mm to the common canaliculus. The area of bone that is ideally removed is shown in Figure 50–22.
M. Attention is now turned to the lacrimal sac. The Goldman retractor is loosened and a No. 0 probe is inserted into either canaliculus. The medial wall of

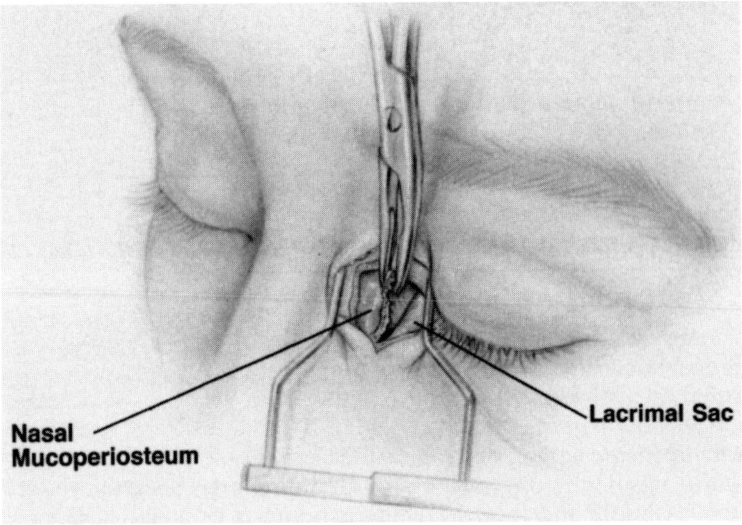

Figure 50–21. Enlarging bony ostium.

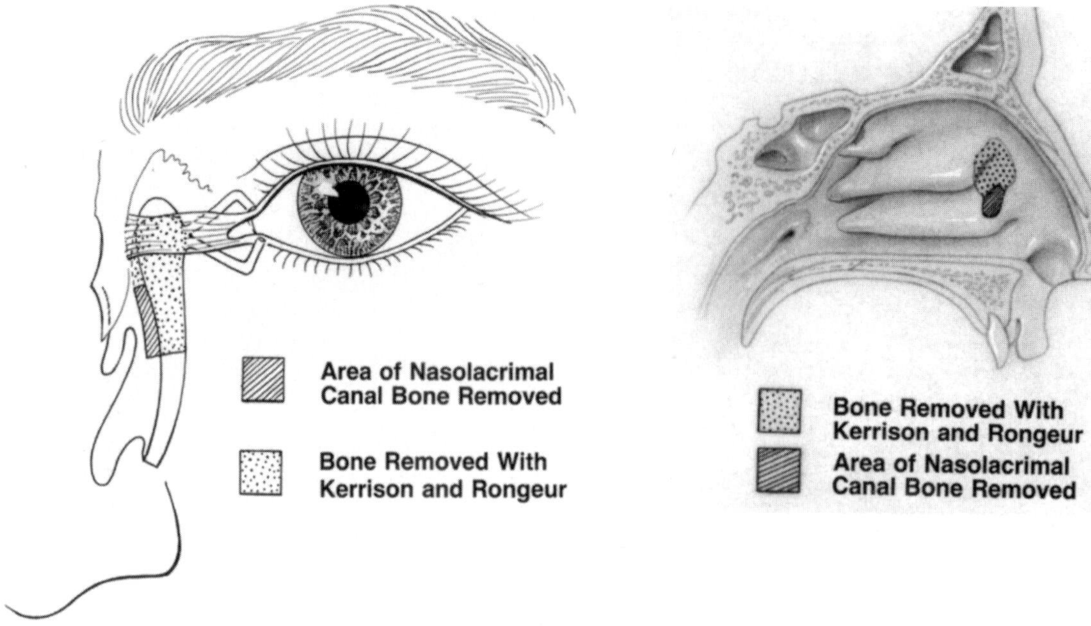

Figure 50–22. Location and extent of bone removal.

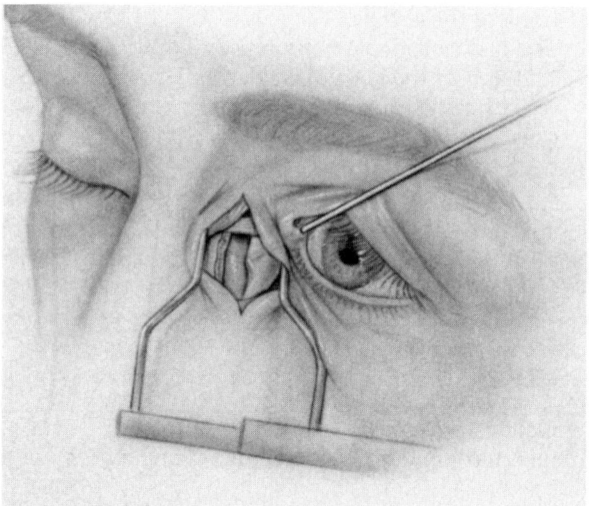

Figure 50–23. "Tenting" lacrimal sac medially to be opened sharply.

the lacrimal sac is then "tented" medially (Fig. 50–23). A No. 11 blade is used to cut through the periosteum and the sac slightly lateral to the probe tip. The incision is then extended using the sharp Stevens scissors. Extend the incision to the top of the fundus and to the opening of the sac into the nasolacrimal duct.

N. Place a Freer elevator into the nares and elevate the nasal mucoperiosteum laterally. Incise the mucoperiosteum with a No. 11 blade, parallel with the lacrimal sac incision. Extend this opening with the sharp Stevens scissors.

O. Cut away the posterior part of both the lacrimal sac and the nasal mucoperiosteum with the sharp Stevens scissors and forceps. There is no need to sew these flaps together.

P. At this point, a Quickert-Dryden probe with a piece of silicone tubing wedged on the sharp end (Crawford, Cline-Guibor) can be inserted in either canaliculus and directed into the open sac, where it can be grasped, under direct visualization through the wound, using a straight hemostat placed into the nose (Fig. 50–24). A straight metal suction tip inserted through the nares into the bony ostium can also be used to guide the probe. The probe is placed into the suction tip and advanced under direct visualization.

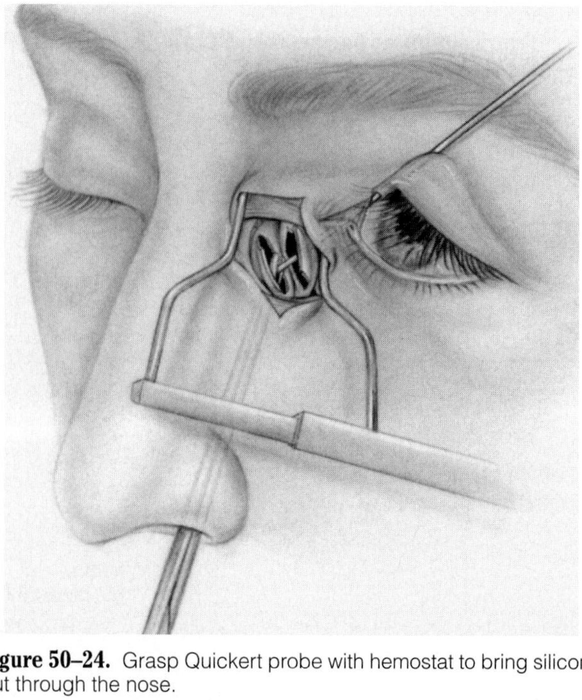

Figure 50–24. Grasp Quickert probe with hemostat to bring silicone out through the nose.

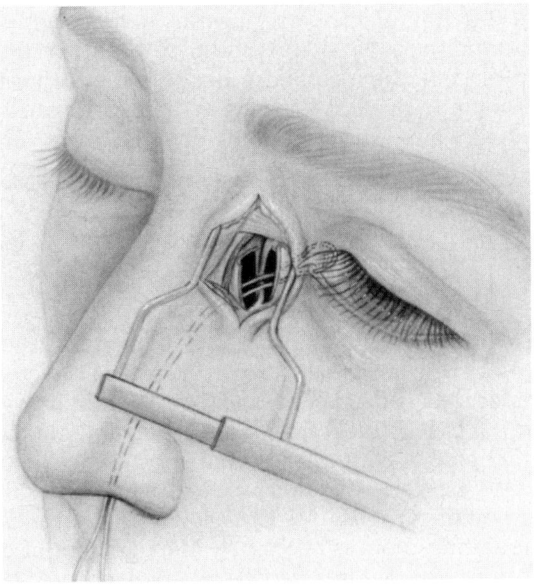

Figure 50–25. Silicone stent in place.

Q. Another probe attached to the opposite end of the silicone tube can then be passed through the opposite canaliculus in the same fashion. It also is brought out through the nares with the help of a forcep or suction tip (Fig. 50–25).
R. If bleeding is a problem or concern, a rolled piece of Instat (Johnson & Johnson) can be placed beneath the flaps, anterior to the tip of the middle turbinate. We use this routinely.
S. The silicone is tied with a square knot after the probes are separated from the tubing. There must be no tension on the punctum (Fig. 50–26).
T. The anterior flap of the lacrimal sac is approximated with anterior-based flap of the nasal mucosa using two interrupted 5-0 polyglactin 910 sutures on a P-2 needle. Remove the retractor.
U. The periosteum and orbicularis muscle are closed with running or interrupted polyglactin 910 suture.
V. The skin can be closed with a running 6-0 fast-absorbing gut or a running subcuticular 6-0 polyglactin 910.
W. Erythromycin or an antibiotic/steroid combination ointment is placed on the incision, which is then covered by a bandage strip cut lengthwise.

Postoperative ice packs are recommended. Patients are cautioned not to blow their nose as this will increase the chance of epistaxis. The silicone tube is usually removed in 6 weeks in the office. The silicone tubing is located in the nose with the use of a nasal speculum and bayonet forceps. The tube is then cut in the medial canthal area, between the upper and lower puncti; the tube is then withdrawn through the nares with the use of the foreceps.

CONJUNCTIVODACRYOCYSTO-RHINOSTOMY (CDCR)

When both canaliculi on the same side are absent or obstructed, there is less than 8 mm of salvagable canaliculus from the punctum, or there is paralysis of the lacrimal pump system with patent canaliculi, a conjunctivodacryocystorhinostomy is indicated.[14]

A. A dacryocystorhinostomy is performed as described, stopping before inserting the silicone tubing and closing the anterior flaps (steps A–O above).
B. Dissect away the caruncle to assure it will not obstruct the tube later, preserving the adjacent conjunctiva.
C. Insert a sharp Stevens scissors into the lacus lacrimalis 2 mm posterior to the cutaneous margin of the commissure (Fig. 50–27). Using blunt and sharp dissection, gently manipulate the scissors into the opened lacrimal sac, being sure the scissors are anterior to the body of the middle turbinate. If the anterior tip of the turbinate interferes, it should be resected (partial turbinectomy). Orientation of the scissors during the maneuver should be medial, posterior, and inferior.

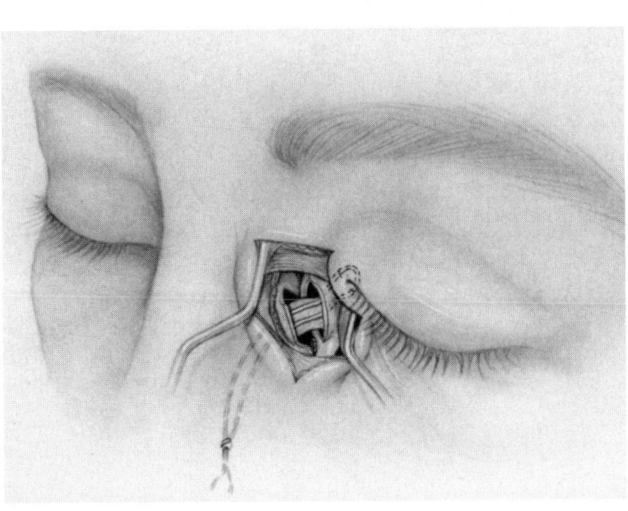

Figure 50–26. Instat place deep to silicone stent for added hemostasis.

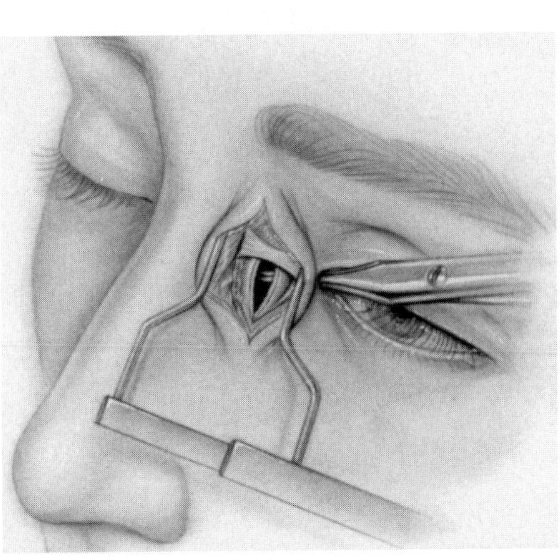

Figure 50–27. Creation of fistula track for placement of pyrex tube (CDCR).

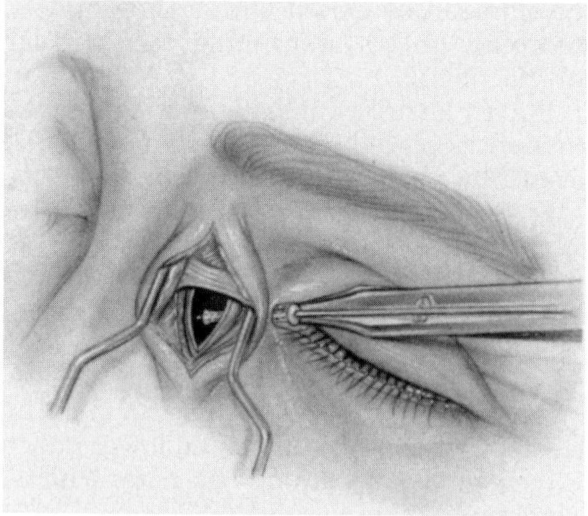

Figure 50–28. Placement of Jones tube on probe in fistula as the scissors is removed.

D. With the blades of the scissors in place, pass a No. 0 probe with appropriate Pyrex tube in place, just above or anterior to the scissors, between the opened blades, and into the sac (Fig. 50–28).
E. Remove the scissors and simultaneously push the Pyrex tube down the course of the probe. Be sure the tip of the Pyrex tube does not touch the nasal septum. If it does, a shorter length of tube must be used. The tube should extend well beyond the lateral wall of the nose.
F. A 5-0 polyglactin 910 suture is then wrapped around the collar of the tube, tied, and then sutured in place in the medial canthus. A 4-mm collar tube is usually used at first. It can be exchanged for a smaller size if needed in the future.
G. Close the anterior flaps, deep tissue, and skin as described for a DCR (steps T–W above).

FAILED DACRYOCYSTORHINOSTOMY

In less than 5% of our external DCR patients, a stricture or outright cicatricial closure of the internally created fistula occurs. If this is noted early postoperatively, dilation of the fistula with successively bigger nasolacrimal probes will avert permanent closure. This can generally be done with topical anesthetic in the office using Bowman probes 0–4. Occasionally a return visit to the operating room is necessary. Management of complete cicatricial closure (Fig. 50–29) involves three steps.

A. Decongesting the nose as previously described for probing.
B. A Bowman probe is placed in one canaliculus and used to "tent" the cicatrix into the nasal passage where it can be removed with a sharp dissection or a front-biting instrument.
C. Silicone intubation is then required to stent the new opening. This can be removed after 6 weeks. We have not found it necessary to use mitomycin C to inhibit gear formation in the majority of cases.

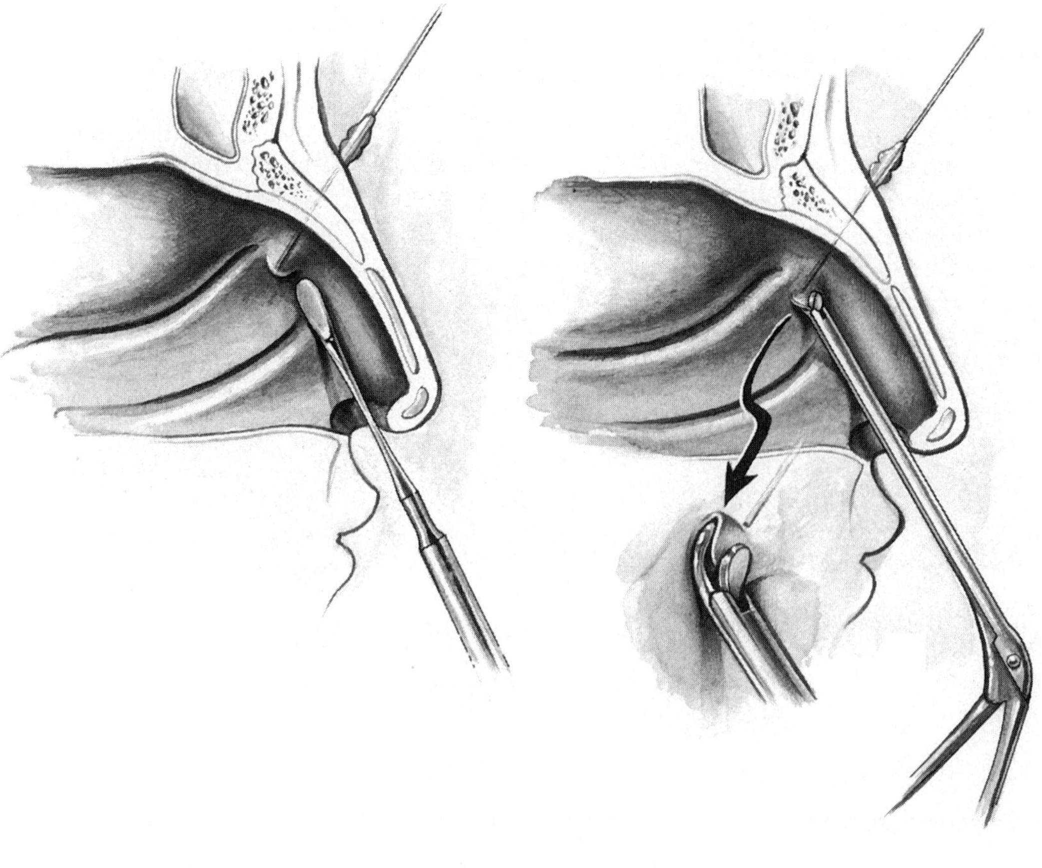

Figure 50–29. Closure of rhinostomy site.

REFERENCES

1. Jones LT, Wobig JL: Surgery of the Eyelids and Lacrimal System. Birmingham, AL, Aesculapius, 1976.
2. Schirmer O: Studies on the physiology and pathology of the secretion and drainage of tears. Arch. Ophthalmol 1903;54:197.
3. Jones LT, Marquis MM, Vincent NJ: Lacrimal function. Am J Ophthalmol 1972;73:658–9.
4. Jones LT, Linn ML: The diagnosis of the causes of epiphora. Ophthalmology 1987;94:698–705.
5. Milder B, DeMorest BH: Dacryocystography II—The pathologic lacrimal apparatus. Arch Ophthalmol 1955;54:410–21.
6. LaPiana FG: Management of occult atretic lacrimal puncta. Am J Ophthalmol 1972;74:32–3.
7. Nowinski TS, Anderson RL: The medial spindle procedure for involutional medial ectropion. Arch Ophthalmol 1985;103: 1750–3.
8. Dortzbach RK, Angrist RA: Silicone intubation for lacerated lacrimal canaliculi. Ophthal Surg 1985; 16:639–42.
9. Hawes MJ, Sigrest DR: Effectiveness of bicanalicular silicone intubation in the repair of canalicular laceration. Opththal Plast Reconstr Surg 1985;1:185–90.
10. Dailey RA, Wobig JL, Loff JH: The bubble test: An atraumatic method for canalicular laceration repair. Ophthal Plast Reconstr Surg 1996;12:61–4
11. Dortzbach RK, France TD, Kushner BJ, et al.: Silicone intubation for obstruction of the nasolacrimal duct in children. Am J Ophthalmol 1982;94:585–90.
12. Katowitz JA, Welsh MG: Timing of initial probing and irrigation in congenital nasolacrimal duct obstruction. Ophthalmology 1987;94:697–705.
13. Wesley RE: Inferior turbinate fracture in the treatment of congenital nasolacrimal duct obstruction and congenital nasolacrimal duct anomaly. Ophthal Surg 1985;16:368–71.
14. Wobig JL, Dailey RA: Surgery of the lacrimal apparatus. Ophthalmic Surgery. St. Louis, CV Mosby, 1993.
15. Mauriello JA, Vadehra VK: Dacryocystectomy: Surgical indications and results in 25 patients. Ophthal Plast Reconstr Surg 1997;13:216–20.
16. Stefanyszyn MA, Hidayat AA, Pe'er JJ, et al.: Lacrimal sac tumors. Ophthal Plast Reconstr Surg 1994;10:169–84.
17. Massaro BM, Gonnering RS, Harris GJ: Endonasal laser dacryocystorhinostomy: A new approach to nasolacrimal duct obstruction. Arch Ophthalmol 1990;108:1172–76.
18. Gonnering RS, Lyon DB, Fisher JC: Endoscopic laser-assisted lacrimal surgery. Am J Ophthalmol 1991;111:152–7.

CHAPTER 51

Trichiasis

DAVID R. MILSTEIN, M.D.

Trichiasis is a descriptive term for an acquired condition characterized by eyelashes that are abnormally directed against the globe. *Distichiasis* refers to a congenital or acquired condition characterized by a second row of eyelashes arising from metaplastic meibomian gland orifices. It is important to distinguish between these conditions to achieve optimum surgical results. It is also important to differentiate trichiasis from cicatricial entropion, in which not only the eyelashes but also keratinized skin and the entire eyelid margin are turned against the cornea. Manual epilation, ophthalmic ointments, or a therapeutic contact lens may be used prior to surgical therapy. Surgical therapy for trichiasis or distichiasis requires a follicle destructive procedure such as electrolysis, argon laser, radiofrequency tissue ablation, cryotherapy or direct excision. A localized group of abnormally directed eyelashes may be treated with a full-thickness eyelid excision and reconstruction of the eyelid margin. When eyelashes are directed against the globe from eyelid malrotation or cicatricial causes, surgical therapy is specifically directed towards treatment of the eyelid malrotation.

The hair follicle and its germinal tissue are hardy and may be deprived of its blood supply for extended periods of time and still regenerate. This phenomenon is illustrated by the high success rate of hair-baring autografts for androgenic or traumatic baldness. Hair growth as well as eyelash growth is cyclic and not continuous. The terms Anagen, Catagen, and Telogen phases apply to eyelash growth as well as to hair growth phases elsewhere in the body. Failure of treatment may only mean that an adjacent aberrant eyelash has moved from the Telogen growth phase into the Anagen growth phase. In follicle-destructive procedures, the quantity of tissue damage must be sufficient, or stem cells and possibly other germinal growth tissue will regenerate the eyelash, and trichiasis will recur. In addition, new aberrant eyelashes may arise as part of the natural history of the original disease. Regardless of the follicle destructive procedure chosen, each treatment is roughly 66% to 75% successful. Physicians must therefore expect and anticipate that multiple treatment sessions will be necessary. They must plan to make the patient comfortable during each encounter and with the overall surgical plan. It is important to inform patients that recurrence is an expected event and that treatment is performed in stages.

ANESTHESIA

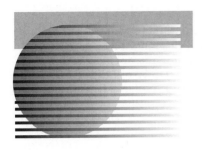

To minimize the discomfort of transcutaneous injections, topical EMLA cream or ELA-Max cream are applied to the eyelid skin. The cream should be kept away from the ocular surface. If the cream does come in contact with the eye, a mild stinging sensation may occur. This side effect is self-limited and relieved by irrigation with a balanced salt solution. The topical skin anesthetics are hindered only by their delayed onset of action and their cost. Transconjunctival anesthesia is rapid and well tolerated, with many advantages for purposes of electrolysis anesthesia. Transconjunctival injections are more comfortable than transcutaneous injections of buffered and warmed lidocaine. A lower incidence of ecchymosis has been observed with the use of transconjunctival injections when compared to transcutaneous anesthesia. The technique of transconjunctival anesthesia is not limited to electrolysis, but may also be used for a wide variety of disorders including chalazion excision, full-thickness excision of aberrant lash-bearing eyelid tissue, entropion repair, and cryotherapy.

TECHNIQUE OF TRANSCONJUNCTIVAL EYELID ANESTHESIA

a. Anesthetize the surface with topical anesthetic.
b. Apply two sets of 4% unpreserved lidocaine-soaked pledgets to the conjunctival injection site for 30 seconds.
c. In the upper eyelid, inject anesthetic solution through a 30-gauge needle just proximal to the junction of Mueller's muscle and tarus and advance the needle into the subcutaneous tissues. Infiltration of up to 2 cc's of fluid may be needed. If the needle is passed too far superficially, the injection will sting somewhat more than if infiltration occurs more deeply, although the sensation of discomfort appears to be better than a transcutaneous injection.
d. In the lower eyelid, the vertical dimension of tarsus is shorter and the anesthetic solution may be infiltrated closer to the eyelid margin.
e. Allow sufficient time for the anesthetic to diffuse through tissue, usually 5 to 10 minutes.
f. If transconjunctival anesthesia is incomplete, the above procedure may be repeated, or supplemented with a transcutaneous injection.

FULL-THICKNESS EYELID EXCISION

Discrete localized areas of trichiasis may be corrected with full-thickness eyelid excision and plastic repair of the resultant defect. When trichiasis results from an abnormal position of the eyelid margin, it should be corrected with surgery directed toward correcting the eyelid position. Trichiasis due to cicatricial entropion, as in Stevens-Johnson syndrome, requires a lid-splitting approach since ablative treatments such as cryotherapy and extensive electrolysis actually worsen the condition.

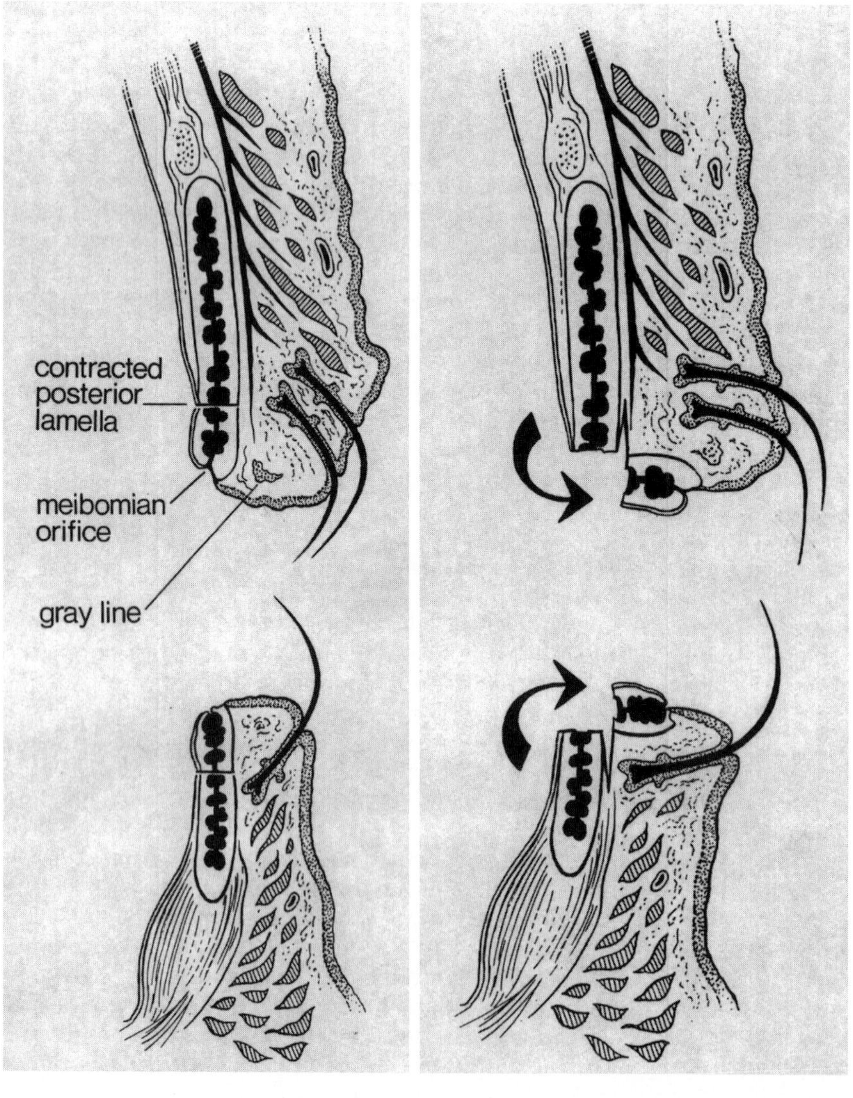

Figure 51–1. In cicatricial entropion, the entire eyelid margin is rotated against the cornea. The tarsus is split longitudinally 2 mm posterior to the gray line, and the distal segment is rotated 180 degrees. A nasal turbinate mucosal graft is sutured into position to act as a new eyelid margin, and as a buttress for the rotated distal segment. (© Copyright 1999, Regents of the University of California)

TECHNIQUE OF SURGICAL EYELID REVISION FOR CICATRICIAL ENTROPION[1]

a. A horizontal tarsectomy is performed in the upper and lower eyelid approximately 2 to 3 mm posterior to the gray line.
b. The distal tarsal segments are then dissected and a rotation of 180 degrees is attempted (Fig. 51–1).
c. A graft of nasal turbinate mucosa or hard palate mucosa measuring 1.5 × 3 cm is harvested.
d. The graft is sutured to the cut edge of tarsus in the upper and lower eyelid using a serpentine externalized suture such as 6-0 polypropylene.
e. The rotated distal tarsus segment is stabilized against the graft using 5 mattress sutures of 6-0 in both the upper and lower eyelids.
f. After 3 weeks, the graft is split by sharp dissection between the upper and lower eyelids.

CRYOTHERAPY

Cryotherapy is an acceptable procedure when tarsus and conjunctiva are normal. Eyelash follicles are usually more sensitive to the effects of a double freeze–thaw cycle than skin, tarsus, orbicularis and other skin appendages. However, this sensitivity is not entirely predictable. Permanent loss of skin pigmentation should be expected and is particularly noticeable in darkly pigmented skin. Eyelid margin deformity has also been reported from the use of cryotherapy. Cryotherapy produces significant postoperative swelling and, possibly, blistering of the skin. Patients should be counseled regarding this inflammatory response. As noted above, cryotherapy is contraindicated in the management of trichiasis associated with cicatricial conditions such as those seen in Stevens-Johnson syndrome because it worsens the condition. Transcutaneous cryotherapy is an acceptable means of delivery, but fewer eyelid deformities result when the eyelid is surgically divided into anterior lamellae and posterior lamellae, with cryotherapy being applied to the posterior lamella in treatment for conditions such as distichiasis. Treatment failures occur and areas of abnormal eyelashes may be retreated using cryotherapy.

TECHNIQUE

a. Instill topical anesthetic eye drops and then anesthetize the eyelid.
b. Protect the ocular surface and globe with a nonmetallic scleral contact lens. A plastic coffee spoon is acceptable.
c. Insert the thermocouple needle of the cryotherapy unit anterior to tarsus and posterior to the orbicularis in the region of the eyelashes to be treated.
d. Place the cryoprobe against the tissue and perform two freeze–thaw cycles to −20° C. The best success is obtained by rapidly freezing and slowly thawing the tissues. Allow near-complete re-thawing of tissue between cycles.
e. An antibiotic ointment is used for 5 days. Oral analgesics are prescribed as needed.

ELECTROLYSIS AND ARGON/ DIODE LASER TREATMENT

If isolated lashes are symptomatic and cause corneal irritation, they may be removed using radiofrequency needle ablation, argon or diode laser, or needle electrolysis. Regardless of the modality used, the objective is to destroy the eyelash and its germinal tissue at the base of the hair follicle canal. Within the eyelid, the base of this canal may lie up to 3 mm deep to the eyelid margin. The canal may not take a straight course, particularly in various cicatricial, metaplastic, or post-inflammatory conditions.

ELECTROLYSIS

There are several excellent electrolysis units available. The Perma-Tweeze unit (Fig. 51–2) has several advantages. It is reasonably priced, portable, battery-operated, and has a flexible fine needle that minimizes false passages and facilitates placement within the depths of the follicular canal. Parts are easy to obtain and inexpensive. However, any electrolysis machine is adequate as long as it has an adjustable power source. This feature is important because current delivery can be adjusted to just above the threshold where bubbles appear at the follicle opening. This is the minimum current that will effectively ablate the eyelash follicle and produce minimal scarring of the eyelid margin.

TECHNIQUE

a. The patient is comfortably seated at the slit-lamp biomicroscope.
b. Anesthetize the ocular surface with a topical anesthetic and then anesthetize the eyelid segment to be treated.
c. Leave the aberrant eyelash intact prior to treatment. Do not epilate.
d. Insert the electrolysis needle into the lash follicle canal under slit-lamp magnification in the direction of lash growth without creating a false passage. The plastic tweezer tips of the Perma Tweeze unit may be removed for more precise use in removing eyelashes.
e. Slowly increase the current until bubbles are seen at the opening of the hair follicle. Use the minimum amount of current that generates bubbles at the skin surface. With the Perma-Tweeze unit, having the patient increase contact with, or squeeze harder against the hand held electrode increases the amount of current delivered.
f. The electrolysis needle provided by the Perma-Tweeze unit is flexible and is suspended by a spring. The surgeon may use a trick to assure placement of the needle tip at the base of the follicular canal. Once the needle has been properly advanced to maximum

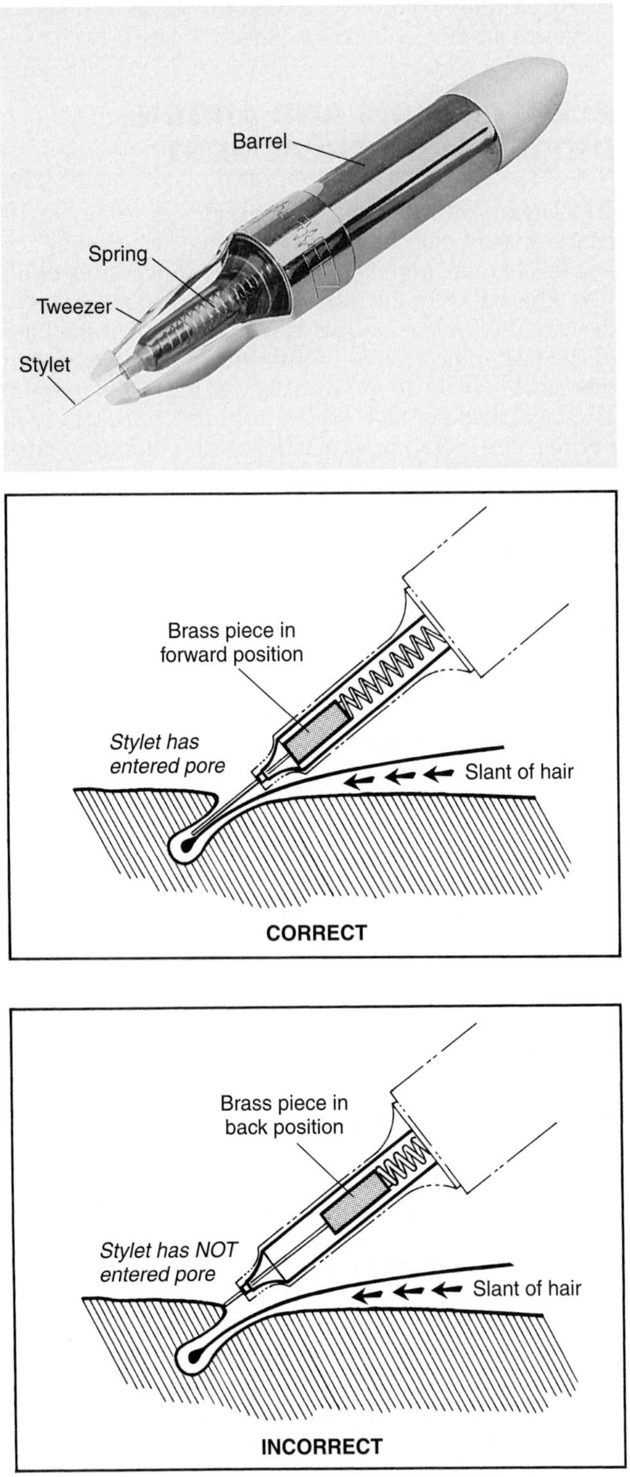

Figure 51–2. Perma-Tweeze electrolysis instrument. (© Copyright General Medical Company).

depth, maintain the needle at this depth and use the flexible property of the needle to bend it gently in circular movements as though it is "orbiting" or "jump-roping" around the eyelash. If the surgeon observes that the electrolysis needle successfully completes one or two orbits of the eyelash it is more likely that the needle has been inserted to the correct depth and direction and is fully advanced into the follicular canal. The application of sufficient power is confirmed when bubbles are seen emanating from the tissues. Loosening of the eyelash from its attachments appears to be the best clinical method of determining the proper endpoint of the procedure. Manual epilation of the eyelash following treatment should not be met with any resistance; otherwise continue the procedure.

g. Antibiotic eyedrops or ointment may be prescribed for one or two days postoperatively

ARGON/DIODE LASER

Argon laser eyelash destruction has been shown to be an effective, although expensive, means of eyelash destruction. Argon or diode laser works by heat uptake of the laser light frequency within the target tissue, in this case the eyelash and adjacent skin. For this reason, current lasers have not proven useful for non-pigmented eyelashes, or distichiasis with lanugo or velus lashes. Nonetheless, a high degree of success has been reported using argon and diode laser for pigment-containing eyelash destruction. Experience with the technique suggests that it is not any less painful than conventional electrolysis, and may also produce tiny eyelid margin deformities. Moreover, the treatment may require more than 200 applications per eyelash.

TECHNIQUE

a. Anesthetize the corneal surface and eyelid.
b. Protect the globe by having the patient direct their gaze away from the laser light or use a protective contact lens.
c. Select a 100 to 200 micron spot size and increase the power until eyelash tissue is ablated with each laser pulse.
d. Direct the laser or manipulate the eyelid so that the treatment is directed along the axial length of the eyelash.
e. Treatment must be carried out to a depth of 2 to 3 mm, and up to several hundred laser applications may be necessary for each eyelash.
f. Apply postoperative antibiotic eye drops or ointment for 3 days.

SUMMARY

Surgical treatment of aberrant eyelashes is highly successful but must be considered a multistage process. Patients will accept the concept of multiple treatments, if the treatment sessions are as comfortable as possible. The use of transconjunctival eyelid anesthesia is well suited to this process.

The above-described methods are not the only means for eyelash removal. Direct excision of eyelashes through a lid crease incision and also by direct transcutaneous dissection have been used successfully. Noninvasive devices marketed as electronic tweezers claim to permanently remove unwanted body hair. A clinical trial by the author (unpublished data) of one of these devices was conducted by modifying a fine jewelers forceps and adjusting the energy output to conform to FDA requirements. Although the treatment was virtually painless and well tolerated, within the study period 100% regrowth of aberrant eyelashes was seen within 6 to 8 weeks.

Recently noninvasive hair removal "laser" devices have been employed for treatment of unwanted pigmented body hair. Newer laser units employ an expanded frequency of light and coupling gels that have claimed to make it possible to treat blond and gray hair as well. This is a relatively new modality, and the past few years have shown this modality to be capable of retarding hair growth but not entirely eliminating it. At the present time, handpieces for the delivery of laser energy to the eyelid have not yet been adapted for the treatment of the eyelashes. The goal of "non-invasive" permanent hair and eyelash removal has not yet been realized. This field of research currently awaits validation by clinical study.

CHAPTER 52

Temporal Artery Biopsy

DAVID A. WEINBERG, M.D. and BRIDGET SUNDELL, M.D.

Temporal artery biopsy (TAB) is a commonly performed procedure that involves removal of a segment of the superficial temporal artery, usually for the purpose of finding histopathologic evidence of giant cell arteritis (GCA), also known as *temporal arteritis* or *cranial arteritis.* Most ophthalmologists and general surgeons are familiar with this surgery, which generally carries low morbidity. A detailed understanding of the anatomy of the temporal region and the course of the facial nerve is essential in avoidance of complications.

TAB remains the "gold standard" for the definitive diagnosis of GCA, although other diagnostic tests have been proposed, including ocular pneumoplethysmography,[1] temporal gallium uptake,[2] and fluorescein angiography.[3] A recent study by Schmidt and associates[4] investigated the use of color duplex untrasonography of the superficial temporal artery (STA) and reported findings characteristic of GCA: a dark halo around the lumen of the involved vessel. The authors suggest that color duplex ultrasonography may supplant the need for TAB in certain cases of GCA with a more typical presentation.

INDICATIONS

The primary indication for TAB is clinical suspicion of GCA. Occasionally, TAB is used to diagnose other conditions[5,6] because temporal artery inflammation has also been reported in polyarteritis nodosa, Wegener's granulomatosis, and Churg-Strauss syndrome.[7] The STA is biopsied because it is easily accessible and frequently involved in GCA.[8] Temporal artery biopsy is performed to provide confirmation of the diagnosis of GCA because management of this condition involves a very long course of oral prednisone (usually for at least 1 year), and prolonged oral corticosteroid therapy carries the risk of numerous minor and major adverse effects.[9] Furthermore, other immunosuppressive agents, such as methotrexate, may be needed.

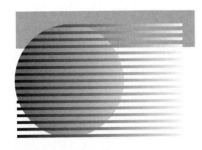

TAB is recommended for patients suspected of having GCA, particularly when the diagnosis is unclear. There are a number of physicians who believe that TAB is probably unnecessary for patients in whom the diagnosis of GCA is clinically "obvious."[10–12] In patients in whom the underlying diagnosis is particularly vague, TAB will have a strong impact on whether to subject the patient to the lengthy course (often 1 to 2 years) of systemic corticosteroids. However, in patients with strong clinical evidence for GCA, the physician–patient team may decide to treat the patient regardless of the biopsy results. It may then be asked: Why biopsy if you plan to treat the patient regardless of whether the biopsy is positive or negative? The reason is to provide substantiation of the diagnosis should the primary care physician and the patient consider prematurely discontinuing the prednisone in the event that the patient suffers a fracture due to osteoporosis, develops overt or poorly controlled diabetes mellitus, has an exacerbation of peptic ulcer disease, or encounters another serious adverse reaction to the systemic corticosteroid therapy. With a clearly positive TAB, there can be little or no doubt about the need for protective immunosuppressive therapy. For this reason, many physicians advocate pursuing TAB in *every* patient in whom GCA is suspected, and this has traditionally been the standard of care.[8,13–16]

BRIEF OVERVIEW OF GIANT CELL ARTERITIS

Giant cell arteritis is a systemic vasculitis involving medium- and large-sized arteries, which contain an internal elastic lamina.[17] This disorder may result in blindness, stroke, or myocardial infarction, making it a potentially fatal condition. The disease is more common in Caucasian women, especially those living in northern latitudes, such as Scandinavians.[18–20] The incidence of GCA in women is two to three times that in men, and both incidence and prevalence increase with age and vary by geographic region. The age-specific incidence rate increases from 2.3/100,000 in the sixth decade of life to 44.7/100,000 in the ninth decade, with an average age at onset of 71 years.[21] Ninety percent of patients are over the age of 60.[18] Giant cell arteritis is uncommon among African Americans and Asians[16,22–25] and very rare in patients under the age of 50 years.[23,26]

The etiology of GCA is unknown, although the pathophysiologic mechanisms involve the cell-mediated immune response. Most of the infiltrating lymphocytes in TAB specimens have been found to be T cells.[27] In addition, immunoglobulin deposits have been detected in biopsy samples, suggesting a possible autoimmune mechanism.[28] One study that used the polymerase chain reaction found evidence of parvovirus B19 in TAB specimens from GCA patients indicating a possible role for this virus in the pathogenesis of GCA.[29] Another group of investigators recently discovered varicella-zoster virus DNA in 26% of biopsied temporal arteries that showed histologic evidence of GCA.[29a]

The diagnosis of GCA should be considered in patients with any of the typical symptoms, particularly if they are over the age of 55. Constitutional symptoms include headache, generalized malaise, fatigue, anorexia, unintentional weight loss, fever of unknown origin, scalp tenderness and hyperesthesia, jaw claudication, and diffuse muscle aching (polymyalgia rheumatica), as well as sweats and arthralgias in some patients. Temporal headaches and tenderness are common, sometimes with a prominent, firm, and cordlike superficial temporal artery. The most specific signs and symptoms of GCA are jaw or tongue claudication, transient or permanent visual loss, diminished pulse or tenderness of the superficial temporal artery, scalp tenderness, neck pain, and elevated C-reactive protein (above 2.45 mg/dl) and/or Westergren erythrocyte sedimentation rate (ESR) above 46 mm/h.[18,30–32]

When GCA is suspected, a prompt ESR should be obtained, preferably by the Westergren method.[33] An elevated Westergren ESR, typically greater than 50 mm/hour and not uncommonly over 90 mm/hour, supports the diagnosis. The approximate upper limits of "normal" for the Westergren ESR are [age divided by two] in men and [(age + 10) divided by two] in women[34]. Patients with biopsy-proven GCA may have a normal ESR[35–42] in some cases because of prior systemic corticosteroid therapy for conditions such as polymyalgia rheumatica or rheumatoid arthritis. At the same time, there are numerous patients with an elevated ESR who do not have GCA.[6,15,43,44] While Hedges and colleagues[15] found that patients with biopsy-proven GCA tended to have a higher ESR than patients without GCA, Roth and associates[6] observed no significant difference in the ESR between these two groups and suggested that the ESR "was of little value in predicting the ultimate diagnosis." In patients found to have a negative TAB and in whom there was low clinical suspicion of GCA, there was an increased incidence of cancer (21%), diabetes mellitus (20%), and various chronic systemic inflammatory diseases (16%), and most had an elevated ESR (some >100).[6,15] Polymyalgia rheumatica, vascular or muscle contraction headaches, viral or bacterial infections, and a variety of other conditions have also been described as the ultimate diagnoses in patients who had negative TABs.[14] Some authorities believe that the C-reactive protein may be a more sensitive and reliable test than ESR in GCA,[12,30,31] although a normal C-reactive protein in the face of an elevated ESR and clinically obvious GCA has been reported.[45]

Whereas some patients have a classic presentation, i.e., with many of the typical symptoms of GCA listed above, other cases may be ambiguous. There are numerous reports of patients with "occult" GCA in whom there are no constitutional symptoms,[33,46–48] representing 21.2% (18/85) of patients with GCA in one series.[46] These patients pose a significant diagnostic challenge, and TAB is essential in making the diagnosis. It is extremely important to at least entertain the diagnosis of GCA in any elderly patient who presents with visual loss or vague constitutional symptoms.

In terms of the ophthalmologic manifestations, patients with GCA may complain of transient or permanent visual loss, diplopia, or eye pain. Ocular complications of GCA may include anterior (or infrequently posterior) ischemic optic neuropathy, ischemic retinopathy, central retinal artery occlusion, choroidal ischemia, ocular motility disturbances, and, more rarely, scintillating scotomata, anterior segment ischemia, ocular ischemic syndrome, ocular hypotony, autonomic pupillary abnormalities, and orbital ischemia or infarction.[35,49,50] Anterior ischemic optic neuropathy (ALON) is the cause of permanent visual loss in approximately 90% to 95% of patients with temporal arteritis, while ischemic retinopathy (including cilioretinal artery occlusion) and central retinal artery occlusion are much less common.[50,51] Permanent visual loss is preceded by episodes of transient visual loss (amaurosis fugax) in 10% to 30% of patients.[33,50,51] Ocular motility disorders, due to orbital, cranial nerve, or brain stem ischemia, are found in 10% to 15% of patients with GCA, although a larger number of patients (44%) have ophthalmoparesis without diplopia.[33,52] Giant cell arteritis may also produce myocardial infarction, stroke, neuropsychiatric syndromes, transient ischemic attacks, neuro-otologic syndromes, and peripheral neuropathy, among other signs and symptoms.[33,53,54]

Early diagnosis and treatment are essential because severe and bilateral visual loss is common when treatment is delayed or withheld. Severe visual loss develops in approximately one third of untreated cases of GCA, and two thirds of patients with untreated arteritic AION suffer bilateral involvement.[33] In sequential bilateral cases of arteritic AION, the second eye tends to become involved within 24 hours in one third of patients and within one week in two thirds of patients.[8] Therefore, as soon as there is clinical suspicion of GCA, the patient should immediately be started on systemic corticosteroids, even before the TAB is done. To reduce the chances of a false-negative biopsy because of corticosteroid therapy, TAB has been recommended within 1 week after initiation of treatment.[8,55] Adequate dosage of systemic corticosteroids often, but not always, protects the contralateral eye against visual loss when the corticosteroids are initiated prior to the onset of visual loss. It is unclear, however, what constitutes adequate dosage. Once visual loss begins, it frequently will progress despite the initiation of therapy.[56–58] Thus, the emphasis is on *prevention* of ocular involvement.

There is a long history of controversy regarding whether the corticosteroids should be administered orally or intravenously and at what dosage. Oral prednisone is commonly initiated at a dosage of 60 to 100 mg daily, while intravenous methylprednisolone is frequently given in the range of 1 to 2 g daily in divided doses.[8,49] Although some studies have shown clinical response to lower doses of oral prednisone (in the range of 20 to 40 mg daily),[59–61] this lowered dose does carry some risk, particularly in patients who have experienced some visual loss. For this reason, more aggressive, high-dose intravenous corticosteroid therapy is widely advocated in patients who present with recent visual loss,[58] although some authors believe that intravenous corticosteroid therapy may be no more protective against visual loss than oral therapy.[62] In addition to visual signs or symptoms, other serious signs of vascular compromise, such as myocardial or cerebral ischemia, may necessitate high-dose intravenous corticosteroids for several days before initiating oral therapy.[63] Alternate day corticosteroid regimens should be avoided because they may not be as protective.[64]

After the ESR has reached its nadir and the patient has become relatively asymptomatic, a slow taper of the prednisone may be initiated, while closely monitoring the ESR and the clinical symptomatology. Various tapering schedules have been suggested,[16,60,63] but the basic tenet is gradual reduction in dosage over months. An increase in ESR during the corticosteroid taper should be carefully monitored, but it does not always indicate relapse. Kyle and Hazleman[60] suggest that clinical symptoms and signs of GCA, rather than the ESR or C-reactive protein, should be the major gauge of disease control. Systemic corticosteroid therapy usually needs to be maintained for at least 12 to 18 months, with a mean duration of treatment of 16 months in one study.[63] Other studies report significantly longer courses of therapy being required, sometimes lifelong. Persistent GCA symptoms or intolerance to the prednisone sometimes requires initiation of another immunosuppressive agent, such as methotrexate or azathioprine, to control the disease or to safely terminate the corticosteroid.

Although not all physicians believe that TAB should be performed in cases where there is strong clinical evidence for GCA,[11] it is helpful to have a positive biopsy to support the need for corticosteroids because systemic corticosteroid therapy carries numerous potential complications, some of which are life-threatening. If the biopsy is positive, corticosteroid therapy is continued, with the physician remaining vigilant for an increase in the ESR and signs and symptoms of GCA. A negative TAB does *not* rule out GCA; the false-negative rate with TAB ranges from 9% to 61%.[32] Temporal artery biopsy has been reported to carry a sensitivity of 56% to 97% in the detection of GCA,[14,32] and the "maximum possible sensitivity" of unilateral TAB is said to be approximately 85%.[32] One large study found a TAB sensitivity of 94%. The authors attribute the high predictive value of TAB in their hands to the length of artery biopsied (5.4 cm on average) and to the usual practice of performing bilateral TAB when the first side was negative.[14] Other investigators have also suggested that the likelihood of demonstrating GCA is probably increased by bilateral TAB and removal of longer segments of artery. Biopsy of the contralateral STA (when a unilateral TAB is negative) has been reported to increase the chances of finding pathologic evidence of GCA by as much as 15%,[16,65] although a recent study by Boyev and associates found only a 3% increase in diagnostic yield with bilateral TAB compared with unilateral TAB.[66] Even if bilateral TABs are negative, the physician must trust his or her clinical instincts. With a high degree of clinical suspicion of GCA, one may decide to treat the patient despite a negative biopsy. The patient and the primary care physician should be involved in the decision-making process, and it may be desirable, in certain cases, to seek the input of a rheumatologist.

Histopathologic findings in GCA-involved arteries include intimal thickening; inflammatory infiltrates of lymphocytes, macrophages, multinucleated giant cells; and disruption of the internal elastic lamina, all indicative of active arteritis. Healed arteritis is suggested by intimal thickening, fibrosis, vascularization, fragmentation of the internal elastic lamina, and foci of lymphocytes. With prolonged systemic corticosteroid use, the inflammatory cells may be sparse or absent, making the diagnosis more challenging, but certain histopathologic features (i.e., healed arteritis) of GCA will usually persist. It may be difficult to differentiate healed arteritis from arteriosclerosis and atherosclerosis. Arteriosclerosis causes intimal thickening with elastosis and a preserved internal elastic lamina. Atherosclerosis, on the other hand, shows intimal thickening with plaque deposition of atheromatous material and a disrupted internal elastic lamina in the region of the plaque. It may require an experienced pathologist to make the correct diagnosis in less straightforward cases, and a second pathologic opinion may be appropriate at times. McDonnell and associates[67] studied 48 patients who underwent TAB for a clinical diagnosis of GCA. They found active arteritis in 65%, healed arteritis in 19%, and atherosclerosis in 17%. Skip lesions, i.e., focal and segmental arterial inflammation with intervening non-inflamed areas, were rare, and they recommended processing the biopsy specimen in multiple-step cross sections at 0.25- to 0.5-mm intervals. Cohen and Smith[68] also found skip lesions to be rare, although they have been described in up to 28% of TAB specimens.[67,69,70] Although skip lesions may contribute to false-negative results, it has been suggested that suboptimal biopsy and processing techniques may be more often responsible.[32]

The above is a condensed overview of GCA. A more detailed review of this topic may be found elsewhere.[32,33]

RELEVANT ANATOMY

ARTERIAL ANATOMY

The external carotid artery gives rise to the STA and the maxillary artery within the parotid gland. The STA initially lies between the deep and superficial lobes of the parotid gland, where it is crossed by the temporal and zygomatic branches of the facial nerve and one or two veins. Coursing superiorly, the STA is bounded by the cartilage of the acoustic meatus posteriorly and the capsule of the temporomandibular joint medially before giving rise to the middle temporal artery, as well as the transverse facial artery, which travels anteriorly just below and parallel to the zygomatic arch. Along its proximal segment, the STA is covered only by skin and fascia and can be easily palpated. As the STA crosses the zygomatic process, it is covered by the auricularis anterior muscle and dense fascia. Immediately above the zygomatic arch, the STA enters the superficial temporal fascia and can be found *within* this layer, whereas the facial nerve branches are found along the deep surface of the superficial temporal fascia. The proximal STA gives rise to the transverse facial, middle temporal, zygomatico-orbital, and anterior auricular arteries. The STA then usually bifurcates into the frontal (anterior) and parietal (posterior) branches, which occurs 2 to 5 cm above the zygomatic arch. The remainder of the vascular arborization is more variable. Three major terminal branching patterns (Figs. 52–1 and 52–2) of the STA were observed in a dissection study of 161 temporal arteries.[71] In 95% of the patients, there were two terminal branches (frontal and parietal). In 2.5%, there were three terminal branches, and in another 2.5%, there was one major tributary that gave rise to a parietal branch more distally. Ethnic variation has been described.[72]

All of these vessels branch extensively, richly supplying the superficial temporal fascia and overlying skin. The frontal branch follows a tortuous course onto the forehead, where it supplies skin and scalp, muscle (frontalis), and pericranium, and it anastomoses with the supraorbital and supratrochlear branches of the ophthalmic artery. Typically, at least 70 mm of the frontal branch are available for biopsy.[73] However, it has been reported that the frontal branch is atrophic or absent in approximately 16% of patients.[74] The larger parietal branch courses posteriorly along the side of the head, anastomosing anteriorly with the frontal branch and posteriorly with the posterior auricular and occipital branches of the external carotid and with the parietal branch of the contralateral STA.

The superficial temporal vein follows the course of the STA and terminates near the origin of the STA, where it joins the maxillary vein, forming the retromandibular vein and then the external jugular vein. The STA runs within the superficial temporal fascia, but the venous branches tend to be found along the outer surface of the superficial temporal fascia, just below the hair follicles. A more detailed description of the STA anatomy may be found elsewhere.[74,75]

FASCIAL LAYERS OF THE TEMPORAL REGION

The STA is usually biopsied above the zygomatic arch, where the artery ascends within the superficial temporal fascia. The anatomy of the temporal region is somewhat confusing because varied and inconsistent nomenclature is used in the literature. A good review is provided by Abul-Hassan and co-workers.[76] Although the STA and frontal branch of the facial nerve are found to have variable patterns of branching, they are consistent with regard to the fascial layer in which they course.[77] Therefore, it is important to understand the fascial layers of the temporal region.

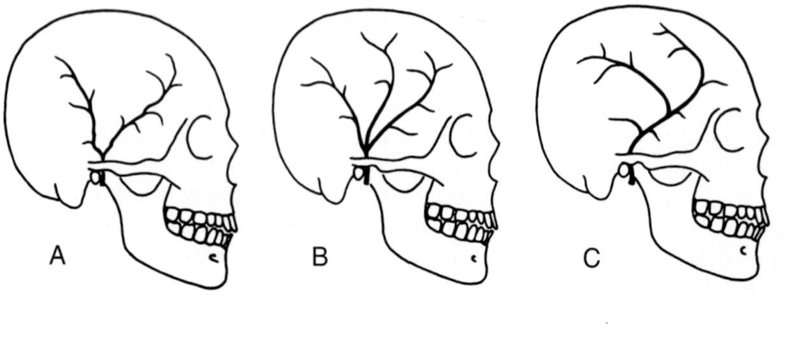

Figure 52–1. Patterns of branching of the superficial temporal artery found on dissection of 161 cadaver half-heads. *A.* Type I (present in 94.6%), two terminal branches. *B.* Type 2 (2.5%), three terminal branches. *C.* Type 3 (2.5%), a single terminal branch. (From Daumann C, Putz R, Schmidt D: The course of the superficial temporal artery: Anatomical studies as a prerequsite to arterial biopsy. Klin Monatsbl Augenheilkd 1989;194:37–41.)

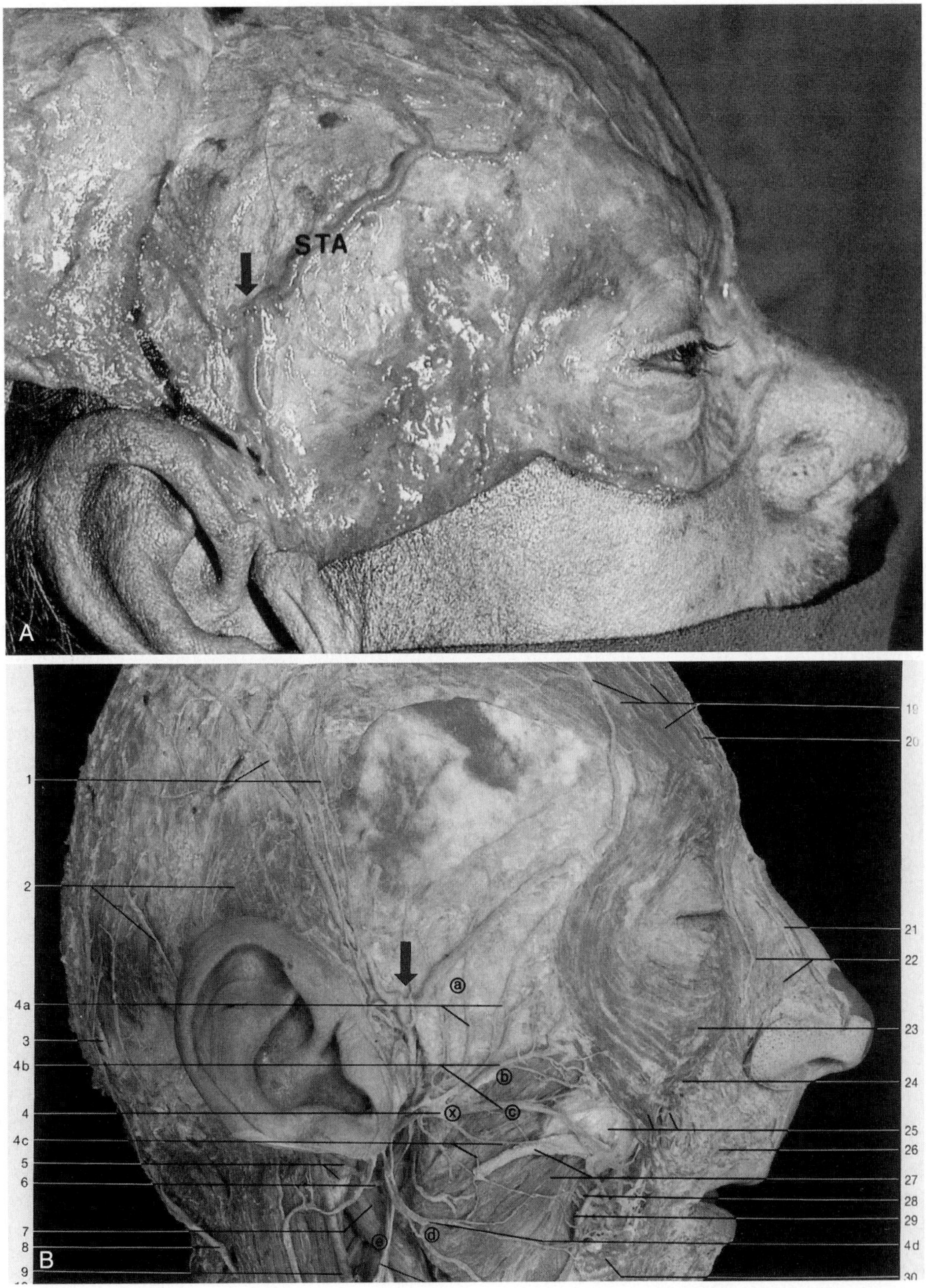

Figure 52–2. Photographs from two anatomy atlases demonstrating the variable location of the terminal bifurcation (arrow) of the superficial temporal artery. *A*. Higher bifurcation. *B*. Lower bifurcation. Note the frontal branches of the facial nerve (see label "4a" in *B*), which are anterior to the main trunk of the superficial temporal artery and cross under the frontal branch of the artery because of the low artery bifurcation. (*A* from Zide BM, Jelks GW: Surgical Anatomy of the Orbit. New York, Raven Press; 1985:16. *B* from Rohen JW, Yokochi C: Color Atlas of Anatomy: A Photographic Study of the Human Body, 3rd Edition. New York: Igaku-Shoin; 1993, p. 78. Copyright 1993 © Lippincott Williams & Wilkins, with permission.)

The superficial temporal fascia (also known as the temporoparietal fascia, epicranial aponeurosis, and galeal extension) is the temporal component of the superficial musculoaponeurotic system (SMAS). It lies just below the hair follicles and subdermal fibrofatty layer, to which it is loosely attached. Beneath the superficial temporal fascia, a subaponeurotic plane of loose areolar tissue is found overlying the deep temporal fascia. No vessels cross this plane over the deep temporal fascia. This loose areolar layer provides the scalp its natural mobility. The superficial temporal fascia is continuous with the galea aponeurotica superiorly, the frontalis muscle anteriorly, the occipitalis muscle posteriorly, and the auricularis muscles inferiorly, all of which are components of the SMAS. Inferiorly and anteriorly, in the zygomatico-frontal area, the superficial temporal fascia is less substantial, offering only a thin layer of protection over the frontal (temporal) branch of the facial nerve. The superficial temporal fascia is a highly vascular structure, supplied by many branches of the superficial temporal artery and vein.

The deep temporal fascia (also know as the temporal fascia, temporalis fascia, and investing fascia of temporalis) is a dense whitish layer of connective tissue lying directly over and adherent to the temporalis muscle from the temporal line down to the zygomatic arch. As it approaches the superior orbital rim, the deep temporal fascia splits into a deep and a superficial layer, separated by a fat pad termed the *superficial temporal fat pad* (it has also been called *Yasargil's fat pad* or the *intermediate temporal fat pad* by others who have reserved the designation *superficial temporal fat pad* for the less substantial fatty tissue lying on the outer surface of the deep temporal fascia). Inferior to this fat pad dividing the two layers of the deep temporal fascia is the zygomatic arch. On the "internal" side of the deep temporal fascia inferiorly, the deep temporal (buccal) fat pad is found.

FACIAL AND AURICULOTEMPORAL NERVES

The frontal (temporal) branch of the facial nerve, which is motor in function, arises from the main nerve trunk within the parotid gland and emerges from the anterosuperior pole of the parotid gland. It crosses the zygomatic arch approximately one finger-breadth behind the posterior edge of the zygomatic process of the frontal bone and the takeoff of the zygomatic arch, usually dividing into three to five rami.[78] These branches can be found along the deep surface of the superficial temporal fascia, within the loose areolar layer. The frontal branches of the facial nerve innervate the frontalis, the superior portion of the orbicularis oculi, the corrugator supercilii, and the procerus muscles, entering the muscles from their posterior surface. The nerve passes approximately 1.5 cm lateral to the temporal edge of the brow and enters the frontalis muscle within 2 cm above the superior orbital rim. A surgical incision at least 2 cm above the brow is likely to avoid the facial nerve, although inferiorly oriented dissection may place the nerve at risk. The facial nerve is particularly vulnerable to injury along the surface of the zygomatic arch and up to several centimeters above the arch.[77,79–81]

Scott and co-workers[82] reviewed a number of anatomical studies of the facial nerve and described the following "danger zone" based on consistent anatomical landmarks. The facial nerve is most at risk in the region bounded by (1) the tragus of the ear; (2) the junction of the zygomatic arch and the lateral orbital rim; (3) 2 cm above the level of the superior orbital rim and in a line directly superior to (2); and (4) superior to the tragus and in horizontal alignment with (3). Within this roughly square region, the facial nerve lies at a relatively superficial depth and closely follows the STA. It would be best to avoid biopsy in this area unless this appears to be the only segment of the STA clinically involved by GCA.

The auriculotemporal nerve crosses over the zygomatic arch just posterior to the STA. Its branches travel within the superficial temporal fascia, giving sensory supply to the skin of the superior temporal region.

CHOOSING A BIOPSY SITE

In selecting the specific site for biopsy, one should "go where the money is," that is find an accessible segment of the external carotid artery that appears to be clinically involved (on the basis of tenderness, absent pulsations, overlying erythema, or arterial nodularity and swelling). Biopsy may be performed on the parietal branch of the STA or the occipital artery if either of these vessels are palpably swollen, tender, or inflamed. Temporal artery biopsy is traditionally done on the same side as the visual symptoms, and this is what has been recommended in numerous texts and articles on GCA and TAB. However, some authorities suggest that the biopsy site need not be limited to the side of ocular involvement or a segment of clinically involved STA and that the vascular inflammation tends to be diffuse.[8]

Tomsak[83] recommends biopsy of the main trunk of the STA because of easier localization of the artery, but he does not discuss the facial nerve. The preauricular region is considered a "danger zone" for the facial nerve in TAB because the frontal branch of the facial nerve lies in relatively close proximity to the STA there.[82] This is the main reason for exercising extreme caution in this region. Although it has been suggested that the main trunk of the STA should be spared for possible future anastomosis with the middle cranial artery in patients with carotid artery disease,[84] STA-to-middle-cerebral-artery bypass surgery was determined to be ineffective in stroke prevention.[85] Therefore, that is likely not to be an important issue for most patients.

Before the surgeon makes the incision, the course of the STA should be evaluated by palpating for a pulse or a thickened vascular cord. Frequently, the frontal branch of the STA can be identified throughout its course, and the distal frontal branch can be biopsied with less risk to the facial nerve. If the vessel cannot be palpated, a Doppler ultrasound probe may be used (Fig. 52–3).[86,87]

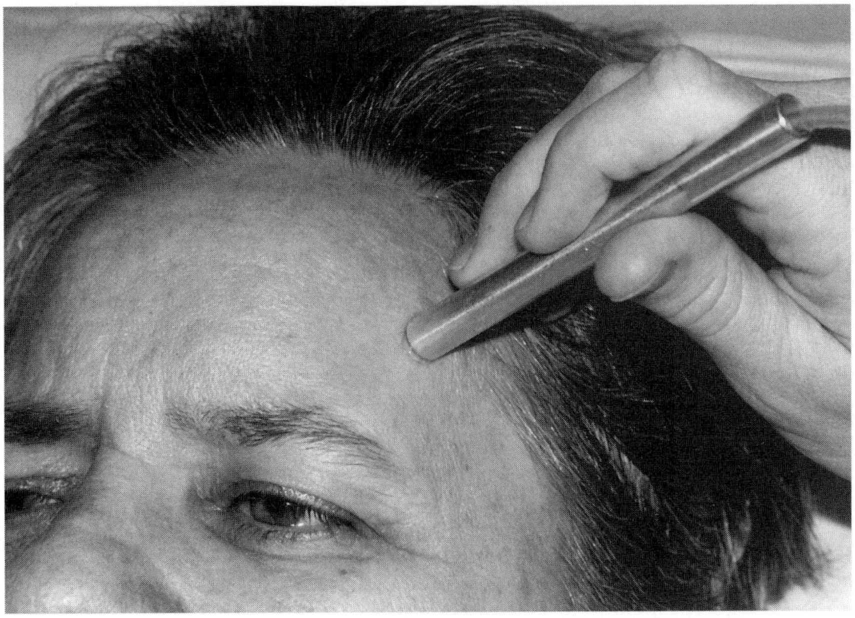

Figure 52–3. A Doppler ultrasound probe may be used to locate the superficial temporal artery when the vessel cannot be palpated.

Elaborate schemes have been proposed for localization of the STA for biopsy. In a study of 161 STAs, Daumann and colleagues[71] used a grid pattern for surface analysis and determined an incision site and orientation that would encounter the frontal branch of the STA in approximately 85% of the patients they examined (Fig. 52–4). The incision location is based on the following anatomical landmarks: The German horizontal line (DH) extends from the inferior orbital rim to the external acoustic meatus. A more superior horizontal line, along the superior orbital rim (OH), is fashioned parallel to the German horizontal line. A 2.5-cm incision line is created along a line oriented at a 45-degree angle to the upper horizontal line (OH). This 45-degree line originates at the intersection of the upper horizontal line (OH) and a vertical line along the lateral orbital rim (LOB). The incision line begins 1 to 1.5 cm away from the superior-lateral orbital rim and extends superiorly and posteriorly. This is a rather complicated scheme for placement of the incision in TAB when the STA cannot be palpated. The incision line is perpendicular to the relaxed skin tension lines, which will often create a more noticeable scar, and the location places the incision in the region of the frontal branch of the facial nerve.

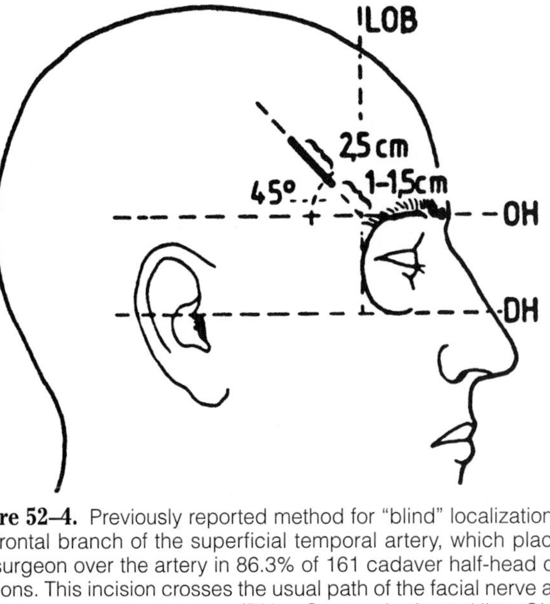

Figure 52–4. Previously reported method for "blind" localization of the frontal branch of the superficial temporal artery, which placed the surgeon over the artery in 86.3% of 161 cadaver half-head dissections. This incision crosses the usual path of the facial nerve and produces a conspicuous scar. (DH = German horizontal line, OH = upper horizontal line, LOB = lateral orbital border). (From Daumann C, Putz R, Schmidt D: The course of the superficial temporal artery: Anatomical studies as a prerequsite to arterial biopsy. Klin Monatsbl Augenheilkd 1989;194:37–41.)

SURGICAL TECHNIQUE

The scalp may be shaved around the biopsy site, although this is usually unnecessary. Mapping the course of the STA on the overlying skin with a surgical marking pen before local anesthetic injection is extremely helpful (Fig. 52–5). This aids in planning the location and orientation of the skin incision, which should be directed parallel to the relaxed skin tension lines, whenever possible, for optimal cosmesis.

Local anesthetic solution is injected subcutaneously with a long 25- or 27-gauge needle along both sides of the STA. This carries less risk of perforating the vessel and causing a hematoma than trying to inject over the vessel. Local anesthetics commonly used are 1% to 2% lidocaine with 1:100,000 or 1:200,000 epinephrine, and hyaluronidase can aid in diffusion of the anesthetic. This facilitation of tissue diffusion provided by hyaluronidase permits the surgeon to inject the anesthetic from fewer sites, further reducing the chances of

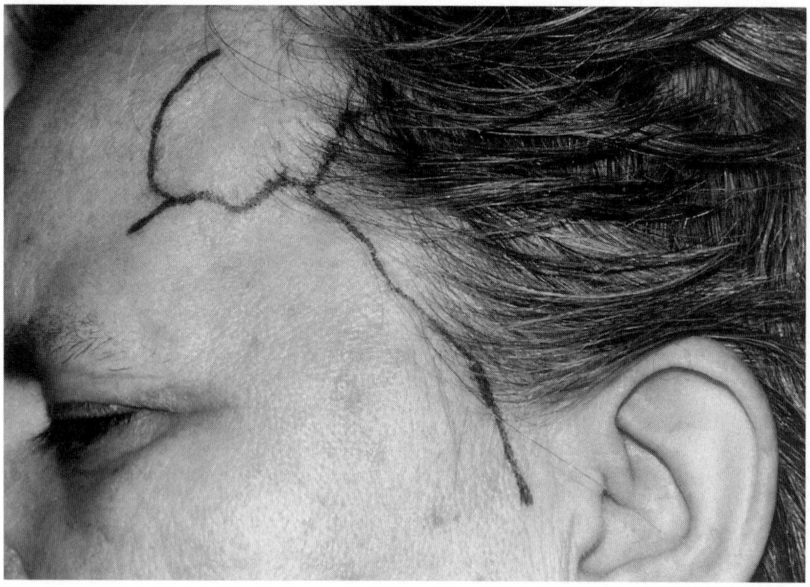

Figure 52–5. The course of the superficial temporal artery has been marked on the skin preoperatively.

producing a hematoma. Slow injection of the anesthetic tends to be less painful. Other methods for reducing discomfort of anesthetic injection have been described, including buffering the lidocaine with sodium bicarbonate or injecting dilute (0.1%) lidocaine first. Some surgeons use 0.5% to 0.75% bupivicaine to reduce postoperative pain, although, in my experience, patients do not describe much discomfort postoperatively when lidocaine is used. It is best to wait 10 minutes after local anesthetic injection to allow for epinephrine effect. Sedation is usually unnecessary, but it may be reserved for particularly nervous patients. Cardiovascular monitoring is generally prudent, even in patients receiving local anesthesia alone.

Orienting the wound along the axis of the artery facilitates obtaining the longest artery segment through the smallest possible incision. It has been recommended that the incision line actually cross over the STA to avoid "missing" the artery and inadvertently dissecting too deeply, into the plane of the facial nerve.[82] Most important is taking the time needed to identify and mark the course of the STA prior to making the incision so that, regardless of the location of the incision, the surgeon will know where to find the artery, even if there is vasospasm due to epinephrine in the local anesthetic. This is time well spent. It reduces the chances of needing to go on a "fishing expedition" for the STA, which greatly increases the probability of injuring a facial nerve branch. Vasospasm caused by epinephrine may reduce the STA vessel caliber and pulsations,[88,89] but it usually does not interfere with vessel identification when the course of the STA has been marked along the skin *prior* to local anesthetic injection. In fact, good hemostasis aided by the epinephrine allows for optimal visualization of the STA and facial nerve, if encountered. Surgical loupes may be helpful in identifying the fine branches of the STA and facial nerve.

The biopsy site is prepped and draped according to sterile process. Care must be taken during the skin prep to avoid wiping away the skin markings that show the course of the STA. A plastic, self-adhesive drape offers the advantage of being transparent, permitting wide visualization of surrounding anatomical structures, such as the ear and brow. This helps to keep the surgeon anatomically oriented and may aid in avoidance of facial nerve branches. An incision approximately 3 to 4 cm long is made alongside and relatively parallel to the STA with a scalpel blade (Fig. 52–6). Although a biopsy segment 4 to 6 cm long is generally recommended, a longer incision is generally unnecessary because retraction of the wound will usually provide exposure of a longer segment of artery. The incision should be through skin only and no deeper than the subcutaneous fat. An overly aggressive cut can easily reach one of the branches of the STA and produce bleeding that will make the dissection and vessel isolation more difficult. Every attempt should be made to avoid having to cauterize sites of bleeding along the STA, which could complicate histopathologic interpretation of the biopsy specimen. If necessary, a ligation suture can be placed around the proximal end of the STA to reduce bleeding from the distal vessel once a segment of the vessel is exposed and isolated.

The skin edge is then elevated. With careful blunt and sharp dissection, the wound is undermined in the direction of the adjacent STA, spreading parallel to skin in the subcutaneous fatty layer. The subdermal fatty layer is incised with blunt scissors as it is lifted away from the underlying superficial temporal fascia and STA. With the use of epinephrine in the local anesthetic solution, there is usually little bleeding unless the STA is inadvertently cut. If the incision is made just adjacent to or crossing over the STA, the vessel is usually immediately visible through the thin, diaphanous, outer layers of the superficial temporal fascia at this point. These transparent overlying tissue lamellae are incised with scissors while grasping them with forceps and tenting them away from the STA, as was done with the subdermal

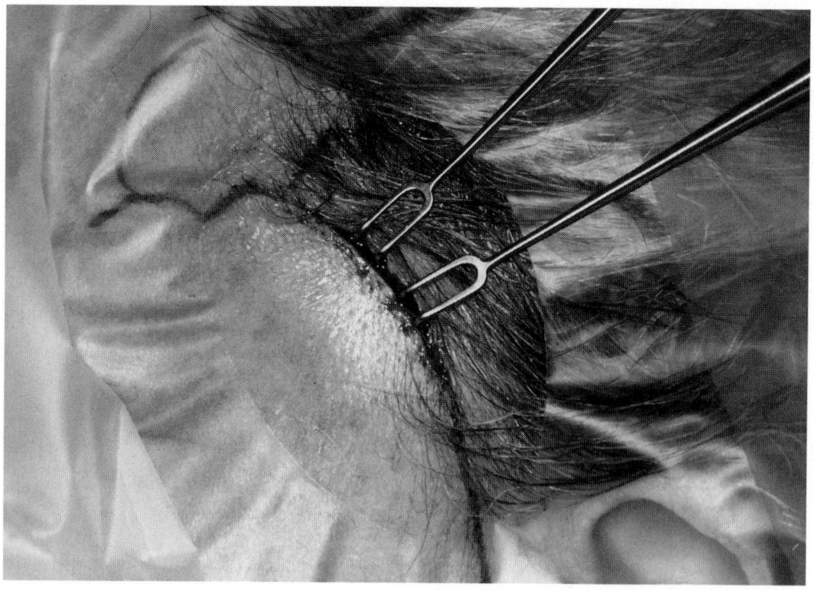

Figure 52–6. An incision has been made through skin only, immediately posterior to the marked location of the artery. This wound is positioned away from the facial nerve branches (which are more anterior) and is parallel to the relaxed skin tension lines.

fatty layer. Once the plane of the STA is reached, the vessel may be isolated by gently spreading blunt scissors, or a fine hemostat, adjacent and parallel to the vessel, aiming the tips of the scissors beneath the vessel until the artery is freed up on both sides and along its deep surface. The surgeon must continue to watch for fine branches of the STA and try to stay within the superficial temporal fascia, because the facial nerve branches lie just beneath this layer. For exposure, a self-retaining retractor may be used after the superficial temporal fascia is exposed.

The superficial temporal vein rarely courses alongside the artery. It is usually superficial to the artery, and it may be cauterized if necessary. If there is any difficulty locating the artery, finger palpation may help. This will aid in differentiating the artery from the vein, which is thinner walled and nonpulsatile. When the STA is involved by GCA, the artery may be thickened and nodular, although that is often not the case.

Once the artery is identified, the surgeon performs blunt and sharp dissection along each side of the vessel in both directions (Fig. 52–7), watching for arterial branches, which may be cauterized if small or ligated if they are large. After exposing the length of artery that is to be excised and freeing it up on all sides, the surgeon isolates this segment by ligating the artery with sutures proximally and distally. A closed hemostat is passed beneath the artery, and a suture tie is retrieved from the other side. This tie is initially used as a traction suture and then as a ligature (Fig. 52–8). Traditionally, 4-0 silk suture ties have been used,[82,90] although absorbable suture, such as polyglactin, is sometimes recommended because it is unnecessary to leave a permanent suture in place. Permanent foreign bodies, e.g., silk suture, run the risk of late exposure, inflammation, or abscess formation. The first throw of the knot is loosely tied, and the sutures are advanced toward the proximal and distal ends of the wound as far as possible before the suture is firmly tied. This maximizes the length of the specimen. Two suture ligatures may be placed proximally along the STA to provide additional protection against bleeding, which is one of the major potential complications of this procedure. Clamping the vessel with a hemostat may also aid in suture placement or hemostasis. The vessel is then cut just inside the proximal and distal sutures, leaving a 1- to 2-mm stump of artery to prevent the sutures from slipping off the vessel. The proximal and distal vessel stumps may be lightly cauterized. Excessive cautery could compromise the stability of the ligatures.

The biopsy specimen should be handled very gently to avoid crush artifact, which, like cautery burns, could complicate histologic interpretation. The specimen should be stored in a preservative, such as formalin, unless it will be rapidly transported to the pathology lab and immediately processed. A specimen length of at least 2 cm has been recommended because of "skip lesions" on histopathologic examination,[33] and a 4 to 6 cm specimen is advised in cases where the artery does not appear clinically involved (Fig. 52–9).[16] Chambers and Bernardino,[91] on the other hand, found that an artery segment as short as 4 mm was sufficient to make the pathologic diagnosis of GCA, with a false-negative rate less than 1%, assuming proper serial sectioning of the specimen.

After ensuring good hemostasis, the wound is closed in a layered fashion. Buried, interrupted 5-0 absorbable, e.g., polyglactin, subcutaneous sutures approximate the subcutaneous tissue, without any tension on them. The skin is closed with a 5-0 or 6-0 absorbable, e.g., mild chromic or fast-absorbing gut, or nonabsorbable, e.g., prolene or nylon, suture, placed either as a continuous suture or as multiple interrupted sutures with the skin edges slightly everted (Fig. 52–10). Antibiotic ointment is applied, and a light pressure dressing may be placed for one day to several days to inhibit the development of a postoperative hematoma. A pressure dressing is usually unnecessary, however, and is no replacement

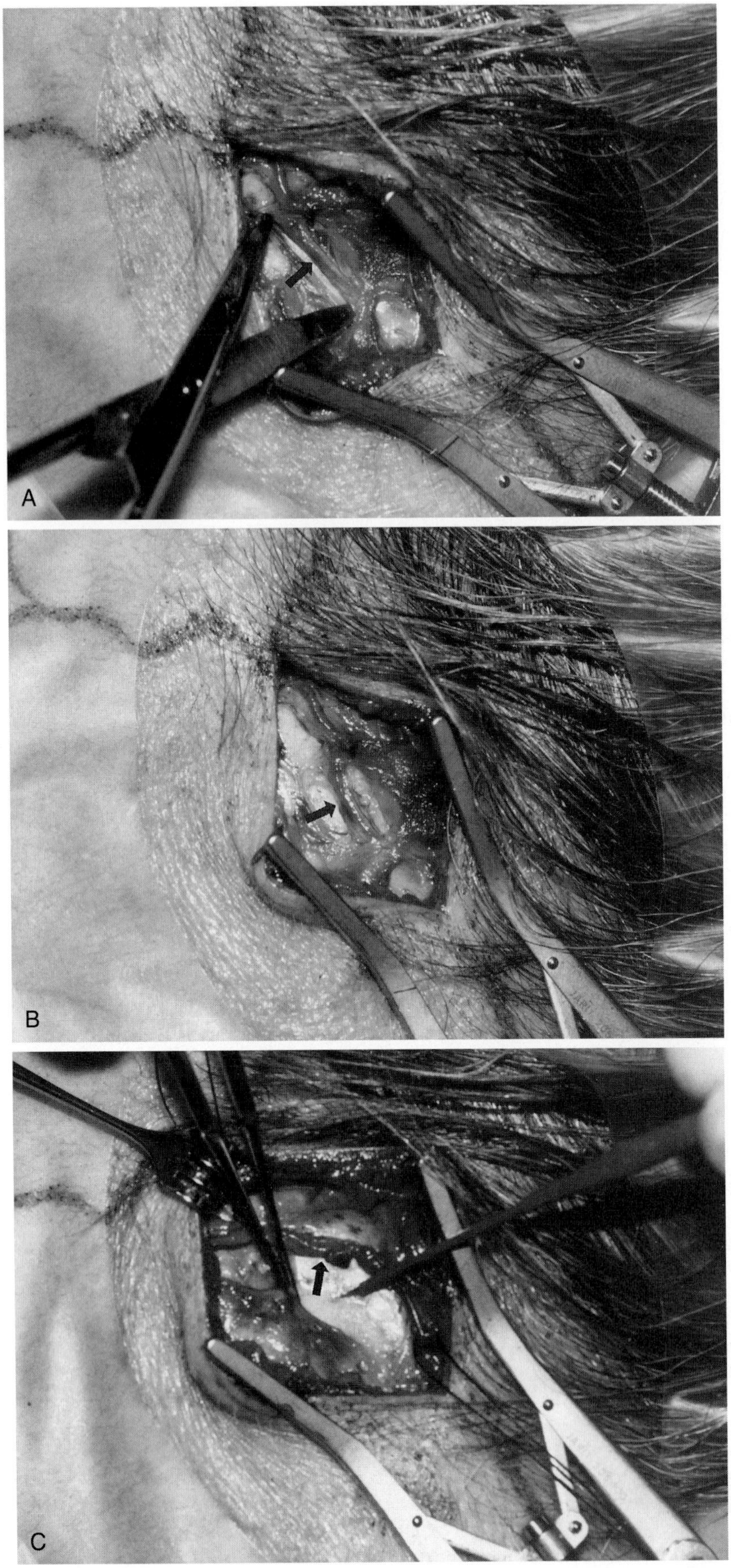

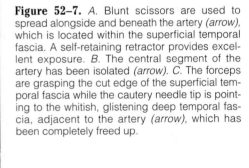

Figure 52–7. *A.* Blunt scissors are used to spread alongside and beneath the artery *(arrow),* which is located within the superficial temporal fascia. A self-retaining retractor provides excellent exposure. *B.* The central segment of the artery has been isolated *(arrow). C.* The forceps are grasping the cut edge of the superficial temporal fascia while the cautery needle tip is pointing to the whitish, glistening deep temporal fascia, adjacent to the artery *(arrow),* which has been completely freed up.

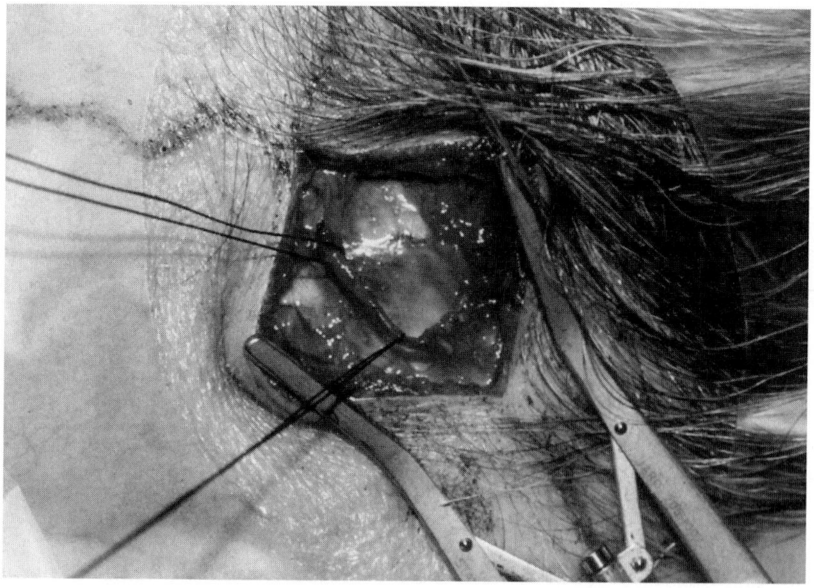

Figure 52–8. Silk sutures have been passed around the artery and are being used as traction sutures. These sutures will then be advanced as far proximally and distally as possible and securely tied, isolating as long of a vessel segment as possible.

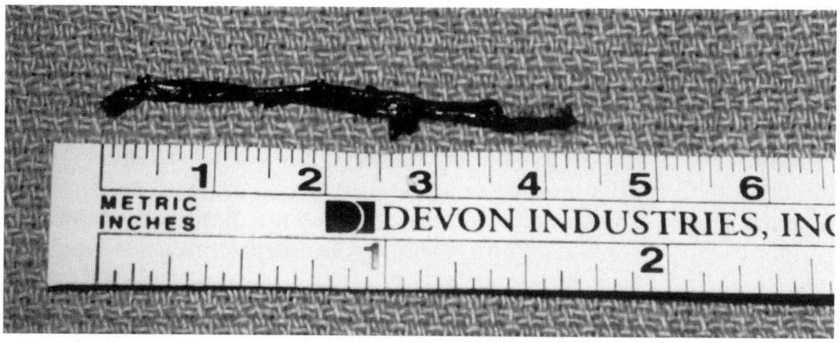

Figure 52–9. An artery segment slightly longer than 4 cm is sent for histopathologic examination.

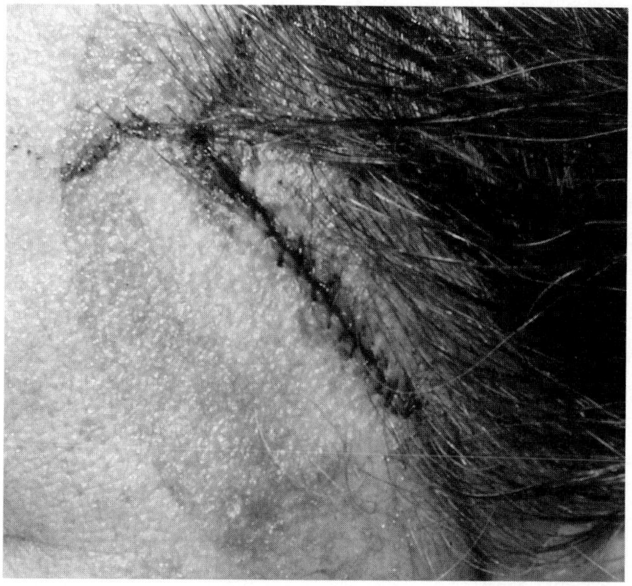

Figure 52–10. The wound has been closed in a layered fashion, with a running 6-0 fast-absorbing gut suture for skin edge approximation. The result was a cosmetically acceptable scar.

for good hemostasis prior to closing the wound, but it may be especially helpful in patients prone to bleeding (due to coagulopathies or the use of anticoagulants or platelet inhibitors). Antibiotic ointment is applied to the wound three times per day, and any nonabsorbable skin sutures are removed 5 to 7 days postoperatively.

COMPLICATIONS AND HOW TO AVOID THEM

Temporal artery biopsy generally carries a very low morbidity rate. Bleeding and damage to the facial nerve, the two major potential complications of this procedure, are usually avoidable. Intraoperative hemorrhage can result from an excessively deep skin incision that inadvertently cuts the STA or vein. The initial scalpel incision should be through skin only. Tenting up the subcutaneous fat and superficial temporal fascia during the dissection further protects the STA and facial nerve. Vigilance should be maintained for any branches of the STA, which should be cauterized or ligated before they are cut. Postoperative hemorrhage may result from poor hemostasis at the end of the procedure or inadequate ligature of the proximal and distal STA stumps. The patient may also be taking an anticoagulant or antiplatelet drug. Because the STA forms multiple anastomoses with other facial and scalp arteries, the distal STA ligature is as important as the proximal one. Late slippage of the ligatures may be prevented by leaving at least a 1- to 2-mm vessel stump outside the ligature and avoiding excessive cautery of the stump.

Inability to find the STA may be especially frustrating. Time spent at the beginning of the procedure localizing and marking the position of the artery (before local anesthetic injection) is invaluable. Arteries involved by GCA are not always easy to palpate. Occasionally, a Doppler ultrasound probe may be helpful preoperatively or intraoperatively. Knowledge of the regional anatomy is essential, but significant anatomical variation exists from person to person with regard to the pattern of vascular arborization. Two very consistent aspects of the STA anatomy are the location of the main trunk of the STA[74,83] and the plane in which the frontal branch of the STA travels (within the superficial temporal fascia). Although it is theoretically possible that one could accidentally biopsy the superficial temporal vein instead of the STA, the appearance and pulsatility of the two vessels are so different that it is unlikely the artery and vein would be confused.

One of the most feared complications of TAB is damage to the facial nerve. Invariably it is the frontal branch of the facial nerve that is involved, resulting in brow ptosis due to paralysis of the frontalis muscle[92] and, potentially, lagophthalmos due to superior orbicularis oculi weakness. Although these nerve fibers may be observed intraoperatively and obviously should be avoided, detailed understanding of the anatomy of the facial nerve and temporal fascial layers and careful selection of the biopsy site will usually keep the surgeon out of trouble. There are certain areas where the facial nerve fibers are particularly vulnerable to injury, such as along the surface of the zygomatic arch. Tissue dissection within 1.5 cm lateral to the brow and less than 2 cm above the superior orbital rim should be avoided, if possible.

Stroke[93] or blindness can result from TAB, on rare occasions, when the internal carotid artery is severely stenotic or occluded and the external carotid artery is responsible for blood supply to the globe and the intracranial internal carotid artery via branches of the ophthalmic artery. Those patients at risk for stroke or blindness following TAB frequently demonstrate ocular ischemic syndrome, and reversal of flow in the ophthalmic artery may be seen on orbital color Doppler imaging.[94] In these patients, a bounding STA pulse may be felt, and interrupting the flow of the STA could result in immediate loss of vision or cerebrovascular compromise. If there is concern that the patient may be at risk, then noninvasive vascular studies of the carotid arteries and orbital vasculature can be performed preoperatively. However, a simple "bedside" test is to externally locate and occlude the STA with digital palpation for one to several minutes[88] and observe the patient for any visual or neurologic signs or symptoms. If any problems are encountered, then a more distal branch of the STA or the contralateral STA may be utilized (assuming "finger occlusion" causes no symptoms). Proximal STA biopsy is unlikely to significantly compromise blood supply to the distal branches of the STA because of the rich collateral supply from other facial and scalp vessels.

Scalp necrosis is quite rare, and it has generally been attributed to extensive arterial involvement by GCA and not to the performance of the TAB.[16,95,96] Infection is also rare. A prominent scar can be avoided by adherence to certain basic rules of facial plastic surgery: Try to orient the incision along the relaxed skin tension lines; close the wound in a layered fashion in order to minimize tension on the skin edges and prevent wound dehiscence in those individuals who are "slow healers." If biopsy is performed through a hair-bearing portion of the scalp, cautery of vessels along the superficial layers of the scalp wound carries a risk of hair follicle damage and resultant hair loss.

SUMMARY

Giant cell arteritis may present with a wide variety of clinical manifestations, potentially causing blindness, stroke, or myocardial infarction. Most of the vascular complications are probably preventable with prompt initiation of adequate systemic corticosteroid therapy. This requires maintaining a high index of suspicion of GCA in any patient over the age of 50 years who presents with any of the signs and symptoms known to be associated with GCA.

If there is any clinical suspicion of temporal arteritis, then systemic corticosteroids should immediately be initiated, and TAB should be performed soon thereafter (within 1 to 2 weeks). Temporal artery biopsy remains the gold standard for GCA diagnosis. When performed carefully, with knowledge of the anatomy of the temporal region, TAB is a very safe and quick procedure that can be performed in the office setting.[97]

REFERENCES

1. Bosley TM, Savino PJ, Sergott RC, et al.: Ocular pneumoplethysmography can help in the diagnosis of giant-cell arteritis. Arch Ophthalmol 1989;107:379–81.
2. Genereau T, Lortholary O, Guillevin L, et al.: Temporal 67-gallium uptake is increaed in temporal arteritis. Rheumatology (Oxford) 1999;38:709–13.
3. Siatkowski RM, Gass JDM, Glaser JS, et al.: Fluorescein angiography in the diagnosis of giant cell arteritis. Am J Ophthalmol 1993;115:57–63.
4. Schmidt WA, Kraft HE, Vorpahl K, et al.: Color duplex ultrasonography in the diagnosis of temporal arteritis. N Engl J Med 1997;337:1336–42.
5. Behari M, Mishra NK, Sarkar C, et al.: Contralateral hemiplegia in herpes zoster ophthalmicus. Role of temporal artery biopsy. J Assoc Physicians India 1989;37:606–9.
6. Roth AM, Milsow L, Keltner JL: The ultimate diagnoses of patients undergoing temporal artery biopsies. Arch Ophthalmol 1984;102:901–3.
7. Haugeberg G: Vasculitis in the temporal artery—found not only in temporal arteritis. Tidsskr Nor Laegeforen 1998;118:598–9.
8. Burde RM, Savino PJ, Trobe JD: Clinical Decisions in Neuro-Ophthalmology, 2nd Edition. St. Louis: Mosby; 1992:51-6.

9. Nadeau SE: Temporal arteritis: A decision-analytic approach to temporal artery biopsy. Acta Neurol Scand 1988;78:90–100.
10. Hollenhorst RW, Brown JR, Wagener HP, et al.: Neurologic aspects of temporal arteritis. Neurology 1960;10:490–8.
11. Kachroo A, Tello C, Bais R, Panush RS: Giant cell arteritis: Diagnosis and management. Bull Rheum Dis 1996;45:2–5.
12. Paice EW: Giant cell arteritis: Difficult decisions in diagnosis, investigation and treatment. Postgrad Med J 1989;65:743–7.
13. Buchbinder R, Detsky AS: Management of suspected giant cell arteritis: A decision analysis. J Rheumatol 1992;19:1220–8.
14. Hall S, Lie JT, Kurland LT, et al.: The therapeutic impact of temporal artery biopsy. Lancet 1983;2:1217–20.
15. Hedges TR III, Gieger GL, Albert DM: The clinical value of negative temporal artery biopsy specimens. Arch Ophthalmol 1983;101:1251–4.
16. Hunder GG: Giant cell arteritis and polymyalgia rheumatica. Hosp Pract (Off Ed) 1992;27:75–93.
17. Wilkinson IMS, Russell RWR: Arteries of the head and neck in giant cell arteritis: A pathological study to show the pattern of arterial involvement. Arch Neurol 1972;27:378–98.
18. Hunder GG, Bloch DA, Michel BA, et al.: The American College of Rheumatology 1990 Criteria for the Classification of Giant Cell Arteritis. Arthritis Rheum 1990;33:1122–8.
19. Hunder GG, Michet CJ: Giant cell arteritis and polymyalgia rheumatica. Clin Rheum Dis 1985;11:471–83.
20. Machado EBV, Michet CJ, Ballard DJ, et al.: Trends in incidence and clinical presentation of temporal arteritis in Olmsted County, Minnesota, 1950-1985. Arthritis Rheum 1988;31:745–9.
21. Hunder GG: Giant cell arteritis and polymyalgia rheumatica. In Kelly WN, Harris ED, Ruddy S, et al (eds.), Textbook of Rheumatolog, Philadelphia: WB Saunders; 1989:1200.
22. Ballou SP, Khan MA, Kushner I: Giant-cell arteritis in a black patient. Ann Intern Med 1978;88:659–60.
23. Cullen JF, Coleiro JA: Ophthalmic complications of giant cell arteritis. Surv Ophthalmol 1976;20:247–60.
24. Dimant J, Farmer PM, Sobol N: Giant cell arteritis in a black person. Arthritis Rheum 1978;21:391–3.
25. Sanford RG, Berney SN: Polymyalgia rheumatica and temporal arteritis in blacks—clinical features and HLA typing. J Rheum 1977;4:435–42.
26. Eshaghian J: Controversies regarding giant cell (temporal, cranial) arteritis. Doc Ophthalmol 1979;47:43–67.
27. Banks PM, Cohen MD, Ginsburg WW, et al.: Immunohistologic and cytochemical studies of temporal arteritis. Arthritis Rheum 1983;26:1201–7.
28. Wells KK, Folberg R, Goeken JA, et al.: Temporal artery biopsies: Correlation of light microscopy and immunofluorescence microscopy. Ophthalmology 1989;96:1058–64.
29. Gabriel SE, Espy M, Erdman DD: The role of parvovirus B19 in the pathogenesis of giant cell arteritis: A preliminary evaluation. Arthritis Rheum 1999;42:1255–8.
29a. Mitchell BM, Font RL: Detection of varicella-zoster virus DNA in some patients with giant cell arteritis. Invest Ophthalmol Vis Sci 2001;42:2572–7.
30. Hayreh SS: Masticatory muscle pain: An important indicator of giant cell arteritis. Spec Care Dentist 1998;18:60–5.
31. Hayreh SS, Podhajsky PA, Raman R, et al.: Giant cell arteritis: Validity and reliability of various diagnostic criteria. Am J Ophthalmol 1997;123:285–96.
32. Mizen TR: Giant cell arteritis: Diagnostic and therapeutic considerations. Ophthalmol Clin North Am 1991;4:547–56.
33. Keltner JL: Giant cell arteritis: Signs and symptoms. Ophthalmology 1982;89:1101–10.
34. Miller A, Green M, Robinson D: Simple rule for calculating normal erythrocyte sedimentation rate. Br Med J 1983;286:266.
35. Glutz von Blotzheim S, Borruat FX: Neuro-ophthalmic complications of biopsy-proven giant cell arteritis. Eur J Ophthalmol 1997;7:375–82.
36. Grodum E, Petersen HA: Temporal arteritis with normal erythrocyte sedimentation rate. J Intern Med 1990;227:279–80.
37. Jundt JW, Mock D: Temporal arteritis with normal erythrocyte sedimentation rates presenting as occipital neuralgia. Arthritis Rheum 1991;34:217–9.
38. Kansu T, Corbett JJ, Savino P, Schatz NJ: Giant cell arteritis with normal sedimentation rate. Arch Neurol 1977;34:624–5.
39. Nelsh PR, Sergent JS: Giant cell arteritis: A case with unusual neurologic manifestations and a normal sedimentation rate. Arch Intern Med 1991;151:378–80.
40. Wise CM, Agudelo CA, Chmelewski WL, McKnight KM: Temporal arteritis with low erythrocyte sedimentation rate: A review of five cases. Arthritis Rheum 1991;34:1571–4.
41. Wong RL, Korn JH: Temporal arteritis without an elevated erythrocyte sedimentation rate. Case report and review of the literature. Am J Med 1986;80:959–64.
42. Zweegman S, Makkink B, Stehouwer CD: Giant cell arteritis with normal erythrocyte sedimentation rate: Case report and review of the literature. Neth J Med 1993;42:128–31.
43. Boyd RV, Hoffbrand BI: Erythrocyte sedimentation rate in elderly hospital inpatients. Br Med J 1966;1:901–2.
44. Sharlond DE: Erythrocyte sedimentation rate: The normal range in the elderly. Am J Geriatr Soc 1980;28:346.
45. Eshaghian J, Goeken JA: C reactive protein in giant cell (cranial, temporal) arteritis. Ophthalmology 1980;87:1160–6.
46. Hayreh SS, Podhajsky PA, Zimmerman B: Occult giant cell arteritis: Ocular manifestations. Am J Ophthalmol 1998;125:521–6.
47. Jonasson F, Cullen JF, Elton RA: Temporal arteritis: A 14-year epidemiological, clinical and prognostic study. Scott Med J 1979;11:111–9.
48. Simmons RJ, Cogan DG: Occult temporal arteritis. Arch Ophthalmol 1962;68:8–13.
49. Hayreh SS: Anterior ischaemic optic neuropathy. Eye 1990;4:25–41.
50. Hayreh SS, Podhajsky PA, Zimmerman B: Ocular manifestations of giant cell arteritis. Am J Ophthalmol 1998;125:509–20.
51. Wagener HP, Hollenhorst RW: The ocular lesions of temporal arteritis. Am J Ophthalmol 1958;45:617–30.
52. Dimant J, Grob D, Brunner NG: Ophthalmoplegia, ptosis, and miosis in temporal arteritis. Neurology 1980;30:1054.
53. Collado A, Santamaria J, Ribalta T, et al.: Giant-cell arteritis presenting with ipsilateral hemiplegia and lateral medullary syndrome. Eur Neurol 1989;29:266–8.
54. Reich KA, Giansiracusa DF, Strongwater SL: Neurologic manifestations of giant cell arteritis. Am J Med 1990;89:67–72.
55. Allison MC, Gallagher PJ: Temporal artery biopsy and corticosteroid treatment. Ann Rheum Dis 1984;43:416–7.
56. Aiello PD, Trautmann JC, McPhee TJ, et al.: Visual prognosis in giant cell arteritis. Ophthalmology 1993;100:550–5.
57. Clearkin LG, Watts MT: Ocular involvement in giant cell arteritis. Br J Hosp Med 1990;43:373–6.
58. Liu GT, Glaser JS, Schatz NJ: Visual morbidity in giant cell arteritis: Clinical characteristics and prognosis for vision. Ophthalmology 1994;101:1779–85.
59. Delecoeuillerie G, Joly P, De Lara AC, et al.: Polymyalgia rheumatica and temporal arteritis: A retrospective analysis of prognostic features and different corticosteroid regimens (11 year survey of 210 patients). Ann Rheum Dis 1988;47:733–9.
60. Kyle V, Hanzleman BL: Treatment of polymyalgia rheumatica and giant cell arteritis. I. Steroid regimens in the first two months. Ann Rheum Dis 1989:48:658–61.
61. Nesher G, Rubinow A, Sonnenblick M: Efficacy and adverse effects of different corticosteroid dose regimens in temporal arteritis: A retrospective study. Clin Exp Rheumatol 1997;15:303–6.
62. Cornblath WT, Eggenberger ER: Progressive visual loss from giant cell arteritis despite high-dose intravenous methylprednisolone. Ophthalmology 1997;104:854–8.
63. Lundberg I, Hedfors E: Restricted dose and duration of corticosteroid treatment in patients with polymyalgia rheumatica and temporal arteritis. J Rheumatol 1990;17:1340–5.
64. Hunder GG, Sheps SG, Allen GL, et al.: Daily and alternate-day corticosteroid regimens in treatment of giant cell arteritis: Comparison in a prospective study. Ann Intern Med 1975:82:613–8.
65. Hall S, Hunder GG: Is temporal artery biopsy prudent? Mayo Clin Proc 1984;59:793–6.
66. Boyev LR, Miller NR, Green WR: Efficacy of unilateral versus bilateral temporal artery biopsies for the diagnosis of giant cell arteritis. Am J Ophthalmol 1999;128:211–5.
67. McDonnell PJ, Moore GW, Miller NR, et al.: Temporal arteritis: A clinicopathologic study. Ophthalmology 1986;93:518–30.
68. Cohen DN, Smith TR: Skip areas in temporal arteritis: Myth versus fact. Trans Am Acad Ophthalmol Otolaryngol 1974;78:772–83.

69. Klein RG, Campbell RJ, Hunder GG, et al.: Skip lesions in temporal arteritis. Mayo Clin Proc 1976;51:504–10.
70. Mehler MF, Rabinowich L: The clinical neuro-ophthalmologic spectrum of temporal arteritis. Am J Med 1988;85:839–44.
71. Daumann C, Putz R, Schmidt D: The course of the superficial temporal artery: Anatomic studies as a prerequisite to arterial biopsy. Klin Monatsbl Augenheilkd 1989;194:37–41.
72. Chen TH, Chen CH, Shyu JF, et al.: Distribution of the superficial temporal artery in the Chinese adult. Plast Reconstr Surg 1999;104:1276–9.
73. Ikard RW: Clinical efficacy of temporal artery biopsy in Nashville, Tennessee. South Med J 1988;81:1222–4.
74. Marano SR, Fischer DW, Gaines C, Sonntag VKH: Anatomical study of the superficial temporal artery. Neurosurgery 1985;16: 786–90.
75. Stock AL, Collins HP, Davidson TM: Anatomy of the superficial temporal artery. Head Neck Surg 1980;2:466–9.
76. Abul-Hassan HS, von Drasek Ascher G, Acland RD: Surgical anatomy and blood supply of the fascial layers of the temporal region. Plast Reconstr Surg 1986;77:17–24.
77. Stuzin JM, Wagstrom L, Kawamoto HK, Wolfe SA: Anatomy of the frontal branch of the facial nerve: The significance of the temporal fat pad. Plast Reconstr Surg 1989;83:265–71.
78. Zide BM, Jelks GW: Surgical Anatomy of the Orbit. New York: Raven Press; 1985:16.
79. De Castro Correia P, Zani R: Surgical anatomy of the facial nerve as related to ancillary operations in rhytidoplasty. Plast Reconstr Surg 1973;52:549–52.
80. Liebman EP, Webster RC, Berger AS, Della Vecchia M: The frontalis nerve in the temporal brow lift. Arch Otolaryngol 1982;108:232–5.
81. Rudolph R: Depth of the facial nerve in face lift dissections. Plast Reconstr Surg 1990;85:537–44.
82. Scott KR, Tse DT, Kronish JW: Temporal artery biopsy technique: A clinico-anatomical approach. Ophthalmic Surg 1991;22:519–25.
83. Tomsak RL: Superficial temporal artery biopsy: A simplified technique. J Clin Neuro-ophthalmol 1991;11:202–4.
84. Clearkin LG, Watts MT: How to perform a temporal artery biopsy. Br J Hosp Med 1991;46:172–4.
85. The EC-IC Bypass Study Group: Failure of extracranial-intracranial arterial bypass to reduce the risk of ischemic stroke: Results of an international randomized trial. N Engl J Med 1985;313:1191–200.
86. Beckman RL, Hartmann BM: The use of a Doppler flow meter to identify the course of the temporal artery (letter). J Clin Neuro-ophthalmol 1990;10:304.
87. Bienfang DC: Use of the Doppler probe to detect the course of the superficial temporal artery. Am J Ophthalmol 1984;97:526–7.
88. Brennan J, McCrary JA III: Diagnosis of superficial temporal arteritis. Ann Ophthalmol 1975;7:1125–9.
89. O'Connor PS: Ancillary clinical procedures. In Kline LB, Bajandas FJ (eds.), Neuro-ophthalmology Review Manual, 3rd Edition. Thorofare, N.J.: Slack, Inc.; 1988:175–7.
90. Servais EG, Hayreh SS: Temporal artery biopsy. In Phelps CD, Kolder HEJW (eds.), Manual of Common Ophthalmic Surgical Procedures. New York: Churchill Livingstone; 1986.
91. Chambers W, Bernardino V: Specimen length in temporal artery biopsies. J Clin Neuro-ophthalmol 1988;8:121–5.
93. Fisher CM: Giant cell arteritis—discussion. Trans Am Neurol Assoc 1971;96:12.
92. Slavin ML: Brow droop after superficial temporal artery biopsy. Arch Ophthalmol 1986:104:1127.
94. Ho AC, Lieb WE, Flaharty PM, et al.: Color Doppler imaging of the ocular ischemic syndrome. Ophthalmology 1992;99:1453–62.
95. Currey J: Scalp necrosis in giant cell arteritis and review of the literature. Br J Rheumatol 1997;36:814–6.
96. Dummer W, Zillikens D, Schulz A, et al.: Scalp necrosis in temporal (giant cell) arteritis: Implications for the dermatologic surgeon. Clin Exp Dermatol 1996;21:154–8.
97. Hofmann RJ: In-office temporal artery biopsy. Rhode Island Med 1995;78:356–8.

SECTION VI

Creig S. Hoyt, M.D.

Extraocular Muscle Surgery

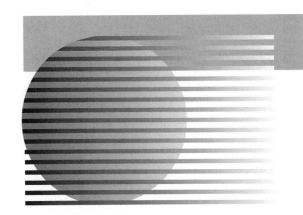

CHAPTER 53

Strabismus Surgery

DOUGLAS R. FREDRICK, M.D. and CREIG S. HOYT, M.D.

As with every ophthalmic operation, it is necessary to understand the functional goals of the procedure before performing strabismus surgery. Strabismus surgery is performed to (1) restore binocular vision, (2) improve ocular alignment, (3) enlarge the field of single binocular vision, (4) alleviate abnormal head position, and (5) improve the aesthetic appearance of the patient. To achieve these goals, a rigorous preoperative assessment should be performed on all patients with strabismus, making certain that all steps of the exam are addressed and not overlooked (Table 53–1). Attention to the sensory and motor components of the strabismus examination will ensure that the correct procedure is performed and that the functional goals are achieved.

PREOPERATIVE ASSESSMENT

OCULAR HISTORY

The date of the onset of strabismus should be obtained through the patient or the patient's parents. It is always helpful to have the parents bring photographs of the child dating from infancy onward, as these can be used to document the date of onset as well as the presence of anomalous head position. In adults with strabismus, such photographs are also useful. The duration of strabismus as well as the variability should be noted. Factors that exacerbate or alleviate the strabismus should be identified. Progression of strabismus and the presence of associated neurologic symptoms should be

TABLE 53–1. Strabismus Evaluation Checklist

Ocular history	Ocular examination
Family history of strabismus	Visual acuity
Family history of eye disease	Facial features (plagiocephaly, microsomia)
Pregnancy, delivery complications	Head position
Medical illnesses	Face position
Prior facial trauma or surgery	Nystagmus (type, amplitude, frequency and null point)
Neurological disorder	Ductions
Prior ocular trauma	Versions
Prior ocular illness	Accommodative amplitude
Prior ocular surgery	Convergence amplitude
Prior strabismus therapy	Near point of convergence
Prior orthoptic therapy	AC/A ratio
Strabismus features	Stereoscopic measurement
Onset	Suppression testing
Duration	Heterotropia
Progression	Heterophoria
Diplopia	The 9 diagnostic fields of gaze measurement method
Reading difficulties	Diplopic fields
Exacerbating features (fatigue, illness)	Pupil reaction
Associated features (squint, headache)	Funduscopic exam (cyclotortion, fundus health)
	Cycloplegic refraction/retinoscopy
	Cranial nerve exam

ascertained in all patients. Family history of strabismus should be questioned, as there is a strong predisposition for strabismus within families.[1]

Special attention should be paid to the medical history in children, including possible complications of pregnancy and delivery. Knowledge of developmental milestones is important, as failure to attain milestones or loss of milestones may indicate neurologic abnormality. Children with genetic syndromes or multiple anomalies often have specific associated patterns of strabismus or ocular anomalies that can aid in the diagnosis of the syndrome.

In older children or in adults, prior history of patching therapy, spectacle use, or orthoptic therapy vs. surgical therapy must be ascertained, and any prior operative reports should be obtained. Adults with acquired strabismus should be questioned about underlying medical conditions such as thyroid disease, diabetes, hypertension, carcinoma, myasthenia gravis, and other neurologic disorders. Any previous ocular, orbital, facial, or cranial trauma or surgery should be noted, and old computed tomography (CT), magnetic resonance imaging (MRI) or x-ray films obtained and personally reviewed.

OCULAR EXAMINATION

Visual Acuity

Visual acuity must be assessed in all patients and the method of testing clearly documented. Neonates should fixate and follow a face by 2 months of age. Brightly colored, high-contrast toys can be used to assess fixation. Visual acuity can be quantitated using forced choice preferential looking techniques. Between the age of 2 and 3 years, acuity can be quantitated using the HOTV cards, Lea cards, Allen figures, or tumbling E-game.[2] Full horizontal lines of figures should be used, as single optotypes may overestimate acuity in children with amblyopia due to the crowding phenomenon. Full-line Snellen letters is the gold standard of visual acuity assessment. Patients with nystagmus often have better visual acuity when tested binocularly than when tested monocularly, as the nystagmus will increase during occlusion.[3,4] These patients should have vision tested and recorded monocularly by using a +5 diopter lens to fog the eye. Binocular acuity should be tested in all positions, allowing the patient to assume their null point to maximize acuity.

Fixation

Poorly acquired and maintained fixation in one eye in infants may be due to refractive errors, organic lesions, or amblyopia. Wright has described a useful technique to uncover amblyopia in preverbal children.[5] In the 10-diopter fixation test a vertically held prism is placed in front of an eye to induce a vertical deviation. Fixation preference is then assessed by the ability of the child to fixate with each eye. Children with amblyopia will choose to maintain fixation through the prism and manifest vertical eye movement. This technique allows screening for amblyopia in preverbal children with straight eyes.

If amblyopia is detected in infants or children, occlusion therapy must be initiated to reverse the amblyopia prior to any surgical therapy. Occlusion therapy may be part-time or full-time, but caution must be taken in full-time occlusion to prevent occlusion amblyopia from occurring in the sound eye. Noncompliant patients can be treated by penalization of the sound eye with atropine or by the use of occlusion foils on the spectacle lenses.[6]

Appearance of the Eyes

Prior to any measurement or testing for heterotropias, notation should be made of the appearance of the eyes and the face. Head tilts, head bobbing, or face turning will be seen by observing the child at play or during the introduction phase of the examination.[7] Facial asymmetry will be apparent by the relationship of the palpebral fissures to brows, nose, ears, maxilla, mouth, and chin. Epicanthal folds or ptosis may create the appearance of pseudostrabismus or microphthalmos. Finally, the position of the globes themselves may create the appearance of strabismus, with hypertelorism simulating exotropia and close-set eyes simulating esotropia.

Light Reflex

The corneal light reflex is commonly used to estimate the angle of deviation in patients with strabismus. This light reflex will vary depending on where the light source is held and the degree compliance of fixation upon the light. Where the light reflex falls on the cornea is dependent on the alignment and the angle kappa. Angle kappa is the angle formed by the pupillary axis and the visual axis. Most people have positive angle kappa, which results in the light reflex appearing slightly nasal to the center of the pupil. Temporal displacement of the macula by conditions such as retinopathy of prematurity can lead to large positive angle kappas and the appearance of exotropia. Only by performing cover tests can heterophorias and heterotropias be determined and quantitated.

Ductions, Versions, and Nystagmus

Ductions and versions should be tested in all patients. Ductions refer to the movements of one eye when the fellow eye is occluded. Versions are performed and recorded by having both eyes open and observed together. Brightly colored objects should be used to get the child's attention. In infants, vestibular evoked nystagmus can be used to assess both horizontal and vertical eye movements. This is performed by rotating the child and observing subsequent induced nystagmus. Attention should be paid to the smoothness of pursuits as well as the initiation, accuracy, and speed of saccades. Overaction or underaction of the oblique muscles as well as the rectus muscles should be recorded. Overshoots, nystagmus, and apraxic eye movements should be noted as well. Once versions have been assessed, the presence of a heterophoria or heterotropia should be detected and quantitated using the alternate cover fixation test. Fixation must be assured and the accommodation controlled, and the measurements should be performed in the nine diagnostic positions of gaze (Fig. 53–1). It is important to remember that primary and reading positions are the most important in the patient, and other positions should be assessed for

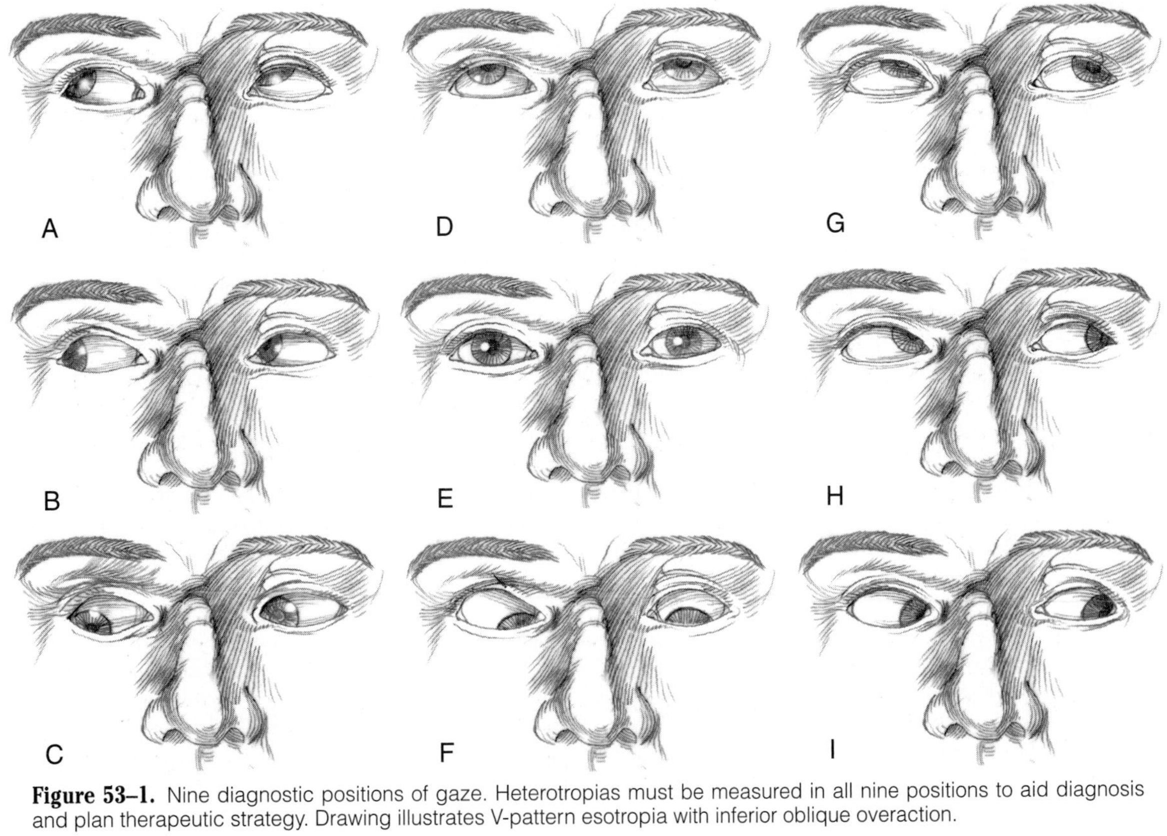

Figure 53–1. Nine diagnostic positions of gaze. Heterotropias must be measured in all nine positions to aid diagnosis and plan therapeutic strategy. Drawing illustrates V-pattern esotropia with inferior oblique overaction.

the sake of diagnostic and therapeutic decisions. Measurements should be made using both the distance and near fixation targets. The alternate cover test is performed by having the patient fixate on a target then alternately occluding each eye and observing eye movements that occur to maintain fixation. Prisms are then used to offset these refixation movements until the movement is neutralized. This amount of prism is the total magnitude of the deviation, the full amount of heterotropia.

By measuring heterotropias in the nine diagnostic fields of gaze, A- and V-patterns will be uncovered.[8,9] These patterns are vertically incomitant horizontal deviations that change in magnitude with upgaze and downgaze. Measurements of the horizontal deviation are made in primary gaze, 25 degrees up, and 25 degrees down. A V-pattern is described when there is increasing esotropia in downgaze or increasing exotropia in upgaze, with a difference of 15 prism diopters or more.[10] V-patterns are commonly seen in esotropia, with overaction of the inferior oblique muscles. A-patterns occur when there is an increase in convergence (esotropia) in upgaze, or increasing divergence (exotropia) in downgaze, with a difference measuring 10 prism diopters or more. A-patterns are more frequently associated with superior oblique overaction.[11] Other patterns, such as Y- and X-pattern have been described. Patterns of strabismus can point to the etiology of strabismus and should not be overlooked. For example, V-pattern exotropia can be seen in Brown's syndrome, whereas A-pattern exotropia can be seen in hydrocephalus.[12]

Accommodative and Convergence Amplitudes

Accommodative and convergence amplitudes and relationships must be evaluated. Accommodative amplitude should be measured using method of spheres or an accommodation rule. Convergence amplitude should be measured using prism bars. Near point of convergence should be measured as well as convergence amplitude. The accommodative convergence/accommodation ratio must be measured using the gradient or heterophoria methods. The measurement of these amplitudes is critical in the therapeutic decisions made in treating accommodative esotropia and in all forms of exo deviation.[13] This should be done prior to instillation of cycloplegic eye drops.

Once a heterotropia has been detected it must be quantitated in reproducible fashion. The best way to quantitate the angle of deviation is by the alternate cover test, as described above. This test measures total deviation, both latent and manifest. Measurements should be made at distance and near, with and without glasses. A complete dissociation is required to determine the entire deviation, and this may require prolonged occlusion prior to the measurement, especially in patients with exodeviations. When a patient cannot maintain fixation on an object well, the angle of deviation can be estimated by using a light reflex. The angle of strabismus can be estimated using the Hirschberg corneal light reflex test.[14,15] In this test, a light source is held 14 inches from the patient and the reflex is observed on the patient's cornea. In an esotropic eye, the reflex is displaced temporarily, and in an exotropic eye the reflex is displaced nasally. It has been estimated that each millimeter of decentration equals approximately 20 prism diopters of misalignment, so that a corneal reflex at pupil margin indicates a 30 prism diopter deviation and a reflex at the limbus indicates a 90 prism diopter deviation.

The Krimsky test is useful for measuring angles of deviation in densely amblyopic eyes that cannot pick up fixation. The test is performed by using a prism to reposition the displaced corneal light reflex back to the center of the pupil. For both the Hirschberg and the Krimsky tests interobserver variability has been shown to be quite high and one alternative cover prism test should always be used when possible to quantitate the angle of deviation.

Sensory Testing

Stereo acuity testing has been used as an initial screening for amblyopia and strabismus. The presence of stereopsis must be assessed as its presence will help guide therapeutic decisions. Stereopsis can be tested by the Randot test or the Titmus test. Distance stereo vision can be measured using the BVAT system. Suppression should be evaluated using the Worth four-dot test, 4 prism diopter test, Bagolini lenses, or projector vectograph. Adult patients with diplopia can have diplopia quantitated using a Hess screen, Lancaster screen, or measurement of singular binocular field using a Goldmann perimeter.

Pupils

Pupils should be examined closely to make certain that there is no anisocoria and no sign of aberrant third cranial nerve regeneration. Assessment for Marcus-Gunn pupils due to optic atrophy in association with strabismus points to a central nervous system lesion. Ptosis can be seen in patients with cranial nerve three palsy, Horner's syndrome, myasthenia gravis, or myopathies, all conditions that can be associated with strabismus.

Refraction

All adults and children should have a cycloplegic refraction. Cyclopentolate 1% instilled twice provides adequate cycloplegia in most patients, and allows refraction to be performed 30 to 40 minutes after instillation of the eye drops.[16] Patients with dark irides can be dilated with atropine 1% ointment instilled nightly for 3 nights prior to the examination. Cyclopentolate should be used with caution in patients with seizure disorders, and this agent can cause unusual psychologic effects in some children. Retinoscopy in children should be performed using loose lenses, as children often have a difficult time remaining in position behind a phoropter. For patients with esotropia or exotropia, treatment of refractive errors with spectacles can often control the strabismus.

Optical therapy for strabismus should always be considered prior to recommended surgical therapy. In both infantile and accommodative esotropia, full correction of any hyperopic refractive error greater than +1.50 should be attempted. Patients with accommodative esotropia with a high accomodative conversence accomodation (AC/A) ratio should be placed in bifocal spectacles with the executive style or wide flat top segment to be placed so that the segment bisects the pupil. Progressive bifocals should not be used in this form of therapy.

Children with intermittent exotropia can be placed in minus sphere lenses in order to stimulate accommodation and convergence. Up to −2.00 diopters can be prescribed and this may control the exotropia and maintain fusion at both distance and near.

Every child with strabismus should have any significant underlying refractive error corrected with spectacles, as improved visual acuity and reversal of amblyopia can reduce or eliminate many forms of strabismus.

Surgery should not be performed until a second motility examination is conducted. This will allow assessment of the effectiveness of spectacles and patching therapy, allow confirmation of stability and type of ocular deviation, and confirm the stability of the angle of deviation.[17]

SPECIAL TESTS

Forced Duction/Force Generation Testing

In cases of restrictive or incomitant strabismus, use of forced duction testing is critical for both proper diagnosis and planning surgical correction. Forced duction testing should be performed intraoperatively in all strabismus cases and preoperatively in cooperative adults. The technique, first described in the 1900s, has been well described by Jampolsky.[18] The eye is anesthetized with a tetracaine-soaked cotton-tipped applicator applied to the conjunctiva at the area to be grasped. A toothed forceps is used to grasp the conjunctiva and the Tenon's capsule insertion opposite the side of gaze limitation. The patient is then asked to look into the field of restriction. When the patient cannot move the eye anymore, the examiner attempts to further rotate the globe, taking care not to retropulse the globe (which would give a false negative result). If the eye cannot be rotated, restriction is present. If it can be passively rotated paresis is present.

Forced duction testing should be done intraoperatively in all strabismus cases. Depolarizing paralytic anesthetics should be avoided and local, peribulbar or retrobulbar anesthetics could alter results. The test should be performed prior to beginning surgery, after the muscle has been moved to make certain restriction has been freed and at the end of the case to make certain that the conjunctiva has not recreated restriction.

Forced generation testing is performed in the office in cooperative adult patients with incomitant strabismus. This technique will help differentiate a restrictive from a paretic form of strabismus. An example is a patient who cannot depress an eye following a blowout fracture. The limitation may be due to a paretic or restricted entrapped inferior rectus muscle. After anesthetizing the conjunctiva as for forced duction testing, the surgeon uses forceps to grasp the conjunctiva and Tenon's capsule at the 6 o'clock position, and the patient is asked to slowly look down. If the muscle is paretic, no force will be felt on the forceps. Forced duction testing can then be performed to evaluate for restriction.

Orbital Imaging

Recent advances in imaging technology have changed our understanding of extraocular muscle anatomy and physiology. High-resolution MRI and dynamic MRI have yielded images that delineate the relationship between extraocular muscles and surrounding connective tissues to produce a new model of functional anatomy of the extraocular muscles.[19] By combining clinical data from preoperative and postoperative ocular alignment with data from high-resolution MRI and CT scanning, a computer model has been created that predicts the effect of muscle surgery, given a variety of different clinical scenarios.[20] Such high-resolution imaging is also useful in cases of slipped or lost extraocular muscle or orbital trauma.[21]

SURGICAL ANATOMY

Although carefully performed preoperative examination and a thoughtfully developed operative plan usually yield a good surgical result, the surgeon must be prepared for anatomic anomalies that will necessitate a change in plans. Congenital anomalies and previous muscle surgery will disrupt the normal appearance and relationship of the extraocular muscles. For this reason, a thorough understanding of the normal anatomic relationships of the extraocular muscles is important.

POSITION OF THE GLOBE

When a patient is under general anesthesia the eye may assume any position. When the patient is lightly anaesthetized, the eyes are often elevated and extorted. Deeper anesthesia will bring the eyes to midline, but usually they will remain slightly extorted. Instillation of local anesthesia by retrobulbar or peribulbar injection may lead to partial paralysis of the extraocular muscles, often sparing the superior oblique, leading to an intorted eye.

CONJUNCTIVA

Even if strabismus surgery results in perfectly aligned eyes, the patient may be unhappy if left with unattractive, scarred conjunctiva. Careful handling and attention to detail will result in a quiet-appearing eye that makes any necessary reoperations easier. Prior to surgery, the conjunctiva will provide landmarks to properly orient the eye and the underlying muscles. The position of the caruncle and plica should be noted so that both can be placed in the same position postoperatively. The lateral limbal triangle is formed by decreased conjunctival and scleral overlay, and it provides the surgeon with the proper orientation prior to making any incisions. When conjunctival incisions are made, the surgeon must allow for adequate exposure to avoid tearing of the tissues during dissection. When closing the conjunctiva, the surgeon must make certain that conjunctiva is opposed to conjunctiva, not Tenon's capsule; poor closure can lead to excessive scarring and epithelial inclusion cysts. In turn, scarring may lead to restriction of eye movements or reverse leash restrictions simulating paretic eye muscles. It is also important to avoid dragging the plica toward the limbus, as this will give a poor aesthetic result to any strabismus surgery.

TENON'S CAPSULE

Tenon's capsule is the underappreciated envelope of elastic connective tissue that serves two vital roles to ensure smooth and accurate ocular rotations. First, it acts as a collagenous sleeve through which extraocular muscles pass and become invested (Fig. 53–2). These sleeves have connections to other structures within the orbit, which allow the muscles to maintain a stable relationship within the orbit. Maintenance of these sleeves, or pulleys, is vital to maintaining ocular alignment, and disruption of this connective tissue by trauma or previous ocular surgery will disrupt function of the muscles. The second function is to provide a physical separation of the orbital fat from the muscles and sclera. If Tenon's capsule is violated, it may lead to adherence of orbital fat or extraocular muscle to the sclera, and a subsequent restrictive strabismus. Tenon's capsule arises from the apex and separates fat from sclera posterior to the equator. The extraocular muscles penetrate Tenon's capsule at the equator, separating them from sclera and conjunctiva. Tenon's inserts into the sclera at a point 3 mm posterior to the limbus at the intermuscular membrane.

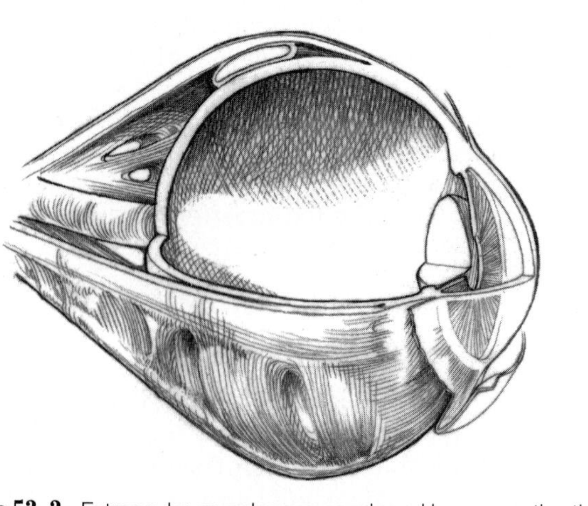

Figure 53–2. Extraocular muscles are enveloped by connective tissue and Tenon's capsule, tissues that may cause adhesions to the globe when subjected to trauma or poor surgical technique.

When isolating an extraocular muscle, the surgeon should treat Tenon's capsule with particular care to avoid complications that can ruin the surgical outcome. This tissue should always be dissected sharply, not pushed aside with a cotton-tipped applicator. The membrane should be dissected from the surface of the muscle, and should never be stripped from the muscle itself. When placing scleral sutures, care should be taken to avoid incorporating Tenon's capsule in these bites, as Tenon's cysts may develop underneath the recessed or resected muscle.

EXTRAOCULAR MUSCLES

The six extraocular muscles involved in eye movements insert into the sclera with remarkable predictability. The rectus muscles insert progressively posterior to the limbus in the following order: medial rectus, 5.5 mm (average distance from limbus); inferior rectus, 6.5 mm; lateral rectus, 6.9 mm; and superior rectus, 7.7 mm (Fig. 53–3). The orientation of the insertions differ between the horizontal and vertical recti, as the horizontal recti insert parallel to the limbus, while the temporal portion of the vertical recti insert more posterior than the medial portion (Fig. 53–4). Inspection of this insertion angle will help distinguish vertical and horizontal muscles.

Blood supply to the extraocular muscles is provided by the anterior ciliary arteries. Each rectus muscle has two arteries, except the lateral rectus muscle, which has

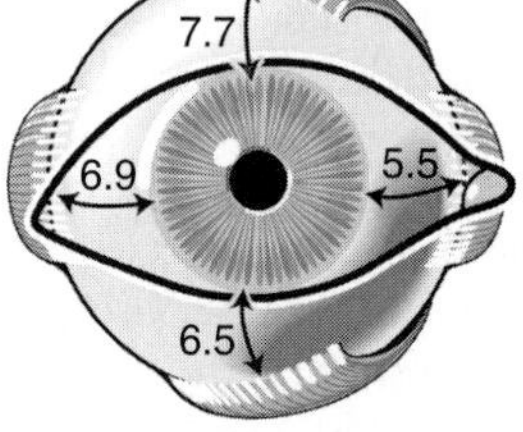

Figure 53–3. Insertions of rectus muscles are predictably located (medial: 5.5, inferior: 6.5, lateral: 6.9, superior: 7.7) millimeters from the limbus.

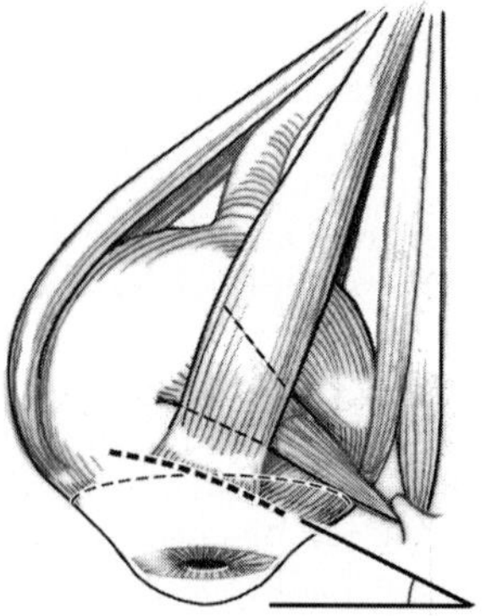

Figure 53–4. Insertions of the vertical rectus muscles are slanted, with the temporal insertion being more posterior than the nasal insertion.

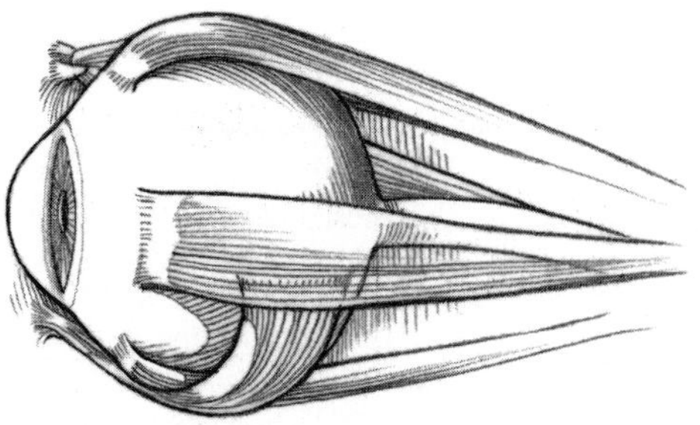

Figure 53–5. The inferior oblique insertion lies underneath the lateral rectus muscle, making it susceptible to trauma during lateral rectus surgery.

one. The vessels are found in the body of the muscle and penetrate to the anterior surface at the muscle–tendon junction. They stay on the muscle surface until they penetrate the sclera anterior to the point of muscle insertion. These vessels supply 70% of the blood supply to the anterior segment, and therefore ischemia may result when multiple muscles are operated upon simultaneously.

The oblique muscles, especially the superior oblique, display more anatomic variability than the rectus muscles, but they still maintain reliable relationships to the rectus muscles. The inferior oblique passes inferior to the inferior rectus after originating lateral to the lacrimal fossa. It then passes under the lateral rectus muscle before forming a broad insertion in the posterior lateral globe (Fig. 53–5). A common error is to incorporate fibers of the inferior oblique muscle during lateral rectus resection procedures, leading to unexpected vertical deviations. The superior oblique muscle has the longest tendon, which passes underneath the superior rectus muscle (remember "rectitude over obliquity") before inserting into the sclera at the lateral edge of the superior rectus (Fig. 53–6). The tendon is thin at the point of insertion and care must be taken not to cut it at the time of isolation and resection of the superior rectus muscle.

The inferior oblique muscle is unique in that only weakening or transposition procedures are performed on this muscle. Strengthening procedures are not performed. Overaction of the inferior oblique muscle may be primary, as seen in association with horizontal strabismus, or secondary, as seen in superior oblique

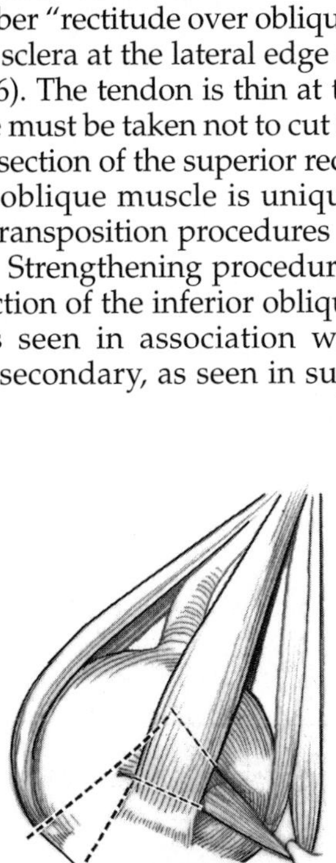

Figure 53–6. The insertion of the superior oblique muscle is broad, and the fibers are thin and diaphanous in appearance.

paresis. The degree of overaction has been graded according to various schemes, but the important consideration is to determine the amount of hypertropia in the adducting eye with the fellow eye fixating. A 1 to 4+ scale is commonly used to quantitate the deviation.

While strabismologists argue at length about the surgical indications for weakening procedures, there are three common clinical situations that require inferior oblique weakening. First, in the presence of a unilateral fourth nerve palsy with a deviation (hypertropia) of 10 prism diopters or less, an ipsilateral inferior oblique myectomy is recommended. Larger deviation may require either concurrent or subsequent vertical rectus surgery. The second indication for weakening procedure is a V-pattern horizontal strabismus with oblique overaction. The oblique muscles must be weakened at the time of horizontal muscle surgery, or the vertical incomitancy will not be collapsed. The final indication involves dissociated vertical deviation associated with overaction of the inferior oblique muscle. In these cases, anterior transposition of the inferior oblique muscle may correct both conditions.

INDICATIONS FOR STRABISMUS SURGERY

The goal of any strabismus surgeon is to improve binocular function or improve the appearance of the patient. All nonsurgical modalities should be used prior to undertaking strabismus surgery.[22] These include spectacle therapy, occlusion therapy, prism therapy, and in some instances orthoptic therapy. When these modalities fail, surgery should be considered. There is no rigid minimum number of prism diopter deviations one must have to consider surgical therapy. In fact, incomitancy may be causing the greatest degree of functional difficulty in the patient with straight eyes in the primary position. Unlike any other subspecialty in ophthalmology, there are many different approaches to the same problem, and an equal number of opinions concerning the timing of intervention. The two central questions regarding the patient with strabismus are "what should be done?" and "how much should be done?" The first question is answered from the information given in Table 53–2 and the related discussions. The references are provided for further review of the individual strabismus conditions. The question of how much is to be done is difficult to answer, as it is highly variable from surgeon to surgeon. Table 53–3 provides guidelines based on Parks, which should provide predictable results for most surgeons. Each surgeon will develop his or her own technique, and these surgical numbers should be modified based on the results of the individual surgeon.

OPERATIVE TECHNIQUE

PREPARATION OF THE PATIENT

Preparation of the patient involves providing information and obtaining consent. As with any surgical pro-

TABLE 53–2. Common Forms of Strabismus: Features and Treatment

Condition	Definition	Features	Treatment
Infantile esotropia	Esotropia occurring before 6 months of age	Large angle, cross-fixation, alternate fixation, dissociated vertical deviation, inferior oblique overaction, low hyperopia	1. If refractive error is greater than +150 sphere, place infant in a trial of spectacles. 2. If not freely alternating, patch until amblyopia reversed. 3. Bimedial recession when angle is stable. Controversy exists regarding optimal timing of surgery. 4. If greater than 40 prism diopter esotropia, perform bimedial recession with resection of one lateral rectus muscle. 5. Advise parents of approximately 50% risk of need for second strabismus procedure some time in the child's life as intermittent esotropic deviation becomes constant with time.
Accommodative esotropia	Accommodative esotropia presenting at age 1 to 5 as intermittent esodeviation that becomes constant over time	Amblyopia frequently occurs	1. Spectacles with full cycloplegic refraction. 2. Amblyopia therapy. 3. If eyes straight with spectacles, do not do surgery, for high risk of consecutive exotropia.
Accommodative esotropia with AC/A ratio	Acute onset of esotropia between the ages of 1.5 and 5 years	Hyperopic refractive error; angle of deviation increases at near point of fixation; high AC/A ratio when measured by gradient/heterophoria technique.	1. Bifocals with add segment to bisect pupil. 2. Phospholine iodide if not compliant with bifocal. 3. Bimedial recession. 4. Posterior fixation procedure.
Partly accommodative esotropia	Acute onset of esotropia between the ages of 1.5 and 4 years	Hyperopic refractive error; Esotropia is reduced but not eliminated by full hyperopic correction therapy.	1. Surgery for nonaccommodative component. 2. Recession/resection procedure if amblyopia or prefers fixation. 3. Bimedial recession if freely alternating fixation. 4. Instruct parents that spectacles will be necessary postoperatively.
Basic esotropia	Acute onset of esotropia with no hyperopia (hyperopia less than 1.5 sphere)	Usually unilateral with associated amblyopia.	1. Rule out abducens palsy or central nervous system disorder. 2. Reverse amblyopia with occlusion therapy. 3. Recession/resection procedure.
Sensory esotropia	Unilateral esotropia in a poorly seeing eye due to optic nerve, retinal, lenticular, or corneal pathology	Usually a longstanding deviation in children or adults; commonly associated with tight medial rectus muscle.	1. Identify cause of poor vision. 2. Intraocular forced duction testing. 3. Recession/resection procedure with medial rectus on adjustable suture if possible.
Consecutive esotropia	Esotropia following previous surgical correction for exotropia	Usually occurs in immediate postoperative period in children or adults undergoing surgery for exotropia. If child is less than 5 years of age, may develop amblyopia quickly.	1. Occlusion therapy to treat or prevent amblyopia. 2. + lenses. 3. Phospholine iodide. 4. Prism spectacles. 5. Reoperation with advancement of lateral rectus muscle.
Infantile exotropia	Constant exotropia occurring within the first 2 months of life	Deviation same at distance and near; usually large angle deviation with poor ability to adduct the eye commonly associated with A or V patterns; all patients should be evaluated for underlying neurologic disorder.	1. Neurology consultation and neuroimaging. 2. Amblyopia therapy. 3. Large bilateral lateral rectus recessions.

Table continued on opposite page

TABLE 53–2. Common Forms of Strabismus: Features and Treatment *Continued*

Condition	Definition	Features	Treatment
Basic exotropia	Constant exotropia; same measurement at near vs. distance fixation	Can be associated with amblyopia with a dominant eye fixating.	1. Recession/resection procedure. 2. Lateral rectus recessions if alternating.
Divergence excess exotropia	Exotropia greater at distance than at near fixation	Patients often can fuse at near with good stereopsis.	1. Bilateral lateral rectus recession. 2. Adjustable suture technique. 3. Aim for 4 to 8 prism diopters esotropia postoperatively.
Convergence insufficiency	Exotropia at near with decreased convergence amplitude	Patient presents with low convergence amplitude.	1. Convergence exercises. 2. Prism therapy for near vision. 3. Bimedial resection.
Dissociated vertical deviation (DVD)	Elevation with excyclotortion occurring during cover test or when fusion is disrupted	Commonly seen in patients with infantile esotropia.	1. Superior rectus recession, 8 to 12 mm. 2. Faden procedure with superior rectus recession. 3. Anteriorization of inferior oblique muscle if DVD present with oblique overaction.
Double elevator palsy	Inability to elevate the eye in either adduction or abduction	Patients commonly present with chin-up position and pseudoptosis.	1. Forced duction testing under anesthesia. 2. If positive, forced duction large inferior rectus recession with conjunctival recession. 3. If no restriction on forced duction, perform transposition of lateral and medial rectus to superior rectus (Knapp procedure).
Brown's syndrome	Inability to elevate adducted eye secondary to restriction of passage of superior oblique tendon through trochlea	Patient presents with hypotropia on involved eye associated with V-pattern.	1. If no deviation in primary or reading position, no treatment necessary. 2. If hypotropic, perform ipsilateral superior oblique tenotomy. 3. Consider superior oblique spacer. 4. Consider ipsilateral inferior oblique recession at time of superior oblique tenotomy to prevent hypertropia.
Third cranial nerve palsy	Palsy or paresis of cranial nerve III	Inability to elevate, depress, or adduct eye and may be associated with pupillomotor fibers; aberrant regeneration common after trauma or presenting signs if intracranial meningioma	1. Correction of ptosis necessary in addition to strabismus repair. 2. Large recession resection procedure with traction sutures to prevent abduction. 3. Superior oblique transposition moving superior oblique to medial rectus. Superior oblique may be disinserted from trochlea.
Congenital cranial nerve IV palsy	Palsy or paresis of fourth cranial nerve associated with hypertropia and head tilt	Head tilt present from early in life documented in photographs; characteristic facial features with maxillary hypoplasia on side contralateral to hypertropia; diagnosis confirmed by Park's Three-Step Test.	1. If hypertropia is less than 10 prism diopters in the primary position, perform ipsilateral inferior oblique myectomy. 2. If hypertropia is greater than 10 prism diopters, perform inferior oblique myectomy with contralateral inferior rectus recession. 3. For longstanding deviations with hypertropia greater than 30 prism diopters, consider performing forced duction testing. If ipsilateral superior rectus tight, consider inferior oblique myectomy with superior rectus recession and contralateral inferior rectus recession using adjustable suture technique. 4. If marked underaction of superior oblique muscle, consider strengthening this procedure with superior oblique tuck.

Table continued on following page

TABLE 53–2. Common Forms of Strabismus: Features and Treatment *Continued*

Condition	Definition	Features	Treatment
Cranial IV nerve paresis or palsy often associated with closed head trauma		The patient complains of cyclotortion as well as hypertropia. Must rule out bilateral fourth cranial nerve palsy.	1. As described above. 2. If torsion, strengthen superior oblique.
Bilateral fourth cranial palsy	Alternating hypertropia associated with paresis of superior oblique muscle	Commonly found after closed head trauma associated with V-pattern and excyclotortion greater than 10 degrees.	1. If significant esotropia in downgaze, perform bilateral superior oblique tucks. 2. If cyclotortion primary complaint, perform bilateral Harada-Ito procedures. 3. May require bilateral inferior oblique myectomies.
Sixth cranial nerve palsy	Palsy or paresis of sixth cranial nerve associated with esotropia	Child: may be post-viral or associated with pontine glioma; Adult: microvascular, diabetic, clivus chordoma.	1. If complete paresis with no resolution after 6 months, (a) transposition procedure with a full tendon transfer or split tendon transfer associated with ipsilateral medial rectus weakening procedure (intraoperative botulinum toxin or medial rectus recession performed prior to transposition procedure), (b) large recession/resection procedure. 2. If partial sixth cranial nerve palsy, recession/resection procedure ipsilaterally using adjustable suture on medial rectus muscle.
Duane's syndrome type I	Restricted strabismus with inability to abduct the eye	Commonly associated with face turn toward affected side; small angle esotropias are common.	1. Ipsilateral medial rectus recession using hang-back technique. 2. For upshoots or down shoots, Faden procedure on lateral rectus muscle.
Thyroid eye disease	Enlarged extraocular muscles associated with thyroid eye disease; restricted strabismus and tight extraocular muscles[137]	Most commonly affects inferior rectus muscle with medial superior less commonly affected than lateral rectus.	1. Treatment of underlying hyperthyroid state. 2. Treatment of optic nerve compression by orbital decompression procedure if optic neuropathy present. 3. Once patient euthyroid and measurement stable, perform recession of restricted muscle. Leave patient undercorrected as late slippage of tight muscles is well documented.
Strabismus following blowout fracture	Orbital floor fracture with subsequent entrapment of inferior rectus muscle or paresis of muscle secondary to neuromuscular trauma	Patient presents with either hypotropia on involved side secondary to entrapment and inability to elevate the eye or hypertropia on involved side due to posterior fracture and posterior fixation of inferior rectus muscle or paresis due to damage to the neurovascular bundle.	1. Treatment of orbital fracture if significant enophthalmos, entrapment, or large bony defect. 2. If hypotropic eye with restricted inferior rectus, perform inferior rectus recession. 3. If hypertropic eye with weak inferior rectus, perform Faden procedure on contralateral inferior rectus muscle.
Strabismus surgery for nystagmus	Nystagmus associated with null point achieved by taking abnormal head position	Patient may have more than one null point, and strabismus surgery may simply shift the patient to secondary null point.	1. For significant deviation, perform Kestenbaum-Anderson procedure (see Table 53–3).

TABLE 53–3. Surgical Guidelines

Esodeviation
Symmetrical Surgery

ET angle	Recess MR OU	or	Resect LR OU
15 PD	3.0 mm		4 mm
20 PD	3.5 mm		5 mm
25 PD	4.0 mm		6 mm
30 PD	4.5 mm		7 mm
35 PD	5.0 mm		8 mm
40 PD	5.5 mm		8 mm
50 PD	6.0 mm		9 mm
60 PD	6.0 mm and unilateral		LR resection 6.0 mm

Esodeviation
Monocular recess-respect procedures

ET angle	Recess MR	and	Resect LR
15 PD	3.0 mm		4 mm
20 PD	3.5 mm		5 mm
25 PD	4.0 mm		6 mm
30 PD	4.5 mm		7 mm
35 PD	5.0 mm		8 mm
40 PD	5.5 mm		8 mm
50 PD	6.0 mm		9 mm

Exodeviation
Symmetrical Surgery

XT angle	Recess LR OU	or	Resect MR OU
15 PD	4 mm		3 mm
20 PD	5 mm		4 mm
25 PD	6 mm		5 mm
30 PD	7 mm		6 mm
35 PD	7.5 mm		
40 PD	8 mm		

These guidelines for exodeviation are designed to give an initial overcorrection.

Exodeviation
Monocular recess-resect procedures

XT angle	Recess LR	and	Resect MR
15 PD	4 mm		3 mm
20 PD	5 mm		4 mm
25 PD	6 mm		5 mm
30 PD	7 mm		6 mm
35 PD	7.5 mm		6 mm
40 PD	8 mm		6.5 mm

Exotropia with profound amblyopia

XT angle	Recess LR	and	Resect MR
40 PD	8 mm		6 mm
50 PD	9 mm		7 mm
60 PD	10 mm		8 mm
70 PD	10 mm		9 mm
80 PD	10 mm		10 mm

Vertical Deviations (always use adjustable)

Hypertropia (PD)	Vertical Muscle Recession	Vertical Resection/Recession
5 mm	3 mm	
10 mm	5 mm	
15 mm		3 mm/3 mm
20 mm		4 mm/4mm
25 mm		5 mm/5 mm
30		5 mm/6 mm

Nystagmus Surgery
Nystagmus surgery for anomalous head posture
40% augmented Kestenbaum procedures
(if null point with right face turn/left gaze)
Nystagmus surgery for face turn

Left eye		Right Eye	
Recess LR	Resect MR	Recess MR	Resect LR
10 mm	8.0 mm	7 mm	11 mm

Nystagmus surgery for improved visual acuity, 4 muscle recession, left
Lateral rectus recession 10 mm
Medial rectus recession 7.5 mm

Above figures modified from basic and clinical science course. American Academy of Ophthalmology, 1996.

cedures, the patient or the parent should be informed of all risks involved. These include loss of life due to anaesthetic complication, which occurs approximately in one in every 250,000 operative procedures. Loss of vision is also extremely rare whether a consequence of inadvertent ocular perforation or from secondary endophthalmitis. Certainly the most common complications of strabismus surgery are overcorrection and undercorrection. The rate of surgical success quoted depends on the form of strabismus being corrected. For example, patients with infantile esotropia are instructed that they have an 80% to 90% chance of adequate postoperative alignment after one surgery, but they are also advised that there is a 30% to 40% chance the patient will develop strabismus in the future, requiring a second operation sometime in their lifetime. Use of adjustable suture technique reduces the risk of overcorrection or undercorrection and need for subsequent strabismus surgery. Patients should also be warned that there will be some postoperative discomfort, redness of the eye, and perhaps diplopia. Prism spectacles may be necessary for a short time after the surgery if diplopia develops postoperatively. Patients operated upon for partly accommodative esotropia must be told that they will still require spectacles postoperatively. They are also advised that occlusion therapy may be required if amblyopia develops after the strabismus surgery. Prior to induction of anesthesia, the patient or parent must be asked which eye or eyes will be operated upon. If there is any chance of bilateral surgery, the patient must be properly informed and give consent for unexpected intraoperative findings affecting treatment decisions.

CHOICE OF ANESTHESIA

General anesthesia is used for infants, children, and young adults. Usually, infants do not require preoperative sedation, as separation anxiety does not develop until after the age of 18 months. After that time, preoperative midazolam is commonly used to sedate the child, which makes separation easier for child and parent alike. Masked induction using nitrous oxide and halothane or sevoflurane allows for smooth induction and endotracheal intubation. Laryngeal mask airways can be used in infants and children, and these lessen both postoperative discomfort and the incidence of postoperative nausea and vomiting. Nausea can also be controlled through the use of propofol anesthesia and odansetron, a powerful antiemetic. The oculocardiac reflex occurs almost universally in children undergoing strabismus repair. Slowing of the heart rate and asystole may occur, and atropine should be given to prevent this life-threatening condition.

Adults may have surgery performed using either general anesthesia, retrobulbar, peribulbar anesthesia, or topical anesthesia. General anesthesia is required when bilateral surgery is being performed. It is also helpful to use general anesthesia in a patient with previous ocular surgery, where scarring of the extraocular muscles is expected. General anesthesia is also indicated when a surgical decision will be influenced by the forced duction testing. The use of retrobulbar anesthesia can cause only partial paresis and can change the intraorbital pressure, leading to false findings on forced duction testing and use of the spring-back test. Adult patients who are having monocular surgery can be readily operated on using retrobulbar or peribulbar anesthesia. Supplemental anesthesia can be given during the procedure using a gently curved irrigating cannula and infiltrating 2% lidocaine along the sides of the muscle. Infiltration with sharp needles should be avoided because of the risk of inadvertent ocular perforation. It is possible to perform strabismus surgery using topical anesthesia with either topical cocaine or 4% lidocaine soaking the muscle insertions with a pledget to provide local anesthesia. This has the advantage of allowing suture adjustment interoperatively or soon after surgery.

Some surgeons have advocated the use of propofol, a fast-acting intravenous anaesthetic, to allow intraoperative adjustment of muscles. This is best used in a patient who is a poor candidate for suture adjustment postoperatively. With propofol, the patient can be aroused on the operating table, so that a cover test can be performed to ensure ocular alignment. Then, after the patient is resedated with additional propofol, the desired adjustment can be made. This requires a cooperative patient, a cooperative anesthesiologist, and increased operating room time.

PREPARATION IN THE OPERATING ROOM

The anesthesiologist should be asked to use a Rae type endotracheal tube, which will be directed away from the patient's eyes, allowing the surgeon full access to the periocular region. The operating bed should be rotated 90 degrees, so that there is room for the surgeon to be seated on either side at the patient's head, providing for access to all extraocular muscles. A shoulder roll should be placed under the patient to extend the neck and place the chin pointing slightly upward. A small cushion donut placed under the patient's head will provide stabilization. The patient's surgical prep should include Betadine placed in the patient's eyes and irrigated with balanced saline solution. Although this may cause mild irritation of the conjunctiva and cornea, it significantly reduces bacterial colonization of these tissues. The lids and lashes should be scrubbed with Betadine solution, and the periocular region painted with Betadine solution. Special care should be taken to carefully drape the patient's nasal bridge and malar region with a plastic drape. Children are prone to large amounts of secretion, which can make their way under the drape and enter the ocular field.

Strabismus surgery is best performed using loupe magnification and headlamp illumination. Magnification helps when placing scleral bites into thin sclera, and headlights are essential when working the oblique muscles.

Forced duction testing should be performed on all patients as a matter of routine. Using two toothed forceps, the eye is grasped at the limbus, first at the 6 o'clock and 12 o'clock positions, rotating the eye into abduction and adduction, then at 3 o'clock and 9 o'clock, rotating the eye into superduction and infraduction. Care should be taken not to depress the globe during the rotation, as this may result in an overestimation of ductions. The oblique muscles can also be tested with a traction test. The findings of the forced duction testing should be dictated in the operative report, as this will aid in future decision making if additional strabismus surgery is required. After forced duction testing is performed, traction sutures may be placed at the limbus. Using 6-0 silk on a taper needle, traction sutures are placed at the limbus. For horizontal rectus muscles, the sutures are placed at 6 o'clock and 12 o'clock; for vertical muscle surgery and oblique muscle surgery, the sutures are placed at 3 o'clock and 9 o'clock. Hemostats can be placed on the ends of both silk sutures, and the eye rotated to provide excellent exposure of the muscle to be operated upon.

SURGICAL PROCEDURES

THE RECTUS MUSCLES

While both limbal and fornix conjunctival incisions have been recommended for exposure of the rectus muscles, limbal incisions are most commonly used because they provide certain advantages. First, they allow the best exposure of the rectus muscles, especially when a surgical assistant is not available. Second, it is possible to recess the conjunctiva and prevent conjunctival contracture. Finally, peritomies performed at the limbus will provide excellent exposure of the suture knot when the adjustable suture technique is performed.[22]

For surgery on the medial, inferior, lateral, and superior recti, the peritomies are performed at the limbus, with winged incisions made in the quadrants surrounding the muscle (Fig. 53–7).

After the peritomy has been performed and bare sclera is exposed, Wescott scissors or Stevens tenotomy scissors are used to dissect the quadrants surrounding the rectus muscle. The scissors should be held perpendicular to the globe, spreading Tenon's capsule away from the globe using direct visualization (Fig. 53–8). The goal is to perforate Tenon's capsule to provide an opening for the muscle hook to slide easily behind the muscle insertion without catching Tenon's capsule. After the quadrants have been dissected with either Wescott scissors or tenotomy scissors, a von Graefe muscle hook is used to isolate the rectus muscle. Care should be taken to avoid splitting the muscle insertion. A Green, Jameson, or square muscle hook is then passed in the opposite direction, ensuring that all muscle fibers are firmly secured on the muscle hook. A bent or enlarged tip will keep the muscle secure during additional manipulation. The muscle hook is grasped by the surgical assistant, and the eye is rotated toward the surgeon. Wescott scissors are used to sharply dissect conjunctiva and Tenon's away from the muscle sheath. A vein retractor or a small Desmarres retractor is placed between the conjunctiva and the muscle surface (Fig. 53–9). This provides excellent exposure of the rectus muscle. The vessels on the surface of the rectus muscle will be plainly visible and should be avoided. Blood vessels inadvertently cut should be cauterized. Using direct visualization, the intermuscular septum is isolated on a .5 Castroviejo forceps, and the Wescott scissors are used to sharply dissect the intermuscular septum away from the muscle until the muscle is cleanly exposed. Dissection should be carried out only until the white condensation of Tenon's capsule is visualized. Tenon's should not be perforated posterior to this point as this may result in prolapse of orbital fat and restrictive strabismus.

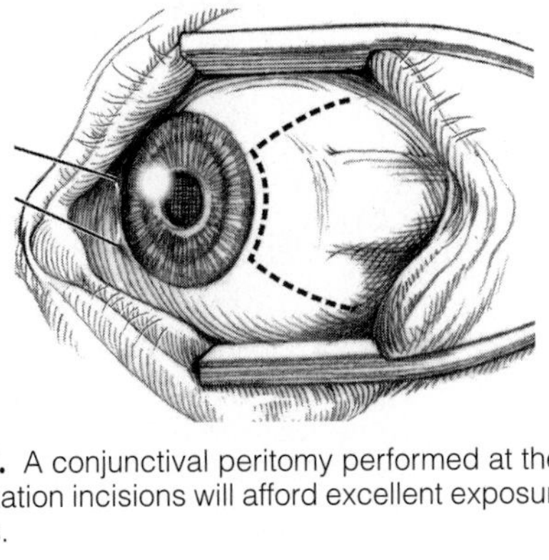

Figure 53–7. A conjunctival peritomy performed at the limbus with winged relaxation incisions will afford excellent exposure of extraocular muscles.

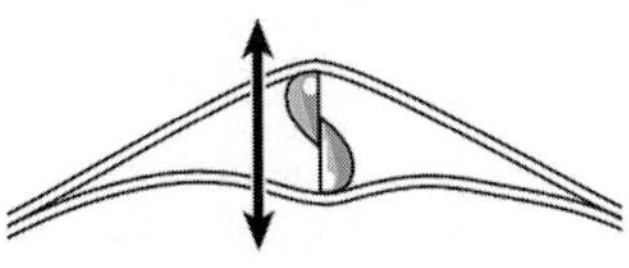

Figure 53–8. When dissecting in the quadrants above and below the rectus muscle, spread the scissor blades vertically to avoid damage to the muscle.

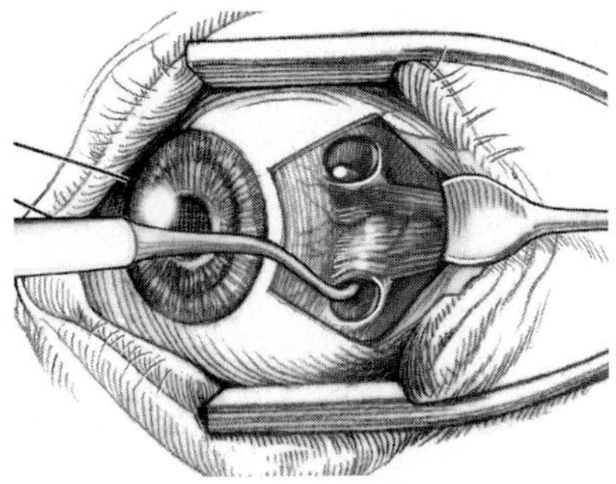

Figure 53–9. A Jameson muscle hook is used to isolate the entire width of the rectus muscle, and a small Desmarres retractor provides exposure for dissection of the intermuscular septum.

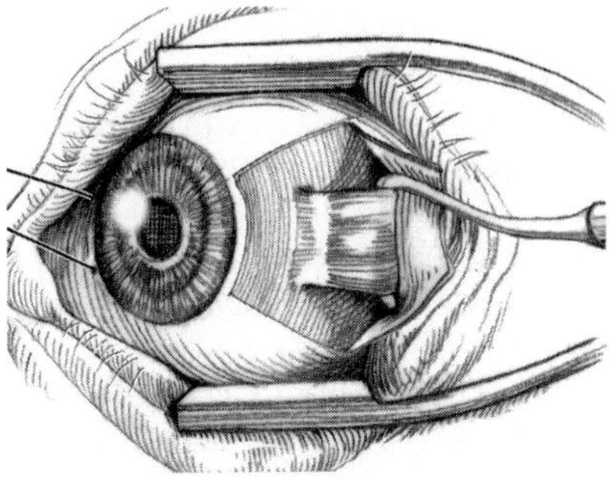

Figure 53–10. Dissection of intermuscular septum and facial attachments will enable easy imbrication of suture into muscle.

After dissection is complete, the muscle insertion is identified. The surgeon then lifts the muscle hook, drawing it away from the scleral surface, so that the muscle is easily splayed out on the muscle hook and a space is created between the muscle insertion and the underlying sclera (Fig. 53–10).

Rectus Muscle Recession

Approximately one millimeter from the insertion, a double-armed 6-0 Vicryl suture is to be imbricated through the muscle insertion (Fig. 53–11). The suture is

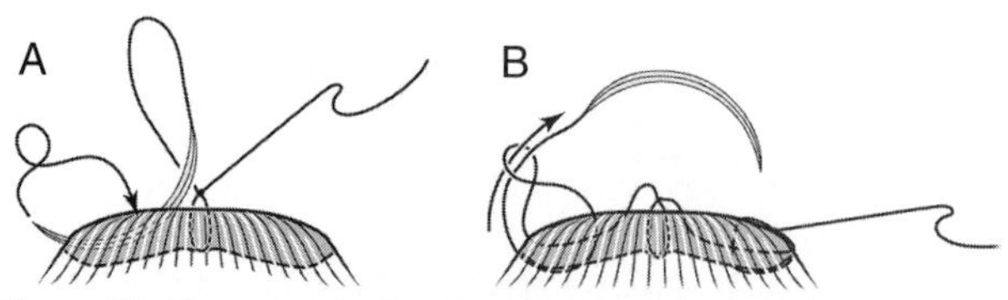

Figure 53–11. The 6-0 suture is imbricated and locked into the muscle centrally and at the edges. Imbrication passes should be partial depth, and locking bites should be full thickness.

left double-armed. One needle is used to create a full-thickness pass through the muscle in the center of the muscle at the insertion. This suture is tied securely at this point with a 3-1-1 knot, which provides added security and prevents central sag during the recession procedure. One needle is then placed in the center of the muscle and passed toward the edge of the muscle at a depth of 50% of the thickness of the muscle insertion. It is important that this not be a full-thickness pass, but should incorporate one-half of the muscle width. At this point, the surgeon grasps the needle and makes a full-thickness pass incorporating the outer quarter of the muscle fibers. It is critical to make this a full-thickness pass encompassing the posterior capsule to prevent postoperative muscle slippage. The suture is locked after this bite is taken. This forms a locking imbricated purchase on the muscle. The other end of the suture is then passed through the remaining half of the muscle in a similar fashion. This secures the muscle to the suture in three positions, at both edges and in the center. Some surgeons use a muscle clamp to fixate the muscle and disinsert the muscle from the globe before placing the suture into the muscle.

After the muscle is firmly secured on the suture, the muscle is disinserted from the globe using the Wescott scissors. Small bites should be taken with the scissors, making certain not to cut the suture or "buttonhole" the sclera. Hand-held cautery is used for hemostasis (Fig. 53–12). At this time, the suture and muscles should be inspected to make certain that there is adequate purchase of suture on the muscle. If there is any question about the security of the pass, additional imbricating passes should be made in the muscle. After adequate security is assured, calipers are used to measure the amount of recession from the original insertion site. The muscle can be recessed in either the scleral fixation fashion, or in the hangback fashion (see below). For scleral fixation, calipers (Fig. 53–13) are used to measure the desired amount of recession, and the suture needles are passed through partial-depth sclera 0.1 mm deep, using the crossed-swords technique (Fig. 53–14). The needle should always be visible within the sclera to avoid inadvertent perforation. After measurement is reconfirmed, measuring the amount of recession both from the original insertion site and from the limbus, the suture knot is secured with a 3-1-1 knot. If adjustable sutures will be used, use the hangback technique.

In the hangback technique, the suture needles are passed back through the original insertion site, and a triple throw is placed temporarily in the knot. Calipers

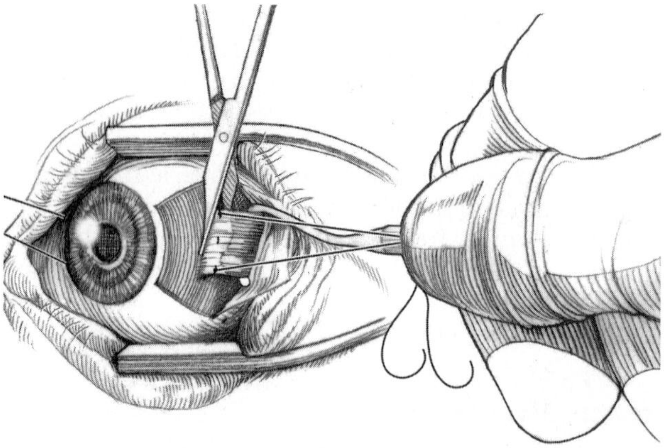

Figure 53–12. The rectus muscle is disinserted by taking small bites with the Wescott scissors, holding the stitch away from the scissor blades to avoid accidental cutting.

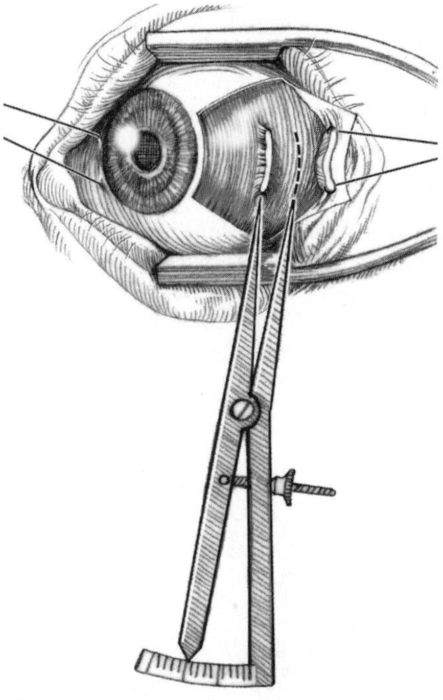

Figure 53–13. Calipers are used to measure from original insertion site as well as from the limbus.

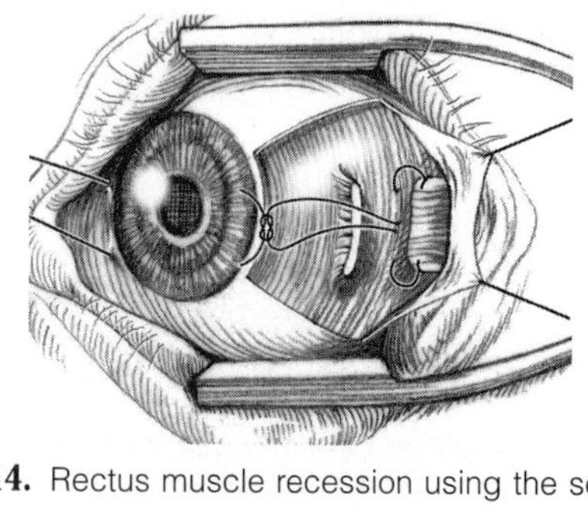

Figure 53–14. Rectus muscle recession using the scleral fixation technique.

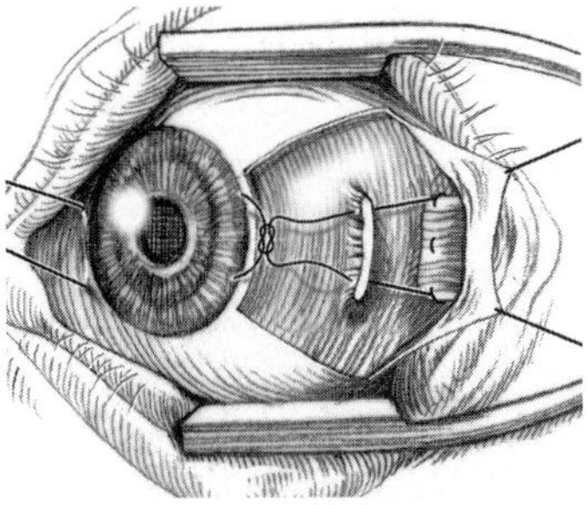

Figure 53–15. Rectus muscle recession using the "hangback" technique.

are used to measure from the site of insertion to the point where the muscle is recessed on the scleral surface. After measurement is confirmed, the knot is secured with additional single throws (Fig. 53–15). The hangback technique is always used when adjustable suture technique will be used, but it may be used in other circumstances, such as with very large recessions or when exposure is difficult and scleral refixation is dangerous.[23–25] When using adjustable suture technique, it is important to make long intrascleral passes so that the suture will not pull out of the sclera during the adjustment phase.

After the muscle is securely reattached to the sclera, the overlying conjunctiva is closed with interrupted 6-0 plain gut suture (Fig. 53–16). Care should be taken to reapproximate the conjunctiva precisely to avoid inclusion cysts and dellen formation. If the conjunctiva is tight, it should be recessed to avoid development of postoperative restrictions (Fig. 53–17).

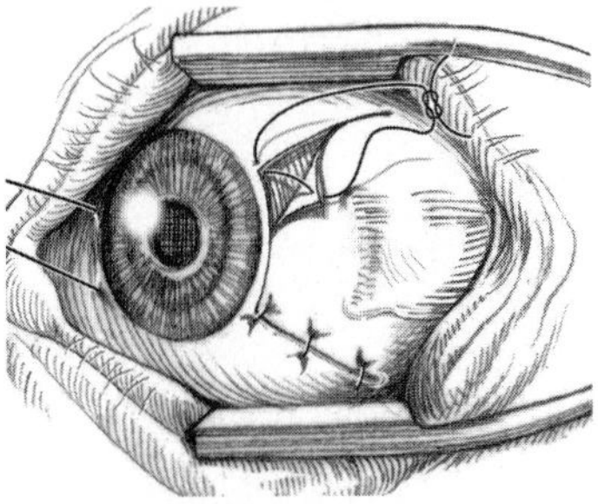

Figure 53–16. Closure of the conjunctival using 6-0 gut.

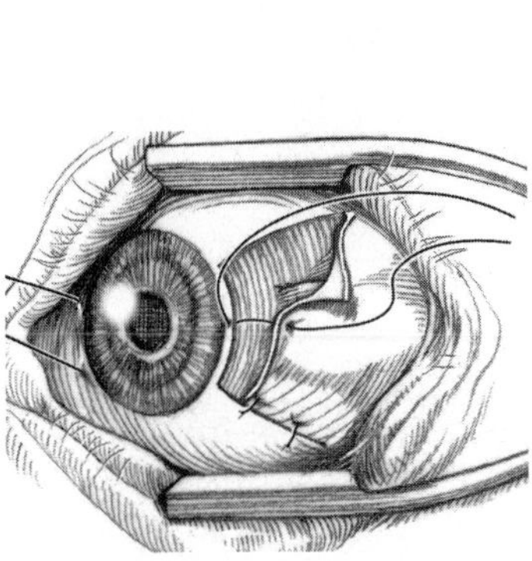

Figure 53–17. Recession of the conjunctiva should be performed when the conjunctiva is tight and when placement back to the limbus would result in a positive forced duction test.

Conjunctival Fornix Incision

It is possible to approach the horizontal rectus muscles using a fornix-based incision rather than a limbal incision (Figs. 53–18 through Fig. 53–25). This technique hides the incision in the inferior cul de sac. An incision is made through the conjunctiva and Tenon's capsule to bare sclera along the inferior border of the medial rectus muscle. A muscle hook engages the rectus muscle and a smaller hook is used to drape the conjunctiva over the tip of the muscle hook. The superior edge of the muscle hook is cleaned freely, isolating the muscle. The procedure proceeds in the standard fashion. This technique is useful in contact lens wearers but requires a skilled assistant and is not suitable for reoperation.

Rectus Muscle Resection

Exposure of the rectus muscle is performed as described for the recession technique. After the muscle is isolated on the Greene muscle hook, an additional muscle hook is placed behind the muscle insertion, and the hook spread out in the opposite direction. This splays out the muscle and elevates it away from the sclera. A 6-0 double-armed Vicryl suture is used for resection technique. Calipers are used to measure the desired amount of resection, measuring from the insertion site posterior on the muscle surface. Low-temperature cautery can be used to mark the location of the desired resection on the muscle surface. At this point, a full-thickness bite is placed in the 3-1-1 knot secured in the Vicryl suture (Fig. 53–26). This knot prevents central sag and assures appropriate measurement of the amount of resection necessary. The muscle is then imbricated as described for recession, placing the first throw from the center of the muscle laterally to the edge of the muscle at 50% muscle depth, the locking bite being full thickness on the lateral one-quarter of the muscle width (Fig. 53–27). After the suture is firmly secured on the muscle, a straight hemostat is used to crush the muscle anterior to the suture. The muscle is then transected at this point (Fig. 53–28). The muscle stump is removed from the globe with Wescott scissors, and disposable cautery is used for hemostasis. At this time, the surgeon passes the suture needles through the original insertion site, taking care to prevent inadvertent perforation behind the muscle insertion site, where the sclera is at its thinnest (Fig. 53–29). The suture is drawn up securely, which reapproximates the resected muscle to the original insertion site. The suture is secured with a 3-1-1 knot (Fig. 53–30), the overlying conjunctiva is closed with 6-0 plain gut suture. Many surgeons use two separate sutures for muscle resections in order to prevent slipped or lost muscles, and some surgeons use muscle clamps when performing resection procedures (Figs. 53–31 through Fig. 53–33).

Vertical Transposition of the Horizontal Rectus Muscles

Transposition of the horizontal rectus muscles may be performed during either monocular or bilateral strabismus surgery. To collapse A- and V-patterns, it should

Text continued on p. 567.

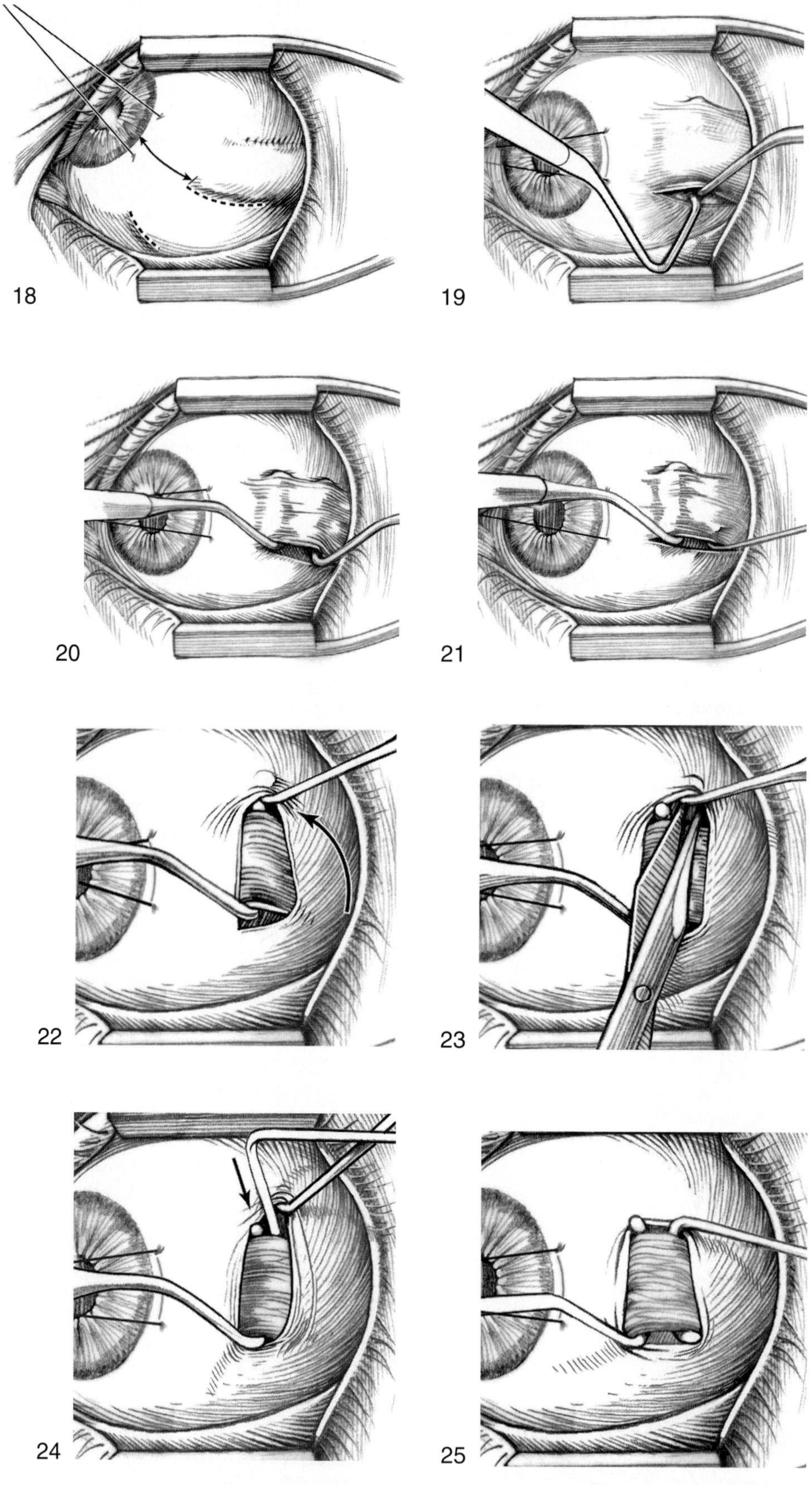

Figures 53–18 through 53–25. Surgical approach to horizontal rectus muscle using a fornix incision.

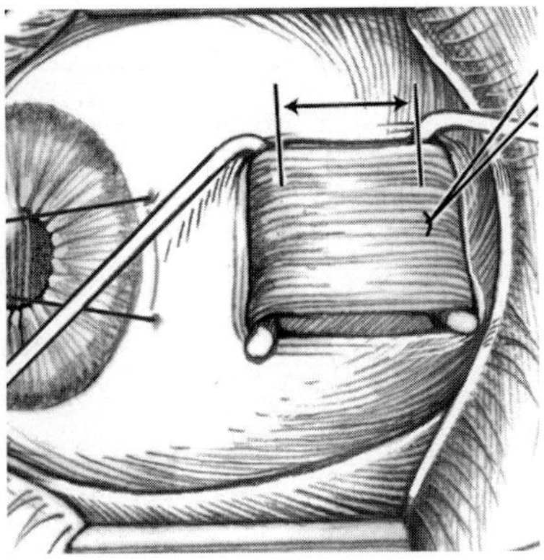

Figure 53–26. Preparation of the horizontal rectus muscle for resection using a fornix incision. Suture is imbricated at location on muscle belly, measured, and marked with calipers.

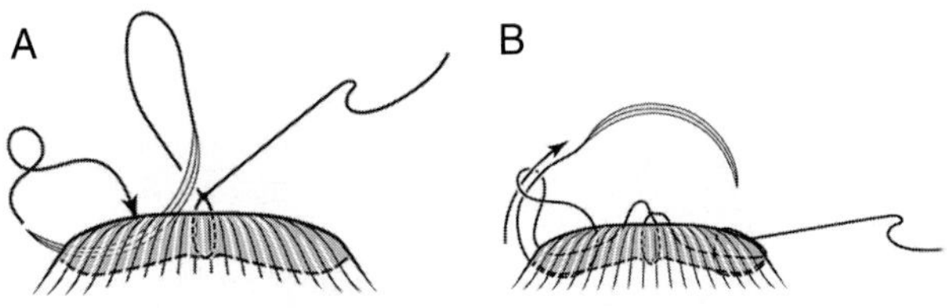

Figure 53–27. Standard imbrication technique.

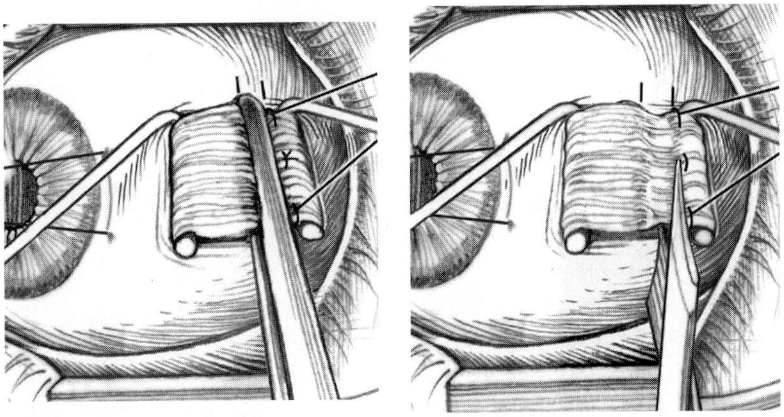

Figure 53–28. A straight hemostat is used to crush the muscle anterior to suture placement. Wescott scissors are used to transect the muscle at this point.

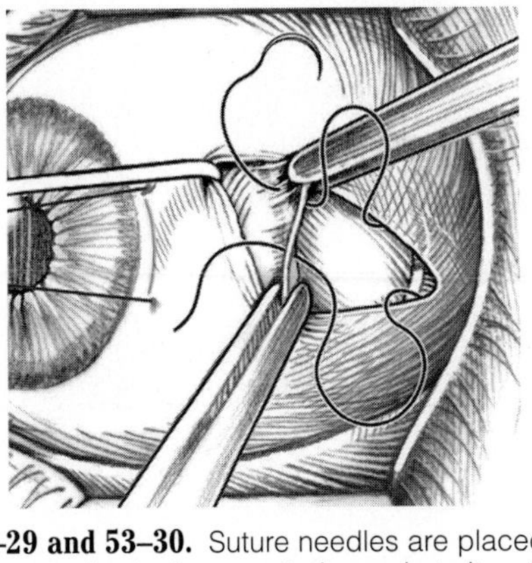

29

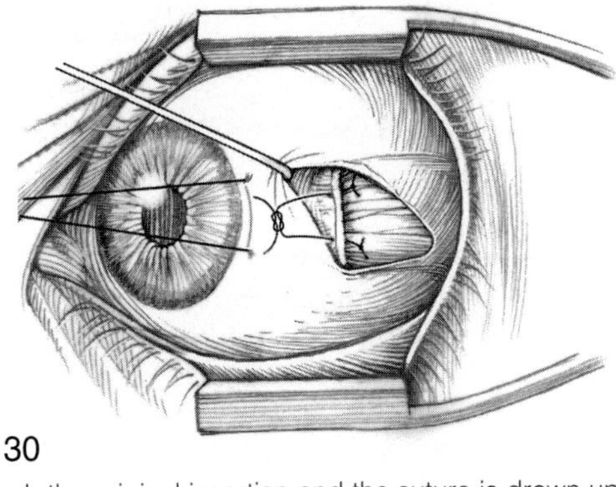

30

Figures 53–29 and 53–30. Suture needles are placed through the original insertion and the suture is drawn up securely to snugly reapproximate the resected muscle to its original insertion.

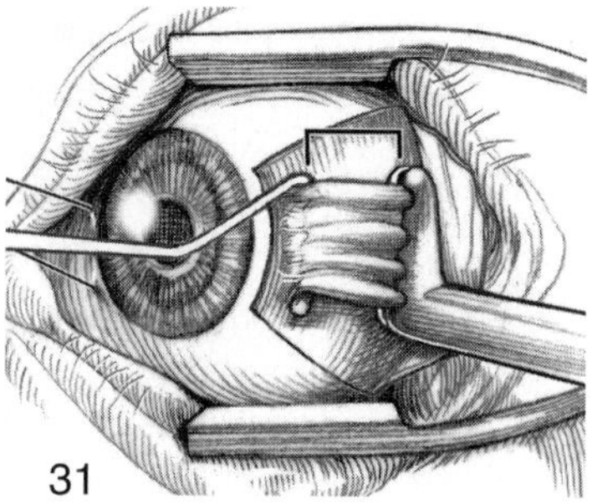

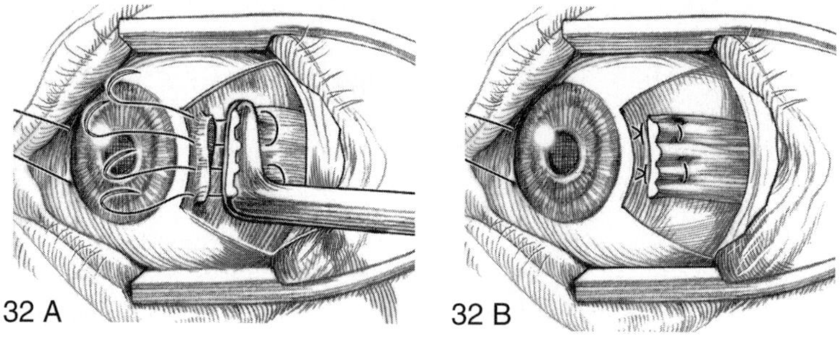

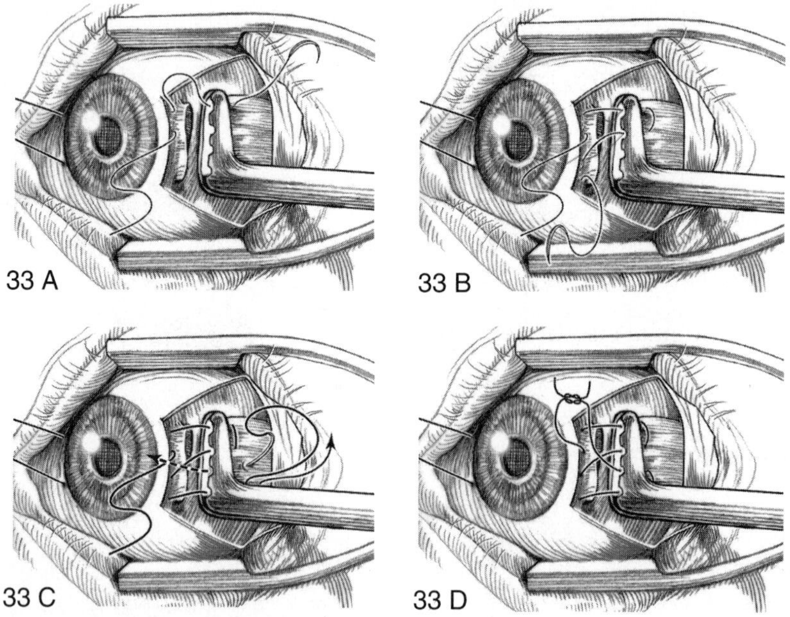

Figures 53–31 through 53–33. Recession or resection procedures may be performed with specially designed muscle clamps. When clamps are used, the sutures are placed in the muscle after the muscle has been transected from the globe. Clamps are useful in re-operations and when placement of sutures is difficult in scarred or tight muscles.

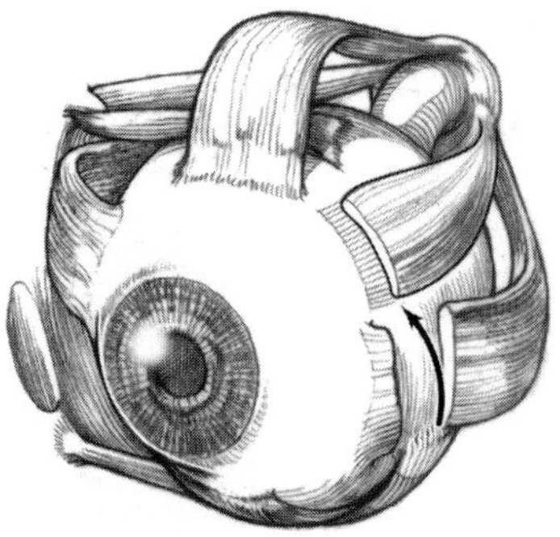

Figure 53–34. Superior transposition of lateral rectus muscle combined with recession. When performing transposition, measure from the limbus to maintain the desired weakness or strengthening effect.

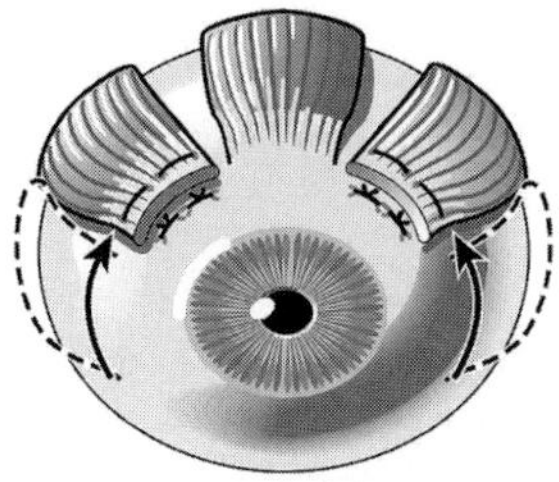

Figure 53–35. The Knapp procedure.

be remembered that the horizontal rectus muscles are moved in the direction in which weakening is required. For example, in a V-pattern esotropia, the medial rectus muscles are transposed inferiorly, whereas in an A-pattern esotropia, they are transposed superiorly. If a patient here undergoing bilateral lateral rectus recessions for a V-pattern exotropia, the muscles would be moved transposed superiorly after they had been recessed.[26,27]

When transposing a horizontal rectus muscle, the hangback technique should be avoided if possible, and the muscle should be sutured directly to the sclera. It is important to measure the amount of recession from the limbus rather than from the original insertion site. This will ensure that the muscle insertion remains parallel to the limbus and that the amount of recession or resection affected is not inadvertently altered. The muscle should be transposed one muscle tendon width, approximately 10 mm in the desired direction in order to achieve maximum effect to collapse A- or V-patterns (Fig. 53–34). Lesser amounts of transposition have lesser effect in collapsing patterns.

The horizontal muscles can also be transposed to convert horizontal forces to generate either elevating or depressing forces in a paretic eye (Fig. 53–35). For example, in a case of superior rectus palsy or double elevator palsy, both the lateral and the medial rectus muscles can be transposed superiorly to the insertion of the superior rectus muscle to elevate the eye. This procedure, known as the Knapp procedure, is useful in cases of double elevator palsy where there is not coexistent contracture or restriction of the inferior rectus muscle.

Horizontal muscle transposition can also be used for the treatment of small hypertropias when there is coexistent esotropia or exotropia. The appropriate amount of horizontal muscle surgery is performed, and the muscle is transposed one-half tendon width to one tendon width inferiorly or superiorly to treat vertical deviations measuring from zero to eight prism diopters.

Marginal Myotomy of the Horizontal Rectus Muscles

Most often, horizontal rectus muscles are weakened by recession procedures. On occasion, it may be necessary to further weaken the effect of a horizontal rectus muscle that has been maximally recessed.[28] This can be achieved by performing a marginal myotomy. In this procedure, a clamp is used to crush the superior one third of the muscle and the inferior one third of the muscle, with an intervening offset. The muscle is then transected at these positions, which allows it to lengthen, thereby weakening its contractile efficiency of the muscle (Fig. 53–36). Care should be taken not to weaken the muscle so much that it inadvertently becomes transected. The technique is limited by the fact that its predictability is variable, depending on the appearance of the muscle and the presence of previous strabismus surgery.

Posterior Fixation Suture (Faden Operation) or Retroequatorial Myopexy

The posterior fixation suture is a procedure used to weaken a horizontal rectus muscle. In this procedure, first described by Cuppers, the muscle belly is sutured

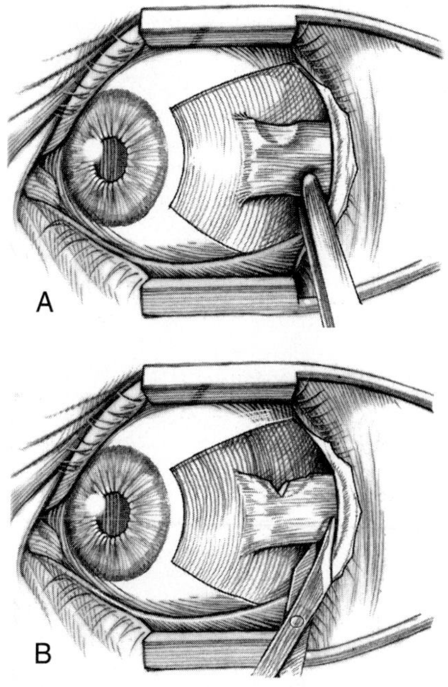

Figure 53–36. Marginal myotomy is performed to weaken a muscle.

to the sclera at a location posterior to the equator.[29] It may be combined with a concurrent recession of the muscle. The posterior fixation suture combined with concurrent recession is indicated for weakening of the muscle when the eye is in the field of action rather than in a primary position. Posterior fixation suture without the recession is useful in cases of desired weakening when the eye is straight in the primary position. This allows weakening of the muscle without changing alignment of the eye in the primary position. This technique is most useful in treating conditions where weakening of a yoke muscle is required. It is also useful in cases of nystagmus blockage syndrome, dissociated vertical divergence, the treatment of incomitance secondary to orbital floor fractures, and cases of convergence excess esotropia with or without high AC/A ratio.[30,31] A final indication is in the treatment of Duane's syndrome with significant upshoots or downshoots; where placing a posterior fixation suture on the lateral rectus muscle may prevent these vertical deviations.

Figure 53–37 demonstrates recession combined with posterior fixation suture. Posterior fixation is usually 12 to 14 mm posterior to the original insertion. A nonabsorbable suture (5.0 Dacron on a T5 [Alcon] needle) is used for placing the posterior fixation suture. The nonabsorbable suture is placed through the sclera and then placed through the undersurface of the rectus muscle, incorporating the superior 25% of the muscle fibers. The previously imbricated rectus muscle is then recessed the desired amount in the standard fashion. Finally, the nonabsorbable suture is tied securely, thus forming a recession with the posterior fixation suture (Fig. 53–38).

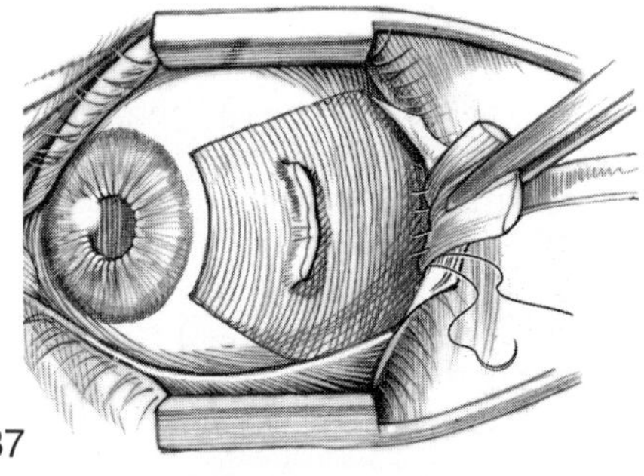
37

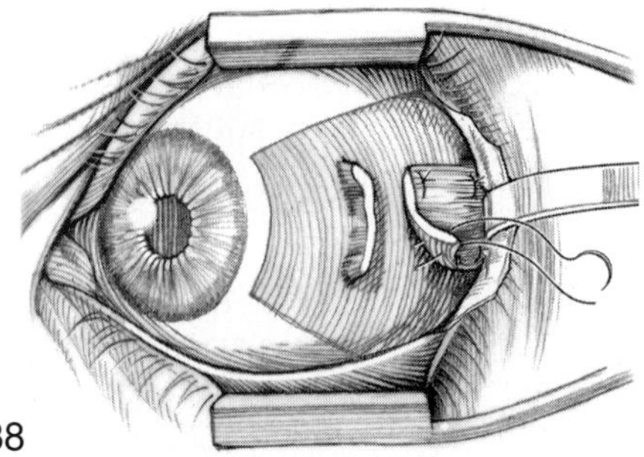
38

Figures 53–37 and 53–38. Placement of a Faden suture (posterior fixation suture) may be performed with or without concurrent recession.

When a posterior fixation suture is placed without recession, the same nonabsorbable suture is placed through the sclera 12 mm posterior to the original insertion site. The superior 25% of the muscle and the inferior 25% of the muscle are fixed to the sclera using two separate nonabsorbable sutures.

To perform this procedure safely, the surgeon should use a headlight, and malleable retractors are often helpful in the exposure. The sutures are placed very far posteriorly, increasing the risk of inadvertent perforation. Care must be taken not to involve more than 50% of the muscle fibers, as ischemia and necrosis of the muscle have been described.

At the completion of the procedure, forced duction testing should be performed, and there should be no passive restriction of eye movements. Restriction indicates inadvertent entrapment of tissue other than the muscle, which is acting as a leash, preventing passive rotation of the eye. If such resistance is encountered, the muscle should be explored and adherent tissue removed.

THE SUPERIOR OBLIQUE MUSCLE

Of all extraocular muscles, the superior oblique muscle is the most difficult to treat surgically. Surgical exposure is difficult because of upper eyelid tissue. Further, the anatomy of the superior oblique tendon can be highly variable. The surgical result can be highly variable. The superior oblique muscle can be approached from the nasal aspect, the temporal aspect, or via disinsertion of the superior rectus muscle.[32] The safest approach involves a temporal approach to the superior oblique tendon. This approach can be used for either weakening or strengthening procedures, and it is desirable because it allows continuous direct observation of the superior rectus tendon and will avoid inadvertent damage to the superior rectus muscle (Figs. 53–39 through Fig. 53–42).

A conjunctival incision is made in the superior temporal fornix 8 mm posterior to the limbus. The temporal border of the superior rectus is directly identified, and a Green muscle hook is placed around the superior rectus muscle. The eye is rotated downward by traction on the Green muscle hook, and, under direct observation, the superior oblique tendon is identified where it passes underneath the superior rectus muscle. Care should be taken not to dissect tissue between the superior rectus muscle and the superior oblique muscle, as inadvertent transsection of the superior oblique tendon can occur. The tendon insertion is thin and diaphanous in many cases, and can be mistaken for connective tissue. A Desmarres retractor can be placed underneath the conjunctiva to give better exposure to the superior oblique tendon insertion. If exposure of the superior oblique tendon is desired nasal to the superior rectus muscle, the Desmarres retractor can be used to pull the conjunctiva nasally, thereby exposing the medial aspect of the superior rectus muscle. Intramuscular septum can be carefully dissected away from the medial aspect of the superior rectus tendon, taking care not to transect the more

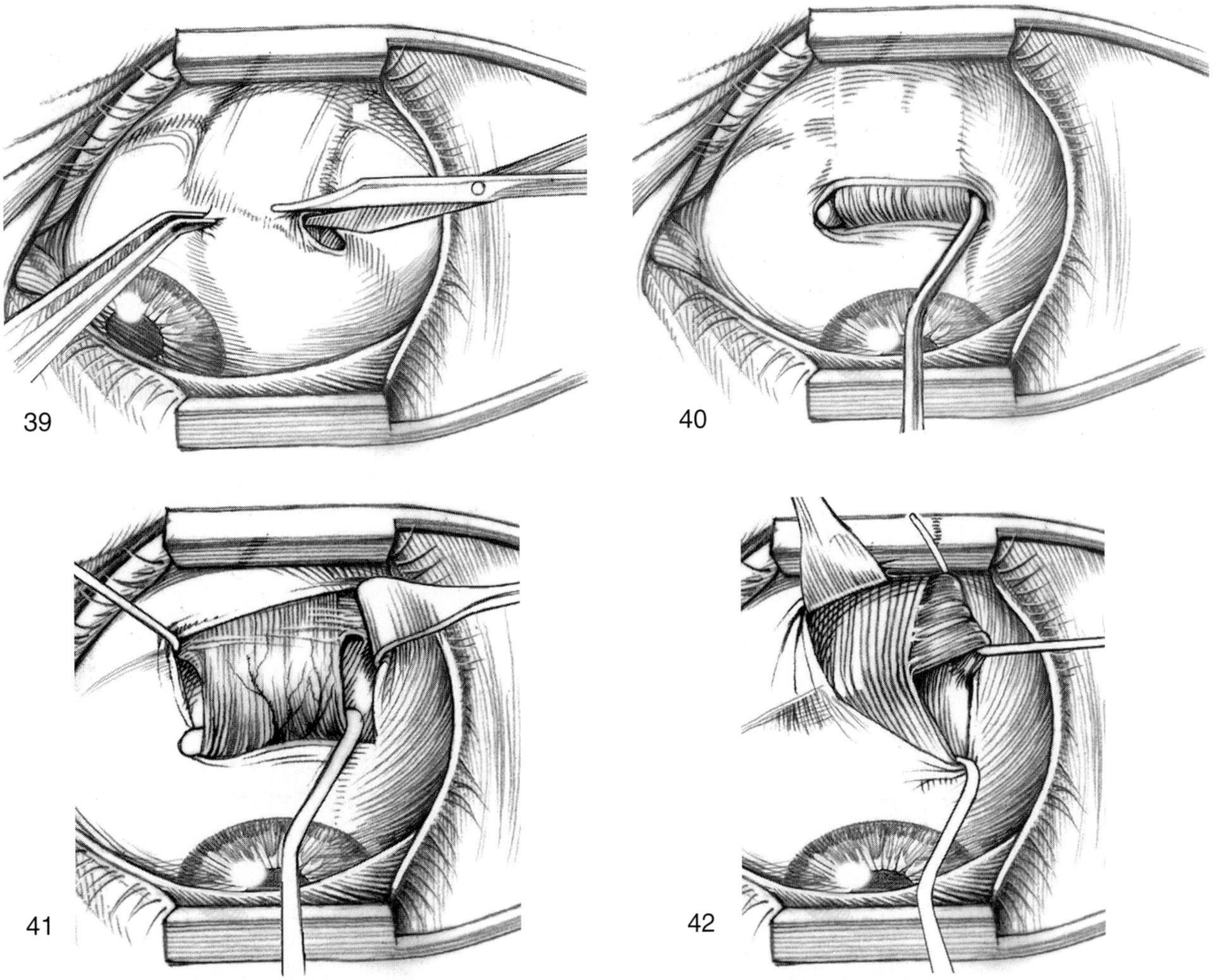

Figures 53–39 through 53–42. Surgical isolation and exposure of the left superior oblique tendon using a temporal approach.

collagenous tendon on the nasal aspect of the superior rectus muscle. Care should be taken in exposure of the superior oblique muscle, as there is often a vortex vein anterior to the insertion of the superior oblique muscle.

Superior Oblique Muscle Strengthening

The superior oblique muscle most commonly requires strengthening in cases of superior oblique muscle palsy.[33,34] As stated earlier, in cases of small deviation in the primary position measuring less than 10 prism diopters, an ipsilateral inferior oblique muscle weakening procedure can be performed. When there is severe superior oblique underaction with minimal inferior oblique overaction and hyperdeviation that is greatest in downgaze, an ipsilateral superior oblique tuck may be indicated.[35] The other indication for superior oblique tuck is the presence of bilateral superior oblique palsy, which can be determined by 10 prism diopters of esotropic shift in downgaze, and the presence of greater than 10 degrees of excyclotortion in the primary position. These bilateral cases often require bilateral full tendon tucks.[36]

The superior oblique muscle is isolated in the standard fashion using the temporal approach. The surgeon then isolates superior oblique tendon on a Jameson muscle hook, taking care to incorporate all posterior fibers. The posterior intramuscular septum is dissected so that the tip of the muscle hook can freely pass along the posterior border of the superior oblique tendon. A tendon tucker is placed around the superior oblique muscle (Figs. 53–43 and 53–44). The amount of muscle tucked varies between 8 mm and 15 mm, and the tuck is held with a 5-0 Mersiline suture placed in a double mattress fashion (Fig. 53–45). If a tendon tucker is not available, a tuck may be taken simply using a muscle hook (Fig. 53–46). The nonabsorbable Mersiline suture is placed 8 to 10 mm proximal to the insertion site in a double-locking fashion. The suture needles are then placed at the original insertion site and the suture is drawn up securely. This creates a knuckle of tendon, which may be affixed to the sclera. After performing a tucking procedure, it is important to conduct a traction test to make certain that Brown's syndrome has been induced. It should be difficult to elevate the eye in adduction, indicating tightening of the superior oblique muscle.

Cases of acquired fourth cranial nerve palsy are often characterized by torsional diplopia. Torsional diplopia of 10 prism diopters or more in the primary position often requires bilateral Harada-Ito procedures.[37] In the

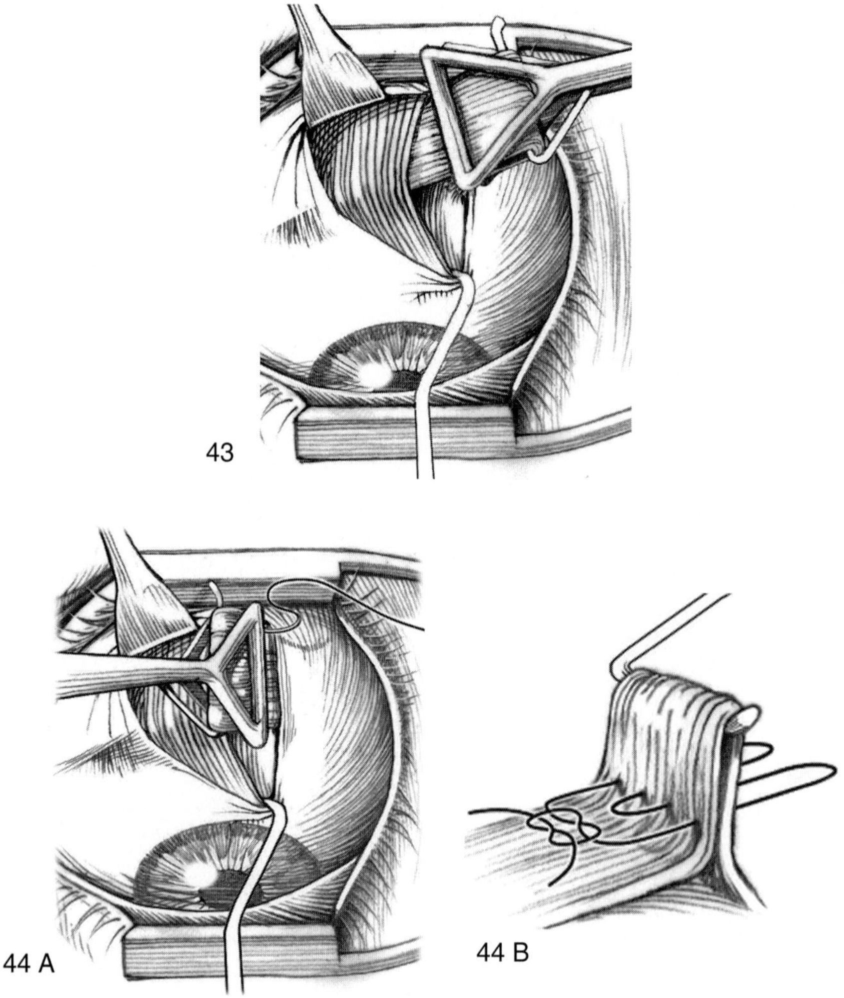

Figures 53–43 through 53–44. Use of a tendon tucker to strengthen the superior oblique muscle.

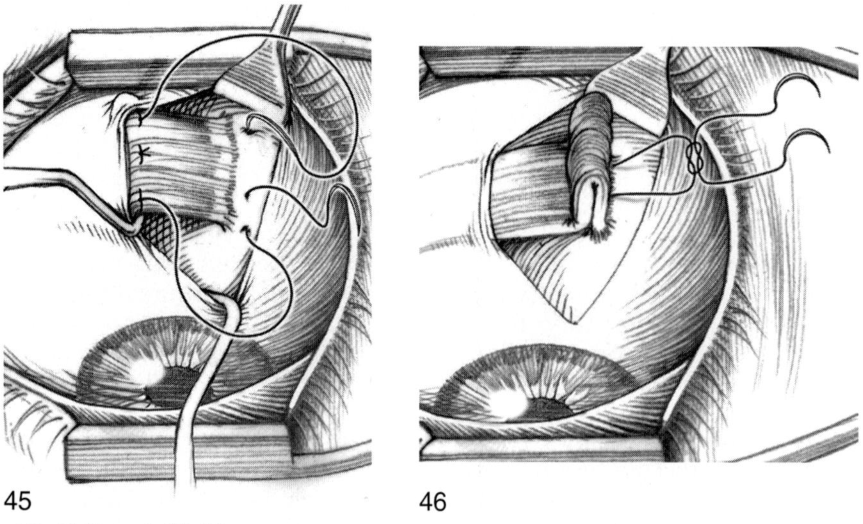

Figures 53–45 through 53–46. Use of a muscle hook to touch and strengthen a superior oblique muscle.

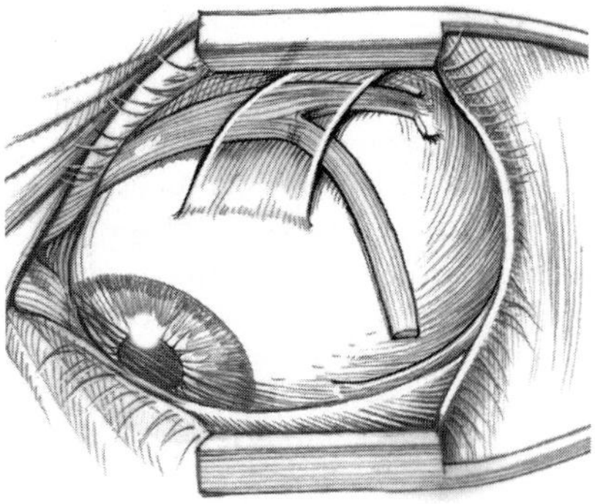

Figure 53–47. Harada-Ito procedure via disinsertion technique used to strengthen incyclotorsion. The procedure may be used with adjustable suture to allow variable degrees of incyclotorsion.

Harada-Ito procedure, the anterior superior oblique tendon fibers are tightened, inducing incyclotortion without significantly affecting posterior tendon functions of abduction and depression. The Harada-Ito procedure may be performed using either a disinsertion technique or a non-disinsertion technique (Fig. 53–47). In the disinsertion technique, the superior oblique muscle is isolated as described above for the tucking procedure. The muscle is then split along its length, isolating the anterior 4 mm of the tendon, the fibers responsible for cyclotortion. These fibers are secured on a 6-0 Vicryl suture in the fashion described for recession of a muscle. After the muscle is firmly secured on the suture, the anterior fibers are disinserted from the insertion using Wescott scissors. The suture needles are then passed at a location along the superior border of the lateral rectus muscle 8 mm posterior to the insertion. The suture may be tied securely at this point, or the sutures left long in the adjustable suture fashion, and the suture adjusted postoperatively. It is possible to assess the degree of induced intortion by viewing the change in the fundus using the indirect ophthalmoscopy intraoperatively. In the classic Harada-Ito procedure, the muscle fibers are isolated as described above, but rather than transecting the oblique muscle fibers from the point of insertion, a 5-0 Mersiline suture is placed around the isolated anterior muscle fibers, and then the needle is placed at the location 8 mm posterior to the insertion of the lateral rectus muscle along its superior border. The sutures are drawn up securely, tightening the anterior fibers and inducing encyclotortion as in the disinsertion technique. Again, intraoperative adjustment can be performed using the Guyton technique, or postoperative adjustment can be used using adjustable suture technique.

Superior Oblique Muscle Weakening

Superior oblique weakening procedures are most commonly indicated in the treatment of Brown's syndrome, which is characterized by an inability to elevate the eye in adduction or for the treatment of superior oblique overaction. Brown's syndrome is best treated by ipsilateral superior oblique tenotomy, with consideration of a concurrent inferior oblique myectomy to prevent secondary hypertropia. Other techniques for superior oblique weakening include posterior 7/8 tenotomy and tenotomy with silicon expander as described by Wright.

In superior oblique tenotomy, the superior oblique tendon is approached from the temporal aspect. A muscle hook is used to isolate the superior rectus muscle, and then additional muscle hooks and Desmarres retractors are used to retract the conjunctiva nasally to expose the superior oblique tendon in its fascial sheath. Once the tendon has been directly identified, a small incision can be made in the fascial sheath, and then a small muscle hook can be used to isolate the superior oblique tendon (Fig. 53–48). Two Stevens hooks are placed around the superior oblique tendon and spread apart to allow a full-thickness tenotomy to be performed. The location of the tenotomy will determine the degree of weakening. The closer the tenotomy is performed to the trochlea, the greater the effect of muscle weakening.

One complication of complete tenotomy of the superior oblique muscle is induction of superior oblique palsy with resultant hypertropia.[38] Wright has described a technique to prevent complete palsy of the superior oblique tendon. In this procedure, a silicone expander is placed between the two cut ends of the superior oblique tendon (Fig. 53–49). This allows a graded weakening procedure of the superior oblique tendon to be performed.[39,40]

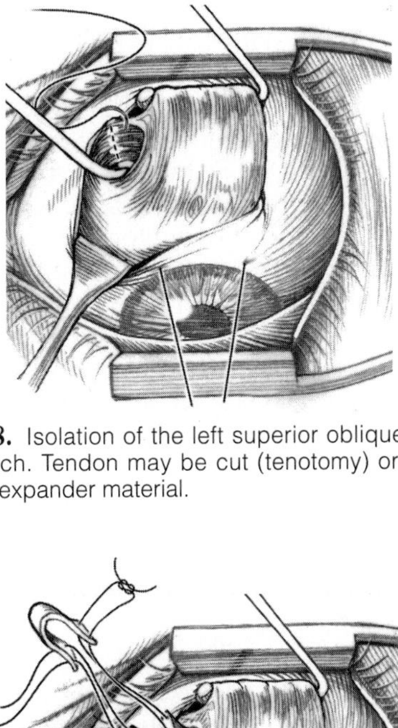

Figure 53–48. Isolation of the left superior oblique tendon from nasal approach. Tendon may be cut (tenotomy) or prepared for placement of expander material.

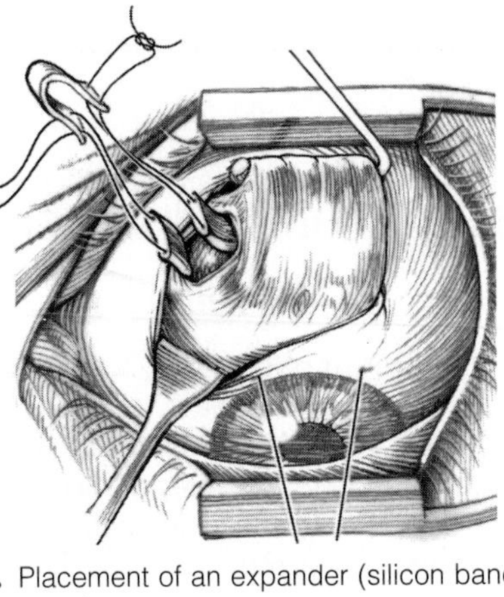

Figure 53–49. Placement of an expander (silicon band) in the left superior oblique tendon.

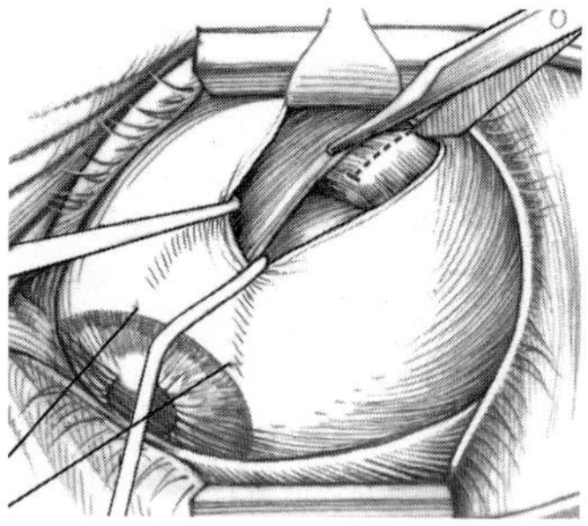

Figure 53–50. Posterior 7/8 in tenotomy of the left superior oblique tendon.

Two final weakening procedures should be mentioned. In the posterior 7/8 tenotomy, the posterior fibers are weakened selectively, sparing the anterior fibers (Fig. 53–50). This is a useful procedure that is performed when weakening of abduction in downgaze is desired but induced torsion is to be avoided. This is particularly useful in patients who are fusing, in whom the induction of torsion and resultant diplopia needs to be avoided. In this procedure, the superior oblique tendon is approached from the temporal aspect and the superior oblique muscle is identified along the temporal aspect of the superior rectus muscle. Using direct observation, the posterior 7/8 fibers are transected using the Wescott scissors, sparing the anterior 1/8 of the fibers. This selective weakening is useful to collapse A-patterns associated with superior oblique overaction. By preserving the anterior fibers, torsion is not induced.

The final procedure which has been described is recession of the superior oblique muscle.[41] The muscle is isolated in the standard fashion, and a Vicryl suture is placed through the muscle in its insertion. The muscle is then transected and allowed to recess along its pathway. Recessions can be graded depending on the degree of superior oblique overaction.

Complications of superior oblique surgery include misidentification of the muscles, leading to inadvertent transection of the superior rectus muscle. Temporal approaches to the superior oblique tendon make this complication highly unlikely. Additional complications include fat adherence syndrome due to prolapse of orbital fat after an extensive posterior dissection. Induced Brown's syndrome will occur in strengthening procedures. The patient should be forewarned of limitation of elevation of the eye.

THE INFERIOR OBLIQUE MUSCLE

Inferior Oblique Recession

Although the inferior oblique muscle may be recessed, myectomized,[42] denervated and extirpated,[43] or anteriorized,[44] inferior oblique recession and myectomy are the most common procedures performed.[45–47] Careful isolation of the muscle based on knowledge of the anatomy of the inferior oblique muscle is necessary if recession surgery is to be successful. Traction sutures of 6-0 silk are placed at the 6 o'clock position and in the temporal limbus (Fig. 53–51). The eye is then rotated into elevation and adduction (Fig. 53–51). Calipers are used to measure 8 mm from the limbus in the inferotemporal quadrant. When the eye is rotated, the inferior oblique muscle can be seen beneath the conjunctival surface as a pink elevated mass. At this location, 8 mm from the limbus, an incision is made through the conjunctiva and Tenon's capsule down to bare sclera. Care must be taken not to make this incision too far posteriorly, as an incision over the inferior oblique muscle will cause excessive bleeding. After the incision is made, it is extended 3 mm in circumferential fashion. Headlight illumination is useful in inferior oblique muscle surgery. With direct illumination and careful dissection, the inferior oblique muscle fibers can be seen and isolated on a small von Graefe muscle hook. Care should be taken to include all muscle fibers on this dissection. It is often necessary to pass several muscle hooks around the inferior oblique muscle to make certain that all fibers have been incorporated. Care should be taken to avoid excessive passes of the muscle hooks, as inadvertent disruption of posterior Tenon's can lead to prolapse of orbital fat and fat adherence syndrome. Also, the vortex vein is located near the inferior oblique muscle, and care must be taken not to transect it.

After the inferior oblique muscle is isolated on a von Graefe muscle hook, the inferior oblique muscle can be fully dissected. A muscle hook should be placed around the inferior rectus and lateral rectus muscles to

A

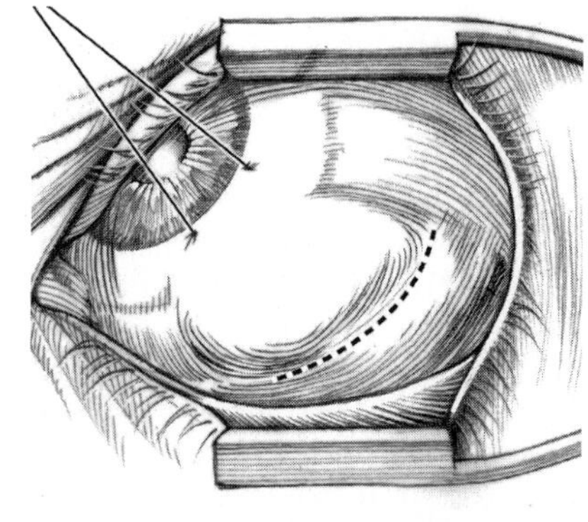

B

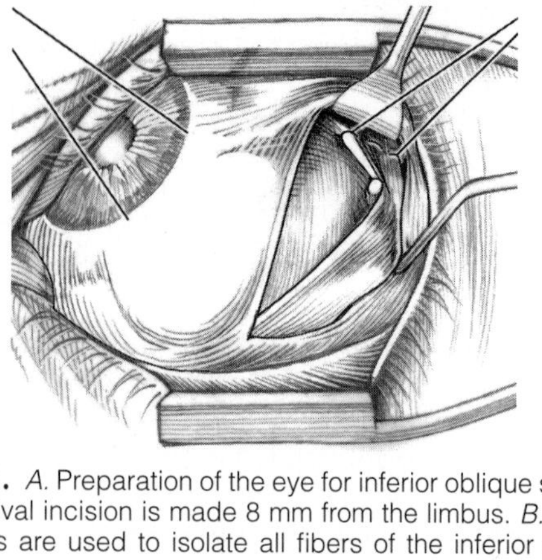

Figure 53–51. *A.* Preparation of the eye for inferior oblique surgery. The conjunctival incision is made 8 mm from the limbus. *B.* Graefe muscle hooks are used to isolate all fibers of the inferior oblique muscle. Direct visualization of the muscle will prevent inadvertent fat prolapse and missed fibers.

avoid inadvertent transection of either of them. The inferior oblique muscle is dissected using the Wescott scissors and forceps. If the inferior oblique muscle is to be recessed, a 6-0 double-armed Vicryl suture is interwoven through the muscle in a double-locking fashion as described for rectus muscle surgery. After the muscle is firmly secured in the suture, the muscle can be disinserted at its insertion posteriorly. Care should be taken to avoid dissection too close to the insertion of the inferior oblique muscle, as its insertion is near the macula, and ocular perforation at this point would be catastrophic. Some surgeons prefer to place a Jameson muscle clamp around the inferior oblique muscle, transect the muscle, and then imbricate the Vicryl suture through the muscle, after the muscle is safely removed from the sclera. After the Vicryl suture is imbricated through the inferior oblique muscle, the muscle can be recessed the desired amount. Recessions are generally classified as mild, moderate, and large, the amount of recession being determined by the location from the lateral edge of the inferior rectus muscle.

Inferior Oblique Myectomy

When an inferior oblique myectomy is to be performed, the inferior oblique muscle is isolated on two muscle hooks (Fig. 53–52). The muscle hooks are splayed apart 8 mm. At this point, straight hemostats are used to crush the muscle, after which the intervening 8 mm segment of muscle is transected and removed. Care must be taken to cauterize the cut ends of the muscles fully, as inadequate cautery will lead to bleeding. After the muscle is adequately cauterized, the hemostats are removed. The oblique muscle should be seen to quickly retract it into the orbit, indicating that all muscle fibers have been transected. If the muscle fibers do not retract briskly into the orbit, there should be a suspicion that there are additional muscle fibers that were not incorporated on the muscle hook prior to transection.

Anteriorization of the inferior oblique muscle is useful in cases of inferior oblique overaction and dissociated vertical deviation.[48,49] In inferior oblique anterior transposition, the inferior oblique muscle is isolated and imbricated on a double-armed 6-0 Vicryl suture. Rather than recessing the muscle 4 to 6 mm posterior to the insertion of the inferior rectus muscle, the inferior oblique muscle is reapproximated immediately adjacent to the lateral

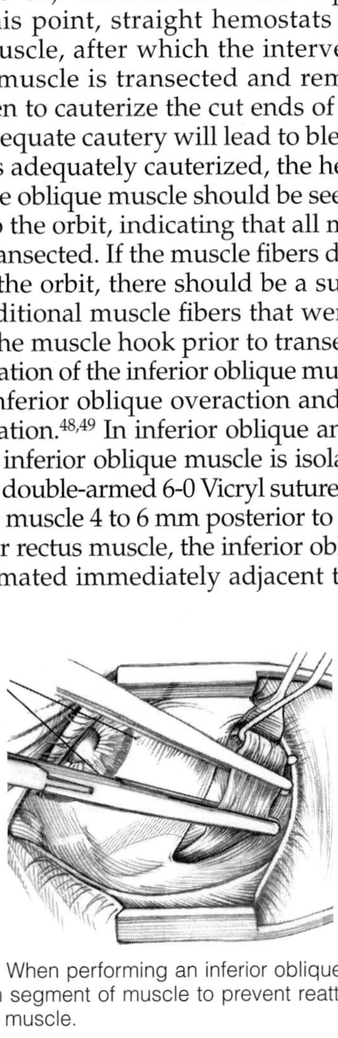

Figure 53–52. When performing an inferior oblique myectomy, remove an 8 mm segment of muscle to prevent reattachment of the cut ends of the muscle.

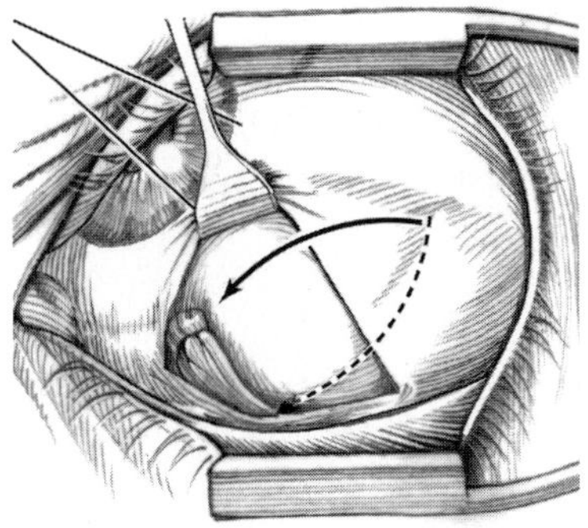

Figure 53–53. Anterior transposition of the left inferior oblique muscle. The insertion of the inferior oblique is placed immediately adjacent to the temporal border of the inferior rectus insertion.

border of the inferior rectus muscle. The insertion should be bunched up to prevent a deficiency of elevation in abduction (anti-elevation syndrome).[50] Anteriorization changes the mechanical action of the inferior oblique muscle from an elevator to a depressor (Fig. 53–53).

Inferior Oblique Myectomy/Nasal Approach

One final procedure involving the inferior oblique muscle is inferior oblique myectomy using a nasal approach. This procedure was described by Stager and is useful in cases of inferior oblique overaction in the presence of a previously recessed or anteriorized inferior oblique muscle. The inferior oblique muscle is approached nasally rather than temporally. An incision is made in the conjunctival nasal to the inferior rectus muscle. The inferior rectus muscle is isolated on a muscle hook, and the inferior oblique muscle is isolated as it crosses inferior to the inferior rectus insertion. The inferior oblique muscle is isolated by direct visualization and isolated on muscle hooks. The capsule of the inferior oblique muscle is transected and dissected toward its insertion on the nasal inferior orbital rim. The inferior oblique muscle is transected at this point. This leaves the inferior oblique muscle suspended at the posterior orbital apex by its neurovascular bundle. This changes the vector forces of the inferior oblique muscle from an abductor and elevator to a depressor.

Complications unique to inferior oblique muscle surgery include fat prolapse secondary to perforation of the posterior Tenon's capsule, significant hemorrhage from disruption of the vortex veins, and internal ophthalmoplegia as the result of traction on the pupillary oculomotor fibers.

MUSCLE TRANSPOSITION FOR RECTUS PALSY

Double Elevator Palsy

In double elevator palsy, there is an inability to elevate the eye, from weakness of the superior rectus muscle or from contraction of the inferior rectus muscle.

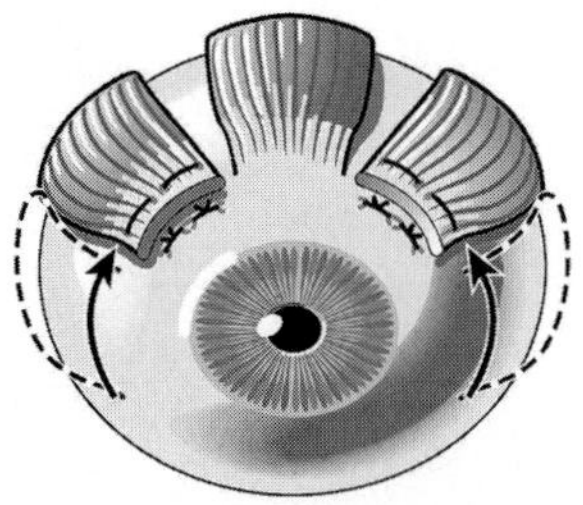

Figure 53–54. The Knapp procedure is used for double elevator palsy.

Forced duction testing should be performed to differentiate the cause. If forced duction testing reveals a restriction of elevation and tight inferior rectus, a large inferior rectus recession should be performed with conjunctival resection. If there is no restriction, then a Knapp procedure should be performed (Fig. 53–54). In this procedure, a full tendon transfer of the lateral and medial rectus muscle is performed at the insertion of the superior rectus muscle.[51] It is important to perform a large posterior dissection of the intermuscular septum and fascial attachments to allow mobilization of these muscles to give maximum elevating capacity to the horizontal rectus muscles. It is also important to maintain the muscle insertions of the transposed medial and lateral rectus muscles so that they follow the spiral of Tillaux and thereby avoid inducing vertical deviations.

Lateral Rectus Palsy

Operative Procedures

When a sixth cranial nerve palsy is complete and shows no sign of spontaneous resolution, a transposition procedure will be required to develop abducting forces. Procedures may be full tendon transfers or split tendon procedures. In the Jensen procedure, the inferior and superior rectus muscles are isolated, as well as the lateral rectus muscle. Dissection is carried out 14 mm posterior to the insertion, and all intermuscular septum and fascial attachments are dissected away from the muscles until they are exposed (Fig. 53–55). The muscles are then split one-half tendon width by separating two small Stevens muscle hooks. This split is made 14 mm posterior to the insertion. Care is taken not to traumatize the anterior ciliary arteries. After the inferior, superior, and lateral rectus muscles have been split, a 5-0 Mersiline suture is placed between the adjacent muscle halves, and the sutures are tied together relatively loosely to avoid anterior ciliary artery strangulation.

In the Hummelsheim procedure, the muscles are split as described in the Jensen procedure, along the superior and inferior rectus, but the lateral rectus muscle is not split.[52] The lateral halves of the inferior and superior rectus muscles are isolated on Vicryl sutures, transected from the globe, and transposed to the insertion of the lateral rectus muscle.

For maximum abduction effect, a full tendon transfer is advocated. Here, the superior inferior rectus muscles are isolated in the standard fashion on absorbable Vicryl sutures, disinserted from the globe, and transposed to the lateral rectus muscle insertion. In a modification of this procedure, a full tendon transfer as described by Foster,[53] additional nonabsorbable posterior fixation sutures are placed 8 to 10 mm posterior, along the inferior border of the superior rectus muscle and the superior border of the inferior rectus muscle, and attached to the sclera at this posterior site (Fig. 53–56). Placement of these posterior fixation sutures changes the vector forces on the vertical muscles and gives them more horizontal abducting effect. Transposition procedures often require a concurrent weakening procedure of the medial rectus muscle. Because the risk of anterior segment ischemia is high when three muscles are operated on concurrently, muscle procedures should be performed in a staged fashion, or botulinum toxin should be injected into the medial rectus muscle to avoid compromise of the ciliary circulation.

Anterior segment ischemia has been reported in every transposition procedure. McKeown has described a procedure in which the ciliary vessels are spared, and anterior segment ischemia is avoided.[54]

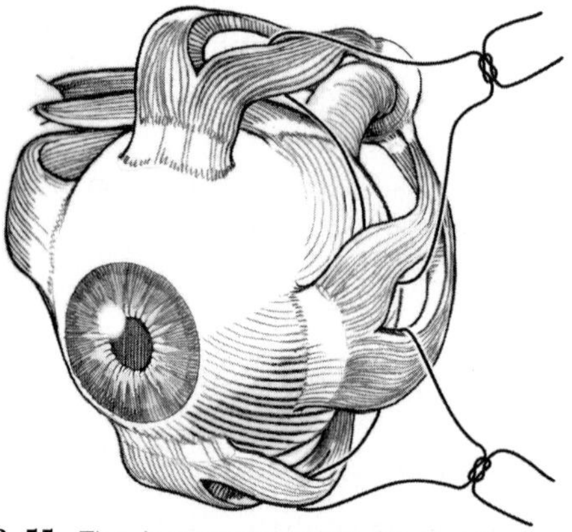

Figure 53–55. The Jensen procedure for abducens palsy. The muscles are split and the muscle bellies joined using nonabsorbable suture.

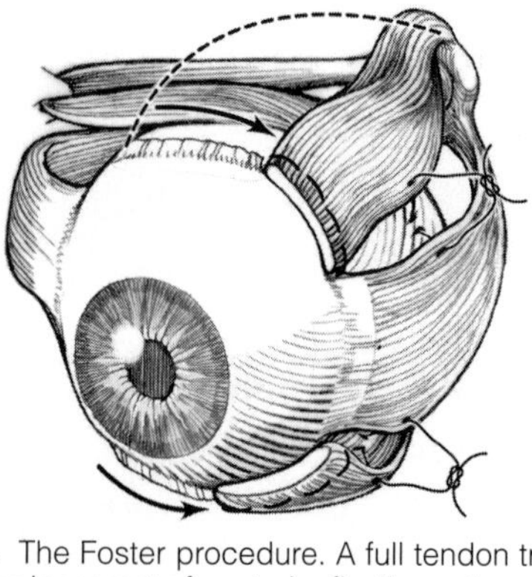

Figure 53–56. The Foster procedure. A full tendon transposition is augmented by placement of posterior fixation sutures.

ADJUSTABLE SUTURE TECHNIQUE

In adult patients and cooperative children, it is possible to perform postoperative adjustment of extraocular muscles using the adjustable suture technique.[55] This technique is most useful in cases of reoperation, complicated strabismus, large-angle strabismus, and thyroid myopathy. In these cases the predicted results are less reliable and unexpected results can be minimized postoperatively with the adjustable suture technique. Some patients cannot tolerate this procedure. To determine whether a patient may be a suitable candidate, it is recommended to perform the cotton tip applicator test preoperatively. In this test the patient's eye is anesthetized and a cotton-tipped applicator is used to touch and manipulate the conjunctiva. A patient who can tolerate this manipulation without significant eyelid squeezing or discomfort, should be able to handle the postoperative suture adjustment.

Adjustable suture technique can be performed under general anesthesia or local anesthesia. If local anesthesia is used, a short-acting anesthetic, such as 1% or 2% lidocaine should be used. Suture adjustment should be performed 5 to 6 hours postoperatively or the day after surgery, when it is certain that all local anesthetic has worn off. With general anesthesia adjustment can be performed shortly after awakening. It is important to avoid the use of narcotics in the postoperative or intraoperative period as this will interfere with a patient's cognition, and decrease the reliability of the patient's responses postoperatively. A technique of interoperative adjustment has been described: The patient is aroused during the procedure and measurements are taken. Then anesthesia is reinduced using Propofol, and the suture adjustment performed.

Most postoperative adjustment is made in the afternoon of the day of surgery or the following morning. Although it is possible to adjust a muscle 2 or 3 days postoperatively, healing often occurs rapidly, and the adjustment may be difficult.

Adjustment can be made in the examining room using clean surgical technique. It is helpful to have a suture adjustment tray, which contains Wescott scissors, two needle holders, Castroviejo forceps, and 6-0 plain gut suture. It is important to have the patient remove the eye patch and be allowed to use the eyes with full optical correction for 10 to 15 minutes prior to adjusting a suture. All eyes will demonstrate postoperative drift, even after adjustment, and for this reason small overcorrections are usually the desired result. Patients with exotropia are generally left 6 to 10 prism diopters esotropic to allow for postoperative drift. The eyes of patients with esotropia and amblyopic eyes should be left straight.

The Procedure

It is possible to perform the adjustable suture technique from either a limbal or a fornix-based approach. Muscle isolation and identification is performed in the standard fashion. The muscle is imbricated on an double arm 6-0 Vicryl suture. In recession procedures the muscle is imbricated at its insertion in the standard fashion, whereas in resection procedures, the muscle is also imbricated with a single, double-armed Vicryl suture in the double-locking fashion. After the muscle has been either transected or disinserted from the globe, it is then reattached to the eye using the hangback technique. The "bow-tie" technique is advocated (Fig. 53–57). In this technique the needles from the Vicryl suture are passed through the original insertion site using long interscleral passes, with the tips and angle in a cross-swords fashion. A triple throw is placed on the suture. Calipers are used to measure the muscle insertion and determine the appropriate amount of recession. At this time a single bow-knot is placed on the triple throw, and the ends of the suture are left long. The ends of the sutures are then steri-stripped to the patient's cheek, and the eye is patched. Antibiotic solution is placed in the eyes prior to patching the eye, and ointments are avoided as this can lead to difficulty in suture manipulation during the adjustment phase.

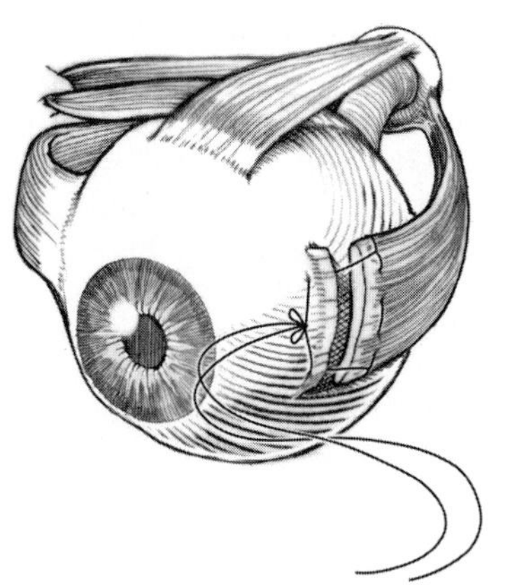

Figure 53–57. Adjustable suture technique using bow-knot over triple throw and leaving the suture ends long, steri-stripped to the cheek for later adjustment.

In resection procedures a similar method is employed. In general it is better to resect 1 or 2 mm more than planned and to leave the muscle recessed 1 to 2 mm. This will allow for additional advancement if necessary, or for relaxation of the muscle if it has been over-resected.

In general it is easier to pull a muscle up than it is to relax a muscle. To facilitate further recession of a muscle, preplacement of a 5-0 silk traction suture at the muscle insertion is useful. This traction suture can be used to pull on the eye if the patient cannot cooperate and move the eye during the adjustment phase.

During the adjustment phase the steri-strip is removed from the Vicryl suture, and ocular alignment is established. If the eyes are well aligned, the bow can simply be cut and the unattached end removed. Two additional single throws are then placed over the triple throw to secure the muscle in position. If the muscle needs to be recessed further, the bow is pulled free, the triple throw is relaxed, the muscle is allowed to recess back, and the measurement is reconfirmed. Once the eye is orthotopic or in the desired position, the muscle is tied securely with three single throws placed over the triple throw. Similarly, if the muscle needs to be advanced, the suture is simply pulled up before it is cinched tight. After the muscle is firmly secured, the conjunctiva can be reapproximated over the suture knot with 6-0 plain gut suture. This suture can be preplaced at the time of original surgery, or it can be added after suture adjustment.

There are a few complications associated with the adjustable suture technique. Because a suture knot is often left exposed and incompletely closed or covered by conjunctiva, small granulomas often form at the site of the Vicryl suture. These granulomas respond well to topical corticosteroids and rarely require surgical intervention. It is not uncommon for patients to feel faint and have vagal reactions during suture adjustment. The physician should be prepared to allow the patient to lie supine during the course of the adjustment. In addition, patients should be monitored during that adjustment phase to make certain they do not become hypertensive or develop cardiac irregularities.

SURGICAL DECISIONS

INFANTILE ESOTROPIA

Esotropia occurring in a child younger than six months of age is defined as *infantile esotropia*.[56] Its features include a large angle of deviation, dissociated vertical deviation, inferior oblique overaction, cross fixation, and low hyperopic refractive error. This form of esotropia usually requires surgical correction.[57] However, cases of spontaneous resolution have been described. The timing of surgical correction is controversial.[58–60] Some authors have advocated early surgery to stimulate fusional centers.[61] Others have recommended deferring surgery for 1 to 2 years, until stability of measurement is obtained and association of oblique dysfunction identified.[62,63] If patients have greater than 1.5 diopters of refractive error, spectacles should be tried. If there is no improvement with spectacles, surgery should be undertaken. The amblyopia must be reversed prior to strabismus surgery. In a child who alternates fixation equally, a bimedial recession is the preferred mode of therapy. When the deviation is greater than 45 prism diopters, it is often necessary to perform lateral rectus muscle resection at the time of bimedial recession. Parents must be cautioned that there is a 30% to 40% chance that additional surgery will be required later in life for recurrent esotropia or vertical deviations.[64]

ACCOMMODATIVE ESOTROPIA

Esotropia associated with hyperopic refractive errors is accommodative esotropia.[65,66] When the spectacles align the eyes no surgery is indicated. Patients who have strabismus surgery performed to align the eyes and eliminate the need for glasses will often develop consecutive exodeviations later in life. If a patient is only partially corrected with spectacle therapy, it is important to measure AC/A ratio to make certain that the patient does not have a high AC/A ratio with residual esotropia at near fixation.[67] High AC/A ratio should be treated with either phospholine iodide or bifocal therapy. Only in those cases in which the residual esodeviation measurement is greater than 8 prism diopters at either distance or near should undergo bimedial recession to align the eyes. Only the degree of esotropia not corrected with spectacles should be corrected surgically.[68] Patients with amblyopia and a constant esotropia that does not alternate may have a recession resection procedure performed.

DIVERGENCE PARALYSIS

Divergence paralysis usually presents in an elderly patient as esotropia at distance with orthotropia at near. This most likely represents bilateral incomplete sixth cranial nerve paresis. For small deviations, prism therapy is the best treatment. Deviations measuring greater than 10 to 15 prism diopters can be treated with bilateral lateral rectus resections.

A-PATTERN ESOTROPIAS

Treatment of horizontal deviations associated with vertical patterns involve two steps. First, the appropriate horizontal muscle surgery should be performed to eliminate the deviation in the primary position. Second, the pattern must be collapsed, either by transposition of the horizontal rectus muscles or by weakening of the overacting oblique muscles. If the oblique muscles are overacting, they must be weakened or the pattern will not be collapsed by transposition of the horizontal rectus muscles. Only if there is no oblique muscle dysfunction should transposition of the horizontal rectus muscles be contemplated. Patients with A-patterns often have overaction of the superior oblique muscles. Weakening of the superior oblique muscles should be contemplated only in patients who have significant superior oblique overaction, and it should be used carefully to avoid induced torsion in patients who are able to fuse.[69] An ideal operation to weaken the muscle without causing significant torsion is the posterior 7/8 tenotomy. This maintains the anterior fibers, which are important in cyclotortion function. Patients with A-pattern esotropias should have a bimedial recession accompanied by superior oblique muscle weakening. If there is no superior oblique muscle dysfunction, the bimedial recession could be accompanied by superior transposition of the medial rectus muscles one tendon width.

V-PATTERN ESOTROPIA

V-pattern esotropia is usually associated with inferior oblique overaction. As with A-patterns, the goal is to treat the horizontal deviation and collapse the vertical incomitancy. V-pattern esotropia should be treated by bimedial recession. If there is overaction of the inferior oblique muscles, a bilateral inferior oblique weakening procedure should be performed. If there is not inferior oblique overaction, then inferior transposition of the medial rectus one tendon width should be performed at the time of recession of the muscle.

NYSTAGMUS BLOCKAGE SYNDROME—CIANCIA'S SYNDROME

Nystagmus blockage syndrome is characterized by large-angle infantile esotropia with significant nystagmus on attempted abduction. Treatment includes large bimedial recession with consideration of posterior fixation suture of the medial rectus muscle.

DIVERGENCE EXCESS EXOTROPIA

Exotropia worse at distance than near is best treated with a bilateral lateral rectus recession, though some surgeons recommend a unilateral recession/resection procedure.[70–77] The adjustable suture technique should be used in adults. Postoperative overcorrection is desired, as the eye tends to deviate outward after the initial correction.

CONSTANT EXOTROPIA

Patients with constant exotropia with one dominant eye can be treated with a recession/resection procedure of the exotropic eye. The procedure is also useful for patients with amblyopia associated with exotropia.[78,79]

SIXTH CRANIAL NERVE PALSY

Acute cranial nerve six palsies must be investigated to determine their cause.[80–82] Traumatic sixth cranial nerve palsies can often be treated with botulinum toxin injected into the medial rectus muscle to prevent medial rectus contraction and to allow increased field of single binocular vision.[83] If function does not fully return and patients are left with a partial paresis, recession/resection procedures can be performed to provide alignment of the eye. If a patient is left with a complete cranial nerve six palsy, a transposition procedure is necessary.[84–86] Transposition procedures may involve muscle splitting or full tendon transfer. Care should be taken to limit muscle surgery to only two extraocular muscles to avoid anterior segment ischemia. Our preferred mode of therapy is an augmented full tendon transfer as described by Foster (Fig. 53–56). The superior and inferior rectus muscles are transposed to the lateral rectus muscle insertion, and are function augmented by the placement of a posterior fixation suture. Botulinum toxin is injected into the medial rectus muscle at the time of surgery.

THIRD CRANIAL NERVE PALSY

Third cranial nerve palsies are often accompanied by ptosis, which must be corrected before any attempt is made to straighten the eye.[87–89] Even with surgical intervention, prognosis is poor, and diplopia free fields are often limited after treatment for a third cranial nerve palsy.[90] Therapies include large recession/resection procedures accompanied by transposition of the superior oblique muscle to the medial rectus muscle.

FOURTH CRANIAL NERVE PALSY

Unilateral fourth cranial nerve palsies with hypertropia less than 10 prism diopters should be treated by ipsilateral inferior oblique myectomies.[91] Larger deviations often require recession of the contralateral inferior rectus muscle in addition to inferior oblique myectomy. If forced duction testing at the time of surgery reveals a contracture of the superior rectus muscle on the side of the hypertropic eye, this muscle may need to be recessed using adjustable suture technique. Patients with significant underaction of the superior oblique muscle and those with significant torsion in acquired fourth cranial nerve palsies may require strengthening of the superior oblique muscle.[92] This can be performed by tucking of the superior oblique muscle. When only torsion is the significant complaint, torsional surgery such as the Harada-Ito procedure is recommended.

RESTRICTIVE STRABISMUS

Duane's Syndrome

Most cases of Duane's syndrome do not require surgical treatment, as they produce only a minimal face turn to allow binocular vision without diplopia.[93–96] There are, however, three conditions that require surgical treatment: development of a large associated esotropia, significant upshoots or downshoots, and significant enophthalmos caused by retraction.[97] Esotropia can be treated using recession of the restricted medial rectus muscle on the involved side. The transposition procedure as described by Foster has also been used for treatment of Duane's syndrome with significant face turn associated with esotropia. The upshoots or downshoots are best treated by placement of a posterior fixation suture on the lateral rectus muscle.[98–100] Finally, significant enophthalmos can be treated by recession of both the medial rectus muscle and the lateral rectus muscle performed concurrently.[101]

Double Elevator Palsy

Inability to elevate one eye is described as a *double elevator palsy.* This may be due to elevational weakness of the eye or to restriction of the inferior rectus muscles.[102,103] Only by performing forced duction at the time of surgical repair can the differentiation be made.[104] When forced duction testing reveals significant restriction, the inferior rectus muscle should be maximally recessed, with recession of the conjunctiva performed concurrently. If there is no significant restriction, the Knapp procedure should be performed, transposing the horizontal rectus muscles superiorly to the superior rectus, thereby increasing the elevating ability of the eye. It is often necessary to recess the contralateral superior rectus muscle to match the deficit of the eye that does not elevate well.

Superior Oblique Tendon Sheath Syndrome—Brown's Syndrome

Only when there is a significant hypotropia of the involved eye should surgical therapy be undertaken. Treatment involves superior oblique tenotomy,[105–108] which can be performed either by free tenotomy, introduction of a spacer within the superior oblique tendon, or tenotomy associated with concurrent inferior oblique weakening procedure.[109–112]

Dissociated Vertical Deviation

Dissociated vertical deviation is most commonly seen in patients with a history of infantile esotropia. When dissociated vertical deviation occurs in the presence of overaction of the inferior oblique muscles, inferior oblique anterior transposition is the desired procedure.[113–116] If there is no inferior oblique overaction or if the inferior oblique muscle has already been recessed or weakened, large recessions of the superior rectus muscle should be performed.[117–119]

INTRAOPERATIVE COMPLICATIONS

Intraoperative complications include anesthetic complications such as malignant hyperthermia, which is most common in children undergoing strabismus surgery, and ocular cardiac reflex with dysrhythmias. Children undergoing strabismus surgery should have a temperature probe in place, and the anesthesiologist should be aware of the high risk of malignant hyperthermia in patients with strabismus. Prompt recognition and intervention will prevent disastrous consequences. Both the surgeon and the anesthesiologist should be aware of the ocular cardiac reflex, and the presence of a slowed heart rate should cause the surgeon to stop pulling on the muscle until the heart rate has resumed normal.[120] Intravenous atropine or glycopyrrolate will prevent the ocular cardiac reflex.

ANATOMIC VARIATIONS

The superior oblique muscle is most commonly seen in abnormal positions with abnormal laxity. Patients with cranial facial disorders often have abnormal extraocular muscles, and absence of the superior rectus muscles has been well described. Muscle insertions are often found in slightly abnormal places, and occasional adhesions may cause restrictive strabismus or paresis.

LOST EXTRAOCULAR MUSCLES

Extraocular muscles can be lost during strabismus surgery, especially during resection procedures. When a muscle is not adequately secured on the suture, it may pull away from the suture prior to its reinsertion into the sclera. The muscle will quickly retract into the orbit. The strabismus surgeon should always have a muscle clamp or hemostat at hand so that if the muscle begins to pull away from the suture, a clamp can be placed around the muscle to prevent it from slipping and retracting into the orbit. If a muscle does retract into the orbit the surgeon should proceed in a deliberate and calm fashion.[121] A headlight should be worn for maximum visibility, and balanced saline solution should be used for delineation of tissue planes. If a small conjunctival incision had been made, it should be enlarged to provide maximum exposure. Traction sutures should be placed through either the limbus or the muscle stump, and the eye rotated away from the lost muscle. It is important to remember the anatomic pathways of the extraocular muscles, and to remember that the muscles travel within collagenous muscle sleeves, and penetrate Tenon's capsule. Balanced saline solution should be applied frequently; it causes Tenon's capsule and connective tissue to appear white, whereas muscle tendon and fiber will remain pink. Smooth forceps should be used so that Tenon's capsule is not inadvertently ripped, allowing fat prolapse. If fat prolapse does occur it will lead to restrictive strabismus. Once adequate light, magnification, and exposure have been obtained, and the use of Desmarres retractors is available, the quadrant should be inspected carefully. Very often it is possible to see the perforation in Tenon's capsule through which the muscle has passed. With smooth forceps picking up the edge of this perforation in Tenon's capsule will usually reveal the cut end of muscle fiber. Remember that the muscle passes toward the orbital apex and does not follow the edge of the globe closely. Once the muscle has been identified, it can be grasped with a fine-tooth forceps and pulled gently. If atropine has not previously been given to the patient, the ocular cardiac reflex will confirm the presence of muscle tissue.[122] If the muscle has not been paralyzed by anesthetic agents, then a muscle stimulator can be used to see if there is contraction in the isolated tissue. Very often it is possible to isolate a muscle by tracing its intermuscular septum from the adjacent rectus muscles. If the muscle can be isolated and identified it should be imbricated on a 6-0 Vicryl suture and reattached to the globe. If it is not possible to identify the muscle, the most prudent course is to stop the case, consult with a strabismus surgeon who has a large degree of experience in locating lost muscles, and refer the patient promptly for re-exploration and isolation of the extraocular muscle.

BLEEDING

Bleeding can result from insufficient cautery or lack of ligation of vessels at the time of imbrication on muscle sutures. It also may result from transection of vortex veins. Bleeding can be controlled by the use of handheld or wetfield cautery. Bleeding is to be avoided because excessive bleeding can lead to heavy scarring and restrictive strabismus.

Scleral Perforation

Scleral perforation is more common in cases that involve posterior fixation sutures, in patients with high myopia and thin sclera, and in patients with previous strabismus surgery or other ocular surgeries.[23,123–125] If perforation is suspected, the pupil should immediately be dilated and the retina inspected at the time of surgery.[126] If no retinal hemorrhage is seen no treatment is necessary. The presence of a retinal hole should be treated with either cryotherapy or laser therapy applied by the indirect ophthalmoscope. Retinal detachment should be evaluated by a vitreoretinal surgeon and treated appropriately. Patients with documented perforation at the time of strabismus surgery should be placed on oral antibiotics, and periocular antibiotics should be instilled at the time of closure of the conjunctiva.

OPERATION ON THE WRONG MUSCLE

Surgery on the wrong muscle results from misidentification at the time of surgery. If the error is recognized at the time of surgery, the muscle can be replaced at its original insertion, and the planned procedure can be performed. If the error is discovered postoperatively, the patient should be fully informed of the complication, and reoperation performed as soon as possible to prevent contracture.

POSTOPERATIVE PROBLEMS

INFECTION

Infections are rare after strabismus surgery, they occur in less than 1 in 1,500 patients. Patients with infection will present with conjunctival injection and pain. It is important to treat infections promptly as a panophthalmitis can result from an extraocular infection. Cultures should be taken, and patients should be tested for sensitivity of conjunctival swabs, placed on a broad-spectrum antibiotic, and followed closely. If the patient does not respond promptly hospitalization will be necessary for intravenous therapy to prevent endophthalmitis.

SLIPPED OR LOST EXTRAOCULAR MUSCLE

Muscle slippage usually occurs within the first 24 to 48 hours after surgery, but it can occur as late as 2 to 3 weeks postoperatively.[127,128] The result is overcorrection leaving the patient unable to perform ductions in the affected field of gaze of the operated muscle. The presence of a slipped muscle requires reoperation to identify the lost extraocular muscle and reapproximate it securely to the sclera.

ANTERIOR SEGMENT ISCHEMIA

Anterior segment ischemia is more common in older patients, and is more likely after muscle surgery involving three or more extraocular muscles.[129,130] It has been described in patients with operation on two of the extraocular muscles, and it is more common when two adjacent muscles are treated.[131] Patients will present with intraocular inflammation, pain, and redness. Treatment involves topical and systemic corticosteroid therapy.

OVERCORRECTION AND UNDERCORRECTION

Overcorrection and undercorrection can be seen in 5% of postoperative strabismus patients, and require treatment with occlusion, spectacles, patching therapy, prism therapy, or orthoptic exercises. Most overcorrections or undercorrections can be treated by conservative therapy, but if a significant deviation persists the patient will need to undergo reoperation. The patient should be told of this possibility before the initial muscle surgery.

POSTOPERATIVE CARE

Children undergoing bilateral surgery should not receive bilateral patches. Topical antibiotic ointment should be placed in the eyes and used twice per day for two weeks. Adult patients also have antibiotic placed in the eyes at the time of discharge, but go on to use topical antibiotic solutions postoperatively. Patches are required only to prevent the patient from inadvertently pulling on an adjustable suture. Patients should be instructed not to eat for several hours postoperatively, because nausea is the most common complication. Antibiotic steroid solution should be used 3 times per day for 2 weeks. The patient should be seen within 5 days postoperatively, and within 1 to 2 weeks after the first postoperative visit. They should be instructed not to swim for two weeks' time. Patients are followed closely to make certain they do not develop infection, dellen formation, or recurrent strabismus.

CHEMODENERVATION THERAPY

Chemodenervation therapy using type A botulinum toxin (Botox, Allergan) was first described by Scott and coworkers in the 1980s.[132] Botulimun toxin binds to nerve terminals and prevents release of acetylcholine, inducing denervation paralysis. The paralysis lasts from 4 weeks to several months in a dose-dependent fashion. The mechanism of Botox is due to internal sarcomere reorganization with resultant changes in the length of the muscles that have been paralyzed.

Botulinum toxin injection has been used or attempted in almost every strabismus situation where weakening of a muscle is indicated. Its greatest utility is in treatment of paralytic strabismus, childhood strabismus, and strabismus following previous ocular surgery. The chief advantage of this technique is that it can be to performed in an outpatient setting with topical anesthesia. The disadvantage is its inherent decreased predictability and lower correction rate compared to incisional surgery. It is most successful when correcting small deviations; large-angle deviations often require multiple repeated injections. It has been estimated that there is a 30% to 40% chance that one botulinum injection will correct deviation to 10 prism diopters or less.[133]

One commonly encountered situation in which botulinum toxin can be used is in acute sixth nerve palsy. If there is no sign of spontaneous recovery within one month of onset, injection of botulinum toxin into the medial rectus muscle can eliminate diplopia and face turn. In ischemic sixth nerve palsies, botulinum toxin had no long-term effect on spontaneous recovery compared to a control group in which the patients achieved single binocular vision and reduced abnormal head turn and diplopia earlier than would have been achieved otherwise.[134] In cases of traumatic sixth nerve palsy, when spontaneous recovery may be delayed or prolonged, injection of the medial rectus muscle with botulinum toxin will prevent contracture of the muscle and may decrease the requirement for extraocular muscle surgery in the future. When sixth nerve paralysis is permanent and complete, botulinum toxin is useful as an adjunct to the surgical management of this large-angle esotropia. Full tendon transposition of the superior inferior rectus to the lateral rectus muscle provides the greatest degree of exo shift and results in the largest area of single binocular vision. Injection of the ipsilateral medial rectus muscle with botulinum toxin will decrease the risk of anterior segment ischemia and again prevents medial rectus contracture from occurring or may decrease the amount of contracture present at the time of strabismus surgery.

Infantile esotropia has been treated by simultaneous bimedial botulinum toxin injection with a success rate between 60% and 80%, with repeated injections usually being required.[134]

Acute acquired comitant esotropia, which is not due to a neurologic cause, has also been successfully treated with botulinum toxin A injection, which when performed early yielded a high degree of return of binocular function.[136]

Other indications for botulinum A injection include inferior rectus contracture following cataract surgery, following traditional incisional surgery when either undercorrection or overcorrection has resulted, and in large-angle deviation accompanied by poor vision when the patient would like to avoid incisional surgery but seeks to achieve a more aesthetically pleasing appearance.

When used in extraocular muscles, botulinum toxin should be injected either with guidance by any electromyographic control or by direct visualization. The patient should be informed of the risks of the procedure, including ocular perforation; partial ptosis which can occur in approximately 25% of cases; temporary overcorrection and subsequent diplopia lasting 1 to 2 months; and the need for possible reinjection or incisional surgery. Botulinum toxin A is a labile material and must be reconstituted with non-preserved saline and used within 2 hours of reconstitution. The amount of saline injected into the vial will determine the number of units per 0.1 ml, with a dosage ranging from 2.5 units to 10 units; most initial injections are 2.5 units. Injection is made using a specially-prepared Emg guided, Teflon-coated needle attached to an injection amplifier, which provides auditory feedback as the needle is placed into the extraocular muscle. Anesthesia includes topical proparacaine to anesthesize the conjunctiva with a cotton-tipped applicator applied over the injection site. After a ground lead has been placed to the patient's forehead, injection is made into the extraocular muscle entering the conjunctiva 10 mm posterior to the limbus and slowly advancing the needle into the extraocular muscle using the electromyographic auditory signal. When the signal is at its maximum, injection of the botulinum toxin is performed slowly, and the needle is left in place for 15 to 30 seconds so that the botulinum toxin does not flow back through the needle track. Children can be injected using either intravenous ketamine, nitrous oxide sedation, or physical restraint. All patients should have had their pupils dilated and the fundus inspected to make certain that inadvertent perforation did not occur. The patient is advised to not lie down for one hour after the procedure to prevent spread of the material to the levator muscle and thus decrease the risk of ptosis. Onset of paresis occurs within 48 to 72 hours and reaches a maximum within 5 days. The effect is quite variable, with paresis lasting from 4 weeks to 3 months. Full contractile force of the muscle will return, but reorganization of the sarcomeres will result in permanent realignment of the eye.

REFERENCES

1. Aurell E, Norkell K: A longitudinal study of children with a family history of strabismus. Factors determining the incidence of strabismus. Br J Ophthalmol 1990;74:589.
2. Mayer DL, Fulton AB, Rodier D: Grating and recognition activities in pediatric patients. Ophthalmology 1984;91:947.
3. Dell'Osso LF, Flynn JT: Congenital nystagmus surgery. A quantitative evaluation of the effects. Arch Ophthalmol 1979;97: 462–469.
4. Dell'Osso LF, Schmidt D, Daroff RB: Latent, manifest latent and congenital nystagmus. Arch Ophthalmol 1979;97:1877–1885.
5. Wright KW, Walonker F, Edelman P: 10-diopter fixation test for amblyopia. Arch Ophthalmol 1981;99:1242–1246.
6. Repka MX, Ray JM: The efficacy of optical and pharmacological penalization. Ophthalmology 1993;100:769–775.
7. Parks MM: Ocular Motility and Strabismus. Hagerstown, MD: Harper & Row, 1975; pp 1–12.
8. Guyton DL, Weingarten PE: Sensory torsion as the cause of primary oblique muscle overaction/underaction in A- and V-pattern strabismus. Binocular Vision Q 1994;9:211–235.
9. Knapp P: Vertically incomitant horizontal strabismus: The so-called "A" and "V" syndromes. Trans Am Ophthalmol Soc 1959; 57:666–699.
10. Magee AJ: Minimal values for the A and V syndromes. Am J Ophthalmol 1960;50:753–756.

11. Kushner BJ: The role of ocular torsion in the etiology of A and V patterns. J Pediatr Ophthalmol Strabismus 1985;22:171–179.
12. France TD: The association of A pattern strabismus with hydrocephalus. In Moore S, Mein J (eds.), Orthoptics: Past, Present and Future. New York: Grune & Stratton, 1976; pp 287–292.
13. Hardesty HH, Boynton JR, Keenan JP: Treatment of intermittent exotropia. Arch Ophthalmol 1978;96:268–274.
14. Hirschberg J: Uber die Messung des Schieldgerades und die Dosierung der Schieloperation. Zentralbl Prakt Augenheilkd 1885;8:325.
15. DeRespinis PA, Naidu E, Brodie SE: Calibration of Hirschberg test photography under clinical conditions. Ophthalmology 1989;96:944.
16. Rosenbaum AL, Bateman JB, Bremer DL, et al.: Cycloplegic refraction in esotropic children: Cyclopentolate versus atropine. Ophthalmology 1981;88:1031.
17. Hiles DA, Davies GT, Costenbader FD: Long term observations on unoperated intermittent exotropia. Arch Ophthalmol 1968;80:436–442.
18. Jampolsky A: Surgical leashes and reverse leashes in strabismus surgical management. In Symposium on Strabismus. Transactions of the New Orleans Academy of Ophthalmology. St. Louis: CV Mosby, 1978; pp 244–268.
19. Miller JM. Demer JL: Biomechanical analysis of strabismus. Binocular Vision Eye Muscle Surg Q 1992;7:233.
20. Demer JL, Miller JM, Koo EY, Rosenbaum AL: Quantitative magnetic resonance morphometry of extraocular muscles: A new diagnostic tool in paralytic strabismus. J Pediatr Ophthalmol Strabismus 1994;31:177–188.
21. Shin G, Demer JL, Rosenbaum AL: High resolution dynamic magnetic resonance imaging in complicated strabismus. J Pediatr Ophthalmol Strabismus 1996;33:282–290.
22. Parks MM: Rectus muscle surgery. In Parks MM (ed.), Atlas of Strabismus Surgery. Philadelphia: Harper & Row, 1983.
23. Nelson LB, Ervin-Mulvey LD, Calhoun JH, et al.: Surgical management for abnormal head position in nystagmus: The augmented modified Kestenbaum procedure. Br J Ophthalmol 1984;68:796–800.
24. Repka MX, Fishman PJ, Guyton DL: The site of reattachment of the extraocular muscle following hang-back recession. J Pediatr Ophthalmol Strabismus 1990;27:286–290.
25. Repka MX, Guyton DL: Comparison of hang-back, medical rectus recession with conventional recession. Ophthalmology 1988;95:782–787.
26. Metz HS, Schwartz L: The treatment of A and V patterns by monocular surgery. Arch Ophthalmol 1977;95:251–253.
27. Jampolsky A: Oblique muscle surgery of the A-V patterns. J Pediatr Ophthalmol 1965;2:31–36.
28. Helveston EM, Cofield DD: Indications for marginal myotomy and technique. Am J Ophthalmol 1970;70:574.
29. Cuppers C: The so-called "faden operation" (surgical correction by well-defined changes in the arc of contact). In Fells P (ed), Proceedings of the Second Congress of the International Strabismological Association, Marseilles, Diffusion Générale de Librairie, 1976; pp 395–400.
30. Harley RD: Surgical management of persistent diplopia in blowout fractures of the orbit. Am Ophthalmol 1975;7: 1621–1626.
31. Emery JM, von Noorden GK, Schlernitzauer DA: Orbital floor fractures: longterm follow-up of cases with and without surgical repair. Trans Am Acad Ophthalmol Otolaryngol 1971;75: 802–812.
32. Knapp P, Moore S: Diagnosis and surgical options in superior oblique surgery. Int Ophthalmol Clin 1976;16:137–149.
33. Knapp P: Classification and treatment of superior oblique palsy. Am Orthop J 1974;24:18–22.
34. Mitchell PR, Parks MM: Surgery for bilateral superior oblique palsy. Ophthalmology 1982;89:484–488.
35. Helveston EM: Classification of superior oblique muscle palsy. Ophthalmology 1992;99:1609–1615.
36. Pratt-Johnson JA, Tillson G: The investigation and management of torsion preventing fusion in bilateral superior oblique palsies. J Pediatr Ophthalmol Strabismus 1987;24:145–150.
37. Harada M, Ito Y: Visual corrections of cyclotropia. Jpn J Ophthalmol 1964;8:88.
38. Berke R: Tenotomy of superior oblique muscle for hypertropia. Arch Ophthalmol 1947;38:605–644.
39. Wright K: Superior oblique silicone expander for Brown syndrome and superior oblique overaction. J Pediatr Ophthalmol Strabismus 1991;28:101–107.
40. Wright KW, Min BM, Park C: Comparison of superior oblique tendon expander to superior oblique tenotomy for the management of superior oblique overaction and Brown syndrome. J Pediatr Ophthalmol Strabismus 1992;29:92–97.
41. Buckley EG, Flynn JP: Superior oblique recession versus tenotomy: A comparison of surgical results. J Pediatr Ophthalmol Strabismus 1983;20:112–117.
42. Davis G, McNeer KW, Spencer RF: Myectomy of the inferior oblique. Arch Ophthalmol 1986;104:855–858.
43. Del Monte MA, Parks MM: Denervation and extirpation of the inferior oblique: An improved weakening procedure for marked overaction. Ophthalmology 1983;90:1178–1183.
44. Stager DR, Weakley DR, Stager DR: Anterior transposition of the inferior oblique: Anatomic assessment of the neurovascular bundle. Arch Ophthalmol 1992;110:360–362.
45. Parks MM: Inferior oblique weakening procedures. Int Ophthalmol Clin 1985;25:107–117.
46. Parks MM: The weakening surgical procedures for eliminating overreaction of the inferior oblique muscle. Am J Ophthalmol 1972;73:107.
47. Stager DR, Parks MM: Inferior oblique weakening procedures. Effect on primary position horizontal alignment. Arch Ophthalmol 1973;90:15–16.
48. Bacal DA, Nelson LB: Anterior transposition of the inferior oblique muscle for both dissociated vertical deviation and/or inferior oblique overaction: Results of 94 procedures in 55 patients. Binocular Vision Eye Muscle Surg Q 1992;17:219–225.
49. Elliott RL, Nankin SJ: Anterior transposition of the inferior oblique. J Pediatr Ophthalmol Strabismus 1981;18:35–38.
50. Kushner BJ: Restriction of elevation in abduction after inferior oblique anteriorization. J Am Assoc Pediatr Ophthalmol Strabismus 1997;1:55.
51. Burke JP, Ruben JB, Scott WE: Vertical transposition of the horizontal recti (Knapp procedure) for the treatment of double elevator palsy: Effectiveness and long-term stability. Br J Ophthalmol 1992;76:734–737.
52. Helveston EM: Muscle transposition procedures. Surv Ophthalmol 1971;16:92–97.
53. Foster RS: Vertical muscle transposition augmented with lateral fixation. J AAPOS 1997;1:20–30.
54. McKeown CH, Shore JW, Lambert HM: Preservation of the anterior ciliary vessels during extraocular muscle surgery. Ophthalmology 1989;96:498.
55. Nelson LB, Wagner RS, Calhoun JH: The adjustable suture technique in strabismus surgery. Int Ophthalmol Clin 1985;25:4.
56. Costenbader FD: Infantile esotropia. Trans Am Ophthalmol Soc 1961;59:397–429.
57. Helveston EM, Ellis FD, Schott J, et al.: Surgical treatment of congenital esotropia. Am J Ophthalmol 1983;96:218–228.
58. Birch BB, Stager DR: Monocular acuity and stereopsis in infantile esotropia. Invest Ophthalmol Vis Sci 1985;26:1624–1630.
59. Parks MM: Early operations for strabismus. In Transactions of the First Congress of the International Strabismological Association, London, 1971; pp 29–36.
60. Von Noorden GK, Isaza A, Parks ME: Surgical treatment of congenital esotropia. Trans Am Acad Ophthalmol Otolaryngol 1972;76:1465–1478.
61. Charles SJ, Moore AT: Results of early surgery for infantile esotropia in normal and neurologically impaired infants. Eye 1992;6:603–606.
62. Friendly DS: Management of infantile esotropia. Int Ophthalmol Clin 1985;25:37–52.
63. Von Noorden GK: Current concepts of infantile esotropia. Eye 1988;2:343–357.
64. Good WV, deSa LCF, Lyons CF, Hoyt CS: Monocular visual outcome in untreated, early-onset esotropia. Br J Ophthalmol 1993; 77:492–495.
65. Baker JD, Parks MM: Early onset accommodative esotropia. Am J Ophthalmol 1980;90:11–18.
66. Parks MM: Management of acquired esotropia. Br J Ophthalmol 1974;58:240–247.

67. Breinin GM: Accommodative strabismus and the AC/A ratio. Am J Ophthalmol 1971;71:303.
68. Keenan JM, Willshaw HE: The outcome of strabismus surgery in childhood esotropia. Eye 1993;7:341–345.
69. Fierson WM, Boger WP III, Diorio PC, et al.: The effect of bilateral superior oblique tenotomy on horizontal deviation in A-pattern strabismus. J Pediatr Ophthalmol Strabismus 1980;17: 364–371.
70. Bielchowsky A: Divergence excess. Arch Ophthalmol 1934;12: 157–166.
71. Burian HM, Spivey BE: The surgical management of exodeviations. Am J Ophthalmol 1965;59:603–620.
72. Burian HM: Exodeviations: Their classification, diagnosis and treatment. Am J Ophthalmol 1966;62:1161.
73. Caltrider N, Jampolsky A: Overcorrecting minus lens therapy for treatment of intermittent exotropia. Ophthalmology 1983;90: 1160–1165.
74. Carlson MR, Jampolsky A: Lateral incomitancy in intermittent exotropia. Cause and surgical therapy. Arch Ophthalmol 1979; 97:1922–1925.
75. Cooper J, Medow N: Intermittent exotropia, basic and divergence excess type. Binoc Vis Eye Muscle Surg Q 1993;8(Suppl 3):185–216.
76. Freeman RS, Isenberg SJ: The use of part-time occlusion for early onset unilateral exotropia. J Pediatr Ophthalmol Strabismus 1989;26:94–96.
77. Jampolsky A: Management of Exodeviation. Transactions of the New Orleans Academy of Ophthalmology. New York: Raven, 1962; pp 140–156.
78. Cooper EL: The surgical management of secondary exotropia. Trans Am Acad Ophthalmol Otolaryngol 1961;65:595.
79. Rubin SE, Nelson LB, Wagner RS, et al.: Infantile exotropia in healthy children. Ophthalmic Surg 1988;19:792–794.
80. Ernest JT, Costenbader FD: Lateral rectus muscle palsy. Am J Ophthalmol 1968;65:721.
81. Robertson DM, Hines JD, Rucker CW: Acquired sixth nerve paresis in children. Arch Ophthalmol 1970;83:574.
82. Rush JA, Younge BR: Paralysis of cranial nerves III, IV and VI: Cause and prognosis in 1,000 cases. Arch Ophthalmol 1981;99: 76–79.
83. Fitzsimmons R, Lee JP, Elston J: Treatment of sixth nerve palsy in adults with combined botulinum toxin chemodenervation and surgery. Ophthalmology 1988;95:1535–1542.
84. Reinecke RD: Surgical management of third and sixth cranial nerve palsies. Int Ophthalmol Clin 1985;25:4.
85. Rosenbaum AL, Foster RS, Ballard E, et al.: Complete superior and inferior rectus transposition with adjustable medial rectus recession for abducens palsy. Strabismus 1984;2:599–605.
86. Rosenbaum AL, Kushner BJ, Kirschner D: Vertical rectus muscle transposition and botulinum (Oculinum) to medial rectus for abducens palsy. Arch Ophthalmol 1989;107:820–823.
87. Balkan R, Hoyt CS: Associated neurologic abnormalities in congenital third nerve palsies. Am J Ophthalmol 1984;97:315–319.
88. Good WV, Barkovich AJ, Nickel BL, Hoyt CS: Bilateral congenital oculomotor nerve palsy in a child with brain anomalies. Am J Ophthalmol 1991;111:555–558.
89. Gottlob I, Catalano RA, Reinecke RD: Surgical management of oculomotor nerve palsy. Am J Ophthalmol 1991;111:71–76.
90. Miller NR: Solitary oculomotor nerve palsy in childhood. Am J Ophthalmol 1977;83:106–111.
91. Ellis FD, Helveston EM: Superior oblique palsy: Diagnosis and classification. Int Ophthalmol Clin 1976;16:127–135.
92. Kraft SP, Scott WE: Masked bilateral superior oblique palsy: Clinical features and diagnosis. J Pediatr Ophthalmol Strabismus 1986;23:264–267.
93. Duane A: Congenital deficiency of abduction associated with impairment of adduction retraction movements, contraction of the palpebral fissure and oblique movements of the eye. Arch Ophthalmol 1905;34:133.
94. Elsas P: Occult Duane's syndrome: Co-contraction revealed following strabismus surgery. J Pediatr Ophthalmol Strabismus 1991;28:328–335.
95. Huber A: Duane's retraction syndrome: consideration of pathogenesis and aetiology of the different forms of Duane's retraction syndrome. In Hugonnier R, Hugonnier S (eds.), Strabismus, Heterophoria, Ocular Motor Paralysis: Clinical Ocular Muscle Imbalance. St. Louis: CV Mosby, 1969; 62.63, p 36.
96. Isenberg S, Urisi MJ: Clinical observations in 101 consecutive patients with Duane's syndrome. Am J Ophthalmol 1977;84: 419–424.
97. Kraft SP: A surgical approach for Duane's syndrome. J Pediatr Ophthalmol Strabismus 1988;25:119–130.
98. Molarte AB, Rosenbaum AL: Vertical rectus muscle transposition surgery for Duane's syndrome. J Pediatr Ophthalmol Strabismus 1990;27:171–177.
99. Rogers GL, Bremer DL: Surgical treatment of the upshoot and downshoot in Duane's retraction syndrome. Ophthalmology 1984;91:1380–1383.
100. Von Noorden G, Murray E: Up- and downshoot in Duane's retraction syndrome. J Pediatr Ophthalmol Strabismus 1986;23: 212–215.
101. Von Noorden G: Recession of both horizontal recti muscles in Duane's retraction syndrome with elevation and depression of the adducted eye. Am J Ophthalmol 1992;114:311–313.
102. Knapp P: The surgical treatment of double elevator paralysis. Trans Am Ophthalmol Soc 1969;67:304.
103. Metz HS: Double elevator palsy. Arch Ophthalmol 1979;97: 901–903.
104. Scott WE, Jackson OB: Double elevator palsy: The significance of inferior rectus restriction. Am Orthop J 1977;27:5–10.
105. Brown HW: Congenital structural muscle anomalies. In Allen JA (ed.), Strabismus Ophthalmic Symposium. I. St. Louis: CV Mosby, 1950; pp 205–236.
106. Brown HW: True and simulated superior oblique tendon sheath syndrome. Doc Ophthalmol 1973;34:123–136.
107. Crawford JS, Orton RB, Labow-Daily L: Late results of superior oblique muscle tenotomy in true Brown's syndrome. Am J Ophthalmol 1980;89:824–829.
108. Crawford JS: Surgical treatment of true Brown's syndrome. Am J Ophthalmol 1976;81:289–295.
109. Eustis HS, O'Reilly C, Crawford JA: Management of superior oblique palsy after surgery for true Brown's syndrome. J Pediatr Ophthalmol Strabismus 1987;24:10–16.
110. Parks MM, Eustis HS: Simultaneous superior oblique tenotomy and inferior oblique recession in Brown's syndrome. Ophthalmology 1987;94:1043–1048.
111. Santiago AP, Rosenbaum AL: Grave complications after superior oblique tenotomy or tenectomy for Brown syndrome. AAPOS 1997;1:8–15.
112. Scott AB, Knapp P: Surgical treatment of superior oblique tendon sheath syndrome. Arch Ophthalmol 1972;88:282.
113. Braverman DE, Scott WE: Surgical correction of dissociated vertical deviations. J Pediatr Ophthalmol Strabismus 1977;14: 337–342.
114. Sargent R: Dissociated hypertropia: Surgical treatment. Trans Am Acad Ophthalmol Otolaryngol 1979;86:1428–1438.
115. Mims JL, Wood RC: Bilateral anterior transposition of the inferior obliques. Arch Ophthalmol 1989;107;41–44.
116. Wright KW: Inferior oblique surgery. In Wright KW (ed.), Color Atlas of Ophthalmic Surgery, Strabismus. Philadelphia: JB Lippincott, 1991; pp 173–174.
117. Esswein MB, von Noorden GK, Coburn A: Comparison of surgical methods in the treatment of dissociated vertical deviation. Am J Ophthalmol 1992;113:287–290.
118. Kushner BJ, Price RL: Correcting an ipsilateral manifest hypotropia and dissociated hypertropia (dissociated hypertropia, DVD). Binoc Vis 1988;3:41–45.
119. Magoon E, Cruciger M, Jampolsky A: Dissociated vertical deviation: An asymmetric condition treated with large bilateral superior rectus recession. J Pediatr Ophthalmol Strabismus 1982;19:152–156.
120. Apt TL, Isenberg S, Gaffney WL: The oculocardiac reflex in strabismus surgery. Am J Ophthalmol 1973;76:533.
121. MacEwen CJ, Lee JP, Fells P: Aetiology and management of the "detached" rectus muscle. Br J Ophthalmol 1992;76:131–136.
122. Apt L, Isenberg SJ: The oculocardiac reflex as a surgical aid in identifying a slipped or "lost" extraocular muscle. Br J Ophthalmol 1980;64:362–365.
123. Apple DJ, Jones GR, Reidy JJ, Loftfield K: Ocular perforation and phthisis bulbi secondary to strabismus surgery. J Pediatr Ophthalmol Strabismus 1985;22:184–187.
124. Gottlieb F, Castro JL: Perforation of the globe during strabismus surgery. Arch Ophthalmol 1970;84:151–157.

125. McLean JM, Galin M, Baras I: Retinal perforation during strabismus surgery. Am J Ophthalmol 1960;50:1167.
126. Havener WH, Kimball OP: Scleral perforation in strabismus surgery. Am J Ophthalmol 1960;50:807.
127. Plager DA, Parks MM: Recognition and repair of the "lost" rectus muscle. A report of 25 cases. Ophthalmology 1990;97:131–137.
128. Plager DA, Parks MM: Recognition and repair of the "slipped" rectus muscle. J Pediatr Ophthalmol Strabismus 1988;25:270–274.
129. Olver JM, Lee JP: Recovery of anterior segment circulation after strabismus surgery in adult patients. Ophthalmology 1992;99:305–315.
130. Saunders RA, Bluestein EC, Wilson M, Berland JE: Anterior segment ischemia after strabismus surgery. Survey Ophthalmol 1994;38:456–466.
131. Von Noorden GK: Anterior segment ischemia following the Jensen procedure. Arch Ophthalmol 1976;94:845.
132. Scott, AB, Magoon EH, McNeer KW, et al.: Botulinum treatment of strabismus in children. Trans Am Ophthalmol Soc 1989;87:174.
133. Biglan AW, Burnstene RA, Rogers GL, et al.: Management of strabismus with boutlinum A toxin. Ophthalmology 1989;96:935.
134. Lee J, Harris S, Cohen J, et al.: Results of a prospective randomized trial of botulinum toxin therapy in acute unilateral sixth nerve palsy. J Pediatr Ophthalmol Strabismus 1994;31:283.
135. McNeer KW, Spencer RF, Tucker MG: Observations on bilateral stimultaneous botulinum toxin injections in infantile esotropia. J Pediatr Ophthalmol Strabismus 1994;31:214.
136. Dawson EL, Marshman WE, Adams GG: The role of botulinum toxin A in acute onset esotropia. Ophthalmology 1999;106:1727–1730.
137. Scott WE, Thalacker JA: Diagnosis and treatment of thyroid myopathy. Ophthalmology 1981;88:493–498.

SECTION VII

William S. Tasman, M.D.

Vitreoretinal Surgery

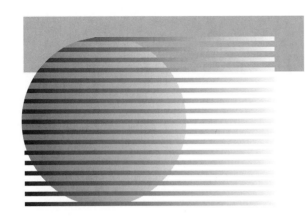

CHAPTER 54

Proliferative Diabetic Retinopathy

DAVID A. QUILLEN, M.D., THOMAS W. GARDNER, M.D., GEORGE W. BLANKENSHIP, M.D., and KIMBERLY A. NEELY, M.D., Ph.D.

Among the most dramatic improvements in modern medicine are those accomplished by the vitreoretinal surgeon. In the last half of the 20th century, causes of blindness that afflicted a major portion of the worlds' population started being able to be prevented: diabetic retinopathy, retinal detachment secondary to severe trauma, and various types of macular degeneration. The technique of vitreoretinal surgery has become increasingly specialized. Nonetheless, comprehensive ophthalmologists can benefit their patients more completely by knowing about these techniques. Here we present those procedures believed to be of most importance.

Management of proliferative diabetic retinopathy is guided by the findings and recommendations of the Diabetic Retinopathy Study (DRS),[1–3] Early Treatment Diabetic Retinopathy Study (ETDRS),[4] Diabetic Retinopathy Vitrectomy Study (DRVS)[5,6] and the Diabetes Control and Complication Trial (DCCT).[7] The combination of successful results achieved with the DRS, ETDRS, DRVS, and DCCT have clearly established the indications, techniques, and benefits of photocoagulation and pars plana vitreous surgery, and intensive control of blood sugars for people with diabetes.

CLINICAL FEATURES

The severity of diabetic retinopathy is strongly related to the duration of diabetes: the prevalence of proliferative diabetic retinopathy ranges from 0% in individuals with fewer than 5 years of diabetes to as high as 50% in individuals with 20 or more years of diabetes.[8] In addition to duration of diabetes, other factors are influential in the development and progression of proliferative diabetic retinopathy. These include puberty, pregnancy, poor metabolic control, hypertension, hypercholesterolemia, renal disease, and intraocular surgery.

Proliferative diabetic retinopathy is characterized by the presence of newly formed blood vessels arising from the retina or optic disc. The risk of proliferative diabetic retinopathy is related to the extent of ischemia within the retina.[9,10] Clinically, the most important findings in predicting progression to proliferative diabetic retinopathy include intraretinal hemorrhages and microaneurysms, venous beading, and intraretinal microvascular abnormalities (IRMA).[11] The "four-two-one rule" is helpful in assessing the severity of diabetic retinopathy and predicting the progression to proliferative retinopathy (Fig. 54–1). Severe nonproliferative diabetic retinopathy is defined as the presence of either *four* quadrants of dot/blot hemorrhages or microaneurysms, *two* quadrants of venous beading, or *one* quadrant of IRMA. In eyes with severe nonproliferative diabetic retinopathy, approximately 50% will progress to proliferative diabetic retinopathy within 1 to 3 years.

Most eyes with neovascularization will have neovascularization on the disc itself or within one disc diameter of the disc (NVD). Neovascularization of the disc appears as fine lacy vessels lying on the surface of the disc or bridging the physiologic cup. As the NVD pro-

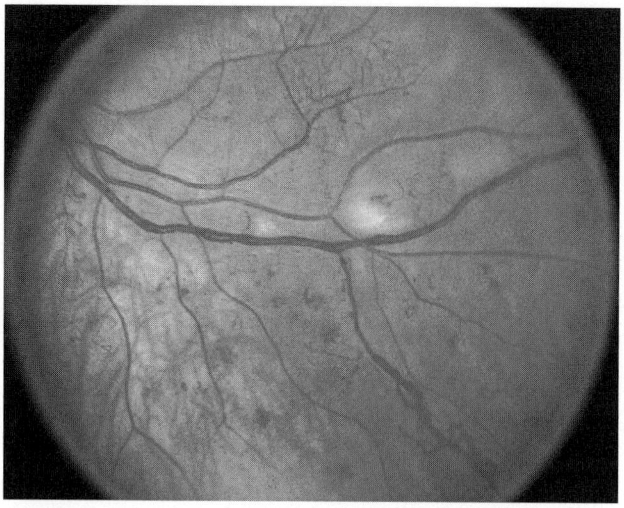

Figure 54–1. Severe nonproliferative diabetic retinopathy. Severe nonproliferative diabetic retinopathy is defined as the presence of either four quadrants of dot/ blot hemorrhages or microaneurysms, two quadrants of venous beading, or one quadrant of IRMA.

gresses, the vessels become more prominent and extend into the vitreous cavity or along the vascular arcades; the new vessels may be associated with significant fibrous proliferation. Neovascularization elsewhere (NVE) is defined as new vessels located at retinal sites other than on or within one disc diameter of the optic disc. Neovascularization elsewhere is usually associated with the retinal veins and arteriovenous crossing sites between areas of perfused and nonperfused retina.

The vitreous plays a critical role in the development and progression of proliferative diabetic retinopathy.[12] It appears that the posterior vitreous surface provides a "scaffold" for the progression of neovascularization. As the posterior vitreous detachment progresses, there is increased traction on the fibrovascular tissue. This may result in recurrent preretinal/vitreous hemorrhage or traction retinal detachment, or both.

Iris neovascularization or rubeosis may develop during the course of proliferative diabetic retinopathy. Iris neovascularization is characterized by the proliferation of fine lacy vessels on the iris surface; progressive iris neovascularization may result in angle-closure and neovascular glaucoma.

MAJOR DIABETIC RETINOPATHY STUDIES

The DRS and ETDRS provide clear guidelines for the management of proliferative diabetic retinopathy. Definitions used by the DRS and ETDRS are listed in Table 54–1.

DIABETIC RETINOPATHY STUDY

Does photocoagulation surgery reduce the risk of severe visual loss in diabetic retinopathy? The DRS evaluated individuals with proliferative diabetic retinopathy in at least one eye or severe nonproliferative diabetic retinopathy in both eyes.[1,2] One eye was randomly selected for photocoagulation, while the other eye was observed. Extensive scatter panretinal photocoagulation (PRP) and focal laser of new vessels on the surface of the retina was performed using either argon laser or xenon arc. Typical argon laser parameters included: 800 to 1600 burns, 500 micron spot size, 0.1 second duration, and intensity to obtain definite whitening.

The DRS identified four retinopathy risk factors for severe visual loss in diabetic retinopathy: new vessels

TABLE 54–1. Diabetic Retinopathy Study (DRS) and Early Treatment Diabetic Retinopathy Study (ETDRS) Definitions

Moderate visual loss	Loss of 15 or more letters on the ETDRS reading chart (equivalent to a doubling of the initial visual angle, e.g., 20/20 to 20/40 or 20/50 to 20/100)
Severe visual loss	Visual acuity less than 5/200 on two consecutive follow-up visits scheduled at 4-month intervals
Severe nonproliferative retinopathy:	Any one of the following: Hemorrhages and/or microaneurysms in four quadrants Venous beading in two quadrants Intraretinal microvascular abnormalities (IRMA) in one quadrant
Early Proliferative Retinopathy	Proliferative retinopathy without DRS high-risk characteristics
Less Severe Retinopathy	Mild or moderate nonproliferative retinopathy
More Severe Retinopathy	Severe nonproliferative or early proliferative retinopathy
High Risk Proliferative Diabetic Retinopathy	At least three of the following risk factors: New vessels present New vessels located on or within 1 disc diameter of the disc (NVD) Vitreous and/or preretinal hemorrhage Moderate to severe new vessels NVD greater than standard photo 10a (⅓ disc area) (Fig. 54–2) In absence of NVD, neovascularization elsewhere (NVE) greater than ½ disc area

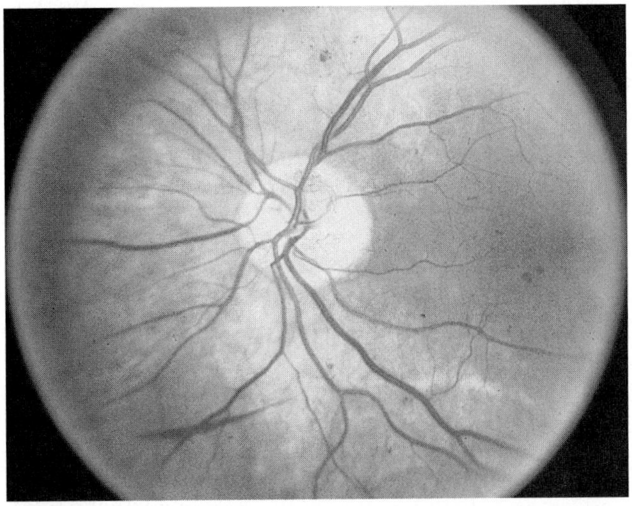

Figure 54–2. Severe neovascularization of the disc (NVD). Standard fundus photograph 10A from the modified Airlie classification of diabetic retinopathy demonstrating the lower limit of moderate- severe NVD.

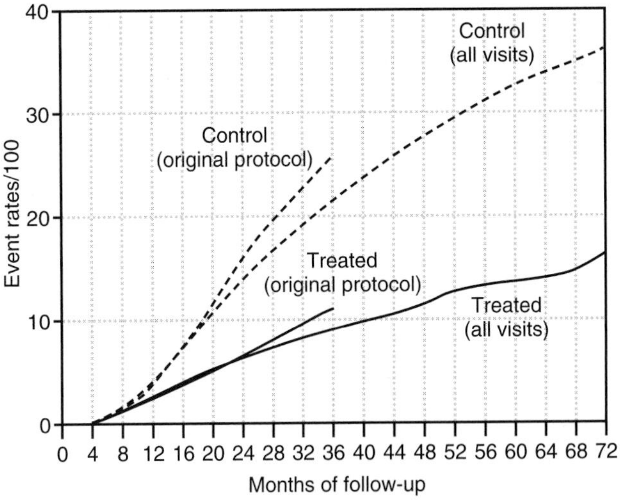

Figure 54–3. Severe visual loss. Cumulative rates of severe visual loss, including and excluding observations made after the 1976 Diabetic Retinopathy Study protocol change, argon and xenon groups combined. Extensive scatter photocoagulation reduces the risk of severe visual loss by 50% or more. (From The Diabetic Retinopathy Study Research Group: Photocoagulation treatment of proliferative diabetic retinopathy. Clinical application of Diabetic Retinopathy Study [DRS] findings. DRS Report Number 8. Ophthalmology 1981;88:583-600.)

present, new vessels located on or within one disc diameter of the disc, vitreous or preretinal hemorrhage, and moderate to severe new vessels (NVD greater than standard photo 10a [Fig. 54–2] or, in the absence of NVD, NVE greater than one half the disc area).[3] The risk of severe visual loss increased progressively as more risk factors were added: the risk of severe visual loss remained relatively low with two or fewer risk factors (roughly 5% at 2 years) but increased considerably with three or more risk factors (roughly 25% at 2 years). Therefore, the presence of three or four of these retinopathy risk factors indicates "high risk" for severe visual loss.

Extensive PRP reduced the risk of severe visual loss by greater than 50% regardless of the baseline severity of retinopathy (Fig. 54–3). After two years, severe visual loss occurred in 16.3% of all untreated eyes compared to only 5.3% of eyes that received xenon arc and 7.4% of eyes treated with argon laser.

Although xenon arc was slightly more effective than argon laser in reducing the risk of severe visual loss, this advantage was outweighed by the greater adverse effects of xenon arc. Visual field constriction attributable to PRP occurred in 10% of argon-treated eyes compared to 35% of xenon arc–treated eyes. Persistent decreases of one or more lines of vision occurred in approximately 10% of argon-treated eyes compared to 20% of xenon arc–treated eyes.

The DRS findings strongly indicate that prompt panretinal laser PRP should be performed in eyes with high-risk proliferative diabetic retinopathy. In these eyes, the risk of severe visual loss is high. Laser surgery effectively reduces the risk of severe visual loss by greater than 50%. In high-risk proliferative retinopathy, the beneficial effects of PRP clearly outweigh the adverse effects. In eyes with severe nonproliferative or proliferative diabetic retinopathy without high-risk characteristics, the DRS does not provide a clear choice between prompt treatment and careful follow-up with deferral of PRP until high-risk characteristics develop. The risk of severe visual loss in these eyes is relatively low. Although laser surgery reduces the risk of severe visual loss, the beneficial effects of PRP must be weighed against the adverse effects.

EARLY TREATMENT DIABETIC RETINOPATHY STUDY

When, during the course of diabetic retinopathy, is it most appropriate to initiate photocoagulation therapy? The ETDRS enrolled patients with mild to severe nonproliferative diabetic retinopathy or early proliferative retinopathy without high-risk characteristics in both eyes.[4] One eye of each patient was assigned randomly to early full or mild PRP and the other to deferral. For eyes assigned to deferral, full PRP was performed immediately if high-risk proliferative diabetic retinopathy developed. Eyes with macular edema were also randomized to immediate or delayed focal laser surgery.

The ETDRS provided very important information on the natural history of diabetic retinopathy. For eyes with mild or moderate nonproliferative retinopathy, the risk of progression to high-risk proliferative diabetic retinopathy was low: approximately 10% over 3 years. For eyes with more severe retinopathy, the risk of progression to high-risk proliferative retinopathy increased to about 50% over 3 years. Early PRP effectively reduced the rate of developing high-risk proliferative retinopathy by over 50% regardless of baseline severity of retinopathy.

The development of severe visual loss for all baseline categories of retinopathy was low for both the treatment and the deferral groups (2.6% vs 3.7%, respectively).

Adverse effects of PRP on visual acuity and visual field were observed. Eyes assigned to immediate full PRP had significantly greater loss of visual field as measured by the Goldmann 1/4e test object than those eyes assigned to deferral. Treated eyes were more likely to have early moderate visual loss than untreated eyes, particularly when early PRP was applied in eyes with preexisting macular edema. In eyes with macular edema, immediate focal photocoagulation with delayed PRP—added only if more severe retinopathy developed—was the most effective strategy for reducing the risk of moderate visual loss.

Although early PRP reduces the risk of developing high-risk proliferative retinopathy by more than 50%, the ETDRS demonstrated that the risk of severe visual loss for all eyes studied is low, whether treated with early PRP or followed closely and treated as soon as high-risk proliferative retinopathy developed. Early full PRP is associated with higher rates of moderate visual loss and visual field loss than deferral. Provided careful follow-up can be maintained, PRP is not recommended for eyes with less severe retinopathy. As retinopathy approaches the high-risk stage, the benefits and risks of early PRP may be roughly balanced. Initiating PRP early in at least one eye seems particularly appropriate when both of a patient's eyes are approaching the high-risk stage. Once high-risk proliferative diabetic retinopathy develops, PRP should not be delayed. Focal treatment should be considered for eyes with clinically significant macular edema, preferably before PRP for high-risk proliferative retinopathy becomes urgent.

PERFORMING PANRETINAL PHOTOCOAGULATION

Eyes with high-risk proliferative diabetic retinopathy are at significant risk for severe visual loss and should undergo PRP without delay. Recall that high-risk proliferative diabetic retinopathy is defined as the presence of three or four of the following risk factors: new vessels present, new vessels on the disc, preretinal or vitreous hemorrhage, and moderate to severe new vessels (new vessels on the disc greater than one third disc area or new vessels elsewhere greater than one half disc area).[3] The presence of three or four high-risk characteristics translates into essentially three clinical situations (Fig. 52–4). These include moderate to severe neo-

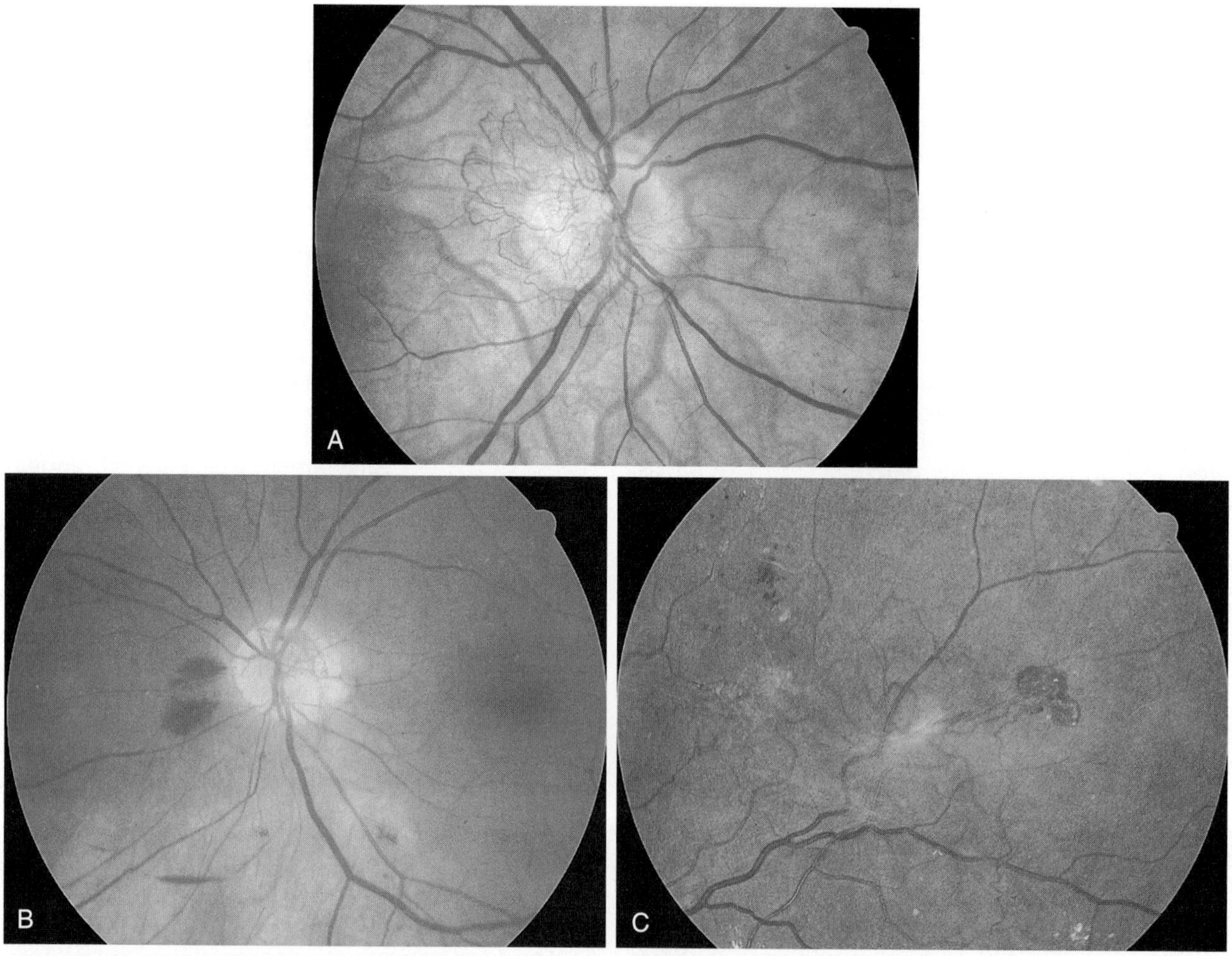

Figure 54–4. High risk proliferative diabetic retinopathy. Examples of high risk proliferative diabetic retinopathy including *(A)* severe NVD (greater than standard photograph 10*A*), *(B)* any NVD with preretinal/ vitreous hemorrhage, and *(C)* severe NVE with preretinal/ vitreous hemorrhage.

vascularization on the disc in the presence or absence of preretinal or vitreous hemorrhage, less severe neovascularization on the disc associated with preretinal or vitreous hemorrhage, or moderate to severe neovascularization elsewhere associated with preretinal or vitreous hemorrhage. Iris neovascularization is another indication for prompt PRP, whether or not high-risk characteristics are present.

In eyes with less severe proliferative diabetic retinopathy or severe nonproliferative diabetic retinopathy, the treating ophthalmologist must weigh the benefits of early PRP versus the potential risks.

Panretinal photocoagulation is tolerated well by many individuals with topical anesthesia alone. However, retrobulbar, peribulbar, sub-Tenon's, or subconjunctival anesthesia may be necessary.

Panretinal photocoagulation may be performed in one or multiple sessions. Eyes undergoing treatment in one session are more likely to have transient adverse effects than eyes treated in multiple sessions.[13] These adverse effects include exudative retinal detachment, choroidal detachment, and angle closure. However, the long-term beneficial effects of laser are equal whether laser is administered in one or multiple sessions. In eyes with macular edema, extensive fibrovascular proliferations, or traction retinal detachments, it is advisable to perform PRP in two or more sessions separated by 2 to 3 weeks.

The type or wavelength of laser may vary. Studies have demonstrated similar efficacies of argon, krypton, diode, and dye lasers.[14–17] In cases of dense cataract or vitreous hemorrhage, the red wavelength may be more useful.

Several wide-field funduscopic lenses are available for PRP. These lenses allow visualization to the ora serrata and give an inverted, reversed view of the retina. Most of the available lenses magnify the laser spot size 1.5 to 2 times at the retina.

With the retina in focus, the laser power is increased until slight whitening of the retina is achieved. One method is to start with the power set at 0.2 watts, the exposure time at 0.2 second, and spot size 200 micron pole in a lightly pigmented patient and 0.13 watts, 0.2 second and 200 microns in a pigmented patient. If the treatment causes pain the intensity is increased and the power decreased. If it is not possible to obtain a satisfactory burn with a power setting of one watt or less, a smaller spot size or longer exposure time may be used.

Laser burns are spaced one-half to one spot-width apart (Fig. 54–5). Peripheral PRP is advocated to reduce the risk of visual loss, exacerbation or development of macular edema, and extensive visual field loss.[18] The posterior fundus is demarcated with two to three rows of laser to reduce the risk of extension into the macula or optic disc. The burns are placed one disc diameter from the optic disc and the major temporal vascular arcades. Special care must be used when demarcating the posterior extent of treatment of the temporal retina. Generally, laser should not extend posterior to an imaginary line drawn at two fovea-disc diameters from the optic disc. Panretinal photocoagulation is then extended peripherally to the equator and beyond.

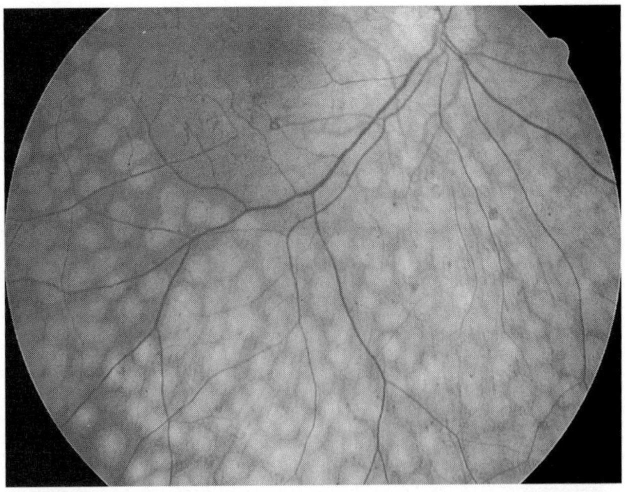

Figure 54–5. Panretinal Photocoagulation. 500 micron spots using enough energy to obtain slight whitening of the RPE are placed one-half to one burn width apart to the retina.

Approximately 1600 burns of 500 microns or larger are common for eyes with high-risk proliferative diabetic retinopathy. However, the extent of PRP—not necessarily the number of burns placed—is important in assessing the completeness of surgery.

A follow-up visit is scheduled in 2 or 3 weeks for additional laser, if divided sessions are used, or in 1 month following completion of PRP. In eyes that fail to regress despite standard PRP, supplemental laser may be helpful.

REGRESSION OF PROLIFERATIVE DIABETIC RETINOPATHY

The efficacy of PRP is related to the induced regression of retinopathy risk factors (Fig. 54–6).[19,20] Regression of high-risk characteristics may take several forms: complete regression of new vessels, marked reduction in the severity of new vessels, or resolution of preretinal and vitreous hemorrhage.

A subset of eyes fail to show regression of retinopathy risk factors despite standard PRP; failure to demonstrate regression of high-risk characteristics may be associated with a poorer prognosis.[19–22] Supplemental laser may induce regression of high-risk retinopathy in eyes that fail to respond to initial therapy.[21–26] The DRS and the ETDRS did not evaluate the efficacy of supplemental PRP in eyes that fail to respond to standard therapy. However, the DRS showed that the risk of severe visual loss decreased with an increasing amount of initial treatment as measured by treatment density in the post-treatment photographs.[27]

In addition to regression of retinopathy risk factors, manifest changes in the retinal vascular system are associated with a favorable response to laser treatment. There is a significant increase in the venous caliber as the stage of diabetic retinopathy progresses.[28] Panreti-

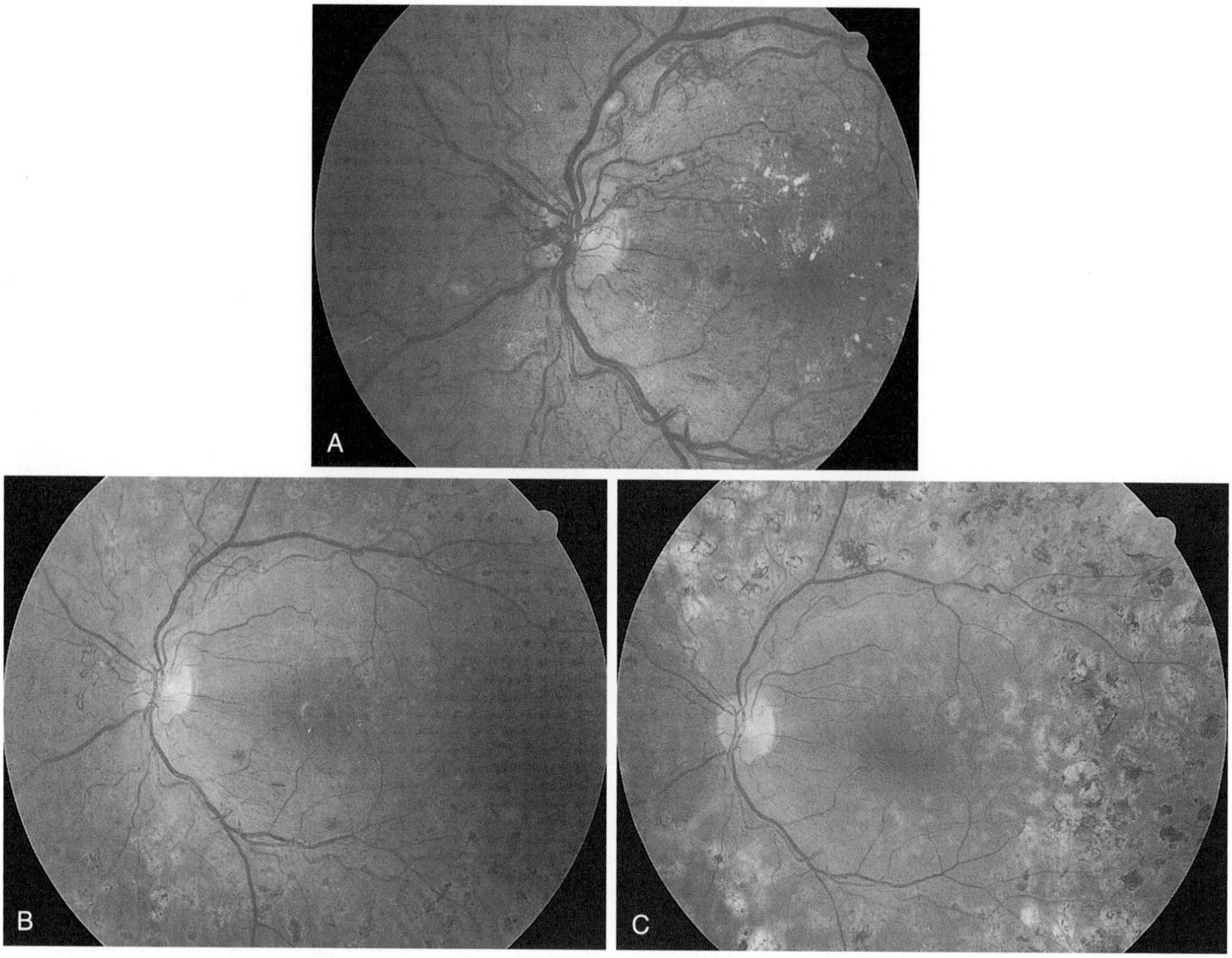

Figure 54–6. Regression of Proliferative Diabetic Retinopathy. Panretinal photocoagulation induces a rapid and stable reduction of retinopathy risk factors in most eyes. *(A)* High risk proliferative diabetic retinopathy; *(B)* one month following PRP; *(C)* six months following PRP.

nal photocoagulation has been shown to reduce retinal blood flow and retinal vessel diameter.[29–32] The diameter of the retinal vessels is correlated to the amount of regression of proliferative diabetic retinopathy.[33,34]

HOW DOES PANRETINAL PHOTOCOAGULATION WORK?

Photocoagulation destroys the photoreceptor–retinal pigment epithelial (RPE) complex and produces significant thinning of the outer retina.[35] By decreasing the oxygen consumption at the photoreceptor–RPE complex, more oxygen is available to diffuse into the inner retina and vitreous.[35–38] Enhanced oxygen diffusion into the inner retina and vitreous reduces inner retina ischemia and the stimulus for neovascularization.

Vascular endothelial growth factor (VEGF), an angiogenic molecule whose expression is markedly induced by retinal hypoxia,[39] is the leading candidate linking retinal ischemia and intraocular neovascularization. Vitreous VEGF levels are significantly higher in eyes with proliferative diabetic retinopathy than in eyes without proliferative diabetic retinopathy.[40] Vascular endothelial growth factor concentrations in vitreous fluid decline significantly after successful PRP, suggesting that PRP reduces retinal ischemia and the hypoxia-induced expression of VEGF.[41]

In addition, photocoagulation may inhibit neovascularization by inducing changes in the RPE. Retinal pigment epithelial cells have the ability to inhibit vascular endothelial cell proliferation and induce regression of new blood vessels.[42] Photocoagulation of RPE cells may induce changes in the production of growth factors. In particular, it appears that photocoagulated RPE cells may release potential inhibitors of neovascularization.[43]

COMPLICATIONS OF PANRETINAL PHOTOCOAGULATION

Laser photocoagulation effectively reduces the risk of severe visual loss in eyes with high-risk proliferative diabetic retinopathy. However, adverse effects may occur (Table 54–2).

TABLE 54–2. Complications of Panretinal Photocoagulation

Blurred vision
Nyctalopia
Visual field constriction
Poor color discrimination
Transient myopia
Accommodation defects
Corneal abnormalities
Intraocular pressure alterations
Narrow-angle glaucoma
Iris and pupillary abnormalities
Lens opacities
Inadvertent macular/foveal burns
Macular edema
Exudative macular detachment
Ciliochoroidal effusion
Cilioretinal/choriovitreal neovascularization
Optic neuropathy
Complications of local anesthesia

Subjective changes in vision after PRP include blurred vision, decreased accommodation, difficulty adjusting to changing levels of illumination, color vision abnormalities, constriction of peripheral visual fields, and poor night vision.[44] Adverse effects to the cornea include corneal burns, erosions, and superficial punctate keratitis.[45,46]

Panretinal photocoagulation may affect intraocular pressure. Blondeau and associates noted transient intraocular pressure elevations soon after treatment, which resolved within several hours.[47] Conversely, transient decreases in intraocular pressure may occur.[48,49] Elevation of intraocular pressure may be associated with anterior chamber shallowing and frank angle-closure glaucoma.

Iris and pupillary abnormalities include pupillary border hyperpigmentation or atrophy, posterior synechiae, reduced pupillary reactivity, mydriasis, miosis, accommodative palsy, light-near dissociation, and sector palsies of the iris sphincter.[50]

Stable, nonprogressive lens opacities may occur after laser treatment.[51,52]

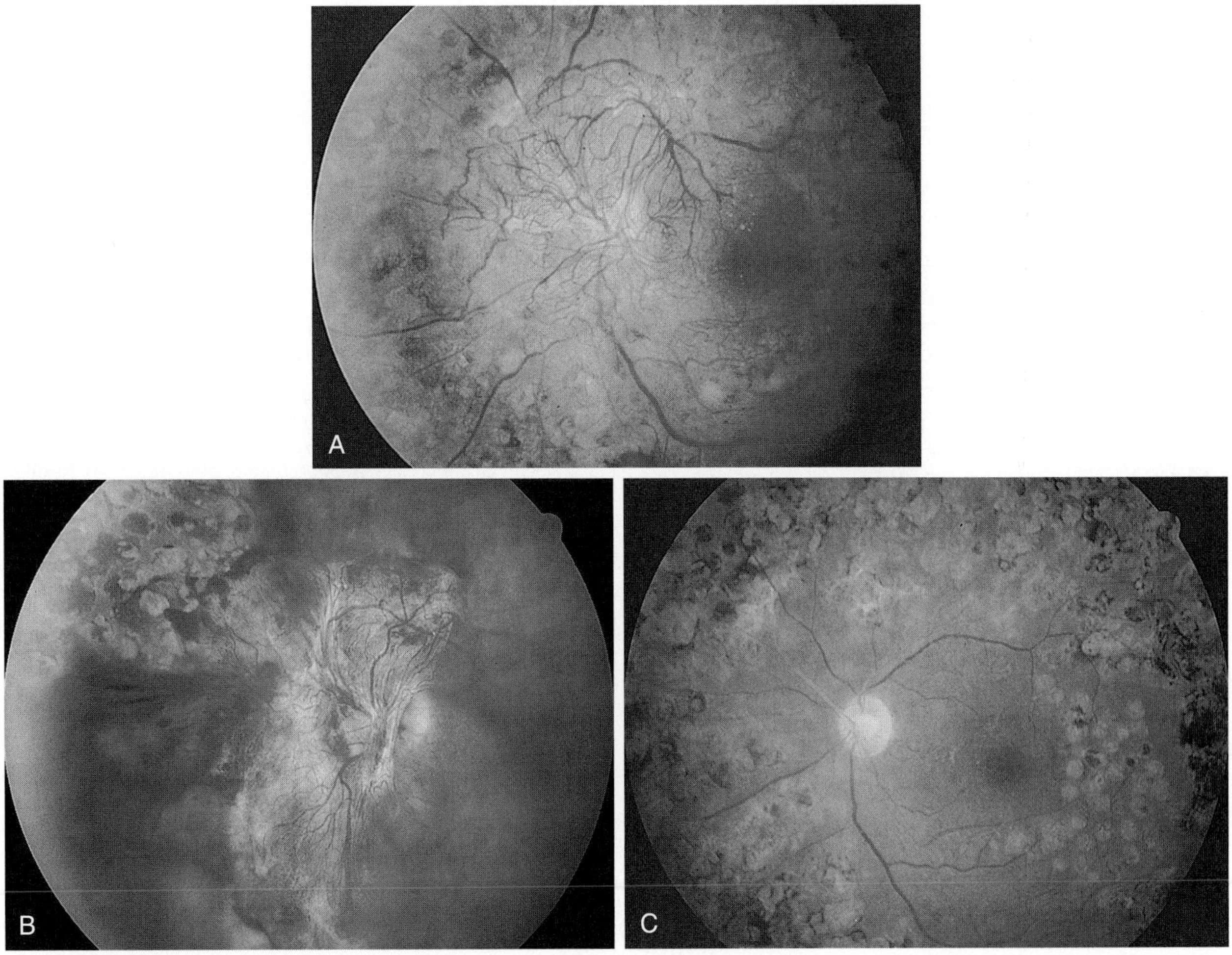

Figure 54–7. Pars Plana Vitrectomy. Pars plana vitrectomy is indicated for eyes with vitreous hemorrhage and active neovascularization despite extensive panretinal laser. *A.* This 24-year-old woman developed severe proliferative diabetic retinopathy during pregnancy. *B.* She developed preretinal and vitreous hemorrhage despite extensive photocoagulation. *C.* She underwent pars plana vitrectomy with vision stabilizing at 20/40.

Posterior segment complications of laser surgery include inadvertent macular/foveal burns, exacerbation or development of macular edema, exudative macular detachment, ciliochoroidal effusion, hemorrhage, rupture of RPE/ Bruch's membrane, cilioretinal and chorioitreal neovascularization, extension of tractional retinal detachment, and optic neuropathy.[4,53–65]

Retrobulbar anesthesia may be employed safely to reduce the discomfort of PRP.[66,67] Risks of retrobulbar anesthesia include penetration or perforation of the globe, retrobulbar hemorrhage, central retinal artery or central retinal vein occlusion, optic neuropathy, Purtscher's retinopathy, central nervous system depression, or even respiratory arrest.

CRYOSURGERY

Peripheral retina ablation with cryosurgery may be useful in proliferative diabetic retinopathy when media opacities such as severe cataract or vitreous hemorrhage prevent PRP, or in individuals who fail to demonstrate regression despite extensive laser surgery.[68–73] This method of surgery may be particularly helpful for individuals who are not candidates for pars plana vitrectomy with intraoperative PRP.

PARS PLANA VITRECTOMY

Pars plana vitrectomy is an important surgical option for complicated proliferative diabetic retinopathy (Fig. 54–7). Indications include nonclearing vitreous hemorrhage, retinal detachment, premacular fibrosis, macular heterotopia, proliferative diabetic retinopathy/iris neovascularization unresponsive to conventional therapy, hemolytic glaucoma, and dense cataract impeding photocoagulation.

REFERENCES

1. Diabetic Retinopathy Study Research Group: Preliminary report on effects of photocoagulation therapy. Am J Ophthalmol 1976; 81:383–96.
2. The Diabetic Retinopathy Study Research Group: Photocoagulation treatment of proliferative diabetic retinopathy. Clinical application of Diabetic Retinopathy Study (DRS) findings. DRS Report Number 8. Ophthalmology 1981;88:583–600.
3. Diabetic Retinopathy Study Research Group: Four risk factors for severe visual loss in diabetic retinopathy: The third report from the Diabetic Retinopathy Study. Arch Ophthalmol 1979;97:654–5.
4. Early Treatment Diabetic Retinopathy Study Research Group: Early photocoagulation for diabetic retinopathy. ETDRS Report Number 9. Ophthalmology 1991;98:766–85.
5. Diabetic Retinopathy Vitrectomy Study Research Group (Appended): Early vitrectomy for severe vitreous hemorrhage in diabetic retinopathy. Arch Ophthalmol 1985;103:1644–52.
6. The Diabetic Retinopathy Vitrectomy Study Research Group: Early vitrectomy for severe proliferative diabetic retinopathy in eyes with useful vision: Results of a randomized trial—Diabetic Retinopathy Vitrectomy Study Report 3. Ophthalmology 1988;95:1307–20.
7. The Diabetes Control and Complications Trial Research Group: The effect of intensive treatment of diabetes on the development and progression of long-term complications in insulin-dependent diabetes mellitus. N Engl J Med 1993;329:977–86.
8. Klein R: The epidemiology of diabetic retinopathy: Findings from the Wisconsin epidemiologic study of diabetic retinopathy. Int Ophthalmol Clin 1987;27:230–8.
9. Shimizu K, Kobayashi Y, Muraoka K: Midperipheral fundus involvement in diabetic retinopathy. Ophthalmology 1981;88: 601–12.
10. Early Treatment Diabetic Retinopathy Study Research Group: Fluorescein angiographic risk factors for progression of diabetic retinopathy. ETDRS Report 12. Ophthalmology 1991;98:834–40.
11. Early Treatment Diabetic Retinopathy Study Research Group: Fundus photographic risk factors for progression of diabetic retinopathy. ETDRS Report 12. Ophthalmology 1991;98:823–33.
12. Davis MD: Vitreous contraction in proliferative diabetic retinopathy. Arch Ophthalmol 1965;74:741–51.
13. Doft BH, Blankenship GW: Single versus multiple treatment sessions of argon laser panretinal photocoagulation for proliferative diabetic retinopathy. Ophthalmology 1982;89:772-9.
14. The Krypton Argon Regression Neovascularization Study Research Group: Randomized comparison of krypton versus argon scatter photocoagulation for diabetic disc neovascularization. The Krypton Argon Regression Neovascularization Study Report 1. Ophthalmology 1993;100:1655–64.
15. Blankenship GW, Gerke E, Batle JF: Red krypton and blue–green argon laser diabetic panretinal photocoagulation. Graefe's Arch Clin Exp Ophthalmol 1989;227:364–8.
16. Bandello F, Brancato R, Trabucchi G, et al.: Diode versus argon–green laser panretinal photocoagulation in proliferative diabetic retinopathy: A randomized study in 44 eyes with a long follow-up time. Graefe's Arch Clin Exp Ophthalmol 1993;231: 491–4.
17. Seiberth V, Schatanek S, Alexandridis E: Panretinal photocoagulation in diabetic retinopathy: Argon versus dye laser coagulation. Graefe's Arch Clin Exp Ophthalmol 1993;231:318–22.
18. Blankenship GW: A clinical comparison of central and peripheral arson laser panretinal photocoagulation for proliferative diabetic retinopathy. Ophthalmology 1988;95:170–7.
19. Doft BH, Blankenship GW: Retinopathy risk factor regression after laser panretinal photocoagulation for proliferative diabetic retinopathy. Ophthalmology 1984;91:1453–7.
20. Vander JF, Duker JS, Benson WE, et al.: Long-term stability and visual outcome after favorable initial response of proliferative diabetic retinopathy to panretinal photocoagulation. Ophthalmology 1991;98:1575–9.
21. Vine AK: The efficacy of additional argon laser photocoagulation for persistent, severe proliferative diabetic retinopathy. Ophthalmology 1985;92:1532–7.
22. Doft BH, Metz DJ, Kelsey SF: Augmentation laser for proliferative diabetic retinopathy that fails to respond to initial panretinal photocoagulation. Ophthalmology 1992;99:1728–35.
23. Rogell GD: Incremental panretinal photocoagulation. Results in treating proliferative diabetic retinopathy. Retina 1983;3:308–11.
24. Theodossiadis GP, Ismiridis KJ: Time span of regression or disappearance of optic disk neovascularization in proliferative diabetic retinopathy after panretinal argon laser photocoagulation and results over a two-year follow-up. Fortschr Ophthalmol 1987;84:465–7.
25. Reddy VM, Zamora RL, Olk RJ: Quantitation of retinal albation in proliferative diabetic retinopathy. Am J Ophthalmol 1995;119: 760–6.
26. Aylward GW, Pearson RV, Jagger JD, Hamilton AM: Extensive argon laser photocoagulation in the treatment of proliferative diabetic retinopathy, Br J Ophthalmol 1989;73:197–201.
27. Kaufman SC, Ferris FL, Seigel DG, et al.: Factors associated with the visual outcome after photocoagulation for diabetic retinopathy. Diabetic Retinopathy Study Report 13. Invest Ophthalmol Vis Sci 1989;30:23-8.
28. Yoshida A, Feke GT, Morales-Stoppello J, et al.: Retinal blood flow alterations during progression of diabetic retinopathy. Arch Ophthalmol 1983;101:225–7.
29. Feke GT, Green GJ, Goger DG, McMeel JW: Laser doppler measurements of the effect of panretinal photocoagulation on retinal blood flow. Ophthalmology 1982;89:757-62.
30. Oswald B, Oswald VH, Jutte A, et al.: Measurement of flow—Physiologic parameters of retinal blood circulation in type 1 and 2 diabetics before and after photocoagulation. Graefe's Arch Clin Exp Ophthalmol 1985;223:154–7.

31. Grunwald JE, Riva CE, Brucker AJ, et al.: Effect of panretinal photocoagulation on retinal blood flow in proliferative diabetic retinopathy. Ophthalmology 1986;93:590–5.
32. Fujio N, Feke GT, Goger DG, McMeel JW: Regional retinal blood flow reduction following half fundus photocoagulation treatment. Br J Ophthalmol 1994;78:335–8.
33. Wilson CA, Stefansson E, Clombers L, et al.: Optic disk neovascularization and retinal vessel diameter in diabetic retinopathy. Am J Ophthalmol 1988;106:131–4.
34. Grunwald JE, Brucker AJ, Petrig BL, Riva CE: Retinal blood flow regulation and the clinical response to panretinal photocoagulation in proliferative diabetic retinopathy. Ophthalmology 1989;96:1518–22.
35. Molnar I, Poitry S, Tsacopoulas M, et al.: Effect of laser photocoagulation on oxygenation of the retina in miniature pigs. Invest Ophthalmol Vis Sci 1985;26:1410–4.
36. Alder VA, Cringle SJ, Brown M: The effect of regional retinal photocoagulation on vitreal oxygen tension. Invest Ophthalmol Vis Sci 1987;28:1078–85.
37. Stefansson E, Machemer R, deJuan E, et al.: Retinal oxygenation and laser treatment in patients with diabetic retinopathy. Am J Ophthalmol 1992;113:36–8.
38. Novack RL, Stefansson E, Hatchell DL: The effect of photocoagulation on the oxygenation and ultrastructure of avascular retina. Exp Eye Res 1990;50:289–96.
39. Pe'er J, Shweiki D, Itin A, et al.: Hypoxia-induced expression of vascular endothelial growth factor by retinal cells is a common factor in neovascularizing ocular diseases. Lab Invest 1995;72: 638–45.
40. Adamis AP, Miller JW, Bernal MT, et al.: Increased vascular endothelial growth factor levels in the vitreous of eyes with proliferative diabetic retinopathy. Am J Ophthalmol 1994:118:445–50.
41. Aiello LP, Avery RL, Arrigg PG: Vascular endothelial growth factor in ocular fluid of patients with diabetic retinopathy and other retinal disorders. N Engl J Med 1994;331:1480–7.
42. Glaser BM, Campochiaro PA, Davis JL, Sato M: Retinal pigment epithelial cells release and inhibitor of neovascularization. Arch Ophthalmol 1985;103:1870–5.
43. Yoshimura N, Matsumoto M, Shimizu H: Photocoagulated human retinal pigment epithelial cells produce an inhibitor of vascular endothelial cell proliferation. Invest Ophthalmol Vis Sci 1995;36:1686–91.
44. Russell PW, Sekuler R, Fetkenhour C: Visual function after panretinal photocoagulation: A survey. Diabetes Care 1985;8:57–63.
45. Kanski JJ: Anterior segment complications of retinal photocoagulation. Am J Ophthalmol 1975;79:424–7.
46. Little HL: Complications of argon laser photocoagulation: A five-year study. Int Ophthalmol Clin 1976;16:145–59.
47. Blondeau P, Pavan PR, Phelps CD: Acute pressure elevation following panretinal photocoagulation. Arch Ophthalmol 1981;99:1239–41.
48. Schiodte SN: A pressure-lowering effect of retinal xenon photocoagulation in normotensive diabetic eyes. Acta Ophthalmol 1980;58:369–76.
49. Schiodte SN: Changes in eye tension after panretinal xenon arc and argon laser photocoagulation in normotensive diabetic eyes. Acta Ophthalmol 1982;60:692-700.
50. Lobes LA, Bourgon P: Pupillary abnormalities induced by argon laser photocoagulation. Ophthalmology 1985;92:234–6.
51. Lankhanpal V, Schocket SS, Richards RD, Nirankari VS: Photocoagulation-induced lens opacity. Arch Ophthalmol 1982;100: 1068–70.
52. McCanna P, Chandra SR, Stevens TS, et al.: Argon laser-induced cataract as a complication of retinal photocoagulation. Arch Ophthalmol 1982;100:1071–3.
53. Ferris FL, Podgor MJ, Davis MD: The DRS Research Group: Macular edema in diabetic retinopathy study patients. DRS Report 12. Ophthalmology 1987;94:754–60.
54. Francois J, Cambie E: Further vision deterioration after argon laser photocoagulation in diabetic retinopathy. Ophthalmologica 1976;173:28–39.
55. McDonald HR, Schatz H: Visual loss following panretinal photocoagulation for proliferative diabetic retinopathy. Ophthalmology 1985;92:388–93.
56. Seiberth V, Alexandridis E, Feng W: Function of the diabetic retina after panretinal argon laser coagulation. Graefe's Arch Clin Exp Ophthalmol 1987;225:385–90.
57. Kleiner RC, Elman MJ, Murphy RP, Ferris FL: Transient severe visual loss after panretinal photocoagulation. Am J Ophthalmol 1988;106:298–306.
58. Elliott A, Flanagan D: Macular detachment following laser treatment for proliferative diabetic retinopathy. Graefe's Arch Clin Exp Ophthalmol 1990;228:438–41.
59. Benson WE, Townsend RE, Pheasant TR: Choriovitreal and subretinal proliferations: Complications of photocoagulation. Ophthalmology 1979;86:283–9.
60. Chandra SR, Bresnick GH, Davis MD, et al.: Choroidovitreal neovascular ingrowth after photocoagulation for proliferative diabetic retinopathy. Arch Ophthalmol 1980;98:1593–9.
61. Wallow I, Johns K, Barry P, et al.: Chorioretinal and choriovitreal neovascularization after photocoagulation for prolifertaive diabetic retinopathy. A clinicopathologic correlation. Ophthalmology 1985;92:523–32.
62. Diabetic Retinopathy Study Research Group: Photocoagulation treatment of proliferative diabetic retinopathy: Relationship of adverse treatment effects to retinopathy severity. Diabetic Retinopathy Study Report Number 5. Dev Ophthalmol 1981;2:248–61.
63. D'Amico DJ: Diabetic traction retinal detachments threatening the fovea and panretinal argon laser photocoagulation. Semin Ophthalmol 1991;6:11–17.
64. Wade EC, Blankenship GW: The effect of short versus long exposure times of argon laser panretinal photocoagulation on proliferative diabetic retinopathy. Graefes Arch Clin Exp Ophthalmol 1990;228:226–31.
65. Swartz M, Apple DJ, Creel D: Sudden severe visual loss associated with peripapillary burns during panretinal argon photocoagulation. Br J Ophthalmol 1983;67:517–9.
66. Smith JL: Retrobulbar bupivacaine can cause respiratory arrest. Ann Ophthalmol 1982;14:1005–6.
67. Hay A, Flynn HW, Hoffman JI, Rivera AH: Needle penetration of the globe during retrobulbar and peribulbar injections. Ophthalmology 1991;98:1017–24.
68. Schimek RA, Spencer R: Cryopexy treatment of proliferative diabetic retinopathy: Retinal cryoablation in patients with severe vitreous hemorrhage. Arch Ophthalmol 1979;97:1276–80.
69. Hilton GF: Panretinal cryotherapy for diabetic rubeosis. Arch Ophthalmol 1979;97:776–9.
70. Daily MJ, Gieser RG: Treatment of proliferative diabetic retinopathy with panretinal cryotherapy. Ophthalmic Surg 1984;15:741–5.
71. Segato T, Piermarocchi S, Midena E, Bertoja H: Retinal cryotherapy in the management of proliferative diabetic retinopathy. Am J Ophthalmol 1984;98:240–1.
72. Mosier MA, Del Piero E, Gheewala SM: Anterior retinal cryotherapy in diabetic hemorrhage. Am J Ophthalmol 1985;100:440–4.
73. Benedett R, Olk RJ, Arribas NP, et al.: Transconjunctival anterior retinal cryotherapy for proliferative diabetic retinopathy. Ophthalmology 1987;94:612–9.

CHAPTER 55

Diabetic Macular Edema

THOMAS W. GARDNER, M.D., DAVID A. QUILLEN, M.D.,
KIMBERLY A. NEELY, M.D., Ph.D., and
GEORGE W. BLANKENSHIP, M.D.

Macular edema is the leading cause of visual impairment in people with diabetes and affects approximately 25% of those with type I and type II diabetes. Each year approximately 95,000 people with diabetes are estimated to develop macular edema.[1]

This chapter will discuss the pathogenesis and treatment of diabetic macular edema in terms of ocular and systemic factors (Tables 55–1 and 55–2).

PATHOPHYSIOLOGY

SYSTEMIC FACTORS

Macular edema manifests clinically as retinal thickening that results from chronic breakdown of the blood-retinal barrier. Extracellular fluid accumulates in the outer plexiform layer and extends into the inner retina with increasing severity. The pathophysiologic factors that govern the formation of edema in the macula are similar to those that contribute to edema elsewhere, such as in the brain. That is, tissue edema occurs when the ability of the blood vessels and the surrounding tissue to regulate leakage are overcome either by increased intralumenal hydrostatic pressure or increased extravascular (tissue) concentration of solutes. This relationship is classically described in the Starling equation, which states that fluid filtration is related to the forces that drive fluid across the vessel wall (blood pressure, intravascular fluid volume, and interstitial fluid osmotic pressure) minus the forces that promote fluid reabsorption (plasma oncotic pressure). The importance of this concept has been recently related to macular edema in diabetes by Kristinsson and co-workers.[2]

The primary systemic factor that contributes to disruption of the normal autoregulatory process of the retinal vasculature is systemic arterial hypertension. Epidemiologic studies have confirmed that hypertension aggravates existing retinopathy and increases the risk of developing retinopathy.[3] This point is illustrated in Figure 55–1. The patient whose eye is illustrated is a 65-year-old woman with 10 years of type II diabetes; and her blood pressure was 150/105 mm Hg. The eye has diffusely narrowed retinal arterioles, nerve fiber layer infarcts, and hemorrhages. The right macula is thickened, and lipid exudates threaten the fovea. Visual acuity was 20/40. The left eye had a similar appearance.

In addition to hypertension, intravascular fluid overload from congestive heart failure or renal failure increases the pressure across the vascular wall and the propensity to edema formation. The ophthalmologist should ask patients with diabetic macular edema about symptoms of fluid overload, such as orthopnea and dyspnea, and should observe whether those patients have pitting edema of their ankles.

Patients with hyperlipidemia may also have an increased tendency for macular edema formation when serum lipoproteins accumulate in the retina and exert the osmotic influences that draw water out of retinal vessels and cause retinal thickening. Data from the Early Treatment Diabetic Retinopathy Study (ETDRS) have shown a twofold increase in risk of macular edema in visual loss in patients with total serum cholesterol greater than 240 mg/dl.[4]

The issue of glycemic control as an isolated factor in the development of macular edema is difficult to determine because insulin affects numerous aspects of cellular metabolism. However, in the Diabetes Control

TABLE 55–1. Risk Factors for Development of Diabetic Macular Edema

Systemic Factors
Hypertension
Intravascular fluid overload (congestive heart failure, renal failure)
Hyperlipidemia
Poor metabolic control
Nephropathy
Ocular Factors
Cataract extraction
Intensive panretinal photocoagulation
Posterior hyaloid contraction

and Complications Trial (DCCT), the risk of macular edema was approximately 50% greater in the conventional treatment group than in the intensive treatment group. The overall risk of developing macular edema in the intensively treated patients in the secondary intervention group (those patients who had mild to moderate retinopathy at the beginning of the study) was 27%.[5]

Diabetic nephropathy is also associated with increased incidence and progression of retinopathy in general and macular edema in particular. This correlation of diabetic nephropathy and retinopathy is known as the diabetic "renal-retinal syndrome." The risk of macular edema is greatest in patients with overt proteinuria.[6] Nephropathy may aggravate macular edema via hypertension, fluid overload, hypoproteinemia, hyperlipidemia, or increased difficulty with metabolic control.

Taken together, poor metabolic (glycemic) control, increased blood pressure and serum lipids, and nephropathy all contribute to the development of retinopathy and macular edema.

OCULAR RISK FACTORS

In addition to systemic influences on the retinal circulation, several ocular conditions may also increase the risk of macular edema.

The combination of cataract and diabetic retinopathy is a common and clinically challenging problem. Cataract extraction, even with an intact posterior capsule and a posterior chamber intraocular lens, frequently increases the severity of retinopathy and macular edema.[7] The reasons for this are unclear, but may relate to release of inflammatory mediators around the time of cataract extraction. The risk of macular edema after cataract extraction increases with increasing severity of overall retinopathy, and with increasing age of the patients. In their series of 109 patients, Benson and co-workers found that only 48% achieved 20/40 or better final acuity and that 28% tested at 20/200 or less. Only 65% improved two or more lines of Snellen acuity.

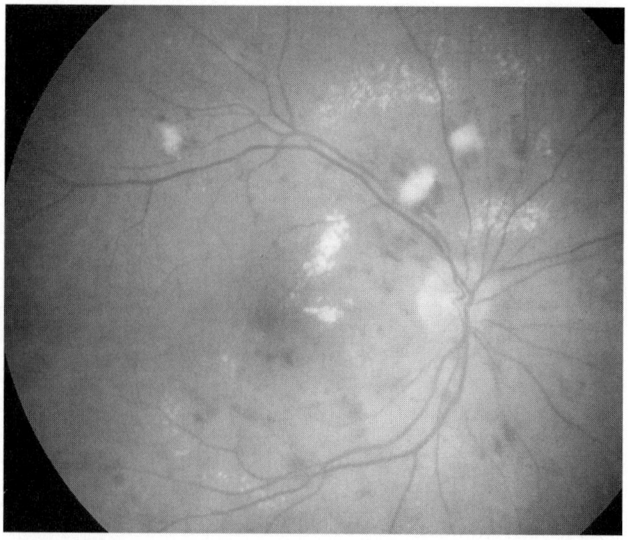

Figure 55–1. Effect of uncontrolled hypertension on diabetic macular edema. The right eye of a 65-year-old female with 10 years of type II diabetes whose blood pressure was 150/105 mm Hg. Note the diffusely narrowed retinal arterioles, the nerve fiber layer infarcts and hemorrhages. Her right macula is thickened with lipid exudates threatening the fovea, and her visual acuity was 20/40. The macular edema did not respond well to focal laser because her blood pressure remained elevated.

An additional risk factor for the development of macular edema is intensive panretinal photocoagulation.[8] Macular edema is particularly likely to be increased after panretinal photocoagulation when the treatment is applied in a single session or close to the macula.

Uncommonly, contraction of the posterior hyaloid face of the vitreous can exert traction on the macula, and this traction may contribute to the formation of macular edema.

TREATMENT OF MACULAR EDEMA

The evaluation of both systemic and ocular factors must be included for optimal management of diabetic macular edema (Table 55–2).

TABLE 55–2. Treatment of Diabetic Macular Edema

Systemic Factors
1. Optimize metabolic control (hemoglobin A_1C <6%)
2. Blood pressure < 130/80 mm Hg
3. Total cholesterol < 240 mg/dl and triglycerides < 200 mg/dl
4. Exclude congestive heart failure, nephropathy
Ocular Factors
1. Photocoagulation

SYSTEMIC TREATMENT

The primary factor to address is metabolic control. As mentioned above, the risk of macular edema was significantly lower in the intensively treated group than in the conventional treatment group in the DCCT. No study has directly addressed the issue of metabolic control in patients with existing macular edema. In general, the glycemic levels should be as low as can be achieved and tolerated by the patient without undue risk of hypoglycemia. A hemoglobin A_1C value less than or equal to 6% is a desirable goal, even if a difficult one for many patients to attain. In patients who have poor metabolic control, it is generally advisable to improve the metabolic control gradually over 6 to 12 months, because rapid tightening of control can cause transient worsening of retinopathy, usually made manifest by increasing "cotton wool" spots or intraretinal microvascular abnormalities; rarely, neovascularization develops. In the DCCT transient worsening occurred in 22% of the intensively treated group and 13% of the conventionally treated group.[9]

Blood pressure in persons with diabetes should be 130/80 mm Hg or less.[10] This value has been identified and significantly lowers the risk of progression of incipient diabetic nephropathy to overt nephropathy and is reasonable to apply in patients with retinopathy as well. Serum lipids should also be evaluated and treated in accordance with guidelines for the reduction of stroke and myocardial infarction.[11] That is, total cholesterol should be lower than 240 mg/dl, and triglycerides should be below 200 mg/dl. The availability of improved medications for the control of hyperglycemia, hyperlipidemia, and hypertension over the last several years makes this possible. Identification and treatment of systemic risk factors can have substantial benefits in macular edema, even that which is clinically significant, as demonstrated in Figure 55–2. By identifying these systemic risk factors, the ophthalmologist has the opportunity not only to improve the visual prognosis, but the prognosis for life as well. To have this impact, the ophthalmologist must view diabetic macular edema as a systemic as well as ocular disease. This approach can facilitate collaboration with primary care physicians, diabetologists and other specialists involved in the care of persons with diabetes.

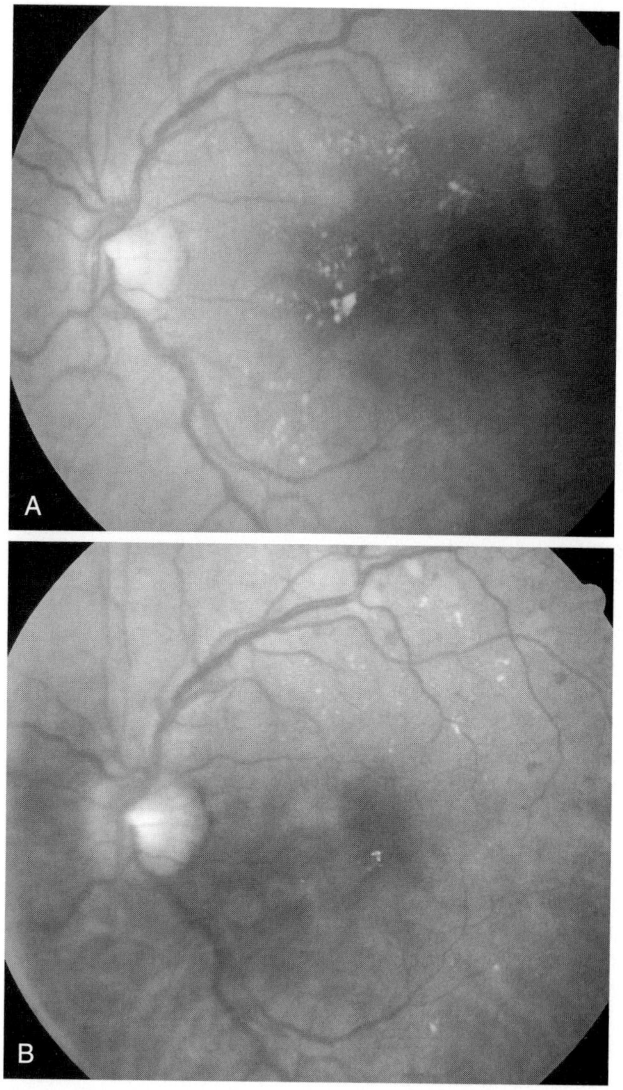

Figure 55–2. Effect of improved metabolic control on diffuse macular edema. *A*. The left eye of a 47-year-old woman with poorly controlled type II diabetes (hemoglobin A_1C 12.5%), hyperlipidemia (total cholesterol 250 mg/dl), and triglycerides (542 mg/dl). Visual acuity was 20/60. Note the diffuse macular lipid exudates and thickening. *B*. The same eye 9 months later when the patient's cholesterol level was 200 mg/dl, her triglycerides were 240 mg/dl, and her hemoglobin A_1C was 10.2%. The macular lipid exudates and thickening have almost completely regressed without photocoagulation and visual acuity is 20/30.

OCULAR TREATMENT

The ETDRS[12] established the role of macular photocoagulation for patients with "clinically significant macular edema." *Clinically significant* macular edema is defined as "retinal thickening at or within 500 microns of the center of the macula, hard exudate at or within 500 microns of the center of the macula associated with retinal thickening, or retinal thickening one disc area or larger within one disc diameter of the center of the macula." Focal laser surgery reduces the risk of moderate visual loss (doubling of the visual angle) by approximately 50%. The benefit of this treatment was independent of the initial visual acuity, from 20/20 to 20/200. Treatment involves direct ablation of microaneurysms with or without a "grid" pattern to areas of retinal thickening. Because foveal ischemia may coexist with macular edema and contribute to visual loss, and because it is associated with a worse visual prognosis, a preoperative fluorescein angiogram helps in the assessment of the foveal circulation. Patients with mild irregularity or enlargement of the foveal avascular zone may benefit from macular photocoagulation, but those with highly irregular avascular zones or greater than one disc diameter of foveal ischemia often will have less benefit, and their vision may be more likely to deteriorate after photocoagulation.

For focal treatment of diabetic macular edema, the spot size should generally range from 50 to 100 microns in diameter. The burns should be intense enough to cause light blanching of the microaneurysms or underlying pigment epithelium.[13] The power setting will necessarily be higher in patients with hazy media or light fundus pigmentation. The required power may also vary with the degree of retinal thickening. A burn duration of 0.1 second usually allows an adequate burn and is short enough to prevent spread of the lesion if the patient moves the eye. The wavelength of the laser light has not been shown to result in clinically important differences in results, despite theoretical considerations of absorption of blue-green light by macular xanthophyll pigment. The ophthalmologist should try to treat all of the detectable sites of leakage but avoid involvement of the foveal avascular zone. Two to three months may have to elapse before it is possible to determine the response of an eye to macular photocoagulation, and if clinically significant thickening remains after 3 to 6 months, then additional treatment is probably indicated. In eyes that have coexisting proliferative diabetic retinopathy or severe nonproliferative retinopathy, panretinal photocoagulation may be applied concurrently. If the risk of immediate severe visual loss from vitreous hemorrhage appears low, then it is probably reasonable to apply macular photocoagulation first. Eyes that have vitreous hemorrhage or active neovascularization, however, may be treated with concurrent panretinal and macular photocoagulation. Panretinal photocoagulation improves retinal vascular autoregulation[14] and macular edema in selected cases.[15] Panretinal photocoagulation applied initially in the midperiphery and then to the more posterior retina if needed is associated with a lower risk of macular edema than panretinal photocoagulation applied to the entire retina simultaneously.[16]

This discussion points out that diabetic macular edema is often multifactorial in origin, so effective treatment should include consideration of both systemic and ocular factors.

REFERENCES

1. Klein R, Klein BEK: Vision disorders in diabetes. In National Diabetes Data Group: Diabetes in America, 2nd Edition. Bethesda, MD: National Institutes of Health. NIH Publication 95-1465, 1995:293–338.
2. Kristinsson JK, Gottfredsdottir MS, Stefansson EA: Retinal vessel dilatation and elongation precedes diabetic macular oedema. Br J Ophthalmol 1997;81:274.
3. Klein R, Klein BEK, Moss SE, et al.: Is blood pressure a predictor of the incidence or progression of diabetic retinopathy? Arch Intern Med 1989;149:2427.
4. Chew EY, Klein ML, Ferriss FL III, et al.: Association of elevated serum lipid levels with retinal hard exudates in diabetic retinopathy. Early Treatment Diabetic Retinopathy Study Group (ETDRS) Report 22. Arch Ophthalmol 1996;114:1079.
5. Diabetes Control and Complications Trial Research Group: Progression of retinopathy with intensive versus conventional treatment in the Diabetes Control and Complications Trial. Ophthalmology 1995;102:647.
6. Klein R, Moss SE, Klein BEK: Is gross proteinuria a risk factor for the incidence of proliferative diabetic retinopathy? Ophthalmology 1993;100:1140.
7. Benson WE, Brown GC, Tasman W, et al.: Extracapsular cataract extraction with placement of a posterior chamber lens in patients with diabetic retinopathy. Ophthalmology 1993;100:730.
8. Meyers SM: Macular edema after scatter laser photocoagulation for proliferative diabetic retinopathy. Am J Ophthalmol 1980;90:210.
9. Diabetes Control and Complications Trial Research Group: The effect of intensive treatment of diabetes on the development and progression of long-term complications in insulin-dependent diabetes mellitus. N Engl J Med 1993;329:977.
10. Parving H-H: Initiation and progression of diabetic nephropathy. N Engl J Med 1996;335:1682-3.
11. Expert Panel on Detection, Evaluation, and Treatment of High Blood Cholesterol in Adults: Summary of the second report of the National Cholesterol Education Program (NCEP) Expert Panel on Detection, Evaluation, and Treatment of High Blood Cholesterol in Adults (Adult Treatment Panel II). JAMA 1993;269:3015.
12. Early Treatment Diabetic Retinopathy Study Research Group: Photocoagulation for macular edema. ETRDR Report 1. Arch Ophthalmol 1985;103:1796.
13. Early Treatment Diabetic Retinopathy Study Research Group: Treatment techniques and clinical guidelines for photocoagulation of diabetic macular edema. ETDRS Report 2. Ophthalmology 1987;94:761.
14. Grunwald JE, Brucker AJ, Petrig BL, et al.: Retinal blood flow regulation and the clinical response to PRP in proliferative diabetic retinopathy. Ophthalmology 1989;96:1518.
15. Gardner TW, Eller AW, Friberg TR: Reduction of severe macular edema in eyes with poor vision after panretinal photocoagulation for proliferative diabetic retinopathy. Graefe's Arch Clin Exp Ophthalmol 1991:229:323.
16. Blankenship GW: A clinical comparison of central and peripheral argon laser panretinal photocoagulation for proliferative diabetic retinopathy. Ophthalmology 1988;95:170.

CHAPTER 56

Retinal Detachment

CARL D. REGILLO, M.D., F.A.C.S. and WILLIAM E. BENSON, M.D.

PRIMARY RETINAL DETACHMENT

A primary retinal detachment is a rhegmatogenous (Greek *rhegma:* break) detachment that is spontaneous in nature and not the result of an exogenous force such as trauma or a specific underlying retinal disease process such as diabetic retinopathy. In the general population, such detachments occur with a frequency of approximately 1 in 10,000 persons per year.[1–4] Current options for management of uncomplicated primary retinal detachment will be discussed in this chapter.

PREOPERATIVE EVALUATION—POSTERIOR VITREOUS DETACHMENT

The possibility of retinal detachment should be considered in any patient complaining of light flashes or "floaters," which are the symptoms of posterior vitreous detachment (PVD). When the vitreous liquefies, collapses, and moves forward, traction on the retina causes the sensation of brief flashes of light in the periphery of the visual field. Glial tissue torn free from the epipapillary area is the source of a single centrally located circular opacity called a Weiss ring.

More ominous, however, are the symptoms of vitreous hemorrhage: a myriad of small floaters or blurred vision. Retinal tears or detachment are rarely found in patients who have PVD without vitreous hemorrhage, whereas they are found in approximately two thirds of those with vitreous hemorrhage.[5–9] Up to 50% of cases have more than one tear.[10]

Although nearly all retinal detachments are preceded by PVD, 50% of all patients have no symptoms prior to the visual field loss or decreased visual acuity caused by the detachment itself.[10–12]

Anterior Findings

The intraocular pressure is usually lower in an eye with retinal detachment (RD) than it is in the fellow eye.[13–15] In patients with glaucoma, an unexpected drop in intraocular pressure may signify that retinal detachment is present. On the other hand, a few patients with long-standing detachments have increased intraocular pressure (with or without cells in the anterior chamber), and are often mistakenly treated for uveitis or glaucoma.[16–18] When the RD is found and repaired, the intraocular pressure often returns to normal.

Clumps of pigment ("tobacco dust" appearance) in the vitreous of patients without previous ocular surgery are virtually pathognomonic of a retinal tear or detachment.[19,20]

Media opacities such as cataract and cortical remnants may interfere with surgery, influencing the surgeon to do a vitrectomy rather than a scleral buckling procedure or a pneumatic retinopexy. If the pupil will not dilate, the surgeon can plan to use iris hooks.

Differential Diagnosis

The most common entities that are confused with rhegmatogenous retinal detachment are intraocular neoplasms with or without secondary RD, inflammatory diseases such as Harada's disease and posterior scleritis, idiopathic central serous chorioretinopathy with bullous RD, RD caused by an optic pit, traction RD caused by diabetic retinopathy, juvenile and senile retinoschisis, and choroidal detachment. The differential diagnosis of RD is beyond the scope of this chapter and has been covered elsewhere.[21]

Indirect Ophthalmoscopy

We use the 20 diopter large, aspheric lens, which is easy to use and provides adequate magnification (2.3×). In patients with small pupils, some surgeons prefer the 28 or 30 diopter lenses. The lens is held with the more convex surface toward the observer and is tilted to move the light reflexes away from the center of the lens (Fig. 56–1).

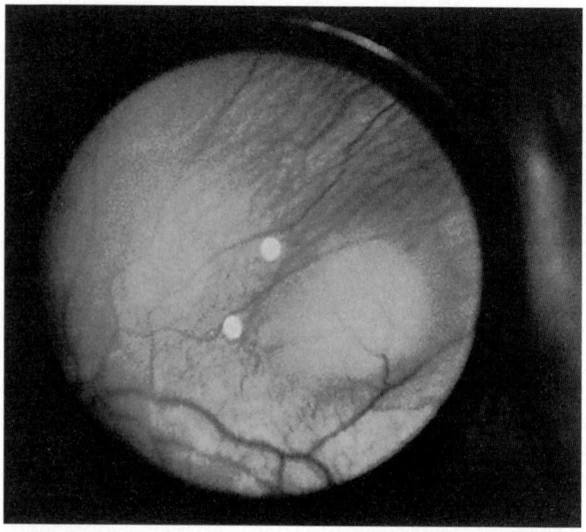

Figure 56–1. The lens is slightly tilted to separate the light reflections on its surface. (Courtesy of Dr. Jerry Shields.)

The patient should be reclining comfortably for the examination. Bilateral cycloplegia combined with topical anesthesia reduces photopsia and enhances cooperation. Bell's phenomenon is avoided if the patient keeps both eyes open. A fixation target, such as the patient's own thumb or a mark on the ceiling, is helpful (Fig. 56–2).

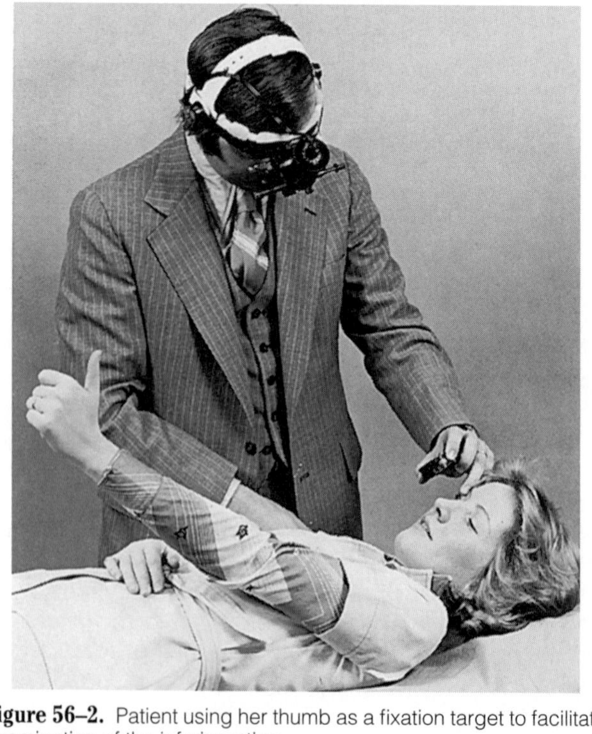

Figure 56–2. Patient using her thumb as a fixation target to facilitate examination of the inferior retina.

The superior periphery should be examined first, because patients with photophobia find it easier to look up than down and because the periphery is less sensitive to light than is the posterior pole. Initially the transformer rheostat should be set at a low voltage. Higher light intensities can be used later as the patient becomes less light sensitive.

The ophthalmologist performing the examination should hold his head so that he looks directly into the quadrant being examined. To examine the temporal periphery, he should stand on the side opposite the eye being examined (Fig. 56–3); for the nasal periphery, on the same side (Fig. 56–4). To avoid awkward maneuvering, especially during scleral depression, the exam-

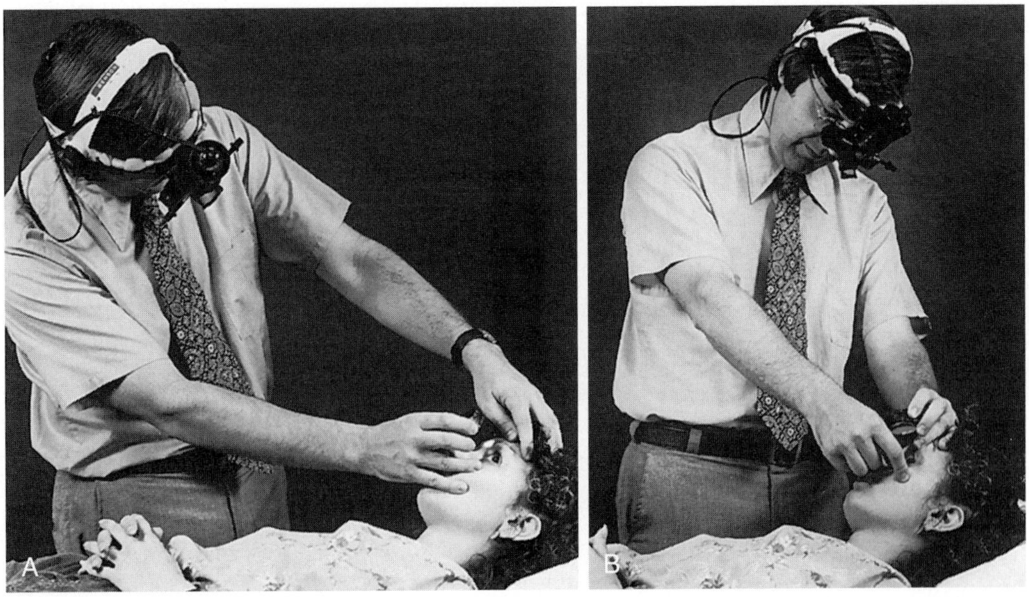

Figure 56–3. *A*. Examination of the left eye, superotemporal periphery. The lens is held in the examiner's right hand. The patient looks up and to the left. *B*. Examination of the left eye, inferotemporal periphery. The lens is held in the examiner's left hand. The patient looks down and to the left.

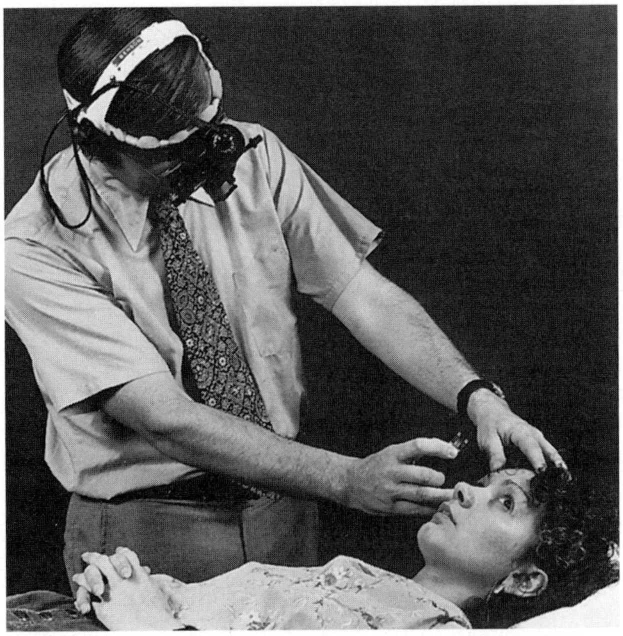

Figure 56–4. Examination of the right eye, superonasal periphery. The lens is held in the examiner's right hand. The patient looks up and to the left.

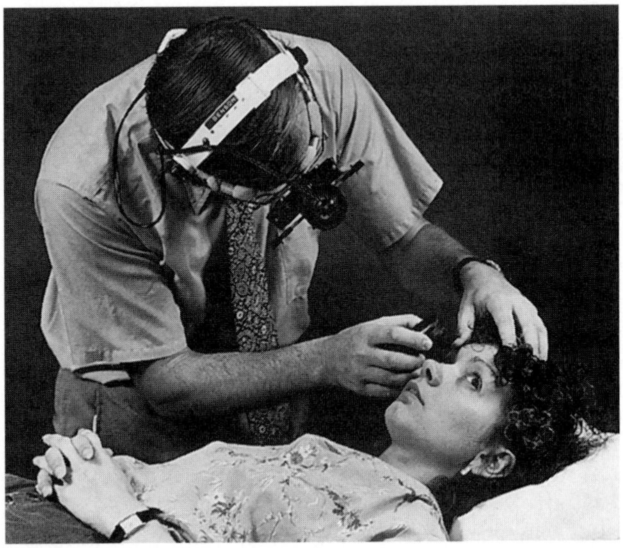

Figure 56–5. Examiner standing too close to the patient. Focusing is difficult, and it is difficult to get sufficient light into the eye while viewing the fundus.

iner should shift the hand lens from the right to left hand as necessary. The patient's nose becomes less of an obstacle to viewing the temporal periphery when the patient rolls his head toward the observer while looking temporally.

Beginners frequently make the error of standing too close to the patient (Fig. 56–5). It is much easier for the examiner to obtain a clear fundus image if the arm holding the lens is extended. This is especially important if the pupil is small.

A detailed drawing of the fundus should be made. Such drawings may help the ophthalmologist locate the retinal tears during surgery if the media become opaque or if the pupil constricts. Retinal hemorrhages, pigment, blood vessels, and folds should all be represented in the drawing.

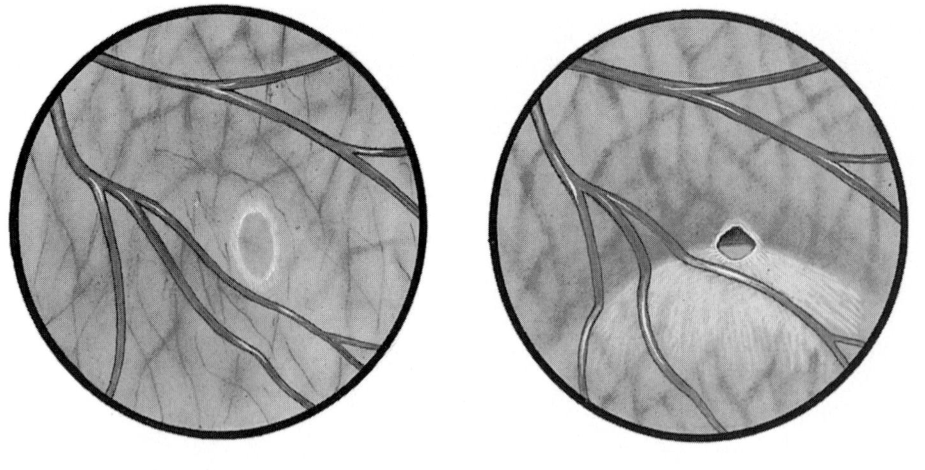

Figure 56–6. *Left,* A retinal break that can barely be seen because of little contrast between the retina and the underlying choroid. *Right,* Scleral depression darkens the underlying choroid. The break is more easily seen as dark spot. Also, the posterior edge of the break is more easily seen because it is viewed at a more acute angle.

There are two ways to correct for the inverted image of the indirect ophthalmoscope. The first is to observe the retina, then mentally correct for the inverted image, drawing the findings as they are, not as they are seen. The second method is to invert the drawing pad and then to draw the findings as they are seen. When the drawing is finished, the findings will be correctly positioned.

After the limits of the detachment have been sketched, all retinal breaks must be found.[22] To this end, the examiner may start at the optic nerve and follow each of the retinal vessels to the periphery. A scanning technique should also be used. Keeping his eyes and the hand lens aligned, the examiner swings his gaze along the periphery, examining 90 degrees of retina in one swing.

Scleral Depression

All patients are examined with scleral depression preoperatively except those who have had recent intraocular surgery. At retinal detachment surgery, any recently created surgical wounds can be inspected and reinforced if needed before the scleral depressed examination. Scleral depression helps in three ways to detect small breaks. First, it increases the contrast between the intact retina and the break; the indented choroid retinal epithelium being darker than the unindented choroid/retinal pigment epithelium and darker still than the intact retina. The break then appears as a dark spot (Fig. 56–6). Second, as the depressor tilts the retina downward, the retina appears more opaque because it is seen at a more acute angle. This increases the contrast between the hole and the retina and makes the hole more visible. Also, as the examiner looks at a more acute angle, he or she can sometimes see the posterior edge of a break (Fig. 56–6). Third, the flaps of tiny breaks at the posterior vitreous base can sometimes be seen as the eye is indented. In all cases, constant movement of the scleral depressor maximizes the chances of finding a small break.

Stretching and compressing the patient's eyelids can cause pain. Therefore, because the upper lid is looser and more flexible than the lower, scleral depression should be started superiorly. We ask the patient to look down, place the depressor near the lid margin (Fig. 56–7), and then follow the eyelid up as the patient is asked to look up (Fig. 56–8). Again, if the depressor is held vertically, it should be easy to locate the indentation on the inside of the eye. If the indentation is not readily seen, the beginner should make a scanning movement from side to side. If the indentation is still not seen, he should begin all over again. If the ora serrata is to be viewed, the patient should be asked to look as far superiorly as possible (Fig. 56–8). Beginners will see the ora serrata most easily in highly myopic eyes. If areas posterior to the equator are to be examined, the patient must look slightly inferiorly (Fig. 56–9).

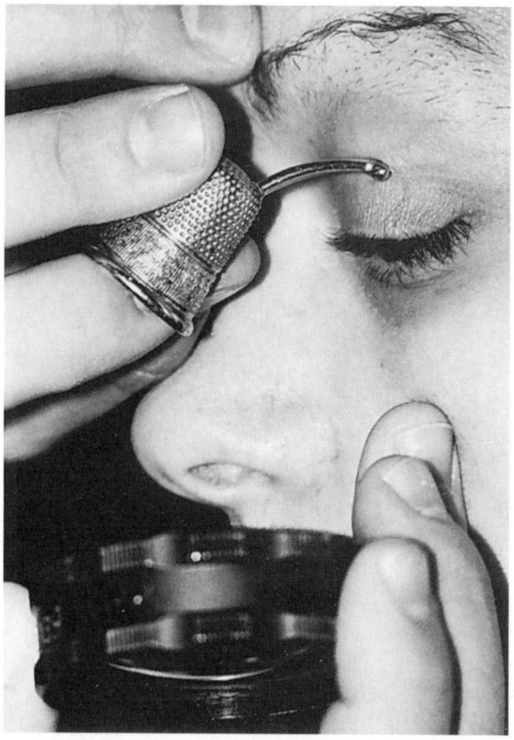

Figure 56–7. Scleral depression of the superior retina. The patient looks down, and the depressor is placed on the lid fold.

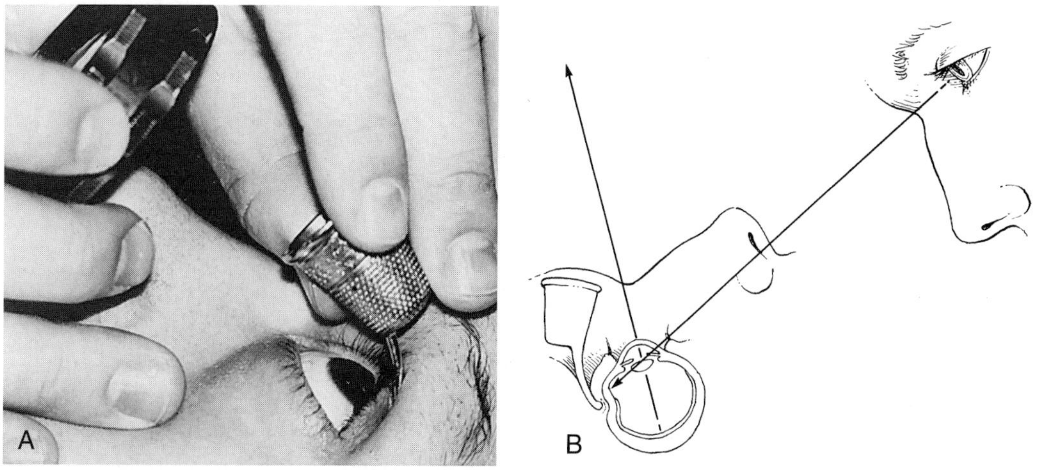

Figure 56–8. *A.* Scleral depression of the ora serrata of the superior retina. *B.* Viewing the ora serrata. The patient looks up as far as possible.

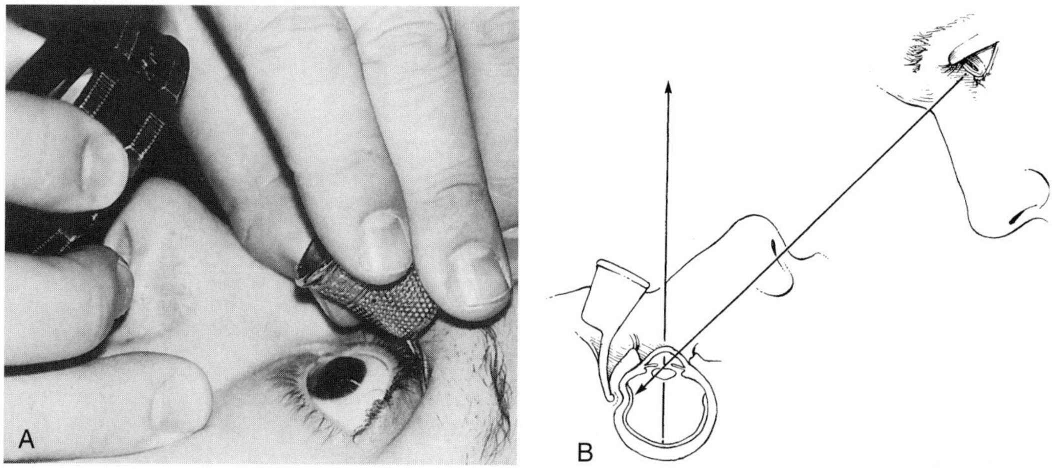

Figure 56–9. *A.* Examination of the midperiphery. The patient looks downward. *B.* Viewing the midperiphery.

Scleral depression is most difficult at the 9 o'clock and 3 o'clock positions because the canthal ligaments resist posterior movement of the depressor. Direct scleral depression at the canthus is painful. Moreover, the depressor may slip off the eyelid and strike the patient's eye. The following techniques help to avoid these problems. First, the depressor is placed on the superior eyelid down to the horizontal meridian (Fig. 56–10). The lid becomes more slack when the patient, his head rolled away from the examiner, is not looking into an extreme position of gaze. Second, a cotton-tipped applicator, being blunter and softer than the scleral depressor, may be better tolerated. Finally, after topical anesthesia, one can easily depress directly on the conjunctiva (Fig. 56–11).

After a thorough examination by indirect ophthalmoscopy and scleral depression, we sometimes use the slit lamp and the Goldmann three-mirror lens to search for small breaks and to evaluate vitreous traction. Finally, because the bilateral incidence of retinal detachment in phakic eyes is approximately 10%, it is essential that the fellow eye be carefully examined for retinal breaks or other abnormalities that might require prophylactic treatment.

PREOPERATIVE MANAGEMENT

It has been shown that emergency late-night surgery for retinal detachment does not result in better surgical results than does surgery performed the next day.[23,24] However, because detachment of the macula may lead to permanent visual loss, when the detachment is close to the center of the macula, surgery on the day the patient presents is sometimes recommended. If the macula has been detached for less than a day, surgery is nearly always done on the next day, as prompt retinal reattachment can often restore much of the central vision. There is essentially no difference in the visual result if the macula has been detached for 2 to 7 days, so waiting a day or two does not make a difference.[23,24] If the macula has been detached for more than 2 to 7 days, there is considerably less urgency, but surgery should be done within a few days. If the macula has been detached for more than a week, the timing of the surgical repair is still less critical.[25–27]

In patients who will be undergoing lengthy surgical procedures, a careful medical examination is important. Some retinal detachment procedures last 2 or more

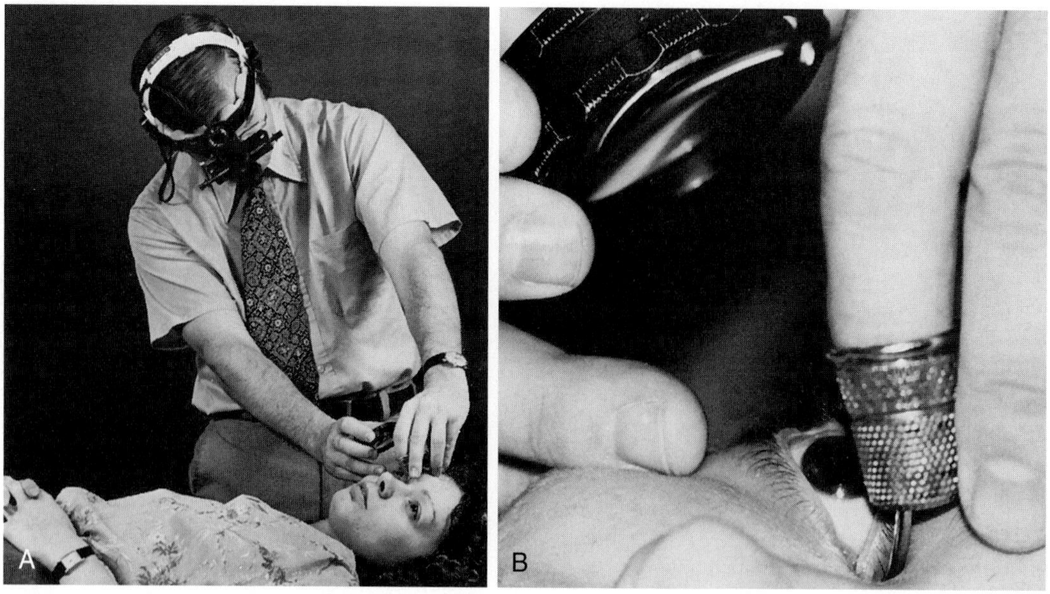

Figure 56–10. *A.* Scleral depression of the horizontal meridian. The patient rolls her head away from the examiner and looks straight ahead. *B.* The eyelid is pushed down so that the horizontal periphery can be examined.

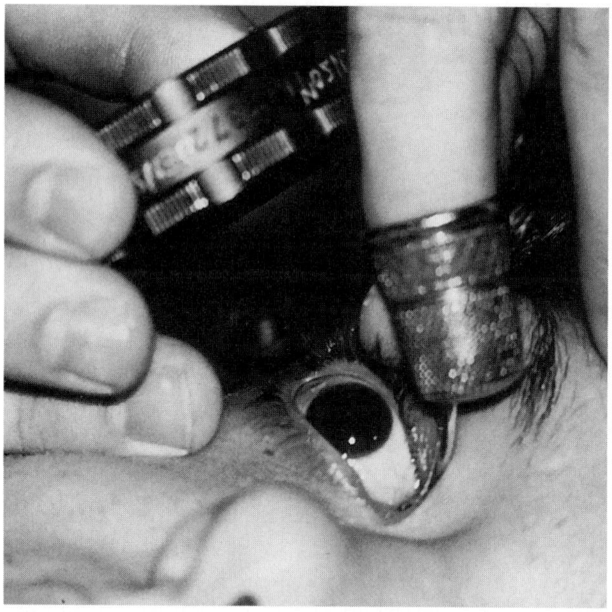

Figure 56–11. After topical anesthesia, one can easily depress directly on the conjunctiva.

hours and may be performed under general anesthesia. Allergic reactions must also be avoided.

SCLERAL BUCKLING PROCEDURES

Ernst Custodis made a great contribution to retinal detachment surgery when he introduced the scleral buckling procedure. He sutured a synthetic material onto the sclera to "buckle" (indent) it toward the retinal breaks. The goal is to indent the sclera and choroid enough to closely reapproximate the edges of the retinal tear to the retinal pigment epithelium. The first benefit of scleral buckling is that it makes retinal reattachment possible without the necessity of draining subretinal fluid. The "buckle" reduces vitreous traction and vitreous currents, so that even if the retinal break is not closed at the time of surgery, it will often settle onto the buckle later. When the retinal break is closed, the remainder of the subretinal fluid is absorbed.

The second benefit of scleral buckling is that it reduces strong vitreous traction, which impedes the development of a firm chorioretinal scar. Even after thorough drainage of subretinal fluid plus proper treatment with cryotherapy or diathermy, unrelieved vitreous traction can reopen a retinal break before the sealing scar has developed. Custodis's scleral buckle allows the scar to form.

ANESTHESIA

Local anesthesia has three advantages: total operating-room time is decreased, the patient recovers quickly postoperatively, and operative morbidity and mortality are slightly decreased. Disadvantages include possible retrobulbar hemorrhage, central retinal artery occlusion, respiratory arrest, and more difficult exposure during surgery. In addition, the patient may experience pain during the procedure, may become disoriented and restless if over-sedated, and may have discomfort from having to lie still during a long procedure. Obviously, the choice is individualized depending on the patient and the projected complexity of surgery. We perform about three quarters of our scleral buckles with local anesthesia.

OPENING

In primary operations, the peritomy can be made either at the limbus or 3 to 5 mm from it. Between two rectus muscles and near the limbus, the conjunctiva and Tenon`s capsule are tented up with toothed forceps and are incised with blunt scissors down to the sclera (Fig. 56–12). Blunt dissection separates Tenon's capsule from the sclera so that a 360-degree incision can be made (Fig. 56–13). When a single radial sponge is to be placed, a 180-degree incision suffices. Two relaxing incisions, 180 degrees apart, serve to avoid tearing the conjunctiva (Fig. 56–14). Additional blunt dissection is used posteriorly to further separate Tenon's capsule from the sclera so that the muscles can be hooked and bridled. A 4-0 black silk suture is passed under the muscle and tied. Before proceeding further, the surgeon must search the sclera for thinning or staphylomas. In the rare cases in which adequate exposure cannot be obtained, a lateral canthotomy is performed, and one or more muscles are disinserted. A traction suture is placed into the stump of the tendon.

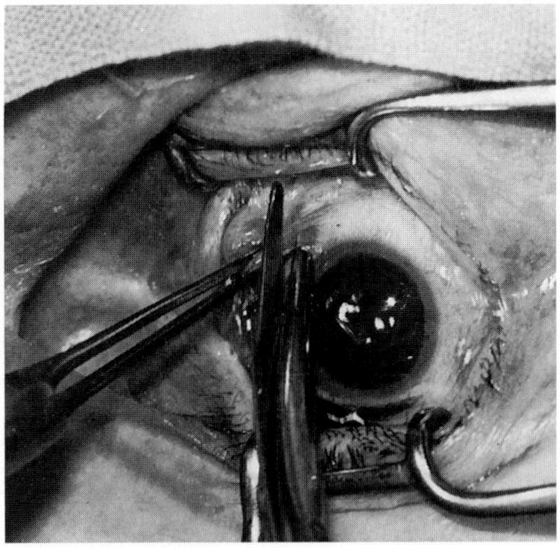

Figure 56–14. Radial relaxing incision.

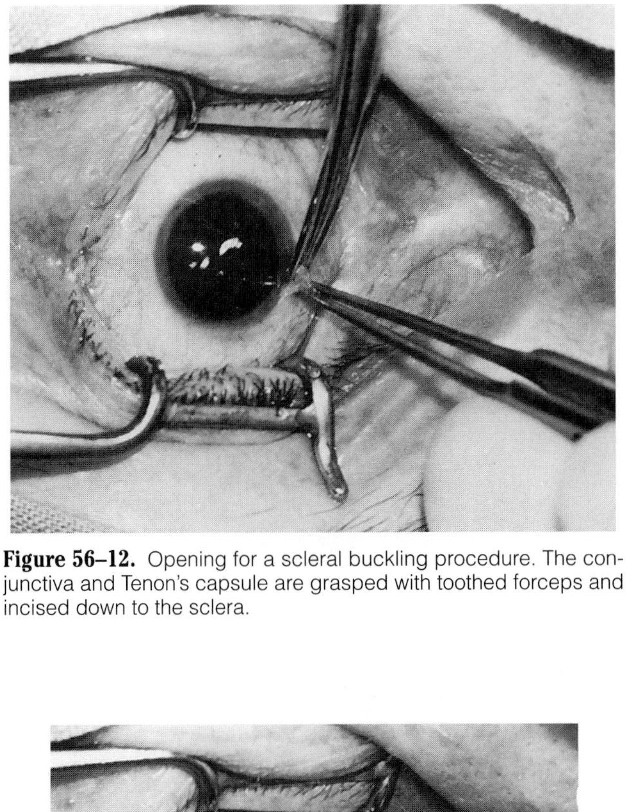

Figure 56–12. Opening for a scleral buckling procedure. The conjunctiva and Tenon's capsule are grasped with toothed forceps and incised down to the sclera.

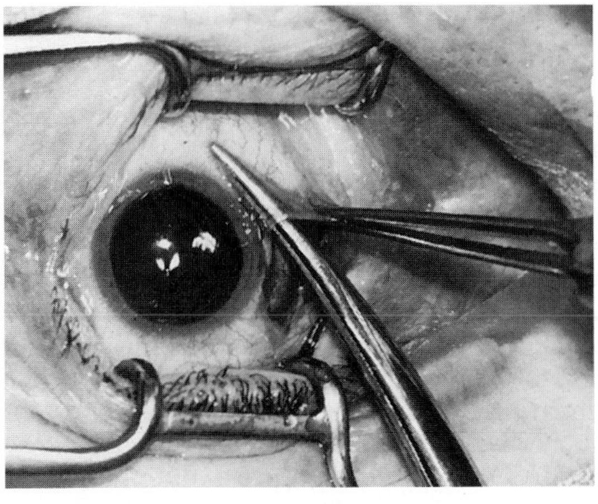

Figure 56–13. Blunt dissection to free Tenon's capsule from the episclera.

LOCALIZATION OF THE BREAK(S)

To place the scleral buckle correctly, the surgeon must localize all breaks within the detachment (i.e., the sclera underlying each break must be marked). We localize with a blunt-tipped diathermy electrode. First, the intensity of the diathermy is tested on anterior sclera. The assistant then steadies the eye by holding two bridle sutures while the surgeon, using a cotton-tipped applicator for scleral depression, locates the meridian of the break. The diathermy electrode is introduced into this meridian and is used to localize the breaks precisely under indirect ophthalmoscopic control (Fig. 56–15*A* and *B*). The surgeon cocks his wrist to ensure that only the tip of the instrument indents the sclera. A few gentle applications of diathermy are made on the sclera underlying the retinal break. The eye is then rolled forward and additional diathermy is applied to make a permanent mark.

For small breaks, the posterior edge alone is localized; for large flap tears, the posterior edge and both anterior horns (Fig. 56–15C); for lattice degeneration with holes, both ends of the degeneration; for dialysis, the ends of the dialysis as well as the point in the center of the dialysis where the surgeon estimates that the retina will fall when the subretinal fluid is drained or is absorbed. Anterior and posterior localization of long tears is important, because many are not radial in direction.

If either a staphyloma or very thin sclera is present in the area of the hole, the diathermy technique is dangerous because the electrode may penetrate the globe. Instead, the surgeon can use the blunt end of a cotton-tipped applicator or can make a mark in thicker adjacent sclera. Once the apparent breaks have been localized, the retina should be examined once again for any

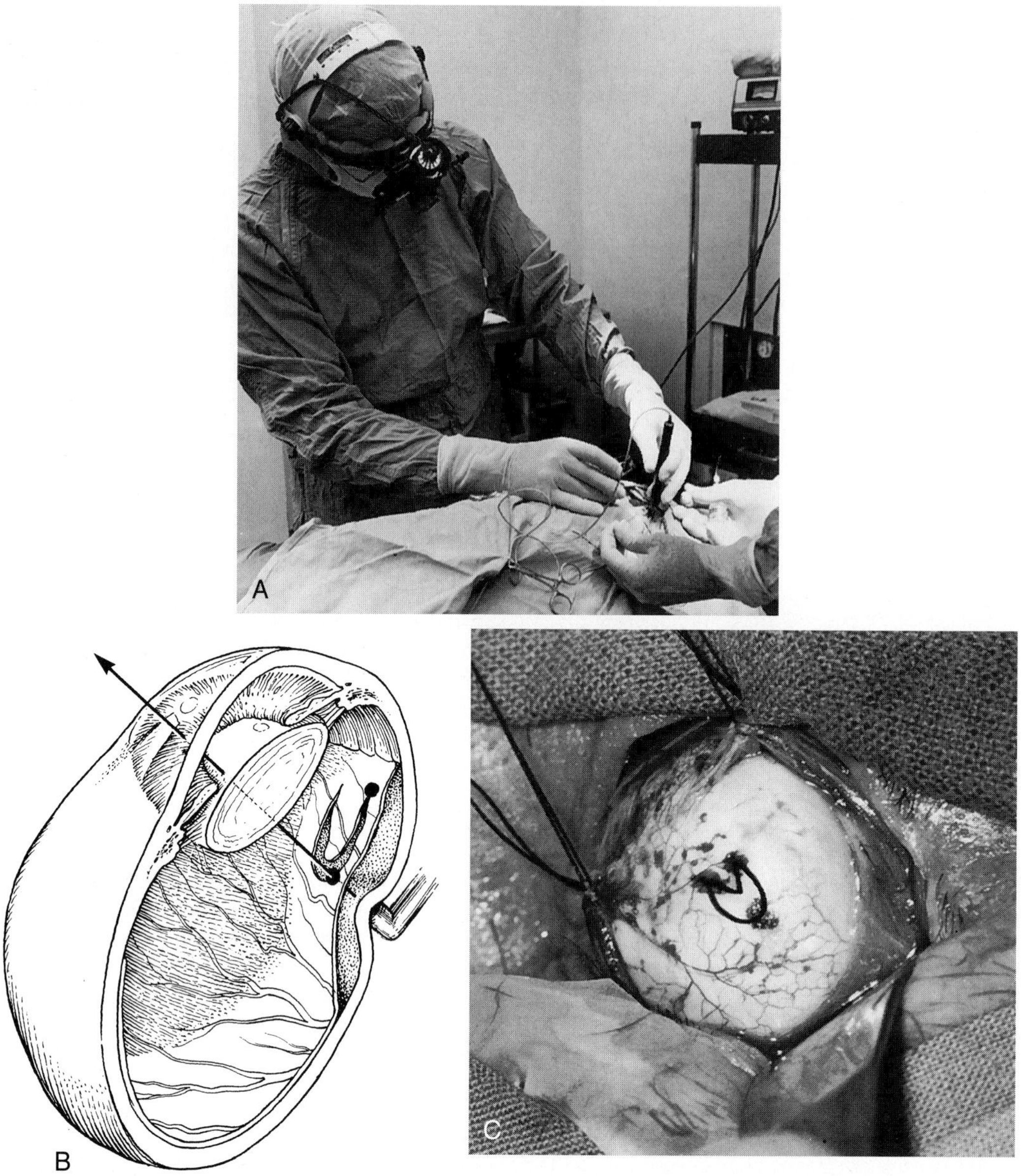

Figure 56–15. *A.* Using the blunt diathermy probe, the surgeon indents and marks the sclera under the retinal break. *B.* The localizing instrument, functioning as a scleral depressor, is slid posteriorly under indirect ophthalmoscopic control until the surgeon determines that the apex has been reached. He marks the sclera at this point. *C.* Localizing marks on the sclera overlying both anterior horns and the apex of a flap tear. (Methylene blue has been dabbed on the marks for purposes of illustration.)

overlooked break. A cotton-tipped applicator serves as a scleral depressor for this final check, which is especially important if the preoperative examination has been difficult.

CRYOTHERAPY

When the retina is too highly elevated for laser photocoagulation, most retinal surgeons use cryotherapy to make a firm adhesion between the retina and the retinal pigment epithelium or Bruch's membrane.[28–30] Some surgeons believe that an adequate adhesion results from cryotherapy of the pigment epithelium surrounding a break, even if the overlying detached retina is not frozen. Experimental evidence indicates, however, that such treatment results in a relationship between the sensory retina and the pigment epithelium similar to the relatively weak adhesion found in eyes without detachment.[31] A histopathologically strong adhesion results when the pigment epithelium and the sensory retina are both frozen during treatment, for tight junctions are later seen between Muller cells and the pigment epithelium or Bruch's membrane.[31,32]

The pressure of the cryoprobe on the sclera forces fluid from the eye. As the eye softens, high indentation by the probe is possible. Therefore, breaks in attached retina should be frozen first; breaks in highly detached retina, last. As the assistant steadies the eye with the rectus muscle bridle sutures, the surgeon, viewing with the indirect ophthalmoscope (Fig. 56–16), surrounds the tears with 2 to 3 mm of retinal freezing to ensure adequate adhesion. It is important that the surgeon keep his wrist cocked outward so that only the tip of the cryoprobe indents the eye. Beginners tend to indent the eye with the shaft of the probe, which may cause severe posterior freezing to occur beyond the areas of visualization. Most cryoprobes have a small knob 180 degrees away from the freezing tip to aid the surgeon in orienting the probe. The freezing portion of the tip must be pressed squarely against the globe. After the first application, the surgeon waits for the iceball to thaw, and then, watching retinal landmarks, gently slides the probe sufficiently to place the next contiguous lesion. Obviously, freezing the pigment epithelium within the hole does not increase the strength of the adhesion. Such freezing only releases more pigment into the vitreous, increasing postoperative glare and possibly contributing to proliferative vitreoretinopathy.[33,34]

The firmer the indentation, the faster the rate of freezing, because choroidal blood flow (an insulator) is stopped. If a break is so highly elevated that the retina cannot be frozen, the surgeon should not indent excessively or try to reach the retina with a huge ice ball, but should wait until the subretinal fluid has been drained before applying the cryotherapy.

When the sensory retina has been frozen, it becomes slightly opaque, helping the surgeon to verify that the treatment applications have been contiguous. Scleral depression makes this opacity easier to see. The opaqueness also aids in differentiating small retinal breaks from small patches of thin retina. Normal and thin retina both turn white where frozen. Full-thickness retinal breaks appear dark in contrast to the adjacent frozen retina.

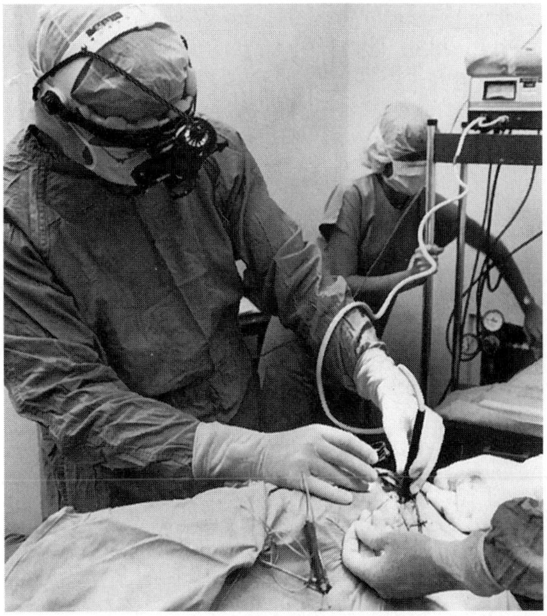

Figure 56–16. Cryotherapy of a retinal tear under direct visualization.

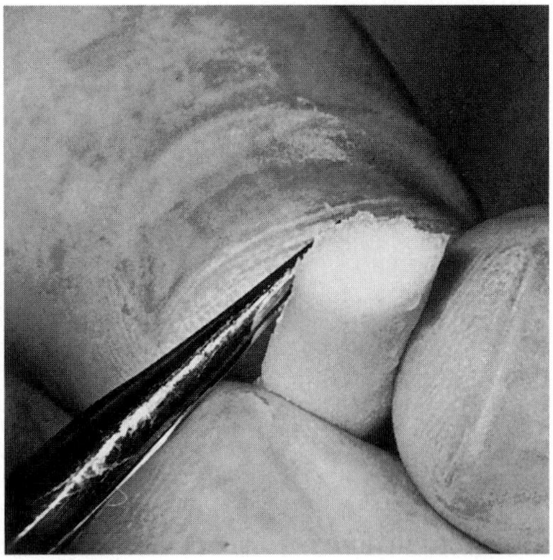

Figure 56–17. The sponge is cut in half lengthwise to reduce its bulk.

PLACEMENT OF THE SCLERAL BUCKLE

Explant Materials

Explants may be radial (perpendicular to the ora serrata) or circumferential (parallel to the ora serrata). All explant material currently in use is made of silicone. There are two varieties, silicone sponge and solid silicone. Both come in a large variety of sizes and shapes. We usually trim sponges to a height of 2 to 3 mm to reduce their bulk (Fig. 56–17).

Suture Technique

Mattress sutures of 5-0 monofilament nylon hold explants in place. Thinner sutures tend to erode out of the sclera. The assistant provides exposure and steadies the globe by gently pulling on the bridle sutures adjacent to the break and by holding back Tenon's capsule with a Fisher or a Schepens retractor. The surgeon further prevents movements of the globe by grasping the tendon of a rectus muscle. It is difficult to place deep scleral sutures in a hypotonic eye without accidental penetration of the choroid. If the eye is soft, the assistant must increase the pressure to a nearly normal level by gentle indentation. If the break is located under a rectus muscle, the assistant can aid in the placement of sutures by retracting the muscle with a muscle hook. Alternatively, a circumferential explant can be used instead of a radial one.

Scleral bites should be both deep and long, so that the suture will not erode out of the sclera postoperatively. A spatula needle must be used. Its tip is introduced slowly into the sclera. When the proper depth has been reached, the needle is carefully pushed along between scleral lamellae. Proper depth can be verified by gently lifting the needle while keeping it parallel to the sclera. The needle must not be allowed to lose its depth, because it is difficult and dangerous to regain depth once it has been lost.

Radial Explants

Silicone sponge is usually used for radial explants. They are preferred over circumferential explants for closing wide horseshoe tears because the latter often cause fishmouthing of the break's posterior edge (see below).[35,36] In addition, for very posterior breaks, it is easier to place the sutures necessary for a radial explant than those required for a circumferential explant.

The indentation of the radial buckle should extend 1 to 2 mm beyond the margins of the break. A 5-mm sponge will adequately close a break 3 mm wide; a 7.5 × 5.5 mm sponge, a break 5-mm wide. Larger breaks are treated with a circumferential explant or by vitrectomy and gas. The height of the indentation is determined not only by the diameter of the explant but also by the distance between the arms of the mattress suture. How tightly the mattress suture is tied is also important. We place the arms of the suture 1 mm further apart than the width of the sponge (Fig. 56–18). For small breaks, one suture is adequate. For larger ones, two are needed. To reduce the risk of the fishmouth phenomenon (see below), we begin the posterior bite at the level of the apex of the tear and carry it 3 mm posteriorly. The anterior suture starts 2 mm anterior to the horns of the tear.

Circumferential Explants

Circumferential explants can be either sponge or solid silicone. They are indicated for wide retinal breaks, for multiple breaks at different distances from the ora serrata (Fig. 56–19), and for detachments in which no break is found. The sutures are asymmetrically placed so that the hole will lie on the crest or anterior slope of the buckle. The posterior bite of the mattress suture usually must be made 4 mm posterior to the localizing mark of the apex of the tear. The anterior bite is 1 mm anterior to the anterior marks. The width of the explant is 2 mm less than the width of the mattress.

Encircling Procedures

The introduction of silicone bands for encircling procedures is one of Schepens' many contributions to retinal surgery.[35–39] A silicone band or sponge is used to encircle and constrict the eye to permanently reduce vitreous traction. Encircling is indicated if there is evidence of early proliferative vitreoretinopathy, such as fixed folds or strong vitreous traction. Encircling can also be used when no break is found. In these cases, the posterior vitreous base is treated with cryotherapy for the whole length of the detached retina and is buckled with an encircling silicone band. Pseudophakic retinal detachments usually are treated with encircling, both because of their higher incidence of proliferative vitreoretinopathy and because they characteristically have small breaks, some of which may be missed.

The encircling element, usually a 2-mm-wide silicone band, is anchored to the sclera by mattress sutures (Fig. 56–20). The ends are tied with a suture or with a Watzke sleeve. If additional indentation is needed (e.g., to close large breaks), solid silicone or sponge explants are placed under the encircling band. The surgeon should try to obtain an encircling indentation of 1 to 2 mm. Excessive indentation may cause severe postoperative pain or anterior segment necrosis.

DRAINAGE OF SUBRETINAL FLUID

Despite its complications, drainage of subretinal fluid must be performed in some cases. Eyes with poor retinal circulation, staphylomatous sclera, or recent intraocular surgery require a drainage procedure because the indentation of the scleral buckle causes a rise in intraocular pressure, and this pressure rise can close the central retinal

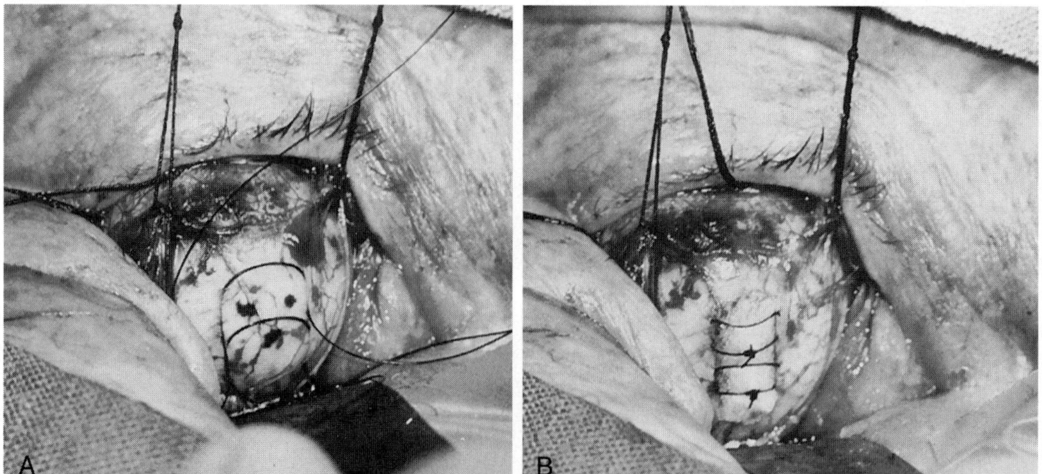

Figure 56–18. *A.* Suture placement for a flap tear. *B.* Sutures tied over the sponge.

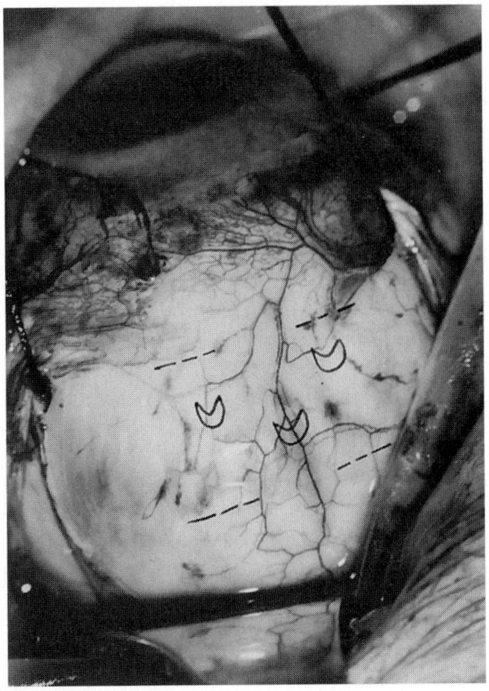

Figure 56–19. Three retinal breaks at different levels. A circumferential explant is required. Dashed lines indicate the location for the mattress sutures.

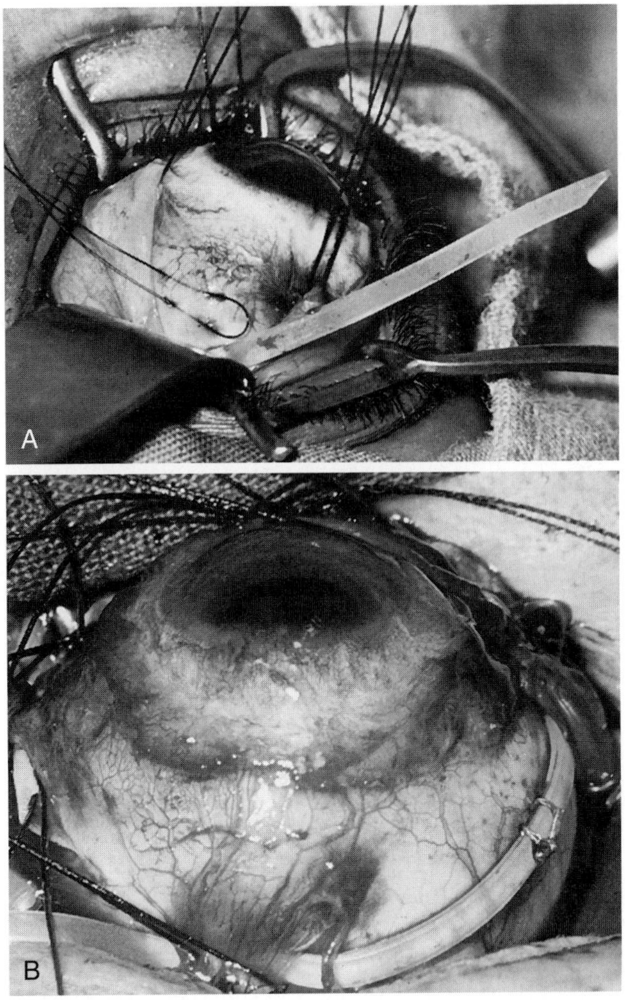

Figure 56–20. *A*. Mattress suture placed in the sclera to anchor an encircling band. *B*. Encircling band in place.

artery or rupture the globe. Drainage of the fluid softens the eye and allows it to accommodate the indentation without a precipitous rise in pressure. Because of their poor outflow facility, glaucomatous eyes also require a drainage procedure; without drainage, they may sustain damage before the intraocular pressure returns to normal. When the retinal break cannot be closed at surgery and it is apparent that vitreous traction (as in proliferative vitreoretinopathy) will prevent postoperative settling of the retina, the subretinal fluid should be drained.

Although Lincoff and others[40–43] believe that most other cases can be managed without drainage of subretinal fluid, most retinal surgeons choose to drain in a high percentage of cases.[44] The reason for this choice is that nondrainage procedures have a higher rate of reoperation.[45] Common causes of failure in nondrainage procedures are inadequate indentation, inaccurate placement of the scleral buckle, vitreous traction, and meridional folds (fishmouthing). In reoperations the risks of complication are increased: if drainage is required, the inflammation caused by the initial operation increases the likelihood of choroidal bleeding; postoperative infection and explant extrusion are more common following reoperations; the patient has to face again the danger of anesthesia and the inconvenience and psychic trauma of surgery; some patients refuse the reoperation.

Technique

Because there are few large choroidal blood vessels immediately adjacent to the rectus muscles, these are prime drainage sites. The chances of hemorrhage are further minimized if the choroid is perforated anteriorly. It is best to drain through sclera that will be buckled by the intended explant. Then, should the retina be perforated or incarcerated at the drainage site, the repair will not entail placing additional sutures in a soft eye. Drainage under a large bulla of subretinal fluid allows a good quantity of fluid to drain before the retina settles over the drainage site and closes it. It also helps to avoid retinal perforation by the drainage needle. One final consideration is that the stiff retina of a fixed fold will rarely incarcerate.

The surgeon must be especially careful with the occasional rhegmatogenous retinal detachment with shifting fluid. The fluid may move away from the selected drainage site and the retina may be perforated accidentally.[46]

It is important that the eye be normotensive for drainage. If the intraocular pressure is too high, it must be lowered by administration of mannitol, or by anterior chamber paracentesis. Otherwise, when the choroid is perforated, sudden decompression can cause choroidal hemorrhage or rapid evacuation of the subretinal fluid followed by retinal or vitreous incarceration. If the intraocular pressure is too low, the assistant must indent the eye with a cotton-tipped applicator to

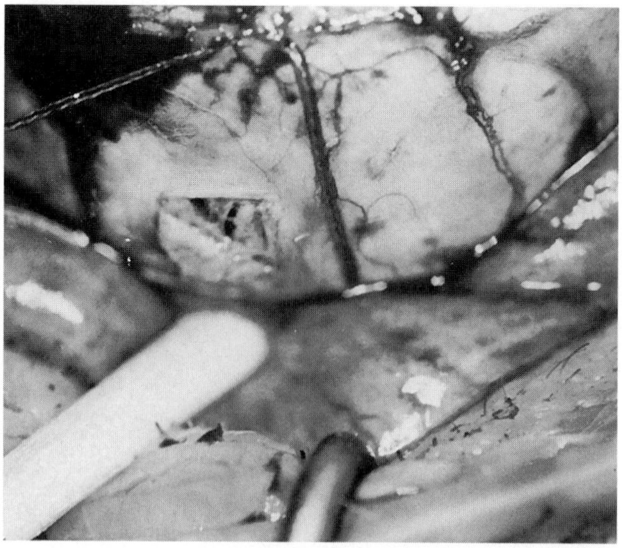

Figure 56–21. Drainage in an explant procedure. The choroid is exposed in the base of a triangular scleral flap.

restore the pressure nearly to normal, thus facilitating scleral dissection and choroidal perforation. The best drainage is obtained if no scleral fibers overlie the choroid at the drainage site.

There are many techniques for drainage of subretinal fluid. Some surgeons simply perforate the sclera and choroid with a hollow needle and observe the drainage with the indirect ophthalmoscope. In our technique, we first expose the choroid in the bed of a small triangular scleral flap (Fig. 56–21) or simply through a radial cut down. A longer cut down provides better exposure, allowing safe removal of the deep scleral fibers. The thicker the sclera, the longer the cut down should be. Prior to choroidal perforation, a suture is pre-placed for later closure. If the drainage site will be under an explant, the scleral flap or cut down is closed with an absorbable suture (Fig. 56–22) or left unsutured. If not, it should be closed with a nonabsorbable suture. Next, to further reduce the possibility of hemorrhage, the exposed choroid is treated with applications of low-intensity diathermy with a blunt conical electrode.

The choroid is then perforated with a diathermy needle electrode, a 27-gauge hypodermic needle, or a tapered suture needle. Perforation by the argon laser has also been described.[47] Prior to the perforation, the surgeon must again verify that the pressure in the eye is not elevated. A gentle thrust penetrating 2 mm is sufficient.

When the subretinal fluid begins to drain, gentle indentation of the globe away from the drainage site helps to shift subretinal fluid toward it. Excessive pressure on the eye to force out subretinal fluid must be avoided because it might cause retinal incarceration (Fig. 56–23). Traction on the edge of the scleral flap with a small forceps helps to hold the sclera and choroid away from the retina, reducing the chances of incarceration.

When little or no subretinal fluid remains, a small hemorrhage or pigment granules frequently appear at the drainage site. When the drainage stops, the fundus must be inspected to see if there is subretinal fluid over the drainage site. If there is, gentle lateral traction on the scleral flap may allow further drainage. Occasionally, another choroidal perforation is required. It is almost never necessary to drain until all of the subretinal fluid is gone or even until the break is flat on the buckle, so long as the buckle is properly placed and of adequate height. When adequate fluid has been drained, the suture over the drainage site is tied immediately. This prevents the retinal incarceration that

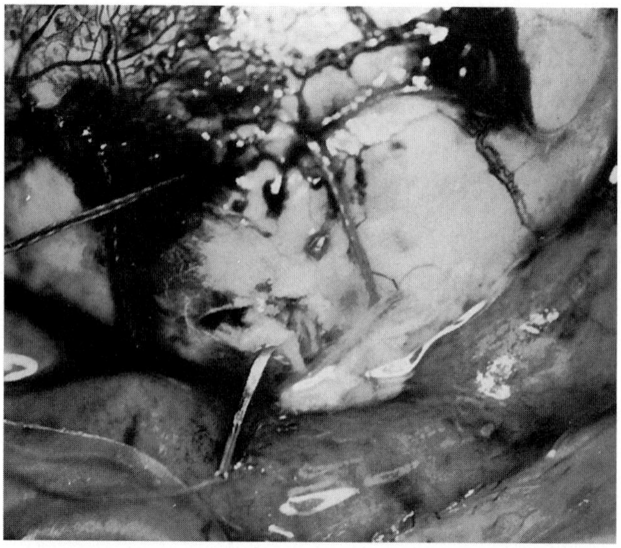

Figure 56–22. A suture is pre-placed for later closing of the drainage site.

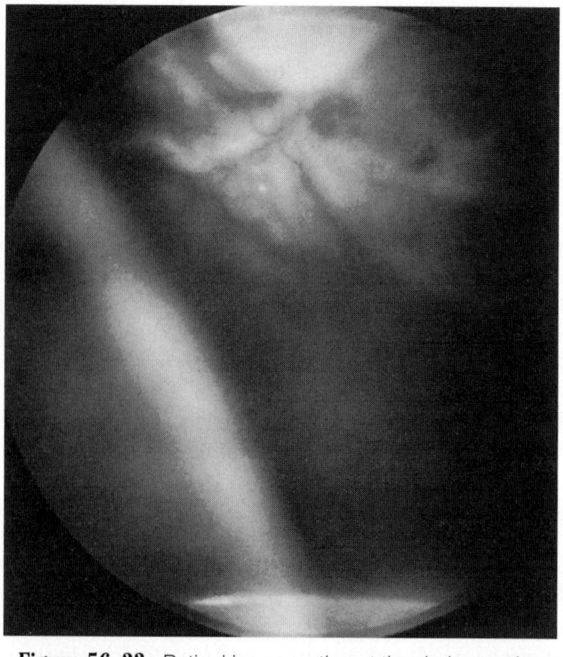

Figure 56–23. Retinal incarceration at the drainage site.

might otherwise result from a sudden elevation in intraocular pressure caused by manipulation of the globe.

Complications

Complications of drainage result in postoperative loss of vision in 1% to 2% of the cases in which it is performed. The four major complications are retinal perforation, subretinal hemorrhage, retinal incarceration, and loss of formed vitreous. A retinal break caused by the drainage instrument usually does not cause postoperative visual loss, but it does require treatment and buckling. Subretinal hemorrhage, if subfoveal, can cause permanent visual loss. Retinal incarceration can keep a nearby break open. Vitreous loss is followed by a high incidence of proliferative vitreoretinopathy (PVR).[48]

INTRAOCULAR AIR OR GAS

Tamponade of a retinal break with air or gas temporarily closes a break as effectively as a scleral buckle does. The choroid/pigment epithelium then absorbs the subretinal fluid, effecting contact between the treated retinal pigment epithelium and the sensory retina, allowing formation of a firm chorioretinal scar. Intraocular air or gas is also useful in treating tears showing the fishmouthing phenomenon. In some cases in which drainage of subretinal fluid is attempted near large tears, liquid vitreous can pass through the tear and out of the eye. The eye becomes very soft, but the amount of fluid under the retina remains the same. In these cases, we close the drainage site, place the scleral buckle, and inject air or gas to tamponade the retinal hole. Once the hole has been closed in this way, the subretinal fluid is absorbed.

Technique

Sterile air is obtained by drawing room air through a Millipore filter. After the filter is removed, the air is injected into the vitreous cavity through a 30-gauge needle placed over the pars plana (4 mm from the surgical limbus).

When the tamponading effect will be needed for longer than 2 days, a long-lasting gas is used. Sulfur hexafluoride (SF_6) remains in the vitreous for 7 to 10 days.[49,50] Perfluoropropane (C_3F_8) lasts approximately 5 weeks.[51,52] In their undiluted states, these gases also expand, approximately 2.5- and 4-fold, respectively. (See Pneumatic Retinopexy, below.) As an adjunct to scleral buckling procedures, usually only 0.25 to 0.35 cc of pure gas is required.

Complications

Prior to injection of the air or gas, if nitrous oxide is being used for general anesthesia, it must be turned off for at least 15 minutes prior to injection. Nitrous oxide rapidly diffuses into the injected air or gas bubble, and can cause a marked elevation in the intraocular pressure. Needless to say, the surgeon must be very careful not to strike the lens with the needle as it enters the eye. If the needle does not pass cleanly through the pars plana epithelium before the air or gas is injected, a dialysis may occur. If too much air or gas is injected, an excessive rise in intraocular pressure may occlude the central retinal artery, rupture the globe, or tear out scleral sutures.

INTRAOPERATIVE PROBLEMS

Small Pupil

If the pupil will not dilate, it can be stretched with iris hooks. If these are not available, a sector iridectomy can be made.

Corneal Edema

Prolonged or excessive scleral depression during localization or cryotherapy may cause epithelial edema. A clearer view of the fundus can be obtained if the corneal epithelium is removed with a rounded blade. The epithelium usually heals postoperatively in 1 to 2 days, though healing may take longer in patients with diabetes mellitus.

Posteriorly Located Breaks

It is sometimes difficult to place sutures for posteriorly located breaks. Adequate exposure can usually be provided by a lateral canthotomy. If this does not suffice, disinsertion of a rectus muscle may be necessary. A traction suture placed through the stump of the muscle enables the surgeon to manipulate the eye to obtain the desired exposure. In many cases, however, posterior breaks are best managed by vitrectomy.

Oblique Muscles

To place an explant correctly, it may be necessary to place a scleral suture where the superior or inferior oblique muscle inserts into the globe. If the muscle cannot be retracted far enough, it should be partially disinserted to give the surgeon an unobstructed view of the sclera.

Staphyloma

Placing sutures into very thin sclera is dangerous because the choroid may accidentally be perforated. Moreover, the sutures may pull out postoperatively. The scleral sutures should be placed in adjacent thicker sclera, which usually means that a circumferential explant must be used. Because the mattress suture is then wider than actually required, a larger explant will be needed to close the break. If the scleral bites must be shallow, the risk of late suture extrusion is reduced if an encircling band is added. Silicone sponges should be used over staphylomatous sclera because they are less likely to intrude into the eye than is solid silicone. When a true staphyloma exists, the surgeon must be

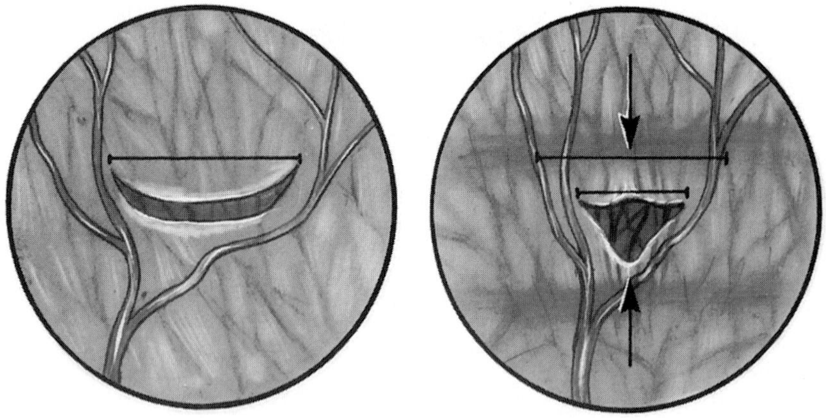

Figure 56–24. The "fishmouth" phenomenon. *Left,* Flap tear in detached retina. *Solid line* indicates the width of the tear. *Right,* A circumferential buckle *(between arrows)* compresses the tear (*large line* indicates original width), keeping its posterior edge open.

very careful not to raise the intraocular pressure too high during the procedure, or the globe may rupture.

Needle Perforation of the Sclera

If the needle accidentally penetrates the choroid while sutures are being placed, subretinal fluid may drain, causing the eye to become markedly hypotonous. The suture should be removed and its replacement suture positioned so that the accidental drainage site will later fall under the buckle. Pressure with a cotton-tipped applicator over the accidental drainage site can be used to make the eye firm enough for proper placement of the remaining sutures. If too much fluid has drained, even this will not suffice, and an intraocular injection of saline solution will be necessary to restore the intraocular pressure. If a deep suture perforates attached retina, the area should be treated with cryotherapy and scleral buckling.

Increased Intraocular Pressure

As the surgeon ties the scleral sutures or pulls up the encircling band, he must constantly monitor the intraocular pressure. An estimate can be obtained by palpation (finger tension) or by indentation with a muscle hook. More accurate readings can be taken with the Schiotz tonometer or Tonopen. If the pressure is high, the surgeon must inspect the optic disc to see if the central retinal artery is pulsating or occluded. If the pressure is too high and all of the scleral sutures cannot be tied because of increased intraocular pressure, several maneuvers are possible. First, if the eyelids have been pushed behind the globe, decreasing the available orbital space, they should be pulled forward and the globe reposited. Second, an anterior chamber paracentesis is helpful. Third, the surgeon can loosen some of the sutures or loosen the encircling band. A last resort is vitreous aspiration.

The "Fishmouth" Phenomenon

Scleral buckling may result in a meridional fold formed by redundant retina on the posterior slope of the buckle. The buckle, in this case, actually prevents reattachment (Fig. 56–24) by keeping the break open and allowing free passage of subretinal fluid posteriorly. This phenomenon, called "fishmouthing," is more likely to occur with circumferential buckling than with radial buckling.[35,36] If the break is superiorly located, an intravitreal injection of air or gas will usually close the break. If not, the meridional folding can be reduced by decreasing the height of the buckle (by loosening the sutures). Another approach is to place a radial element under the circumferential buckle.

FINAL INSPECTION AND ADJUSTMENTS

If all of the subretinal fluid has been drained, it is easy to determine if the scleral buckle has been placed correctly (Fig. 56–25). If subretinal fluid remains under the break, the surgeon can push gently on the scleral buckle. The increased indentation helps to assess the

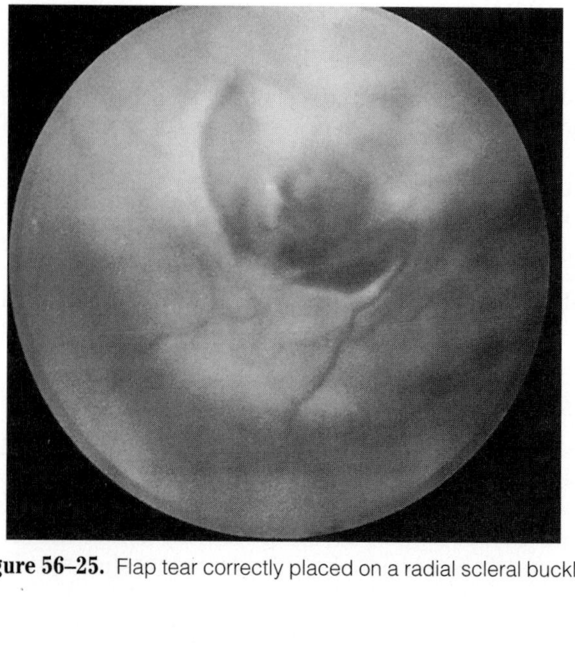

Figure 56–25. Flap tear correctly placed on a radial scleral buckle.

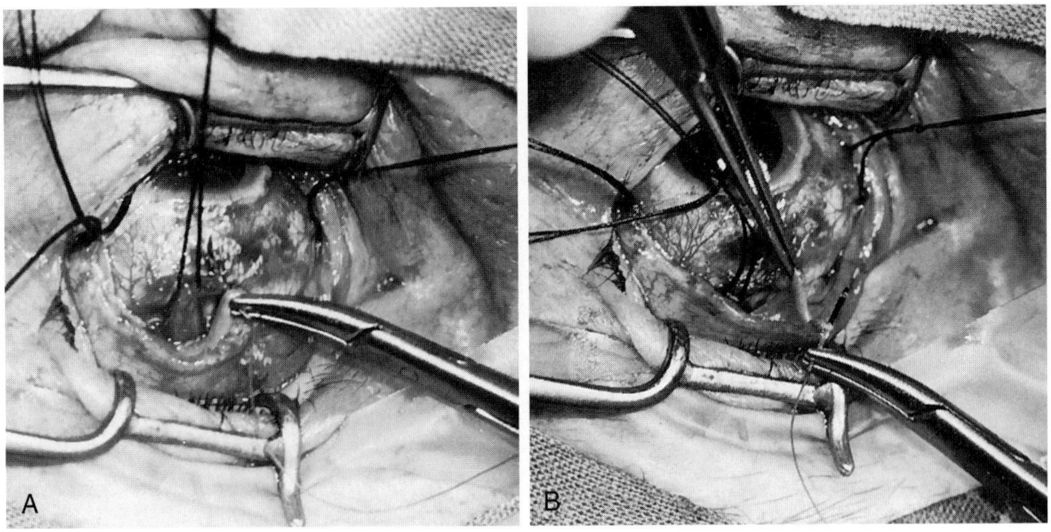

Figure 56–26. *A.* Closure of the peritomy. The posterior flap is stretched forward by a suture needle so that Tenon's capsule can be firmly grasped. *B.* Tenon's capsule is anchored to the rectus muscle tendon in all four quadrants.

buckle's relationship to the break. If an explant is not properly placed, the surgeon must place a new scleral suture and remove the old one. It is important not to trim an explant too close to its mattress sutures until adequate closure of the retinal break has been confirmed. If the explant has not been properly placed, an additional suture can be easily placed. The conjunctiva is closed with plain catgut or 8-0 Vicryl (Fig. 56–26). Atropine and antibiotic ointment are then applied, and the eye is patched with a semi-pressure dressing to reduce postoperative eyelid edema.

POSTOPERATIVE MANAGEMENT

If there is air or gas in the vitreous cavity, the patient is positioned so that the bubble rises against the break to tamponade it. Atropine 1% or scopolamine 0.25% is given twice daily, and an antibiotic–corticosteroid mixture is given 4 times daily. Most patients require only mild analgesics. They are usually discharged on the day of surgery. All patients are seen on the day after surgery.

Early Complications

Acute Angle-Closure Glaucoma

Choroidal congestion resulting from the surgery can cause forward rotation of the ciliary body and closure of the filtration angle. The consequent increased intraocular pressure causes pain and corneal edema. This condition may be misdiagnosed, because the central portion of the anterior chamber may remain deep. The diagnosis is made by applanation tonometry. Schiotz tonometry may give a falsely low reading because of decreased scleral rigidity. Because pupillary block is not a contributing factor, treatment with pilocarpine or with iridectomy is not effective. Proper management includes the use of aqueous suppressants (acetazolamide, dorzolamide, brimonidine, timolol), topical or systemic corticosteroids, and, if necessary, mannitol. It is sometimes necessary to loosen the encircling band.

Anterior Segment Necrosis

Anterior segment necrosis is common following operations in which three muscles have been disinserted, three vortex veins have been occluded,[53] diathermy has been applied over the long ciliary arteries, or a tight, posteriorly located encircling band has been used.[13,54–56] Patients

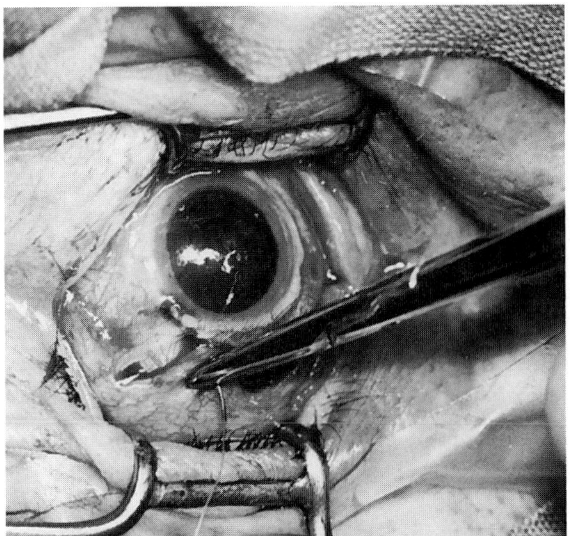

Figure 56–27. The relaxing incision is closed with an absorbable suture.

with sickle cell disease are especially prone to this condition.[57] The earliest finding is striate keratopathy. Later, corneal edema develops, without elevated intraocular pressure. Many patients have marked chemosis. A diagnostic finding is white flakes floating in the anterior chamber or deposited on the lens. Large keratic precipitates may be present. Late findings are hypotony due to atrophy of the ciliary processes, an irregularly dilated pupil, iris atrophy, posterior synechiae, and cataract. If anterior segment necrosis is suspected, the patient should be treated with high doses of topical and systemic corticosteroids. The encircling band should be loosened.

Infection

The incidence of buckle infections is approximately 1% to 3%. The risk can be decreased by soaking the sponges in an antibiotic solution prior to suturing them to the globe. The best indicator is unusually severe pain. In addition, there is marked chemosis and injection of the conjunctiva, mucopurulent discharge, and progressive swelling of the eyelids. Some patients have numerous inflammatory cells in the vitreous. A localized exudate over a scleral buckle is a particularly ominous sign, for it may indicate early scleral necrosis and endophthalmitis.

The most common bacteria involved are *Staphylococcus aureus, Pseudomonas,* and *Proteus.*[58] Treatment with systemic and topical broad-spectrum antibiotics is started in severe infections, but they cannot be cured with antibiotics alone: the explant must be removed. If removal is done soon after the original surgery there is a high risk of redetachment.[59] If the retina redetaches, after the orbit has been sterilized, either the buckle must be placed again or the detachment must be repaired internally with vitrectomy techniques.

Choroidal Detachments

Choroidal detachments are common after retinal detachment surgery, especially in elderly or aphakic patients. They are also seen in patients with broad or posteriorly located buckles and in the patients who have undergone reoperations.

Late Complications

Refractive Error

Encircling procedures usually elongate the globe, with a consequent increase in myopia. On average, this shift is usually in the range of 1 to 2 diopters, but it may be higher. Segmental buckling procedures can cause regular or irregular astigmatism. Spectacle or contact lens changes should be deferred for about 2 months after surgery, when the induced refractive errors are usually stable.

Muscle Imbalance

Disturbances in ocular motility are especially common if a vertical muscle has been disinserted, if a large implant or explant has been placed under a rectus muscle,[60–62] or if Tenon's capsule has been broken. This most commonly occurs in the muscle sheath 10 mm posterior to the limbus.[63,64] Scarring then causes loss of elasticity in the extraconal septae. Excessive scarring following reoperations is another important contributing factor. Because many patients have temporary diplopia after a scleral buckling procedure, it is advisable to wait at least 6 months before considering corrective muscle surgery.[65] It is then important to determine whether the diplopia is due to scar tissue preventing rotation of the eye or to the underaction of a muscle that is adherent to the globe. Forced ductions aid greatly in this determination.[60]

Extrusion of Implants or Explants

Sometimes when a sponge erodes through the conjunctiva, the patient has either no symptoms or minimal irritation. In other cases, such erosion is followed by infection, with pain and mucopurulent discharge. If the retina was repaired with a sponge explant and an encircling band, we generally remove the sponge and easily reached sutures and leave the band in place. It has been reported that approximately one third of the retinas will redetach after removal of the scleral buckle,[66] but many surgeons believe that the incidence of redetachment is much lower, especially if the original buckling procedure was performed more than 6 weeks earlier.[59]

Macular Pucker

Macular pucker, which usually occurs 6 to 8 weeks after surgery, can ruin an otherwise good visual result.[67] The macular pucker is thought to be the result of breaks in the internal limiting membrane through which glial cells migrate or of membranes formed by intravitreal, metaplastic retinal pigment epithelial cells. The risk is highest in eyes with loss of formed vitreous at surgery, retinal incarceration, subretinal hemorrhage, or vitreous hemorrhage.

Cystoid Macular Edema

Angiographically demonstrable cystoid macular edema has been found in as many as 25% of phakic eyes and 60% of aphakic eyes.[68,69] It may cause visual loss whether or not the macula was detached preoperatively, but it usually resolves within several months. Persistent, visually significant edema is rare.

OUTCOMES

Early Causes of Failure

If any break in the detached retina has been missed, the surgery will not be successful. In nondrainage and partial-drainage procedures, the retina will not settle. Even if the subretinal fluid was drained and the retina was flat at the time of surgery, new fluid often will accumulate. The only remedy is a reoperation to close the missed break.

Reoperation is also necessary if the cause of the failure is an inaccurately placed buckle. If the break remains elevated over a properly placed scleral buckle, however, reoperation may be avoided. If the hole is nearly closed, argon laser or xenon arc photocoagulation may seal the break.[70] If the break is superiorly located, an intravitreal gas injection may tamponade it so that the subretinal fluid can be absorbed. If these remedies fail, drainage of the subretinal fluid is indicated.

If a scleral buckle is revised within 2 weeks, opening the conjunctiva and Tenon's capsule is swiftly accomplished, because these tissues have not yet scarred down to the sclera. The surgeon must take great care not to inadvertently penetrate the eye through a drainage site.

If the sensory retina has been thoroughly frozen in the first operation, tight junctions will probably form between the pigment epithelium and Muller's cells without retreatment (see above). However, if only the pigment epithelium was frozen in the original operation, retreatment probably is indicated after 4 to 5 days. By this time, the treated pigment epithelium will have been replaced by pigment epithelial cells sliding over from untreated areas, and a firm adhesion will not result.

The most common cause of failure of retinal detachment surgery is proliferative vitreoretinopathy (PVR). Metaplastic pigment epithelial and glial cells proliferate on the retina and on vitreous strands and then contract, preventing settling of the retina or causing its redetachment.[33,71–73] Risk factors include vitreous hemorrhage, large tears, choroidal detachment, long duration of detachment, total detachment, and inflammation.[74] The goal of the reoperation is to relieve vitreous traction. If a properly placed scleral buckle with adequate indentation is unsuccessful, vitrectomy is indicated.

Late Causes of Redetachment of the Retina

In patients observed at the Wills Eye Hospital, the most common cause of late redetachment of the retina has been found to be a new break posterior to an encircling band. New breaks can also be seen overlying an encircling band or in quadrants without a buckle.

In the past, patients with successfully reattached retinas had a high risk of redetachment if they subsequently underwent an intracapsular cataract extraction. With current extracapsular and phacoemulsification techniques, however, the risk is now very low. One series of 47 cases had no redetachments.[75] Late redetachments caused by new breaks have an excellent prognosis for successful repair. Extensive operations are not necessary; all that is required is to close the new breaks with a local explant or even by pneumatic retinopexy.

Final Success Rates

Reattachment success rates are dependent on their preoperative characteristics. Sometimes two or more operations are required, but the following generalizations can be made:

- *Excellent prognosis (nearly 100%):* detachments due to dialysis, or to small or round holes; detachments with demarcation lines; detachments with minimal subretinal fluid.
- *Good prognosis (98% to 99%):* pseudophakic detachments, total detachments, detachments with associated detachment of nonpigmented epithelium of pars plana, detachments with early proliferative vitreoretinopathy.[74,76,77]
- *Fair prognosis (75% to 85%):* Detachments that present with associated choroidal detachment or with advanced PVR have a poor prognosis if treated with scleral buckling alone. When treated with advanced vitrectomy techniques in combination with scleral buckling, however, the success rate is 90% to 95%.

Postoperative Visual Acuity

Overall, some 50% of patients will regain a visual acuity of 20/50 (6/15) or better, 25%, 20/60 to 20/100; and 25%, 20/200 or worse. Postoperative visual acuity chiefly depends on whether and how long the macula was detached before surgery. When the macula has detached, necrosis of photoreceptors may prevent good postoperative visual acuity. Seventy-five percent of patients with a macular detachment of less than 1 week's duration will obtain a final visual acuity of 20/70 (6/21) or better, as opposed to 50% with a macular detachment of 1 to 8 weeks' duration.[23–26,78]

The prognosis for vision is far better in cases in which the macula has not detached, though 10% to 15% of these patients lose vision from macular pucker or cystoid macular edema.[79–81] Obviously, intraoperative complications (see above) also affect the final visual acuity.

SUMMARY

Advantages

Scleral buckling makes nondrainage procedures possible and permanently reduces vitreous traction on retinal breaks. Of all the techniques for retinal detachment repair, scleral buckling has the longest track record. It has been used since the late 1950s. With a single operation success rate of about 85% to 90% and a reattachment rate of 98% to 99% in uncomplicated cases, it remains the standard against which all other approaches are measured.

Disadvantages

The risk of complications of scleral buckling procedures, described in detail above, is low, but when they do occur they may be devastating.

PNEUMATIC RETINOPEXY

Rosengren was the first to inject air into the vitreous to tamponade retinal breaks.[82] Fineberg and Norton introduced sulfur hexafluoride (SF_6) as an adjunct to scleral buckling.[49,83] SF_6 is a relatively insoluble gas, which has the advantage of expanding within the eye, so that a small injection results in a large bubble. Further, the bubble remains in the eye, helping to keep the break(s) closed for up to 2 weeks. In the 1980s, Dominguez and Hilton independently described the use of gas to treat and cure retinal detachments *without* a scleral buckle.[84,85] The procedure, called "pneumocausis" by Dominguez and "pneumatic retinopexy" by Hilton, is relatively simple. The break is treated with cryotherapy and is tamponaded with gas injected into the vitreous cavity. Postoperatively, the patient is positioned so that the gas bubble rises against the retinal break. The subretinal fluid is absorbed and a chorioretinal adhesion forms around the break.

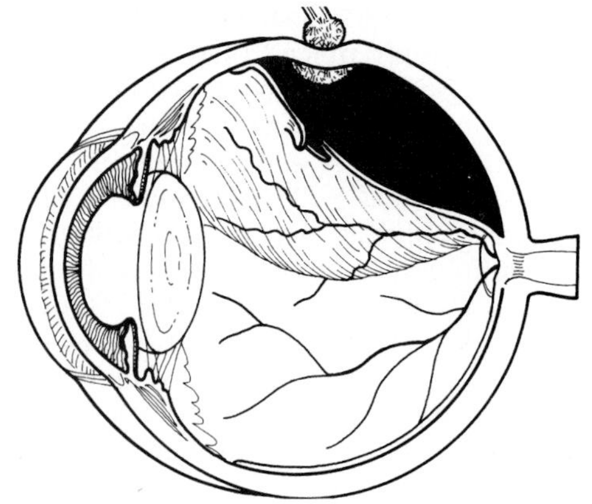

Figure 56–28. Pneumatic retinopexy. The retinal tear is treated with cryotherapy.

PATIENT SELECTION

The chorioretinal scar has the best chance of healing if the retinal break can be kept flat by prolonged patient positioning for 5 to 7 days. Therefore, pneumatic retinopexy should not be attempted in people who cannot adhere to the postoperative positioning requirements. The best results are obtained if the breaks are located in the superior 8 clock hours and are less than 1 clock hour in size or, if multiple, subtend less than 1 clock hour of retina. Relative contraindications to pneumatic retinopexy include greater than 3 clock hours of lattice degeneration, breaks with bridging blood vessels or incompletely torn lattice degeneration, moderate vitreous hemorrhage, proliferative vitreoretinopathy, extensive retinal detachment, and media opacities that preclude finding all of the retinal breaks.[86–89] Some surgeons have reported lower success rates in pseudophakic eyes, especially those with open posterior capsules,[87,88,90,91] but a large controlled trial found that this was a minor factor.[77,92] If we include pseudophakic eyes, one third to one half of all patients with primary retinal detachments are potential candidates.

ANESTHESIA

Retrobulbar anesthesia can be used, but peribulbar anesthesia is quite acceptable. If preservation of ocular motility is desired to facilitate examination and treatment and the amount of retinopexy is not too extensive, sub-Tenon's anesthesia is usually preferred.

RETINOPEXY

The retinal breaks are treated with cryotherapy (Fig. 56–28). An alternative is to wait for flattening of the retinal break and to use laser photocoagulation. Any retinal breaks seen in uninvolved, attached retina must also be treated.

PARACENTESIS

Anterior chamber paracentesis is performed to make room for the injected gas and prevent a marked rise in intraocular pressure. Also, because there is less risk of getting multiple small gas bubbles or "fish-eggs" in the softened eye (see below), there is less risk of subretinal gas migration.

GAS INJECTION

The gas bubble must be large enough to completely cover the break(s) and must last at least 1 week to allow effective healing of the chorioretinal scar. This usually means injecting 0.4 to 0.5 ml of pure sulfur hexafluoride (SF_6). The bubble will double in size within the first 36 hours after injection and lasts about 10 to 14 days. For multiple breaks, breaks located around the horizontal meridian, and breaks in larger (highly myopic) eyes, 0.3 to 0.4 ml of perfluoropropane (C3F8) is used. It quadruples in volume within the first 3 days and lasts 4 to 6 weeks.

In preparation for the gas injection, several drops of 5% povidone-iodine solution should be instilled to reduce the risk of subsequent endophthalmitis. The selected gas is then drawn-up in sterile fashion through a 0.22 micron Millipore filter into a 1 ml syringe. A 30-gauge, one-half-inch needle is placed on the syringe and the excess gas is discarded. The injection site is 3.5 to 4.0 mm posterior to the limbus. A large, single intraocular gas bubble is ideal, and subretinal gas must be avoided. The patient's head is tilted to place the injection site higher and the break(s) lower (Fig. 56–29). A brisk injection is less likely to result in multiple small bubbles (fish eggs) than is a slow one. Another technique for avoiding fish eggs is to let them coalesce before asking the patient to sit up, and to gently flick the eye with your finger to break the surface tension between the bubbles.

After injecting, the surgeon must inspect the fundus to verify that the gas bubble is freely mobile in the vitreous and not trapped at the injection site or anterior hyaloidal space. At the same time central retinal artery patency is confirmed. An antibiotic-steroid ointment is instilled and the eye is patched.

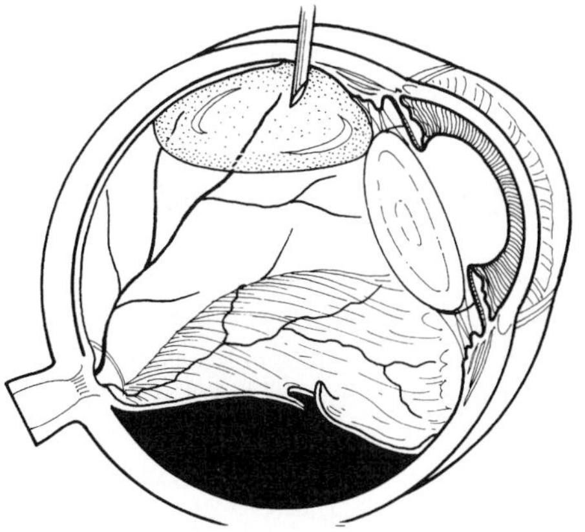

Figure 56–29. Pneumatic retinopexy. The gas is injected into the most superior part of the globe and away from large retinal breaks.

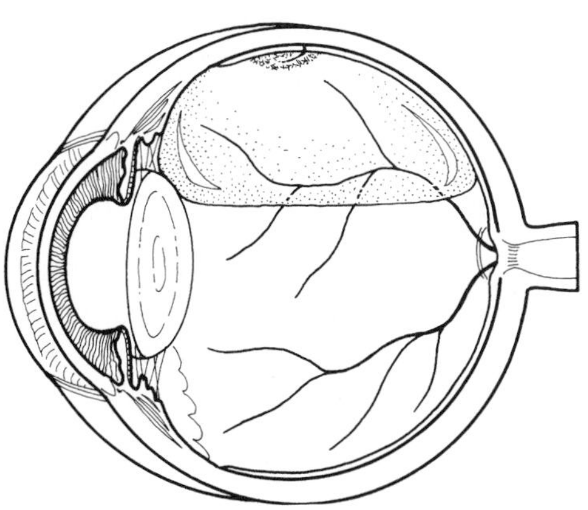

Figure 56–31. Pneumatic retinopexy. As the gas is absorbed, a firm chorioretinal scar forms.

POSTOPERATIVE MANAGEMENT

It is important that the patient maintain the correct head position to tamponade the break for the first 3 to 5 postoperative days in order to promote absorption of the subretinal fluid (Fig. 56–30) and keep the retina flat until the cryotherapy scar develops (Fig. 56–31). After the gas bubble is absorbed, a firm chorioretinal scar will remain (Fig. 56–32). Unless there has been extensive cryotherapy, the degree of ocular discomfort is usually minimal, and acetaminophen or another oral nonsteroidal anti-inflammatory agent will suffice for pain control. Until the gas bubble is gone (or very small), the patient is restricted from any high-altitude (greater than 4,000 feet) travel.

Relatively close follow-up is recommended. The eye should be examined the first postoperative day, 3 to 4 days later, and then every 2 to 4 weeks for the first 3 months. Subretinal fluid should start to resorb within the first 24 to 48 hours and the retina is usually completely attached within the first week. The subretinal fluid of chronic detachments can take longer to resorb. As long as the retinal breaks are sealed and the quantity of fluid remains unchanged, reoperation is not indicated. However, if the fluid increases, either the original break is open or there are new or missed breaks, and another procedure is necessary.

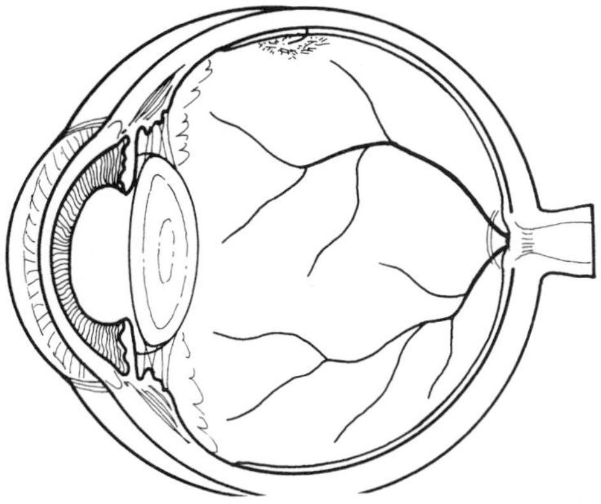

Figure 56–32. Pneumatic retinopexy. After the gas is absorbed, a firm chorioretinal scar remains.

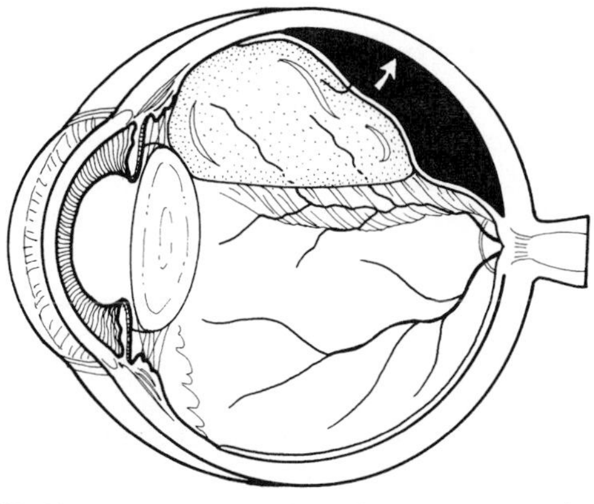

Figure 56–30. Pneumatic retinopexy. The gas tamponades the retinal break so that subretinal fluid can be absorbed.

CAUSES OF FAILURE

Initial Failure

The main reason for failure to close the original break is strong vitreoretinal traction, as is seen in cases of tears with bridging retinal blood vessels or tears with incompletely torn lattice degeneration, and in cases with early proliferative retinopathy. Strong traction can also reopen an initially closed break.

New or Missed Tears

New or missed tears have been reported in 6% to 20% of cases. They are usually found in the first postoperative month and are more common after pneumatic retinopexy than they are after scleral buckling procedures.[77,92] They can often be successfully treated by laser photocoagulation, cryotherapy, or by a repeat pneumatic retinopexy, but approximately one half of eyes with new tears eventually need a scleral buckling procedure.

Late Failure

The risk of proliferative vitreoretinopathy is about the same as it is after scleral buckling procedures: 3% to 5%.[77,92]

SUCCESS RATE

Initial Success

The initial success rate for pneumatic retinopexy is 69% to 84%.[77,88,92] In a large, prospective, multicenter trial it was 73% for pneumatic retinopexy versus 84% for scleral buckling.[77,92] Success rates in pseudophakic eyes appear to be improved with 360 degrees of peripheral laser treatment.[76]

Final Success

Initially it was feared that if pneumatic retinopexy failed, a high rate of proliferative vitreoretinopathy would lead to a high ultimate failure rate. Fortunately, this has been proved to not be the case, and the final success rate in cases that meet the guidelines for pneumatic retinopexy is 98% to 99% for both pneumatic retinopexy and scleral buckling procedures, and the visual outcomes are similar. However, reoperation rates are higher in eyes first treated with pneumatic retinopexy rather than in those treated with scleral buckling.[77,92,93]

SUMMARY

Advantages

The main advantage of this procedure is that it is minimally invasive. Furthermore, because it can be performed in an office setting, the costs of repairing retinal detachment with pneumatic retinopexy are significantly lower than they are with scleral buckling.[76] Pneumatic retinopexy is an excellent technique and is becoming more popular all the time. Younger surgeons especially favor it.[94] In addition, complications of scleral buckling such as submacular hemorrhage, retinal perforation, myopic shift, and diplopia are avoided. Finally, there is considerably less postoperative pain.

Disadvantages

The main disadvantage of pneumatic retinopexy is that patients are delayed in getting back to work because of the need for postoperative positioning and because of the higher reoperation rate. A minor disadvantage is that they cannot fly in airplanes until the gas bubble has been largely resorbed.

THE LINCOFF BALLOON

The technique is an improvement on nondrainage scleral buckling procedures, which Lincoff has long championed. The difference is that no foreign material is sutured to the eye and the buckle is temporary. The Lincoff balloon is an inflatable device that is placed under Tenon's capsule and under the retinal break, which is removed after 7 to 12 days.[95,96]

PATIENT SELECTION

Patients must have a single break or a closely clustered group of breaks, as for pneumatic retinopexy, but the breaks can be in any meridian. Because the buckle is temporary, it is not advised for patients with proliferative vitreoretinopathy.

ANESTHESIA

Retrobulbar anesthesia can be used, but both subconjunctival or peribulbar anesthesia are satisfactory.

TECHNIQUE

Retinopexy

The retinal break(s) is treated with cryotherapy. An alternative is to use laser photocoagulation on the first postoperative day or even later, after the retina is flat. Laser or cryotherapy also should be applied to any retinal breaks seen in uninvolved, attached retina.

Localization

The conjunctiva is marked with a marking pen at the site of the final cryotherapy application, which is deliberately made at the posterior margin of the tear.

Placement of the Balloon

Several drops of 5% povidone-iodine solution are instilled to reduce the risk of orbital infection. A 1- to 2-mm opening down to bare sclera is made 3 to 4 mm anterior to the localization mark. Blunt dissection is then used to make a posterior tunnel. The deflated balloon is first inserted and then partially inflated with 0.5 ml of sterile water to confirm placement. When placement is seen to be correct, another 1 to 1.5 ml is injected. The patency of the central retinal artery is confirmed. The inflated balloon is self-retaining. The tube is taped to the skin, antibiotic ointment is instilled, and the eye is patched.

POSTOPERATIVE MANAGEMENT

On the first postoperative day, the height of the balloon is sometimes augmented with an additional injection of water. It is removed after 7 to 12 postoperative days.

CAUSES OF FAILURE

Initial Failure

The initial success rate is reported to be about 90% in most series.[97–99] Causes of early failure include failure to close the break, reopening of the break after removal of the balloon, and new retinal breaks.

Late Failure

Fortunately, the risk of proliferative vitreoretinopathy is about the same as it is after scleral buckling procedures and pneumatic retinopexy.[97–99]

SUCCESS RATE

Patients in whom the procedure is not successful are treated with conventional techniques. The final success rate is the same as for pneumatic retinopexy and scleral buckling procedures.[97–99] However, there is no controlled trial comparing these procedures.

SUMMARY

Advantages

The Lincoff balloon is an excellent technique for repairing selected retinal detachments. It has several advantages. First, it is entirely extraocular, thereby avoiding scleral buckling complications such as submacular hemorrhage, retinal perforation, and endophthalmitis. Second, because the balloon is removed, late complications of scleral buckling such as myopic shift and diplopia are avoided. Third, it can be used to treat not only superior retinal breaks, but also inferior ones for which pneumatic retinopexy is inappropriate. Finally, it is minimally invasive and can be performed in an office setting. Its costs are significantly lower than the costs with scleral buckling.

Disadvantages

The complications are mostly minor and include corneal abrasion and mild patient discomfort.

PRIMARY VITRECTOMY

Pars plana vitrectomy without scleral buckling was introduced by Kloti in Europe[100] and by Escoffery and colleagues in the United States.[101] The current procedure consists of a pars plana vitrectomy with careful excision of the vitreous base. Subretinal fluid is removed during an air–liquid exchange through a retinotomy. The breaks are treated with laser photocoagulation. In addition, some surgeons place several rows of laser posterior to the entire circumference of the vitreous base.

RESULTS

In a series of 29 cases, Escoffery reported a success rate of 79% (23/29) with one operation and 93% (27/29) with two.[101] Campo and colleagues successfully repaired the detachment in 88% of pseudophakic eyes, but routinely used 360-degree laser photocoagulation of the vitreous base.[102]

SUMMARY

Advantages

The advantages over scleral buckling procedures are similar to those of pneumatic retinopexy. In addition, all vitreous debris is removed, and patients have minimal or no postoperative floaters or glare.

Disadvantages

This procedure has all of the disadvantages of pneumatic retinopexy plus the complications of vitrectomy itself, including cataract formation. In addition, it is at least as time-consuming as scleral buckling procedures, and it is more expensive.

REFERENCES

1. Laatikainen L, Tolppanen EM, Harju H: Epidemiology of rhegmatogenous retinal detachment in a Finnish population. Acta Ophthalmol 1985;63:59–64.
2. Sasaki K, Ideta H, Yonemoto J, et al.: Epidemiologic characteristics of rhegmatogenous retinal detachment in Kumamoto, Japan. Graefes Arch Clin Exp Ophthalmol 1995;233:772–6.
3. Tornquist R, Stenkula S, Tornquist P: Retinal detachment. A study of a population-based patient material in Sweden 1971–1981. I. Epidemiology. Acta Ophthalmol 1987;65:213–22.
4. Wilkes SR, Beard CM, Kurland LT, et al.: The incidence of retinal detachment in Rochester, Minnesota, 1970–1978. Am J Ophthalmol 1982;94:670–3.
5. Diamond JP: When are simple flashes and floaters ocular emergencies? Eye 1992;6:102–4.
6. Hikichi T, Trempe CL: Relationship between floaters, light flashes, or both, and complications of posterior vitreous detachment [see comments]. Am J Ophthalmol 1994;117:593–8.
7. Lindner B: Acute posterior vitreous detachment. Am J Ophthalmol 1975;80:44–8.
8. Tabotabo M, Karp L, Benson W: Posterior vitreous detachment. Ann Ophthalmol 1980;12:59.
9. Tasman W: Posterior vitreous detachment and peripheral retinal breaks. Trans Am Acad Ophthalmol Otolaryngol 1968;72:217.
10. Morse PH, Scheie HG, Aminlari A: Light flashes as a clue to retinal disease. Arch Ophthalmol 1974;91:179.
11. Delaney WV Jr, Oates RP: Retinal detachment in the second eye. Arch Ophthalmol 1978;96:629–34.
12. Morse P, Scheie H: Prophylactic cryoretinopexy of retinal breaks. Arch Ophthalmol 1974;92:204.

13. Dobbie J: A study of the intraocular fluid dynamics in retinal detachment. Arch Ophthalmol 1963;69:159.
14. Langham M, Regan C: Circulatory changes associated with the onset of primary retinal detachment. Arch Ophthalmol 1969;81:820.
15. Moses R, Becker B: Clinical tonography: the scleral rigidity factor. Am J Ophthalmol 1958;45:196.
16. Linner E: Intraocular pressure in retinal detachment. Arch Ophthalmol 1966;84:101.
17. Netland P, Mukai S, Covington H: Elevated intraocular pressure secondary to rhegmatogenous retinal detachment. Surv Ophthalmol 1994;39:234.
18. Schwartz A: Chronic open-angle glaucoma secondary to rhegmatogenous retinal detachment. Am J Ophthalmol 1973;75:205.
19. Hamilton A, Taylor W: Significance of pigment granules in the vitreous. Br J Ophthalmol 1972;56:700.
20. Shafer D: Comment. In Schepens C, Regan C (eds.), Controversial Aspects of the Management of Retinal Detachment. Boston: Little, Brown; 1965:51.
21. Regillo CR, Benson WE: Retinal Detachment, Diagnosis and Management. Philadelphia: Lippincott-Raven; 1998.
22. Lincoff H, Gieser R: Finding the retinal hole. Arch Ophthalmol 1971;85:565.
23. Hartz AJ, Burton TC, Gottlieb MS, et al.: Outcome and cost analysis of scheduled versus emergency scleral buckling surgery [see comments]. Ophthalmology 1992;99:1358–63.
24. Ross W, Kozy E: Visual recovery in macula-off rhegmatogenous retinal detachment. Ophthalmology 1998;105:2149–53.
25. Burton T: Recovery of visual acuity after retinal detachment surgery. Trans Am Ophthalmol Soc 1982;80:475.
26. Grupposo S: Visual results after scleral buckling with silicone implant. Arch Ophthalmol 1975;93:327.
27. Gundry MF, Davies EW: Recovery of visual acuity after retinal detachment surgery. Am J Ophthalmol 1974;77:310–4.
28. Lincoff H, Bloch OCPD, Nadel A, et al.: The cryosurgical adhesion. II. Trans Am Acad Ophthalmol Otolaryngol 1970;74: 98–107.
29. Lincoff H, Baras AI, McLean J: Modifications to the Custodis procedure for retinal detachment. Arch Ophthalmol 1965;73:160.
30. Lincoff HA, McLean JM: Cryosurgical treatment of retinal detachment. II. Am J Ophthalmol 1966;61:1227–34.
31. Laqua H, Machemer R: Repair and adhesion mechanisms of the cryotherapy lesion in experimental retinal detachment. Am J Ophthalmol 1976;81:833–46.
32. Feman SS, Smith RS, Ray GS, Long RS: Electron microscopy study of cryogenic chorioretinal adhesions. Am J Ophthalmol 1976;81:823–32.
33. Campochiaro PA: Pathogenic mechanisms in proliferative vitreoretinopathy. Arch Ophthalmol 1997;115:237–41.
34. Campochiaro PA, Kaden IH, Vidaurri-Leal J, Glaser BM: Cryotherapy enhances intravitreal dispersion of viable retinal pigment epithelial cells. Arch Ophthalmol 1985;103:434–6.
35. Lincoff H: Radial buckling in the repair of retinal detachment. Int Ophthalmol Clin 1976;16:127–34.
36. Lincoff H, Kreissig I: Advantages of radial buckling. Am J Ophthalmol 1975;79:955–7.
37. Schepens CL: Scleral buckling with circling element. Trans Am Acad Ophthalmol Otolaryngol 1964;68:959.
38. Schepens CL, Acosta F: Scleral implants: an historical perspective. Surv Ophthalmol 1991;35:447–53.
39. Schepens CL, Okamura ID, Brockhurst RJ: The scleral buckling procedures. I. Surgical techniques and management. Arch Ophthalmol 1957;58:797–811.
40. Chignell AH: Retinal detachment surgery without drainage of subretinal fluid. Am J Ophthalmol 1974;77:1–5.
41. Hilton GF: The drainage of subretinal fluid: a randomized controlled clinical trial. Trans Am Ophthalmol Soc 1981;79:517–40.
42. Kreissig I, Rose D, Jost B: Minimized surgery for retinal detachments with segmental buckling and nondrainage. An 11-year follow-up. Retina 1992;12:224–31.
43. Scott JD: A rationale for the use of liquid silicone. Trans Ophthalmol Soc UK 1977;97:235–7.
44. Wilkinson CP, Bradford RH Jr: The drainage of subretinal fluid. Trans Am Ophthalmol Soc 1983;81:162–71.
45. Chignell A, Fison L, Davies E, et al.: Failure in retinal detachment surgery. Br J Ophthalmol 1973;57:525.
46. Kirkby GR, Chignell AH: Shifting subretinal fluid in rhegmatogenous retinal detachment. Br J Ophthalmol 1985;69:654–5.
47. Ibanez H, Bloom S, Olk R, et al.: External argon laser choroidotomy versus needle drainage technique in primary scleral buckling procedures. Retina 1994;14:348–50.
48. Humphrey W, Schepens C, et al.: The release of subretinal fluid and its complications. In Pruett R, Regan C (eds.), Retina Congress. New York: Appleton-Century-Crofts; 1974;383–90.
49. Fineberg E, Machemer R, Sullivan P, et al.: Sulfur hexafluoride in owl monkey vitreous cavity. Am J Ophthalmol 1975;79:67–76.
50. Kelley F, Edelhauser H, Aabergt T: Intraocular sulfur hexafluoride and octofluorocyclobutane. Arch Ophthalmol 1978;96:511.
51. Lincoff H, Coleman J, Kreissig I, et al.: The perfluorocarbon gases in the treatment of retinal detachment. Ophthalmology 1983;90:546–51.
52. Lincoff H, Mardirossian J, Lincoff A, et al.: Intravitreal longevity of three perfluorocarbon gases. Arch Ophthalmol 1980;98: 1610–1.
53. Hayreh S, Barnes J: Occlusion of the vortex veins: an experimental study. Br J Ophthalmol 1973;57:217.
54. Diddie K, Ernest J: Uveal blood flow after 360 degrees constriction in the rabbit. Arch Ophthalmol 1980;98:719.
55. Regillo CD, Sergott RC, Brown GC: Successful scleral buckling procedures decrease central retinal artery blood flow velocity. Ophthalmology 1993;100:1044–9.
56. Wilson DJ, Green WR: Histopathologic study of the effect of retinal detachment surgery on 49 eyes obtained post mortem. Am J Ophthalmol 1987;103:167–79.
57. Ryan SJ, Goldberg MF: Anterior segment ischemia following scleral buckling in sickle cell hemoglobinopathy. Retina 1986;6:146.
58. Smiddy WE, Miller D, Flynn HW Jr: Scleral buckle removal following retinal reattachment surgery: clinical and microbiologic aspects. Ophthalmic Surg 1993;24:440–5.
59. Hilton GF, Wallyn RH: The removal of scleral buckles. Arch Ophthalmol 1978;96:2061–3.
60. Portney GL, Campbell LH, Casebeer JC: Acquired heterotropia following surgery for retinal detachment. Am J Ophthalmol 1972;73:985–90.
61. Sewell JJ, Knobloch WH, Eifrig DE: Extraocular muscle imbalance after surgical treatment for retinal detachment. Am J Ophthalmol 1974;78:321–3.
62. Theodossiadis G, Chatzoulis D, Patelis J, Velissaropoulos P: Extraocular observations in episcleral sponge implants. Ophthalmologica 1975;171:439–50.
63. Parks M: Discussion of Wright KW: The fat adherence syndrome and strabismus after retina surgery. Ophthalmology 1986;93:411.
64. Wright K: The fat adherence syndrome and strabismus after retina surgery. Ophthalmology 1986;93:411.
65. Mets MB, Wendell ME, Gieser RG: Ocular deviation after retinal detachment surgery. Am J Ophthalmol 1985;99:667–72.
66. Lindsey PS, Pierce LH, Welch RB: Removal of scleral buckling elements. Causes and complications. Arch Ophthalmol 1983; 101:570–3.
67. Lobes LA Jr, Burton TC: The incidence of macular pucker after retinal detachment surgery. Am J Ophthalmol 1978;85:72–7.
68. Lobes LA Jr, Grand MG: Incidence of cystoid macular edema following scleral buckling procedure. Arch Ophthalmol 1980;98: 1230–2.
69. Sabates NR, Sabates FN, Sabates R, et al.: Macular changes after retinal detachment surgery. Am J Ophthalmol 1989;108:22–9.
70. Curtin VT, Norton EWD, Gass JDM: Photocoagulation: its use in the prevention of reoperation after scleral buckling operations. Trans Am Acad Ophthalmol Otolaryngol 1967;71:432–41.
71. Elner SG, Elner VM, Diaz-Rohena R, et al.: Anterior proliferative vitreoretinopathy. Clinicopathologic, light microscopic, and ultrastructural findings. Ophthalmology 1988;95:1349–57.
72. Laqua H, Machemer R: Clinical-pathological correlation in massive periretinal proliferation. Am J Ophthalmol 1975;80:913–29.
73. Machemer R, Laqua H: Pigment epithelium proliferation in retinal detachment (massive periretinal proliferation). Am J Ophthalmol 1975;80:1–23.
74. Grizzard WS, Hilton GF, Hammer ME, Taren DL: A multivariate analysis of anatomic success of retinal detachments treated with scleral buckling. Graefes Arch Clin Exp Ophthalmol 1994;232: 1–7.

75. Kerrison JB, Marsh M, Stark WJ, Haller JA: Phacoemulsification after retinal detachment surgery. Ophthalmology 1996;103:216–9.
76. Tornambe P: Pneumatic retinopexy: the evolution of case selection and surgical technique. A twelve-year study of 302 eyes. Trans Am Ophthalmol Soc 1997;95:551–78.
77. Tornambe PE, Hilton GF, Brinton DA, et al.: Pneumatic retinopexy. A two-year follow-up study of the multicenter clinical trial comparing pneumatic retinopexy with scleral buckling. Ophthalmology 1991;98:1115–23.
78. Guidry C, McFarland RJ, Morris R, et al.: Collagen gel contraction by cells associated with proliferative vitreoretinopathy. Invest Ophthalmol Vis Sci 1992;33:2429–35.
79. Tani P, Robertson DM, Langworthy A: Prognosis for central vision and anatomic reattachment in rhegmatogenous retinal detachment with macula detached. Am J Ophthalmol 1981;92:611–20.
80. Tani P, Robertson DM, Langworthy A: Rhegmatogenous retinal detachment without macular involvement treated with scleral buckling. Am J Ophthalmol 1980;90:503–8.
81. Wilkinson CP: Visual results following scleral buckling for retinal detachments sparing the macula. Retina 1981;1:113–6.
82. Rosengren B: Uber die Behandlung der Netzhautablosung mittelst Diathermie und Luftijektionen in den Glaskorper. Acta Ophthalmol (Kbh) 1938;16:3.
83. Norton EWD: Intraocular gas in the management of selected retinal detachments. Trans Am Acad Ophthalmol Otolaryngol 1973;77:OP85–98.
84. Dominguez D: Cirugia precoz y ambulatoria del desprendimiento de retina. Arch Soc Esp Oftal 1985;48:47–54.
85. Hilton GF, Grizzard WS: Pneumatic retinopexy. A two-step outpatient operation without conjunctival incision. Ophthalmology 1986;93:626–41.
86. Algvere PK, Hallnas K, Palmqvist BM: Success and complications of pneumatic retinopexy. Am J Ophthalmol 1988;106:400–4.
87. Boker T, Schmitt C, Mougharbel M: Results and prognostic factors in pneumatic retinopexy. Ger J Ophthalmol 1994;3:73–8.
88. Grizzard WS, Hilton GF, Hammer ME, et al.: Pneumatic retinopexy failures. Cause, prevention, timing, and management. Ophthalmology 1995;102:929–36.
89. Hilton GF, Kelly NE, Salzano TC, et al.: Pneumatic retinopexy. A collaborative report of the first 100 cases. Ophthalmology 1987;94:307–14.
90. Ambler JS, Meyers SM, Zegarra H, et al.: Reoperations and visual results after failed pneumatic retinopexy. Ophthalmology 1990;97:786–90.
91. McAllister IL, Meyers SM, Zegarra H, et al.: Comparison of pneumatic retinopexy with alternative surgical techniques. Ophthalmology 1988;95:877–83.
92. Tornambe PE, Hilton GF: Pneumatic retinopexy. A multicenter randomized controlled clinical trial comparing pneumatic retinopexy with scleral buckling. The Retinal Detachment Study Group [see comments]. Ophthalmology 1989;96:772–83; discussion 784.
93. Han D, Mahsin N, Guse C, et al.: Comparison of pneumatic retinopexy and scleral buckling in the management of primary rhegmatogenous retinal detachment. Am J Ophthalmol 1998;126:658–68.
94. Benson WP, Chan S, Sharma S, et al.: Current popularity of pneumatic retinopexy. Retina 1999;19:238–41.
95. Lincoff H, Kreissig I: Results with a temporary balloon buckle for the repair of retinal detachment. Am J Ophthalmol 1981;92:245–51.
96. Lincoff H, Kreissig AI, Hahn YS: A temporary balloon buckle for the treatment of small retinal detachments. Ophthalmology 1979;86:586–96.
97. Green S, Yarian D, Masciulli L, Leff S: Office repair of retinal detachment using a Lincoff temporary balloon buckle. Ophthalmology 1996;103:1804–10.
98. Kreissig I, Failer J, Lincoff H, Ferrari F: Results of a temporary balloon buckle in the treatment of 500 retinal detachments and a comparison with pneumatic retinopexy [see comments]. Am J Ophthalmol 1989;107:381–9.
99. Schoch LH, Olk RJ, Arribas NP, et al.: The Lincoff temporary balloon buckle. Am J Ophthalmol 1986;101:646–9.
100. Kloti R: Amotio-Chirurgie Ohne Skleraeindellung. Primare Vitrektome. Klin Monatsbl Augenheilkd 1983;182:474.
101. Escoffery RF, Olk RJ, Grand MG, Boniuk I: Vitrectomy without scleral buckling for primary rhegmatogenous retinal detachment. Am J Ophthalmol 1985;99:275–81.
102. Campo R, Sipperley J, Sneed S, et al.: Pars plana vitrectomy without scleral buckling for pseudophakic retinal detachment. Ophthalmology 1999;106:1811–6.

CHAPTER 57

Vitreoretinal Surgery, Principles: Age-Related Macular Degeneration

THOMAS A. CIULLA, M.D.

Age-related macular degeneration (AMD) is the leading cause of irreversible visual loss in the United States, occurring in over 10% of the population aged 65 to 74 years and over 25% of the population over the age of 74 years.[1] More specifically, nonexudative AMD occurs in approximately 27% of patients over 75 years of age, and exudative AMD occurs in nearly 5% of that group.[2] Overall, 10% to 20% of patients with nonexudative AMD progress to the exudative form, which is responsible for most of the estimated 1.2 million cases of severe visual loss from AMD.[3] Also, AMD is a bilateral disorder; choroidal neovascular membranes (CNVM) develop in over one fourth (26%) of fellow eyes that are initially free of exudative AMD over a 5-year period.[4] As the population in the United States ages, visual loss from AMD will become even more prevalent.

Although the exudative form is treatable, treatment efficacy is currently low. The only widely accepted method of treatment is laser photocoagulation of the CNVM. However, only a minority of patients with exudative AMD show well-demarcated "classic" CNVM amenable to laser treatment, and at least half of those patients suffer persistent or recurrent CNVM formation within 2 years. In addition, because the treatment itself causes a blinding central scotoma when the CNVM is located subfoveally, many clinicians do not treat subfoveal CNVM. With these treatment limitations, there has been a great deal of interest in alternative therapies for exudative AMD, including surgical therapy.

PATHOPHYSIOLOGY OF AMD AND CNVM BIOLOGY

Theories for AMD pathogenesis include primary retinal pigment epithelium (RPE) and Bruch's membrane senescence, primary genetic defects, and primary ocular perfusion abnormalities and oxidative insults. Traditionally, senescence of the RPE, which metabolically supports and maintains the photoreceptors, is thought to lead to AMD.[5,6] Senescent RPE accumulates metabolic debris as remnants of incomplete degradation from phagocytosed rod and cone membranes. Progressive engorgement of these RPE cells in turn leads to drusen formation, with further dysfunction of the remaining RPE.[5,6] Bruch's membrane, thickened with drusen, could be predisposed to crack formation.[7,8] Calcification and fragmentation of Bruch's membrane is more prominent in eyes with exudative AMD, and it is thought that these defects in Bruch's membrane could facilitate development of CNVM.[9]

This theory is supported by findings in myopic degeneration and angioid streaks in which CNVM develop through breaks in Bruch's membrane. The well-known primate-laser model developed by Ryan may also support this theory for CNVM.[10–19] In this model, high-intensity laser burns are used to create ruptures in the Bruch's membrane/RPE complex to initiate a repair process in the fundus that results in the development of subretinal neovascularization.[13] The exact stimulus for CNVM formation is unclear; it is possible that macrophages involved in the initial response to Bruch's membrane injury secrete angiogenic growth factors.[20]

A mechanism by which CNVM could develop in response to fragmentation of Bruch's membrane could relate to matrix metalloproteinases (MMP), which are extracellular matrix degrading enzymes that may play a key role in angiogenesis and CNVM formation.[21] Bruch's membrane has been shown to contain tissue inhibitor of metalloproteinases (TIMP)-3,[22] and eyes with AMD have been shown to have abnormal levels of TIMP-3 compared to normal age-matched control eyes[23]; calcification and fragmentation observed in Bruch's membrane may represent a breach in this antiangiogenic barrier, facilitating CNVM development. Whatever the initial stimulus for CNVM formation, it is clear that angiogenic growth factors are ultimately involved. Surgically excised and post mortem CNVM tissue, as well as RPE cells, have been shown to be immunoreactive for various growth factors thought to be angiogenic, including vascular endothelial growth factor (VEGF), transforming growth factor-beta (TGF-β), platelet derived growth factor (PDGF), and basic fibroblast growth factor (FGF).[24–27]

The morphology of the CNVM complex plays a significant role in the surgical management of exudative AMD and its prognosis. According to Gass, through normal senescence and the presence of degenerative disorders such as AMD, the normal firm attachment of the RPE to the underlying Bruch's membrane becomes weakened.[28] When this occurs, the CNVM that penetrates Bruch's membrane encounters little mechanical resistance to further growth and can displace the RPE, growing beneath it and spreading laterally in the sub-RPE space.[29] This sub-RPE CNVM, which Gass categorizes as type I CNVM, initially exhibits slow blood flow and little exudation during an early "occult" phase, but later it grows and exhibits increased blood flow, result-

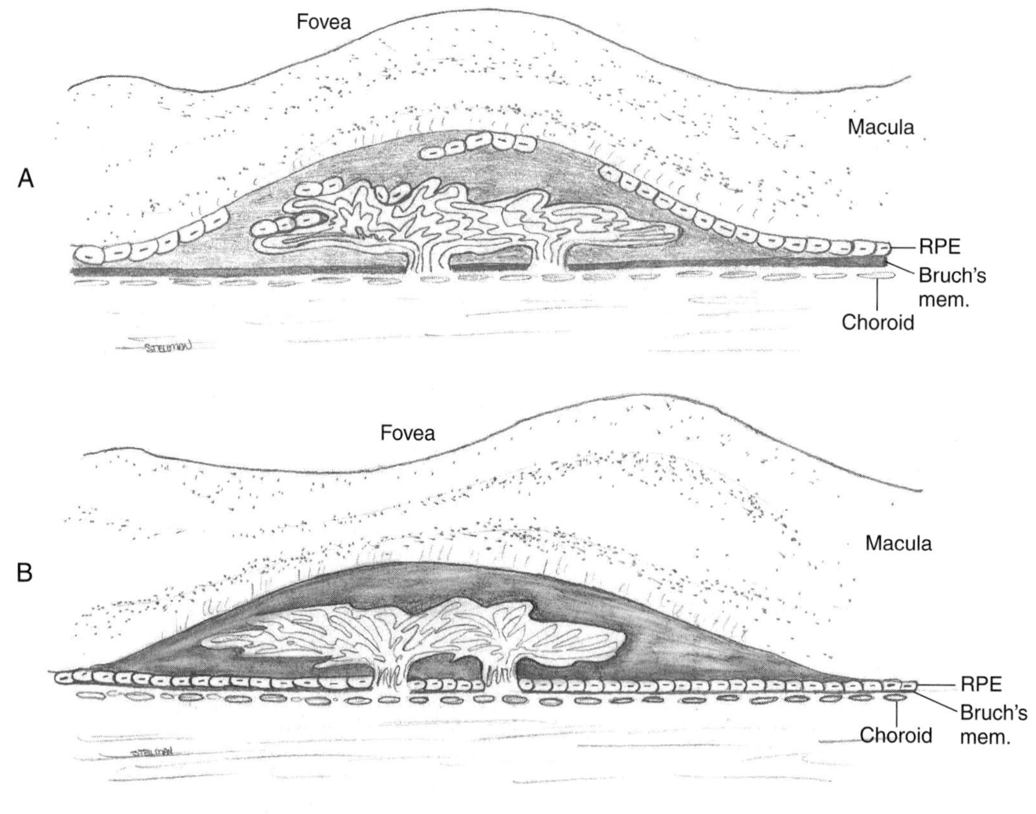

Figure 57–1. Choroidal neovascular membrane (CNVM) morphology. *A.* Type 1 CNVM grows in the subretinal space. According to Gass, the CNVM that originally penetrates Bruch's membrane encounters little mechanical resistance to further growth in age-related macular degeneration (AMD) and can displace the senescent, poorly adherent RPE, growing beneath it and spreading laterally in the sub-retinal pigment epithelium (RPE) space. It initially exhibits slow blood flow and little exudation during an early "occult" phase, but it later grows and exhibits increased blood flow, resulting in decompensation of the CNVM endothelium, exudation into the subretinal space, and an RPE detachment. *B.* Type 2 CNVM grows in the subretinal space. In contrast to patients with AMD, younger patients typically have firm attachment of the RPE to Bruch's membrane. According to Gass, when CNVM forms in response to damaged Bruch's membrane (e.g., focal choroiditis as in the presumed ocular histoplasmosis syndrome [POHS], or focal trauma as in choroidal rupture), the CNVM encounters significant resistance to subretinal growth and is generally directed anteriorly through Bruch's membrane/RPE, where it can then spread laterally in the subretinal space.

ing in decompensation of the CNVM endothelium, exudation into the sub-RPE space and an RPE detachment (Fig. 57–1).[28] The CNVM is generally firmly adherent to the RPE. In contrast to AMD, younger patients typically exhibit firm attachment of the RPE to Bruch's membrane; when CNVM forms in response to damaged Bruch's membrane (e.g., focal choroiditis as in the presumed ocular histoplasmosis syndrome [POHS], or focal trauma as in choroidal rupture), the CNVM encounters significant resistance to sub-RPE growth and is generally directed anteriorly through Bruch's membrane/RPE, where it can then spread laterally in the subretinal space.[28,29] This subretinal CNVM, which Gass categorizes as type 2 CNVM, is associated with reactive RPE proliferation at the advancing border of the CNVM, resulting in a hyperpigmented ring that can be visualized ophthalmoscopically, as well as by subretinal exudation (Fig. 57–1).[28] Consequently, surgical excision of the type 1 sub-RPE CNVM, which is often encountered in AMD, would lead to concurrent excision of the RPE because of the firm attachments of the CNVM to the overlying RPE.[30–34] In contrast, surgical excision of the type 2 subretinal CNVM, which is often encountered in younger patients with POHS, could facilitate retention of the RPE and a better visual prognosis.[29,35] A recent histopathologic study by Grossniklaus and Gass confirmed several clinical features characteristic of type 2 CNVM, including a subretinal pigment halo and sharply defined borders, as well as younger age (average 53 years versus 76 years).[36]

PRESENTATION

Patients with nonexudative AMD are typically mildly symptomatic with minimally blurred central vision, difficulty reading, color and contrast disturbances, and mild metamorphopsia. If geographic atrophy develops in the foveal region, they may complain of a corresponding central scotoma, which can progress over a period of months to years. Patients with exudative AMD typically describe painless progressive blurring of central vision, which can be acute or insidious in onset. Patients who develop subretinal hemorrhage from a classic CNVM, for example, will typically note an acute onset. Patients with occult CNVM may experience insidious blurring secondary to shallow subretinal fluid or pigment epithelial detachments. They also complain of relative or absolute central scotomas, metamorphopsia, and difficulty reading.

On examination, visual acuity is variably reduced. Amsler grid testing typically reveals relative central scotomas or metamorphopsia. Patients with nonexudative AMD present with drusen, RPE hypertrophy, and RPE atrophy. Those with exudative AMD present with subretinal fluid, pigment epithelial detachments (PED), subretinal lipid, or flecks of subretinal hemorrhage in the affected eye, in addition to RPE changes and drusen. Macular contact lens examination facilitates identification of subtle signs, such as shallow subretinal fluid. Flecks of subretinal lipid often demarcate the peripheral edge of the subretinal fluid, where reabsorption takes place. The CNVM itself may be seen as yellow-green subretinal discoloration, sometimes surrounded by a pigment ring, due to reactive RPE proliferation as noted above. Subretinal hemorrhage typically develops at the margins of the CNVM initially and can sometimes obscure the entire complex. Occasionally, the subretinal hemorrhage can "break through" the retina and cause vitreous hemorrhage that is dense enough to obscure visualization of the posterior pole (Fig. 57–2). Consequently, patients who present with vitreous hemorrhage with findings of AMD in the fellow eye should be suspected of harboring a CNVM, especially if there is no preceding history of diabetes or other causes of vitreous hemorrhage.

Other signs of CNVM include subretinal pigment proliferation, hemorrhagic PEDs, RPE tears, and subretinal fibrosis; rarely the actual choroidal neovascular vessels can be visualized. Hemorrhagic PEDs present clinically with dark blood under the RPE; when they are large, they can mimic the appearance of a choroidal melanoma, but ultrasonography will reveal higher internal echodensity than a melanoma. A tear of the RPE can occasionally develop spontaneously or during laser photocoagulation and presents as a collection of subretinal pigmented tissue, representing retracted and scrolled RPE, adjacent to an absolute defect in the RPE. In advanced cases, a central collection of subretinal fibrosis, in the form of disciform scarring is commonly observed, and this is associated with severe visual loss. Disciform scarring, the common end-stage morphology, is often associated with variable degrees of pigmentation related to proliferating RPE cells, as well as findings associated with active CNVM, which is often located at the peripheral edge of the scar. For example, there can be associated subretinal fluid, hemorrhage, and lipid exudates often peripheral to the subretinal fibrosis.

IMAGING STUDIES

RAPID SEQUENCE FLUORESCEIN ANGIOGRAPHY

Rapid sequence fluorescein angiography (RSFA) is performed to evaluate for CNVM in patients who present with symptomatic visual loss or any signs of exudation. Angiography is customarily performed no longer than 72 hours prior to laser photocoagulation, because CNVM morphology and resulting treatment parameters can evolve rapidly. Lesions that stain include regions of RPE atrophy and drusen. Drusen can also block the underlying choroidal fluorescence, as can subretinal hemorrhage and lipid. Serous PED often present as discrete accumulations or pooling of dye uniformly within the lesion without leakage (enlargement in size or intensity) in the later frames of the angiogram. Leakage is a hallmark of CNVM.

The Macular Photocoagulation Study Group (MPS) defined two basic angiographic patterns for CNVM. The classic form presents as discrete early hyperfluorescence with late leakage of dye into the overlying neurosensory retinal detachment (Fig. 57–3). A lacy pat-

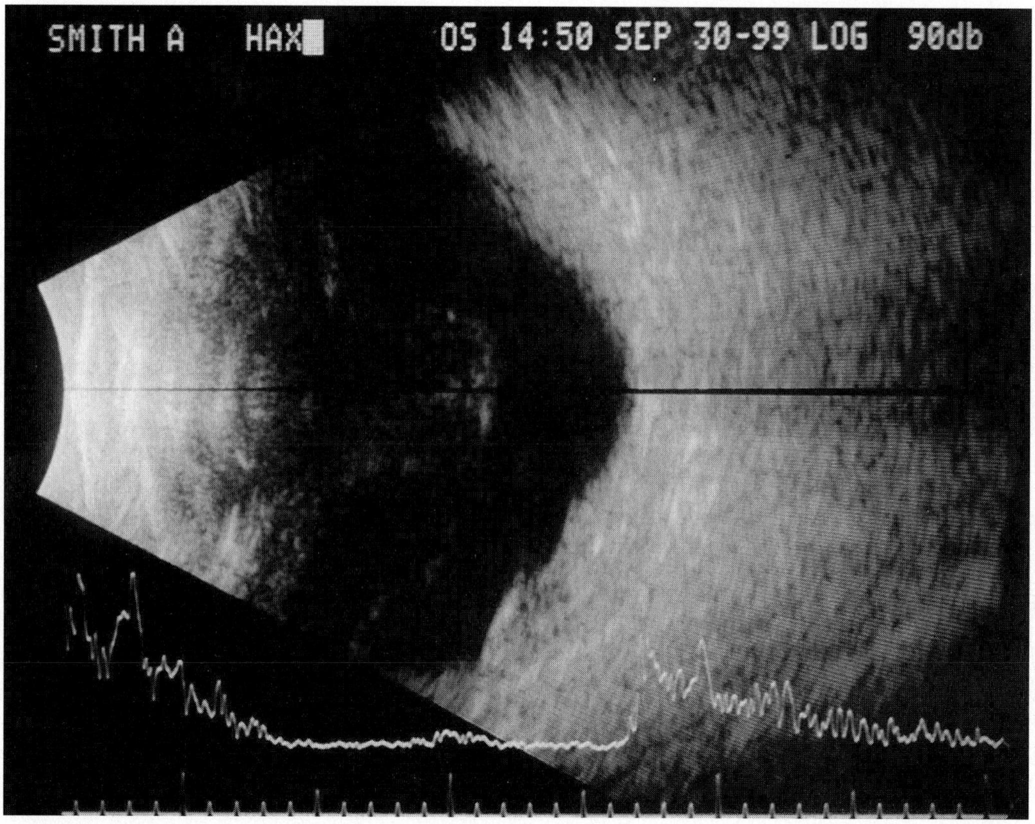

Figure 57–2. Vitreous hemorrhage from AMD-associated CNVM. On B-scan ultrasonography, macular elevation with moderately high echodensity may be noted, which is consistent with submacular hemorrhage and/or disciform scarring. The macular elevation is seen in the lower portion of this horizontal axial view. The opacities in the vitreous cavity represent vitreous hemorrhage. (Ultrasonography by Lissa McNulty, B.S., R.D.M.S.)

tern within the CNVM is not typically observed in exudative AMD, but is more commonly observed in POHS and other causes of CNVM. Occult CNVM are categorized into two basic forms, late leakage of undetermined source, or fibrovascular PEDs. Late leakage of undetermined source manifests as regions of stippled or ill-defined leakage into an overlying neurosensory retinal detachment, without a distinct source focus identified on the early frames of the angiogram. Fibrovascular PEDs present as irregular elevation of the RPE associated with stippled leakage into an overlying neurosensory retinal detachment in the early and late frames of the angiograms (Fig. 57–3).

Fibrovascular PEDs are to be differentiated from serous PEDs, which show more rapid homogeneous filling of the lesion in the early frames without leakage in the late frames of the angiogram. Serous PEDs typically show smooth and sharp hyperfluorescent contours. Unlike fibrovascular PEDs, serous PEDs may not necessarily result from occult CNVM, as senescent impermeable Bruch's membrane or impaired choroidal circulation could limit transfer of fluid across the RPE, which would in turn detach the RPE, creating a serous PED. Other causes of RPE elevation that are to be differentiated from these entities include hemorrhagic PEDs, RPE hyperplasia, and confluent soft drusen. Hemorrhagic PEDs present clinically with dark sub-RPE blood that blocks choroidal fluorescence on angiography. Retinal pigment epithelium hyperplasia will also block choroidal fluorescence. Confluent soft drusen, which often present in the fovea, typically show cruciate pigment clumping. Confluent soft drusen will show angiographic findings similar to those of serous PEDs, with homogeneous pooling of dye and no leakage, but they typically exhibit only faint fluorescence. Tears of the RPE will present as regions of intense staining of the visible scleral region from which the RPE is torn, adjacent to sharply demarcated blockage of the choroidal fluorescence by the redundant scrolled RPE. There may be CNVM associated with the RPE tear, and this will cause leakage in addition to the findings noted above.

Disciform scarring shows diverse angiographic characteristics owing to the varying degrees of fibrosis, pigmentation from proliferating RPE, and active CNVM, which is often located at the peripheral areas of the scar. Angiographically, the fibrotic component will block the choroidal fluorescence in the early frames of the angiogram followed by late staining. Hyperpigmented regions as well as subretinal hemorrhage will block the choroidal fluorescence throughout the angiogram. Regions of active CNVM will show leakage.

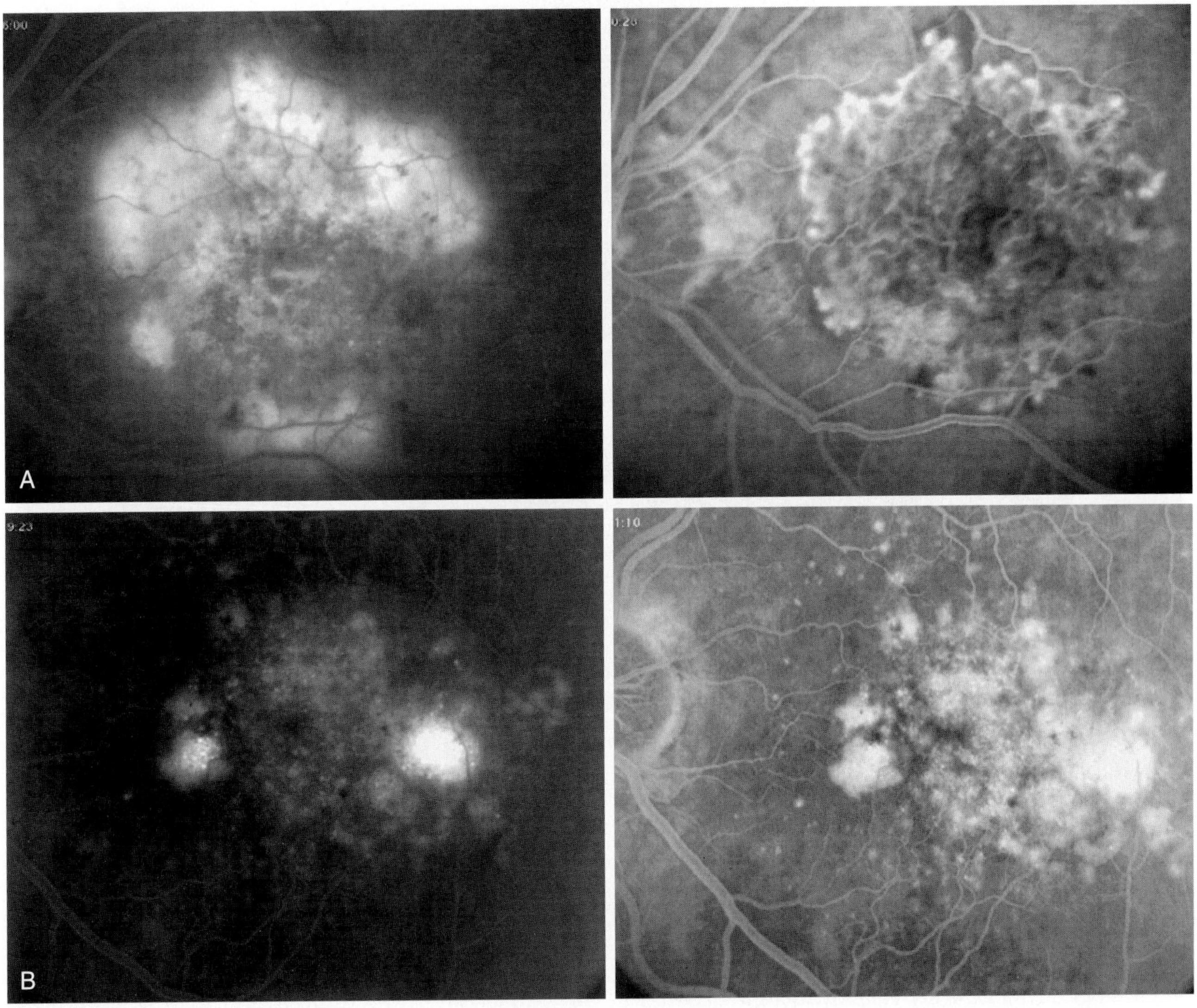

Figure 57–3. The CNVM subtypes on flourescein angiography. *A.* Classic CNVM presents as discrete early hyperfluorescence *(right)* with late leakage of dye into the overlying neurosensory retinal detachment *(left)*. A lacy pattern within the CNVM is not typically observed in exudative AMD, but is more commonly observed in POHS and other causes of CNVM. (Photographs by Tim Steffens, B.S., C.R.A.) *B.* Occult CNVM are categorized into two basic forms, late leakage of undetermined source, or fibrovascular pigment epithelium detachments (PED). Fibrovascular PED, shown here, present as irregular elevation of the RPE on the earlier frames of the angiogram *(top)* associated with stippled slow leakage into an overlying neurosensory retinal detachment in the late frames of the angiograms *(bottom)*. (Photographs by Tim Steffens, B.S., C.R.A.)

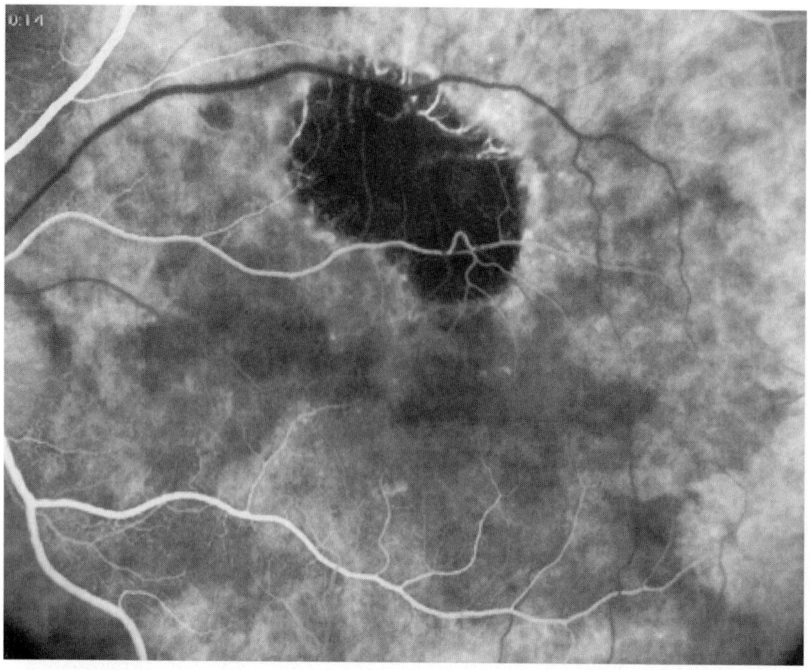

Figure 57–4. Fluorescein angiography after laser photocoagulation. Laser scars are generally hypofluorescent in the early frames of the angiogram due to photocoagulation and subsequent nonperfusion of the choriocapillaris and CNVM. On the late frames of the angiogram, there is variable staining, particularly at the edge of the scar. (Photographs by Tim Steffens, B.S., C.R.A.)

Long-standing laser scars are generally atrophic and show staining throughout the angiogram sequence. Recent laser scars can be hypofluorescent in the early frames of the angiogram due to blockage by pigment and/or obliteration of the choriocapillaris and CNVM. On the late frames of the angiogram, there is variable staining, particularly at the edge of the scar (Fig. 57–4). Persistent or recurrent CNVM generally manifests as leakage at the margin of the laser scar.

INDOCYANINE GREEN ANGIOGRAPHY

Indocyanine green (ICG) angiography facilitates study of the choroidal circulation for several reasons. First, ICG better delineates the choroidal circulation than fluorescein because the near-infrared light absorbed by ICG (795–810 nm) penetrates the retina pigment epithelium better than the shorter wavelength absorbed by fluorescein. Also, unlike fluorescein, ICG is strongly bound to plasma proteins, which prevents diffusion of the compound through the fenestrated choroidal capillaries, and permits better delineation of choroidal details. Finally, ICG can facilitate visualization of choroidal vasculature and CNVM through hemorrhage. Generally, ICG angiography can show CNVM as localized "hot spots" or as diffuse hyperfluorescent "plaques." Guyer and others reported the largest series of digital ICG videoangiography of occult choroidal neovascularization as determined by fluorescein angiography; in their 1000 consecutive cases, they found that ICG could better image the occult choroidal neovascular membrane (CNVM) over fluorescein angiography with ICG angiography yielding 283 cases (29%) of focal hyperfluorescent spots; 597 cases (61%) of hyperfluorescent plaques (consisting of 265 cases [27%] of well-defined plaques and 332 cases [34%] of poorly defined plaques); and 84 cases (8%) of combination lesions (consisting of 35 cases [3%] of marginal spots, 37 cases [4%] of overlying spots, and 12 cases [1%] of remote spots).[37]

LASER PHOTOCOAGULATION

THE MACULAR PHOTOCOAGULATION STUDIES

The macular photocoagulation studies (MPS) showed that photocoagulation of well-demarcated CNVM effectively prevented large decreases in visual acuity compared to observation for extrafoveal, juxtafoveal, and subfoveal CNVM (200–2500 microns, 1–199 microns, and directly under the geometric center of the foveal avascular zone [FAZ] respectively). In these studies, patients were deemed eligible for laser photocoagulation if they manifested well-defined CNVM with some classic morphology. Poorly defined or occult-only CNVM were not eligible for photocoagulation.

In the extrafoveal CNVM studies, the proportion of eyes with severe visual loss (SVL; 6 or more lines of vision loss) in control eyes compared to treated eyes was 41% versus 24% at 1 year, 63% versus 45% at 3 years, and 64% versus 46% at 5 years.[38,39] Similar results were obtained in a British randomized clinical trial of laser photocoagulation for extrafoveal CNVM.[40]

In the juxtafoveal CNVM studies, laser photocoagulation showed similar benefits; the proportion of eyes experiencing SVL in control compared to treated eyes was 45% versus 31% at 1 year, 61% versus 50% at 3 years, and 57% versus 54% at 5 years.[41,42] The protocol differed somewhat in the juxtafoveal CNVM studies to avoid iatrogenic laser injury to the foveal center. Whereas the CNVM was overlapped by 100 microns at all borders in the extrafoveal studies, the CNVM was not treated beyond its border at the foveal edge, if an overlapping laser burn were to coincide with the foveal center in the juxtafoveal studies.[41] In addition, laser wavelength differed. In the extrafoveal studies, argon blue-green was used, because it was most readily available in the late 1970s when these studies were initiated. In the later juxtafoveal studies, krypton red was used because it penetrates hemorrhage better than argon blue-green and it potentially avoids thermal injury to the yellow macular xanthophyll, which absorbs in the blue range of the argon blue-green laser wavelengths. However, the later subfoveal studies, which randomized patients into argon green and krypton red laser photocoagulation, demonstrated no significant advantage of one wavelength over the other.[43] This conclusion was independently confirmed in a 3-year Canadian multicentered randomized trial of argon green versus krypton red laser photocoagulation for well-defined extrafoveal CNVM.[44] It is also important to note that subgroup analysis of the juxtafoveal studies, but not the extrafoveal or subfoveal studies, showed that there was no treatment benefit in patients with hypertension (elevated systolic or diastolic blood pressure, or a history of antihypertensive use).[42] Consequently, although hypertension may represent a poor prognosticator for laser photocoagulation, the discrepancy in study findings suggests that hypertension should not exclude a patient from laser photocoagulation.

In the subfoveal studies, which included only classic well-demarcated CNVM less than 3.5 disc areas, laser photocoagulation (which included the foveal center) was associated with SVL in the short term but proved beneficial in the long term compared to observation.[45–47] Specifically, at 3 months, the proportion experiencing SVL in control compared to treated eyes was 11% versus 20%.[45,46] However, at 2 years, the proportion of eyes experiencing SVL was 37% versus 20% in the control versus laser-treated eyes.[45–47] Laser-treated eyes in the subfoveal studies also experienced treatment benefit with respect to reading speed and contrast sensitivity.[45–47] Subgroup analysis demonstrated diminishing treatment benefit with larger lesions.

Persistence and recurrence after laser photocoagulation are common. According to the MPS definition, persistence denotes leakage from the peripheral edge of the laser scar within 6 weeks of treatment, whereas recurrence denotes new leakage after 6 weeks from treatment. Persistence was observed in 10% and 32% of treated eyes in the extrafoveal and juxtafoveal studies, respectively.[39,48,49] Possible explanations for this difference include different biologic behaviors of extrafoveal and juxtafoveal CNVM, differences in laser wavelengths (argon green versus krypton red), or the failure to completely cover the foveal edge of the juxtafoveal CNVM. This latter explanation is most likely. For example, in the extrafoveal studies, the CNVM was not completely covered in 14% of lesions compared to 41% in the juxtafoveal studies.[49] The reluctance of the treating ophthalmologist to treat very close to the foveal center is understandable.

Recurrence of CNVM is also very common. In the extrafoveal studies, recurrence occurred in 41% of treated eyes by 1 year and 54% of treated eyes by 5 years.[39] In the juxtafoveal studies, recurrence occurred in 54% of treated eyes by 1 year and 79% of treated eyes by 5 years.[49] In both the extrafoveal and juxtafoveal studies, persistence and recurrence had deleterious effects on visual acuity, with over one half of these eyes experiencing SVL by 2 years in both studies. In contrast, although persistence and recurrence were also very common in the subfoveal studies (51% at 2 years), it did not adversely affect visual acuity, because the foveal center had already been photocoagulated.[45]

To address treatment efficacy of laser photocoagulation for extrafoveal or juxtafoveal CNVM that had recurred through the foveal center, the subfoveal recurrent studies included patients with classic well-demarcated CNVM that had recurred through the foveal center. The entire lesion, including the prior laser scar, measured less than six disc areas with sparing of some retina within 1500 microns of the foveal center. These studies showed similar results to the subfoveal new CNVM studies as noted above. Specifically, laser photocoagulation (which included the foveal center) was associated with SVL in the short term, but it proved beneficial in the long term, compared to observation.[50,51] For example, at 3 months, the proportion experiencing SVL in control eye compared to treated eyes was 9% versus 14%.[50] However, at 2 years, the proportion experiencing SVL was 28% versus 9% in the control versus laser-treated eyes.[50] Laser-treated eyes in the subfoveal recurrent studies also experienced treatment benefit with respect to reading speed and contrast sensitivity.[50,51]

TECHNIQUE

As noted previously, angiography is customarily performed within 72 hours of laser photocoagulation, because CNVM morphology and resulting treatment parameters can evolve rapidly. An early frame of the angiogram is enlarged, projected, or displayed in the laser suite to provide landmarks for photocoagulation. Retrobulbar anesthesia is generally used for juxtafoveal CNVM to immobilize the eye during treatment and is particularly recommended for inferior juxtafoveal CNVM, where a Bell's phenomenon movement could cause "foveation" of the laser beam. Akinesia from the retrobulbar anesthesia facilitates careful treatment of juxtafoveal CNVM borders since undertreatment may facilitate persistence and overtreatment can lead to foveal injury and iatrogenic vision loss. As already noted, patients with a history of hypertension may be at higher risk for persistence or recurrence. The juxtafoveal MPS, but not the extrafoveal or subfoveal studies, showed that there was no treatment benefit in patients with hypertension (elevated systolic or diastolic blood pressure, or a history of antihypertensive use).[42] However, hypertension should not exclude a patient from laser photocoagulation.

Generally, guidelines developed for the MPS are followed.[38,41,45,46,50,52] Only well-defined lesions are eligible for laser photocoagulation. Poorly defined lesions, such as those almost completely obscured by subretinal hemorrhage, or purely occult lesions, are not eligible for laser photocoagulation based on MPS criteria. The end point of laser photocoagulation is to create a uniform white treatment lesion. As noted, the MPS showed no significant advantage of krypton red over argon green laser photocoagulation.[43] Theoretically, however, red may cause less thermal injury to the macular xanthophyll in the juxtafoveal region. Also, red theoretically penetrates subretinal hemorrhage better than green, sparing the overlying retina from thermal injury while facilitating photocoagulation of any underlying CNVM. The treatment area is initially demarcated with overlapping spots, typically using a spot size of 200 microns, duration of 0.2 seconds, and increasing power to achieve a white burn. Small spots and short durations are to be avoided, to limit the risk of Bruch's membrane rupture, hemorrhage, and iatrogenic CNVM. Once the edges of the treatment area are demarcated, the central portions are treated with larger spots (up to 500 microns), longer durations (up to 1 second), and appropriate power to achieve a uniform white treatment lesion. According to the MPS, areas to be treated include the CNVM and any adjacent regions of blocked fluorescence from subretinal hemorrhage or pigment. It is important to treat the entire lesion, including any occult component in addition to the classic component. Treatment of only the classic component, without treatment of any adjacent defined occult component, could potentially "seed" the CNVM, causing more aggressive growth. Treatment is extended 100 microns beyond the borders of the lesion to be treated, except when this would result in treatment of the geographic center of the fovea in the case of juxtafoveal CNVMs. In these cases, treatment is extended to the foveal edge of the CNVM only. Peripapillary treatment should generally extend no closer than 100 microns from the optic nerve head. Treatment in the areas of major retinal vessels should generally straddle the vessels to avoid iatrogenic vascular injury.

Although MPS techniques and parameters are commonly used for laser photocoagulation of CNVM in AMD, other techniques have been successfully employed. For example, several investigators have described successful diode laser photocoagulation (infrared, 810 nm) of CNVM.[53–55] This wavelength is thought to penetrate into the choriocapillaris and CNVM more deeply.[53–55] In addition, as noted, ICG angiography can be very helpful in delineating CNVM that is not well defined on fluorescein angiography.[37,56–68]

Subfoveal CNVMs are eligible for laser photocoagulation based on MPS criteria.[45,46] As noted, the subfoveal studies included only classic well-demarcated CNVM less than 3.5 disc areas, and subgroup analysis demonstrated increasing treatment benefit with smaller lesions, particularly those less than 2 disc areas. Consequently, the best candidates are patients with small lesions and poor vision, and the worst candidates are patients with large lesions and good vision. Patients with subfoveal recurrent CNVM are also eligible for laser photocoagulation based on MPS criteria if the entire lesion, including the prior laser scar, measures less than 6 disc areas with sparing of some retina within 1500 microns of the foveal center. For these subfoveal recurrent CNVM, treatment is extended 300 microns into the prior laser scar. Since laser photocoagulation of the fovea in these cases leads to an immediate decrease in vision, many clinicians refrain from treating patients with subfoveal CNVM or subfoveal recurrent CNVM.

To ensure complete treatment of the lesion, posttreatment photographs can be compared to the pretreatment angiogram. Areas harboring CNVM that have not been completely covered by photocoagulation burns can be treated. After all sessions of laser photocoagulation, patients are asked to return at 2 to 3 weeks for best-corrected visual acuity, slit-lamp biomicroscopy, and fluorescein angiography. As noted, laser scars are generally hypofluorescent in the early frames of the angiogram because of photocoagulation and subsequent nonperfusion of the choriocapillaris and CNVM. On the late frames of the angiogram, there is variable staining, particularly at the edge of the scar (Fig. 57–4). Persistence generally manifests as leakage at the margin of the laser scar. Patients who show areas of persistence undergo repeat laser photocoagulation and are reassessed in 2 to 3 weeks. Patients who show no angiographic evidence of persistence are also asked to return in 2 to 3 weeks for reassessment, at which time the treating physician may perform fluorescein angiography because the risk of persistence is high in the initial 6 weeks after laser photocoagulation. Patients are then reassessed periodically and are asked to return immediately if they note any changes in central vision, particularly if they experience new metamorphopsia or scotomas on Amsler grid testing. They are also followed closely for CNVM development in the fellow eye, as the risk varies from approximately 10% for fellow eyes with small drusen, to approximately 30% for fellow eyes with either large drusen or RPE clumping, to as high as approximately 60% for fellow eyes with both large drusen and RPE clumping.[4] The technique for laser photocoagulation is summarized in Table 57–1.

LIMITATIONS AND ALTERNATIVE LASER TECHNIQUES

As reviewed above, only 13% to 26% of patients with exudative AMD show well-demarcated classic CNVM eligible for laser treatment based on MPS criteria, and at least half of these patients suffer from persistent or recurrent CNVM formation within 2 years.[39,48,52] Patients with poorly demarcated or occult-only CNVM make up the majority of patients with exudative AMD, and it is unclear whether laser photocoagulation is beneficial, as these patients were not eligible for laser therapy in the MPS.[38,39,52,69,70]

In addition, laser treatment itself irreversibly damages the retinal pigment epithelium and retina, causing an absolute scotoma correlating with the site of the laser photocoagulation scar. Because the treatment itself causes a blinding central scotoma when the CNVM is located subfoveally, many clinicians do not treat subfoveal CNVM, although the subfoveal portion of the MPS suggested that laser photocoagulation for subfoveal CNVM in AMD is better than observation under certain circumstances (small CNVM associated with poor visual acuity, e.g., size less than 1 disk area and acuity lower than 20/125, or size greater than 1 disk area and acuity lower than 20/200).[45–47]

To avoid photocoagulating the foveal center, some investigators have attempted to photocoagulate feeder vessels to subfoveal CNVM.[71] Other investigators have evaluated grid or scatter laser treatment, avoiding photocoagulation of the fovea when the CNVM is located subfoveally.[72–75] In one recent study, however, 51 patients with occult subfoveal CNVM were randomized to macular scatter laser photocoagulation (with confluent laser photocoagulation of classic CNVM in 8 of these patients) and showed a visual acuity decrease from baseline that was greater than that of the control group of 52 patients who were observed for up to 24 months.[73] This difference was greatest within the first year after randomization; at 24 months, approximately 40% of eyes in each group lost 6 or more lines of visual acuity.[73] It therefore appears that this technique provides no large benefit, and it is unlikely that a large randomized prospective study will be carried out to further evaluate this modality.[76]

TABLE 57–1. Laser Photocoagulation of AMD-Related CNVM

- Perform angiography within 72 hours of laser photocoagulation.
- Display an early frame of the angiogram in the laser suite for landmarks.
- Consider retrobulbar anesthesia, especially for juxtafoveal CNVM.
- Consider krypton red for juxtafoveal CNVM (less thermal injury to the macular xanthophyll than argon green) and for subretinal hemorrhage (better penetration than argon green).
- Initial settings: argon green, spot size of 200 microns, duration of 0.2 seconds, and increasing power to achieve a white burn.
- Demarcate treatment area with overlapping spots, then treat central portions with larger spots (up to 500 microns), longer durations (up to 1 second), and appropriate power to achieve a uniform white treatment lesion.
- Include both the classic and any occult CNVM, as well as any adjacent regions of blocked fluorescence from subretinal hemorrhage or pigment.
- Extend treatment 100 microns beyond the borders of the lesion, except when this would result in treatment of the geographic center of the fovea in the case of juxtafoveal CNVM.
- Apply peripapillary treatment no closer than 100 microns from the optic nerve head.
- Reassess patients in 2 to 3 weeks with angiography to rule out persistence.

SURGICAL THERAPY

Given the limitations of laser photocoagulation, investigators have pursued alternative treatments for exudative AMD, including photodynamic therapy (PDT), transpupillary thermotherapy (TTT), antiangiogenic therapy, radiation therapy, and surgical therapy. In recent years, there has been a proliferation of surgical therapies for AMD. Most noteworthy, of all therapies for AMD, only surgical therapy (e.g., retinal translocation surgery) can lead to improved vision in AMD, compared to other therapies, which seek to limit loss of vision. At this early stage in the development of surgical therapies for AMD, the risks associated with surgery are obviously greater than those encountered in the alternative therapies for AMD. However, in the future, as these procedures are refined, the risk–benefit ratio may assume a favorable profile.

To study surgical therapies for AMD, the National Eye Institute of the National Institutes of Health awarded funding to the submacular surgery trial (SST) in 1998 to perform a randomized multicenter prospective clinical trial of surgery versus observation for exudative AMD. Two groups of AMD patients are being studied. Group N includes patients with large or poorly demarcated new subfoveal CNVM, and group B includes patients with submacular hemorrhage from either new CNVM or CNVM recurring after prior laser photocoagulation. The SST also includes a cohort of patients with subfoveal CNVM due to the POHS or idiopathic cases (group H), and this study has been active since 1997. Patients will be followed for visual stabilization for at least 2 years in all groups. Health status and visual functioning (quality of life) will be a secondary outcome in all three trials.

SURGERY FOR BREAKTHROUGH VITREOUS HEMORRHAGE

As noted, CNVM can sometimes lead to large subretinal hemorrhages that "break through" the retina and cause vitreous hemorrhage dense enough to obscure visualization of the posterior pole. Patients who present with vitreous hemorrhage and AMD in the fellow eye should be suspected of harboring a CNVM, especially if there is no history of diabetes or other causes of vitreous hemorrhage. On B-scan ultrasonography, macular elevation with moderately high echodensity may be noted, which is consistent with submacular hemorrhage and/or disciform scarring (Fig. 57–2).

The prognosis for central vision is generally guarded with or without surgical therapy. Standard pars plana vitrectomy to excise the vitreous hemorrhage can be combined with extraction of the submacular hemorrhage, and possibly extraction of the CNVM, if intervention is undertaken soon after the vitreous hemorrhage occurs. In eyes with long-standing vitreous hemorrhage, extraction of the submacular hemorrhage or CNVM generally provides little visual benefit, because long-standing submacular hemorrhage is toxic to the foveal photoreceptors,[77] and because long-standing

CNVM generally leads to disciform scarring with photoreceptor disorganization.

SURGERY FOR SUBMACULAR HEMORRHAGE

Submacular hemorrhage from AMD-associated CNVM portends a poor visual prognosis compared to other causes of submacular hemorrhage.[78,79] This may relate to the preexisting widespread RPE dysfunction and ongoing disciform scarring process in AMD compared to other causes of CNVM. In addition, the thickness of the hemorrhage correlates with the final visual acuity in terms of the natural history of this condition.[79] In a rabbit model, subretinal hemorrhage leads to irreversible photoreceptor damage within 24 hours and loss of the photoreceptors at 7 days.[77] The mechanism for photoreceptor injury in this model was postulated to include iron toxicity, impairment of metabolic exchange from the RPE through the hemorrhage, and physical damage to the photoreceptors from clot contraction.[77] A later cat model of subretinal hemorrhage suggested that fibrin within the clot directs early retinal damage, as the fibrin interdigitates with the photoreceptors, causing mechanical injury to them.[80]

There are two approaches to treatment for submacular hemorrhage, pneumatic displacement or pars plana vitrectomy with direct removal of the clot. Pars plana vitrectomy was introduced first, but the relatively poor visual prognosis regardless of management and the greater risks associated with pars plana vitrectomy led to introduction of pneumatic displacement. Because irreversible photoreceptor damage ensues relatively rapidly after submacular hemorrhage, either of these approaches likely yields greatly diminishing benefit when the hemorrhage has been present longer than 1 week.[81,82]

PNEUMATIC DISPLACEMENT

Pneumatic displacement of submacular hemorrhage generally involves intravitreal injection of human recombinant tissue plasminogen activator (t-PA) and expansile gas followed by prone positioning (Fig. 57–5).[83–85] One recent report showed complete displacement of thick submacular hemorrhage from the foveal region in all 15 eyes of 15 patients who underwent this procedure.[83] All patients had preexisting good visual acuity in the study eye, and 13 of the 15 hemorrhages were due to AMD. After a mean follow-up of 10.5 months, the best corrected visual acuity improved by 2 lines or more in 67% of eyes. Complications included breakthrough vitreous hemorrhage in 3 eyes, endophthalmitis in 1 eye, and recurrent vitreous hemorrhage in 4 eyes, 3 of which underwent the procedure once again.

This procedure, described in a report by Hassan and others, is an outpatient procedure using sterile technique.[83] It involves injection of 25 to 100 μg t-PA (25 μg/0.1 ml is recommended by the authors) in balanced salt solution into the midvitreous cavity with a 30-gauge needle at the pars plana 3 to 4 mm posterior to the superior-temporal limbus. An aqueous tap to normalize the intraocular pressure is followed by injection of 0.3 to 0.4 ml 100% C_3F_8 or SF_6 into the vitreous cavity in a similar manner. The patient is asked to lie prone for at least 24 hours and is reexamined at 1 day and 1 week.

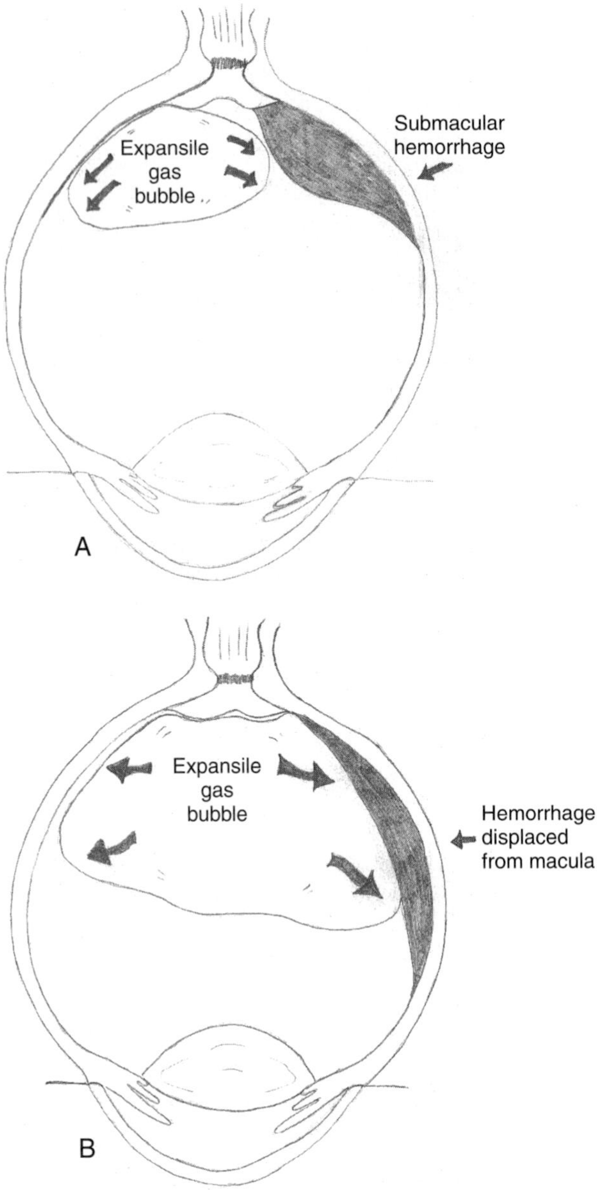

Figure 57–5. Pneumatic displacement of submacular hemorrhage. *A.* An expanding gas bubble is injected into the vitreous cavity and the patient lies prone. *B.* The expanding gas displaces the hemorrhage from the submacular region to a more peripheral region, facilitating examination and angiography of the retina, as well as possible treatment of the underlying CNVM.

Patients should undergo RSFA and ICG angiography within 4 weeks of surgery to delineate any CNVM not previously visualized in the presence of hemorrhage. Extrafoveal or juxtafoveal well-defined CNVM can be photocoagulated according to MPS guidelines. Subfoveal CNVM may be amenable to treatment with new nonsurgical treatments such as PDT, additional surgical procedures as described below, or standard laser photocoagulation according to MPS guidelines, if eligible.

The use of t-PA in this procedure has several controversial aspects. First, t-PA may have some toxic effects on the retina and/or RPE, although the toxicity observed in some studies has been attributed to the arginine-based vehicle of the commercial t-PA solutions and not to the t-PA itself.[86,87] Hassan and others observed no toxicity in the series, even at the highest dose of 100 μg.[83] In addition, t-PA injection may not be necessary as the expanding gas bubble alone may displace the submacular clot.[88,89] It may be reasonable to position the patient prone for 24 hours, and then inject t-PA if the hemorrhage has not been displaced from the macula.[88] Also, injection of t-PA into eyes with recent hemorrhage could theoretically lead to recurrent submacular hemorrhage, and Hassan and others caution against injecting t-PA within 3 days of an acute submacular hemorrhage.[83] Finally, although there are several reports in experimental models that suggest that t-PA can cross the retina to access the subretinal space and yield clot lysis,[90,91] a recent study in a rabbit model using fluorescein isothocyanate labeled t-PA refutes this find.[92]

PARS PLANA VITRECTOMY

As noted above, surgical management of submacular hemorrhage from AMD generally yields varying but generally poor visual outcomes.[93–97] Ultimately, the SST will determine whether surgical evacuation of submacular hemorrhage is beneficial compared to observation with regard to visual stabilization and quality of life.

Pars plana vitrectomy for submacular hemorrhage (Fig. 57–6) includes stripping of the posterior hyaloid from the retinal surface. The posterior hyaloid can be stripped with the silicone-tipped active extrusion cannula or with the vitrectomy probe in suction mode, typically starting in attached cortical vitreous in the peripapillary region, away from the macula. Once the hyaloid is engaged, it can be gently separated from the optic disc and then excised with the vitrector directed toward the vitreous base. A retinotomy site is then chosen, preferably temporally to avoid the maculopapillary bundle and associated visual field defect. The retinotomy can be created adjacent to the submacular hemorrhage, or over large hemorrhages. The intraocular pressure is raised to decrease the risk of additional hemorrhage, and a small retinotomy is created with an MVR blade or any of the commercially available small (33–36)-gauge retinotomy blades. A variety of techniques have been employed to remove the hemorrhage from the subretinal space. The hemorrhage is occasionally liquefied and, in these cases, passive aspiration with a flute needle can be attempted. Alternatively, to express the hemorrhage through the retinotomy site, heavy perfluorocarbon liquids, such as perfluorooctane, can be infused over the retina at an edge of the hemorrhage opposite the retinotomy.[94] The heavy liquid is then removed with a flute needle, followed by gradual normalization of the intraocular pressure with close monitoring for active rebleeding. There is no need to treat small retinotomies in the macular region with the laser, because these are generally self-sealing, as there is no traction once the posterior hyaloid had been stripped from the retinal surface. The periphery is then assessed with scleral depression for retinal tears, and an air–fluid exchange is performed. Just prior to final closure, the air can be exchanged with a short-acting gas such as a nonexpansile concentration of SF_6 (20%), although this may not be necessary because filtered air may suffice. The patient is asked to lie prone for several days.

In many cases, because the hemorrhage is clotted, passive aspiration with a flute needle or infusion of heavy perfluorocarbon liquids will not effectively evacuate the hemorrhage from the subretinal space. Subretinal forceps can be used to mechanically grasp and remove the clot, but this maneuver is traumatic to the retinal photoreceptors adherent to the clot. In addition, the retinotomy is further stretched and traumatically enlarged to accommodate the clot, which can lead to such retinotomy-associated complications as further hemorrhage, nerve fiber injury with associated visual field defects, retinal detachment, and macular pucker. When mechanical removal is employed, it is vital to limit the risk of further hemorrhage by raising the intraocular pressure significantly (above the diastolic pressure of the central retinal artery so that pulsations are observed). In these cases employing mechanical extraction, the CNVM and RPE may be concurrently removed with the clot to which it is often firmly adherent.

To facilitate extraction of clotted submacular hemorrhage, t-PA can be injected into the subretinal space to liquefy the clot.[95,98,99] In a rabbit model of subretinal hemorrhage, 25 to 50 μg/0.1 ml yielded faster clearance of the hemorrhage compared to injection of balanced salt solution as a control, and there was no morphologic evidence of toxicity. In the technique originally described by Lewis, a 33-gauge cannula is used to inject 12 μg t-PA in 0.1 ml balanced salt solution into the subretinal clot, and this is sequentially repeated up to four times for large clots.[95] A small bubble of air is then injected subretinally to tamponade the retinotomies, thereby preventing escape of the t-PA solution; the instruments are removed from the eye; the retinotomies are plugged; the cornea is covered; and 45 minutes is allowed to elapse while the t-PA lyses the clot.[95] A similar technique was described by Lim and others, in which up to three injections of 6 to 12 μg t-PA/0.1 ml were injected subretinally with a 33-gauge cannula, followed by a 40 to 45 minute period for clot lysis, and then subretinal lavage.[96] Other groups have described use of 30-gauge cannulas to perform one or two subretinal injections of 25 μg/0.1 ml t-PA followed by a 20-minute period, during which clot lysis proceeds.[97] In Lewis's technique, a specially designed double-barreled injection-aspirator is used after clot lysis to concurrently inject balanced salt solution while removing the liquefied clot.[95] However, heavy perfluorocarbon liquids, such as perfluoro-octane, can be used to express the hemorrhage from the subretinal space after

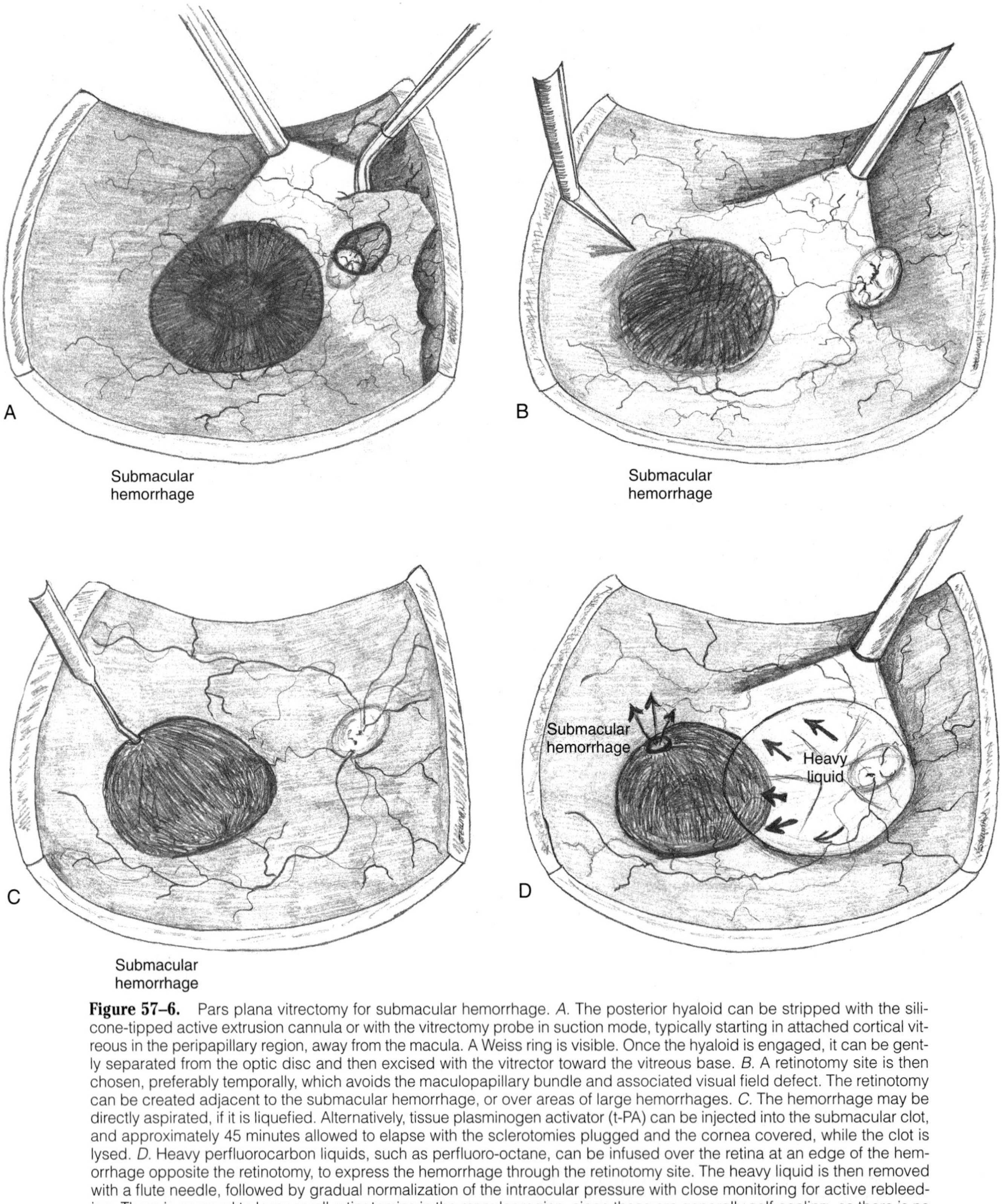

Figure 57–6. Pars plana vitrectomy for submacular hemorrhage. *A.* The posterior hyaloid can be stripped with the silicone-tipped active extrusion cannula or with the vitrectomy probe in suction mode, typically starting in attached cortical vitreous in the peripapillary region, away from the macula. A Weiss ring is visible. Once the hyaloid is engaged, it can be gently separated from the optic disc and then excised with the vitrector toward the vitreous base. *B.* A retinotomy site is then chosen, preferably temporally, which avoids the maculopapillary bundle and associated visual field defect. The retinotomy can be created adjacent to the submacular hemorrhage, or over areas of large hemorrhages. *C.* The hemorrhage may be directly aspirated, if it is liquefied. Alternatively, tissue plasminogen activator (t-PA) can be injected into the submacular clot, and approximately 45 minutes allowed to elapse with the sclerotomies plugged and the cornea covered, while the clot is lysed. *D.* Heavy perfluorocarbon liquids, such as perfluoro-octane, can be infused over the retina at an edge of the hemorrhage opposite the retinotomy, to express the hemorrhage through the retinotomy site. The heavy liquid is then removed with a flute needle, followed by gradual normalization of the intraocular pressure with close monitoring for active rebleeding. There is no need to laser small retinotomies in the macular region, since these are generally self-sealing, as there is no traction after the posterior hyaloid has been stripped from the retinal surface.

the clot is lysed with t-PA.[94,96] Some surgeons inject t-PA intravitreally prior to surgery to avoid the need to wait intraoperatively while the t-PA lyses the subretinal clot.[100] However, as already noted, a recent study using a rabbit model suggests that t-PA may not diffuse across the retina to enter the subretinal space.[92]

One study compared mechanical subretinal clot extraction to t-PA–assisted evacuation in a group of 47 patients undergoing pars plana vitrectomy for submacular hemorrhage extraction.[93] The mean size of the submacular hemorrhage measured 11 disc areas in each group of 23 and 24 eyes, respectively. In the t-PA group, the dose of t-PA ranged from 10 to 40 μg using 10 μg/0.1 ml injections, and the time allowed for clot lysis was 20 to 40 minutes. The hemorrhage was then drained with the Lewis double-lumen subretinal irrigator-aspirator or a single 30-gauge subretinal cannula through the retinotomy site. In the mechanical extraction group, a silicone-tipped extrusion cannula was placed through the retinotomy to aspirate any preexisting liquefied hemorrhage, and then suction was applied to engage and remove subretinal clot. This procedure was followed by use of subretinal forceps to grasp the clot if it could not be removed with the cannula. In this study, the use of t-PA did not improve the visual outcome,[93] but this result could be due, in part, to the uniformly poor visual outcome in AMD patients for the reasons noted above. Another group did not find an acceptable degree of liquefaction of the subretinal clot using 6 to 75 μg t-PA with a 20-minute waiting period, and questioned its benefit in this surgical procedure.[101]

Postoperatively, in addition to the usual postoperative assessments for intraocular pressure, infection, and retinal detachment, patients undergo RSFA and ICG angiography within 4 weeks of surgery to delineate any CNVM not previously visualized in the presence of hemorrhage. As noted, extrafoveal or juxtafoveal well-defined CNVM can be photocoagulated according to MPS guidelines. Subfoveal CNVM may be amenable to treatment with new nonsurgical treatments such as PDT, additional surgical procedures as described below, or standard laser photocoagulation according to MPS guidelines, if eligible.

EXCISION OF SUBFOVEAL CNVM

Direct surgical excision of subfoveal CNVM has become possible. The procedure was introduced in 1988 using a large flap retinotomy technique to access the submacular space,[102] and it was refined in 1991 when a small retinotomy technique was introduced.[103] As noted earlier, this procedure can yield impressive results in histoplasmosis and multifocal choroiditis with type 2 CNVM,[29,35] but the results have been disappointing in age-related macular degeneration, because the type I CNVM typically encountered in AMD develops posterior to the RPE or interdigitates with it, and possibly because of the diffuse dysfunction of the RPE that remains after the procedure.[30–35,104–107] As noted previously, clinical features characteristic of type 2 CNVM include a subretinal pigment halo and sharply defined borders as well as younger age.[36]

Surgical removal of the RPE appears to cause prompt atrophy of the underlying choriocapillaris, with subsequent outer retinal disorganization. The literature suggests that healthy RPE is necessary for maintenance of the choroid and choriocapillaris.[108–114] In primate eyes in which the RPE was selectively damaged by intravitreal ornithine[114] and in porcine eyes in which the RPE was debrided surgically, the choriocapillaris degenerated by 2 months and 1 week, respectively.[108,109] Another group obtained a similar result in a rabbit model in which the RPE was damaged by intravenous sodium iodate, and they also observed absence of the choriocapillaris histopathologically in human eyes with retinitis pigmentosa; they postulated the existence of a diffusible vascular modulation factor, produced by the RPE and responsible for choriocapillaris fenestrae formation and maintenance.[110,111] Some reports suggest that surgical removal of the RPE in humans (during removal of choroidal neovascular membranes) leads to abnormal perfusion of the choriocapillaris, although it is not possible to rule out preexisting atrophy or intraoperative damage.[112,113] These problems highlight the need for successful RPE transplantation after extraction of CNVM and the adherent RPE.

In the largest prospective series of 80 patients with exudative AMD who underwent excision of subfoveal CNVM, the mean visual acuity measured 20/320 at 12 months postoperatively, with an average of one line loss of visual acuity, which may not differ significantly from the visual acuity in untreated subfoveal CNVM in AMD.[104] (The same study showed no significant benefit of subretinal t-PA injection in these cases.[104]) Another large study of 64 patients yielded a mean postoperative visual acuity of 20/400, which was identical to the mean preoperative visual acuity.[105] It is thus unclear if surgical excision of subfoveal CNVM yields a better outcome than the natural history of this disorder, and the ophthalmic community must await the results of the SST to answer this important question.

Excision of subfoveal CNVM (Fig. 57–7) is best suited for patients who show Type 2 CNVM (lying anterior to the RPE), which, as noted earlier, is not commonly encountered in AMD. Patients with occult CNVM are poor candidates for this surgery, whereas patients with classic well-defined ophthalmoscopically apparent CNVM are better suited for this surgery, because the CNVM can be more accurately localized and grasped with the subretinal forceps under direct visualization. A frame of the angiogram is enlarged and hung upside-down in the operating room adjacent to the operating microscope and readily visible to the surgeon, who can confirm landmarks intraoperatively.

The initial portion of the procedure is similar to that described above for evacuation of submacular hemorrhage, with pars plana vitrectomy, stripping and excision of the posterior hyaloid, and creation of a temporal small retinotomy site. The intraocular pressure is also similarly raised to minimize hemorrhage, particularly when the CNVM is separated from its underlying stalks. After the retinotomy is created, balanced salt so-

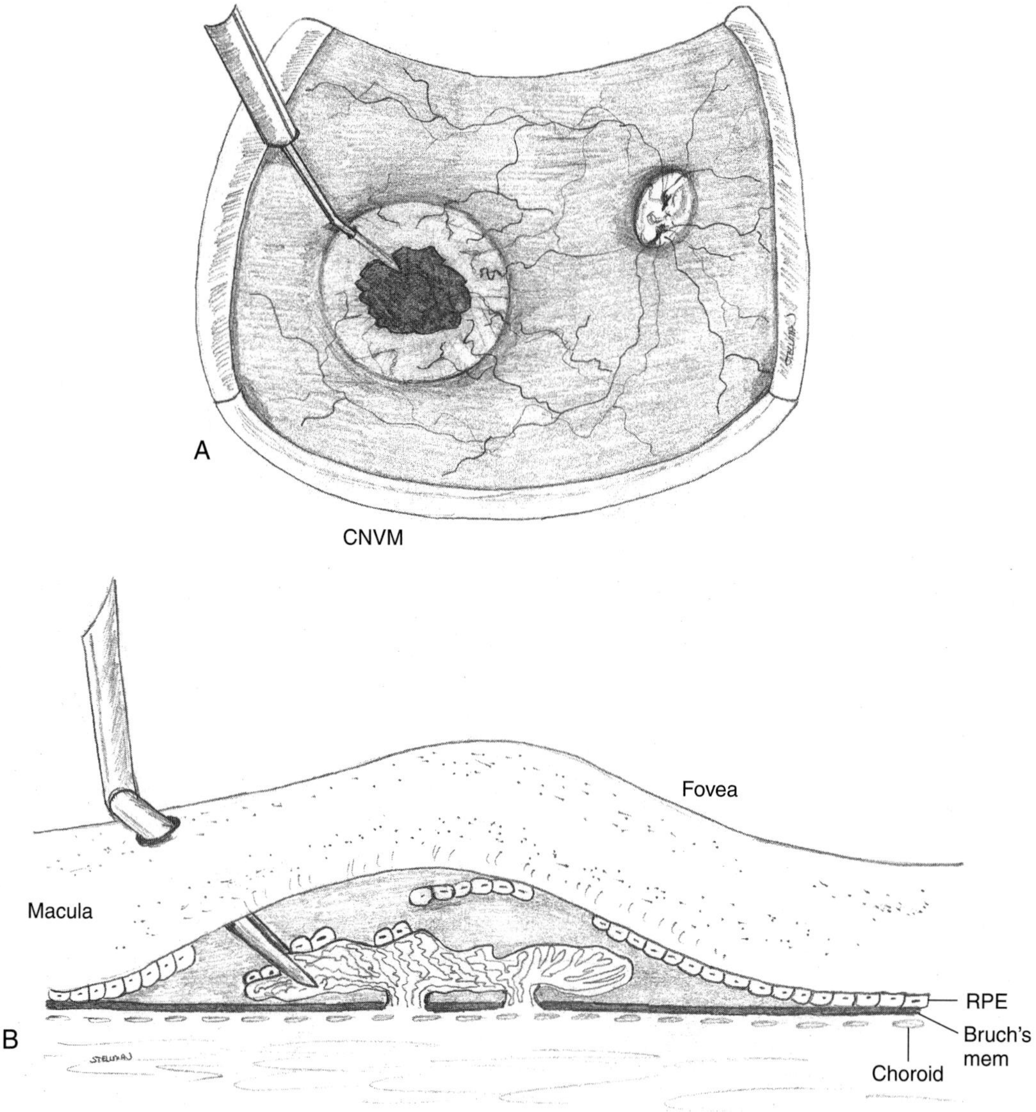

Figure 57–7. Excision of subfoveal CNVM. *A.* After pars plana vitrectomy and stripping and excision of the posterior hyaloid, a temporal small retinotomy site is created, and balanced salt solution is injected gently through the retinotomy to create a shallow macular detachment. Balanced salt solution can be injected through the retinotomy with a 20-gauge silicone-tipped cannula, connected via Silastic tubing to a tuberculin syringe held by an assistant. Alternatively, several commercially available subretinal infusion cannulas and instruments have been designed for this step. An angled subretinal pick is then placed through the retinotomy and gently swept over the CNVM to lyse any adhesions between the CNVM and retina, which may be more common in the presence of a preexisting laser scar. *B.* A subretinal forceps is introduced closed through the retinotomy and then opened in the subretinal space, where it is used to grasp a visible edge of the CNVM without grasping the underlying RPE. The intraocular pressure is raised to minimize hemorrhage, particularly when the CNVM is separated from its underlying stalks. A type 1 CNVM, growing in the sub-RPE space and commonly encountered in AMD, is shown. *C.* The type 1 CNVM complex is gently rocked to further free it from any underlying adhesions. The CNVM complex is then slowly pulled through the retinotomy site, which expands slightly to accommodate the complex. The entire CNVM (typically attached to any laser scar and adherent RPE) is delivered whole through the retinotomy site, with a resulting absolute RPE defect. *D.* In contrast to type 1 CNVM, type 2 CNVM grow anterior to the RPE in the subretinal space and are commonly encountered in younger patients with POHS. The subretinal forceps is introduced through the temporal retinotomy to grasp an edge of the CNVM. *E.* Type 2 CNVM can be extracted with minimal injury to and loss of RPE. Excision of subfoveal CNVM is best suited for patients who show type 2 CNVM, not commonly encountered in AMD.

Illustration continued on opposite page

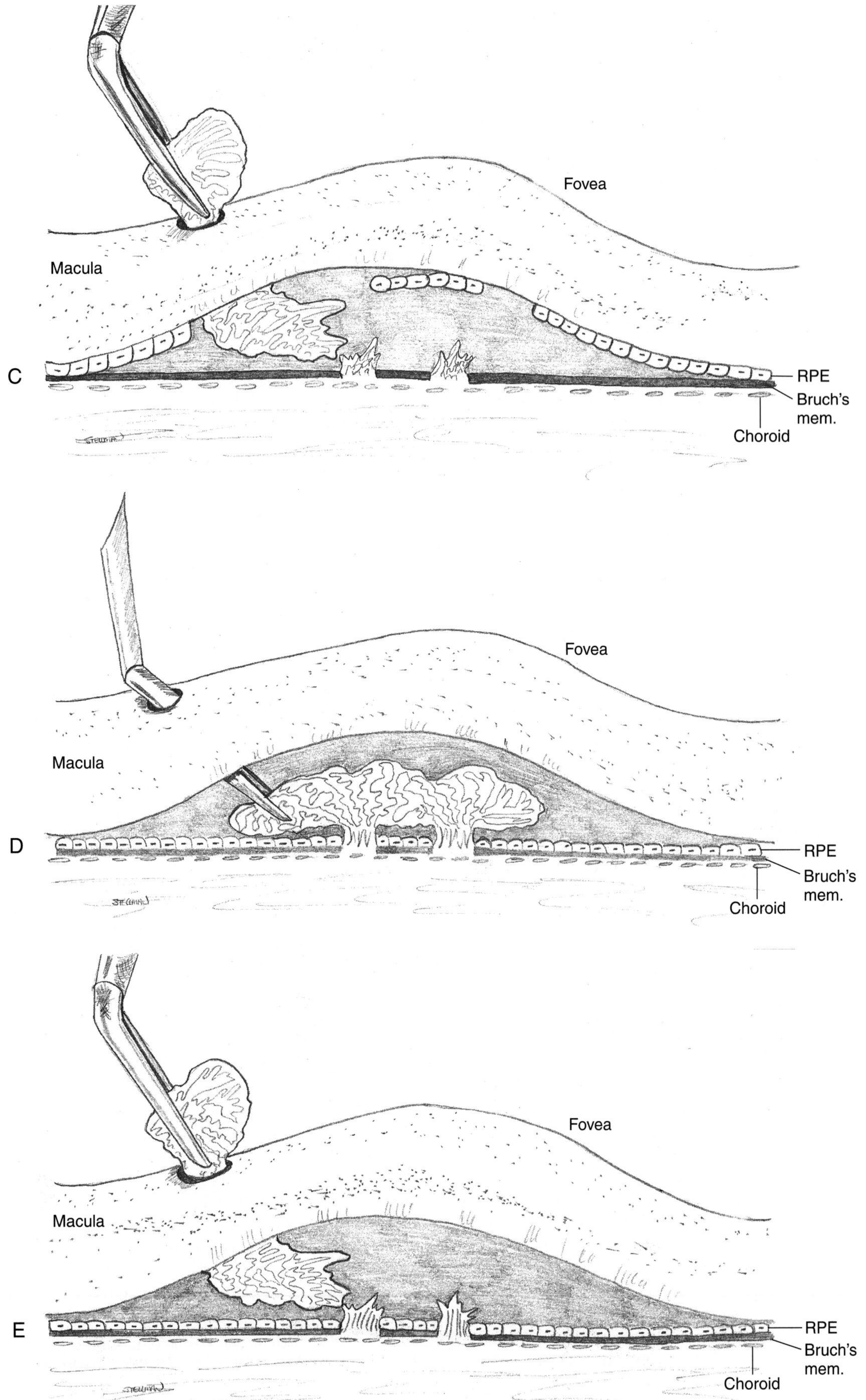

Figure 57–7 ***Continued.*** For legend see opposite page.

lution is injected gently through the retinotomy to create a shallow macular detachment in which the most critical portions of the procedure take place. Balanced salt solution can be injected through the retinotomy with a 20-gauge silicone-tipped cannula that is connected via Silastic tubing to a tuberculin syringe held by an assistant. Alternatively, several commercially available subretinal infusion cannulas and instruments have been designed for this step. An angled subretinal pick is then placed through the retinotomy and gently swept over the CNVM to lyse any adhesions between the CNVM and retina, which may be more common in the presence of a preexisting laser scar. The pick and any other subretinal instruments are always pivoted through the retinotomy site to avoid enlarging it. The angled pick is then used to gently stroke the edge of the CNVM to free it as much as possible from the underlying RPE. In type 2 CNVM, the pick can be used in this fashion to dissect the CNVM from the RPE.

Next, any of the commercially available subretinal forceps is introduced closed through the retinotomy and then opened in the subretinal space, where it is used to grasp a visible edge of the CNVM without grasping the underlying RPE. Subretinal forceps designed for this step range from horizontally closing to vertically closing actions, as well as multifunction forceps that can create the small retinotomy, infuse subretinal fluid, pick the CNVM, and then grasp the CNVM. The CNVM complex is then gently rocked to further free it from any underlying adhesions. The CNVM complex is then slowly pulled through the retinotomy site, which expands slightly to accommodate the complex. The entire CNVM (typically attached to any laser scar and adherent RPE) is delivered whole through the retinotomy site, with a resulting absolute RPE defect. The CNVM complex generally does not fragment. To limit the risk of hemorrhage, the intraocular pressure is raised (above the diastolic pressure of the central retinal artery so that pulsations are observed). Nevertheless, some minor hemorrhage is typically encountered. The intraocular pressure is then gradually normalized with close monitoring for active rebleeding. If hemorrhage is encountered, the pressure is raised again and slowly decreased; this maneuver is repeated until hemostasis is achieved. As noted for evacuation of submacular hemorrhage, there is no need to laser photocoagulate small retinotomies in the macular region, because these are generally self-sealing, as there is no traction because the posterior hyaloid had been stripped from the retinal surface. The periphery is then assessed for retinal tears and an air–fluid exchange is performed. Just prior to final closure, the air can be exchanged with short-acting gas such as a nonexpansile concentration of SF_6 (20%), although this may not be necessary because filtered air may suffice. The patient is asked to lie prone for several days.

Postoperatively, in addition to the usual assessments for intraocular pressure, infection, and retinal detachment, patients undergo RSFA and ICG angiography within 4 weeks of surgery to assess the macular RPE and delineate any CNVM. Typically, an absolute RPE defect may be present. Extrafoveal or juxtafoveal well-defined CNVM may be photocoagulated according to MPS guidelines. Patients are followed closely for recurrence; one study noted leakage 1 year postoperatively on angiography, indicating persistence and/or recurrence, in 18.75% patients.[104] Another study noted a 40% recurrence rate at 2 years.[34]

RETINAL TRANSLOCATION SURGERY

A novel approach to the treatment of subfoveal CNVM includes macular translocation, in which the retina is shifted away from the underlying subfoveal CNVM and moved to a region of healthy RPE. In an early technique, the entire retina is rotated during a procedure consisting of pars plana vitrectomy, 360-degree peripheral retinotomy and retinal detachment, followed by retinal rotation around the optic nerve, and then retinal reattachment to rotate the foveal region away from the diseased underlying choroid and RPE (Fig. 57–8).[115,116] The CNVM can be excised during the procedure or it can be photocoagulated postoperatively to prevent progression to the new foveal location. In an early report by Machemer describing three cases, the retina was rotated between 30 and 80 degrees, the CNVM was excised primarily, and visual acuity improved in all three patients.[116] However, two patients developed proliferative vitreoretinopathy (PVR) postoperatively, and all patients exhibited excyclotorsion.[116] The risk of PVR may be limited by creating retinotomies at the ora serrata.[117] Another group using this technique reported a similarly significant number of complications in a group of seven patients, including retinal detachment in three eyes after silicone oil removal, macular pucker in one eye, and cataract in the phakic eyes.[118] To limit the cyclotropia that can be debilitating after this procedure, one group combines this technique with counter-rotation of the globe by performing torsional muscle surgery.[119]

Another approach involves pars plana vitrectomy with a temporal retinal detachment, 180-degree temporal retinotomy, followed by reattachment of the retina after shifting the fovea superiorly or inferiorly away from the underlying CNVM.[120] Ninomiya described two cases treated with this technique, during which the CNVM was excised and the eye was filled with silicone-oil.[120] One of the patients required reoperation for macular pucker and experienced significant improvement in visual acuity, whereas the other patient required reoperation for retinal detachment and experienced decrease in visual acuity.

With these techniques, as noted above, the patient typically experiences image tilt, diplopia, and risks of retinal detachment and PVR, which may be more likely with larger retinotomies.[115,116,119] To minimize this risk of PVR and retinal detachment, investigators have attempted limited macular translocation without large retinotomies (Fig. 57–9). In this procedure, pars plana vitrectomy is followed by detachment of the temporal retina through one or more small retinotomies and then reattachment of the retina after the sclera has been sur-

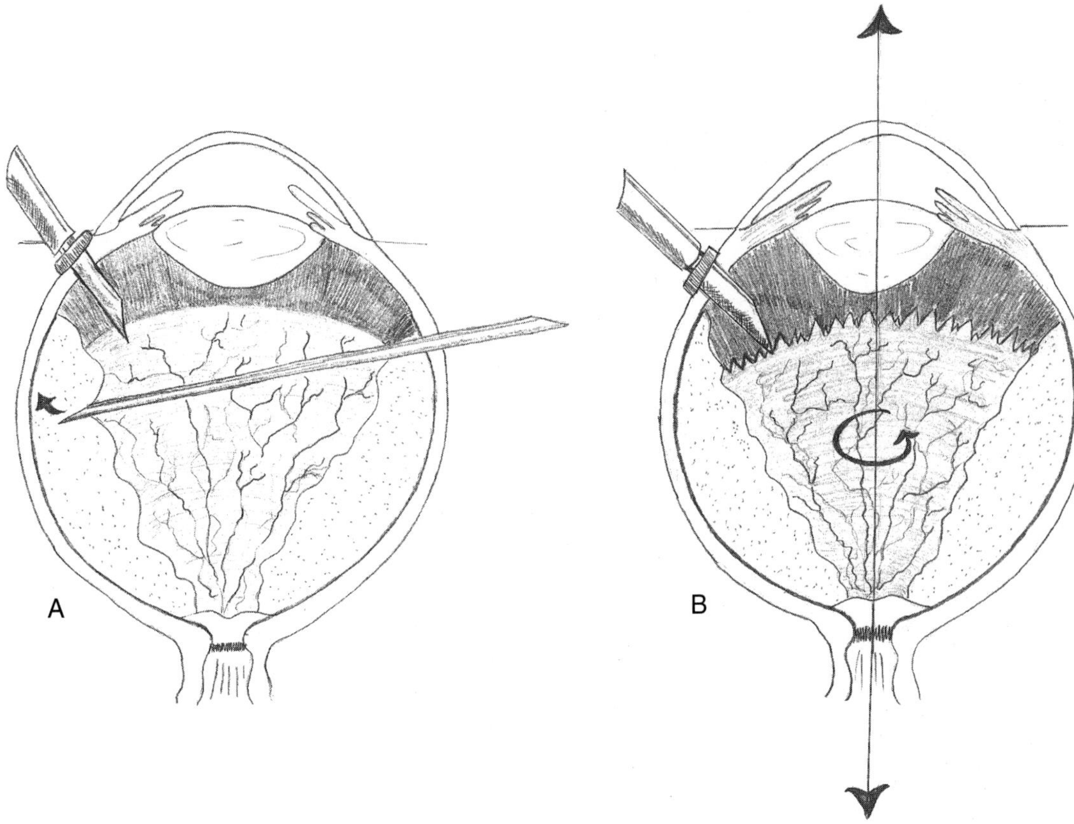

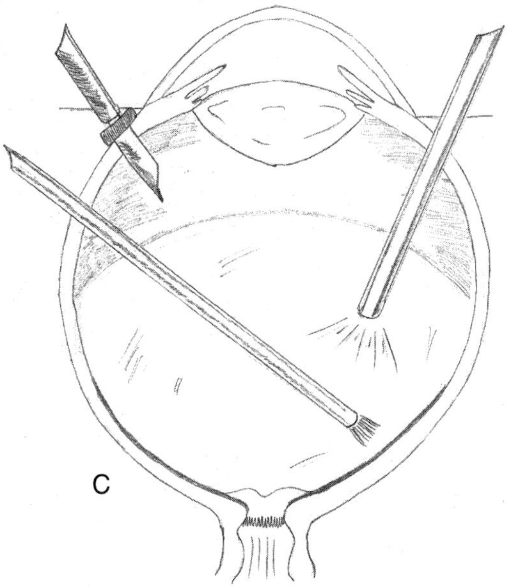

Figure 57–8. Retinal rotation. *A*. The procedure is initiated with pa plana vitrectomy, posterior hyaloid stripping, and meticulous excision the vitreous to the vitreous base. Balanced salt solution is infuse through equatorial retinotomies to create a total retinal detachment. scleral buckle and lensectomy (not shown) is performed by some su geons. *B*. The retina is rotated around the optic nerve, using special designed instruments to handle the retina with minimal trauma, and th retina is reattached with heavy perfluorocarbon liquids. The CNVM ca be excised during the procedure. *C*. Endolaser photocoagulation is ap plied to the peripheral retina for 360 degrees, the heavy liquids are r moved from the vitreous cavity, and silicone-oil is generally used f long-acting tamponade.

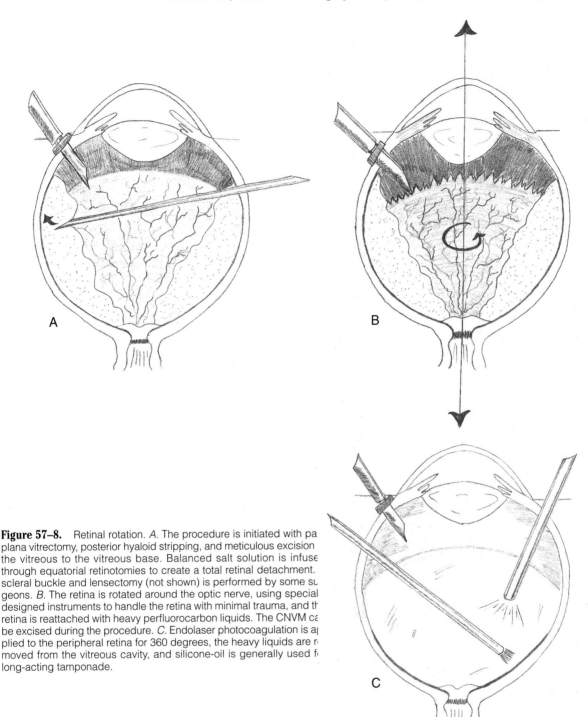

gically foreshortened.[121–124] With reattachment of the retina on the shortened sclera, a retinal fold peripheral to the macula results. These procedures result in limited translocation of the fovea, which may be sufficient for displacing the fovea from small subfoveal CNVM, but the translocation distance is variable and somewhat unpredictable. In the preliminary report of three cases by de Juan and others, the technique included creation of subtotal retinal detachment and reattachment onto infolded sclera, which had undergone crescent-shaped partial-thickness resection and circumferential mattress suturing.[121] In these cases, the fovea was translocated by 350, 1000, and 1500 microns, respectively.[121] The first patient experienced an inferior retinal detachment, which was repaired, and also underwent laser photocoagulation of the CNVM; the visual acuity improved from 20/126 preoperatively to 20/70 at the 8-month postoperative visit. The second and third patients did

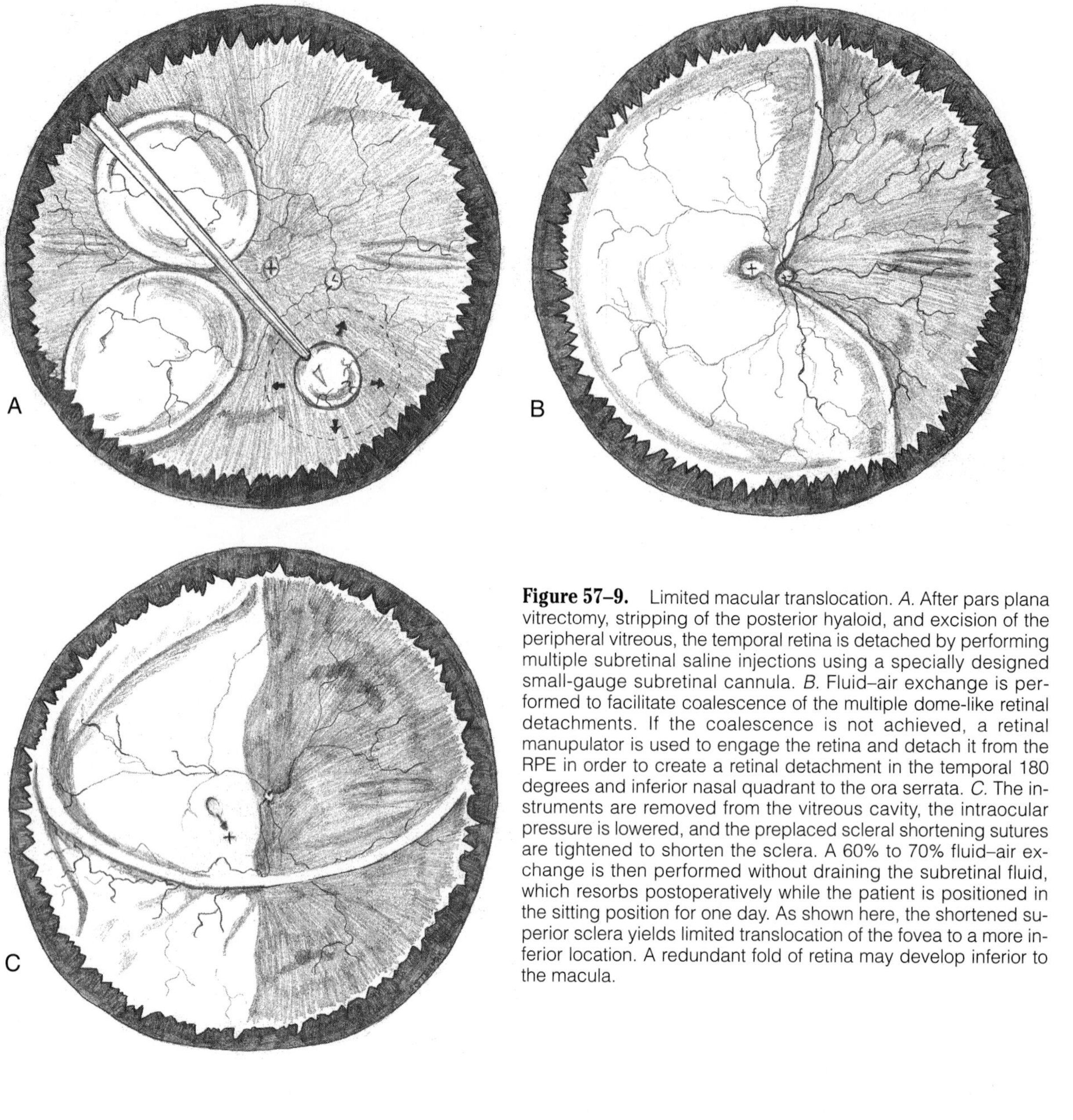

Figure 57–9. Limited macular translocation. *A.* After pars plana vitrectomy, stripping of the posterior hyaloid, and excision of the peripheral vitreous, the temporal retina is detached by performing multiple subretinal saline injections using a specially designed small-gauge subretinal cannula. *B.* Fluid–air exchange is performed to facilitate coalescence of the multiple dome-like retinal detachments. If the coalescence is not achieved, a retinal manupulator is used to engage the retina and detach it from the RPE in order to create a retinal detachment in the temporal 180 degrees and inferior nasal quadrant to the ora serrata. *C.* The instruments are removed from the vitreous cavity, the intraocular pressure is lowered, and the preplaced scleral shortening sutures are tightened to shorten the sclera. A 60% to 70% fluid–air exchange is then performed without draining the subretinal fluid, which resorbs postoperatively while the patient is positioned in the sitting position for one day. As shown here, the shortened superior sclera yields limited translocation of the fovea to a more inferior location. A redundant fold of retina may develop inferior to the macula.

not undergo laser photocoagulation of the CNVM, and experienced an improvement in visual acuity from 20/160 to 20/70 at the 6-month postoperative visit and from 20/160 to 20/30 at the 4-month postoperative visit, respectively. The patients noted tilting of the images, which improved over time.

In the more recent series of ten cases reported by Lewis and others, a similar technique was employed, including partial retinal detachment, scleral infolding but without partial resection, and partial fluid–air exchange.[124] The median foveal displacement measured 1286 microns, with a range of 114 to 1919 microns.[124] In this technique, scleral shortening is achieved by preplacing circumferential 5-0 nylon mattress sutures, with the anterior pass 2 mm posterior to the rectus muscle insertions and the posterior pass 4.5 to 6.0 mm more posteriorly. Placement includes three to four sutures in the superior temporal quadrant, one suture nasal to the superior rectus muscle, and one suture inferior to the lateral rectus muscle. Pars plana vitrectomy with stripping of the posterior hyaloid is performed, and the temporal retina is detached by performing multiple subretinal saline injections using a 39-gauge flexible subretinal cannula. Fluid–air exchange is then performed to facilitate coalescence of the multiple dome-like retinal detachments. If coalescence is not achieved, a retinal manupulator (which resembles a flute needle with three small openings instead of one large opening) is used to engage the retina and detach it from the RPE and thereby create a retinal detachment in the temporal 180 degrees and inferior nasal quadrant to the ora serrata. The instruments are removed from the vitreous cavity, the intraocular pressure is lowered, and the external mattress sutures are tightened and finalized to shorten the sclera. A 60% to 70% fluid–air exchange is then performed without draining the subretinal fluid, which resorbs postoperatively while the patient is positioned in the sitting position for one day. In this series of ten cases, the CNVM was removed intraoperatively in two eyes and photocoagulated postoperatively in seven eyes. In addition, a foveal fold formed in three eyes, requiring reoperation, and one of these eyes experienced a rhegmatogenous retinal detachment. Best-corrected visual acuity improved in four eyes (with a median improvement of 10.5 letters), and decreased in six eyes (with a median decrease of 14.5 letters); the overall median change in best-corrected visual acuity was a decrease of 5 letters.

Limited macular translocation appears promising, as it shows the potential to improve vision, although the technique is in evolution and requires further study and refinement before being adopted as a standard procedure for exudative AMD. In particular, the foveal displacement is limited and unpredictable, as noted. In addition, as a specific complication of this procedure, retinal folds can develop through the macula, necessitating further surgery and limiting the visual recovery.

TRANSPLANTATION OF RPE

Several groups are investigating the possibility of transplanting RPE after surgical excision of CNVM in AMD, as RPE transplantation could theoretically facilitate repair of RPE defects that occur after excision of the CNVM. It is unclear, however, whether functional repair occurs because only a small number of humans have undergone this procedure in pilot studies.[125–133] One group has transplanted patches of human fetal RPE into the subretinal space of five patients after surgical removal of subfoveal fibrovascular membranes, and to four subjects with dry geographic atrophy.[128] Suspensions of RPE cells were transplanted to four other patients with nonexudative AMD.[128] In the exudative AMD patients who underwent initial CNVM removal, RPE transplants developed macular edema and decreased visual acuity after 1 to 6 months, suggestive of host–graft rejection.[128] In geographic atrophy, three of four transplants showed little change in shape and size after 12 months; in non-exudative AMD, RPE suspension transplants showed no evidence of rejection and were associated with the resolution of drusen with stable visual acuity.[128] The investigators suggest that the intact blood–retinal barrier in nonexudative AMD limits rejection.[126–128,134] A more recent report from the same group was consistent with these early findings, with clinical signs of rejection occurring in all cases of exudative AMD and in only five of nine cases of nonexudative AMD, without immunosuppression.[125] Another group, however, found progressive fibrosis in the area of a fetal RPE suspension transplant in a patient with nonexudative AMD who did not take immunosuppressants. This progressive fibrosis, together with leakage on the angiogram and a weakly positive mixed lymphocyte response against phosducin and rhodopsin, was thought to be consistent with rejection.[133]

Various investigators have also evaluated adjunctive modalities in animal models to promote transplant survival. One group, for example, has suggested that cyclosporine promotes survival in xenografts of human fetal neural retina in the subretinal space of rats.[135,136] Another group notes that extracellular matrix plays a major role in the development and regeneration of RPE, and that attachment to extracellular matrix inhibits RPE apoptosis; they have developed a technique in an animal model to harvest and transfer extracellular matrix to inhibit apoptosis and promote survival of the RPE transplant.[137] Other groups are exploring the possibility of autologous iris pigment epithelium transplant.[138]

REFERENCES

1. Leibowitz H, Krueger D, Maunder L, et al.: The Framingham Eye Study monograph: an ophthalmological and epidemiological study of cataract, glaucoma, diabetic retinopathy, macular degeneration, and visual acuity in a general population of 2631 adults, 1973–1975. Surv Ophthalmol 1980;24:335–610.
2. Klein R, Klein B, Linton K: Prevalence of age-related maculopathy. The Beaver Dam Eye Study. Ophthalmology 1992;99:933–43.
3. Tielsch J, Javitt J, Coleman A, et al.: The prevalence of blindness and visual impairment among nursing home residents in Baltimore. N Engl J Med 1995;332:1205–9.
4. Macular Photocoagulation Study Group: Five-year follow-up of fellow eyes of patients with age-related macular degeneration and unilateral extrafoveal choroidal neovascularization. Arch Ophthalmol 1993;111:1189–99.
5. Eagle RJ: Mechanisms of maculopathy. Ophthalmology 1984; 91:613–25.
6. Young R: Pathophysiology of age-related macular degeneration. Surv Ophthalmol 1987;31:291–306.
7. Green WR, McDonnell PJ, Yeo JH: Pathologic features of senile macular degeneration. Surv Ophthalmol 1985;92:615–27.
8. Sarks SH: Ageing and degeneration in the macular region: a clinico-pathological study. Br J Ophthalmol 1976;60:324–41.
9. Spraul C, Grossniklaus H: Characteristics of drusen and Bruch's membrane in postmortem eyes with age-related macular degeneration. Arch Ophthalmol 1997;115:267–73.
10. Ishibashi T, Inomata H, Sakamoto T, et al.: Pericytes of newly formed vessels in experimental subretinal neovascularization. Arch Ophthalmol 1995;113:227–31.
11. Ishibashi T, Miki K, Sorgente N, et al.: Effects of intravitreal administration of steroids on experimental subretinal neovascularization in the subhuman primate. Arch Ophthalmol 1985; 103:708–11.
12. Ishibashi T, Miller H, Orr G, et al.: Morphologic observations on experimental subretinal neovascularization in the monkey. Invest Ophthalmol Vis Sci 1987;28:1116–30.
13. Miller H, Miller B, Ishibashi T, et al.: Pathogenesis of laser-induced choroidal subretinal neovascularization. Invest Ophthalmol Vis Sci 1990;31:899–908.
14. Nishimura T, Goodnight R, Prendergast R, et al.: Activated macrophages in experimental subretinal neovascularization. Ophthalmologica 1990;200:39–44.
15. Ohkuma H, Ryan S: Vascular casts of experimental subretinal neovascularization in monkeys: a preliminary report. Jpn J Ophthalmol 1982;26:150–8.
16. Ohkuma H, Ryan S: Experimental subretinal neovascularization in the monkey. Permeability of new vessels. Arch Ophthalmol 1983;101:1102–10.
17. Ohkuma H, Ryan S: Vascular casts of experimental subretinal neovascularization in monkeys. Invest Ophthalmol Vis Sci 1983;24:481–90.
18. Ryan S: The development of an experimental model of subretinal neovascularization in disciform macular degeneration. Trans Am Ophthalmol Soc 1979;77:707–45.
19. Ryan S: Subretinal neovascularization. Natural history of an experimental model. Arch Ophthalmol 1982;100:1804–9.
20. Ishibashi T, Miki K, Sorgente N, et al.: Effects of intravitreal administration of steroids on experimental subretinal neovascularization in the subhuman primate. Arch Ophthalmol 1985;103:708–11.

21. Steen B, Sejersen S, Berglin L, et al.: Matrix metalloproteinases and metalloproteinase inhibitors in choroidal neovascular membranes. Invest Ophthalmol Vis Sci 1998;39:2194–2200.
22. Faris R, Apte S, Olsen B, et al.: Tissue inhibitor of metalloproteinases-3 is a component of Bruch's membrane of the eye. Am J Pathol 1997;150:323–8.
23. Kamei M, Holleyfield J: TIMP-3 in Bruch's membrane: change during aging and in age-related macular degeneration. Invest Ophthalmol Vis Sci 1999;40:2367–75.
24. Amin R, Puklin J, Frank R: Growth factor localization in choroidal neovascular membranes of age-related macular degeneration. Invest Ophthalmol Vis Sci 1994;35:3178–88.
25. Kvanta A: Expression and regulation of vascular endothelial growth factor in choroidal fibroblasts. Curr Eye Res 1995;14: 1015–20.
26. Lopez P, Sippy B, Lambert H, et al.: Transdifferentiated retinal pigment epithelial cells are immunoreactive for vascular endothelial growth factor in surgically excised age-related macular degeneration-related choroidal neovascular membranes. Invest Ophthalmol Vis Sci 1996;37:855–68.
27. Reddy VM, Zamora RL, Kaplan HJ: Distribution of growth factors in subfoveal neovascular membranes in age-related macular degeneration and presumed ocular histoplasmosis syndrome. Am J Ophthalmol 1995;120:291–301.
28. Gass J: Pathophysiologic and histopathologic bases for interpretation of fluorescein angiography. Stereoscopic Atlas of Macular Diseases: Diagnosis and Treatment. St. Louis: Mosby-Year Book;1997:2–49.
29. Gass J: Biomicroscopic and histopathologic considerations regarding the feasibility of surgical excision of subfoveal neovascular membranes. Am J Ophthalmol 1994;118:285–98.
30. Heimann K: A breakthrough in surgery for age-related macular degeneration? [editorial; comment]. Graefes Arch Clin Exp Ophthalmol 1994;232:706.
31. Hudson H, Frambach D, Lopez P: Relation of the functional and structural fundus changes after submacular surgery for neovascular age-related macular degeneration. Br J Ophthalmol 1995;79:417–23.
32. Lambert H, Capone AJ, Aaberg T, et al.: Surgical excision of subfoveal neovascular membranes in age-related macular degeneration. Am J Ophthalmol 1992;113:257–62.
33. Mandelcorn M, Menezes A: Surgical removal of subretinal hemorrhage and choroidal neovascular membranes in acute hemorrhagic age-related macular degeneration. Can J Ophthalmol 1993;28:19–23.
34. Ormerod L, Puklin J, Frank R: Long-term outcomes after the surgical removal of advanced subfoveal neovascular membranes in age-related macular degeneration. Ophthalmology 1994;101:1201–10.
35. Thomas M, Dickinson J, Melberg N, et al.: Visual results after surgical removal of subfoveal choroidal neovascular membranes. Ophthalmology 1994;101:1384–96.
36. Grossniklaus H, Gass D: Clinicopathologic correlations of surgically excised type 1 and type 2 submacular choroidal neovascular membranes. Am J Ophthalmol 1998;126:59–69.
37. Guyer DR, Yannuzzi LA, Slakter JS, et al.: Classification of choroidal neovascularization by digital indocyanine green videoangiography. Ophthalmology 1996;103:2054–60.
38. Macular Photocoagulation Study Group: Argon laser photocoagulation for senile macular degeneration. Arch Ophthalmol 1982;100:912–23.
39. Macular Photocoagulation Study Group: Argon laser photocoagulation for neovascular maculopathy; five-year results from randomized clinical trials. Arch Ophthalmol 1991;109:1109–14.
40. Moorfields Macular Study Group: Treatment of senile disciform macular degeneration: a single-blind randomised trial by argon laser photocoagulation. Br J Ophthalmol 1982;66:745–53.
41. Macular Photocoagulation Study Group: Krypton laser photocoagulation for neovascular lesions of age-related macular degeneration: Results of a randomized clinical trial. Arch Ophthalmol 1990;108:816–24.
42. Macular Photocoagulation Study Group: Laser photocoagulation for juxtafoveal choroidal neovascularization. Five-year results from randomized clinical trials. Macular Photocoagulation Study Group. Arch Ophthalmol 1994;112:500–9.
43. Macular Photocoagulation Study Group: Evaluation of argon green vs krypton red laser for photocoagulation of subfoveal choroidal neovascularization in the macular photocoagulation study. Macular Photocoagulation Study (MPS) Group. Arch Ophthalmol 1994;112:1176–84.
44. Canadian Ophthalmology Study Group: Argon green vs krypton red laser photocoagulation for extrafoveal choroidal neovascularization secondary to age-related macular degeneration: 3-year results of a multicentre randomized trial. Can J Ophthalmol 1996;31:11–17.
45. Macular Photocoagulation Study Group: Laser photocoagulation of subfoveal neovascular lesions in age-related macular degeneration. Arch Ophthalmol 1991;109:1220–31.
46. Macular Photocoagulation Study Group: Subfoveal neovascular lesions in age-related macular degeneration; Guidelines for evaluation and treatment in the macular photocoagulation study. Arch Ophthalmol 1991;109:1242–57.
47. Macular Photocoagulation Study Group: Laser photocoagulation of subfoveal neovascular lesions of age-related macular degeneration. Arch Ophthalmol 1993;111:1200–9.
48. Macular Photocoagulation Study Group: Recurrent choroidal neovascularization after argon laser photocoagulation for neovascular maculopathy. Arch Ophthalmol 1986;104:503–12.
49. Macular Photocoagulation Study Group: Persistent and recurrent neovascularization after krypton laser photocoagulation for neovascular lesions of age-related macular degeneration. Arch Ophthalmol 1990;108:825–31.
50. Macular Photocoagulation Study Group: Laser photocoagulation of subfoveal recurrent neovascular lesions in age-related macular degeneration; Results of a randomized clinical trial. Arch Ophthalmol 1991;109:1232–41.
51. Macular Photocoagulation Study Group: Visual outcome after laser photocoagulation for subfoveal choroidal neovascularization secondary to age-related macular degeneration. Arch Ophthalmol 1994;112:480–8.
52. Macular Photocoagulation Study Group: Argon laser photocoagulation for neovascular maculopathy; three-year results from randomized clinical trials. Arch Ophthalmol 1986;104:694–701.
53. Friberg T, Karatza E: The treatment of macular disease using a micropulsed and continuous wave 810-nm diode laser. Ophthalmology 1997;104:2030–8.
54. Lanzetta P, Virgili G, Ferrari E, et al.: Diode laser photocoagulation of choroidal hemangioma. Int Ophthalmol 1995;19:239–47.
55. Ulbig M, McHugh D, Hamilton A: Photocoagulation of choroidal neovascular membranes with a diode laser. Br J Ophthalmol 1993;77:218–21.
56. Bartsch DU, Weinreb RN, Zinser G, et al.: Confocal scanning infrared laser ophthalmoscopy for indocyanine green angiography. Am J Ophthalmol 1995;120:642–51.
57. Bischoff P, Speiser P: [Does indocyanine green angiography aid in deciding indications for laser therapy of exudative senile macular degeneration?]. Klin Monatsbl Augenheilkd 1994;204: 298–301.
58. Bischoff PM, Niederberger HJ, Torok B, et al.: Simultaneous indocyanine green and fluorescein angiography. Retina 1995;15:91–100.
59. Dithmar S, Bellmann C, Holz FG, et al.: [Confocal scanning laser indocyanine green angiography of classical choroid neovascularization]. Ophthalmologe 1997;94:343–7.
60. Hartnett ME, Elsner AE: Characteristics of exudative age-related macular degeneration determined in vivo with confocal and indirect infrared imaging. Ophthalmology 1996;103:58–71.
61. Holz FG, Bellmann C, Dithmar S, et al.: [Simultaneous fluorescein and indocyanine green angiography with a confocal laser ophthalmoscope]. Ophthalmologe 1997;94:348–53.
62. Schneider U, Gelisken F, Kreissig I: Retinal choroidal anastomosis in classic choroidal neovascularization demonstrated by indocyanine green angiography. Acta Ophthalmol Scand 1995;73:450–2.
63. Schneider U, Inhoffen W, Gelisken F, et al.: Assessment of visual function in choroidal neovascularization with scanning laser microperimetry and simultaneous indocyanine green angiography. Graefes Arch Clin Exp Ophthalmol 1996;234:612–7.
64. Schneider U, Kuck H, Inhoffen W, et al.: Indocyanine green angiographically well-defined choroidal neovascularization: angiographic patterns obtained using the scanning laser ophthalmoscope. Ger J Ophthalmol 1995;4:67–74.

65. Slakter J, Yannuzzi L, Sorenson J, et al.: A pilot study of indocyanine green videoangiography-guided laser photocoagulation of occult choroidal neovascularization in age-related macular degeneration. Arch Ophthalmol 1994;112:465–72.
66. Staurenghi G, Aschero M, La Capria A, et al.: Visualization of neovascular membranes with infrared light without dye injection by means of a scanning laser ophthalmoscope [letter]. Arch Ophthalmol 1996;114:365.
67. Tang KC, Liu HA: Scanning laser ophthalmoscopy of choroidal neovascularisation using indocyanine green. Aust NZ J Ophthalmol 1995;23:195–202.
68. Wolf S, Remky A, Elsner AE, et al.: Indocyanine green video angiography in patients with age-related maculopathy-related retinal pigment epithelial detachments. Ger J Ophthalmol 1994;3:224–7.
69. Freund KB, Yannuzzi LA, Sorenson JA: Age-related macular degeneration and choroidal neovascularization. Am J Ophthalmol 1993;115:786–91.
70. Moisseiev J, Alhalel A, Masuri R, et al.: The impact of the macular photocoagulation study results on the treatment of exudative age-related macular degeneration. Arch Ophthalmol 1995;113:185–9.
71. Shiraga F, Ojima Y, Matsuo T, et al.: Feeder vessel photocoagulation of subfoveal choroidal neovascularization secondary to age-related macular degeneration. Ophthalmology 1998;105 No.4:662–9.
72. Arnold J, Algan M, Soubrane G, et al.: Indirect scatter laser photocoagulation to subfoveal choroidal neovascularization in age-related macular degeneration. Graefes Arch Clin Exp Ophthalmol 1997;235:208–16.
73. Bressler NM, Maguire MG, Murphy PL, et al.: Macular scatter ('grid') laser treatment of poorly demarcated subfoveal choroidal neovascularization in age-related macular degeneration. Results of a randomized pilot trial. Arch Ophthalmol 1996;114:1456–64.
74. Cardillo PF, Ghiglione D, Allegri P: Grid laser treatment of occult choroidal neovascularization in age related macular degeneration. Int Ophthalmol 1993;17:77–83.
75. Tornambe P, Poliner L, Hovey L, et al.: Scatter macular photocoagulation for subfoveal neovascular membranes in age-related macular degeneration: a pilot study. Retina 1992;12: 305–14.
76. Ferris F, Murphy R: The peril of a pilot study. Arch Ophthalmol 1996;114:1506–7.
77. Glatt H, Machemer R: Experimental subretinal hemorrhage in rabbits. Am J Ophthalmol 1982;94:762–73.
78. Avery R, Fekrat S, Hawkins B, et al.: Natural history of subfoveal hemorrhage in age-related macular degeneration. Retina 1996;16:183–9.
79. Bennet S, Folk J, Boldt C, et al.: Factors prognostic of visual outcome in patients with subretinal hemorrhage. Am J Ophthalmol 1990;109:33–7.
80. Toth CA, Morse LS, Hjelmeland LM, et al.: Fibrin directs early retinal damage after experimental subretinal hemorrhage. Arch Ophthalmol 1991;109:723–9.
81. Vander J, Federman J, Greven C, et al.: Surgical removal of massive subretinal hemorrhage associated with age-related macular degeneration. Ophthalmology 1991;98:23–27.
82. Wade EC, Flynn HW, Olsen KR, et al.: Subretinal hemorrhage management by pars plana vitrectomy and internal drainage. Arch Ophthalmol 1990;108:973–8.
83. Hassan A, Johnson M, Schneiderman T, et al.: Management of submacular hemorrhage with intravitreous tissue plasminogen activator injection and pneumatic displacement. Ophthalmology 1999;106:1900–7.
84. Hesse L, Kroll P: Successful treatment of acute subretinal hemorrhage in age-related macular degeneration by combined intravitreal injection of recombinant tissue plasminogen activator and gas. Adv Ther 1997;14:275–80.
85. Hesse L, Schmidt J, Kroll P: Management of acute submacular hemorrhage using recombinant tissue plasminogen activator and gas. Graefes Arch Clin Exp Ophthalmol 1999;237:273–7.
86. Benner J, Morse L, Toth C, et al.: Evaluation of a commercial recombinant tissue-type plasminogen activator preparation in the subretinal space of the cat. Arch Ophthalmol 1991;109:1731–6.
87. Johnson M, Olsen K, Hernandez E, et al.: Retinal toxicity of recombinant tissue plasminogen activator in the rabbit. Arch Ophthalmol 1990;108:259–63.
88. Heriot W: Discussion: management of submacular hemorrhage with intravitreous tissue plasminogen activator injection and pneumatic displacement. Ophthalmology 1999;106:1906–7.
89. Ohji M, Saito Y, Hayashi A, et al.: Pneumatic displacement of subretinal hemorrhage without tissue plasminogen activator. Arch Ophthalmol 1998;116:1326–32.
90. Boone D, Boldt H, Ross R, et al.: The use of intravitreal tissue plasminogen activator in the treatment of experimental subretinal hemorrhage in the pig model. Retina 1996;16:518–24.
91. Coll G, Sparrow J, Marinovic A, et al.: Effect of intravitreal tissue plasminogen activator on experimental subretinal hemorrhage. Retina 1995;15:319–26.
92. Kamei M, Misono K, Lewis H: A study of the ability of tissue plasminogen activator to diffuse into the subretinal space after intravitreal injection in rabbits. Am J Ophthalmol 1999;128: 739–46.
93. Ibanez H, Williams D, Thomas M, et al.: Surgical management of submacular hemorrhage. A series of 47 consecutive cases. Arch Ophthalmol 1995;113:62–9.
94. Kamei M, Tano Y, Maeno T, et al.: Surgical removal of submacular hemorrhage using tissue plasminogen activator and perfluorocarbon liquid. Am J Ophthalmol 1996;121:267–75.
95. Lewis H: Intraoperative fibrinolysis of submacular hemorrhage with tissue plasminogen activator and surgical drainage. Am J Ophthalmol 1994;118:559–68.
96. Lim J, Drews-Botsch C, Sternberg PJ, et al.: Submacular hemorrhage removal. Ophthalmology 1995;102:1393–99.
97. Moriaty A, McAllister I, Constable I: Initial clinical experience with tissue plasminogen activator (tPA) assisted removal of submacular hemorrhage. Eye 1995;9:582–8.
98. Lewis H, Resnick S, Flannery J, et al.: Tissue plasminogen activator treatment of experimental subretinal hemorrhage. Am J Ophthalmol 1991;111:197–204.
99. Peyman G, Nelson NJ, Alturki W, et al.: Tissue plasminogen activating factor assisted removal of subretinal hemorrhage. Ophthalmic Surg 1991;22:575–82.
100. Chaudhry N, Mieler W, Han D, et al.: Preoperative use of tissue plasminogen activator for large submacular hemorrhage. Ophthalmic Surg Lasers 1999;30:176–80.
101. Hesse L, Schmidt J, Kroll P: Little effect of tissue plasminogen activator in subretinal surgery for acute hemorrhage in age–related macular degeneration. Ger J Ophthalmol 1996;5:479–83.
102. DeJuan E, Machemer R: Vitreous surgery for hemorrhagic and fibrous complications of age-related macular degeneration. Am J Ophthalmol 1988;105:25–9.
103. Thomas M, Kaplan H: Surgical removal of subfoveal neovascularization in the presumed ocular histoplasmosis syndrome. Am J Ophthalmol 1991;111:1–7.
104. Lewis H, VanderBrug Medendorp S: Tissue plasminogen activator-assisted surgical excision of subfoveal choroidal neovascularization in age-related macular degeneration: a randomized double-masked trial. Ophthalmology 1997;104:1847–51.
105. Merrill P, LoRusso F, Lomeo M, et al.: Surgical removal of subfoveal choroidal neovascularization in age-related macular degeneration. Ophthalmology 1999;106:782–9.
106. Roth D, Downie A, Charles S: Visual results after submacular surgery for neovascularization in age-related macular degeneration. Ophthalmic Surg Lasers 1997;28:920–5.
107. Scheider A, Gundisch O, Kampik A: Surgical extraction of subfoveal choroidal new vessels and submacular haemorrhage in age-related macular degeneration: results of a prospective trial. Graefes Arch Clin Exp Ophthalmol 1999;237:10–15.
108. Del Priore L, Hornbeck R, Kaplan H, et al.: Debridement of the pig retinal pigment epithelium in vivo. Arch Ophthalmol 1995;113:939–44.
109. Del Priore L, Kaplan H, Hornbeck R, et al.: Retinal pigment epithelial debridement as a model for the pathogenesis and treatment of macular degeneration. Am J Ophthalmol 1996;122: 629–43.
110. Henkind P, Gartner S: The relationship between retinal pigment epithelium and the choriocapillaris. Trans Ophthalmol Soc UK 1983;103:444–7.

111. Korte G, Reppucci V, Henkind P: RPE destruction causes choriocapillary atrophy. Invest Ophthalmol Vis Sci 1984;25:1135–45.
112. Nasir M, Sugino I, Zarbin M: Decreased choriocapillaris perfusion following surgical excision of choroidal neovascular membranes in age-related macular degeneration. Br J Ophthalmol 1997;81:481–9.
113. Pollack J, Del Priore L, Smith M, et al.: Postoperative abnormalities of the choriocapillaris in exudative age-related macular degeneration. Br J Ophthalmol 1996;80:314–18.
114. Takeuchi M, Itagaki T, Takahashi K, et al.: Changes in the intermediate stage of retinal degeneration after intravitreal injection of ornithine. Nippon Ganka Gakkai Zasshi 1993;1:17–28.
115. Machemer R, Steinhorst U: Retinal separation, retinotomy, and macular relocation, I: experimental studies in the rabbit eye. Graefes Arch Clin Exp Ophthalmol 1993;231:629–34.
116. Machemer R, Steinhorst U: Retinal separation, retinotomy, and macular relocation. A surgical approach for age-related macular degeneration. Graefes Arch Clin Exp Ophthalmol 1993;231: 635–41.
117. Machemer R: Macular translocation. Am J Ophthalmol 1998; 125:698–700.
118. Wolf S, Lappas A, Weinberger A, et al.: Macular translocation for surgical management of subfoveal choroidal neovascularizations in patients with AMD: first results. Graefes Arch Clin Exp Ophthalmol 1999;237:51–7.
119. Eckardt C, Eckardt U, Hans-George C: Macular rotation with and without counter rotation of the globe in patients with age-related macular degeneration. Graefes Arch Clin Exp Ophthalmol 1999;237:313–25.
120. Ninomiya Y, Lewis JM, Hasegawa T, et al.: Retinotomy and foveal translocation for surgical management of subfoveal choroidal neovascular membranes. Am J Ophthalmol 1996;122: 613–21.
121. De Juan E Jr, Loewenstein A, Bressler NM, et al.: Translocation of the retina for management of subfoveal choroidal neovascularization II: a preliminary report in humans. Am J Ophthalmol 1998;125:635–46.
122. Fujikado T, Masahito O, Yoshihiro S, et al.: Visual function after foveal translocation with scleral shortening in patients with myopic neovascular maculopathy. Am J Ophthalmol 1998;125: 647–56.
123. Imai K, Loewenstein A, de Juan EJ: Translocation of the retina for management of subfoveal choroidal neovascularization, I: Experimental studies in the rabbit eye. Am J Ophthalmol 1998;125:627–34.
124. Lewis H, Kaiser PK, Lewis S, et al.: Macular translocation for subfoveal choroidal neovascularization in age-related macular degeneration: a prospective study. Am J Ophthalmol 1999;128: 135–46.
125. Algvere P, Gouras P, Dafgard Kopp E: Long-term outcome of RPE allografts in non-immunosuppressed patients with AMD. Eur J Ophthalmol 1999;9:217–30.
126. Algvere PV: Clinical possibilities in retinal pigment epithelial transplantations [editorial]. Acta Ophthalmol Scand 1997;75:1.
127. Algvere PV, Berglin L, Gouras P, et al.: Transplantation of fetal retinal pigment epithelium in age-related macular degeneration with subfoveal neovascularization. Graefes Arch Clin Exp Ophthalmol 1994;232:707–16.
128. Algvere PV, Berglin L, Gouras P, et al.: Transplantation of RPE in age-related macular degeneration: observations in disciform lesions and dry RPE atrophy. Graefes Arch Clin Exp Ophthalmol 1997;235:149–58.
129. Berglin L, Gouras P, Sheng Y, et al.: Tolerance of human fetal retinal pigment epithelium xenografts in monkey retina. Graefes Arch Clin Exp Ophthalmol 1997;235:103–10.
130. Jiang LQ, Jorquera M, Streilein JW: Immunologic consequences of intraocular implantation of retinal pigment epithelial allografts. Exp Eye Res 1994;58:719–28.
131. Peyman G, Blinder K, Paris C, et al.: A technique for retinal pigment epithelium transplantation for age-related macular degeneration secondary to extensive subfoveal scarring. Ophthalmic Surg 1991;22:102–8.
132. Sheng Y, Gouras P, Cao H, et al.: Patch transplants of human fetal retinal pigment epithelium in rabbit and monkey retina. Invest Ophthalmol Vis Sci 1995;36:381–90.
133. Weisz J, Humayun M, De Juan EJ, et al.: Allogenic fetal retinal pigment epithelial cell transplant in a patient with geographic atrophy. Retina 1999;19:540–5.
134. Gouras P, Algvere P: Retinal cell transplantation in the macula: new techniques. Vision Res 1996;36:4121–5.
135. DiLoreto D Jr, del Cerro C, del Cerro M: Cyclosporine treatment promotes survival of human fetal neural retina transplanted to the subretinal space of the light-damaged Fischer 344 rat. Exp Neurol 1996;140:37–42.
136. Little CW, Castillo B, DiLoreto DA, et al.: Transplantation of human fetal retinal pigment epithelium rescues photoreceptor cells from degeneration in the Royal College of Surgeons rat retina. Invest Ophthalmol Vis Sci 1996;37:204–11.
137. Ho TC, Del Priore LV, Kaplan HJ: En bloc transfer of extracellular matrix in vitro. Curr Eye Res 1996;15:991–7.
138. Thumann G, Bartz-Schmidt K, El Bakri H, et al.: Transplantation of autologous iris pigment epithelium to the subretinal space in rabbits. Transplantation 1999;68:195–201.

CHAPTER 58

Pars Plana Lensectomy

MITCHELL S. FINEMAN, M.D.

The most common indication for pars plana lensectomy is crystalline lens or lens fragment dislocation into the vitreous cavity as a complication of cataract surgery.[1–3] As phacoemulsification cataract extraction now accounts for most of the cataract surgery performed in the United States, it is not surprising that dislocated lens fragments commonly result from a complication of phacoemulsification cataract extraction.[2,4] Dislocation of the lens or lens fragments is caused by loss of posterior capsular support, and is most commonly due to dehiscence of the zonule or a posterior extension of an imperfect capsulorrhexis.[5] Retained lens material has been reported to complicate between 0.4% and 4% of cataract extractions and occurs more commonly with inexperienced surgeons.[3,6–9] Other indications for pars plana lensectomy include crystalline lens dislocation associated with traumatic injury[10] and lens subluxation caused by a variety of systemic conditions, including Marfan's syndrome, homocystinuria, and pseudoexfoliation syndrome.[11–13]

PREOPERATIVE EVALUATION

INITIAL DIAGNOSIS

The diagnosis is most often noted by the cataract surgeon in the course of cataract surgery. Information that may be helpful to the vitreoretinal surgeon performing the secondary lensectomy includes the amount and type of retained lens material, any maneuvers performed in an attempt to retrieve them, the hardness of the lens, the presence or absence of an intraocular lens (IOL), and the amount of capsular support.

INITIAL DIAGNOSTIC EXAMINATION

The cataract incision should be identified and evaluated for leakage. The intraocular pressure should be assessed, because secondary glaucoma is present in about 50% of patients. Corneal edema may be present as early as the first postoperative day and may create difficulty visualizing posterior pathology. The application of topical glycerin ophthalmic solution and the reduction of elevated intraocular pressure may be effective in temporarily reducing corneal edema and facilitating anterior segment and fundus examinations. Anterior chamber inflammation can range from mild cell and flare to a severe fibrinous reaction simulating infectious endophthalmitis.[14] Slit-lamp biomicroscopy and gonioscopy may identify small lens fragments in the anterior chamber angle.[15]

Visualization of the crystalline lens or lens fragments within the vitreous cavity by indirect ophthalmoscopy confirms the diagnosis. Cortical material appears white and fluffy (Fig. 58–1), and nuclear material appears yellowish-brown and has sharper borders, unless it is surrounded by cortex (Fig. 58–2). The examination should include indirect ophthalmoscopy of the peripheral

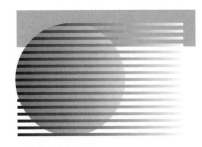

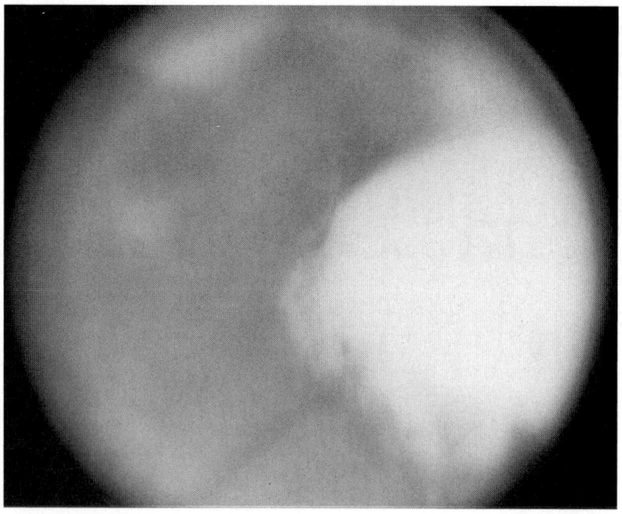

Figure 58–1. Fundus photograph illustrating retained lens cortex in the mid-vitreous after cataract surgery.

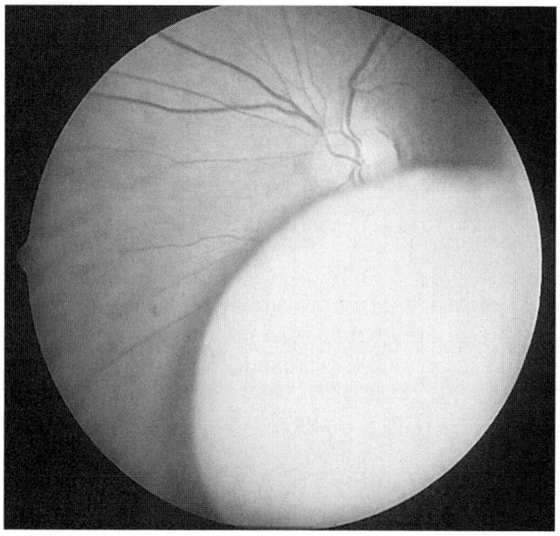

Figure 58–2. Fundus photograph illustrating a crystalline lens nucleus with surrounding cortex that has posteriorly dislocated as a complication of cataract surgery.

retina, specifically looking for retinal tears or detachment and serous or hemorrhagic choroidal effusions. Such complications are more likely to occur if the cataract surgeon attempted to extract posterior lens fragments by irrigation or insertion of instruments into the posterior vitreous.[16,17]

ANCILLARY TESTING WITH ULTRASONOGRAPHY

Ultrasonography is indicated if direct visualization of the fundus is not possible because of anterior or posterior segment pathology (Fig. 58–3). Lens material appears hyperechoic and may demonstrate acoustic shadowing and mobility with eye movement. The number

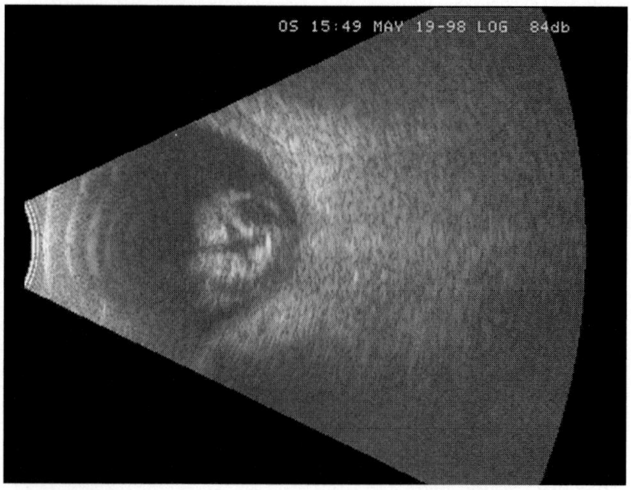

Figure 58–3. B-scan ultrasound demonstrating a posteriorly dislocated crystalline lens. Note the hypoechoic grooves in the nucleus produced during the phacoemulsification cataract surgery. (Photo courtesy of Elizabeth L. Affel, MS, Wills Eye Hospital, Philadelphia, PA.)

and size of the fragments and the presence or absence of a retinal detachment and choroidal effusion should be determined. Hypotony and intraocular inflammation may result in secondary choroidal thickening.

PREOPERATIVE COMPLICATIONS

CORNEAL EDEMA

Approximately 50% of eyes with retained lens fragments present with corneal edema or corneal decompensation.[2,4,18–21] This probably results from a combination of surgical trauma, prolonged phacoemulsification times related to the complicated cataract removal, intraocular inflammation, and increased intraocular pressure. Fortunately, the corneal edema is usually transient and resolves with conservative treatment. Less commonly, retained nuclear fragments sequestered in the anterior chamber may traumatize the corneal endothelium and cause substantial corneal edema and reduced visual acuity, which is reversible only after surgical removal of the fragments.[15] Approximately 3% to 10% of eyes with retained lens material will develop chronic corneal decompensation and bullous keratopathy that requires penetrating keratoplasty.[2,9,19]

UVEITIS

An inflammatory response to retained lens fragments occurs in 56% to 87% of eyes with retained lens material.[2,18,19] Initially, the affected eye may appear quiet, with severe inflammation not developing until weeks later.[14] Treatment with topical cycloplegic agents and corticosteroids should be instituted preoperatively. Rarely, the uveitis may be so severe that it is clinically confused with infectious endophthalmitis.[14]

GLAUCOMA

Secondary glaucoma occurs in approximately 50% of eyes with retained lens material.[2,18–20] The elevation in intraocular pressure may result from lens fragments, heavy molecular weight soluble lens proteins, and macrophages that obstruct the trabecular meshwork.[22–24] A steroid-induced elevation in intraocular pressure may be the responsible mechanism in some eyes, creating a confusing clinical picture. Removal of the lens particles usually results in resolution of the secondary glaucoma.[25] However, as many as one-third of eyes with retained lens fragments treated by vitrectomy and lensectomy demonstrate a persistence of mildly elevated intraocular pressure that requires chronic treatment.[4]

RETINAL DETACHMENT

Cataract surgery complicated by vitreous loss is associated with a 5% incidence of retinal detachment at 4 years, which is 4 to 5 times greater than the risk following uncomplicated cataract surgery.[26] In eyes with retained lens fragments, the incidence of retinal detachment is even greater, affecting from 5% to 16% of eyes (Fig. 58–4).[2,9,19,27,28] About one-half of the retinal detachments are recognized before or during vitrectomy, and one-half develop postoperatively.[2,27,28] The development of proliferative vitreoretinopathy may be more common in eyes with retained lens material, requiring the use of silicone oil for repair and limiting the final visual acuity.[2] Although retinal detachment occurs in the minority of eyes with retained lens material, it is the most common identifiable cause of reduced postoperative visual acuity.[18,21,27]

ENDOPHTHALMITIS

Endophthalmitis may occur concomitantly with retained lens fragments after phacoemulsification.[19,29] B-scan ultrasonography has proved useful in demonstrating the size and type of retained lens material in eyes with endophthalmitis and opaque media.[29] Eyes with retained lens fragments and suspected endophthalmitis should be managed with immediate injection of intravitreal antibiotics in conjunction with pars plana vitrectomy and lensectomy or vitreous tap.[29] The decision of whether to perform pars plana lensectomy should be based on the indications for eyes with retained lens material without endophthalmitis. Although 50% of patients with retained lens fragments have been reported to have positive vitreous cultures, routine vitreous cultures are not recommended because they do not identify eyes at risk for endophthalmitis, nor do they influence the clinical management.[30]

PREOPERATIVE MANAGEMENT

The preoperative management of eyes with retained lens material begins once the surgeon performing the cataract surgery recognizes this complication. After the determination is made that the crystalline lens or lens fragments are posteriorly dislocated into the vitreous cavity, no further attempts should be made to retrieve them. Nuclear fragments remaining in the capsular bag should be phacoemulsified, and residual lens cortex and viscoelastic material should be removed by careful irrigation and aspiration. Anterior vitrectomy may be performed if vitreous has entered the anterior chamber. Attempts to inject fluids or manipulate instruments in the posterior vitreous cavity[31] should be avoided because of the risk of inducing retinal tears or detachments and exacerbating the uveitis.[16,20,32] The preservation of peripheral anterior or posterior lens capsule will allow insertion of a posterior chamber intraocular lens either at the time of the cataract surgery or at a later date. If adequate capsular support is not present, insertion of an anterior chamber intraocular lens may be considered. The cataract wound should be closed with 10-0 nylon sutures even if the wound was constructed to be "self-sealing."

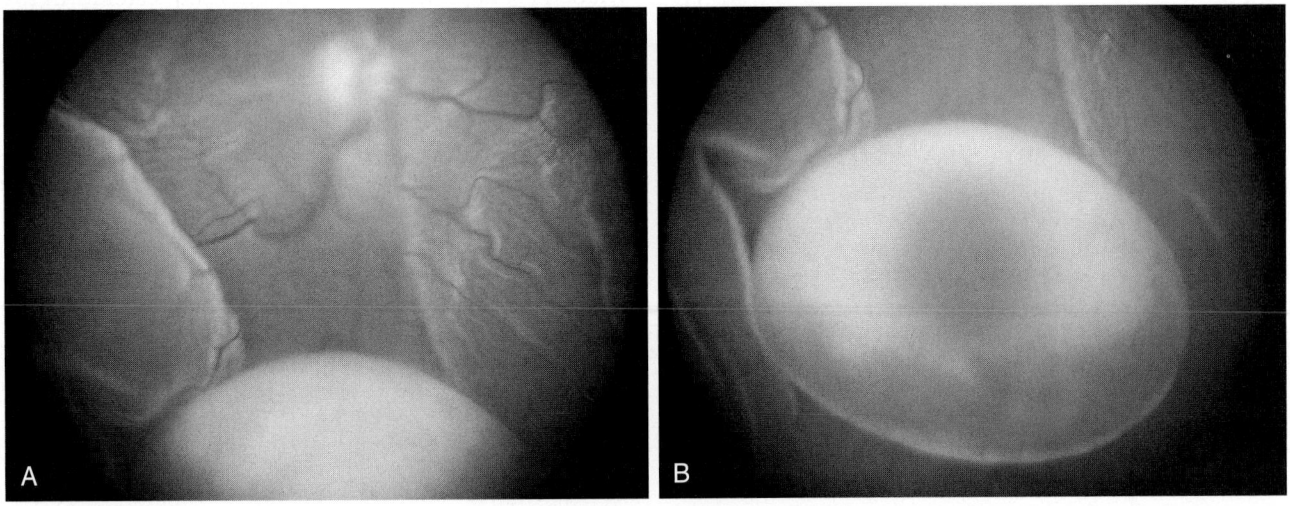

Figure 58–4. *A* and *B*: Fundus photographs illustrating a posteriorly dislocated cataractous crystalline lens associated with a rhegmatogenous retinal detachment. (Photo courtesy of Louis Lobes Jr, MD, Pittsburgh, PA.)

Postoperative treatment with frequent topical corticosteroid and cycloplegic drops should be initiated, and the patient should be evaluated for retained lens material as described in the previous discussion.

INDICATIONS FOR PARS PLANA LENSECTOMY

The indications for pars plana lensectomy in eyes with retained lens material include the presence of large nuclear particles, visual loss from lens particles blocking the visual axis or causing vitreous opacification, persistent and severe uveitis, uncontrollable secondary glaucoma, retinal detachment, and corneal edema caused by retained lens fragments in the anterior chamber.

Eyes with good visual acuity, few lens fragments (especially cortical), and uveitis or glaucoma easily controlled by medication may be treated conservatively. These eyes should be followed until all lens fragments have absorbed, because delayed uveitis, secondary glaucoma, and cystoid macular edema may necessitate late pars plana lensectomy.

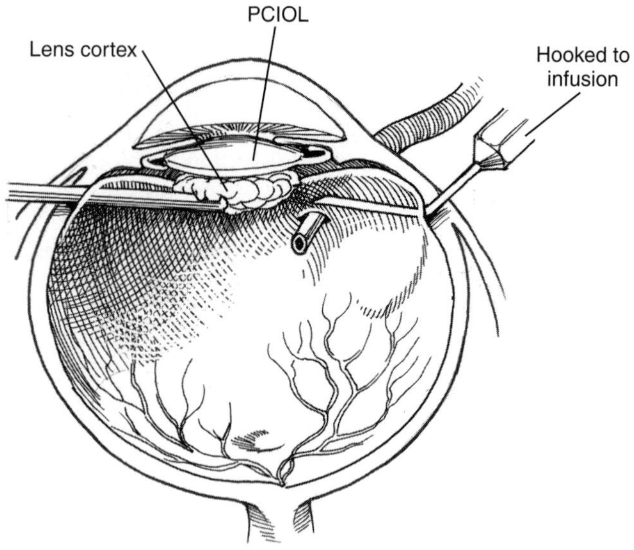

Figure 58–5. The vitrectomy cutter is used to clear lens material from the visual axis. Infusion is provided via a bent 21-gauge needle attached to the infusion fluid bottle. Once the infusion cannula is visualized in the vitreous cavity, the infusion is opened.

TIMING OF PARS PLANA LENSECTOMY

Controversy exists regarding the optimal timing of pars plana lensectomy. Two small series suggested that eyes treated within 3 weeks of lens dislocation had a lower incidence of postoperative glaucoma.[1,4] However, larger and more recent series did not find a statistically significant difference in visual outcomes between eyes treated with early or late pars plana lensectomy.[2,18,19,27] Because pars plana lensectomy has been shown to result in resolution of secondary glaucoma and uveitis, it should not be delayed in eyes that have adequate corneal clarity and that fulfill the criteria for early pars plana lensectomy.[25] In some cases, corneal edema will prevent surgery because it will interfere with visualization by the surgeon. In these cases, aggressive treatment of elevated intraocular pressure and uveitis will usually allow the edema to resolve sufficiently to permit safe vitreoretinal surgery.

OPERATIVE TECHNIQUE

PARS PLANA LENSECTOMY

A standard three-port pars plana vitrectomy, with or without ultrasonic phacofragmentation, is the procedure of choice in eyes with retained lens material. The cataract incision should be inspected, and sutures should be placed if there is evidence of wound leakage.

If lens material in the pupillary axis prevents visualization of the infusion cannula, a bent 21-gauge needle attached to an infusion bottle can be introduced through one of the superior sclerostomy sites, and the vitreous cutter can be placed through the other site (Fig. 58–5). The cannula may be opened only after the lens material has been cleared from the visual axis and the cannula can be directly visualized within the vitreous cavity.

First, lens material that is retained under the iris, within the residual lens capsule, and surrounding the IOL should be removed with the vitreous cutter, in order to improve visualization. If an IOL was not placed, preservation of any residual lens capsule will facilitate placement of an IOL coincident with the vitrectomy or in the future. Lens material that is sequestered in the anterior chamber may be removed by cutting a small opening in the lens capsule or peripheral iris and inserting the cutter into the anterior chamber.

Next, vitreous debris and cortical lens material are cleared from the vitreous cavity with a standard vitrectomy cutter (Fig. 58–6). The vitreous base is trimmed peripherally and the retained lens material is freed from all vitreous attachments. Smaller or softer pieces of nu-

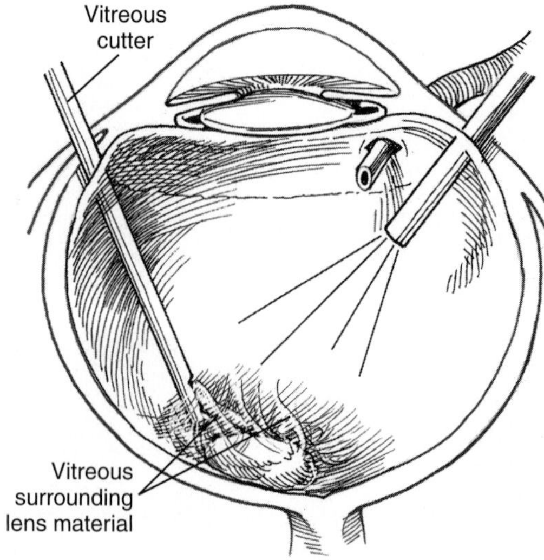

Figure 58–6. The retained lens material is freed of all vitreous adhesions using the vitrectomy cutter.

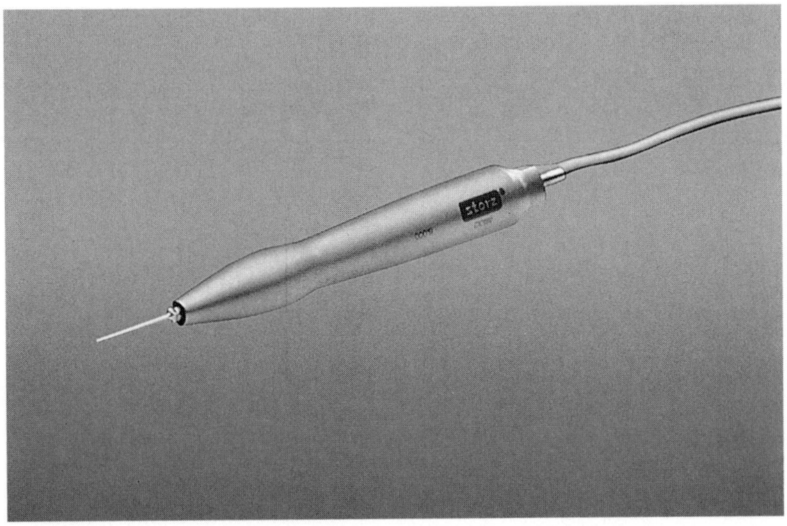

Figure 58–7. The Storz Millennium phacofragmatome handpiece and needle produce ultrasound power at a frequency of 28.5 kHz and vacuum levels up to 400 mm Hg. (Photograph courtesy of Bausch & Lomb Surgical, St. Louis, MO.)

cleus may be removed using the vitreous cutter alone, or by using the light pipe to crush the lens material into smaller pieces and force them into the cutting port. Larger or harder pieces of nucleus require the use of a phacofragmatome, a 20-gauge ultrasound needle capable of phacoemulsifying the lens material (Fig. 58–7). After the phacofragmatome is introduced into the vitreous cavity, aspiration is used to engage the lens material and to elevate it into the midvitreous cavity; only then is phacoemulsification power applied (Fig. 58–8).

Occasionally, hard nuclei may be difficult to phacoemulsify using the phacofragmatome alone. If a lens particle is repeatedly ejected from the tip of the phacofragmatome, several techniques may be used. Lowering the ultrasound power to 5% to 10% of the maximum power, increasing the vacuum, or using the pulse mode option on the phacofragmatome settings may aid in keeping the lens material engaged. A bimanual technique that uses the light pipe or a lighted pick to stabilize the nucleus in the midvitreous cavity is also effective.[33] One potential complication with the use of a lighted pick is the possibility of retained metal shavings if the pick and the phacofragmatome come into contact during lens removal.[33]

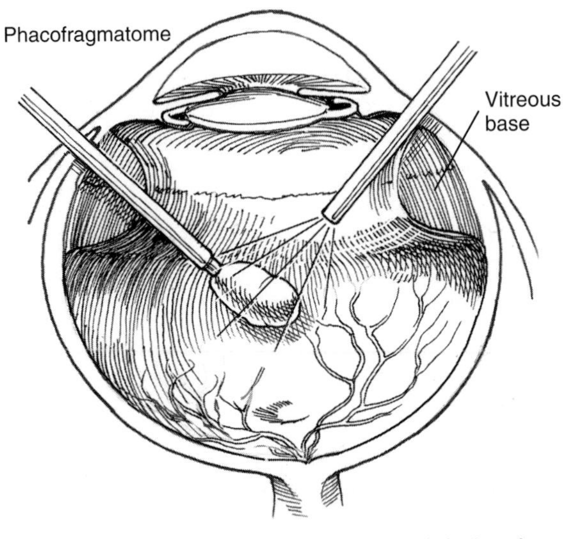

Figure 58–8. The phacofragmatome is used to lift the lens fragment off the surface of the retina by aspiration. Once the lens material is elevated into the midvitreous cavity, phacoemulsification may be performed.

ADJUNCTIVE PERFLUOROCARBON LIQUIDS

Perfluorocarbon liquids may facilitate the safe removal of retained lens material in four ways. First, they provide protection from contusion injuries of the macula caused by lens particles that fall posteriorly or are projected from the tip of the phacofragmatome during emulsification.[34,35] Second, the relative buoyancy of lens material compared to perfluorocarbon liquid causes the lens material to float on the surface, reducing the risk of retinal damage during manipulation and engagement of the particles.[36] Third, perfluorocarbon liquids form a protective layer over the posterior pole, which may reduce the risk of damage to the retinal pigment epithelium and neurosensory retina resulting from the ultrasonic stream of the phacofragmatome.[37] Finally, perfluorocarbon liquids are useful when a retinal detachment occurs concomitantly with retained lens material.[34] The decreased mobility of the retina afforded by the perfluorocarbon liquid bubble reduces the risk of inadvertent retinal injury, floats the lens material above the retinal surface, and aids in repair of the retinal detachment.

Enough perfluorocarbon liquid should be instilled into the eye to extend just outside the arcades (Fig. 58–9). Overfill can complicate the removal of lens ma-

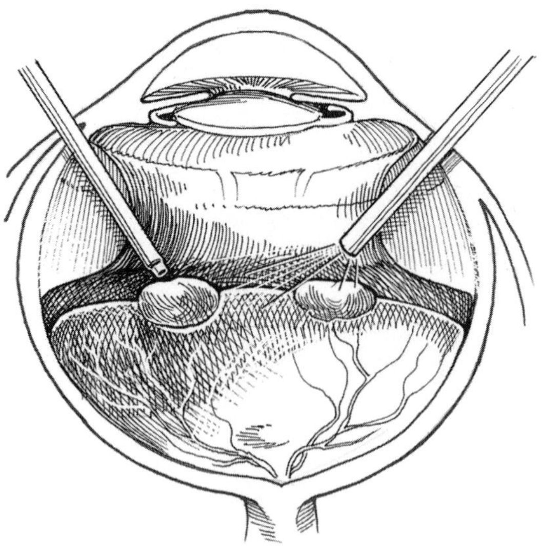

Figure 58–9. Perfluorocarbon liquid may be a useful adjunct in the removal of retained lens material. Enough perfluorocarbon liquid should be instilled to extend just outside the vascular arcades.

terial, because the meniscus of the bubble tends to cause displacement of the lens fragments toward the retinal periphery and vitreous base. Attempts to remove particles that have become trapped in the vitreous base may cause retinal tears or dialyses.

ALTERNATIVE TECHNIQUES

Mechanical crushing of the nucleus between two instruments is a useful technique that complements modern phacofragmentation. If necessary, it may be used as a primary means of removing nuclear lens material if phacofragmentation is not available.

Other techniques have been described for use in the management of extremely hard nuclear lens fragments. They involve mobilizing the retained lens fragments, either into the anterior chamber with delivery through a limbal incision, or into the posterior chamber with delivery through a pars plana incision.[38,39] Both of these techniques require large incisions in either the limbus or pars plana, and the former technique risks corneal endothelial injury. With the development of increasingly better phacofragmentation instruments, the techniques of corneal limbal extraction and phacohydroexpulsion have been largely abandoned.

INTRAOCULAR LENS MANAGEMENT

If an IOL was inserted at the time of cataract surgery, it may require intraoperative repositioning.[40] If an anterior or posterior chamber lens was not inserted at the time of cataract surgery, consideration should be given to placement of an IOL at the time of pars plana lensectomy. Placement at this time is beneficial because it eliminates the need for additional surgery; also, because the IOL is inserted after the pars plana lensectomy, it does not interfere with removal of the retained lens material. If there is significant corneal edema, choroidal detachment or hemorrhage, or lack of capsular support with a contraindication to anterior chamber lens placement, however, then IOL placement should be deferred. If inadequate capsular support is present, and insertion of an anterior chamber intraocular lens is not desirable, a sutured posterior chamber intraocular lens may be considered.[41] There is evidence to suggest that posterior chamber lenses may result in a higher rate of 20/40 or better visual acuity than anterior chamber lenses.[18,19,41]

INTRAOPERATIVE COMPLICATIONS

Major intraoperative complications include cataract incision dehiscence with prolapse of uveal tissue, and choroidal hemorrhage with possible prolapse of uveal tissue and obliteration of the vitreous cavity. Reinforcement of the cataract wound before vitrectomy, direct visualization of the infusion cannula within the vitreous cavity, and the dynamics of the closed system afforded by modern vitrectomy techniques reduce the risk of these complications.

A retinal detachment, tear, or dialysis discovered at the time of pars plana lensectomy should be repaired using the standard operative techniques (see Chapter 56). Intraocular gas tamponade, required for repair of selected retinal detachments, may result in secondary dislocation of a recently inserted sulcus-fixated posterior chamber intraocular lens.

POSTOPERATIVE MANAGEMENT

Treatment with topical corticosteroids and cycloplegia should be continued after vitrectomy and lensectomy. The intraocular pressure should be monitored for evidence of persistent secondary glaucoma. Examination of the peripheral retina for signs of retinal tears or detachment should be performed postoperatively.

POSTOPERATIVE COMPLICATIONS

CORNEAL EDEMA

Corneal decompensation may be worsened as a result of vitrectomy and lensectomy. This further surgical insult to an already traumatized eye can exacerbate corneal edema. Medical management and watchful waiting will usually result in resolution of the edema; however, corneal edema persists in 3% to 10% of eyes with retained lens material.[2,9,19]

RETINAL DETACHMENT

As discussed previously, retinal detachment occurs in 5% to 16% of eyes with retained lens fragments, and

50% of the detachments occur postvitrectomy.[2,9,19,27,28] Proliferative vitreoretinopathy also develops more commonly with retinal detachments that occur in the postvitrectomy period.[1,2,4,42]

CYSTOID MACULAR EDEMA

Postoperative cystoid macular edema (CME) occurs in 3% to 12% of eyes after vitrectomy and lensectomy.[27,43] It is difficult to determine, however, if the cystoid macular edema is a consequence of the complicated cataract surgery, is related to the vitrectomy and lensectomy, or is due to perioperative complications such as retinal detachment or persistent uveitis. Vitrectomy is effective in reducing the inflammatory response and may secondarily reduce the incidence of postoperative CME in otherwise uncomplicated cases.[9,19] In eyes that require repair of a retinal detachment, CME may result in a further decrease in visual acuity.[2,27]

GLAUCOMA

Secondary glaucoma usually resolves promptly after removal of the retained lens material.[25] If the intraocular pressure continues to rise following vitrectomy and lensectomy, the possibility of steroid-induced glaucoma should be considered. As many as one-third of eyes will develop a chronic elevation of intraocular pressure requiring medical treatment.[4]

PROGNOSIS

Pars plana vitrectomy and lensectomy has proved to be effective in restoring vision for eyes with retained lens material. Between 44% and 68% of patients will obtain 20/40 or better acuity after pars plana lensectomy for retained lens fragments.[2,18,19,27] Improved surgical techniques, along with a heightened awareness by surgeons of potential complications and management options, have improved the safety and visual outcome of this procedure.

REFERENCES

1. Fastenberg DM, Schwartz PL, Shakin JL, et al.: Management of dislocated nuclear fragments after phacoemulsification. Am J Ophthalmol 1991;112:535–539.
2. Gilliland GD, Hutton WL, Fuller DG: Retained intravitreal lens fragments after cataract surgery. Ophthalmology 1992;99:1263–1267.
3. Pande M, Dabbs TR: Incidence of lens matter dislocation during phacoemulsification. J Cataract Refract Surg 1996;22:737–742.
4. Blodi BA, Flynn HW Jr, Blodi CF, et al.: Retained nuclei after cataract surgery. Ophthalmology 1992;99:41–44.
5. Chern S, Yung CW: Posterior lens dislocation during attempted phacoemulsification. Ophthalmic Surg 1995;26:114–116.
6. Cotlier E, Rose M: Cataract extraction by the intracapsular methods and by phacoemulsification: the results of surgeons in training. Trans Am Acad Ophthalmol Otolaryngol 1976;81:OP163–182.
7. Fung WE: Phacoemulsification. Ophthalmology 1978;85:46–51.
8. Hurite FG: Symposium: Phacoemulsification. The contraindications to phacoemulsification and summary of personal experience. Trans Am Acad Ophthalmol Otolaryngol 1974;78:OP14–17.
9. Stilma JS, van der Sluijs FA, van Meurs JC, et al.: Occurrence of retained lens fragments after phacoemulsification in The Netherlands. J Cataract Refract Surg 1997;23:1177–1182.
10. Marcus DM,Topping TM, Frederick AR Jr: Vitreoretinal management of traumatic dislocation of the crystalline lens. Int Ophthalmol Clin 1995;35:139–150.
11. Gerding H: Ocular complications and a new surgical approach to lens dislocation in homocystinuria due to cystathionine-beta-synthetase deficiency. Eur J Pediatr 1998;157:S94–S101.
12. Hakin KN, Jacobs M, Rosen P, et al.: Management of the subluxed crystalline lens. Ophthalmology 1992;99:542–545.
13. Koenig SB, Mieler WF: Management of ectopia lentis in a family with Marfan syndrome. Arch Ophthalmol 1996;114:1058–1061.
14. Irvine WD, Flynn HW Jr, Murray TG, et al.: Retained lens fragments after phacoemulsification manifesting as marked intraocular inflammation with hypopyon. Am J Ophthalmol 1992;114:610–614.
15. Bohigian GM, Wexler SA: Complications of retained nuclear fragments in the anterior chamber after phacoemulsification with posterior chamber lens implant. Am J Ophthalmol 1997;123:546–547.
16. Aaberg TM Jr, Rubsamen PE, Flynn HW Jr, et al.: Giant retinal tear as a complication of attempted removal of intravitreal lens fragment during cataract surgery. Am J Ophthalmol 1997;124:222–226.
17. Terasaki H, Miyake Y, Miyake K: Visual outcome after management of a posteriorly dislocated lens nucleus during phacoemulsification. J Cataract Refract Surg 1997;23:1399–1403.
18. Kim JE, Flynn HW Jr, Smiddy WE, et al.: Retained lens fragments after phacoemulsification. Ophthalmology 1994;101:1827–1832.
19. Margherio RR, Margherio AR, Pendergast SD, et al.: Vitrectomy for retained lens fragments after phacoemulsification. Ophthalmology 1997;104:1426–1432.
20. Ross WH: Management of dislocated lens fragments after phacoemulsification surgery. Can J Ophthalmol 1996;31:234–240.
21. Tommila P, Immonen I: Dislocated nuclear fragments after cataract surgery. Eye 1995;9:437–441.
22. Epstein DL: Diagnosis and management of lens-induced glaucoma. Ophthalmology 1982;89:227–230.
23. Epstein DL, Jedziniak JA, Grant WM: Obstruction of aqueous outflow by lens particles and by heavy-molecular-weight soluble lens proteins. Invest Ophthalmol Vis Sci 1978;17:272–277.
24. Filipe JC, Palmares J, Delgado L, et al.: Phacolytic glaucoma and lens-induced uveitis. Int Ophthalmol 1993;17:289–293.
25. Vilar NF, Flynn HW Jr, Smiddy WE, et al.: Removal of retained lens fragments after phacoemulsification reverses secondary glaucoma and restores visual acuity. Ophthalmology 1997;104:787–791.
26. Javitt JC, Vitale S, Canner JK, et al.: National outcomes of cataract extraction. I. Retinal detachment after inpatient surgery. Ophthalmology 1991;98:895–902.
27. Borne MJ, Tasman W, Regillo C, et al.: Outcomes of vitrectomy for retained lens fragments. Ophthalmology 1996;103:971–976.
28. Smiddy WE, Flynn HW Jr, Kim JE: Retinal detachment in patients with retained lens fragments or dislocated posterior chamber intraocular lenses. Ophthalmic Surg Lasers 1996;27:856–861.
29. Kim JE, Flynn HW Jr, Rubsamen PE, et al.: Endophthalmitis in patients with retained lens fragments after phacoemulsification. Ophthalmology 1996;103:575–578.
30. Joondeph BC, Myint S, Joondeph HC: Positive vitreous cultures in eyes with retained lens fragments. Retina 1999;19:354–355.
31. Weinstein GW, Charlton JF, Esmer E: The "lost lens": a new surgical technique using the Machemer lens. Ophthalmic Surg 1995;26:156–159.
32. Monshizadeh R, Samiy N, Haimovici R: Management of retained intravitreal lens fragments after cataract surgery. Surv Ophthalmol 1999;43:397–404.
33. You TT, Arroyo JG: Surgical approaches for the removal of posteriorly dislocated crystalline lenses. Int Ophthalmol Clin 1999;39:249–259.
34. Lewis H, Blumenkranz MS, Chang S: Treatment of dislocated crystalline lens and retinal detachment with perfluorocarbon liquids. Retina 1992;12:299–304.
35. Wallace RT, McNamara JA, Brown G, et al.: The use of perfluorophenanthrene in the removal of intravitreal lens fragments. Am J Ophthalmol 1993;116:196–200.

36. Greve MD, Peyman GA, Mehta NJ, et al.: Use of perfluoroperhydrophenanthrene in the management of posteriorly dislocated crystalline and intraocular lenses. Ophthalmic Surg 1993;24:593–597.
37. Movshovich A, Berrocal M, Chang S: The protective properties of liquid perfluorocarbons in phacofragmentation of dislocated lenses. Retina 1994;14:457–462.
38. Shapiro MJ, Resnick KI, Kim SH, et al.: Management of the dislocated crystalline lens with a perfluorocarbon liquid. Am J Ophthalmol 1991;112:401–405.
39. Fuller D, Jost B: Phacohydroexpulsion: a new technique for removal of luxated sclerotic lens nuclei. Vitreoretinal Surg Tech 1989;4:3,6,8.
40. Campo RV, Chung KD, Oyakawa RT: Pars plana vitrectomy in the management of dislocated posterior chamber lenses. Am J Ophthalmol 1989;108:529–534.
41. Omulecki W, Nawrocki J, Sempinska-Szewczyk J, et al.: Transscleral suture fixation and anterior chamber intraocular lenses implanted after removal of posteriorly dislocated crystalline lenses. Eur J Ophthalmol 1997;7:370–374.
42. Hutton WL, Snyder WB, Vaiser A: Management of surgically dislocated intravitreal lens fragments by pars plana vitrectomy. Ophthalmology 1978;85:176–189.
43. Kapusta MA, Chen JC, Lam WC: Outcomes of dropped nucleus during phacoemulsification. Ophthalmology 1996;103:1184–1187.

CHAPTER 59

Open-Globe Injuries

MITCHELL S. FINEMAN, M.D.

In 1996, Kuhn and associates[1] developed a classification system intended to standardize and simplify the assessment and reporting of ocular trauma and they defined commonly used eye trauma terms. In 1997, The Ocular Trauma Classification Group[2] further refined this classification system by providing a method of categorization during the initial examination or at the time of the primary surgical intervention. The system classifies open-globe injuries according to the type of injury (based upon the mechanism), the grade of injury (defined by visual acuity in the injured eye at initial examination), the status of the pupil (defined as the presence or absence of a relative afferent pupillary defect in the injured eye), and the zone of the injury (based upon the anteroposterior extent of the injury). This chapter will address open-globe injuries in general, defined as any full-thickness wound in the cornea or sclera.

PREOPERATIVE EVALUATION

INITIAL DIAGNOSIS

The diagnosis of open-globe injury should be considered in every patient who has sustained trauma to the eye or orbit. A complete history regarding the details leading up to and following the injury is crucial in the initial assessment. Injuries sustained while hammering metal on metal should be suspected to involve an intraocular foreign body until proven otherwise. Systemic, life-threatening conditions may occur in conjunction with an open-globe injury and should be addressed prior to any further evaluation.

Initial Assessment

An immediate and accurate visual acuity should be assessed using lenses or pin-hole testing prior to any examination of the eye. If formal visual acuity testing is not possible under the circumstances, then the ability to count fingers at a distance or to read fine print should be documented. To reduce the risk of extrusion of intraocular contents, examination of a traumatized eye should be performed in a manner that limits manipulation of the lids or any other maneuver that may put pressure on the globe.

Signs that Suggest Open-Globe Injury

A complete ocular examination, including dilated fundus examination, should be performed when possible. Findings that suggest scleral rupture include a visual acuity of 20/400 or worse, marked chemosis, hyphema, an abnormally deep or shallow anterior chamber (Fig. 59–1), low intraocular pressure or intraocular pressure lower than in the nontraumatized eye, and a relative afferent pupillary defect.[3–5] The Seidel test may reveal an occult penetrating ocular injury. Finally, vitreous hemorrhage may obscure a retained intraocular foreign body.

Most Frequent Sites of Rupture

In eyes that have not undergone prior surgery, the most frequent sites of rupture are at the limbus and parallel to the equator, and between the rectus muscle insertions and the equator.[6] Radially oriented ruptures under the rectus muscles are less common.[4] Eyes that

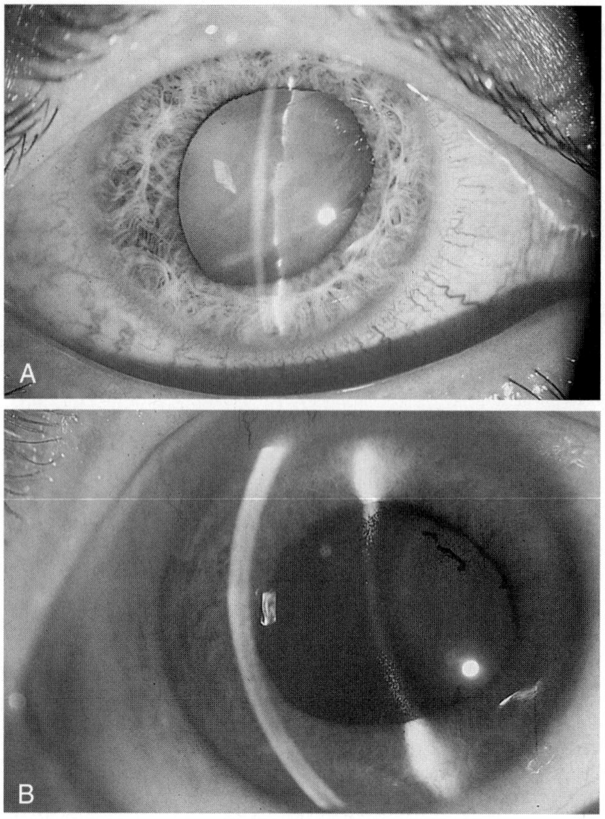

Figure 59–1. *A.* Slit-lamp photograph illustrating shallow anterior chamber in an eye that sustained blunt ocular trauma with scleral rupture. *B.* Slit-lamp photograph illustrating abnormally deep anterior chamber in an eye that sustained blunt ocular trauma with scleral rupture.

have undergone previous surgery tend to rupture at the site of the prior surgical incision. Less frequent sites are in the cornea and at the posterior pole. Posterior ruptures, lying parallel to the equator, are usually found superiorly, in either the nasal or the temporal quadrant.[4]

Imaging Studies

Computed tomography (CT) is the imaging technique of choice for initial assessment after ocular trauma, especially if a retained foreign body is suspected.[7,8] Thin-section axial and coronal CT images at 1.5-mm intervals are recommended for detecting intraocular foreign bodies (IOFB), fractures, and other soft-tissue injuries[8] (Fig. 59–2). The disadvantage of CT is that nonmetallic foreign bodies made of wood or plastic may be missed because they appear hypodense and may be confused with air.[9]

Contact B-scan ultrasonography (US) is also a useful test after ocular trauma because it can diagnose vitreous hemorrhage, retinal detachment, choroidal detachment, IOFB, and ruptured globe when clinical examination is inconclusive or the ocular media are opaque[10–12] (Fig. 59–3). In one study, however, US detected less than 25% of open-globe injuries confirmed by exploration.[4] Whereas CT is superior for detecting most foreign bodies, US can detect intraocular and intraorbital wooden foreign bodies,[9,13] is more useful for localizing foreign bodies relative to the ocular coats,[14] and is superior to CT in demonstrating ocular damage associated with an IOFB.[11]

Ultrasound biomicroscopy is a useful adjunct in evaluating eyes after trauma, especially in patients with media opacities, multiple traumatic injuries, or abnormal anatomy.[15] This high-frequency ultrasound (50 MHz) reveals the appearance of a foreign body and surrounding tissues better than conventional low-frequency ultrasound (10 MHz).[16] Like US, localization of foreign bodies near, or in, the eyewall is possible with ultrasound biomicroscopy.

Nonmetallic objects that are difficult to visualize on CT or US can be visualized with magnetic resonance imaging (MRI).[17] Among the drawbacks of MRI, however, is the potential for movement of ferromagnetic foreign bodies with deleterious effects.[18] Therefore, an

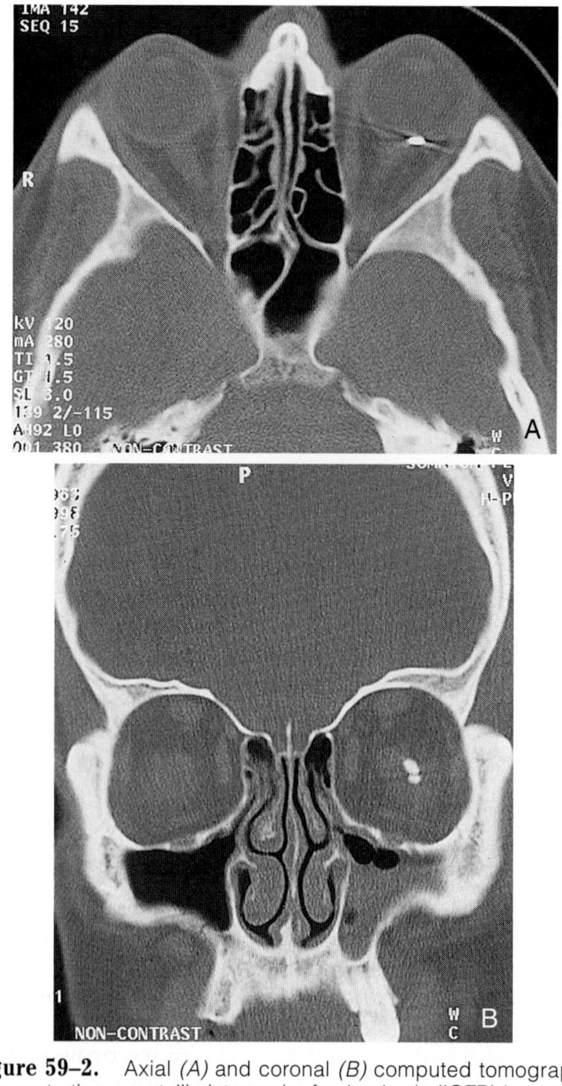

Figure 59–2. Axial *(A)* and coronal *(B)* computed tomography demonstrating a metallic intraocular foreign body (IOFB) located in the posterior pole of the left eye.

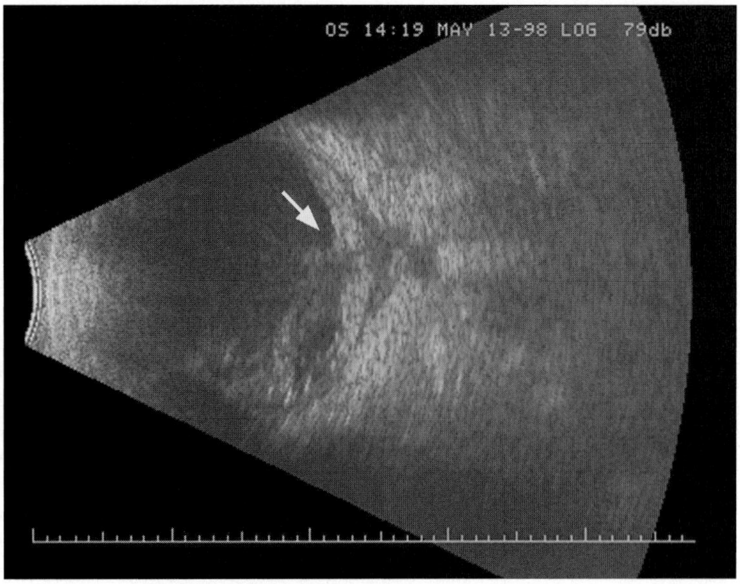

Figure 59–3. B-scan ultrasound demonstrating a posterior scleral rupture in an eye that sustained blunt ocular trauma. The *arrow* identifies the site of scleral rupture.

initial CT is necessary to exclude the presence of an ocular metallic foreign body before performing an MRI. Additionally, MRI is more expensive, not always readily available, and more sensitive to motion artifact than other forms of imaging. An MRI is usually recommended if CT and US are negative, but suspicion of a retained foreign body remains high.[17]

PREOPERATIVE MANAGEMENT

To minimize the delay before general anesthesia can be safely initiated, the patient is instructed to take nothing by mouth. A rigid shield (not a patch) should immediately be placed over the eye to minimize the possibility of extruding intraocular contents. Once the diagnosis of open-globe injury is made, further examination may be postponed until the time of surgical repair, unless management decisions hinge on the results of further examination. Topical medications are used only to facilitate the preoperative assessment, minimizing the risk of toxicity to intraocular contents. Antiemetics are prescribed as needed to control vomiting and reduce the risk of expulsion of the intraocular contents. Tetanus immunity status should be updated. Broad-spectrum intravenous antibiotic therapy should be instituted as soon as possible and continued for a total of 3 days to reduce the risk of posttraumatic endophthalmitis. Because cultures from open-globe injuries reveal a high prevalence of gram-positive bacilli species and polymicrobial infections containing gram-negative species, coverage must be broad.[19] A commonly used regimen includes vancomycin for gram positive-coverage, including *Bacillus* species, and gentamicin or ceftazidime for gram-negative coverage.[20] If the suspicion of an open-globe injury proves to be incorrect after exploration, then the antibiotics may be discontinued.

OPERATIVE TECHNIQUE

ANESTHESIA CONSIDERATIONS

All patients with a suspected or known open-globe injury are managed with general anesthesia, because local anesthesia, and its associated risks of retrobulbar hemorrhage and increased intraocular pressure, may cause further damage to the globe. The goal of anesthesia management involves intubation with full airway protection, while carefully avoiding further damage to the globe. An increase in intraocular pressure is still a concern with the use of general anesthesia because intubation of the trachea raises intraocular pressure, and succinylcholine, the muscle relaxant of choice in patients with a full stomach, also raises intraocular pressure.[21] There are several techniques that minimize the effects of general anesthesia on intraocular pressure, and these are discussed in further detail in Chapter 2. Children with open-globe injuries pose an additional risk, because struggling and crying associated with induction of general anesthesia may increase the intraocular pressure and the subsequent risk of extrusion of intraocular contents. In summary, the life of the patient is the primary concern, but every precaution must be taken to avoid further damage to the injured eye.

EXPLORATION

Scleral exploration is indicated if there is any doubt about the structural integrity of the globe. The risks of this procedure are small and the benefits include producing a primary repair, minimizing extrusion of intraocular contents, and preventing secondary endophthalmitis. Scleral exploration is performed by making a 360-degree conjunctival peritomy, carefully hooking all four rectus muscles, and examining the sclera in all

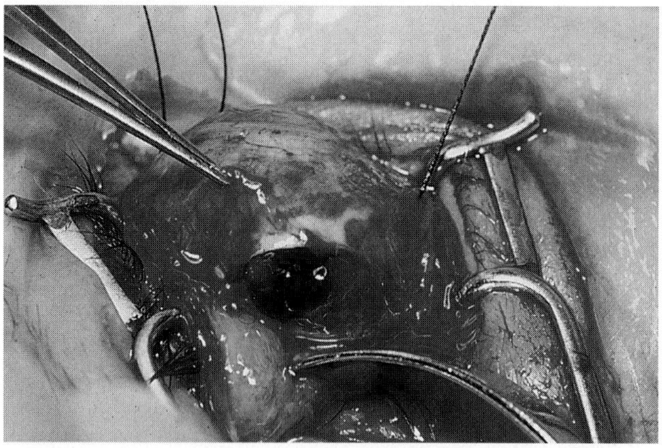

Figure 59–4. Intraoperative photograph demonstrating a scleral rupture evidenced by visible uveal tissue at the equator of the globe.

four quadrants and under the muscles (Fig. 59–4). Lid sutures, instead of a speculum, may be used to increase exposure without applying pressure to the globe. The finding of one rupture site should not preclude the search for others, because multiple scleral ruptures occasionally occur.[22]

REPAIR OF OPEN-GLOBE INJURY

Primary closure of an open-globe injury is the focus of this chapter. For discussion of secondary repair, including anterior segment reconstruction and pars plana vitrectomy, the reader is referred to Chapters 13 and 58. Restoration of the structural integrity of the globe is the primary goal, regardless of the extent or type of wound. Visualization of anterior injuries is aided with the use of the operating microscope, while repair of posterior injuries may be enhanced with the use of surgical loupes.

Corneal Wounds

Fine suture material, such as 10-0 nylon, should be used to suture corneal wounds and the knots should be buried, if possible. Deep, partial-thickness, interrupted corneal sutures should be placed with careful attention to proper tissue alignment. Suture bites of equal depth on opposing edges of the wound will prevent overriding of tissue. To ensure proper alignment, the first suture is placed to bisect the wound lengthwise, and subsequent sutures are placed halfway between the suture and the end of the wound. Viscoelastic material is extremely useful for re-forming a flat anterior chamber or repositing prolapsed iris and is preferentially injected via a paracentesis tract, rather than through the corneal wound.[23] Uveal tissue that remains incarcerated in the wound can be freed by sweeping a cyclodialysis spatula parallel with the iris via a paracentesis port.

Corneoscleral and Scleral Wounds

When repairing corneoscleral wounds, the initial suture should be an interrupted 9-0 nylon suture placed at the anatomic limbus to align the tissues and restore the normal anatomy. After realignment of the limbus, the corneal wound should be repaired (see above). Finally, the extent of the scleral wound should be visualized and then sutured (Fig. 59–5). Posterior scleral wounds may be under tension and may require 8-0 nylon or heavier suture (Fig. 59–6). If the edges of the wound cannot be approximated to allow passage of the suture in one bite, then two separate passes can be made, with tension applied only after the suture is tied. Any prolapsed vitreous is excised with scissors held flush with the sclera or a vitrectomy cutter held at the external aspect of the wound. Traction on the vitreous or blind insertion of the vitrectomy cutter into the wound should be avoided. Prolasped uvea is reposited if it does not appear necrotic or infected. If an extraocular muscle obscures the underlying scleral wound, it may be disinserted from its insertion site after it is secured with a double-armed locking suture. The muscle is sutured back to the original insertion site following closure of the scleral defect.

In some cases, prophylactic cryotherapy around the site of rupture and/or scleral buckling is considered in

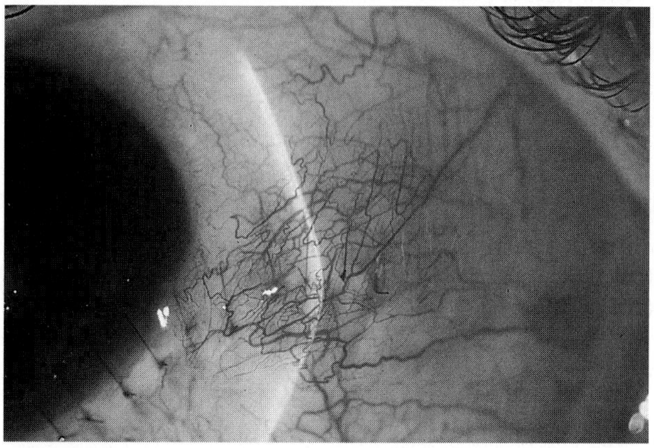

Figure 59–5. Slit-lamp photograph demonstrating a corneoscleral wound repaired with a combination of 9-0 nylon sutures in the limbus and sclera, and 10-0 nylon sutures in the cornea.

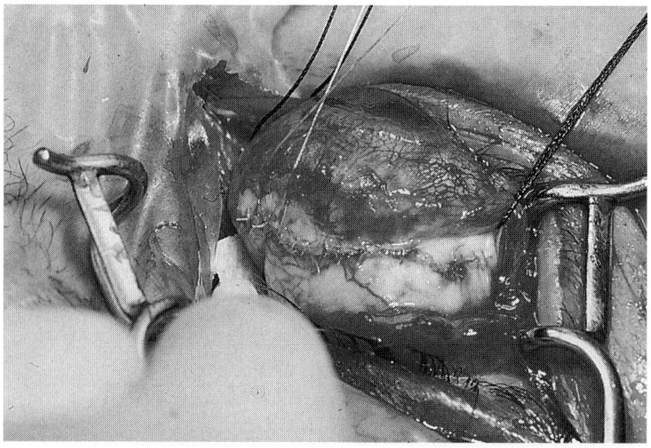

Figure 59–6. Intraoperative photograph of the eye in Figure 59–4 after repair of the scleral rupture.

an attempt to prevent retinal detachment. The indications and technique for primary vitrectomy in the setting of open-globe injury are discussed in Chapter 56. In general, primary vitrectomy is reserved for situations in which a nonmagnetic foreign body, or magnetic foreign body not amenable to removal with a magnet, is encountered.

LENS MANAGEMENT

Controversy exists regarding the proper management of concomitant open-globe injury and traumatic cataract.[24] The management options include primary repair of the open-globe injury without primary removal of the lens, combined primary repair of the globe with primary lensectomy, and combined primary repair of the globe with primary lensectomy and intraocular lens implantation. Factors that must be considered in this decision include the size and location of the open-globe injury and the presence of lens-induced glaucoma and inflammation.[24] Because an exuberant fibrinous reaction can occur on the anterior lens capsule and masquerade as a cataract, conservative management is usually indicated. Even if the lens capsule has been violated, several cases have been described in which lens capsular disruption from an intraocular foreign body resulted in a visually insignificant lens opacity.[25] However, if the lens capsule is significantly disrupted and lens material is present in the anterior chamber in large quantities, then it is reasonable to perform a lensectomy at the time of primary repair.

Implantation of an intraocular lens is not recommended in the setting of an extensive perforating or contaminated injury, because the risk of endophthalmitis is increased.[26] However, in selected cases, intraocular lens implantation at the time of lensectomy and primary repair of a corneal laceration may result in an excellent anatomic and visual outcome.[27]

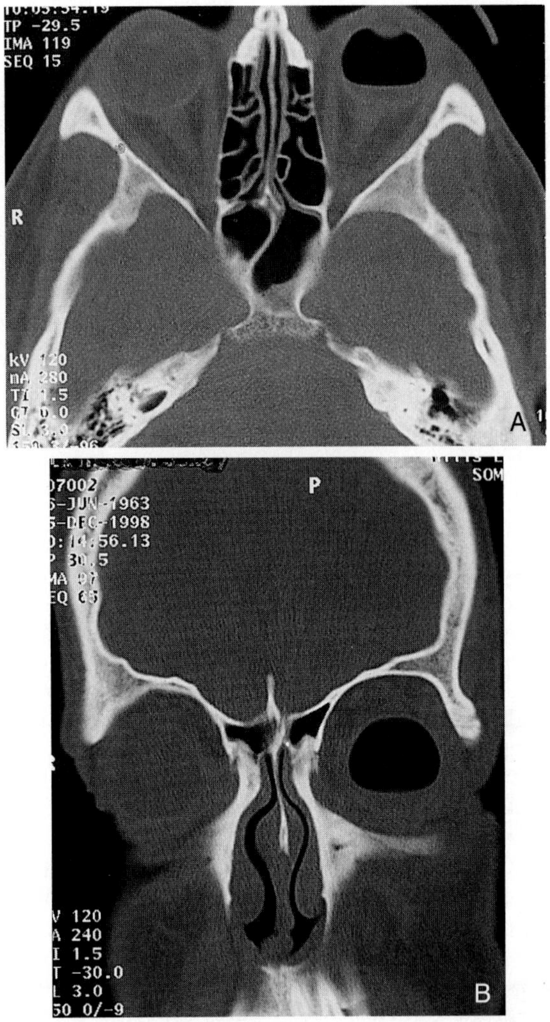

Figure 59–7. Axial *(A)* and coronal *(B)* computed tomography of the eye in Figure 59–2 after pars plana vitrectomy with removal of the IOFB and air–fluid exchange. Note that the IOFB is no longer visualized and the vitreous cavity is filled with air.

INTRAOCULAR FOREIGN BODY

Intraocular foreign bodies are not only potentially damaging to intraocular structures, they also increase the risk of secondary endophthalmitis.[28] Siderosis is also a possible complication of iron-containing foreign bodies. Removal of the foreign body should be performed as soon as possible, because it may reduce the risk of developing infectious endophthalmitis.[29] More importantly, delay in removal allows a capsule to surround the foreign body, making removal more difficult. Magnetic removal of the foreign body may be possible with any ferromagnetic IOFB, and pars plana vitrectomy is indicated for a nonmagnetic IOFB or one not amenable to magnetic removal (Fig. 59–7). Imaging should often be repeated postoperatively.

POSTOPERATIVE MANAGEMENT

Broad-spectrum intravenous antibiotic therapy is continued to complete a 72-hour course of treatment. Treatment with topical antibiotic, cycloplegic eye drops, and corticosteroid eye drops is initiated after the primary repair. Oral or intramuscular analgesic medications are prescribed as needed. The patient is discharged on the third postoperative day.

The timing of vitrectomy after primary repair of open-globe injuries is controversial.[30] There are data to suggest that eyes undergoing early pars plana vitrectomy (within 14 days) have a better visual outcome than those that undergo later vitrectomy.[4,31,32]

COMPLICATIONS

ENDOPHTHALMITIS

Endophthalmitis occurring as a complication of an open-globe injury can cause further devastation to an already traumatized eye (Fig. 59–8). *Bacillus* species, seen more commonly in posttraumatic endophthalmitis, can be particularly destructive.[28,33] Estimates of the

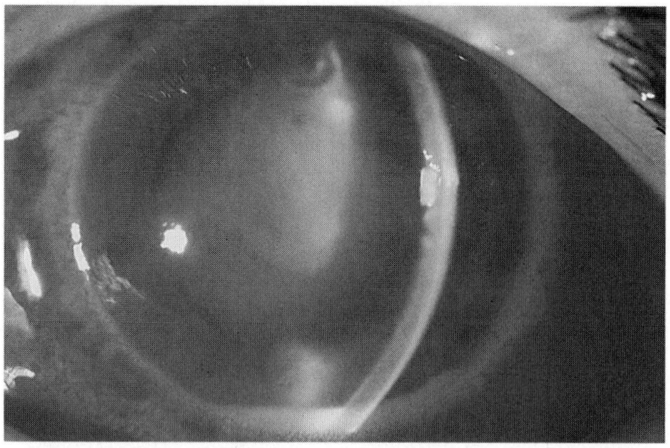

Figure 59–8. Slit-lamp photograph of an eye that sustained an open-globe injury complicated by endophthalmitis. Note the hypopyon and fibrin in the anterior chamber.

rate of posttraumatic endophthalmitis range from 5% to 30% of open-globe injuries.[28,34,35] Factors that appear to increase the risk of endophthalmitis in open-globe injuries include the presence of an IOFB,[28] delay in removal of the IOFB beyond 24 hours,[29] disruption of the crystalline lens,[35] age 50 years or older,[29] and sustaining ocular trauma in a rural setting.[34]

Prevention of posttraumatic endophthalmitis involves early closure of the globe and removal of any IOFB, if applicable. Intravenous antibiotic therapy is instituted as soon as possible. Subconjunctival antibiotics are injected after primary repair and topical antibiotics are used in the postoperative period. Controversy exists regarding the use of intravitreal antibiotics as prophylaxis. In one study[36] examining culture results in open-globe injuries, routine intraoperative cultures were positive in almost 30% of patients; however, they did not help to identify eyes at increased risk for developing endophthalmitis or affect management decisions when there were no clinical signs of endophthalmitis. Another study[37] found positive cultures in 7 of 27 (26%) eyes with retained IOFB, and none of the eyes developed endophthalmitis. However, 3 of the 7 eyes received prophylactic intravitreal antibiotics at the time of surgery. Therefore, intravitreal injections of antibiotics are not recommended except in particular clinical settings such as those with an IOFB that is contaminated with organic matter.[34] In such cases, the authors suggest empiric therapy with intravitreal gentamicin along with either vancomycin or clindamycin.[34]

Successful treatment of posttraumatic endophthalmitis hinges on early diagnosis and aggressive treatment. Once the diagnosis is suspected, pars plana vitrectomy and injection of intravitreal broad-spectrum antibiotics, with coverage against *Bacillus* species and gram-negative organisms, should be performed as soon as possible. Although the prognosis is better when the offending organism is less virulent,[28,35] this aggressive treatment regimen has resulted in preservation of useful visual acuity in several eyes infected with *Bacillus* species.[38] Coverage against fungal organisms should also be considered in the appropriate clinical setting.[19,33]

AMBLYOPIA

The postoperative management of children with open-globe injuries and an immature visual system requires consideration and prevention of amblyopia. Successful surgical repair of an open-globe injury may result in a poor visual outcome if secondary amblyopia is not identified and treated. Aggressive visual rehabilitation is necessary and may include secondary anterior segment reconstruction to clear the visual axis, pars plana vitrectomy to clear vitreous hemorrhage, contact lens fitting to correct aphakia or irregular astigmatism, correction of refractive errors, and patching of the fellow eye.

PROGNOSIS

Although the prognosis for full recovery of vision is poor with major ocular injuries, the potential for preservation of useful vision justifies primary repair in most situations. Despite significant advances in vitreoretinal surgical techniques and a slight improvement in visual outcomes of eyes with open-globe injuries over the past 20 years, the percentage of eyes that achieve a visual acuity of 5/200 or better is still only slightly greater than 50%.[39]

Predictors of good visual outcome after primary repair of an open-globe injury include visual acuity of 20/800 or better on initial examination, a laceration limited to the cornea, absence of an expelled or subluxated lens, lacerations located anterior to the rectus muscle insertions and a rupture length of less than 11 mm.[4,40]

ENUCLEATION

Primary enucleation (performed at the time of the initial surgical procedure) should be reserved for those cases in which the globe is considered irreparable, or when an expulsive choroidal hemorrhage with loss of the intraocular contents has occurred. Primary repair allows further evaluation and assessment of visual potential and preserves the possibility for secondary enucleation in the postoperative period. Secondary enucleation is considered if the eye no longer has light perception and the visual prognosis is hopeless. It is most commonly performed within the 2-week period after the open-globe injury in order to avoid the potential complication of sympathetic ophthalmia.

Approximately 70% of eyes that sustain open-globe injuries resulting in poor visual potential and are not treated with enucleation can be expected to become phthisical over a 5-year period.[41] Enucleation will be required in about 34% of these eyes, most commonly to ameliorate pain.

REFERENCES

1. Kuhn F, Morris R, Witherspoon CD, et al.: A standardized classification of ocular trauma. Ophthalmology 1996;103:240–3.

2. Pieramici DJ, Sternberg P Jr, Aaberg TM Sr, et al.: A system for classifying mechanical injuries of the eye (globe). The Ocular Trauma Classification Group. Am J Ophthalmol 1997;123:820–31.
3. Kylstra JA, Lamkin JC, Runyan DK: Clinical predictors of scleral rupture after blunt ocular trauma. Am J Ophthalmol 1993; 115:530–5.
4. Russell SR, Olsen KR, Folk JC: Predictors of scleral rupture and the role of vitrectomy in severe blunt ocular trauma. Am J Ophthalmol 1988;105:253–7.
5. Werner MS, Dana MR, Viana MA, et al.: Predictors of occult scleral rupture. Ophthalmology 1994;101:1941–4.
6. Benson WE, Jeffers JB: Blunt trauma. In Tasman W, Jaeger EA (eds.), Duane's Clinical Ophthalmology. Vol. 3, Philadelphia: Lippincott-Raven;1997:1–16.
7. Lindahl S: Computed tomography of intraorbital foreign bodies. Acta Radiol 1987;28:235–40.
8. Lustrin ES, Brown JH, Novelline R, et al.: Radiologic assessment of trauma and foreign bodies of the eye and orbit. Neuroimaging Clin North Am 1996;6:219–37.
9. Topilow HW, Ackerman AL, Zimmerman RD: Limitations of computerized tomography in the localization of intraocular foreign bodies. Ophthalmology 1984;91:1086–91.
10. Das T, Namperumalsamy P: Ultrasonography in ocular trauma. Indian J Ophthalmol 1987;35:121–5.
11. McNicholas MM, Brophy DP, Power WJ, et al.: Ocular trauma: evaluation with US. Radiology 1995;195:423–7.
12. Rubsamen PE, Cousins SW, Winward KE, et al.: Diagnostic ultrasound and pars plana vitrectomy in penetrating ocular trauma. Ophthalmology 1994;101:809–14.
13. Coleman DJ: Reliability of ocular and orbital diagnosis with B-scan ultrasound. 2. Orbital diagnosis. Am J Ophthalmol 1972;74: 704–18.
14. Coleman D, Rondeau M: Diagnostic imaging of ocular and orbital trauma. In Shingleton B, Hersh P, Kenyon K (eds.), Eye Trauma. St. Louis: Mosby-Year Book; 1991:25–40.
15. Deramo VA, Shah GK, Baumal CR, et al.: Ultrasound biomicroscopy as a tool for detecting and localizing occult foreign bodies after ocular trauma. Ophthalmology 1999;106:301–5.
16. Nouby-Mahmoud G, Silverman RH, Coleman DJ: Using high-frequency ultrasound to characterize intraocular foreign bodies. Ophthalmic Surg 1993;24:94–9.
17. Green BF, Kraft SP, Carter KD, et al.: Intraorbital wood. Detection by magnetic resonance imaging. Ophthalmology 1990;97:608–11.
18. Kelly WM, Paglen PG, Pearson JA, et al.: Ferromagnetism of intraocular foreign body causes unilateral blindness after MR study. Am J Neuroradiol 1986;7:243–5.
19. Kunimoto DY, Das T, Sharma S, et al.: Microbiologic spectrum and susceptibility of isolates: Part II. Posttraumatic endophthalmitis. Endophthalmitis Research Group. Am J Ophthalmol 1999;128:242–4.
20. Navon SE: Management of the ruptured globe. Int Ophthalmol Clin 1995;35:71–91.
21. Libonati MM, Leahy JJ, Ellison N: The use of succinylcholine in open eye surgery. Anesthesiology 1985;62:637–40.
22. Joondeph BC, Young TL, Saran BR: Multiple scleral ruptures after blunt ocular trauma. Am J Ophthalmol 1989;108:744.
23. Colby K: Management of open globe injuries. Int Ophthalmol Clin 1999;39:59–69.
24. Pieramici DJ: Primary intraocular lens implantation for lens trauma. Ophthalmology 1999;106:643–4.
25. Pieramici DJ, Capone A Jr, Rubsamen PE, et al.: Lens preservation after intraocular foreign body injuries. Ophthalmology 1996;103:1563–7.
26. Koster HR, Kenyon KR: Complications of surgery associated with ocular trauma. Int Ophthalmol Clin 1992;32:157–78.
27. Rubsamen PE, Irvin WD, McCuen BW, et al.: Primary intraocular lens implantation in the setting of penetrating ocular trauma. Ophthalmology 1995;102:101–7.
28. Brinton GS, Topping TM, Hyndiuk RA, et al.: Posttraumatic endophthalmitis. Arch Ophthalmol 1984;102:547–50.
29. Thompson JT, Parver LM, Enger CL, et al.: Infectious endophthalmitis after penetrating injuries with retained intraocular foreign bodies. National Eye Trauma System. Ophthalmology 1993;100:1468–74.
30. Mieler WF, Mittra RA: The role and timing of pars plana vitrectomy in penetrating ocular trauma. Arch Ophthalmol 1997; 115:1191–2.
31. Brinton GS, Aaberg TM, Reeser FH, et al.: Surgical results in ocular trauma involving the posterior segment. Am J Ophthalmol 1982;93:271–8.
32. Coleman DJ: Early vitrectomy in the management of the severely traumatized eye. Am J Ophthalmol 1982;93:543–51.
33. Affeldt JC, Flynn HW Jr, Forster RK, et al.: Microbial endophthalmitis resulting from ocular trauma. Ophthalmology 1987;94:407–13.
34. Boldt HC, Pulido JS, Blodi CF, et al.: Rural endophthalmitis. Ophthalmology 1989;96:1722–6.
35. Thompson WS, Rubsamen PE, Flynn HW Jr, et al.: Endophthalmitis after penetrating trauma. Risk factors and visual acuity outcomes. Ophthalmology 1995;102:1696–701.
36. Rubsamen PE, Cousins SW, Martinez JA: Impact of cultures on management decisions following surgical repair of penetrating ocular trauma. Ophthalmic Surg Lasers 1997;28:43–9.
37. Mieler WF, Ellis MK, Williams DF, et al.: Retained intraocular foreign bodies and endophthalmitis. Ophthalmology 1990;97: 1532–8.
38. Foster RE, Martinez JA, Murray TG, et al.: Useful visual outcomes after treatment of *Bacillus cereus* endophthalmitis. Ophthalmology 1996;103:390–7.
39. Pieramici DJ, MacCumber MW, Humayun MU, et al.: Open-globe injury. Update on types of injuries and visual results. Ophthalmology 1996;103:1798–1803.
40. Sternberg P Jr, de Juan E Jr, Michels RG, et al.: Multivariate analysis of prognostic factors in penetrating ocular injuries. Am J Ophthalmol 1984;98:467–72.
41. Brackup AB, Carter KD, Nerad JA, et al.: Long-term follow-up of severely injured eyes following globe rupture. Ophthalmic Plast Reconstr Surg 1991;7:194–7.

CHAPTER 60

Endophthalmitis: Diagnosis, Treatment, Prevention

HARRY W. FLYNN, Jr., M.D., ROY D. BROD, M.D., DENNIS P. HAN, M.D., and DARLENE MILLER, M.P.H., MT(A.S.C.P.)

Endophthalmitis is defined by marked inflammation of intraocular fluids and tissues. When caused by microbial organisms, infectious endophthalmitis often results in severe visual loss.[1,2] In this chapter, medical and surgical management issues for infectious endophthalmitis are reviewed.

CLASSIFICATION

Infectious endophthalmitis is classified by the events leading to the infection and by the timing of the clinical diagnosis.[1,2] The broad categories include postoperative endophthalmitis (acute-onset, chronic or delayed-onset, conjunctival filtering bleb–associated), posttraumatic endophthalmitis, and endogenous endophthalmitis (Table 60–1). Rare categories include cases associated with microbial keratitis or suture removal. These categories are important in predicting the causative organisms and guiding therapeutic decisions before microbiological confirmation of the clinical diagnosis.

INCIDENCE

Postoperative endophthalmitis is the most frequent category, accounting for greater than 70% of cases.[1,2] In a nosocomial survey (1984–1994) of a university-based hospital reviewing over 41,000 cataract procedures with or without intraocular lens implantation, acute-onset endophthalmitis occurred in 34 cases (0.81%).[3] In this survey of intraocular surgical cases, the rates of endophthalmitis were highest after secondary intraocular lens implantation (0.31% of 5 of 1367 cases) and lowest after pars plana vitrectomy (0.05% or 3 of 6557 cases). There is an increased incidence of endophthalmitis in patients with diabetes mellitus that can possibly be explained by known immune compromise in diabetic patients.[4] Endophthalmitis may also occur infrequently in the setting of a conjunctival filtering bleb,[5–7] suture removal,[8] wound dehiscence, or vitreous wick.[9] Chronic or delayed-onset endophthalmitis may be caused by less virulent bacteria (e.g., *Propionibacterium acnes, Staphylococcus epidermidis*) or by fungi.[10–13]

TABLE 60–1. Classification of Endophthalmitis—Most Frequent Organisms in Various Clinical Settings

1. Postoperative
   a. Acute-onset postoperative endophthalmitis: Coagulase-negative staphylococci, *Staphylococcus aureus, Streptococcus* species, Gram-negative bacteria
   b. Delayed-onset (chronic) pseudophakic endophthalmitis (> 6 weeks postop): *P. acnes*, coagulase-negative staphylococci, fungi
   c. Conjunctival filtering bleb–associated endophthalmitis: *Streptococcus* species, *Haemophilus influenzae, Staphylococcus* species
2. Posttraumatic: *Bacillus* species, Staphylococcus species
3. Endogenous: *Candida* species, *S. aureus*, Gram-negative bacteria
4. Miscellaneous (corneal ulcer perforation): *Pseudomonas, Staphylococcus* species

In reported large clinical series,[14–16] endophthalmitis after penetrating ocular trauma represents approximately 25% of all endophthalmitis cases. In one large study of penetrating ocular trauma, endophthalmitis occurred in 10.7% of cases with a retained intraocular foreign body and 5.2% of cases without a retained intraocular foreign body.[17] The National Eye Trauma System Registry reported an endophthalmitis incidence of 6.9% (34 of 492 cases) after penetrating ocular injuries with retained intraocular foreign bodies.[18] Metallic intraocular foreign bodies were as likely to be associated with infectious endophthalmitis (7.2%) as nonmetallic foreign bodies (7.3%) and organic matter (6.3%) foreign bodies.[18] Rupture of the crystalline lens capsule is also a risk for endophthalmitis in open-globe injuries.[19]

Compared with the postoperative and posttrauma categories, endogenous endophthalmitis cases occur with the least frequency and more often occur in debilitated or immunocompromised patients or in patients with a history of intravenous drug abuse.[20–23]

DIAGNOSTIC FEATURES

The diagnostic features of infectious endophthalmitis can be divided into two aspects: clinical recognition and microbiological confirmation. The clinical signs of endophthalmitis vary depending on the preceding events or surgery, the infecting organism, the associated inflammation, and the duration of the disease. In acute-onset postoperative endophthalmitis when bacteria are the etiologic agents, the hallmark of the clinical diagnosis is marked intraocular inflammation with hypopyon (Fig. 60–1).[1,2] Other signs of acute postoperative bacterial endophthalmitis include fibrin in the anterior chamber and on the intraocular lens (IOL), corneal edema, marked conjunctival congestion, lid edema, and vitreitis. Retinal periphlebitis is another clinical sign that is diagnostically more helpful in eyes with relatively clear media.[24] Endophthalmitis cases caused by fungal organisms generally have less inflammation, a more indolent course, and less ocular pain. Endogenous Candida cases often manifest as isolated white infiltrates in the formed vitreous overlying a focal area of chorioretinitis.[21]

The clinical diagnosis of endophthalmitis is confirmed by obtaining intraocular (aqueous and vitreous) specimens. A vitreous specimen is much more likely to yield a positive culture result than a simultaneously acquired aqueous specimen.[25] The vitreous specimen can be obtained either by needle biopsy or by the use of an automated vitrectomy instrument. A needle biopsy or limited vitrectomy approach can be performed in a treatment room but a three-port pars plana vitrectomy usually requires the use of the operating room and ancillary equipment. One report of 138 culture-proven endophthalmitis cases showed a positive culture result in 34.8% of anterior chamber specimens, 58.2% of vitreous specimens, and 80% of vitrectomy fluid specimens.[25]

The technique for culturing intraocular specimens depends on the volume of the specimen and the suspected clinical diagnosis.[2,25,26] Direct inoculation of the intraocular fluid specimen onto culture media is a traditional approach and remains a very practical technique. The specific media used for direct inoculation are listed in Table 60–2. This approach is especially important when limited specimens (such as a needle vitreous or aqueous aspiration) are obtained. These specimens can be directly inoculated onto the appropriate media, including anaerobic media in cases of suspected *P. acnes* endophthalmitis. Specimens obtained by the use of automated vitrectomy instruments are diluted by the infusion fluid but can be processed by two methods: One method for processing the vitrectomy specimen uses a membrane filter system in which the vitrectomy specimen is passed through 0.45-mm filter paper that concentrates the microorganisms and particulate matter. This filter paper is then sectioned and distributed on the appropriate media. An alternative method involves direct inoculation of the initially aspirated vitrectomy specimen into standard blood culture

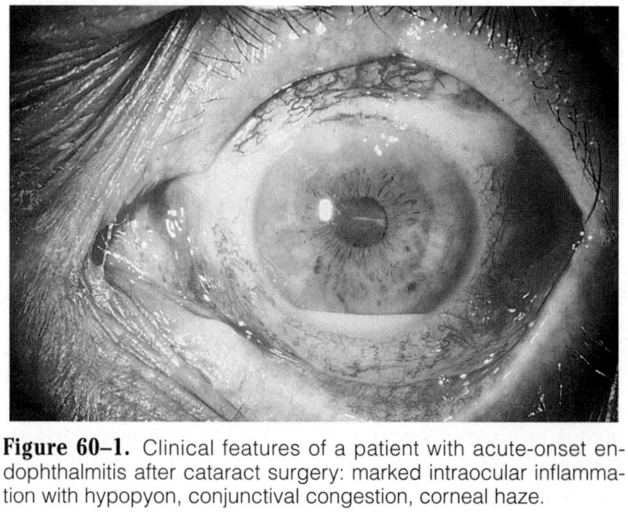

Figure 60–1. Clinical features of a patient with acute-onset endophthalmitis after cataract surgery: marked intraocular inflammation with hypopyon, conjunctival congestion, corneal haze.

TABLE 60–2. Culture Media Used for Endophthalmitis Specimens

1. Chocolate agar: an enriched medium for the recovery of fastidious organisms (i.e., *Neisseria gonorrhoeae* and *Haemophilus influenzae*) from clinical specimens. The chocolate agar should be used as a general purpose medium and as the medium of choice for the recovery of common endophthalmitis isolates when only a few drops of intraocular fluid are available for culture. It must be placed in a CO_2 jar or bag.
2. 5% Sheep blood agar: a general purpose medium for the recovery of the most common bacterial and fungal endophthalmitis isolates. It should be placed in a CO_2 jar or bag.
3. Thioglycollate broth: an enriched medium for the recovery of small numbers of aerobic or anaerobic (including *Propionibacterium acnes*) organisms from ocular fluids and tissues. The broth dilutes the effects of antibiotics and other inhibitory susbstances. The broth should be kept a minimum of 5 days.
4. Anaerobic blood agar: a general purpose medium for the recovery of anaerobic and facultative anaerobic organisms. This medium should be included for all chronic cases of endophthalmitis and/or where *P. acnes* is suspected. The viridans and B-hemolytic streptococci may grow better and faster on this plate. This medium is placed in an anaerobic jar or bag.
5. Sabouraud agar: a selective medium used to promote the growth of fungi (yeasts and molds) from clinical materials.
6. Blood culture bottles: contain specially prepared medium for the recovery of both aerobic and anaerobic bacteria and fungi. Intraocular fluids may be inoculated directly into blood culture bottles. Undiluted fluids should be inoculated into pediatric bottles; diluted fluids (6–12 ml of vitrectomy specimen), into a set of routine (adult) bottles. Identification is made after growth is established.

bottles (Fig. 60–2).[26] The latter technique is particularly useful at night or on the weekend when the microbiology laboratory staff are not available to assist in processing the vitrectomy specimen. In a retrospective review of 83 cases, this blood culture bottle method for processing vitrectomy specimens yielded a 91% incidence of positive culture results.[26] This rate of positive culture results from clinically diagnosed endophthalmitis cases was similar to simultaneously processed specimens using the membrane filter system.

Immunologic as well as molecular genetic technologies enable rapid and specific identification of infectious agents. These techniques have been used in both clinical and experimental settings, and their future use in this area appears promising.[27,28] Molecular genetic technology has made available specific DNA probes that will interact with the unique DNA sequence for a particular pathogen.[27] Polymerase chain reaction (PCR) uses a primer set and DNA polymerase to amplify small amounts of DNA. It shows clinical potential as a rapid and sensitive diagnostic technique to aid in the confirmation of clinical observations.[29] Clinical application of PCR techniques for the more rapid diagnosis of bacterial endophthalmitis is now under investigation.

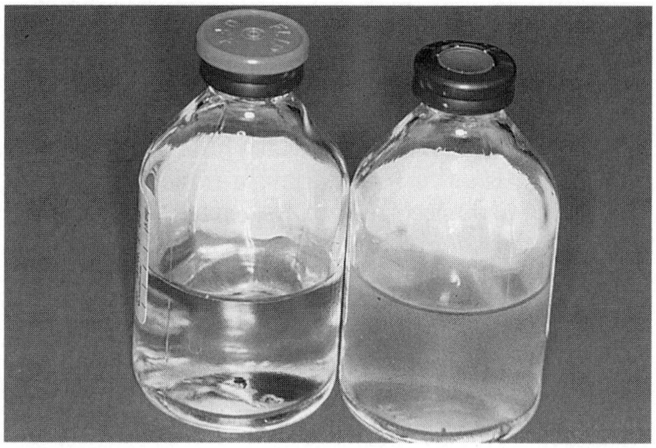

Figure 60–2. Blood culture bottles used for vitrectomy specimens and bacterial growth in right bottle.

DIFFERENTIAL DIAGNOSIS

The differential diagnosis of marked intraocular cellular inflammation after ocular surgery includes sterile inflammation (related to retained lens fragments or vitreous hemorrhage), iris trauma, preexisting uveitis, and foreign material introduced during surgery.[1,2] Retained cortical lens remnants are reported to cause more inflammation than nuclear remnants.[30] Retained lens fragments may occasionally cause a marked inflammatory reaction with hypopyon, which may clinically resemble infectious endophthalmitis (Fig. 60–3).[31] Blood in the anterior chamber or vitreous cavity may also be confused with endophthalmitis, especially when the blood is long-standing and associated with anterior segment trauma during preceding surgery. Similarly, difficult or prolonged surgery, which often includes vitreous loss or vitreous incarceration in the cataract incision, may increase postoperative inflammation.

In eyes with mild to moderate postoperative inflammation without hypopyon, intensive therapy with topical corticosteroids may be used initially. The careful sequential observation of such eyes will allow appropriate diagnostic and treatment approaches to be employed.

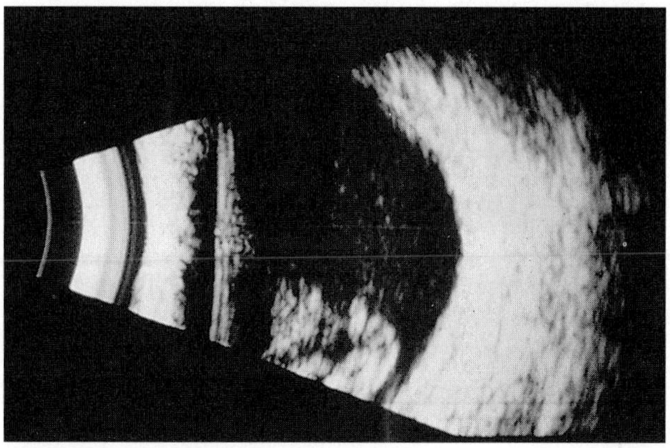

Figure 60–3. Retained lens fragments after phacoemulsification may cause marked intraocular inflammation, which simulates postoperative bacterial endophthalmitis.

Acute-onset postoperative endophthalmitis when caused by more virulent organisms, such as *Streptococcus* species or gram-negative bacteria, will usually present with rapidly progressive clinical signs aiding in the early diagnosis of infectious endophthalmitis. Endophthalmitis caused by the coagulase-negative staphylococci may have less inflammatory signs, often creating difficulty in distinguishing between an infectious and a noninfectious etiology.

TREATMENT MODALITIES

Antibiotics can be delivered to the eye by several routes, including direct intravitreal injection, periocular injection, and topical application (Table 60–3). Endophthalmitis management, like the management of infections elsewhere in the body, requires selection of safe and effective antimicrobial agents. The antibiotics selected should cover the broad range of gram-positive and gram-negative organisms causing clinical endophthalmitis. Systemic antibiotics are not generally used for acute-onset postoperative endophthalmitis but may be considered in other categories depending on the extent of the infection and the causative organisms.

INTRAVITREAL ANTIBIOTICS

Of all the available antimicrobial agents evaluated for intravitreal injection, only a few are used regularly in clinical practice. In the Endophthalmitis Vitrectomy Study (EVS), intravitreal vancomycin 1 mg in combination with amikacin 0.4 mg was used for the initial empiric treatment of acute-onset endophthalmitis.[32–41] An alternative to the aminoglycosides for coverage of gram-negative organisms is the use of intravitreal ceftazidime 2.25 mg, a third-generation cephalosporin.[42,43] These antibiotic combinations provide broad coverage for nearly all of the organisms causing bacterial endophthalmitis, including staphylococci, streptococci, *Bacillus* species, and the gram-negative organisms.

Vancomycin is generally considered to be the drug of choice for gram-positive bacterial coverage. Vancomycin has excellent activity against coagulase-negative staphylococci and other gram-positive organisms. In the EVS, coagulase-negative micrococci were the most commonly cultured bacteria in acute-onset post-cataract surgery cases.[32–41] Vancomycin has been reported to be consistently effective for the broad range of streptococcal organisms as well as nearly all gram-positive organisms.

Repetitive injections of intravitreal antibiotics may cause significant retinal toxicity. In a rabbit model, eyes treated with a second or third intraocular vancomycin/aminoglycoside injection at 48 hour intervals showed progressive toxicity.[44] In view of the low rate of persistent infection after initial combination therapy, repeat injection of intravitreal antibiotics are considered only in those cases with progressive inflammation caused by virulent organisms.[45] Based on the initial culture report, a single intravitreal antibiotic may be selected for this repeat injection.

TABLE 60–3. Antibiotics Considered for Endophthalmitis Treatment: Concentration and Dosages of Principal Agents Used for Treatment of Endophthalmitis*

Agent	Intraocular	Subconjunctival	Topical
Amikacin	0.4 mg	25 mg	20 mg/ml
Ampicillin	0.5 mg	100 mg	50 mg/ml
Ceftazolin	2.25 mg	100 mg	50 mg/ml
Ceftazidime	2.0 mg	100–200 mg	50 mg/ml
Chloramphenicol	1.0 mg	50–100 mg	20 mg/ml
Clindamycin	1.0 mg	15–50 mg	50 mg/ml
Gentamicin	0.1 mg	20 mg	15 mg/ml
Methicillin	2.0 mg	100 mg	100 mg/ml
Tobramycin	0.1 mg	20 mg	15 mg/ml
Vancomycin	1.0 mg	25 mg	25 mg/ml

*Systemic antibiotics generally not used for acute-onset postoperative endophthalmitis.
(Compiled from the *PDR for Ophthalmology*, 2001.)

VITRECTOMY

The potential advantages of vitrectomy for infectious endophthalmitis include the ability to obtain an adequate vitreous specimen without the theoretically harmful tractional effects of needle aspiration on formed vitreous. Vitrectomy also debulks the vitreous cavity, allowing removal of most of the infecting organisms and other inflammatory mediators. Finally, the vitrectomized eye should allow improved drug circulation throughout the vitreous cavity.

Disadvantages of vitrectomy include the requirement for more sophisticated instrumentation, possibly available only in an operating room, a setting that can be associated with a delay in initiating treatment. The view of the posterior segment is frequently obscured by fibrin and inflammatory debris on the surface of the IOL or in the anterior chamber, making vitrectomy surgery difficult and potentially hazardous. The view of the posterior segment can frequently be improved by either aspirating or peeling the inflammatory material from the anterior segment or surface of the IOL.[46]

Another disadvantage of vitrectomy is its effect on reducing the half-life of injected intravitreal antibiotics.[47] Doft and associates studied the ocular clearance of amphotericin B injected into the vitreous in a rabbit model of unmodified phakic eyes, Candida-infected phakic eyes, aphakic eyes, and aphakic vitrectomized eyes. With the use of high-pressure liquid chromatography to assess drug level, the half-lives of drug disappearance after a single amphotericin B 10 μg intravitreal injection were 9.1, 8.6, 4.7, and 4.1 days, respectively. The authors summarized that this rapid disappearance of amphotericin B from vitrectomized eyes must be considered in the clinical management of patients with fungal endophthalmitis.

Vitrectomy for endophthalmitis can be performed using either a two-port (infusion needle and vitreous

{AU: ok or
run-in?}

cutter) or three-port technique (sutured infusion cannula, endoilluminator probe, and vitreous cutter), depending on the surgeon's preference and the clinical circumstances. The advantage of the three-port technique over the two-port approach is the ability to view the retina and to accomplish a more complete removal of the infected vitreous. A pars plana vitrectomy is generally recommended for endophthalmitis cases with moderate (red reflex present and poor view of fundus detail) or severe (no red reflex visible) vitritis. In such cases, preoperative echography should be performed to rule out retinal detachment and to document the presence or absence of a posterior vitreous detachment. When there is a posterior vitreous detachment, the vitrectomy surgeon can remove more opaque vitreous near the posterior pole and have greater confidence in avoiding contact with the retina.

A concentrated undiluted vitreous specimen can be obtained at the beginning of the procedure using manual aspiration into a syringe attached to the aspiration line of the vitrectomy handpiece. The intraocular specimens are evaluated by microbiology laboratory using stained smears and cultures.

THE ENDOPHTHALMITIS VITRECTOMY STUDY

The EVS was a multicenter, National Eye Institute (NEI)-sponsored trial that evaluated pars plana vitrectomy and systemic antibiotics in acute postoperative endophthalmitis.[32–41] The EVS also evaluated a variety of clinical and microbiologic factors relating to endophthalmitis. The study enrolled 420 patients with symptoms and signs of endophthalmitis occurring within 6 weeks of cataract extraction or secondary IOL implantation. Patients were randomized to treatment with pars plana vitrectomy or to vitreous tap/biopsy, and to treatment with or without systemic antibiotics. All patients in the study received intravitreal antibiotic therapy (vancomycin 1 mg and amikacin 0.4 mg), and topical and systemic corticosteroids. Patients who appeared clinically worse after 36 to 60 hours after presentation underwent reinjection of intravitreal antibiotics. Similarly, patients who were initially randomized to tap/biopsy and had worsening, also underwent vitrectomy. The main end point of the study was best corrected visual acuity at 9 to 12 months after presentation. A secondary end point was media clarity.

VISUAL ACUITY RESULTS

The EVS demonstrated that immediate pars plana vitrectomy was beneficial for patients who presented with visual acuity of light perception only.[32] In this subgroup of patients, vitrectomy was associated with a threefold increase in the frequency of achieving 20/40 or better acuity (33% vs. 11%), approximately a twofold chance of achieving 20/100 or better acuity (56% vs. 30%), and a 50% decrease in the frequency of severe visual loss to worse than 5/200 acuity (20% vs. 47%). There was no difference in outcome between immediate pars plana vitrectomy and tap/biopsy for patients with an initial visual acuity of hand motions or better. In this subgroup, patients had about the same chance of achieving 20/40 or better acuity (66% vs. 62%) and 20/100 or better acuity (86% vs. 84%), and a similar risk for severe visual loss to worse than 5/200 acuity (5% vs. 3%), whether they had immediate three-port pars plana vitrectomy or vitreous tap/biopsy. However, there was a possible exception. Diabetic patients with initial visual acuity of hand motions or better obtained somewhat better visual acuity outcome with vitrectomy compared to tap/biopsy. Final visual acuity of 20/40 or better was obtained in 57% of vitrectomy patients and 40% of tap biopsy patients. The difference was not statistically significant. It was suggested that either vitrectomy or tap/biopsy could be considered reasonable for diabetic patients.[32a]

At 9 to 12 months after presentation, clear media, as judged by a 20/40 view of the fundus by indirect ophthalmoscopy, was achieved slightly less frequently in the tap/biopsy eyes (83%) than in the vitrectomized eyes (90%), but this difference was not statistically significant. In no cases were vitreous opacities judged to be a principal cause of impaired vision at the final examination.[36]

Systemic antibiotics were observed to have no effect on visual outcome or media clarity in the EVS, even when subgroup analysis that considered microbiologic susceptibilities was performed.[32,41] The study concluded that systemic antibiotics provided no additional benefit to intravitreally administered antibiotics.

COMPLICATIONS FROM ENDOPHTHALMITIS AND ITS MANAGEMENT

In the EVS, major adverse events included retinal detachment in 5%, phthisis in 3%, significant elevation of intraocular pressure (30 mm Hg or more) in 1%, and enucleation or evisceration in 1%. Compared with vitreous tap/biopsy, vitrectomy was associated with a slightly lower rate of complications. Retinal detachment and phthisis occurred in 2.7% and 2% of vitrectomy eyes, respectively, compared to 7% and 4% of tap/biopsy eyes.[32] Enucleation was performed in three tap/biopsy eyes and in no vitrectomy eyes. The EVS treatment recommendations were based on visual outcome and not small differences in complication rates among treatment modalities.

Macular abnormalities were the most common cause of visual loss in the EVS. These included macular edema, pigmentary degeneration, epiretinal membrane, and ischemia. Such abnormalities were more common with worse presenting visual acuity, occurring in up to 17% of patients with hand motions or better acuity and up to 40% of patients presenting with light perception acuity. In light perception eyes that did not receive vitrectomy (the subgroup that did most poorly), excess visual loss was due to anterior segment media opacification (15%), and phthisis or enucleation (23%). These events were observed much less frequently (0.7% to 7%) in the remaining treatment groups.

Two adverse events during or after endophthalmitis treatment may markedly influence visual acuity outcomes. Antibiotic toxicity and retinal detachment are significant because further visual loss may occur in spite of successful treatment of the infections. Macular infarction after the use of intraocular aminoglycosides is a clinically recognized complication manifesting as a relatively well-defined area of retinal whitening, often in the macula.[49] Reported cases of macular infarction secondary to administration of intraocular aminoglycosides have been observed after excessive intraocular doses and others after apparent injection of a recommended safe dose. A localized increase in the drug concentration in dependent areas of the retina may play a role in aminoglycoside toxicity. If some of the perifoveal capillaries are spared, retention of some central vision is possible.

Retinal detachment may occur before, during, or after endophthalmitis treatment. The visual prognosis for eyes with retinal detachment in the setting of endophthalmitis is generally poor in reported series.[50,51] The rates of postvitrectomy retinal detachment may be reduced by the use of smaller-diameter vitrectomy instrumentation and by performing a partial vitrectomy when the view is compromised by media opacities.

EARLY AND LATE ADDITIONAL PROCEDURES

The EVS also evaluated the frequency of additional intervention following initial treatment.[36] Within 1 week of presentation, additional procedures were required in 8% of vitrectomized eyes versus 13% of those treated with tap/biopsy. Of 44 eyes (10% overall) that required repeat procedures, most (9%) underwent such procedures for worsening inflammation, and the remainder (1.4%, six eyes) for other complications after the initial treatment procedure. These complications included glaucoma, wound leak, and retinal detachment. Eyes that required additional procedures soon after initial presentation had a worse visual outcome, with only 15% of eyes achieving 20/40 or better visual acuity compared to 57% of eyes that did not require such procedures. The poorer outcome in eyes requiring secondary procedures could be attributed to the worse early course in such eyes, rather than to the secondary procedures themselves.

The incidence of late additional surgical procedures was 27% overall, and did not differ whether or not vitrectomy was performed or intravenous antibiotics were administered. Overall, late additional procedures included posterior capsulotomy in 9% of patients, vitrectomy in 7%, retinopexy in 2%, scleral buckling in 1%, and glaucoma procedures in 1%. Macular pucker was operated on in about 2% of patients. Including early additional surgical procedures, approximately one third of EVS patients required repeated surgical intervention after initial treatment.

CLINICAL PRESENTATION AND VISUAL OUTCOME

Clinical factors on presentation can be correlated with final visual outcome in the EVS. The single most important predictor of visual outcome was presenting visual acuity. Patients with LP visual acuity at presentation had twice the risk of decreased vision as to those with hand motions or better. Overall, 23% of patients with light perception acuity achieved 20/40 or better final acuity, compared with 64% of patients who had hand motions or better acuity.[32] The data confirmed that early treatment of endophthalmitis prior to severe visual loss is critical to maximize visual outcome, and that such treatment is more important in influencing outcome than any other factor, including vitrectomy. Other clinical factors that independently predicted decreased final visual acuity were older age, history of diabetes, corneal infiltrate or ring ulcer, abnormal intraocular pressure, rubeosis, an absent red reflex, and an open posterior capsule.[39]

MICROBIOLOGICAL FACTORS

The EVS evaluated the microbiological spectrum and susceptibilities of infecting organisms in acute postoperative endophthalmitis after cataract surgery. The findings provided a basis for choosing initial empiric antibiotic therapy and for evaluating subsequent changes in microbiological spectrum in this disease. The types of organisms and their distribution as observed in the EVS are described in Table 60–4. Visual outcomes by infecting species are also shown in Table 60–4.[3] Because both gram-positive and gram-negative organisms were encountered, antibiotic coverage for both types of organisms is recommended.

Although the infecting organism type predicted visual outcome and response to vitrectomy, the presenting visual acuity was a more powerful, independent, predictor of outcome. Presenting visual acuity appeared to serve as a useful proxy for factors such as duration of infection, host response, and degree of ongoing tissue damage, which are determinants of visual prognosis and response to vitrectomy. Other important EVS observations included the following:

1. A confirmed culture positivity rate of 69% overall; 82% if equivocal cultures were included.[37]
2. A high frequency (approximately 70%) of coagulase-negative staphylococci in culture-positive cases, with a high concordance of intraocular isolates with the patients' periocular skin flora being observed.[34]
3. A 9% rate of polymicrobial infection (infection with two or more strains or species in the same eye).[37]
4. A high rate of susceptibility of infecting organisms (99.4%) to either of two antimicrobial drug combinations available for intravitreal administration, vancomycin plus amikacin, or vancomycin plus ceftazidime.[37]
5. A statistically significant association between secondary IOL implantation and infection with organisms other than coagulase-negative staphylococci,

TABLE 60–4. Visual Outcome by Infecting Organism in the Endophthalmitis Vitrectomy Study*

Infecting Organism	N	>20/40 (%)	>20/100 (%)	<5/200 (%)
Gram-positive, coagulase-negative micrococci	214	58	81	4
Staphylococcus aureus	30	37	50	37
Streptococcus species	23	13	30	39
Enterococcus species	7	0	14	43
Gram-positives, excluding gram-positive coagulase-negative micrococci	69	28	59	33
Gram-negatives	18	39	44	28

*Data obtained from The Endophthalmitis Vitrectomy Study Group. Microbiologic factors and visual outcome in the Endophthalmitis Vitrectomy Study. Am J Ophthalmol 1996;122-837.

such as *Staphylococcus aureus* and streptococci.[37] Such organisms were associated with a much poorer visual prognosis.

6. Virtually identical visual outcome for culture-negative cases and cases infected with coagulase-negative staphylococci, suggesting that many cases of "sterile" endophthalmitis may actually be infectious in origin.[33]
7. Topical preoperative surgical preparation with povidone-iodine had been administered in 85 of 211 (40.3%) of EVS study patients for whom such data were recorded.[37]
8. Prophylactic antibiotics had been administered in the cataract infusion fluid at the initial cataract surgery in 10 of 87 (11.5%) patients in which the data were available.[37]

PITFALLS IN THE IMPLEMENTATION OF THE EVS FINDINGS

Measurement of presenting visual acuity was an important factor in the EVS and its recommendations regarding pars plana vitrectomy. According to the EVS, patients who were unable to perceive hand motions at a distance of 2 feet were designated as having light perception visual acuity. Such patients were shown to benefit from immediate pars plana vitrectomy. Improperly designating such patients with actual light perception acuity as having hand motions acuity would result in their inappropriate exclusion from receiving a potentially beneficial vitrectomy. In the EVS, discrimination between light perception and hand motions acuity required that the illumination source be placed behind (not in front of) the patient, and that the patient correctly identify four of five presentations of hand movements at a distance of 2 feet. A large proportion of patients in the EVS (70%) required such discrimination, having presented with either light perception or hand motions acuity.[32]

The EVS recommendations regarding the use of vitrectomy in acute-onset postoperative endophthalmitis may not be directly applied to other forms of endophthalmitis. The predominant infecting organism in acute-onset postoperative endophthalmitis, coagulase-negative staphylococci, accounted for 70% of the culture positive cases in the study. Other common forms of endophthalmitis are not characterized by such a predominance of this organism. Bleb-related, traumatic, or endogenous endophthalmitis are more likely to harbor organisms of greater virulence such as the toxin-producing *Streptococcus* or *Bacillus* species. In such cases, the benefits of vitrectomy might theoretically be greater because of its presumed ability to physically remove bacteria and toxins from the eye.

SYSTEMIC ANTIBIOTICS

Controversy has existed in the literature whether systemic antibiotics are necessary for successful treatment of infectious endophthalmitis. Intraocular inflammation and/or performance of a vitrectomy may alter the blood–retina barrier in a manner to allow better intravitreal penetration of systemically administered antibiotics. Prior to the EVS, successful treatment results in culture-positive cases of exogenous bacterial endophthalmitis without the use of systemic antibiotic therapy were published.[52] One series included 16 endophthalmitis cases caused by *S. epidermidis* or more virulent organisms. Repeat intravitreal antibiotic injections were performed in seven cases because of suspected initial treatment failure, but in all patients the infection was ultimately cured without the use of systemic antibiotics. Three arguments against the use of intravenous antibiotics are the potential systemic toxicity, the variable intravitreal penetration, and the high cost of some antibiotics.

Certain limitations of the EVS with respect to systemic antibiotic therapy should be recognized. First amikacin and ceftazidime were the only systemic antibiotics evaluated in the EVS. Second, whereas patients with acute-onset endophthalmitis following cataract surgery derived no additional benefit from the EVS systemically administered antibiotics, the study made no recommendations regarding systemic antibiotics for endophthalmitis prophylaxis, or for chronic, traumatic, bleb-related, fungal, or endogenous endophthalmitis.

PERIOCULAR ANTIBIOTIC THERAPY

Conflicting data regarding the intravitreal penetration after periocular antibiotic injection have been reported.[51] Causes for the variability in these experiments include the inflammatory status of the eye and, possibly, sampling technique. The physiochemical properties of the drug may affect transscleral and transcorneal permeability. Of the antibiotics now in use, the third-generation cephalosporins (ceftazidime and ceftriaxone) achieve the highest vitreous levels.

TOPICAL ANTIBIOTIC THERAPY

Most studies concerning the efficacy of topically applied antibiotics pertain to corneal infections. Significant intraocular levels of antibiotics can be achieved with frequent administration of highly concentrated solutions.[53] In eyes with intact corneal epithelium, lipid-soluble antibiotics such as chloramphenicol penetrate better than the less lipid–soluble drugs such as the aminoglycosides. This difference is reduced when the corneal epithelium is damaged. For acute-onset postoperative endophthalmitis, topical vancomycin, 50 mg/ml, in combination with an aminoglycoside or ceftazidime administered hourly is recommended. This regimen can then be adjusted to the specific organism after culture and sensitivity results are available.

CORTICOSTEROID THERAPY

Marked infiltration of the anterior chamber and vitreous cavity by polymorphonuclear neutrophils often occurs in endophthalmitis caused by bacteria. These white blood cells are implicated as mediators of tissue-destructive events by liberating oxygen metabolites such as superoxide and hydrogen peroxide, as well as proteolytic enzymes (elastase, collagenase, gelatinase). Theoretically, corticosteroids should reduce this inflammation-induced ocular damage associated with endophthalmitis.

Corticosteroids can be administered to the eye by several routes (intravitreal, systemic, periocular, and topical). Clinical studies have reported no adverse effect when using intravitreal dexamethasone in conjunction with intraocular antibiotics. In a prospective randomized clinical trial of 63 bacterial endophthalmitis cases, intravitreal dexamethasone was shown to reduce inflammation scores early in the course of treatment but had no independent influence on the final visual outcome.[54] In a series of endophthalmitis cases caused by gram-negative organisms, Irvine and associates[55] reported no adverse effects using intravitreal dexamethasone 400 μg, in conjunction with intravitreal antibiotics. In this report, visual acuity rates of 20/400 or better in eyes treated with adjunctive intraocular dexamethasone (70.0%) were compared with eyes not receiving adjunctive dexamethasone (44.2%). Similarly, Mao and associates[56] reported better visual acuity outcomes after adjunctive treatment with intravitreal dexamethasone 400 μg (87.5% vs. 52.6%) for *Staphylococcus aureus* endophthalmitis.

In addition to intravitreal corticosteroids, periocular corticosteroids are also commonly used in the treatment of endophthalmitis. The periocular dosage may include dexamethasone 12 mg or more, administered together with periocular antibiotics.[1] Topical corticosteroids are usually started on the first morning after the initial treatment of endophthalmitis. These drops may be alternated on an hourly basis with the use of topical antibiotics.

Systemic corticosteroids were used in the EVS in the treatment of all study patients with postoperative endophthalmitis. In one study, a combination of topical and systemic corticosteroids gave better results than no corticosteroids or only topical corticosteroid administration.[57] Because many patients with endophthalmitis also have diabetes mellitus,[4] caution is advised when using higher dosages of systemic corticosteroids.

TISSUE PLASMINOGEN ACTIVATOR

Marked fibrin formation often accompanies endophthalmitis. This fibrin may sometimes cause pupillary block glaucoma or may form a scaffold for cellular proliferation with subsequent traction retinal detachment, cyclitic membrane formation, and/or hypotony.

The use of tissue plasminogen activator (t-PA) for treating severe postvitrectomy intraocular fibrin formation was reported for 23 eyes.[58] In 3 of the 23 eyes, endophthalmitis was the underlying cause for the fibrin production. In all three patients, intraocular t-PA 25 μg resulted in prompt fibrinolysis, although 2 eyes had recurrent fibrin formation. No complications were directly related to the t-PA injection. Only one of these three t-PA–treated patients achieved 20/400 visual acuity. Although t-PA may have a role in the treatment of fibrin formation complicating endophthalmitis, its use should be reserved for severe cases unresponsive to intensive corticosteroid therapy.

MANAGEMENT OF THE CRYSTALLINE LENS AND THE IOL DURING ENDOPHTHALMITIS TREATMENT

An uninvolved crystalline lens can generally be left in place during endophthalmitis treatment (e.g., in endogenous endophthalmitis). Successful treatment of culture-positive cases has been reported using vitrectomy and intravitreal antibiotics while preserving the uninvolved crystalline lens.[59]

In most cases of acute-onset postoperative pseudophakic endophthalmitis, intraocular lens removal is not necessary.[2] There is no evidence that leaving the IOL in place reduces the chance of sterilizing the eye.[60] Removal of the posterior chamber IOL may be hazardous in inflamed eyes and may predispose to anterior and posterior segment complications. In selected cases of fungal endophthalmitis and in cases of *Propionibacterium acnes* not responsive to more conservative therapy, IOL removal should be considered.[11–13] If recurrent infection occurs with pars plana vitrectomy, partial capsulotomy, and intravitreal antibiotics, these cases may require removal of the entire capsular bag and the IOL to achieve a cure.[61]

ENDOPHTHALMITIS CATEGORIES

ACUTE-ONSET POSTOPERATIVE ENDOPHTHALMITIS

Acute-onset endophthalmitis occurs postoperatively within 6 weeks of intraocular surgery. It can occur from a variety of intraocular surgical procedures ranging from radial keratotomy to cataract surgery. Pain is a frequent but inconsistent symptom and was absent in 25% of EVS patients. The visual loss is generally greater than that expected during the usual postoperative course. Organisms most frequently involved are the coagulase-negative staphylococci, *Staphylococcus aureus*, the *Streptococcus* species, and gram-negative organisms.

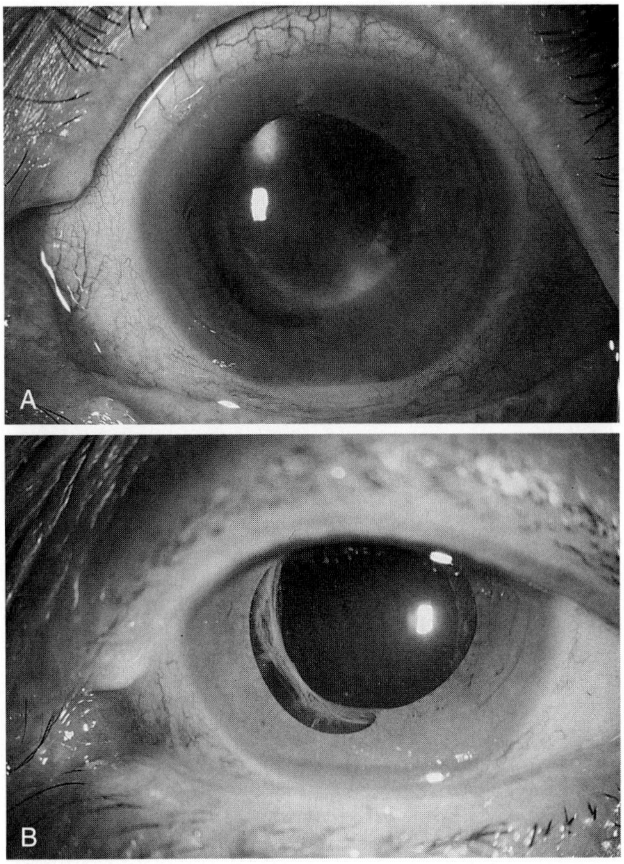

Figure 60–4. *A.* White plaque inside the capsular bag *(P. acnes)*. *B.* After vitrectomy, capsulotomy, and injection of intravitreal antibiotics, the patient had visual improvement and no recurrence.

DELAYED-ONSET OR CHRONIC POSTOPERATIVE ENDOPHTHALMITIS

In this endophthalmitis category, patients may present weeks to months after cataract extraction, often with mild to moderate inflammatory signs and a chronic indolent course.[13,61] *Propionibacterium acnes,* a gram-positive, anaerobic pleomorphic rod, is a common causative organism in this category. The clinical *P. acnes* syndrome of delayed-onset pseudophakic endophthalmitis, first described by Meisler and associates[61] in 1986, typically includes granulomatous inflammation with large keratic precipitates and a white intracapsular plaque that has been shown to be composed of organisms mixed with residual lens cortex. When infection with this slow-growing organism is suspected, anaerobic cultures of both the aqueous and vitreous should be obtained and held at least 2 weeks.

In a review of 19 patients with delayed-onset pseudophakic endophthalmitis (defined as those cases diagnosed 4 weeks or more after cataract surgery and excluding filtering bleb–associated cases), four different etiologic organisms were isolated.[10] These included *Propionibacterium* species (63%), *Candida parapsilosis* (16%), *S. epidermidis* (16%), and *Corynebacterium* species (5%).

In the initial management of *P. acnes* pseudophakic endophthalmitis with a white intracapsular plaque, a pars plana vitrectomy and a central capsulectomy together with intravitreal antibiotics (intravitreal corticosteroids are optional) is generally recommended.[11–13] Selective removal of the observed white plaque using the vitrectomy probe assisted by scleral depression may reduce the frequency of recurrent infection (Fig. 60–4*A* and *B*). Vancomycin 1 mg has been the initial antibiotic of choice because of its broad spectrum of coverage against gram-positive organisms, and because it can be injected into the remaining capsular bag after the vitrectomy.[11–13] Vancomycin has been recommended over other antibiotics, but vancomycin's activity is diminished under anaerobic conditions. *P. acnes* isolates are also sensitive to methicillin, cefazolin, and clindamycin.

In clinically suspected fungal infections characterized by fluffy white vitreous infiltrates (Fig. 60–5), immediate injection of intravitreal amphotericin B 5 μg, should be considered. If the initial treatment approach does not eliminate the infection, total capsulectomy and IOL removal or exchange can be considered in this staged approach.[62,63]

Other categories of delayed-onset endophthalmitis include cases associated with suture removal, severe bacterial keratitis, or exposed glaucoma drainage devices.[63a] Sutures for scleral fixation of IOL haptics may erode through the conjunctiva and allow entry of organisms into the eye.[64]

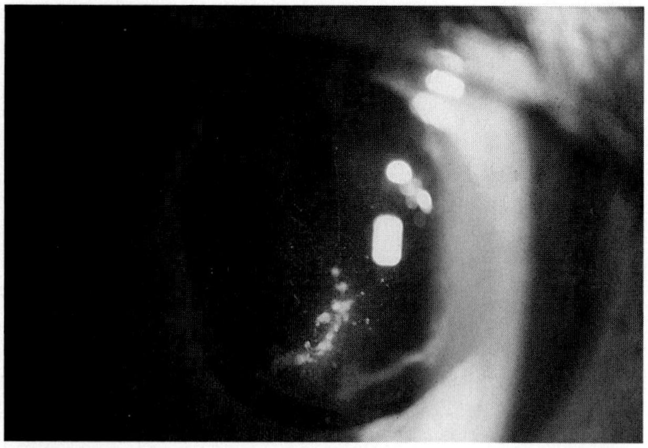

Figure 60–5. Postoperative fungal endophthalmitis *(Candida)* showing "string-of-pearls" appearance.

CONJUNCTIVAL FILTERING BLEB–ASSOCIATED ENDOPHTHALMITIS

This category of endophthalmitis is similar to acute postoperative endophthalmitis in that these patients manifest a sudden onset of pain, visual loss, conjunctival congestion, purulent bleb involvement, and the typical diagnostic features of acute-onset endophthalmitis (Fig. 60–6).[6,7,65] Risk factors for this category of endophthalmitis include a history of conjunctivitis, contaminated topical glaucoma medications, the use of contact lenses, and an inferior filtering bleb.[6,65] The incidence of bleb-related endophthalmitis after a guarded filtration procedure with mitomycin C may be higher than for trabeculectomy without antifibrotic agents.[65] The organisms frequently involved in this type of endophthalmitis include streptococcal species and *Haemophilus influenzae.* Because of the frequency of these virulent organisms and the generally poor visual acuity outcomes, pars plana vitrectomy and intraocular antibiotics are often considered as the initial approach for conjunctival filtering bleb–associated endophthalmitis.

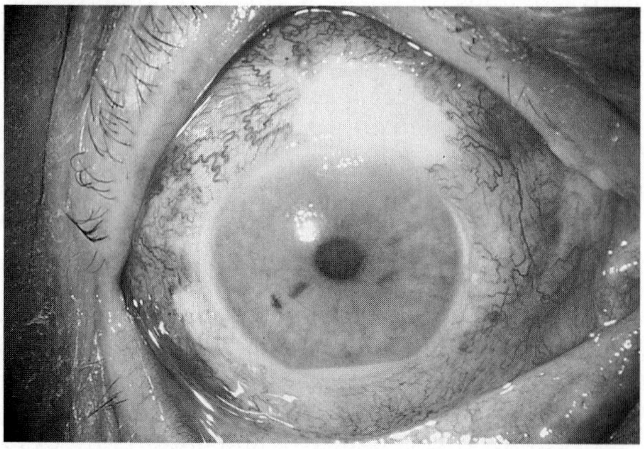

Figure 60–6. Bleb-associated endophthalmitis

It is important to distinguish between a localized bleb infection (blebitis) and true endophthalmitis associated with an infected filtering bleb. The former category can be treated with intensive topical and subconjunctival antibiotics, whereas the latter category can be treated in a manner similar to acute-onset postoperative endophthalmitis.

POSTTRAUMATIC ENDOPHTHALMITIS

The visual outcomes after treatment of posttraumatic endophthalmitis are generally worse than the other endophthalmitis categories. In the National Eye Trauma System[18] review of endophthalmitis after penetrating injuries with retained intraocular foreign bodies, 9 of 22 (40.9%) culture-positive cases achieved 20/400 or better visual acuity. Either *Bacillus* or *Staphylococcus* species were isolated in 21 of these 22 (95%) culture-positive cases. Endophthalmitis was much less likely to develop in eyes with primary repair within 24 hours of the injury (10/287 = 3.5%) than in eyes with primary repair more than 24 hours after the injury (22/164 = 13.4%; $p < 0.0001$). Major reasons for the poor visual acuity outcomes in these cases are the marked structural damage to the eye resulting from the initial injury, the delay in the primary wound repair, and the greater virulence of the organisms commonly associated with the traumatic endophthalmitis. *Bacillus* species, most commonly *B. cereus,* are cultured from 28% to 46% of eyes with posttraumatic endophthalmitis.[17,18] *Bacillus* species are ubiquitous, aerobic, gram-positive, spore-forming rods. Endophthalmitis caused by *Bacillus* species is characterized by a rapidly progressive course, ring corneal infiltrates, and generally a poor visual outcome, even with prompt therapy.[66–70]

A subgroup of trauma-related endophthalmitis is endophthalmitis associated with retained intraocular foreign bodies. Mieler and associates[71] reported 27 consecutive cases of retained intraocular foreign bodies managed by prompt removal of the foreign body using pars plana vitrectomy techniques. Positive vitreous cultures were obtained in 7 of the 19 cases in which cultures were performed. *Bacillus* species were identified in 2 of these 7 culture-positive cases. In spite of the positive intraocular cultures, no patient developed clinical endophthalmitis. In the National Eye Trauma System data, fewer patients with retained foreign bodies (10 of 287 patients [3.5%]) developed endophthalmitis when the primary surgical repair was accomplished within 24 hours after the injury compared with patients in whom the primary surgical repair was delayed more than 24 hours (22 of 164 patients [13.4%]).[18] Signs of infectious endophthalmitis were described at the primary surgical repair in 91.2% (31 of 34 patients), but 8.8% (3 of 34 patients) developed signs of infection after the primary repair. These reports speculate that prompt surgical intervention, use of vitrectomy, and possible use of prophylactic intravitreal antibiotics in selected high-risk cases may reduce the incidence of endophthalmitis or reverse early undiagnosed endophthalmitis in the setting of a retained intraocular foreign body.

The role of prophylactic intravitreal antibiotics in penetrating ocular trauma cases is controversial. However, given the potential for severe visual loss in trauma-related endophthalmitis, it seems prudent to consider their use in selected cases resulting from material such as vegetable matter, foreign body injuries incurred in an outdoor or rural environment, and penetrating ocular injury from eating utensils.[71,72] The combination of vancomycin 1 mg alone or in conjunction with either an aminoglycoside (amikacin, 0.4 mg) or ceftazidime, 2.25 mg, should be considered when prophylactic intraocular therapy seems appropriate. In addition, systemic antibiotics are usually administered.[73]

ENDOGENOUS ENDOPHTHALMITIS

Endogenous endophthalmitis is caused by fungi more often than bacteria.[21] *Candida albicans* is the most common organism causing endogenous fungal endophthalmitis, and *Aspergillus* species are the second most common fungal cause.[22] Endogenous endophthalmitis is more commonly diagnosed in immunocompromised and debilitated patients or intravenous drug abusers (Table 60–5).

The typical clinical features of *Candida* endogenous endophthalmitis include fluffy yellow or white vitreous opacities and creamy white chorioretinal infiltrates (Fig. 60–7*A* and *B*). Anterior uveitis frequently accompanies the posterior segment findings. A large macular abscess and pseudohypopyon formation (layering of inflammatory material under the internal limiting membrane of the retina) is not uncommon in cases of endogenous *Aspergillus* infection.[22]

The management of endogenous endophthalmitis depends on the clinical features (fungal vs. bacterial), the specific organism isolated, and the severity of infection.[21,22] Once a diagnosis of endogenous endophthalmitis is suspected, evidence of other organ involvement must be sought. This is usually accomplished in consultation with an infectious disease specialist or internist. The presumptive clinical diagnosis is made by positive blood or urine cultures or by focal active infection of nonocular tissues.

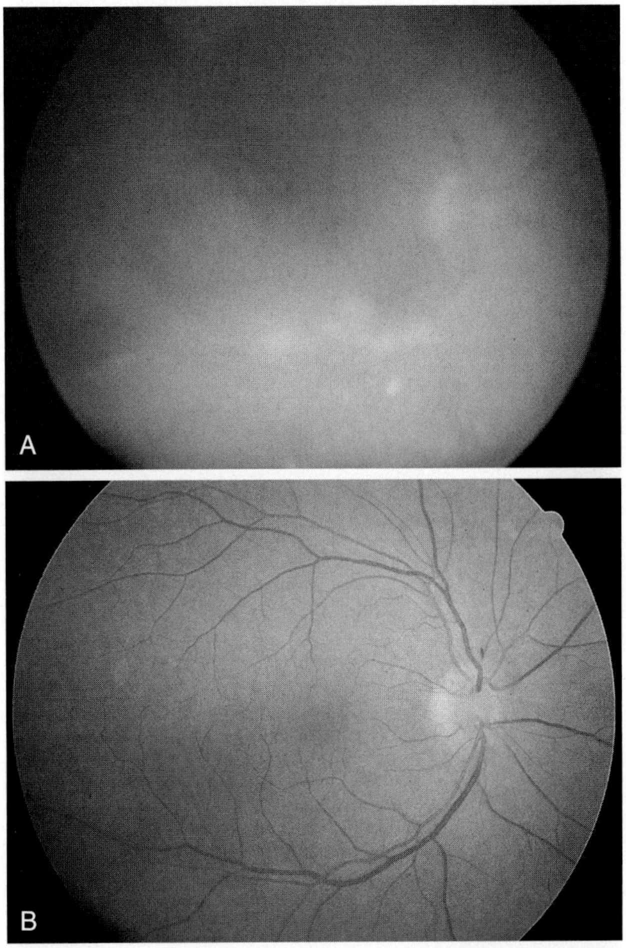

Figure 60–7. *A.* Endogenous Candida endophthalmitis with vitritis and solid infiltrates. *B.* After treatment with vitrectomy and amphotericin B, the infection resolved and the visual acuity returned to 20/20.

TABLE 60–5. Conditions Possibly Predisposing to Endogenous Endophthalmitis

Long-term intravenous line placement	Malignancy
Parenteral hyperalimentation	Diabetes mellitus
Prolonged antibiotic therapy	Pregnancy
Systemic corticosteroids	Massive trauma
Immunosuppressive therapy	Alcoholism
Abdominal surgery	Hepatic insufficiency
Hemodialysis	Post partum
Intravenous drug abuse	Prematurity
AIDS	Genitourinary manipulation

The management approach in cases of suspected endogenous *Candida* endophthalmitis is generally tailored to the clinical situation. When chorioretinal infiltrates are present with no or minimal vitreous involvement, systemic therapy alone is recommended. With moderate to severe vitreous involvement or in cases with a worsening course in spite of systemic therapy, vitrectomy and intraocular amphotericin B are generally recommended.

The choice of systemic antifungal agents is based on several factors.[74] For example, if there is no evidence of disseminated disease or in patients too ill to tolerate the toxicity associated with systemic amphotericin B, other less toxic systemic oral antifungal medications can be used. Such medication is usually administered in conjunction with an infectious disease consultant.

When *Aspergillus* infection is suspected, aggressive local ocular therapy including vitrectomy and intravitreal amphotericin B is usually indicated.[22] Success-

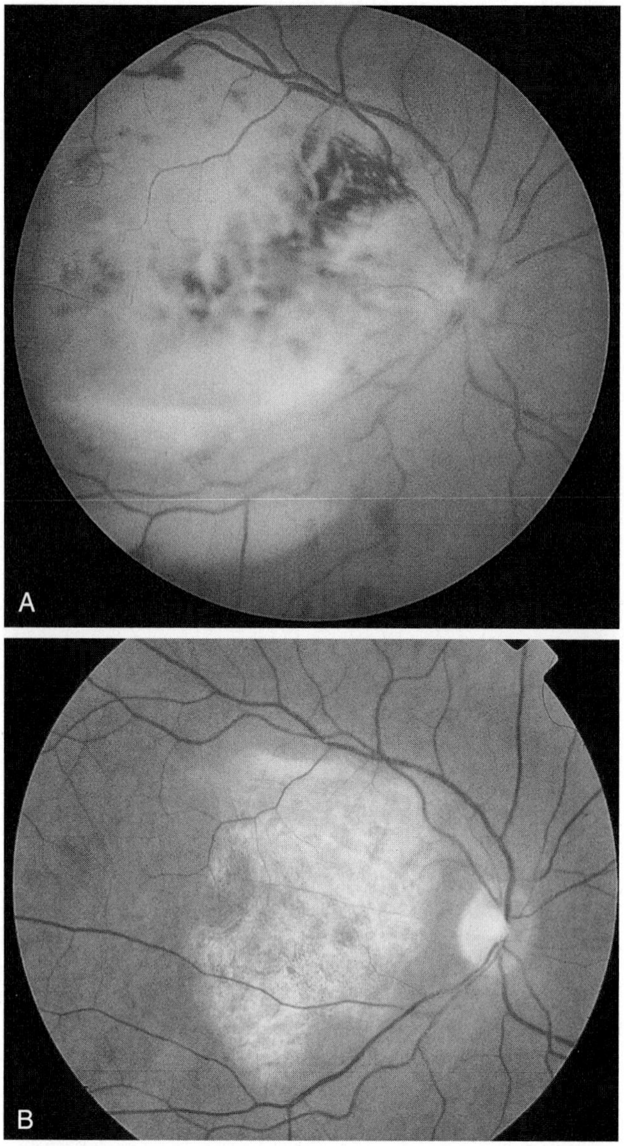

Figure 60–8. *A*. Endogenous Aspergillus endophthalmitis with macular abscess. *B*. After treatment with vitrectomy and intravitreal amphotericin B, the infection resolved, but a macular scar resulted in 20/400 visual acuity. (From Weishaar P, Flynn HW Jr, Murray TG, et al.: Endogenous *Aspergillus* endophthalmitis. Clinical features and treatment outcomes. Ophthalmology 1998;105:57–65.)

ful treatment in *Aspergillus* endophthalmitis cases can be accomplished, but the occurrence of a macular abscess may reduce central vision on a permanent basis (Fig. 60–8*A* and *B*). Because an intraocular *Aspergillus* infection is frequently associated with other organ involvement, particularly cardiac valve vegetation, a comprehensive systemic evaluation is mandatory, and systemic therapy is indicated in most cases.

Endogenous bacterial endophthalmitis is thought to be less common than fungal endophthalmitis. In a 10-year retrospective study of 28 bacterial cases at the Massachusetts Eye and Ear Infirmary,[23] the following organisms were most frequently isolated: *S. aureus*, 25%; *Escherichia coli*, 18%; and *Streptococcus* species, 30%. Sources of infection were identified in 90% of cases. Endocarditis and the gastrointestinal tract were the most common sources.

In a retrospective review of 72 cases of endogenous endophthalmitis from multiple sources, one report reviewed the spectrum of causative bacteria and showed *Bacillus cereus* to be the most frequently reported bacterial agent.[20] This high incidence of endogenous *Bacillus* endophthalmitis was due to its association with intravenous drug abuse. This report also showed an increasing incidence of infections by organisms of low pathogenicity in immunocompromised hosts. The authors of this series proposed a classification scheme for endogenous endophthalmitis based on the location (anterior or posterior segment) and extent (focal or diffuse) of the primary intraocular infection. Focal and anterior cases appear to have a better visual prognosis, whereas posterior diffuse disease nearly always leads to significant loss of vision.[20]

To diagnose endogenous bacterial endophthalmitis, a high index of suspicion is important. All patients with visual loss and progressive intraocular inflammation should undergo indirect ophthalmoscopy looking for evidence of septic foci in the posterior segment. In some cases, the established intraocular inflammation is the initial finding leading to the diagnosis of bacterial endocarditis and sepsis. As with endogenous fungal endophthalmitis, an internist or infectious disease specialist should be involved in both the systemic work-up and the medical therapy. Some patients will present with a known site of infection. In these cases the intraocular organism is almost always the same as that cultured from the other organ site. These findings will help guide the selection of appropriate antibiotic therapy for both the systemic and ocular infection. In cases without a known site of infection other than the eye, a systemic laboratory work-up including cultures of blood, urine, sputum, and other suspicious sites should be obtained.

Systemic antibiotics are often used to treat endogenous endophthalmitis. In cases with focal chorioretinitis but without marked vitreous infiltrates, systemic therapy alone may achieve involution of the lesions. In eyes that fail to respond to systemic antibiotic therapy alone, intraocular therapy may be beneficial. When severe vitritis or marked vitreous infiltrates are present, a vitrectomy and intraocular antibiotic injection are usually recommended.[74]

PREVENTION

Eyelid and ocular surface microflora have been implicated as sources of infection in most cases of postoperative endophthalmitis.[34] Because bacteria can be cultured from the ocular surface of almost all persons, certain risk factors may make patients more susceptible to infection by their ocular surface microflora. Preoperative high-risk factors include chronic bacterial blepharitis, active conjunctivitis, infections of the lacrimal drainage system, tear drainage obstruction, contaminated eye drops, contact lens wear, a prosthesis in the fellow eye, and active nonocular infections.[75–78] These conditions may lead to an abnormally elevated population of ocular surface microbes or colonization of the ocular surface by atypical organisms with greater virulence than the normal microflora. Intraoperative risk factors are prolonged surgery (>60 minutes), surgery complicated by vitreous loss, and contaminated irrigating solutions or intraocular lenses.[3,78] Postoperative entry of ocular surface microflora may be facilitated by mechanical wound problems such as wound leaks or vitreous incarceration in the surgical wound.[9] Host factors that lower resistance to infection such as chronic immunosuppressive therapy and diabetes mellitus have also been reported to be significant risk factors for postoperative endophthalmitis.[3,4]

To reduce the incidence of postoperative endophthalmitis, each of the factors implicated in the pathogenesis should be addressed. First, an attempt should be made to decrease or eliminate eyelid and conjunctival microflora both preoperatively and intraoperatively. This goal may be accomplished by the use of preoperative topical antibiotics and topical antiseptic agents and administration of subconjunctival antibiotic at the time of surgery.

Studies evaluating the effectiveness of preoperative antibiotic administration have reported a significant decrease in conjunctival bacterial colony counts after the use of certain antibiotics.[79–82] Topical antibiotics were reported to be most effective in decreasing conjunctival bacterial colony counts when administered 2 hours before surgery rather than 1 or more days before surgery.[80] Topical application of povidone-iodine has been reported to significantly decrease preoperative conjunctival bacterial colony counts in eyes undergoing ophthalmic surgery.[80–82] Similarly, preoperative povidone-iodine prophylaxis was found to significantly reduce the incidence of postoperative endophthalmitis in retrospective studies. The combination of topical antibiotics and povidone-iodine was found to sterilize the conjunctiva in more than 80% of treated patients.[79]

Subconjunctival antibiotics are commonly administered after intraocular surgery. The rationale for subconjunctival antibiotic administration at the completion of the ocular procedure is to inhibit growth of bacteria that may gain entry into the eye during the operative procedure. Studies performed evaluating the effectiveness of prophylactic subconjunctival antibiotics in reducing the incidence of postoperative endophthalmitis reported conflicting results.[76–78]

Antibiotics in the irrigating fluid for cataract surgery has become a common technique for infection prophylaxis. This technique has many negative associations including potential antibiotic toxicity, the high cost of its general use, and the potential for more rapid emergence of resistant bacteria.[83,84] At least 10 patients in the EVS developed endophthalmitis in spite of receiving antibiotics in the irrigating fluid for cataract surgery. The American Academy of Ophthalmology (2000) has issued a Policy Statement discouraging the routine use of antibiotics in the irrigating fluid for cataract surgery.

The various strategies to prevent postoperative endophthalmitis are based on current knowledge regarding the pathogenic mechanisms of postoperative endophthalmitis. Perhaps of greatest importance, the preoperative ocular examination will help to identify the high-risk patient as previously described. In these patients, eyelid and conjunctival cultures can be performed before performing intraocular surgery. Based on the culture results and the overall clinical evaluation, preoperative antibiotic treatment may be considered. In patients with eye diseases requiring chronic administration of topical medications, new sterile medications should be provided to the patient before and after intraocular surgery.

On the day of cataract surgery, consideration can be given to treating patients with prophylactic topical antibiotics that have activity against organisms commonly causing endophthalmitis. A thorough surgical prep is performed, which includes lid margins. Instillation of 5% povidone-iodine on the conjunctiva followed by irrigation with saline is part of the surgical prep.[85] The eyelids and eyelashes can be draped out of the surgical field with a plastic eye drape. A dry surgical field can be maintained when instruments are passed in and out of the eye. Attention to watertight wound closure is a priority, particularly in complicated surgical procedures, or in reoperations that tend to have a higher incidence of postoperative wound leak. Vitreous incarceration in the wound should be eliminated by anterior vitrectomy techniques. At the conclusion of surgery, subconjunctival antibiotic injection can be considered using a combination of agents effective against the majority of causative gram-positive and gram-negative organisms.

CONCLUSION

Endophthalmitis can be associated with intraocular surgery, penetrating trauma, or endogenous sources and may cause severe visual loss. Early recognition, together with appropriate and timely treatment, can reduce the visual loss. The incidence of endophthalmitis can be reduced by identifying and treating high-risk patients before intraocular surgery and by maintaining careful aseptic techniques during intraocular surgery.

REFERENCES

1. American Academy of Ophthalmology: Basic and Clinical Science Course: Section 9: Intraocular Inflammation and Uveitis, 2001-2002. San Francisco: American Academy of Ophthalmology; 2001.
2. Doft B: Endophthalmitis Management. Focal Points: Modules for Clinicians. San Francisco: American Academy of Ophthalmology; 1997.
3. Aaberg TM Jr, Flynn HW Jr, Newton J: Nosocomial acute-onset postoperative endophthalmitis survey: a 10-year review of incidence and outcomes. Ophthalmology 1998;105:1004–10.
4. Phillips WB, Tasman WS: Postoperative endophthalmitis in association with diabetes mellitus. Ophthalmology 1994;101:508.
5. Mandelbaum S, Forster RK, Gelender H, Culbertson W: Late onset endophthalmitis associated with filtering blebs. Ophthalmology 1985;92:964.
6. Wolner B, Liebmann JM, Sassani JW, et al.: Late bleb-related endophthalmitis after trabeculectomy with adjunctive 5-fluorouracil. Ophthalmology 1991;98:1053.
7. Brown RH, Yang LH, Walker SD, et al.: Treatment of bleb infection after glaucoma filtering surgery. Arch Ophthalmol 1994; 112:57.

8. Gelender H: Bacterial endophthalmitis following cutting of sutures after cataract surgery. Am J Ophthalmol 1982;94:528.
9. Ruiz RS, Teeters VW: The vitreous wick syndrome: a late complication following cataract extraction. Am J Ophthalmol 1970; 70:483.
10. Fox GM, Joondeph BC, Flynn HW Jr, et al.: Delayed onset pseudophakic endophthalmitis. Am J Ophthalmol 1991;111:163.
11. Clark WL, Kaiser PK, Flynn HW Jr, et al.: Treatment strategies and visual acuity outcomes in chronic postoperative *P. acnes* endophthalmitis. Ophthalmology 1999;106:1665–70.
12. Aldave AJ, Stein JD, Deramo VA, et al.: Treatment strategies for postoperative *Propionibacterium acnes* endophthalmitis. Ophthalmology 1999;106:2395–401.
13. Ciulla TA: Update on acute and chronic endophthalmitis. Ophthalmology 1999;106:2237–8.
14. Puliafito CA, Baker AS, Haaf J, Foster CS: Infectious endophthalmitis: review of 36 cases. Ophthalmology 1982;89:921.
15. Rowsey JJ, Newsom MS, Sexton DJ, Harms WK: Endophthalmitis: current approaches. Ophthalmology 1982;89:1055.
16. Bohigian GM, Olk RJ: Factors associated with a poor visual result in endophthalmitis. Am J Ophthalmol 1986;101:332.
17. Brinton GS, Topping TM, Hyndiuk RA, et al.: Posttraumatic endophthalmitis. Arch Ophthalmol 1984;102:547.
18. Thompson JT, Parver LM, Enger C, et al.: Endophthalmitis after penetrating ocular injuries with retained intraocular foreign bodies. Ophthalmology 1993;100:1468.
19. Thompson WS, Rubsamen PE, Flynn HW Jr, et al.: Endophthalmitis after penetrating trauma. Risk factors and visual acuity outcomes. Ophthalmology 1995;102:1696–1701.
20. Greenwald MJ, Wohl LG, Sell CH: Metastatic bacterial endophthalmitis: a contemporary reappraisal. Surv Ophthalmol 1986; 31:81.
21. Brod RD, Flynn HW Jr, Clarkson JG, et al.: Endogenous *Candida* endophthalmitis: management without intravenous amphotericin B. Ophthalmology 1990;97:666.
22. Weishaar P, Flynn HW Jr, Murray TG, et al.: Endogenous *Aspergillus* endophthalmitis. Clinical features and treatment outcomes. Ophthalmology 1998;105:57–65.
23. Okada AA, Johnson RP, Liles C, et al.: Endogenous bacterial endophthalmitis. Ophthalmology 1994;101:832–8.
24. Packer AJ, Weingeist TA, Abrams GW: Retinal periphlebitis as an early sign of bacterial endophthalmitis. Am J Ophthalmol 1983;96:66.
25. Donahue SP, Kowalski RP, Jewart BH, Friberg TR: Vitreous cultures in suspected endophthalmitis: biopsy or vitrectomy? Ophthalmology 1993;100:452.
26. Joondeph BC, Flynn HW Jr, Miller D, Joondeph HC: A new culture method for infectious endophthalmitis. Arch Ophthalmol 1989;107:1334.
27. Rao NA: A laboratory approach to rapid diagnosis of ocular infections and prospects for the future. Am J Ophthalmol 1989; 107:283.
28. DNA technology and rapid diagnosis of infection (editorial). Lancet 1989;2:897.
29. Anand AR, Madhavan HN, Neela V, Lily T: Use of polymerase chain reaction in the diagnosis of fungal endophthalmitis. Ophthalmology 2001;108:326-30.
30. Chandler PA: Problems in the diagnosis and treatment of lens-induced uveitis and glaucoma. Arch Ophthalmol 1958;60:828.
31. Irvine WD, Flynn HW Jr, Murray TG, et al.: Retained lens fragments after phacoemulsification manifesting as marked intraocular inflammation with hypopyon. Am J Ophthalmol 1992; 114:610.
32. Endophthalmitis Vitrectomy Study Group: Results of the Endophthalmitis Vitrectomy Study. A randomized trial of immediate vitrectomy and of intravenous antibiotics for the treatment of postoperative bacterial endophthalmitis. Arch Ophthalmol 1995;113:1479–96.
32a. Doft DH, Wisnisky SR, Kellsy SF, Fitzgerald SG, and the Endophthalmitis Study Group: Diabetes and postoperative endophthalmitis in the Endophthalmitis Vitrectomy Study. Arch Ophthalmol 2001;119:650-6.
33. Endophthalmitis Vitrectomy Study Group: Microbiologic factors and visual outcome in the Endophthalmitis Vitrectomy Study. Am J Ophthalmol 1996;122:830–46.
34. Bannerman TL, Rhoden DL, McAllister M, et al.: The source of coagulase-negative staphylococci in the Endophthalmitis Vitrectomy Study. A comparison of eyelid and intraocular isolates using pulsed-field gel electorphoresis. Arch Ophthalmol 1997; 115:357–61.
35. Braza M, Pavan PR, Doft BH, et al.: Evaluation of microbiological diagnostic techniques in postoperative endophthalmitis in the Endophthalmitis Vitrectomy Study. Arch Ophthalmol 1997;116: 1142–50.
36. Doft BH, Kelsey SF, Wisniewski SR, et al.: Additional procedures after the initial vitrectomy or tap-biopsy in the Endophthalmitis Vitrectomy Study. Ophthalmology, 1998;105:707–16.
37. Han DP, Wisniewski SR, Wilson LA, et al.: Spectrum and susceptibilities of microbiologic isolates in the Endophthalmitis Vitrectomy Study [published erratum appears in Am J. Ophthalmol 1996 Dec 122:920] Am J Ophthalmol 1996;122:1–17.
38. Han DP, Wisniewski SR, Kelsey SF, et al.: Microbiologic yields and complication rates of vitreous needle aspiration versus mechanized vitreous biopsy in the Endophthalmitis Vitrectomy Study. Retina 1999;19:98–102.
39. Johnson MW, Doft BH, Kelsey SF, et al.: The Endophthalmitis Vitrectomy Study. Relationship between clinical presentation and microbiologic spectrum. Ophthalmology 1997;104:261–72.
40. Wisniewski SR, Hammer ME, Grizzard WS, et al.: An investigation of the hospital charges related to the treatment of endophthalmitis in the Endophthalmitis Vitrectomy Study. Ophthalmology 1997;104:739–45.
41. Durand M: Microbiologic factors and visual outcome in the Endophthalmitis Vitrectomy Study. Am J Ophthalmol 1997;124: 127–30.
42. Jay WM, Fishman P, Aziz M, Shickley RK: Intravitreal ceftazidime in a rabbit model: dose and time-dependent toxicity and pharmacokinetic analysis. J Ocul Pharmacol 1987;3:257.
43. Campochiaro PA, Green WR: Toxicity of intravitreous ceftazidime in primate retina. Arch Ophthalmol 1992;110:1625.
44. Oum BS, D'Amico DJ, Wong KW: Intravitreal antibiotic therapy with vancomycin and aminoglycoside: an experimental study of combination and repetitive injections. Arch Ophthalmol 1989; 107:1055.
45. Olson JC, Flynn HW Jr, Forster RK, Culbertson WW: Results in the treatment of postoperative endophthalmitis. Ophthalmology 1983;90:692.
46. Friberg TR: En bloc removal of inflammatory fibrocellular membranes from the iris surface in endophthalmitis. Arch Ophthalmol 1991;109:736.
47. Doft BH, Weiskopf J, Nilsson-Ehle I, Wingard LB Jr: Amphotericin clearance in vitrectomized versus nonvitrectomized eyes. Ophthalmology 1985;92:1601.
48. Campochiaro PA, Conway BP: Aminoglycoside toxicity—a survey of retinal specialists. Arch Ophthalmol 1991;109:946.
49. Campochiaro PA, Lim JL: Aminoglycoside Toxicity Study Group: Aminoglycoside toxicity in the treatment of endophthalmitis. Arch Ophthalmol 1994;112:48.
50. Doft BM, Kelsey SF, Wisniewski SR: EVS study group. Retinal detachment in the endophthalmitis vitectomy study. Arch Ophthalmol 2000;118:1661-5.
51. Foster RE, Rubsamen PE, Joondeph BC, et al: Concurrent endophthalmitis and retinal detachment. Ophthalmology 1994; 101:490.
52. Pavan PR, Brinser JH: Exogenous bacterial endophthalmitis treated without systemic antibiotics. Am J Ophthalmol 1987; 104:121.
53. Barza M: Antibacterial agents in the treatment of ocular infections. Infect Dis Clin North Am 1989;3:533.
54. Das T, Jaleli S, Gothwal V, et al.: Intravitreal dexamethasone in exogenous bacterial endophthalmitis: result of a prospective randomized study. Br J Ophthalmol 1999;83:1050–5.
55. Irvine WD, Flynn HW Jr, Miller DA, et al.: Endophthalmitis caused by gram negative organisms. Arch Ophthalmol 1992;110: 1450–4.
56. Mao LK, Flynn HW Jr, Miller D, et al.: Endophthalmitis caused by *Staphylococcus aureus.* Am J Ophthalmol 1993;116:584.
57. Koul S, Philipson BT, Philipson A: Visual outcome of endophthalmitis in Sweden. Acta Ophthalmol 1989;67:504.

58. Jaffe GJ, Abrams GW, Williams GA, et al.: Tissue plasminogen activator for postvitrectomy fibrin formation. Ophthalmology 1990;97:184.
59. Huang SS, Brod RD, Flynn HW Jr: Management of endophthalmitis while preserving the uninvolved crystalline lens. Am J Ophthalmol 1991;112:695.
60. Hopen G, Mondino BJ, Kozy D, et al.: Intraocular lenses and experimental bacterial endophthalmitis. Am J Ophthalmol 1982; 94:402.
61. Meisler DM, Palestine AG, Vastine DW, et al.: Chronic *Propionibacterium* endophthalmitis after extracapsular cataract extraction and intraocular lens implantation. Am J Ophthalmol 1986;102:733.
62. Stern WH, Tamura E, Jacobs RA, et al.: Epidemic postsurgical *Candida parapsilosis* endophthalmitis: clinical findings and management of 15 consecutive cases. Ophthalmology 1985;92:170.
63. Petit TH, Olson RJ, Foos RY, et al.: Fungal endophthalmitis following intraocular lens implantation. A surgical epidemic. Arch Ophthalmol 1980;98:1025.
63a. Gedde SJ, Scott IU, Tabandeh H, et al.: Late endophthalmitis associated with glaucoma drainage implants. Ophthalmology 2001;108:1323-7.
64. Heilskov T, Joondeph BC, Olsen KR, et al.: Late endophthalmitis after transscleral fixation of a posterior chamber intraocular lens. Arch Ophthalmol 1989;107:1427.
65. Kangas TA, Greenfield D, Flynn HW Jr, et al.: Delayed-onset endophthalmitis associated with conjunctival filtering blebs. Ophthalmology 1997;104:742-52.
66. Boldt HC, Pulido JS, Blodi CF, et al.: Rural endophthalmitis. Ophthalmology 1989;96:1722.
67. Vahey JB, Flynn HW Jr: Results in the management of *Bacillus* endophthalmitis. Ophthalmic Surg 1991;22:681.
68. Kervick GN, Flynn HW Jr, Alfonso E, et al.: Antibiotic therapy for *Bacillus* species infections. Am J Ophthalmol 1990;110:683.
69. Hemady R, Zaltas M, Paton B, et al.: *Bacillus*-induced endophthalmitis: new series of 10 cases and review of the literature. Br J Ophthalmol 1990;74:26.
70. Foster RE, Martinez JA, Murray TG, et al.: Useful visual outcomes after treatment of *Bacillus cereus* endophthalmitis. Ophthalmology 1996;103:390–7.
71. Mieler WF, Ellis MK, Williams DF, et al.: Retained intraocular foreign bodies and endophthalmitis. Ophthalmology 1990;97:1532.
72. Feist RM, Lim JI, Joondeph BC, et al.: Penetrating ocular injury from contaminated eating utensils. Arch Ophthalmol 1991;109:63.
73. Reynolds DS, Flynn HW Jr: Endophthalmitis after penetrating ocular trauma. Current Opin in Ophthalmol 1997;8:32–8.
74. Flynn HW Jr, Essman TF, Brod RD: Endogenous fungal endophthalmitis. In Saer JB (ed.), Vitreous Retinal and Uveitis Update. The Hague, Netherlands: Kugler Publishers; 1998:297–305.
75. Shrader SK, Band JD, Lauter CB, et al.: The clinical spectrum of endophthalmitis: incidence, predisposing factors, and features influencing outcome. J Infect Dis 1990;162:115.
76. Sherwood DR, Rich WJ, Jacob JS, et al.: Bacterial contamination of intraocular and extraocular fluids during extracapsular cataract extraction. Eye 1989;3:308.
77. Speaker MG, Milch FA, Shah MK, et al.: Role of external bacterial flora in the pathogenesis of acute postoperative endophthalmitis. Ophthalmology 1991;98:639.
78. Menikoff JA, Speaker MG, Marmor M, et al.: A case-control study of risk factors for postoperative endophthalmitis. Ophthalmology 1991;98:1761.
79. Isenberg SL, Apt L, Yoshmori R, et al.: Chemical preparation of the eye in ophthalmic surgery: IV comparison of povidone-iodine on the conjunctiva with a prophylactic antibiotic. Arch Ophthalmol 1985;103:1340.
80. Whitney CR, Anderson RP, Allansmith MR: Preoperatively administered antibiotics: their effect on bacterial counts of the eyelids. Arch Ophthalmol 1972;87:155.
81. Apt L, Isenberg S, Yoshimori R, et al.: Chemical preparation of the eye in ophthalmic surgery: III. effect of povidone-iodine on the conjunctiva. Arch Ophthalmol 1984;102:728.
82. Speaker MG, Menikoff JA: Prophylaxis of endophthalmitis with topical povidone-iodine. Ophthalmology 1991;98:1769.
83. Alfonso EC, Flynn HW Jr: Controversies in endophthalmitis prevention. The risk for emerging resistance to vancomycin. Arch Ophthalmol 1995;113:1369–70.
84. Centers for Disease Control and Prevention: Preventing the spread of vancomycin-resistance. Report from the Hospital Infection Control Practices Advisory Committee. 59 Federal Register 1994;25:757.
85. Ciulla TA, Starr MB, Masket S: Bacterial endophthalmitis prophylaxis for cataract surgery. An evidence-based update. Ophthalmology 2002;109:13-26.

CHAPTER 61

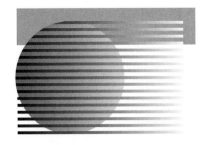

Epiretinal Membrane and Macular Pucker

JENNIFER U. SUNG, M.D. and ALLEN C. HO, M.D.

Macular pucker is a distortion of normal macular anatomy by a proliferation and contraction of a surface membrane. It most commonly affects the elderly and typically causes distortion or a reduction of vision. The etiology of macular pucker may be related simply to a posterior vitreous separation or it may be a secondary consequence of intraocular inflammation, retinal vascular occlusion, or a retinal tear or retinal detachment, among other conditions. Over the past decade and with concomitant advances in vitreous microsurgical instruments and techniques, macular pucker has become amenable to surgical treatment with the potential for improvement in vision.

Iwanoff in 1865 reported the histopathologic description of proliferative membranes overlying the surface of the retina.[1] In 1931, Anderson reported the clinical significance of these proliferative membranes.[2] Removal of epiretinal membranes by surgical delamination was first described by Machemer in 1978.[3] In selected patients, vitrectomy techniques may be employed to improve vision.

Various terminologies have included *macular pucker,*[4] *surface wrinkling retinopathy,*[5] *epiretinal membrane, cellophane maculopathy,*[4] and *preretinal macular gliosis.*[6] The incidence of idiopathic epiretinal membranes has been reported to be 6% in patients over 60 years of age, with 20% occurring bilaterally.[7] In an autopsy series, epiretinal membranes were noted in 2% to 6% of eyes with an increase in frequency corresponding with advanced age.[8]

ETIOLOGY AND CLASSIFICATION

Epiretinal membranes may be idiopathic or may be associated with various ocular conditions including post–retinal detachment repairs, ocular inflammatory disorders, macular holes, trauma with associated vitreous hemorrhage, diabetic retinopathy, retinal vascular occlusive diseases, intraocular tumors, telangiectasis, retinal arteriolar macroaneurysms, and retinitis pigmentosa (Table 61–1).[9] They may also occur after laser photocoagulation or cryotherapy.[10] Congenital epiretinal membranes are rare.[11]

Most idiopathic epiretinal membranes are slowly progressive and cause minor visual disturbances, but some may produce more pronounced visual loss secondary to progressive metamorphopsia and distortion or obscuration of the macula.[10] A classification of epiretinal membranes according to the degree of distortion noted on the underlying retina was described by Gass.[12] According to Gass' classification, cellophane maculopathy, defined as a membrane without associated retinal distortion, is a grade 0. Crinkled cellophane maculopathy, described as membranes that produce minimal distortion of the retina with radiating folds and mild tortuosity of retinal vessels, is classified as a grade 1. Macular pucker is classified as grade 2 and includes membranes that may appear as grayish sheets that are more dense with marked distortion of the underlying retina. These patients may exhibit significant central visual loss and increased metamorphopsia.

HISTOPATHOLOGY

Kampik and associates, using transmission electron microscopy, defined five basic cell types present in epiretinal membranes: retinal pigment epithelial (RPE) cells, macrophages, fibrocytes, fibrous astrocytes, and fibroblast-like cells.[13] The RPE cells were only noted in association with a retinal detachment. In another study of idiopathic macular pucker using electron microscopy techniques, RPE cells appeared to be the main cell

TABLE 61-1. Etiologies of Epiretinal Membranes

Post-retinal detachment repair
Ocular inflammatory disorders
Macular holes
Trauma with associated vitreous hemorrhage
Diabetic retinopathy
Retinal vascular occlusive diseases
Intraocular tumors
Telangiectasis
Retinal arteriolar macroaneurysms
Retinitis pigmentosa
Peripheral retinal neovascularization
Talc maculopathy
Idiopathic

type in 50% of the cases.[14] It is presumed that glial cells, which have direct access to the internal surface of the retina through breaks in the internal limiting membranes, may proliferate or undergo transformation into other cell types, forming epiretinal mebranes.[8,14,15] Another theory suggests that there is transretinal migration of RPE cells in response to chemoattractants.[14] A posterior vitreous detachment, commonly associated with idiopathic epiretinal membranes, may precipitate the formation of these membranes by causing these defects in the internal limiting membrane.[5,16,17]

Epiretinal membranes may contain myofibrocytes, which may exhibit their contractile properties in the clinical feature of prominent retinal striae, especially in younger patients.[14,18] Increased numbers of fibrous cells and collagen may correlate with thicker and whiter membranes, which are more often found in young patients (Fig. 61-1).[18]

CLINICAL FEATURES

Patients with epiretinal membranes range from having no symptoms to complaining of vision loss with metamorphopsia. Epiretinal membranes that do not involve the fovea or disrupt the photoreceptor architecture underlying the fovea are usually asymptomatic. Those proliferative membranes that cause visual symptoms often have a tractional component that may contribute to retinal edema, distortion of retinal vessels and photoreceptors, foveal heterotopia, and tractional retinal detachment (Fig. 61-2).[19] The onset and duration of symptoms are vague in most patients. Visual acuity commonly ranges from 20/30 to 20/70; however, some patients may have vision worse than 20/200.[5,10]

DIAGNOSIS AND ANCILLARY TESTING

Biomicroscopic features of epiretinal membranes vary depending on the thickness, location, and degree of contraction.[19] Macular pucker and epiretinal membranes are best studied with contact lens examination and slit–lamp biomicroscopy. A glistening light reflex may be the only apparent clinical feature in asymptomatic patients. Patients who complain of visual disturbances often exhibit wrinkling of the internal limiting membrane, retinal

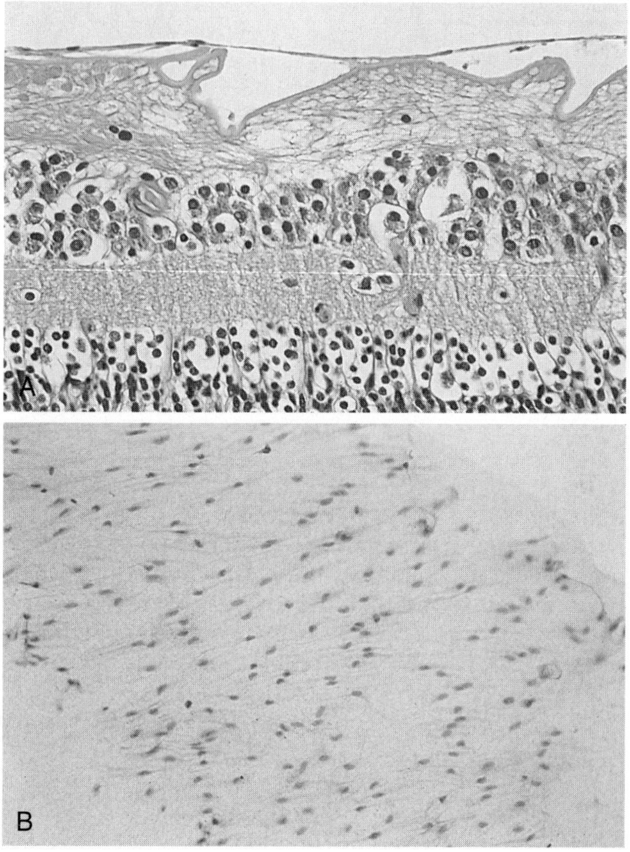

Figure 61–1. *A.* Cross-section of the retina demonstrating an epiretinal membrane with underlying retinal folds. *B.* Epiretinal membrane from a vitrectomy specimen. Note the cellularity of the spindle cells. (H & E stain, 100×; photo courtesy of Ralph Eagle, M.D.)

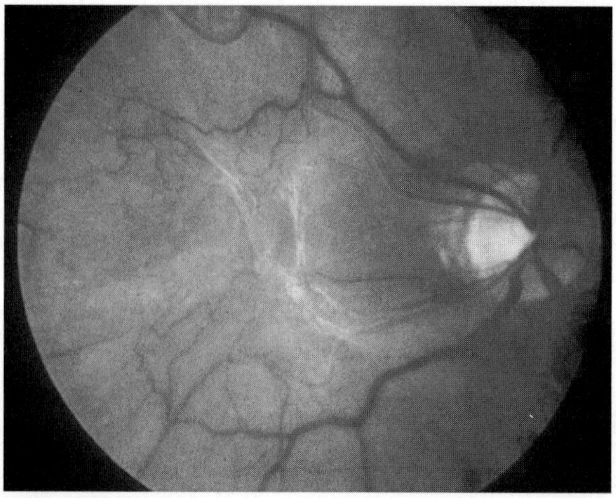

Figure 61–2. Macular pucker demonstrating premacular fibrosis and distortion of the macular retinal vessels.

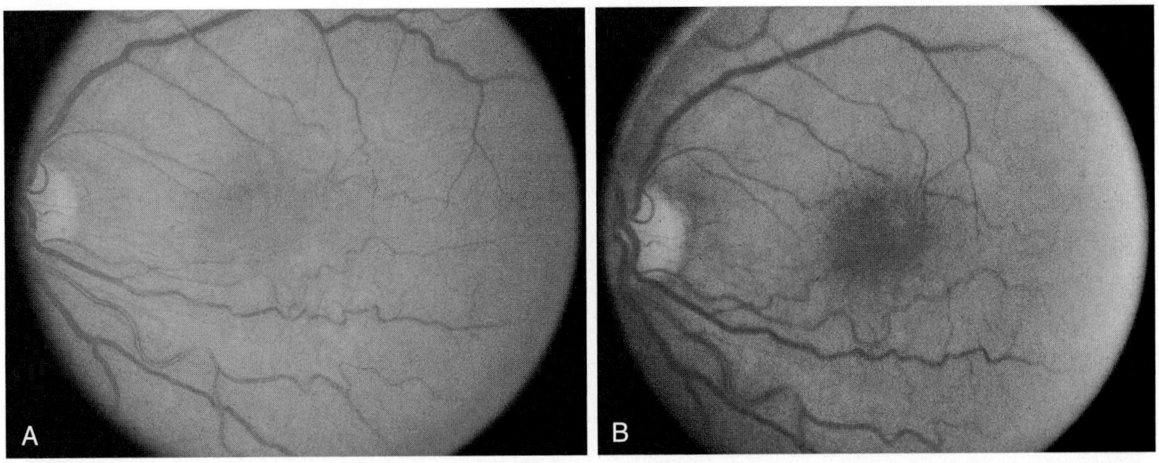

Figure 61–3. *A.* Macular pucker with preoperative visual acuity of 20/70. There is a fine cellophane premacular membrane most prominent inferior and temporal to the fovea. Note the retinal vascular compression and distortion. *B.* Postoperative fundus photograph showing no residual cellophane membrane. A Tano diamond-dusted membrane peeler was used to lift the edge of the macular pucker and the remainder was removed with end-gripping forceps. Postoperative visual acuity was 20/30 with significantly less distortion.

striae, straightening or tortuosity of retinal vessels, punctate intraretinal hemorrhages, retinal edema, macular heterotopia, tractional detachment, and retinal whitening similar to cotton-wool spots (Fig. 61-3).[19] Cystic changes may be evident in the fovea, and both macular holes and pseudoholes may be present (Fig. 61-4). A posterior vitreous detachment is seen in 75% to 100% of patients with idiopathic epiretinal membranes.[8,14,16,20]

Epiretinal membranes vary in their adherence to the retina and may be more pronounced at focal epicenters or along the vascular arcades. In younger patients and in postoperative retinal detachment surgery, the epiretinal membranes may be thick and exhibit pigmentation. Other membranes may be thin, diaphanous, and friable, whereas some may show considerable structural strength.[21] Furthermore, the extent of the membrane may vary from one to two disk diameters in size to 5 mm or more from the center of the macula.[21] These features can sometimes make it difficult to predict the facility of membrane removal with vitrectomy techniques.

Slit–lamp biomicroscopy is an essential diagnostic tool in determining the presence and characteristics of an epiretinal membrane. It is important to check carefully for signs of intraocular inflammation, prior retinal vascular occlusion, or a peripheral retinal tear that may cause a secondary macular pucker (Fig. 61-5). The use of monochromatic red-free illumination may also aid in recognizing the presence of these membranes by enhancing visibility and revealing vascular abnormalities.

Intravenous fluorescein angiography is sometimes helpful in diagnosing epiretinal membranes and excluding other ocular conditions such as the presence of a choroidal neovascular membrane. It may guide in the diagnosis by differentiating a pseudohole associated with an epiretinal membrane from a true macular hole that may exhibit foveal hyperfluorescence. Vascular architecture alterations may become more prominent on the fluorescein angiogram or red-free photographs. Accumulation of dye in late phases may be consistent with the effect of a tractional component of the membrane. Fluorescein angiography may also provide clues to a prior retinal vascular occlusive event that may have precipitated the macular pucker.

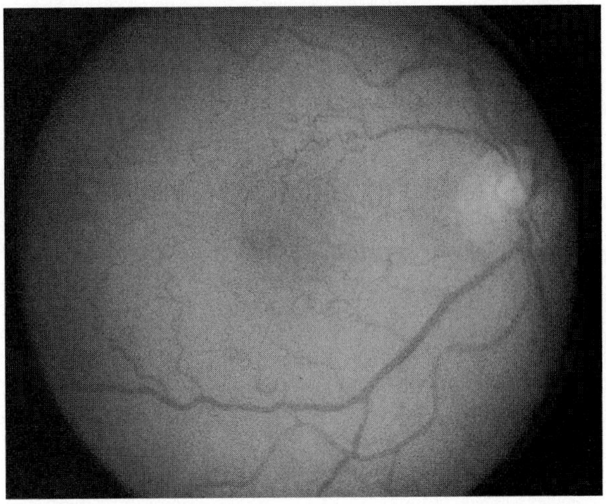

Figure 61–4. Macular pucker with pseudohole. Note the vascular tortuosity. Visual acuity is 20/30.

Optical coherence tomography also aids in differentiating between pseudoholes and full-thickness macular holes.[22] It can determine macular thickness, which may correlate with final visual potential after vitrectomy surgery for removal of the epiretinal membrane.

CLINICAL COURSE AND MANAGEMENT

Most patients with epiretinal membrane do not complain of significant visual symptoms other than mild blurring or distortion. Often these symptoms are only

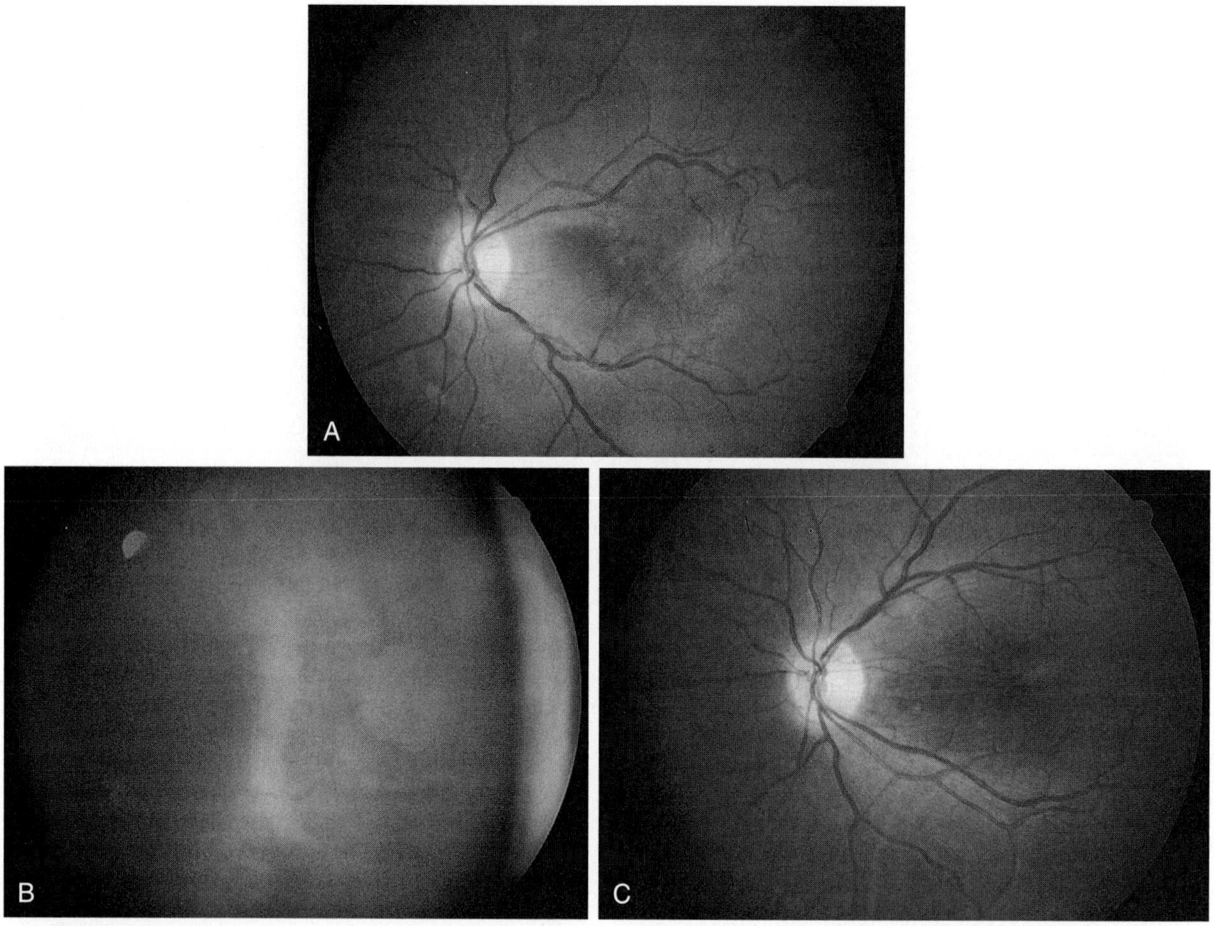

Figure 61–5. *A.* Macular pucker developing after cryoretinopexy for a traumatic retinal tear. Note the macular folds and retinal vascular distortion. The preoperative visual acuity was 20/300. *B.* Peripheral retinal cryoretinopexy with a pigmentary reaction surrounding the peripheral retinal tear. Patients with macular pucker should be carefully examined for peripheral retinal tears. *C.* Postoperative fundus photograph after pars plana vitrectomy with removal of the macular pucker using a bent 22-gauge needle to engage the edge of the membrane. The premacular membrane has been removed and there are still some residual macular folds. Visual acuity has improved to 20/30.

apparent after monocular testing has been performed. Of these patients, fewer that 10% experience progressive visual loss, and 5% progress to visual acuity of 20/200 or worse.[23] The incidence of bilateral idiopathic epiretinal membranes has been reported to be 20%.[7]

Other concomitant conditions may contribute to visual loss such as cystoid macular edema, inflammation, and media opacities. Patients should be evaluated and treated for these conditions prior to consideration for surgical removal of the epiretinal membrane. In patients in whom the epiretinal membrane is the underlying cause of visual loss, a comprehensive preoperative examination should be performed including careful biomicroscopy of the macular region to assess the characteristics of the epiretinal membrane and possible surgical approaches. In addition, careful inspection of the retinal periphery is mandatory to rule out an etiologic retinal tear.

The surgical removal of epiretinal membranes consists of a pars plana vitrectomy with delamination of the membrane with various intraocular picks and forceps

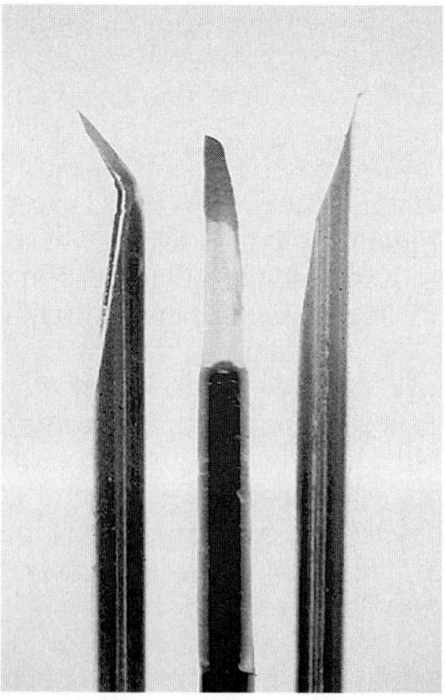

Figure 61–6. Intraocular instruments used in removing epiretinal membranes: bent 22-gauge needle, Tano diamond-dusted membrane peeler, and a barbed 22-gauge needle.

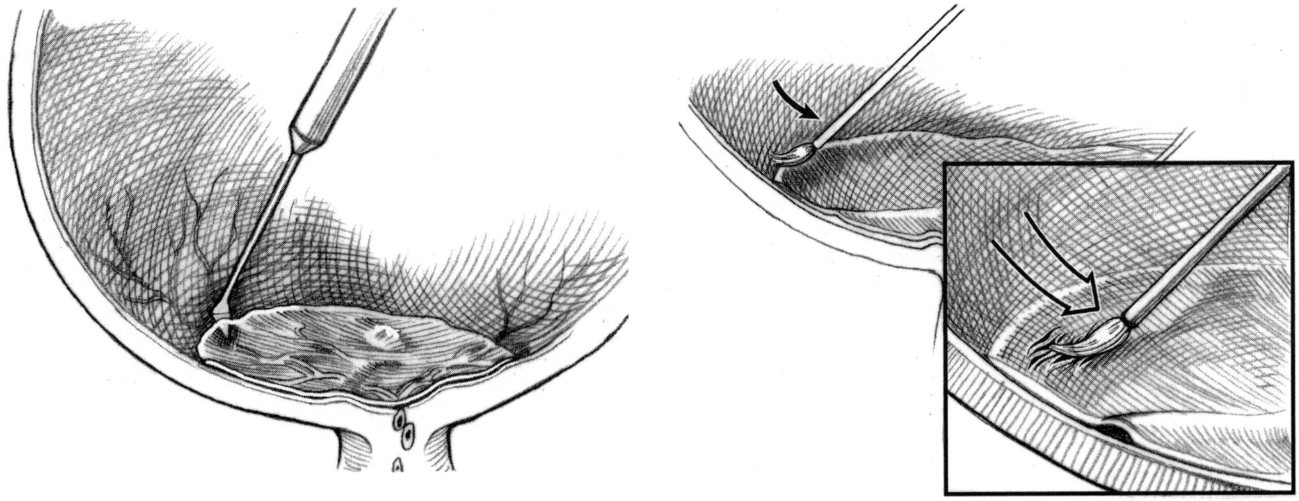

Figure 61–7. Artist's drawing of the surgical technique in delaminating epiretinal membranes.

(Fig. 61-6). It may be useful to create a small bend in the end of micro-vitreoretinal (MVR) blade or a 22–gauge needle on a tuberculin syringe to use as an intraocular tool to engage or to create an edge of the macular pucker. A free edge of the membrane may be evident, which can be engaged to begin the delamination process. In other cases in which a free edge is not identified, the membrane must be incised before delamination; the bent MVR blade or 22–gauge needle may be effective for this. A diamond-dusted flexible brush, such as the Tano membrane peeler, is often useful in removing these membranes. It is used in a sweeping motion that bends the end of the flexible diamond–coated tool over the surface of the macular pucker (Fig. 61–7).

During the delamination process, petechiae may occur. These are visually insignificant and no treatment is necessary. Whitish areas of the retina, which may be apparent preoperatively, may occur after delamination of the epiretinal membrane, and these may represent areas of axoplasmic flow obstruction. It is important to distinguish these areas of axoplasmic obstruction and their translucent appearance intraoperatively so as to avoid further attempts at delamination in these areas. Further manipulation may result in hemorrhage and posterior retinal breaks.[23] With removal of the macular pucker, the areas of axoplasmic obstruction typically fade to a more normal-appearing neurosensory macula.

Post-surgical improvement in visual acuity of at least two lines on the Snellen chart have been reported in 65% to 87% of patients.[10,24,25] Some patients may achieve postoperative visual acuity of 20/20.[24] It is common, however for patients to notice residual symptoms even after dramatic visual improvement from surgical delamination of the epiretinal membranes. Prognostic factors in determining postoperative visual improvements have been inconclusive.[10,21] In one study, preoperative prognostic factors in patients who underwent vitrectomy for idiopathic epiretinal membranes in which final visual acuity was 20/60 or better included (1) initial vision of 20/100 or better, (2) shorter preoperative duration of blurred vision, (3) thin epiretinal membrane, and (4) absence of tractional retinal detachment (Table 61–2).[26] The degree of cystoid macular edema does not appear to bear a relationship to final visual outcome.[10]

Complications of vitrectomy for epiretinal membranes include risks of anesthesia, failure to remove the epiretinal membrane, hemorrhage, posterior or peripheral retinal breaks, retinal detachment, photic maculopathy, progressive nuclear cataract, and endophthalmitis.[10,21,24–26] Peripheral retinal breaks occur in approximately 5% of patients undergoing vitrectomy for epiretinal membrane removal.[24] These breaks can be treated with cryotherapy or laser and intraocular gas injection with or without a local scleral buckle.[24,27] Posterior retinal breaks are much less common and may be treated with intravitreal laser photocoagulation and intraocular gas tamponade.[27] Progressive nuclear sclerosis has been reported in 12.5% to 63% of patients.[10,21,24,26] Patients should be advised of the possible occurrence of cataract within 1 to 5 years of vitrectomy.[19]

Recurrence of epiretinal membranes is uncommon and is reported to occur in 2.5% to 7.3% of patients after successful delamination surgery.[10,21,27] During delamination of the epiretinal membrane, breaks in the internal limiting membrane may occur and be a potential site for epiretinal tissue proliferation.[28] Another possibility is that small remnants of residual epiretinal membrane provide the cellular source for subsequent proliferation.[28] In patients with recurrent epiretinal membranes, visual improvement may be achieved with repeated surgical delamination.[19]

TABLE 61–2. Preoperative Prognostic Factors

Initial vision of 20/100 or better
Shorter preoperative duration of blurred vision
Thin epiretinal membrane
Absence of tractional retinal detachment

REFERENCES

1. Iwanoff A: Beitrage zur normalen und pathologischen anatomie des auges. Graefes Arch Clin Exp Ophthalmol 1865;11:135.
2. Anderson JR: Detachment of the Retina. Cambridge: Cambridge University Press, 1931;94.
3. Machemer, R: Die chirugische entfernung von epiretina en makulamembranen (macular puckers). Klin Monatsbl Augenheilkd 1978;173:36.
4. Gass JDM: Stereoscopic Atlas of Macular Diseases, 4th Edition. St. Louis: CV Mosby, 1997:938.
5. Scudder MJ, Eifrig DE: Spontaneous surface wrinkling retinopathy. Ann Ophthalmol 1975;7:333–341.
6. Nobel KG, Carr RE: Idiopathic preretinal gliosis. Ophthalmology 1982;89:521–523.
7. Pearlstone AD: The incidence of idiopathic preretinal macular gliosis. Ann Ophthalmol 1985;17:378–380.
8. Roth AM, Foos RY: Surface wrinkling retinopathy in eyes enucleated at autopsy. Trans Am Ophthalmol Otolaryngol 1971;75: 1047–1058.
9. Donati G, Kapetanios AD, Pournara CJ: Complications of surgery for epiretinal membranes. Graefes Arch Clin Exp Ophthalmol 1998:236:739–746.
10. Margherio RR, Cox MS, Trese MT, et al.: Removal of epimacular membranes. Ophthalmology 1985;92:1075–1083.
11. Barr CC, Michels RG: Idiopathic neovascularized epiretinal membranes: report of six cases. Ann Ophthalmol 1982;14:335–341.
12. Gass JDM: Stereoscopic Atlas of Macular Diseases, 4th Edition St. Louis: CV Mosby, 1997:940.
13. Kampik A, Kenyon KR, Michels RG, et al.: Epiretinal and vitreous membranes: a comparative study of 56 cases. Arch Ophthalmol 1981;99:1445–1454.
14. Smiddy WE, Michels RG, Green WR: Morphology, pathology, and surgery of idiopathic vitreoretinal macular disorders. Retina 1990;10:288–296.
15. Bellhorn MB, Friedman AH, Wise GN, et al.: Ultrastructure and clinicopathologic correlation of idiopathic preretinal macular fibrosis. Am J Ophthalmol 1975;79:366–373.
16. Hirokawa H, Jalkh AE, Takahas HIM, et al.: Role of the vitreous in idiopathic preretinal macular fibrosis. Am J Ophthalmol 1986;101:166–169.
17. Fine SL: Idiopathic preretinal macular fibrosis. Int Ophthalmol Clin 1977;17:183–189.
18. Smiddy WE, Michels RG, Gilbert HD, Green, WR: Clinicopathologic study of idiopathic macular pucker in children and young adults. Retina 1992;12:232–236.
19. Grand MG: Epiretinal membranes and macular pucker. In Regillo CD, Brown GC, Flynn HW (eds.), Vitreoretinal disease: the essentials. New York: Thieme Medical Publishers, 1999:283–292.
20. Wiznia RA: Posterior vitreous detachment and idiopathic preretinal macular gliosis. Am J Ophthalmol 1986;102:196–198.
21. Michels RG: Vitreous surgery for macular pucker. Am J Ophthalmol 1982;92:628–639.
22. Puliafito CA, Hee MR, Schuman JS: Optical Coherence Tomography of Ocular Diseases. Thorofare, NJ: Slack, Inc., 1996:85–100.
23. McDonald HR, Shatz H, Johnson RN: Introduction to epiretinal membranes. In Ryan SJ (ed.), Retina, 2nd Edition. St. Louis: CV Mosby, 1994:1819–1823.
24. Michels RG: Vitrectomy for macular pucker. Ophthalmology. 1984;92:1384–1388.
25. Crafoord S, Jemt M, Carlsson J, et al.: Long-term results of macular pucker surgery. Acta Ophthalmol Scand 1997;75:85–88.
26. De Bustros S, Thompson JT, Michels RG, et al.: Vitrectomy for idiopathic epiretinal membranes causing macular pucker. Br J Ophthalmol 1988;72:692–695.
27. De Bustros S, Rice TA, Michels RG, et al.: Vitrectomy for macular pucker: use after treatment of retinal tears or retinal detachment. Arch Ophthalmol 1988;106:758–760.
28. Wilkinson CP: Recurrent macular pucker. Am J Ophthalmol 1979; 88:1029–1031.

CHAPTER 62

Macular Hole

ALLEN C. HO, M.D.

A macular hole is a full-thickness defect or tear of retinal tissue involving the anatomic fovea of the eye. Recently, there has been renewed interest in this previously untreatable condition with concomitant refinement of vitreoretinal surgical techniques. Threapeutic approaches to macular hole surgery have ushered in new considerations of pharmacosurgical interventions in vitreoretinal surgery. Although significant progress has been made toward an understanding of macular hole lesions, significant controversy exists regarding the terminology, pathophysiology, diagnosis, natural history, and management of macular holes and precursor lesions.

The first macular hole descriptions were made in the second half of the nineteenth century, and it was not until early in the twentieth century that macular holes were recognized as a clinical entity by most ophthalmologists. Early case descriptions of macular holes focused on young traumatized eyes, but it is now known that "idiopathic," age-related macular holes of the elderly constitute the majority of these lesions. In the beginning of the twentieth century traumatic macular holes were believed to account for one half of all cases of macular holes. In a 1982 series, however, 83% were idiopathic and only 15% were attributable to accidental or surgical trauma.[1]

PATHOGENESIS

There are three basic historical theories concerning the pathogenesis of macular holes: the traumatic theory, the cystic degeneration and vascular theory, and the vitreous theory.[2] In 1869 Knapp provided the first case description of a macular hole in a patient with ocular trauma and an initial diagnosis of a macular hemorrhage. He and most other early observers attributed macular holes to ocular trauma. Two years later Noyes provided the first accurate and detailed ophthalmoscopic description of macular hole which was secondary to blunt trauma in a 13-year-old girl.[3] Noyes noted the difference in depth of focus from the retinal surface to the base of the lesion and probably was the first to recognize that the hallmark of the lesion was a full-thickness defect in retinal tissue within the center of the macula. Blunt ocular trauma could effect immediate macular hole formation from mechanical energy created by vitreous fluid waves and contrecoups macular necrosis or macular laceration.

The first histopathologic descriptions of full-thickness and lamellar macular holes were provided by Fuchs (1907) and Coats (1901), and both supported a cystic degeneration theory of macular hole formation. Coats noted cystic intraretinal changes adjacent to the macular hole and surmised that these changes could be caused by trauma as well as other, atraumatic mechanisms. Intraretinal cyst coalesence could then create a full-thickness macular hole. The major atraumatic theory of macular hole formation was the vascular theory of pathogenesis. Many believed that aging changes of the retinal vasculature lead to cystoid retinal degeneration and subsequent macular hole formation. This vascular theory, sometimes characterized as *ocular angiospasm,* was the basis for a variety of interesting therapies including anxiolytics, vasodilators such as acetylcholine, nicotinic acid, calcium chloride, sodium and potassium iodide, retrobulbar atropine or priscoline, vitamins, minerals, hormones, sedation, and recommendations of abstinence from tobacco.

VITREOUS THEORIES AND CURRENT CONCEPTS OF MACULAR HOLE FORMATION

The vitreous theory of macular hole formation reflects both contemporary and historical perspectives on the pathogenesis of this condition. As early as 1912, the histopathology of overlying premacular vitreous condensation adjacent to foveal cystoid degeneration was recognized.[4] In 1924, Lister was the first of many to implicate antero-posterior vitreous forces in the pathogenesis of macular holes.[5] Several investigators, however, could not completely reconcile this theory of contracting vitreous bands with clinical observations of relatively clear vitreous, devoid of obvious vitreous traction bands.

Other proponents of a vitreous theory emphasized that the process of vitreous separation from the macula was the critical event in the pathogenesis of a macular hole. The problem with this hypothesis is that the incidence of posterior vitreous detachment and macular hole has been reported to have been as variable as 12% to 100%. Data on the vitreous condition as it relates to macular hole formation are muddled by multiple problems, including (1) the definition of vitreous separation (partial versus complete, vitreofoveal separation versus vitreomacular separation), (2) the lack of uniform criteria used for vitreous separation (clinical: Weiss ring, posterior vitreous lacuna, posterior hyaloid; echographic: B-scan ultrasonography; intraoperative: with endoilluminator and retinal pick or silicone-tipped cannula), and (3) the timing of the observation of the vitreous (single versus prospective observation; for example, was vitreous attachment or separation noted before, after, or during the evolution of a macular hole?). Because posterior vitreous detachment is a common event in the age group of those at greatest risk for idiopathic macular hole formation, it is difficult to ascribe a causal relationship to these two events without a prospective evaluation of eyes correlating the status of the vitreous and the evolution of macular holes.

Morgan and Schatz[5] proposed a mechanism of macular hole formation that they described as involutional macular thinning which incorporates vitreous, vascular, and cystic degeneration theories.[6] In the first step of their proposed mechanism, the authors suggested that choroidal vascular changes could lead to altered submacular choroidal vascular perfusion leading to focal foveal and pigment epithelial changes. In their view, these vascular changes then lead to cystic degeneration of the retina which then produce permanent structural changes in the fovea or in the retinal pigment epithelium, leading to involutional macular thinning. The final step in the pathogenesis of a macular hole in this theory is vitreous traction on now susceptible, thinned foveal tissue.[6,7] These authors did not specify the nature of the vitreous traction (anteroposterior forces versus tangential traction) in their theory.

In 1988, Gass and Johnson[8,10] described a classification scheme for idiopathic macular holes and their precursor lesions incorporating their ideas of the pathogenesis of these lesions. (See Gass, 1988, ref. 70 and Johnson, 1988, ref. 67.) From their clinical studies, these authors concluded that attached vitreous appears to move freely and without significant anteroposterior vitreous to macula traction forces. They also believed that an attached vitreous was critical to macular hole formation and that prior observations of macular holes developing despite posterior vitreous separation were incorrect because an optically empty area of a posterior vitreous lacuna may easily be misdiagnosed as a posterior vitreous detachment. Because each of the presumed stages of development of a macular hole caused loss of the normal foveal anatomic depression but no elevation of tissue above the parafoveal retina, they hypothesized that focal shrinkage of the prefoveolar vitreous cortex and tangential retinal traction are responsible for macular hole formation. Tangential vitreous contraction as a factor in the development of macular holes refocused attention on the vitreous and eyes deemed at risk for macular hole formation (premacular hole lesions). In their view, focal shrinkage of the prefoveal vitreous cortex causes anterior traction on the foveolar and then the foveal area, which creates an anterior traction detachment of the fovea.[8] This anterior traction is different from prior theories incorporating ideas on anteroposterior vitreous traction originating from the vitreous base and transmitted by shrinking transvitreal vitreous fibers.

GASS CLASSIFICATION OF PREMACULAR HOLE AND MACULAR HOLE LESIONS

Recently, Gass has updated his biomicroscopic classification and interpretation of macular hole formation (Fig. 62–1 and Table 62–1).[9] Spontaneous tangential traction of the external part of the prefoveolar cortical vitreous detaches foveolar retina, thereby creating an intraretinal yellow spot approximately 100 to 200 μm in diameter (stage 1A).[8–10] The yellow color may result from intraretinal xanthophyll pigment. The foveal retina then elevates to the level of the surrounding perifoveal retina, elongating the foveal retina around the umbo. This transforms the yellow spot to a small donut-shaped yellow ring (stage 1B).[9]

Stage 1 lesions often demonstrate fine radiating retinal striae best observed with retroillumination. Vision is typically in the 20/25 to 20/70 range. Eventually the centrifugal displacement of the retinal receptors, xanthophyll, and radiating nerve fibers leads to a dehiscence of the deeper retinal receptor layer at the umbo (Fig. 62–1).[9] The overlying internal limiting membrane, horizontally oriented Mueller cell processes, and pre-

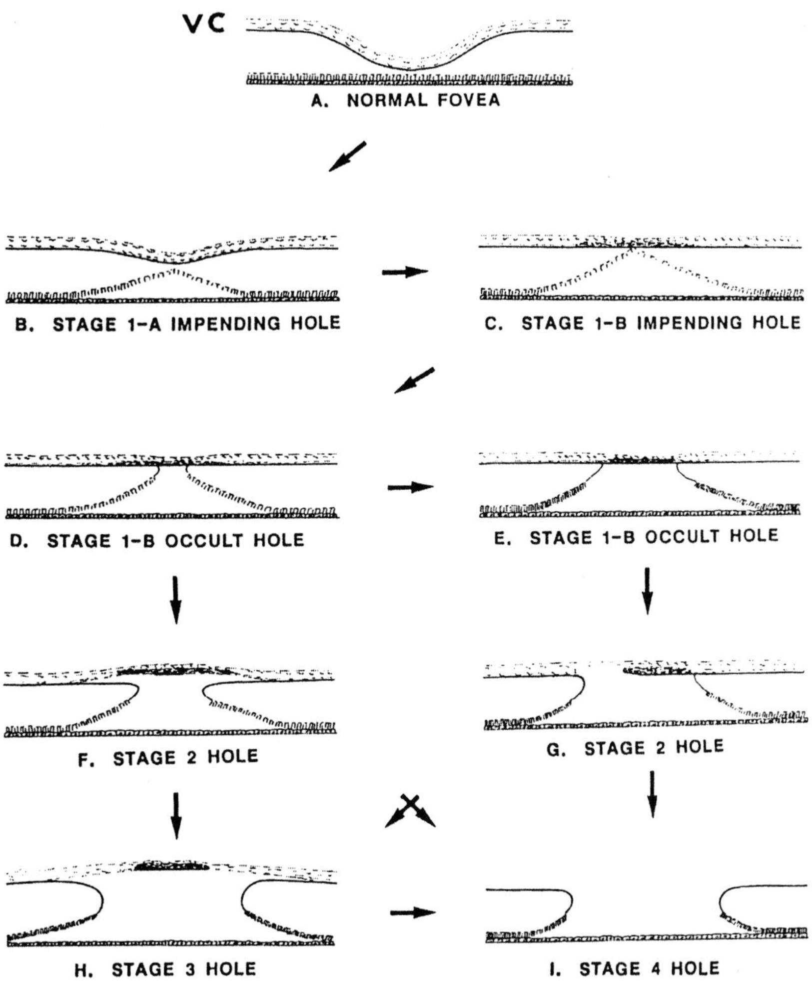

Figure 62–1. 1995 Gass Biomicroscopic Classification of macular hole. *A.* Normal fovea. Layer of vitreous cortex (vc) lying on internal limiting membrane of retina. *B.* Stage 1-A impending hole. Early contraction of outer part of vitreous cortex with foveolar detachment. *C.* Stage 1-B impending hole. Further vitreous contraction and condensation of the prefoveolar vitreous cortex with foveal detachment. *D* and *E.* Stage 1-B occult hole. Dehiscence of the retinal receptor layer at the umbo with centrifugal retraction of the retinal receptors. *F.* Stage 2 hole with early separation of condensed prefoveolar vitreous cortex with formation of pseudo-operculum that is larger than the hole. *G.* Stage 2 hole with tear in vitreous cortex at junction of the prefoveolar vitreous cortex and edge of macular hole. *H.* Stage 3 hole with pseudo-operculum . *I.* Stage 4 hole after posterior vitreous separation. (From Gass JD: Reappraisal of biomicroscopic classification of stages of development of a macular hole. Am J Ophthalmol 1995;119:752-759. Ophthalmic Publishing Company, with permission.)

foveolar vitreous condensation may remain intact (**stage 1B,** occult macular hole; Fig. 62–2) and thereby preclude biomicroscopic detection.[9] An *occult* macular hole is a new concept in Gass's revised classification scheme. The center of the yellow ring may often appear reddish in color, and the yellow ring itself develops a serrated or irregular edge. Spontaneous vitreofoveal separation may then occur, creating a semitranslucent prefoveal opacity (pseudo-operculum) which is often larger than the underlying occult foveolar hole.[9] The yellow ring appears at the edge of the centrifugally displaced retinal receptors and there disappears, presumably because of relief of prefoveolar vitreous traction on the edge of the expanding occult macular hole.[9] The *first biomicroscopically identifiable full-thickness retinal defect is a* **stage 2** *hole (redefined as less than 400 μm in diameter)* and may be obscured by the overlying pseudo-operculum (Fig. 62–3).[9] Most macular hole "opercula" probably do not harbor retinal receptors; they are comprised of vitreous condensation and reactive glial proliferation.[9,11] These generally enlarge to **stage 3** holes (400 μm and greater). Stage 3 holes (partial vitreomacular separation) may then evolve to **stage 4** macular holes (complete separation of the vitreous from the entire macular surface and optic disc).[9] Vision usually varies between 20/70 and 20/400 in stage 3 or stage 4 lesions (Figs. 62–4 and 62–5). An overlying operculum may be observed, and with time, fine radiating retinal striae (26%), drusen, or yellow-white deposits (42%), and atrophy of the retinal pigment epithelium may appear in the base of the hole.[12] Epiretinal membranes, cystic degeneration of the retina, and underlying cuffs of subretinal fluid that effect shallow macular detachments are also observed.

TABLE 62–1. 1995 Gass Biomicroscopic Classification of Macular Hole

		Anatomic Interpretation	
Stage	**Biomicroscopic Findings**	**Old**	**New**
1-A (impending hole)	Central yellow spot, loss of foveolar depression, no vitreofoveolar separation	Early serous detachment of foveolar retina	Same
1-B (impending or occult hole)	Yellow ring with bridging interface, loss of foveolar depression, no vitreofoveolar separation	Serous foveolar detachment with lateral displacement of xanthophyll	Same for small ring. For larger ring, central occult foveolar hole with centrifugal displacement of foveolar retina and xanthophyll, with bridging contracted prefoveolar vitreous cortex. Cannot detect transition from impending to occult hole.
2	Eccentric oval, crescent, or horseshoe retinal defect inside edge of yellow ring	Hole (tear) in peripheral foveolar retina	Hole (tear) in contracted prefoveolar vitreous bridging round retinal hole, no loss of foveolar retina
	Central round retinal defect with rim of elevated retina		
	With prefoveolar opacity	Hole with operculum,* rim of retinal detachment	Hole with pseudo-operculum,† rim of retinal detachment
	Without prefoveolar opacity	Hole, no posterior vitreous detachment from optic disk and macula	Same
3	Central round ≥ 400 μm diameter retinal defect, no Weiss's ring, rim of elevated retina		
	With prefoveolar opacity	Hole with operculum, no posterior vitreous detachment from optic disk and macula	Hole with pseudo-operculum, no posterior vitreous detachment
	Without prefoveolar opacity	Hole, no posterior vitreous detachment from optic disk and macula	Same
4	Central round retinal defect, rim of elevated retina, Weiss's ring		
	With prefoveolar opacity‡	Hole with operculum and posterior vitreous detachment from optic disk and macula	Hole, with pseudo-operculum and posterior vitreous detachment from optic disk and macula
	Without prefoveolar opacity	Hole and posterior vitreous detachment from optic disk and macula	Same

*Operculum contains foveolar retina.
†Pseudo-operculum contains no retinal receptors.
‡Usually found near temporal border of Weiss's ring.
From Gass JDM: Reappraisal of biomicroscopic classification of stages of development of a macular hole. Am J Ophthalmol 1995;119:752-9.

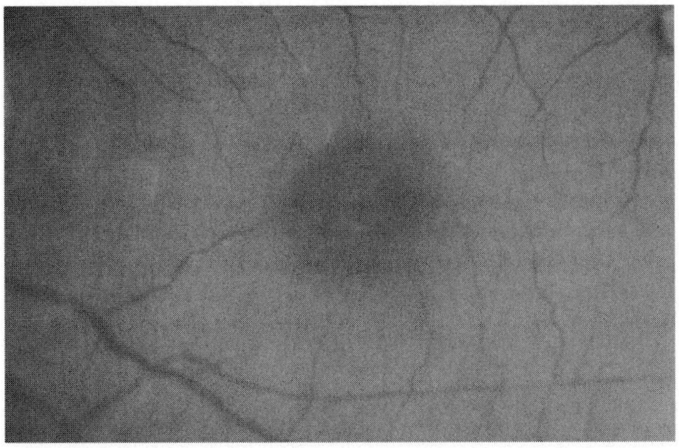

Figure 62–2. Stage 1B presumed occult macular hole. Note the serrated edges of the inner aspect of the yellow ring. Visual acuity is 20/30.

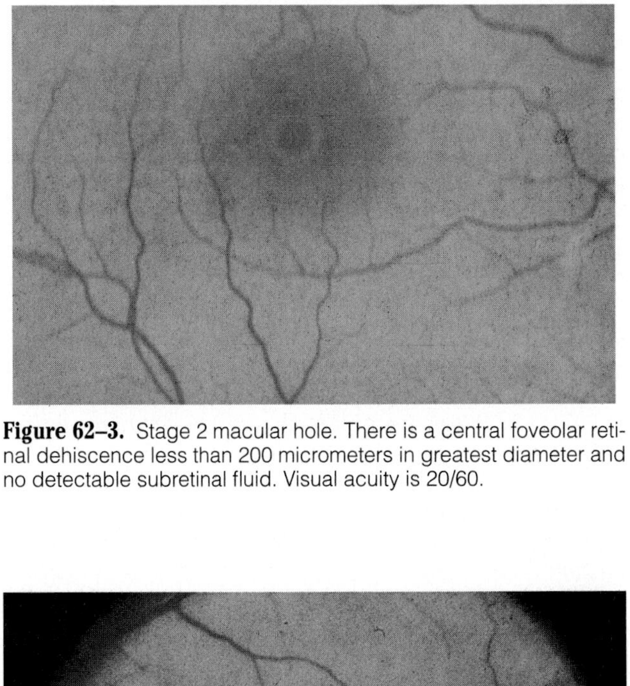

Figure 62–3. Stage 2 macular hole. There is a central foveolar retinal dehiscence less than 200 micrometers in greatest diameter and no detectable subretinal fluid. Visual acuity is 20/60.

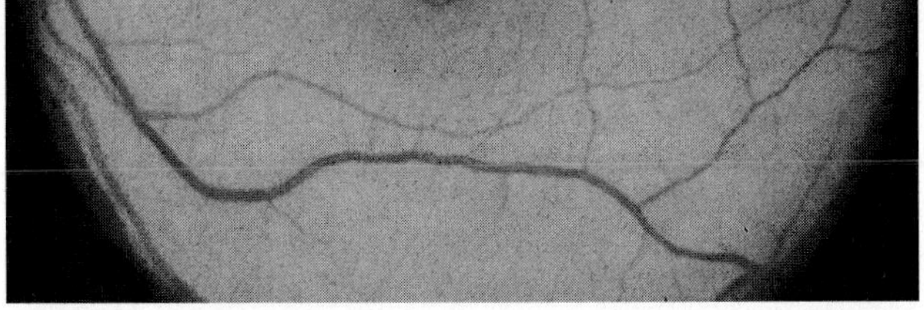

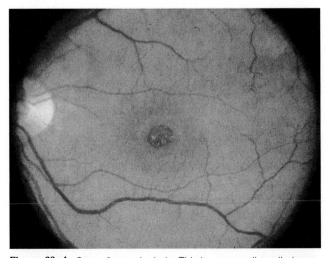

Figure 62–4. Stage 3 macular hole. This is a generally well-circumscribed 300 micron full-thickness retinal defect with an irregular inferotemporal border. Note the yellow clumps of presumed glial cells in the base of the macular hole and the surrounding cuff of subretinal fluid. The posterior hyaloid is attached at the optic nerve and the major temporal retinal arcades. Visual acuity is 20/100.

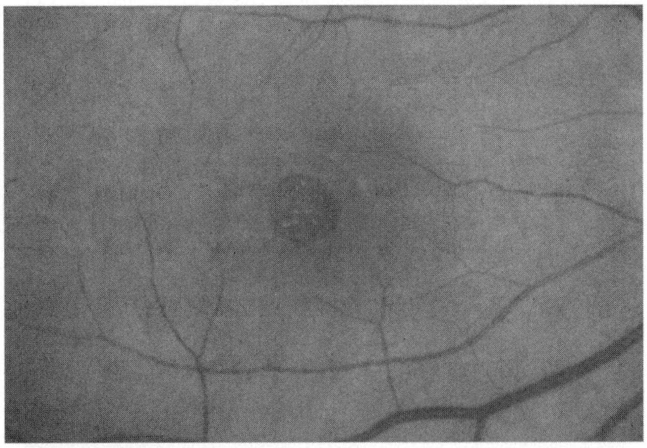

Figure 62–5. Stage 4 macular hole. The full-thickness retinal defect is surrounded by an epiretinal membrane and elevated by a large rim of subretinal fluid. Yellow deposits are noted in the base of the macular hole. Visual acuity is 20/300.

DIFFERENTIAL DIAGNOSIS OF PREMACULAR HOLE AND MACULAR HOLE LESIONS

Macular holes and particularly premacular holes are often misdiagnosed. Careful examination with a contact lens is required to make an accurate diagnosis. In one series, only 1 of 18 subjects referred with the diagnosis of stage 1 macular hole was correct; other cases were actually an aborted stage of macular hole formation (8 cases), stage 2 holes (4 cases), stage 3 holes (1 case), and unrelated lesions (4 cases).[13] Patients with a age-related macular degeneration and a large central druse, central serous retinopathy and a foveal neurosensory detachment, cystoid macular edema, vitreomacular traction syndrome, or a foveal yellow lesion associated with solar retinopathy may all be misdiagnosed for a stage 1 macular hole. In general, macular hole patients are older than most affected by central serous retinopathy and have yellow changes with the retina rather than at the level of the retinal pigment epithelium. Careful contact lens examination of both eyes, together with a medical history to rule out recent solar exposure is helpful. Subretinal fluid is not observed in premacular hole patients, although there is foveal elevation in stage 1 lesions. Patients with cystoid macular edema, vitreomacular traction syndrome, and stage 1B lesions all may have cystic intraretinal features; in patients with stage 1B macular holes, however, the foveola is not elevated above the level of the surrounding retina, as observed in vitreomacular traction.

FULL-THICKNESS MACULAR HOLES

Full-thickness macular holes are also often misdiagnosed. Most commonly, an epiretinal membrane will create a central retinal depression, which simulates a stage 3 macular hole (Fig. 62–6). These pseudoholes do not demonstrate a surrounding cuff of subretinal fluid

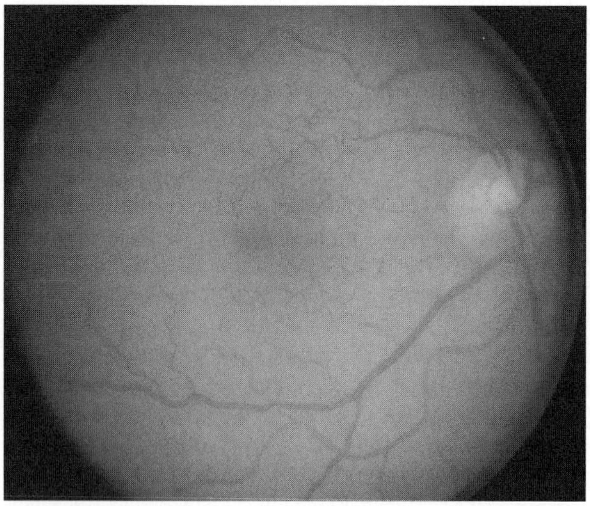

Figure 62–6. Pseudomacular hole. The most common misdiagnosis of a full-thickness macular hole is an epiretinal membrane that creates a circular central depression without any retinal defect. Note the tortuosity of the macular vessels and subtle retinal striae. The Watzke sign was negative and the visual acuity was 20/25.

or drusen-like yellow precipitates on the surface of bare retinal pigment epithelium. Careful contact lens examination should be directed to observe: small eccentric retinal defects, the presence of an associated cuff of subretinal fluid, the status of the vitreoretinal interface, whether the depression is lamellar or full-thickness, and the presence of any drusen-like precipitates on bare retinal pigment epithelium. A positive Watzke sign and the laser-aiming beam test (50 μm laser photocoagulator-aiming beam is directed within and around the macular hole) are more specific than Amsler grid abnormalities for detecting macular holes.[14,15] Visual acuity is typically reduced to 20/60 or worse with macular holes, often at the level of 20/100 to 20/200, while macular pseudoholes fare better.

One condition that may be misdiagnosed as a true macular hole is a lamellar macular hole, which is a partial-thickness defect of macular retina typically described as a red, petal-shaped depression in the inner retinal surface.[13] This is thought to represent a macular lesion created by spontaneous release of vitreous upon an impending macular hole lesion.[8,10] A pseudo-operculum may be observed overlying the lamellar macular hole, which contributes to misdiagnosis of the lesion as a true macular hole.[16] The pseudo-operculum may appear larger than the underlying defect and probably represents condensed cortical vitreous. Newer imaging modalities such as optical coherence tomography (OCT) or laser biomicroscopy may help to distinguish macular holes and precursor lesions from simulating lesions.[17,18]

ASSOCIATED CONDITIONS

Most macular holes are "idiopathic" in origin; however, many other associations have been reported. Full-thickness macular holes have been described in association with a variety of conditions, including proliferative diabetic retinopathy, optic disc coloboma, high myopia, choroidal neovascularization, Best's disease, adult vitelliform macular degeneration, retinal arteriovenous communication, scleral buckling for retinal reattachment, pneumatic retinopexy for retinal reattachment, perforating retrobulbar injections, and topical pilocarpine. Clearly the incidence of macular hole in association with these conditions is small.

Lamellar macular holes (partial-thickness retinal defect) have been described in association with topical pilocarpine, cystoid edema after cataract extraction, and idiopathic parafoveal telangiectasia.

HISTOPATHOLOGY

FULL-THICKNESS MACULAR HOLE

Two large histopathologic series have been reported on macular holes.[19,20] Histopathologic examination of full-thickness macular holes demonstrates round or oval retinal defects surrounded by rounded retinal edges and a cuff of detached neurosensory retina with subretinal fluid. In the most recent series, 79% demonstrated cystoid macular edema and 68% had epiretinal membranes. Photoreceptor atrophy was variable (200 – 750 μm, mean 480 μm from the edge of the retinal margin) in this group of globes, some of which had long-standing macular holes (Fig. 62–7*A* and *B*).[19] In some of the eyes, a thin tapered layer of cortical vitreous is noted that may effect traction on the edges of the macular hole. Two cases of probable resolved macular holes have also been reported.[19] In these specimens, there was no surrounding cuff of subretinal fluid, and the photoreceptors were reapposed to Bruch's membrane. One eye demonstrated hyperplastic retinal pigment epithelium at the margin of the retinal defect, which appeared to seal the macular hole.

LAMELLAR MACULAR HOLE

Histopathology of lamellar macular holes has also been described.[19,21] Lamellar macular holes are characterized by a partial loss of neurosensory retina, which looks like a sharply circumscribed round or petal-shaped red depression in the inner retinal surface. In half of affected eyes, there was evidence of a thin layer of epicortical vitreous membrane causing tangential traction.[19]

PREMACULAR VITREOUS AND OPERCULA

The histopathology of tissue removed during vitreous surgery for impending macular holes has been described.[22,23] In one study, the primary tissue specimen was a thin sheet of acellular premacular vitreous collagen, which is difficult to detect biomicroscopically, and

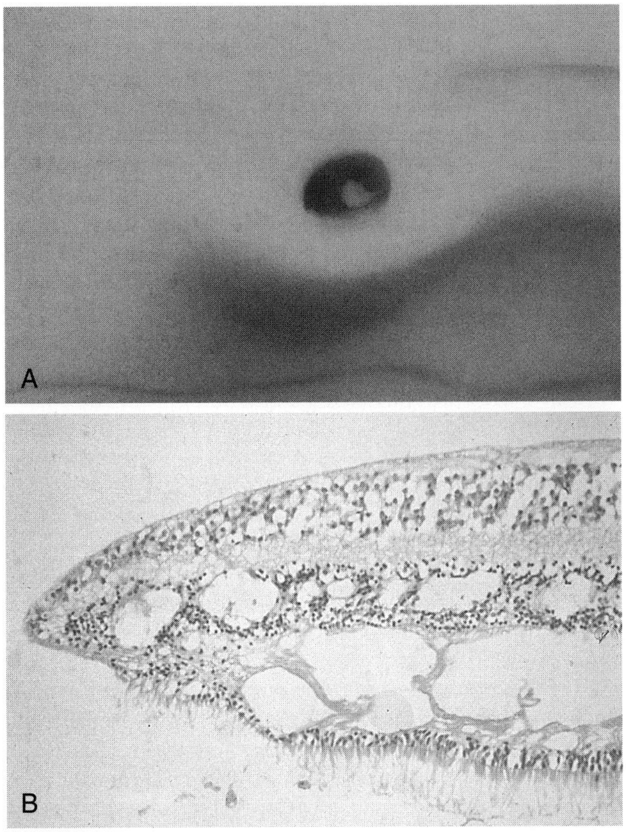

Figure 62–7. *A.* Gross examination of this autopsy eye demonstrates a full-thickness macular hole with an associated operculum. *B.* Histopathologic examination of this macular hole demonstrates rounded edges of retina, intraretinal cystoid macular edema, subretinal fluid, and atrophy of photoreceptors, particularly near the edge of the macular hole. (From Guyer DR, Green WR, de Bustros S, et al.: Histopathologic features of idiopathic macular holes and cysts. Ophthalmology 1990;97:1045–51.)

which may be present even when there is an apparent posterior vitreous detachment.[22] The second report used immunocytochemical labeling of the premacular vitreous sheet and demonstrated cellular, potentially contractile glial and retinal pigment epithelial cells in the surgical specimens,[23] a finding consistent with prior studies on the vitreoretinal interface.[24]

A very interesting report on two surgically retrieved opercula overlying full-thickness macular holes reveals that opercula probably do not represent displaced neurosensory photoreceptors.[11] The opercula were comprised of a proliferation of dislodged, reparative fibrous astrocytes and Mueller cells. This observation is consistent with Gass's revised theory on macular hole pathogenesis, which describes a dehiscence at the umbo, with lateral displacement of photoreceptors; the operculum represents the overlying reparative tissue and not neurosensory retina.

There are two reports on the histopathology of surgically treated macular holes.[25,26] These clinicopathologic studies demonstrated that macular holes can be sealed by fibrous astrocytes and Mueller cells, without significant inflammation, disruption of the underlying retinal pigment epithelium, or cystoid macular edema. There is a closer reapproximation of retinal edges compared with spontaneously resolved macular holes,[19,25] suggesting that surgically treated holes may seal in different ways than spontaneously resolved macular holes. The same fibrous astrocytes and Mueller cells that have been shown to help seal surgically treated macular holes may also contribute to epiretinal membrane formation and recurrent macular holes if the reparative process goes awry.[27]

NATURAL HISTORY

PREMACULAR HOLE LESIONS, STAGE 1A AND 1B

The natural history of stage 1 lesions has been controversial. The best information available on the natural history of stage 1 lesions is derived from the Vitrectomy for Prevention of Macular Hole Study Group, who reported that 14 (40%) of 35 patients randomized to observation progressed to a full-thickness macular hole over a 2-year follow-up period.[28] Generally, a stage 1A lesion progresses to a stage 1B lesion within a few weeks to a few months.[28] Stage 1 lesions progressing to full-thickness lesions do so in an average time of 4.1 months (range 1 to 13 months) after diagnosis.[28] Prior reports estimated the progression rate of stage 1 or other premacular hole lesions to be 10% to 75%.[1,6,10,13,29–35] Several of these studies were limited by their retrospective nature.

In general, resolution of a stage 1 lesion is accompanied by vitreofoveal separation. Sixty percent of stage 1 lesions abort macular hole formation. The resolved fovea may appear normal or may demonstrate the red-faceted, slightly depressed lesion characteristic of a lamellar macular hole. There may be an overlying pseudo-operculum suspended anterior to the fovea, and this may be confused with a stage 1 lesion.[13,16] Lamellar macular holes do not progress to macular holes.[10,13] Moreover, posterior vitreous detachment is generally believed to confer protection against macular hole evolution,[13,29,33,34,36,37] although in one small series of five patients, all were believed to develop macular hole despite a complete posterior vitreous detachment.[38]

The visual acuity of stage 1 lesions ranges between 20/25 and 20/80. Initial visual acuity is believed to predict progression to full-thickness macular hole.[1,39] Recent data from the Vitrectomy for the Prevention of Macular Hole Study Group revealed that eyes with stage I macular holes and best corrected visual acuity between 20/50 and 20/80 had a 66% (10 of 15 eyes) rate of progression to full-thickness macular hole, whereas eyes with best-corrected visual acuity between 20/25 and 20/40 had a 30% (6 of 20 eyes) risk of progression to a full-thickness macular hole. The risk of progression to macular hole is significantly higher in eyes with stage I macular holes with best-corrected visual acuity of 20/50 or worse.[39]

RISK FACTORS

Although the demographic features of age-related macular hole patients are generally widely accepted, risk factors for development of full-thickness lesions are more controversial. The Eye Disease Case-Control Study Group reported on the demographics and risk factors for "idiopathic" macular hole, comparing 198 subjects with macular hole and 1023 matched controls. Seventy-two percent of subjects with macular hole were female[40]; explanations for this female preponderance are speculative. Only 3% of subjects with idiopathic macular hole were less than 55 years of age. This study did not find an association of macular hole with hysterectomy, hypertension, or cardiovascular disease, in contradistinction to prior reports.[1,7] Interestingly, the most significant risk factor for macular hole formation was increased plasma fibrinogen (greater than 2.95 g/liter), which more than doubled the risk of macular hole formation[40]; again, explanations are speculative. Estrogen users were at a reduced risk for hole formation.[40] The Eye Disease Case-Control Study Group did not examine two ocular characteristics that have previously been associated with macular hole formation: macular retinal pigment epithelial changes (involutional macular thinning) and macular vitreous attachment.

STAGE 2 LESIONS

According to the revised Gass classification, stage 1B occult holes become manifest (stage 2 holes) either after early separation of the contracted prefoveolar vitreous cortex from the retina surrounding a small hole or as an eccentric can-opener–like tear in the contracted prefoveolar vitreous cortex at the edge of larger stage 2 holes.[9]

Most stage 2 holes demonstrate progression to stage 3 and 4 macular holes with subsequent loss of vision. The most optimistic study reported a 33% resolution rate with 67% progressing to larger stage 3 and 4 lesions.[35] Hikichi reported a 96% (n = 48 eyes) progression of stage 2 lesions to stage 3 or 4, while only 4% remained in stage 2, with no eyes demonstrating resolution during a median follow-up period of 4 years (range, 2–8 years).[41] Eighty-five percent of stage 2 eyes enlarged their hole size to greater than 400 μm, 64% experienced vitreomacular separation, and visual acuity decreased two or more Snellen lines during the follow-up period in 71% of 48 eyes. These authors concluded that even though vitreomacular separation may improve the prognosis of a macular hole, stage 2 lesions usually will develop an enlarged hole and decreased visual acuity.[29,41] Most stage 2 holes progress and enlarge to stage 3 or 4 within 6 months.

STAGE 3 AND 4 MACULAR HOLES

Most full-thickness macular holes greater than 400 μm retain peripheral vision but suffer loss of central vision to the level of 20/100 and worse. Some stage 3 or 4 lesions will enlarge their hole size, and a minority will undergo progressive loss of central visual acuity. Hikichi reported that 32 (55%) of 58 eyes with a stage 3 lesion, and 5 (16%) of 31 eyes with a stage 4 lesion underwent macular hole enlargement during the median follow-up period of 3 years. Visual acuity decreased two or more lines of Snellen equivalent during the follow-up period in 17 (29%) eyes with a stage 3 lesion, and 4 (13%) eyes with a stage 4 lesion.[29] Visual deterioration may be related to increasing and chronic subretinal fluid, cystoid retinal changes, or photoreceptor atrophy. Less commonly, loss of central and then peripheral vision is related to a progressive retinal detachment. This is most commonly associated with myopia of 6 diopters or greater.[42]

Uncommonly (5% to 12% of stage 3 or 4), spontaneous flattening and improvement in vision may occur.[1,7,35,43] The mechanism of spontaneous flattening is unclear, although two cases have been reported in association with epiretinal membrane formation and vision improving to the 20/20 to 20/30 level.[44,45] Because macular holes demonstrate absolute scotomata on microperimetry within the hole and probable relative scotomata in the surrounding neurosensory detachment,[46,47] spontaneously flattened macular holes may improve their visual function in ways similar to those who have experienced successful surgical repair.[48]

FELLOW EYES

Patients with a unilateral macular hole are understandably concerned about the prognosis for the fellow eye. Most will not develop a macular hole. The risk of fellow eye involvement has been reported to be from 3% to 22%.[31,34] Chew and co-workers of the Eye Disease Case-Control Study estimate the risk to fellow eyes for development of macular hole to be approximately 7%.[49] Normal fellow eyes have a very low incidence (0 to 2%) of macular hole formation, particularly if there is a preexistent posterior vitreous detachment.[6,34–36,49] Fellow eyes with macular cysts or stage 1 lesions and vitreous attachment are probably at a similar risk for hole formation as previously described (about 40%).

MANAGEMENT

Because most patients with macular hole suffer from unilateral loss of central vision with a preserved fellow eye, indications for intervention have been questioned.[51] Nevertheless, many vitreoretinal surgeons offer surgical intervention to afflicted patients because of refinements in surgical technique, better visual outcomes, and up to a 20% chance that the fellow eye will become affected. The first step in the management of a macular hole lesion is to reconfirm the diagnosis, because pseudomacular holes are commonly misdiagnosed as full-thickness macular holes. The management of premacular hole lesions has been guided by the Vitrectomy for Prevention of Macular Hole Study findings.[28]

Historically, therapy for macular holes has evolved from anxiolytics and vasodilator therapies to current day strategies employing intraocular tamponade and vitrectomy surgery. Until recently, most surgeons focused their attention on retinal detachments that were associated with macular hole. Meyer-Schwickerath in 1961 proposed cerclage, subretinal fluid drainage, and light laser photocoagulation employing scleral buckling techniques to flatten a macular hole. Reports in the ensuing two decades advocated variations on this theme including y-shaped plombs, "armed" silicone implants, diathermy, laser photocoagulation, cryotherapy, silicone oil, and intravitreal gas—all without vitrectomy—to flatten the macula and associated retinal detachment. Not surprisingly, many of the subjects of these reports were greater than 6 diopters myopic.

FULL-THICKNESS MACULAR HOLE

In 1991, Kelly and Wendel reported on vitrectomy, removal of cortical vitreous and epiretinal membranes, and strict face-down gas tamponade to stabilize or improve vision in full-thickness macular holes.[52] Their hypothesis was that, by removing tangential vitreous and membrane forces, they could flatten the macular hole and possibly reduce the adjacent cystic retinal changes and neurosensory macular detachment. The overall results were a 58% anatomic success rate and visual improvement of 2 or more lines in 42% of eyes (73% of anatomically successful eyes). A critical surgical step in their technique is the induction of a complete posterior vitreous detachment with a soft-tipped silicone suction needle, which is swept over the retinal surface near the major retinal vascular arcades and temporal to the macula; engagement of cortical vitreous results in the "fish strike" sign, which is then removed to the posterior equatorial zone (Fig. 62–8). Because surface cortical vitreous can be difficult to identify, one report advocates the use of autologous blood to stain this tissue.[53] In addition, fine and often friable epiretinal membranes are removed with a microbarbed microvitreoretinal (MVR) blade and tissue forceps stripping, which often causes small retinal hemorrhages near the macular hole. The peripheral retina is inspected carefully for iatrogenic retinal tears. A total air–fluid exchange is performed to desiccate the vitreous cavity and accumulated posterior retinal fluid, followed by a nonexpansive concentration of long-acting gas. Strict facedown positioning to position the gas bubble against the macular hole for at least 1 week is as important as the technical components of the procedure. Surgical complications include cataract, retinal detachment, retinal trauma, macular light toxicity, and postoperative intraocular pressure rises.

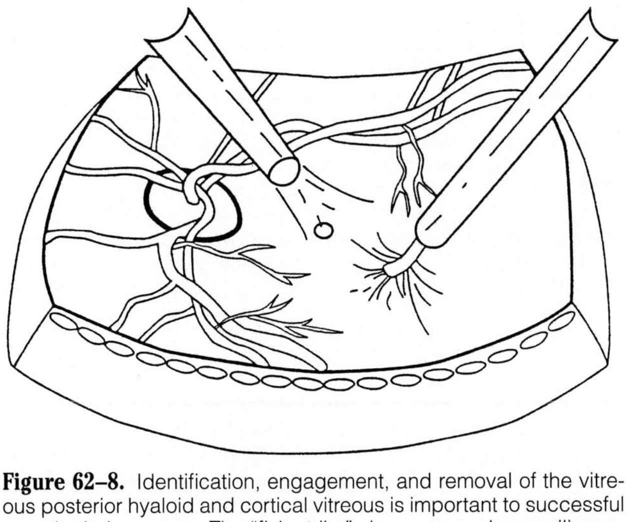

Figure 62–8. Identification, engagement, and removal of the vitreous posterior hyaloid and cortical vitreous is important to successful macular hole surgery. The "fish strike" sign occurs when a silicone-tipped extrusion needle with active suction is swept over the retinal surface and engages cortical vitreous. (From Kelly NE, Wendel RT: Vitreous surgery for idiopathic macular holes. Results of a pilot study [see comments]. Arch Ophthalmol 1991;109:654–9. Copyright © 1991, American Medical Association, with permission.)

More recently, Kelly and Wendel improved their overall results to 73% anatomic success and 55% of patients improving two or more lines of visual acuity.[54] This group and other investigators have noted that macular hole surgery is more successful in patients with macular holes of less than 6 months duration than with those present for 2 years or longer. In a small series, one group noted that surgery on long-standing stage III macular holes (1 year duration) or longer can result in a 58% anatomic success rate with improvement in central visual acuity, although recovery of central vision may be delayed for 6 months or longer.[55] An uncontrolled series of surgery for stage 2 macular holes demonstrated that 61% improved visual acuity, 27% remained stable, and 12% progressed to a stage 3 macular hole with worse vision[56]; 61% of these eyes had a final visual acuity of 20/50 or better. These results compare favorably with prior reports on the natural history progression rates of stage 2 macular holes (67% to 96%).

Glaser and co-workers first reported on the novel use of intravitreal bovine transforming growth factor-beta 2 (TGF-β_2), pars plana vitrectomy, fluid–gas exchange for full-thickness macular hole, with anatomic success rates of about 90%.[57–59] In contradistinction to the surgical technique of Kelly and Wendel, these investigators did not strip surrounding epiretinal membranes in some cases.[59] Longer acting gas tamponade with 16% perfluoropropane gas instead of air improved their surgical success rate but was associated with significant nuclear sclerotic cataract formation (76% requiring cataract extraction with follow-up greater than or equal to 24 months).[12,60] Unfortunately, production recombinant TGF-β_2 (non-bovine-derived) did not yield similarly successful surgical results as bovine TGF-β_2. A variety of other pharmacosurgical adjuvants have been used, including autologous whole blood, plasma, or serum in case series reports. We do not typically use a pharmacosurgical adjuvant for our macular hole surgery.

More recently, peeling of the internal limiting membrane surrounding a macular hole has been controversial, with proponents both for and against this advanced surgical technique. What seems clear is that removal of the internal limiting membrane does not preclude the possibility of improved visual acuity. My technique involves using a fine barb of a bent 22–gauge needle to engage the internal limiting membrane and to lift an edge that can then be grasped with end-gripping forceps and removed in a circular motion around the hole. I use this technique selectively for macular holes with epiretinal membranes or those without membranes, where the edges are everted.

What, then, are the indications for treatment of a full-thickness macular hole? Controversy exists because most of these subjects will not develop a macular hole in their fellow eye, and one investigative group has noted that with careful refraction many eyes with full-thickness macular hole may enjoy better visual acuity than previously believed.[61] The ideal surgical candidate has recent-onset, bilateral, small, full-thickness macular holes and will have no problems maintaining a face-down postoperative position. Perhaps preoperative diagnostic testing, such as laser interferometry, will help select candidates with postoperative visual potential.[62] Potential surgical candidates need to be informed about nuclear cataract progression as well as a host of other posterior segment complications, including but not limited to retinal tears, rhegmatogenous retinal detachment, and retinal pigment epithelial alterations.[63–66] Some patients who have anatomically unsuccessful surgery may undergo another vitrectomy with successful flattening of the macular hole and visual improvement.[67] Other investigators have suggested macular laser photocoagulation with or without intraocular gas tamponade for primary[68] or recurrent macular hole.[69]

PREMACULAR HOLE LESIONS

Because tangential vitreous traction is believed to play a role in the formation of macular holes, removal of cortical vitreous should reduce the rate of progression of stage 1A and 1B premacular hole lesions to full-thickness macular holes. Smiddy and then Jost reported small, uncontrolled pilot series on the technical feasibility of vitrectomy surgery for impending macular holes.[58,70] In another small, uncontrolled series Chan has described intravitreal injection of an expansile gas bubble without vitrectomy surgery to induce a posterior vitreous detachment with resolution of stage 1A (7 of 7) and 1B (3 of 4) premacular hole lesions.[71]

The Vitrectomy for Prevention of Macular Hole Study Group subsequently reported multicenter, prospective, randomized data on vitrectomy surgery and careful peeling of the cortical vitreous for presumed stage 1A and 1B lesions.[28] A full-thickness macular hole developed in 10 (37%) of 27 patients in the vitrectomy group compared with 14 (40%) of 35 patients randomized to observation ($p = 0.81$). This study could not demonstrate a significant benefit of vitrectomy surgery for stage 1A and 1B lesions and the study was terminated because of low recruitment. At this time, I do not recommend vitrectomy surgery for these premacular hole lesions but rather suggest careful follow-up, because a significant proportion will go onto full-thickness macular holes within a year.

Other surgeons question the role of tangential vitreous traction in the pathogenesis of macular hole because surgical peeling of cortical vitreous did not reduce the rate of full-thickness macular hole formation in the Vitrectomy for Prevention of Macular Hole Study.[72] It may be that some premacular hole stage 1 lesions were actually "occult" macular holes as noted intraoperatively by Jost and co-workers, or that the intervention may have been too late in the disease process.[70,73] On the other hand, it may be that tangential traction may only be part of the pathogenesis of this condition and other retinal, retinal pigment epithelial, or choroidal factors may also be important.[6,73]

REFERENCES

1. McDonnell PJ, Fine SL, Hillis AI: Clinical features of idiopathic macular cysts and holes. Am J Ophthalmol 1982;93:777–86.
2. Aaberg TM: Macular holes: a review. Surv Ophthalmol 1970; 15:139–62.
3. Noyes HD: Detachment of the retina, with laceration at the macula lutea. Trans Am Ophthalmol Soc 1871;1:128–9.
4. Zeeman WPC: Uber Loch-und cystenbildung der fovea Centralis. Graefes Arch Ophthalmol 1912;80:259–69.
5. Lister W: Holes in the retina and their clinical significance. Br J Ophthalmol 1924;8:1–20.
6. Morgan CM, Schatz H: Involutional macular thinning. A premacular hole condition. Ophthalmology 1986;93:153–61.
7. Morgan CM, Schatz H: Idiopathic macular holes. Am J Ophthalmol 1985;99:437–44.
8. Gass JDM: Idiopathic senile macular hole. Its early stages and pathogenesis. Arch Ophthalmol 1988;106:629–39.
9. Gass JDM: Reappraisal of biomicroscopic classification of stages of development of a macular hole. Am J Ophthalmol 1995;119:752–9.
10. Johnson RN, Gass JDM: Idiopathic macular holes. Observations, stages of formation, and implications for surgical intervention. Ophthalmology 1988;95:917–24.
11. Madreperla SA, McCuen BW, Hickingbotham D, et al.: Clinicopathologic correlation of surgically removed macular hole opercula. Am J Ophthalmol 1995;120:197–207.
12. Thompson JT, Hiner CJ, Glaser BM, et al.: Fluorescein angiographic characteristics of macular holes before and after vitrectomy with transforming growth factor beta-2. Am J Ophthalmol 1994;117:291–301.
13. Gass JDM, Joondeph BC: Observations concerning patients with suspected impending macular holes. Am J Ophthalmol 1990;109:638–46.
14. Watzke RC, Allen L: Subjective slitbeam sign for macular disease. Am J Ophthalmol 1969;68:449–53.
15. Martinez J, Smiddy WE, Kim J, et al.: Differentiating macular holes from macular pseudoholes. Am J Ophthalmol 1994;117: 762–7.
16. Gass JDM, Van Newkirk NM: Xanthic scotoma and yellow foveolar shadow caused by a pseudo-operculum after vitreofoveal separation. Retina 1992;12:242–4.
17. Kiryu J, Shahidi M, Ogura Y, et al.: Illustration of the stages of idiopathic macular holes by laser biomicroscopy. Arch Ophthalmol 1995;113:1156–60.
18. Puliafito C, Hee M, Lin C, et al.: Imaging of macular diseases with optical coherence tomography. Ophthalmology 1995;102: 217–29.
19. Guyer DR, Green WR, de Bustros S, et al.: Histopathologic features of idiopathic macular holes and cysts. Ophthalmology 1990;97:1045–51.
20. Frangieh GT, Green WR, Engel HM: A histopathologic study of macular cysts and holes. Retina 1981;1:311–36.
21. Gass JD: Lamellar macular hole: a complication of cystoid macular edema after cataract extraction. Arch Ophthalmol 1976;94: 793–800.
22. Smiddy WE, Michels RG, de Bustros S, et al.: Histopathology of tissue removed during vitrectomy for impending idiopathic macular holes. Am J Ophthalmol 1989;108:360–4.
23. Campochiaro PA, Van NE, Vinores SA: Immunocytochemical labeling of cells in cortical vitreous from patients with premacular hole lesions [see comments]. Arch Ophthalmol 1992;110:371–7.

24. Foos RY: Vitreoretinal junction; topographical variations. Invest Ophthalmol 1972;11:801–8.
25. Madreperla SA, Geiger GL, Funata M, et al.: Clinicopathologic correlation of a macular hole treated by cortical vitreous peeling and gas tamponade. Ophthalmology 1994;101:682–6.
26. Funata M, Wendel RT, de la Cruz Z, et al.: Clinicopathologic study of bilateral macular holes treated with pars plana vitrectomy and gas tamponade. Retina 1992;12:289–98.
27. Fekrat S, Wendel RT, de la Cruz Z, et al.: Clinicopathologic correlation of an epiretinal membrane associated with a recurrent macular hole. Retina 1995;15:53–7.
28. De Bustros S: Vitrectomy for prevention of macular holes. Results of a randomized multicenter clinical trial. Vitrectomy for Prevention of Macular Hole Study Group. Ophthalmology 1994;101: 1055–9.
29. Hikichi T, Yoshida A, Akiba J, et al.: Natural outcomes of stage 1, 2, 3, and 4 idiopathic macular holes [see comments]. Br J Ophthalmol 1995;79:517–20.
30. Gass JDM: Risk of developing macular hole [letter; comment] [see comments]. Arch Ophthalmol 1991;109:610–2.
31. Bronstein MA, Trempe CL, Freeman HM: Fellow eyes with macular holes. Am J Ophthalmol 1981;92:757–61.
32. Atmaca LS: Follow-up of macular holes. Ann Ophthalmol 1984;16:1064–5.
33. Akiba J, Yoshida A, Trempe CL: Risk of developing a macular hole [see comments]. Arch Ophthalmol 1990;108:1088–90.
34. Akiba J, Kakehashi A, Arzabe CW, et al.: Fellow eyes in idiopathic macular hole cases. Ophthalmic Surg 1992;23:594–7.
35. Guyer DR, de Bustros S, Diener WM, et al.: Observations on patients with idiopathic macular holes and cysts. Arch Ophthalmol 1992;110:1264–8.
36. Fisher YL, Slakter JS, Yannuzzi LA, et al.: A prospective natural history study and kinetic ultrasound evaluation of idiopathic macular holes. Ophthalmology 1994;101:5–11.
37. Wiznia RA: Reversibility of the early stages of idiopathic macular holes. Am J Ophthalmol 1989;107:241–5.
38. Gordon LW, Glaser BM, Ie D, et al.: Full-thickness macular hole formation with a pre-existing complete posterior vitreous detachment. Ophthalmology 1995;102:1702–5.
39. Kokame GT, de Bustros S: Visual acuity as a prognostic indicator in stage I macular holes. The Vitrectomy for Prevention of Macular Hole Study Group. Am J Ophthalmol 1995;120:112–14.
40. Group TEDC-CS: Risk factors for idiopathic macular holes. Am J Ophthalmol 1994;118:754–61.
41. Hikichi T, Yoshida A, Akiba J, et al.: Prognosis of stage 2 macular holes. Am J Ophthalmol 1995;119:571–5.
42. Aaberg TM: Macular holes. Am J Ophthalmol 1970;69:555–62.
43. Yuzawa M, Watanabe A, Takahashi Y, et al.: Observation of idiopathic full-thickness macular holes: follow-up observation. Arch Ophthalmol 1994;112:1051–6.
44. Bidwell AE, Jampol LM: Macular holes and excellent visual acuity. Arch Ophthalmol 1988;106:1350.
45. Lewis H, Cowan GM, Straatsma BR: Apparent disappearance of a macular hole associated with development of an epiretinal membrane. Am J Ophthalmol 1986;102:172–5.
46. Sjaarda RN, Frank DA, Glaser BM, et al.: Assessment of vision in idiopathic macular holes with macular microperimetry using the scanning laser ophthalmoscope. Ophthalmology 1993;100:1513–8.
47. Acosta F, Lashkari K, Reynaud X, et al.: Characterization of functional changes in macular holes and cysts. Ophthalmology 1991;98:1820–3.
48. Sjaarda RN, Frank DA, Glaser BM, et al.: Resolution of an absolute scotoma and improvement of relative scotomata after successful macular hole surgery. Am J Ophthalmol 1993;116:129–39.
49. Chew EY, Sperduto RD, Hiller R, et al.: Clinical course of macular holes: the Eye Disease Case-Control Study [see comments]. Arch Ophthalmol 1999;117:242–6.
50. Trempe CL, Weiter JJ, Furukawa H: Fellow eyes in cases of macular hole. Biomicroscopic study of the vitreous. Arch Ophthalmol 1986;104:93–5.
51. Fine SL: Vitreous surgery for macular hole in perspective. Is there an indication? [editorial; comment]. Arch Ophthalmol 1991;109: 635–6.
52. Kelly NE, Wendel RT: Vitreous surgery for idiopathic macular holes. Results of a pilot study [see comments]. Arch Ophthalmol 1991;109:654–9.
53. Ryan EA, Lee S, Chern S: Use of intravitreal autologous blood to identify posterior cortical vitreous in macular hole surgery. Arch Ophthalmol 1995;113:822–3.
54. Wendel RT, Patel AC, Kelly NE, et al.: Vitreous surgery for macular holes [see comments]. Ophthalmology 1993;100:1671–6.
55. Orellana J, Lieberman RM: Stage III macular hole surgery. Br J Ophthalmol 1993;77:555–8.
56. Ruby AJ, Williams DF, Grand MG, et al.: Pars plana vitrectomy for treatment of stage 2 macular holes. Arch Ophthalmol 1994; 112:359–64.
57. Glaser BM, Michels RG, Kuppermann BD, et al.: Transforming growth factor-beta 2 for the treatment of full-thickness macular holes. A prospective randomized study. Ophthalmology 1992; 99:1162–72.
58. Smiddy WE, Michels RG, Glaser BM, et al.: Vitrectomy for impending idiopathic macular holes. Am J Ophthalmol 1988;105: 371–6.
59. Lansing MB, Glaser BM, Liss H, et al.: The effect of pars plana vitrectomy and transforming growth factor-beta 2 without epiretinal membrane peeling on full-thickness macular holes. Ophthalmology 1993;100:868–71.
60. Thompson JT, Glaser BM, Sjaarda RN, et al.: Progression of nuclear sclerosis and long-term visual results of vitrectomy with transforming growth factor beta-2 for macular holes. Am J Ophthalmol 1995;119:48–54.
61. Freeman WR: Vitrectomy surgery for full-thickness macular holes. Am J Ophthalmol 1992;2:233–5.
62. Smiddy WE, Thomley ML, Knighton RW, et al.: Use of the potential acuity meter and laser interferometer to predict visual acuity after macular hole surgery. Retina 1994;14:305–9.
63. Park SS, Marcus DM, Duker JS, et al.: Posterior segment complications after vitrectomy for macular hole. Ophthalmology 1995;102:775–81.
64. Duker JS: Retinal pigment epitheliopathy after macular hole surgery [letter; comment]. Ophthalmology 1993;100:1604–5.
65. Poliner LS, Tornambe PE: Retinal pigment epitheliopathy after macular hole surgery [see comments]. Ophthalmology 1992;99:1671–7.
66. Charles S: Retinal pigment epithelial abnormalities after macular hole surgery (letter). Retina 1993;13:176.
67. Ie D, Glaser BM, Thompson JT, et al.: Retreatment of full-thickness macular holes persisting after prior vitrectomy: a pilot study. Ophthalmology 1993;100:1787–93.
68. Schocket SS, Lakhanpal V, Xiaoping M, et al.: Laser treatment of macular holes. Ophthalmology 1988;95:574.
69. Del Priore LV, Kaplan HJ, Bonham RD: Laser photocoagulation and fluid-gas exchange for recurrent macular hole. Retina 1994;144:381–2.
70. Jost BF, Hutton WL, Fuller DG, et al.: Vitrectomy in eyes at risk for macular hole formation. Ophthalmology 1990;97:843–7.
71. Chan CK, Wessels IF, Friedrichsen EJ: Treatment of idiopathic macular holes by induced posterior vitreous detachment. Ophthalmology 1995;102:757–67.
72. Melberg NS, Williams DF: More on macular holes. Ophthalmology 1994;101:1764–5.
73. De Bustros S: Author's reply. Ophthalmology 1994;101:1765.

SECTION VIII

Bertil Damato, M.D., Ph.D., F.R.C.Ophth.

Oncology

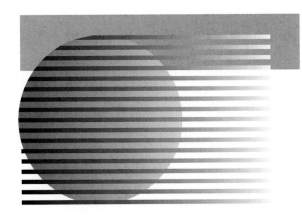

CHAPTER 63

Therapeutic Approaches to Ocular Tumors

BERTIL DAMATO, M.D., F.R.C.OPHTH., Ph.D.,
JAMES J. AUGSBURGER, M.D., PATRICK DE POTTER, M.D., Ph.D.,
NORBERT BORNFELD, M.D., JOHN HUNGERFORD, F.R.C.OPHTH., D.O.,
WILLIAM R. LEE, M.D., F.R.C.PATH., CAROL L. SHIELDS, M.D., and
JERRY A. SHIELDS, M.D.

Ocular tumors are rare and diverse, both in type and presentation.[1a,1b,1c] Many are life-threatening or form part of a potentially lethal syndrome. Furthermore, proper management usually requires specialized facilities and a multidisciplinary team of workers not readily available to a general ophthalmologist. For these reasons, patients with ocular tumors tend to be referred to an ocular oncologist for diagnosis and treatment. This chapter, being written for the general ophthalmologist, aims only to give a brief overview of the various therapeutic approaches to the most common types of tumor so that readers can refer to specialized texts for more detailed information.

Improvement in the treatment of ocular tumors is making rapid progress. In general, radical forms of treatment, such as enucleation and exenteration, are being replaced by less mutilating methods aimed at conserving the eye with as much vision as possible. These consist of radiotherapy, local resection, phototherapy, cryotherapy, and chemotherapy. Previously, these different therapies were regarded as rivaling each other, but now there is an increasing tendency to consider them all as complementary. All the different therapeutic techniques are evolving rapidly, so that there is inevitably much healthy debate about the indications for each technique.

Brief summaries of published data on the therapeutic outcomes are often difficult to interpret meaningfully without taking into consideration a wide range of factors, such as the case mix, the statistical methods used, and the way data have been categorized. The present chapter therefore focuses on the most important factors influencing outcome, we hope in a manner that allows readers to estimate what can realistically be achieved in a particular case. Unlike many other fields in ophthalmic surgery, visual acuity is not always the best measure of success. Other important objectives include the prevention of metastatic disease, retention of the eye, preservation of good cosmesis, avoidance of pain, and restoration of psychological well-being.

UVEAL TUMORS

MELANOMA

INTRODUCTION

Uveal melanomas are conventionally categorized histologically using the modified Callendar Classification into four cell types: spindle B, epithelioid, mixed, and necrotic (spindle A tumors now being regarded as benign).[2] All cell types may be observed within a single tumor. Epithelioid cells behave more aggressively than spindle cells, with regard to spread within the globe and metastasis.

Choroidal tumors tend to cause secondary changes in surrounding tissues, which determine their clinical appearance. The retinal pigment epithelium (RPE) undergoes proliferation, multi-layering, and atrophy, also developing drusen, deposits of lipofuscin ("orange pigment"), and multiple RPE detachments. The retina becomes detached, and eventually the receptors atrophy, causing visual loss. At any stage in its growth, the tumor can rupture Bruch's membrane and RPE, herniating into the subretinal space to develop a collar-stud shape. The tumor may then invade and perforate the retina, then seeding into the vitreous cavity and occasionally causing vitreous hemorrhage. The degree of pigmentation in a melanoma varies from case to case and can be assessed clinically only when the tumor is not obscured by RPE.

Ciliary body tumors tend to impinge on the lens, initially indenting the lens, then causing cataract and subluxation. Growth can occur circumferentially around the ciliary body, posteriorly into the choroid, and anteriorly into the anterior chamber, where annular spread around the angle tends to occur, leading to secondary glaucoma. Most ciliary body melanomas (and indeed all kinds of ciliary body tumor) tend to cause dilatation and tortuosity of overlying episcleral blood vessels ("sentinel vessels").

Iris melanomas account for about 8% of all intraocular melanomas. They tend to occur inferiorly, varying greatly in pigmentation, vascularity, and texture. Growth may extend posteriorly into ciliary body and along the angle, causing secondary glaucoma. Tumor in angle may be difficult to distinguish from an accumulation of melanin-containing macrophages, which may also cause glaucoma.

Intraocular melanomas tend to extend extraocularly along canals for vortex veins, ciliary vessels and nerves, and drainage vessels. Extension along the parenchyma or meninges of the optic nerve is rare.

Some melanomas may spread diffusely throughout the uveal tissue. In the choroid these are difficult to diagnose and are more likely to show extraocular extension than more circumscribed tumors.[3]

Extensive retinal detachment may cause rubeosis iridis, because the outer retina is separated from its blood supply, and this may result in the development of neovascular glaucoma. Infarction of part or all of the tumor can occur at any time, to cause acute uveitis, scleritis, and even a clinical picture mimicking orbital cellulitis.

Metastatic disease usually becomes manifest in the liver[4] and has a poor prognosis, with a median survival of about 6 months.[4a] Recognized prognostic factors for metastatic disease are numerous[5] and include epithelioid cell type, large basal tumor diameter, age greater than 60 years at treatment, anterior tumor extension, transscleral extension, presence of closed vascular loops,[6] intratumoral chromosomal abnormalities such as monosomy 3 and trisomy 8,[7] and variation in nucleolar dimensions.[8]

The overall ten-year survival in patients with uveal melanoma is approximately 50%[9]; however, the chances of survival vary greatly according to the number of risk factors at the time of treatment. After local resection, for example, survival varies from more than 90% at 15 years in patients less than 60 years old with spindle cell melanoma less than 16 mm in diameter, to less than 40% at 4 years if all these risk factors are present.[10] Iris melanomas have a good prognosis for survival,[10a] but it is not known whether this is due to their small size or their location. Ciliary body melanomas have a relatively poor prognosis, and recent studies suggest that this explained by large size and malignant cytology.[11] It is not known when tumor dissemination occurs, what proportion of disseminated cells survive, and how long these cells remain dormant before clinically detectable metastases develop. Such lack of knowledge has contributed to an ongoing controversy about how survival is influenced by treatment of the primary tumor.[12]

PREOPERATIVE ASSESSMENT

As with any other condition, examination is performed in a systematic manner, taking a complete ocular and systemic history, performing full ophthalmic and systemic examinations, and making use of selected ancillary tests as required.

The large majority of intraocular melanomas can be diagnosed by indirect ophthalmoscopy and slit-lamp biomicroscopy, performed by an informed examiner. If the media are opaque or if the tumor is unusual, then other investigations may provide diagnostic clues. For example, echography[13] may show the tumor to have a collar-stud shape, which is almost pathognomonic of a melanoma that has ruptured Bruch's membrane. Tumor diagnosis by standardized echography[14] and acoustic tissue characterization[15] have been described, but both techniques require special equipment and expertise. Fluorescein angiography is not as helpful as previously believed because it only demonstrates surface changes in choroidal tumors, which may be nonspecific if the retinal pigment epithelium is still present.[16] Indocyanine green videoangiography reveals changes in the deeper tissues, but none of these are pathognomonic for any particular type of tumor.[17,18] Magnetic resonance imaging (MRI) reveals the presence of melanin, which has characteristic paramagnetic features, but is also nondiagnostic because many tumor types may share the same MRI appearances as melanoma.[19] Post-contrast-enhanced MRI scans using fat-suppression techniques may demonstrate optic nerve invasion or orbital extension. Computerized tomography is usually less informative than echography or MRI. Although it may demonstrate calcification in an osteoma, it is usually possible to reveal the presence of bone quite adequately by echography.

If the diagnosis is uncertain after completing the clinical assessment or if the patient demands a tissue diagnosis before treatment is started, then most ocular oncologists would proceed to fine-needle aspiration biopsy (FNAB).[20] This procedure is performed under local anesthesia with a 25-gauge needle attached to a 10-ml syringe by flexible tubing. The approach depends on the location of the tumor, and would usually be through the pars plana for choroidal tumors and through the limbus for iris lesions. For best results, the specimens should be examined by a skilled cytopathologist, who should ideally be present in the operating room so that additional material can be obtained if necessary. Tumor seeding in the needle track is thought not to occur if a fine needle is used. Retinal detachment is surprisingly rare, even when a retinal hole is created. Some prefer to use a vitreous cutter so as to improve diagnostic accuracy.[20a]

In some centres, incisional biopsy is preferred to FNAB, either because the pathologist is not confident with needle biopsy specimens or because the surgeon is concerned about ocular complications.[21] The surgical techniques are similar to those described for local resection (below). Examination of frozen section material may result in misdiagnosis because of the poor quality of the specimen, and expedited histology using fixed tissue is preferable. The risk of tumor growth through the scleral defect is minimized by special measures according to the type of treatment that would be indicated if the tumor proved to be a melanoma. If plaque radiotherapy is the treatment of choice, then it is commenced immediately, at a risk of administering unnecessary radiation for a benign lesion. If proton beam radiotherapy or enucleation is indicated, then the wound is sealed with tissue glue, and the appropriate treatment is performed as soon as possible.

Both the location and the extent of the tumor need to be defined precisely for the selection and planning of treatment and for advising the patient on the probable outcome. Centripetal spread is described in terms of invasion or perforation of Bruch's membrane, RPE, and retina, with a specific mention of any vitreous seeding. Distances between posterior tumor margin and both optic disc and fovea are assessed by using binocular indirect ophthalmoscopy, a pre-corneal lens fitted with a graticule, and B-scan echography, and are measured in terms of disc diameters or millimeters. The location of the anterior tumor margin with respect to ora serrata, pars plicata, and angle is identified by indirect ophthalmoscopy, three-mirror examination, ultrasonography with a high-frequency scanner, if possible, and transillumination (bearing in mind the limitations of this technique). Circumferential tumor extension can be documented in clock hours or degrees, whether the measurement is being taken at the optic disc margin, equator of the eye, ciliary body, or angle. Deep tumor extension into orbit or optic disc is assessed by echography or MRI with gadolinium enhancement.

Tumor thickness is measured by A-scan or B-scan echography, with special care to exclude sclera, to scan the tumor through its thickest point and not overestimating thickness by inadvertently scanning the tumor obliquely. Basal dimensions are usually measured along the greatest tumor width and perpendicular to this measurement, taking account of tapering tumor margins and serous retinal detachment, which may lead to underestimation and overestimation, respectively. It is possible to obtain an approximate idea of the basal tumor dimensions by indirect ophthalmoscopy as the field of view is approximately 12 mm with a 20 diopter lens and 13 mm with a 28 D lens. Special charts have also been designed to calculate tumor dimensions.[22]

Secondary effects of the tumor, such as rubeosis and hemorrhage, as well as coincidental conditions such as diabetic retinopathy, cataract, and retinal tears or degenerations are noteworthy as they may influence treatment selection and outcome.

The objectives of systemic examination are to identify any anesthesia risks and to screen for extraocular malignancy, primary or secondary. In most patients with uveal melanoma, detectable liver metastases are much less likely than benign tumors, such as cysts and angiomas. Many ophthalmic oncologists therefore rely on physical examination and biochemical tests of liver function, performing liver ultrasonography or other imaging only if the patient has a large tumor and, hence, an unusually high risk of metastatic disease. Opinions vary as to the value of chest radiography.

COUNSELING

To give informed consent for further management, the patient needs to be aware of all the treatments available, the logistics of each treatment, the complications that may occur, and the likely outcomes in terms of visual acuity, visual field, retention of the eye, and survival.[23] These considerations are meaningful only if the patient has some understanding of the nature of the disease and some knowledge of the anatomy of the eye.

Communication with the patient is complicated by the large amount of information in the explanation and the anxious state that the patient is likely to be in. Interaction is facilitated by quiet and peaceful surroundings, comfortable seating, and a knowledgeable, honest explanation given in an unhurried and sympathetic manner. The patient's ability to create a mental image of the condition is enhanced by the use of a plastic model of the eye, together with actual drawings, photographs and images of the patient's own tumor. It is difficult for patients to remember all that they are told, and information leaflets may be helpful. It is useful to provide patients with an audio cassette tape recording of the actual discussions,[24] and it is helpful if a close friend or relative is present during the consultation. Adequate time should, of course, be allowed for questions.

Selection of the best treatment for a particular patient depends not only on the tumor size and location but also on a wide variety of other factors, such as the patient's psychological, occupational, and recreational requirements. If there is a choice of treatment, the patient's own priorities need to be considered. Most patients will accept a small risk of local tumor recurrence and metastasis in the hope of conserving a useful eye and maintaining a better quality of life. For some individuals, the fear of metastatic death is so great that only enucleation will give peace of mind. The degree of risk that is acceptable varies greatly from person to person, as does the definition of a "useful eye." In some patients, the eye is useful only if there is good central acuity, and for others a temporal visual field is adequate. Many patients do not care about vision as long as they keep their own eye. Much depends on the vision in the fellow eye.

In the first instance, patients are usually given a chance to state their preferred treatment, as patient involvement in decision making enhances psychological well-being in the long term.[25] In most cases, the patient spontaneously selects what the doctor feels to be the best treatment, and all that is necessary is for the doctor to provide reassurance that a reasonable decision has been taken. Patients tend to find it stressful to take responsibility for a decision of such vital importance, in case complications subsequently develop, and it is therefore helpful if the doctor can shoulder this burden. If the patient makes a decision that the doctor considers to be unwise, most practitioners would then reason with the patient, nearly always successfully. It is well understood that lay individuals can gain only a partial understanding of the full implications of their disease and its treatment, so that ultimately it is the doctor's responsibility to give a treatment that is both reasonably safe and well matched to the patient's needs.

Patients tend to ask about heredity. It has been estimated that about 0.6% of patients with uveal melanoma have a positive family history of the disease.[26]

MANAGEMENT

Observation

When Zimmerman and associates cast doubt on the efficacy of enucleation,[12] some ophthalmologists adopted a policy of no treatment. At present, however, observation is generally advocated only for small tumors, as a method of differentiating suspicious nevi from melanomas. Current evidence is insufficient to determine the correctness of this approach, and the metastatic risk involved in not treating small melanomas needs to be balanced against the ocular complications caused by treatment of benign nevi.[27]

When performing sequential examinations, a hand-held, self-illuminated slide-viewer enables baseline photographic transparencies to be compared accurately with funduscopic appearances (Fig. 63–1). Once malignancy is diagnosed, most workers would treat the tumor, except in patients who have both a very limited life expectancy and a small tumor that is not expected to cause an acutely painful eye. Old age is not in itself a reason to withhold treatment, as the subsequent development of acute pain may necessitate urgent enucleation when the patient may be less fit for anesthesia. Further, illness may interfere with follow-up, and also some studies indicate old age to be an independent risk factor for metastatic death, suggesting that tumors are more likely to spread in elderly individuals than in their younger counterparts.

Iris melanomas are relatively believed to be benign and are therefore kept under observation unless they are more than 3 mm in diameter. Growth is regarded as an indication for treatment by most workers.

Plaque Radiotherapy

Introduction

Ionizing radiation displaces electrons from target atoms and produces harmful free radicals, thereby damaging DNA and cell membranes, causing tumor cell death, either immediately or after a delay, when the cell attempts

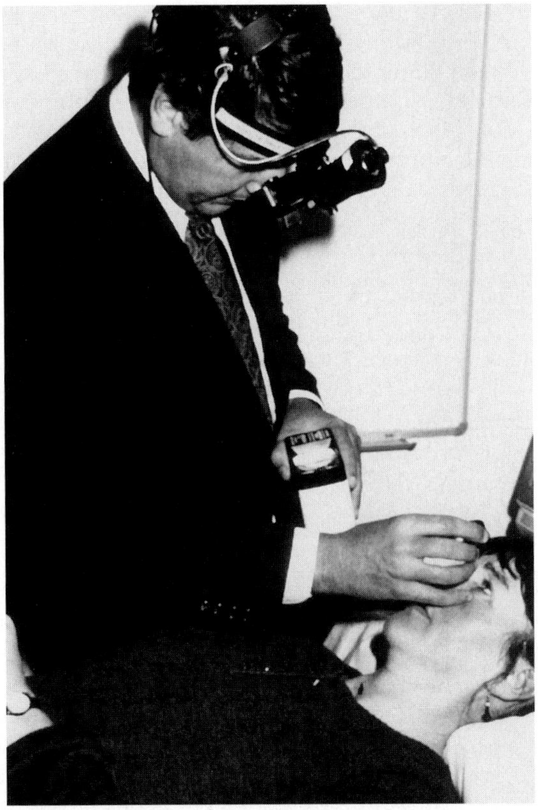

Figure 63–1. Use of hand-held, illuminated slide viewer for comparing ophthalmoscopic findings with previous photographs. (Courtesy of B. Damato, M.D.)

to divide. Radiotherapy kills tumor cells both directly and by depriving them of their blood supply. The unit of absorbed radiation is the Gray (i.e., 1 Gy), which is equal to one joule of energy absorbed per kilogram of target mass, and which is equivalent to 100 rads.

Indications

Brachytherapy is in most oncology centers the first choice of treatment for suitable choroidal tumors (see below) because it is less expensive, less time-consuming, and less difficult than other forms of conservative therapy. Iodine plaque radiotherapy has been advocated for iris lesions, to prevent the complications associated with an iris coloboma and to treat tumors deemed too extensive for surgical excision.[28,28a]

Methods

Previously, the cobalt 60 plaque was popular,[29] but this has largely been abandoned because it is not possible to shield the high-energy gamma irradiation emitted from the outer surface of the plaque so that damage is inevitably caused to adjacent extraocular structures, such as the lacrimal gland and eyelids.

The most widely used isotope today, at least in North America, is iodine 125, which emits low-energy gamma irradiation.[30] The iodine 125 is contained in "seeds," which are held on the inner surface of a concave gold or steel shell by a resin or acrylic insert (Fig. 63–2). It is possible to adjust the dosimetry to suit each tumor by altering the number and distribution of the seeds. The shell, which is 0.3 to 1.0 mm thick, completely shields any radiation emitted away from the eye, and has a marginal lip to reduce side-scatter of radiation to adjacent structures such as optic nerve and fovea. The dose of radiation falls with distance from the plaque, according to the inverse square law, so that the base of the tumor and the sclera receive much higher doses of radiation than the tumor apex. The plastic insert is therefore about 1 mm thick so as to reduce this disparity.

In many European centers, ruthenium 106 is the preferred isotope.[31] This plaque consists of a 0.9-mm-thick silver plate, with its concave surface painted with ruthenium 106 and sealed with a 0.1-mm layer of silver (Fig. 63–3). Most of the radiation emitted consists of electrons, with an energy of approximately 3.5 MEV. This β-irradiation penetrates the ocular tissues much less than the gamma irradiation of iodine plaques, so that if a dose of 100 Gy is delivered at a depth of 5 mm, the dose at 10 mm is only about 15 Gy, as compared to about 30 Gy with iodine plaques (Fig. 63–4). The low penetration of β-irradiation reduces ocular morbidity but also limits this treatment to small tumors. Ruthenium plaques have a longer half-life than iodine plaques (i.e., 1 year as opposed to 60 days).

In one or two centers, other isotopes, such as palladium[32] or strontium are used, but these have not gained wide acceptance.

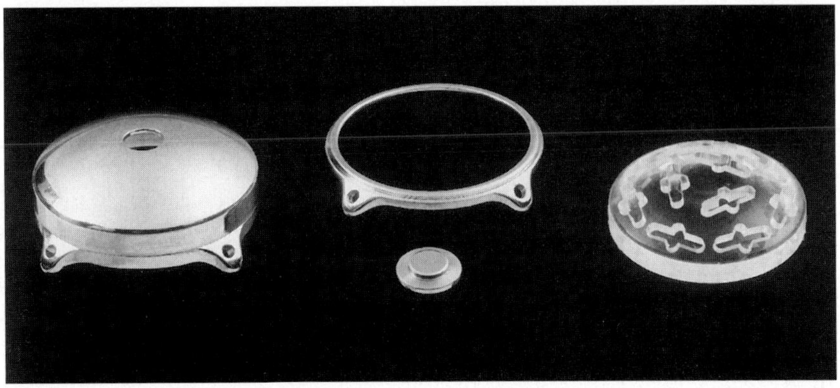

Figure 63–2. The R.O.P.E.S. iodine plaque. (Courtesy of Dr C. Karolis, Radiation Oncology Physics and Engineering Services Pty, Ltd, St Paul's, N.S.W. Australia.)

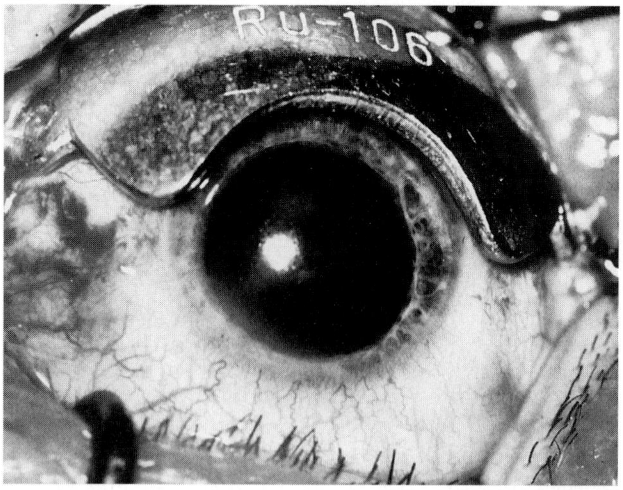

Figure 63–3. A ciliary body ruthenium plaque applicator. (Courtesy of Prof. Dr. N. Bornfeld.)

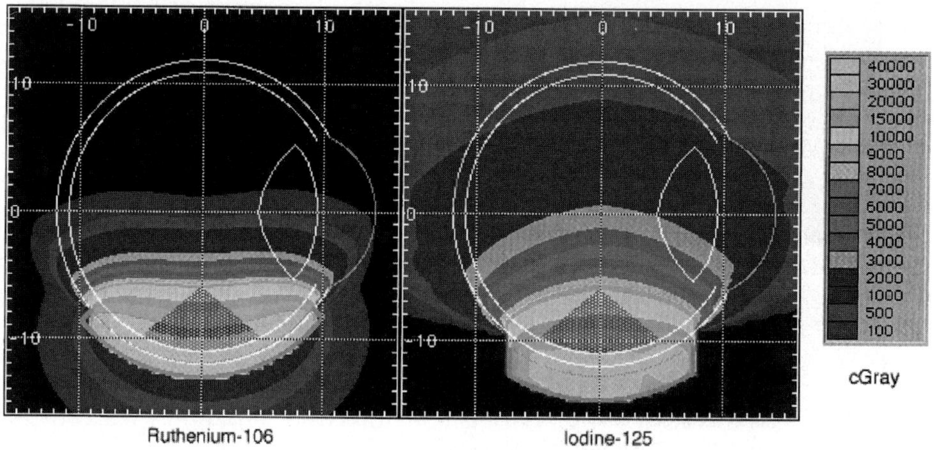

Figure 63–4. Dosimetry of *(A)* iodine, and *(B)* ruthenium plaques. (Courtesy of Prof. Dr. N. Bornfeld.)

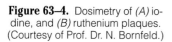

Insertion of the radioactive plaque is performed under local or general anesthesia, according to preference (Fig. 63–5). The sclera overlying the tumor is exposed, disinserting any intervening extraocular muscles, if necessary. The tumor margins are localized, either by transillumination or indentation, and marked on the sclera with ink. An illuminated indentor fitted with a diathermy for marking the sclera, facilitates this part of the operation. A template consisting of a plastic dummy or metal ring is sutured to the sclera to cover the tumor with a safety margin of at least 2 mm. This is replaced with the therapeutic plaque, which is secured with the same sutures. Additional sutures are placed to keep the entire plaque surface tightly apposed to the eye. The muscles are either re-inserted or held in their approximate anatomical positions with slings. Once the desired dose of radiation has been delivered, usually after 3 to 7 days, the plaque is removed, the muscles are re-inserted, and the conjunctiva is closed.

If there is a small, circumscribed nodule of transscleral tumor extension, then this is covered by the plaque, adjusting the dosimetry accordingly. Extrascleral nodules greater than 2 mm in diameter are regarded by some clinicians as a contraindication to plaque radiotherapy but can sometimes be shriveled down to a small size by strong bipolar diathermy so that the plaque can be positioned properly. Another approach is to shave off the tumor flush with the sclera (J. Hungerford) and then to apply an unshielded plaque, which would irradiate the surrounding orbital tissue (J. J. Augsburger).

Most tumors are treated with a minimum apex dose of 80 to 100 Gy. The Collaborative Ocular Melanoma Study protocol suggests that tumors less than 5-mm thick should be treated as if they are 5-mm thick,[33] but this view is not universal. The sclera therefore receives at least 300 Gy, and perhaps as much as 1500 Gy if a very thick tumor is treated (i.e., approximately 10 mm thick). Nevertheless, the sclera seems able to tolerate high doses of radiation remarkably well, except near the limbus, where necrosis and perforation are more likely to occur.

Results

The chances of local tumor control with conservation of good vision are excellent if the tumor is less than 5 to 6 mm thick, less than 15 mm in diameter, and more than 2 DD from disc or fovea.[31,34–38] After treatment, tumors usually regress over months or years into a flat or slightly elevated mass, which is usually more pigmented than the original tumor and surrounded by an area of choroidal atrophy (Fig. 63–6).[39] The rate and extent of tu-

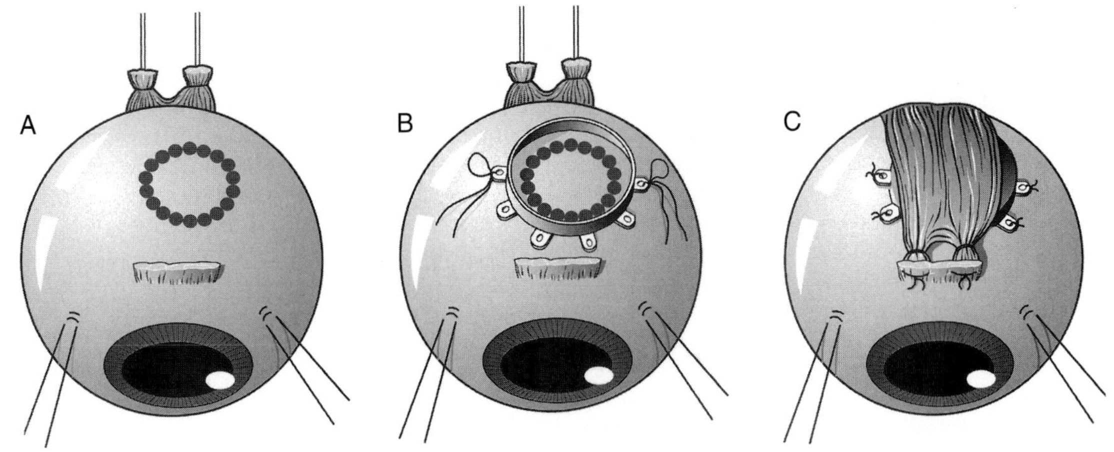

Figure 63–5. Technique for placement of a radioactive plaque. The tumor is localized *(A)*; a template is sutured to the sclera *(B)*; and this is replaced with a therapeutic plaque *(C)*. (Courtesy of B. Damato, M.D.)

mor shrinkage vary greatly. Some tumors remain bulky, being replaced by a fibrous tissue scar. Conversely, a minority of tumors have such a high cell turnover that they regress very rapidly and completely. Not surprisingly, such dramatic regression has been shown to be associated with a poor prognosis for survival.[40]

Tumor recurrence after plaque radiotherapy is rare if the plaque is well positioned, with an adequate safety margin of at least 2 mm all around the tumor, and if the tumor apex is given the recommended dose of radiation.[41] Marginal tumor recurrence is more likely with posterior tumors, which are more difficult to localize. The risk of marginal recurrence is especially high with juxtapapillary tumors, because the optic nerve may prevent proper positioning of the plaque, unless a notched plaque is used.[42] Central tumor recurrence becomes more likely if a tumor more than 10 mm thick is treated with an iodine plaque or if a tumor more than 5 mm thick is treated with a ruthenium plaque. Marginal tumor recurrence is recognized by a progressive, lateral extension of the pigmented margin of the tumor or, rarely, by an amelanotic or pigmented swelling beyond the area of radiational choroidal atrophy. Lack of radiational choroidal atrophy around the entire tumor circumference does not necessarily indicate that a part of the tumor has been inadequately treated. Central recurrence is diagnosed when sequential ultrasonography shows an increase in tumor thickness of more than approximately 1 mm, after taking into account the resolution of the equipment and the repeatability of the examination technique. Sudden growth of surviving tumor may be mimicked by hemorrhage into scar tissue within the tumor and from herniation of necrotic tissue through a defect in Bruch's membrane, so that measurements may need to be repeated two or three times to confirm that progressive tumor growth is indeed occurring.

Survival after plaque radiotherapy of medium-sized tumors does not differ from that after enucleation[33,35]; however, there is evidence that local tumor recurrence after plaque radiotherapy is associated with a relatively high rate of metastatic death.[42,43] Although local tumor recurrence may merely be an indicator of increased tumor aggression, there is also the possibility that metastatic disease has arisen from inadequately treated tumor.

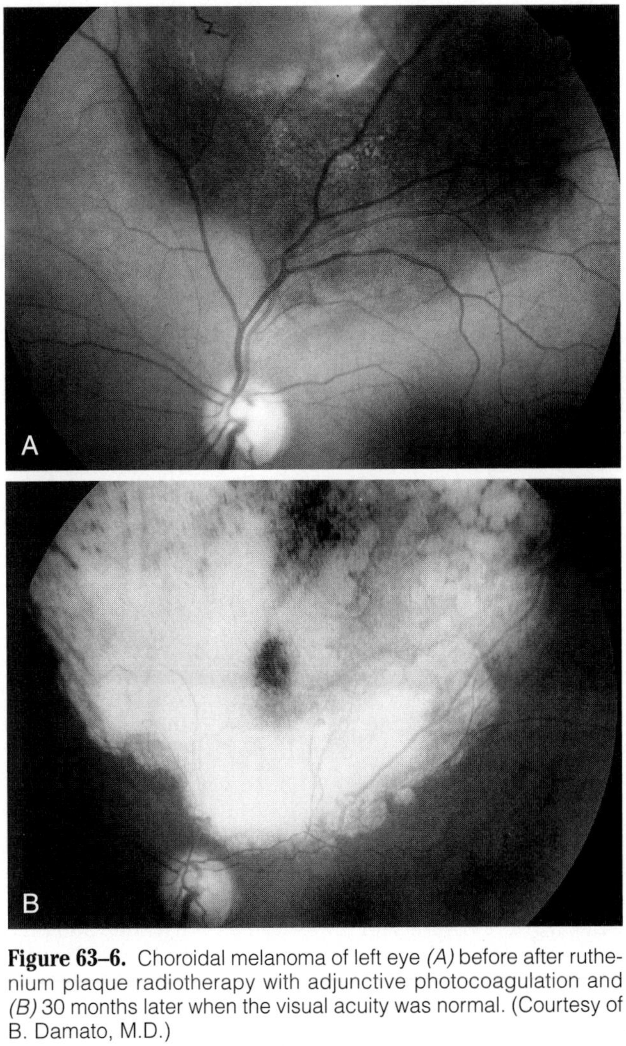

Figure 63–6. Choroidal melanoma of left eye *(A)* before after ruthenium plaque radiotherapy with adjunctive photocoagulation and *(B)* 30 months later when the visual acuity was normal. (Courtesy of B. Damato, M.D.)

Ocular complications of plaque radiotherapy can be related to surgery or radiotherapy. Surgical complications include (1) misplacement of the plaque in relation to the tumor, due to faulty localization or suturing techniques; (2) retinal tears caused when placing scleral sutures, which can result in retinal detachment if not treated adequately; (3) diplopia, caused by inaccurate repositioning of an extraocular muscle; (4) vortex vein compression by the plaque, which may cause choroidal detachment and angle-closure glaucoma; and (5) subretinal hemorrhage, which usually resorbs without any consequence unless the fovea is involved. Early radiational complications include exudative retinal detachment, which usually resolves spontaneously after a few weeks or months but which may rarely persist, with a concomitant risk of neovascular glaucoma. Late complications of radiation usually occur at any time from the second year onwards. These include (1) cataract, if the lens receives a dose greater than 5 to 15 Gy; (2) optic neuropathy, if the optic disc receives more than about 45 Gy, resulting in severe, generalized visual loss and perhaps disc neovascularisation, vitreous hemorrhage, rubeosis iridis, and neovascular glaucoma; and (3) maculopathy, which may be due to leakage of fluid from a superior tumor, cystoid macular edema, radiation retinopathy, or hard exudates. Radiation retinopathy occurs at a dose greater than 40 Gy and is due to depletion of vascular endothelial cells, resulting in microaneurysms, telangiectasia, hemorrhages, exudates, non-perfusion, and neovascularization. Radiation vasculopathy is synergistic with other vasculopathies, such as diabetic retinopathy, vein occlusions, and autoimmune disorders. Troublesome radiation vasculopathy is more likely to occur at the margins of the irradiated area than centrally, where the retina and its vasculature are totally obliterated. An unusual but troublesome complication is recurrent vitreous hemorrhage from the apex of a "collar-stud" tumor that has ruptured retina.

Computer software now allows accurate dosimetry by creating a three-dimensional model of the eye, together with tumor and plaque.[44] Thus, it is possible to estimate preoperatively the doses of radiation that will be received by optic nerve, macula, and lens so that the likely outcome can be predicted.

Contraindications

Plaque radiotherapy is contraindicated when it is not possible to deliver a sufficient dose of radiation to the entire tumor, either because the tumor is too thick or wide, or because the plaque cannot be positioned properly when the tumor extends too far around the optic disc, ciliary body, or angle. When preliminary dosimetry indicates that the chances of retaining useful vision are small, then another form of conservative therapy may be preferable, if good vision is an important priority. Alternatively, the patient may prefer to have the eye removed, thereby eliminating any risk of intraocular tumor recurrence and other ocular complications, and avoiding the need for lifelong follow-up and perhaps repeated surgery.

Charged Particle Teletherapy

Introduction

Heavy charged particles, such as protons and helium ions, cause most atomic ionization as they slow down, so that there is increasing tissue damage with depth up to the point where there is no further penetration (the "Bragg Peak"). The dose of radiation at the distal end of the beam therefore falls from 100% to 10% within 2 mm distally and 3 mm laterally, allowing the entire tumor to receive a uniform dose of radiation, with little spread to surrounding structures. Furthermore, if the tumor is both small and posterior, then superficial tissues can receive as little as 60% of the full dose. Unfortunately, however, many tumors are large or extend anteriorly, so that surface sparing is not clinically significant. Only about a dozen centers worldwide are equipped for charged particle radiotherapy, and most of these deliver a proton beam.

Indications

Most proton beam units receive patients from several ocular oncologists, most of whom tend to reserve charged particle radiotherapy for patients deemed unsuitable for brachytherapy. In one or two centers, charged particle radiotherapy is used exclusively, even with tumors that can be treated with brachytherapy or local resection. A small number of patients with iris and ciliary body melanomas have been treated with proton beam radiotherapy, which is technically easier than with choroidal tumors because there is no need for tantalum markers.

Methods

The first stage of treatment is to suture four or five radio-opaque, tantalum markers to the sclera at known points in relation to the tumor margins and the limbus (Fig. 63–7).[45] These serve to localize the tumor radiographically during the radiotherapy. The surgical techniques for localizing the tumor are the same as those used for plaque radiotherapy.

In the second stage, treatment planning is performed using a simulator. A computerized three-dimensional model of the eye is generated using echographic measurements of the eye and tumor, as well as measurements of marker–marker, marker–tumor, and marker–limbus distances, which are obtained with calipers during marker placement (Fig. 63–8). The software then

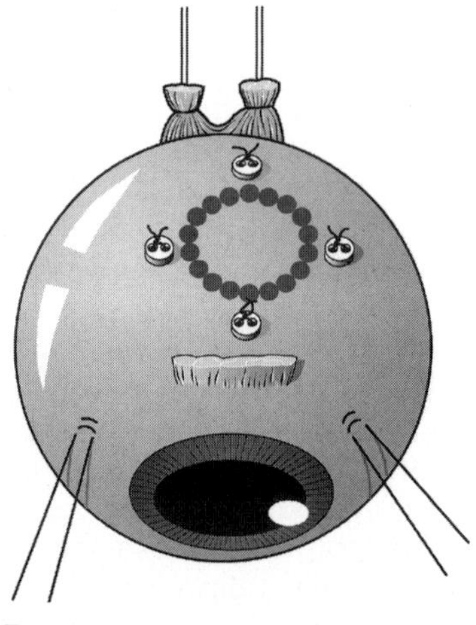

Figure 63–7. Tantalum markers placed at known positions in relation to tumor and limbus. (Courtesy of B. Damato, M.D.)

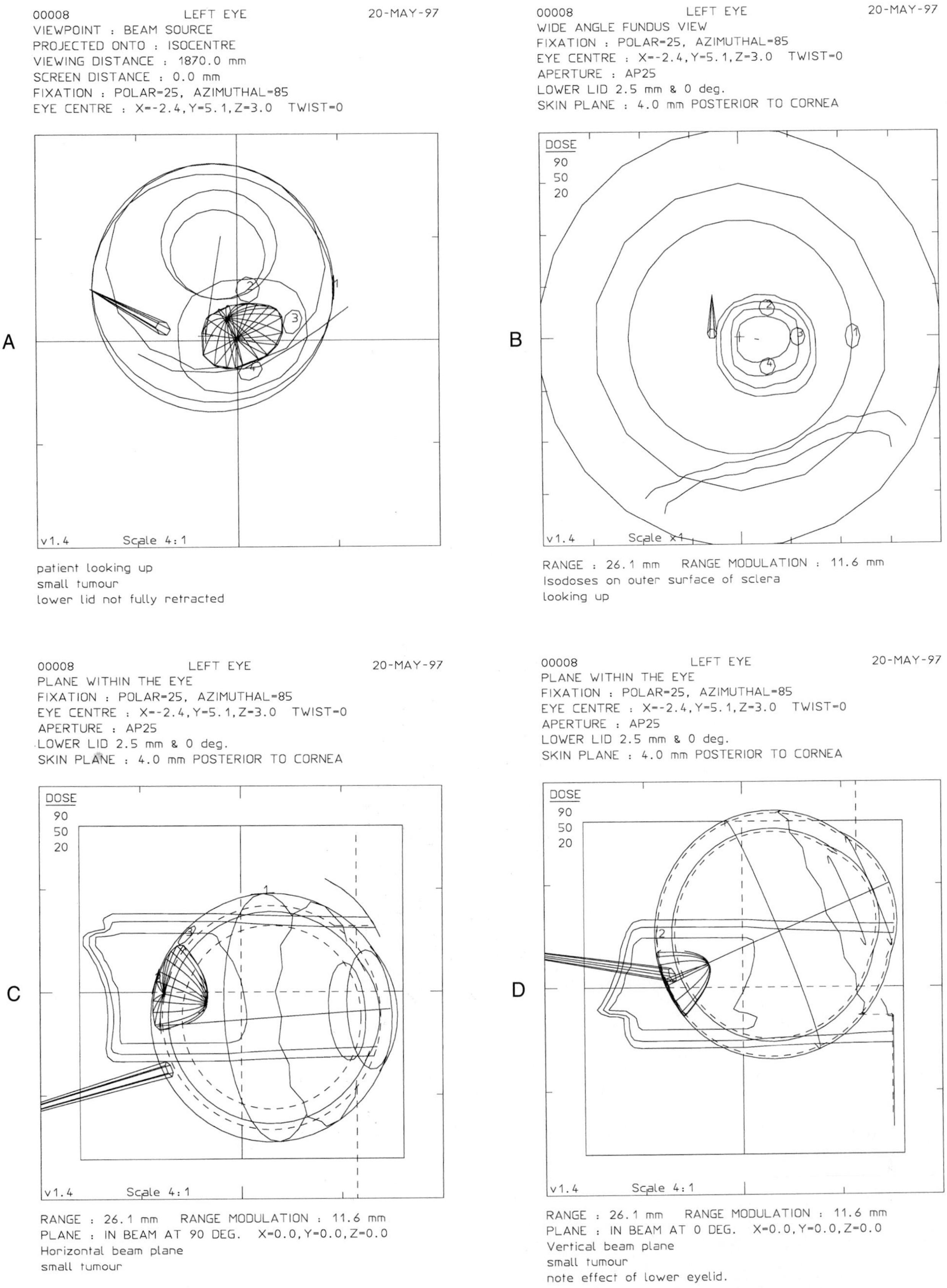

Figure 63–8. Computerized model of the eye, showing the 3-D diagram *(A),* beam view *(B),* fundus view *(C),* horizontal beam plane *(D),* and vertical beam plane. (Courtesy of Dr. A. Kaçperek, Douglas Cyclotron Unit, Clatterbridge Centre for Oncology, Merseyside, UK.)

calculates the optimal range and profile of the beam, the ideal eye position during treatment, and the radiation doses to optic nerve, fovea, lens, ciliary body, and eyelid. The diameter and contour of the beam are shaped for each tumor by a customized brass aperture. The penetration of the beam is adjusted using lucite absorbers and the Bragg peak is modulated into a plateau shape by means of a spinning wedge absorber.

During the radiotherapy, the patient is seated in a mechanized chair, which can be accurately positioned (Fig. 63–9). The head is immobilized in a frame by means of a bite block and an individually contoured face mask. The eye is positioned by asking the patient to look at an adjustable fixation target, preferably with the treated eye or, if this is not possible, with the fellow eye. Before treatment, positioning of the eye is checked radiologically by locating the radio-opaque tantalum markers. During treatment, the eye position is monitored visually, using a high-magnification video camera. Each fraction of radiation is given in 30 to 40 seconds.

Depending on the center, most patients receive 50 to 70 Gray Equivalents (GyE) in four or five fractions over 5 to 10 days, with safety margins of 1.5 to 2.5 mm laterally and distally.

Results

After proton beam radiotherapy, the chances of conserving the eye with good vision are very good if the tumor is small and it if does not extend close to the optic disc or fovea.[46–48] The ocular prognosis can be estimated at the time of treatment planning according to the doses of radiation delivered to disc, macula, and lens, and according to the tumor volume and amount of serous retinal detachment.

Published results show impressive local tumor control rates after charged particle radiotherapy (i.e., more than 95%).[46,48,49] Tumor regression with this form of radiation is slower than after ruthenium plaque brachytherapy (J. D Grange, personal communication, International Symposium on Ocular Tumors, Israel, 1997) but has a similar rate to that after iodine plaque radiotherapy.[34] Regression is sometimes preceded by temporary tumor enlargement after treatment, which is believed to reflect necrosis and edema within the tumor. In some patients, choroidal atrophy around the tumor may unmask hidden lateral tumor extensions, which may be mistaken for active growth.

After proton beam radiotherapy, the survival probability is not significantly worse than after enucleation.[50] With melanomas suitable both for plaque and proton beam radiotherapy, there is probably no significant difference in local control rates between the two types of radiotherapy.[34] As with plaque radiotherapy, local tumor recurrence after proton beam radiotherapy is associated with a poorer prognosis for survival,[51] and it is uncertain whether recurrence actually causes metastatic disease or whether it merely indicates aggressive tumor behavior.

One of the main problems after charged particle teletherapy is persistent exudative retinal detachment. The chances of this complication developing increase with tumor thickness and with the extent of the exudative retinal detachment before treatment.[46] As with any extensive and long-standing retinal detachment, there is a significant incidence of neovascular glaucoma. Exudative retinal detachment after proton beam radiotherapy is generally regarded as untreatable, but it has resolved after local resection of the irradiated tumor (Damato and Bornfeld, unpublished data).

The risk of radiational optic neuropathy after charged particle teletherapy increases as the distance between tumor margin and optic nerve diminishes. Most eyes with tumor extension to within one disc diameter of the optic disc margin eventually develop optic neuropathy, usually within the first 3 or 4 years.[52]

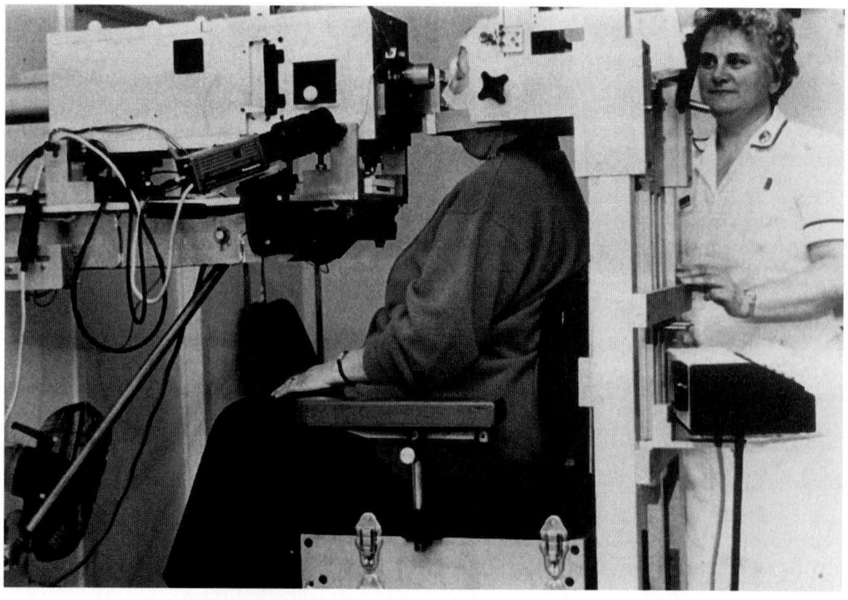

Figure 63–9. Photograph of patient during treatment. Note the face mask, bite block, visual target, closed-circuit TV camera, and the nozzle of the proton beam unit. (Courtesy of Dr. A. Kaçperek, Douglas Cyclotron Unit, Clatterbridge Centre for Oncology, Merseyside, UK.)

The likelihood of developing this complication increases with conditions such as diabetes mellitus, which reduce the functional reserve of the vascular endothelium. As with plaque radiotherapy, optic neuropathy results in severe visual loss and may be associated with neovascular glaucoma.

The treatment plan is adjusted to include in the irradiated field any encapsulated extrascleral tumor nodule.

As with plaque radiotherapy, charged particle radiotherapy of a tumor that has perforated retina may be followed by repeated and persistent vitreous hemorrhage, and occasionally rhegmatogenous retinal detachment.

With charged particle teletherapy, there is little sparing of surface tissues if the tumor is large or anterior, so that patients will inevitably develop external eye complications. These vary according to the location of the tumor.[53] Radiation of the lid margins causes loss of eyelashes and skin de-pigmentation. In addition, if the superior lid margin is damaged, keratinization results in superficial punctate keratopathy. Rarely, if the cornea is anesthetic after receiving a high dose of radiation, then a neurotrophic ulcer may develop and eventually perforate. Radiotherapy of a supero-temporal tumor may be followed by atrophy of the lacrimal gland and keratoconjunctivitis sicca, whereas treatment of an infero-nasal tumor may cause canaliculitis and intractable epiphora. The conjunctival blood vessels may become telangiectatic, and if this occurs in the interpalpebral fissure the patient may develop persistent irritation only partly relieved by artificial tears. As with any radiotherapy, cataract will develop if the lens receives a sufficient dose of radiation.

Contraindications

In most centers, charged particle radiotherapy is contraindicated if it is felt that the tumor can be treated equally well by plaque radiotherapy, which is less expensive and more convenient for the patient. If retention of vision is important, then in some centers additional contraindications would be proximity to the optic disc or fovea, in which case the patient would be treated with phototherapy or, perhaps, endoresection. Another general contraindication is large tumor size, especially if there is an extensive exudative retinal detachment, or if the tumor is anterior, because of the high probability of visual loss, retinal detachment, and neovascular glaucoma. Unless the patient is extremely reluctant to lose the eye, enucleation is the preferred choice of treatment, except in a few centres where trans-scleral local resection is possible.

Stereotactic Radiotherapy

There is increasing interest in treating ocular tumors with stereotactic radiosurgery in which irradiation is delivered to the eye from a large number of directions, with each beam of irradiation being focused on the tumor.[54,55] Long-term results are not yet available, and it remains to be seen whether this technique is superior to charged particle teletherapy.

CRYOTHERAPY

There are anecdotal reports of small choroidal melanomas responding to cryotherapy delivered with a conventional retinal cryoprobe.[55a] Ocular complications included optic atrophy after treatment of a juxtapapillary tumor, retinal vein occlusion, transient exudative retinal detachment and epiretinal membrane.

Choroidectomy

Indications

Trans-scleral local resection of choroidal melanomas is technically difficult and requires profound systemic hypotension, which is also a highly skilled procedure. For these reasons, is performed in only a few centers around the world, and it is reserved for tumors that are considered to be too large for radiotherapy.[56–58]

Surgical Technique

The surgical technique of trans-scleral local resection of posterior segment tumors is described only briefly because this operation is not widely performed (Fig. 63–10). The tumor is localized as for plaque radiotherapy. A lamellar scleral flap is dissected, hinged posteriorly. Any vortex veins in the operative field are cauterized, together with any long posterior ciliary arteries and, if possible, the short posterior ciliary arteries posterior to the tumor. The eye is decompressed by limited pars plana vitrectomy, to prevent prolapse of the ocular contents through the scleral window. The deep sclera is incised with scissors around the tumor, creating a stepped wound edge. The tumor is resected together with the deep scleral lamella, avoiding retinal damage if possible. Using fresh instruments, the scleral window is closed with interrupted sutures. The eye is re-formed with an intravitreal injection of balanced salt solution (BSS). If possible, the margins of the choroidal coloboma are treated with a double row of binocular indirect laser photocoagulation. To treat microscopic residual tumor, some workers recommend adjunctive plaque radiotherapy in all patients, although the long- term results of this additional treatment have yet to be evaluated fully. The plaque is sutured in place to cover the entire scleral flap, and the extraocular muscles are replaced in their anatomical positions. Finally, the conjunctiva is closed and subconjunctival steroids and antibiotics are injected. Postoperatively, patients are treated with topical and systemic steroids and antibiotics. The plaque is removed 2 or 3 days later, once a dose of approximately 100 Gy has been delivered at a depth of 2 to 3 mm.

Preoperative cryotherapy and photocoagulation are unnecessary, as is the use of a Flieringa ring or scleral basket.

Intraoperative hemorrhage is diminished by lowering the systolic blood pressure to approximately 40 mm Hg from the time when the deep sclera is opened until the moment when fluid is injected into the vitreous cavity to raise the intraocular pressure (i.e., usually about 1 hour).

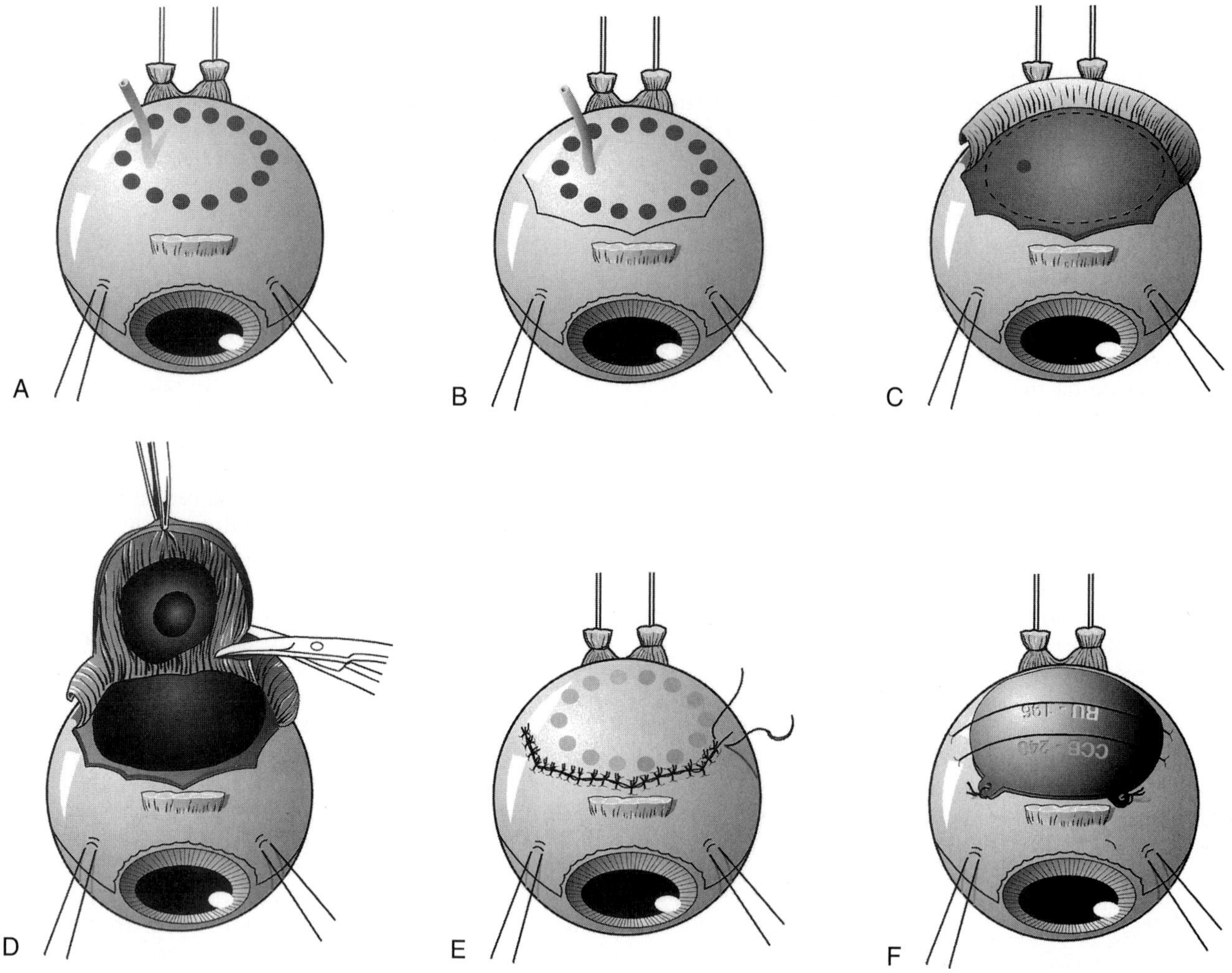

Figure 63–10. Trans-scleral local resection. The tumor is localized *(A)*. Partial-thickness scleral incisions are made *(B)*. A superficial lamellar scleral flap is prepared, cauterizing any intervening vortex veins, and the deep sclera is incised, decompressing the eye to improve access *(C)*. The tumor is removed, together with the deep scleral lamella, avoiding retinal damage *(D)*. The scleral flap is closed with interrupted sutures *(E)*, and a plaque is placed over the operative site *(F)*. (Courtesy of B. Damato, M.D.)

Drugs to induce hypotension are given by an anesthetist who is highly experienced with the technique, using an intra-arterial line to monitor the blood pressure, and with continuous cardiac and cerebral monitoring. If there are any signs of cardiac or cerebral ischemia, the systemic blood pressure is immediately allowed to rise irrespective of the ocular consequences, and the surgeon then needs to decide whether to continue or abandon the procedure in favor of radiotherapy or enucleation.

Most trans-scleral choroidectomies and cyclochoroidectomies take between 2 and 3 hours. Patients are returned to a general ophthalmic ward within 2 hours and are fully mobile on the first postoperative day, usually being discharged from hospital about 3 days postoperatively.

Results

In suitable cases, an experienced surgeon can achieve predictable and satisfactory results, with a low complication rate and good conservation of visual acuity and/or field, depending on the tumor location (Fig. 63–11).[59] When the tumor is located nasally without extending close to optic disc or fovea, most patients retain vision of 6/12 or better. With temporal tumors there is a greater chance of macular damage, with residual vision of 6/36 to 6/60. Posterior tumor extension to within one or two disc diameters of the optic disc or fovea increases the risks of residual tumor, visual loss, and enucleation.

Intraoperative complications include (1) inaccurate tumor localization with malposition of the scleral window, (2) inadvertent buttonholing of the superficial or deep sclera, (3) uncontrolled hemorrhage from vortex veins or uveal margins, (4) lens or retinal damage during vitrectomy, (5) retinal damage during tumor excision, (6) incomplete tumor removal, (7) choroidal rips at the macula, (8) dehiscence of the scleral flap, (9) incorrect positioning of the radioactive plaque, and (10) incorrect repositioning of the extraocular muscles. With experience, most of these complications are avoidable or easily rectified. Complications related to the hypotensive anesthesia include myocardial infarction, cerebral infarction, and death, none of which occurred in a series of more than 300 operations, with the only intraoperative death being caused by a massive pulmonary embolus, which was not believed to be related to the systemic hypotensive anesthesia.[56]

Incomplete tumor excision may result in either clinically visible tumor (i.e., "residual tumor"), or microscopic, subclinical tumor deposits, which may grow to become clinically detectable (i.e., "recurrent tumor").[60] Visible residual tumor is rare and tends to occur only when the posterior tumor margin extends to within one or two disc diameters of the optic disc or fovea. Predictive factors for delayed local tumor recurrence include posterior tumor extension, tumor diameter greater than 16 mm, and epithelioid cell type. Most recurrences occur at the tumor margin, with a small number developing within the coloboma from deposits in sclera or retina, and a tiny minority arise in other parts of the eye. Extraocular recurrences almost always develop from intraocular residual or recurrent tumor. Nearly all tumor recurrences occur within the first 7 years postoperatively and are usually treatable by conservative therapy unless they extend to optic disc or orbit, and unless other complications are present.

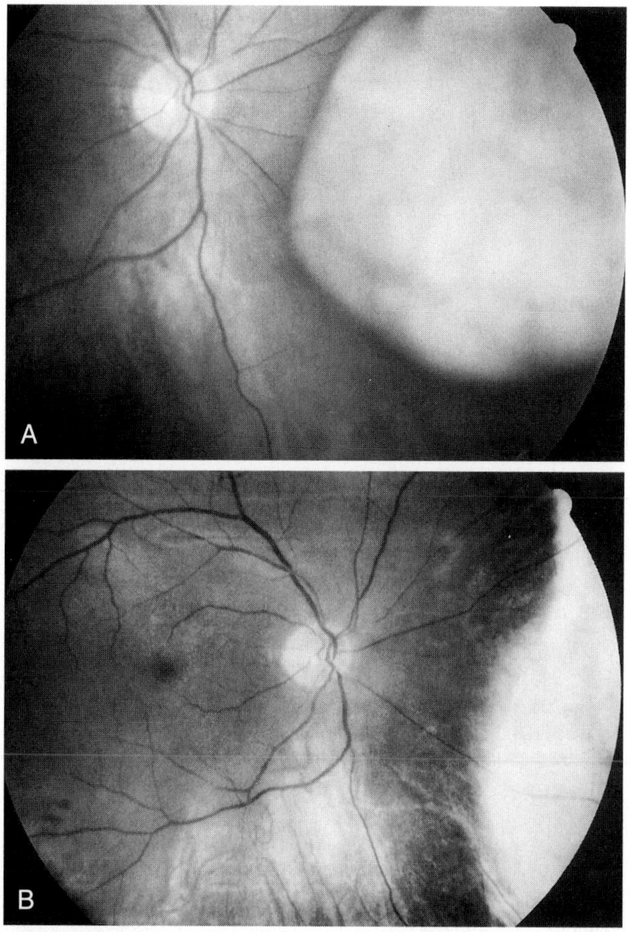

Figure 63–11. Fundus photograph of the right eye, before trans-scleral choroidectomy *(A)* and 9 months later *(B)*. (Courtesy of B. Damato, M.D.)

A study using historical controls suggests that survival after local resection is not significantly worse than after enucleation.[61] Risk factors for metastatic disease are similar to those reported for other forms of treatment.[10] Local tumor recurrence is not associated with a poor prognosis unless the recurrence is large or extends extraocularly. As with radiotherapy, it is not known whether such recurrences are the source of metastases or just an indication of aggressive tumor behavior.

Retinal detachment is the second major complication of trans-scleral local resection, because if it is not treated successfully it causes severe ocular morbidity and prevents recognition and treatment of residual and recurrent tumor. Retinal tears have become uncommon since the introduction of ocular decompression and now tend to occur only if the tumor is very adherent to retina or if there is an extensive retinal dialysis after cyclochoroidectomy. If a retinal tear occurs, immediate vitreoretinal surgery usually prevents retinal detachment from developing.

Vitreous hemorrhage after local resection cannot occur if the retina is intact and suggests that there is an unsealed retinal break. This complication therefore indicates the need for vitrectomy and prophylactic retinal surgery.

Cyclochoroidectomy may also be complicated by ciliary body detachment, ocular hypotension, and phthisis bulbi, especially if more than a third of the ciliary body is excised.

Other ocular complications include cataract, disciform macular scarring due to choroidal neovascularisation arising from the margins of the coloboma, and radiational complications, which depend on the positioning of the plaque.

Contraindications

The main contraindication to trans-scleral local resection is lack of familiarity with the technique. Ocular contraindications include (1) tumor diameter more than 16 mm, because of the increased risk of local tumor recurrence; (2) posterior extension to within one disc diameter of the optic disc or fovea, if this cannot be treated with diathermy and brachytherapy; (3) posterior, trans-scleral tumor extension, because of technical difficulty in placing a full-thickness scleral graft; (4) retinal invasion or perforation, because of the increased risk of retinal detachment; (5) involvement of more than a third of the ciliary body or angle, because of postoperative ocular hypotension and phthisis; and (6) inability to perform hypotensive anesthesia.

Hypotensive anesthesia is contraindicated if there is any history of ischemic heart disease, cerebrovascular disease, or any serious renal, hepatic, or pulmonary insufficiency. Old age is not a contraindication, especially if only iridocyclectomy is being considered, as hemorrhage may cease even at moderate levels of hypotension.

Iridectomy

Indications

Iridectomy is generally regarded as the standard form of treatment for melanomas involving less than about four clock hours of iris and not extending to angle.

Technique

This is performed through a limbal incision using similar techniques to other types of iridectomy. Wide clearance margins are essential as melanomas are often more extensive than is clinically apparent. The adequacy of surgical excision is assessed histologically, although clear surgical margins do not guarantee complete tumor excision.

Contraindications

Broad iridectomy is contraindicated if the tumor is extensive, diffuse, or extending into angle. In view of the problems associated with an iris coloboma, some workers prefer radiotherapy. Problematic photophobia can be treated with painted contact lens or an artificial iris.

Iridocyclectomy

Indications

Iridocyclectomy is indicated if there is tumor involvement of the angle or ciliary body.

Technique

A lamellar scleral flap is prepared, hinged at the limbus and extending posteriorly to the region of the ora serrata (Fig. 63–12). Deep scleral incisions are then made 1 to 2 mm within the superficial scleral incision, so as to create a stepped wound. The anterior chamber is entered anterior to the anterior tumor margin, removing any deep cornea in contact with the tumor *en bloc* with the tumor. Radial iris incisions are made, which are extended posteriorly through ciliary body and around the posterior tumor margin. With the help of a viscoelastic agent, special care is taken to avoid touching the lens and the corneal endothelium. The zonules can usually be separated from the pars plicata by blunt dissection and preserved if the posterior part of the pars plana is left in place. The vitreous cortex is also preserved, by decompressing the eye if necessary,

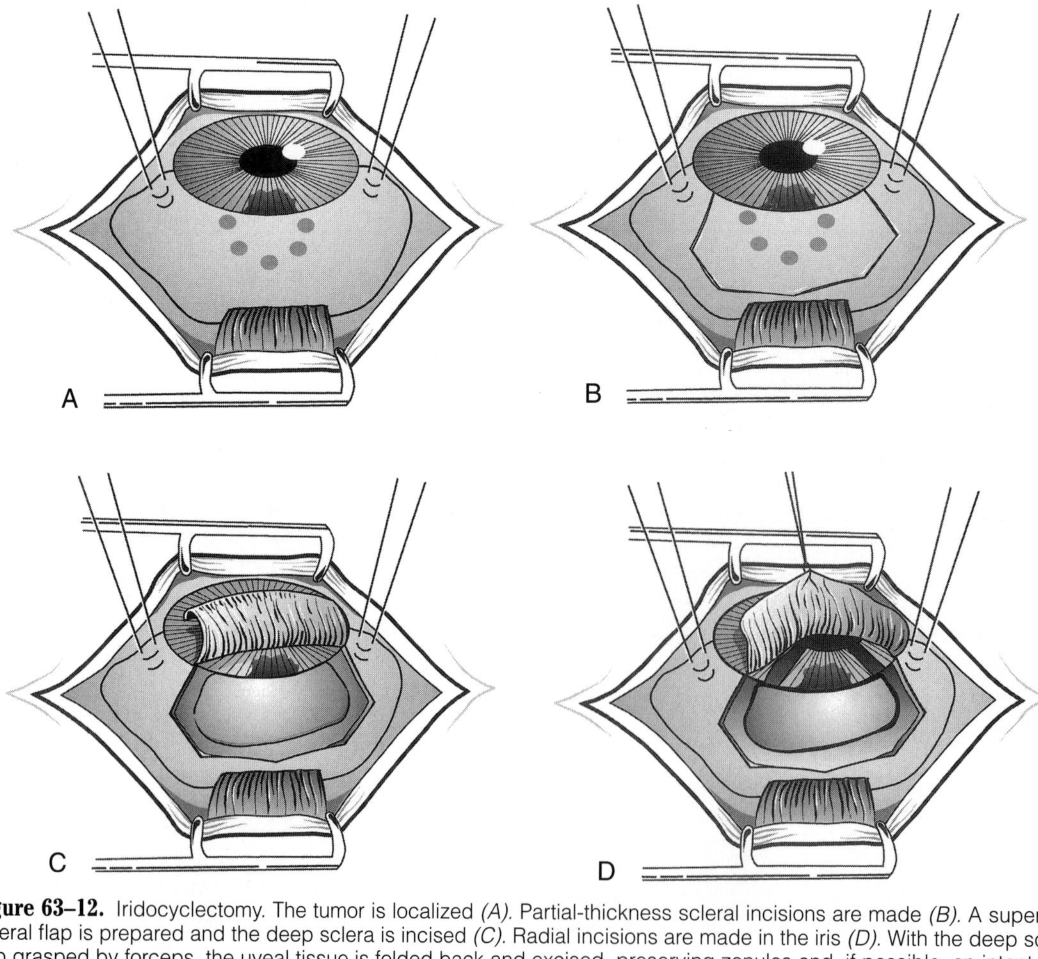

Figure 63–12. Iridocyclectomy. The tumor is localized *(A)*. Partial-thickness scleral incisions are made *(B)*. A superficial scleral flap is prepared and the deep sclera is incised *(C)*. Radial incisions are made in the iris *(D)*. With the deep scleral flap grasped by forceps, the uveal tissue is folded back and excised, preserving zonules and, if possible, an intact vitreous face *(E)*. The scleral flap is closed with interrupted sutures *(F)*. A radioactive plaque is sutured over the operated area *(G)* and the conjunctiva is closed *(H)*. (Courtesy of B. Damato, M.D.) *Illustration continued on opposite page*

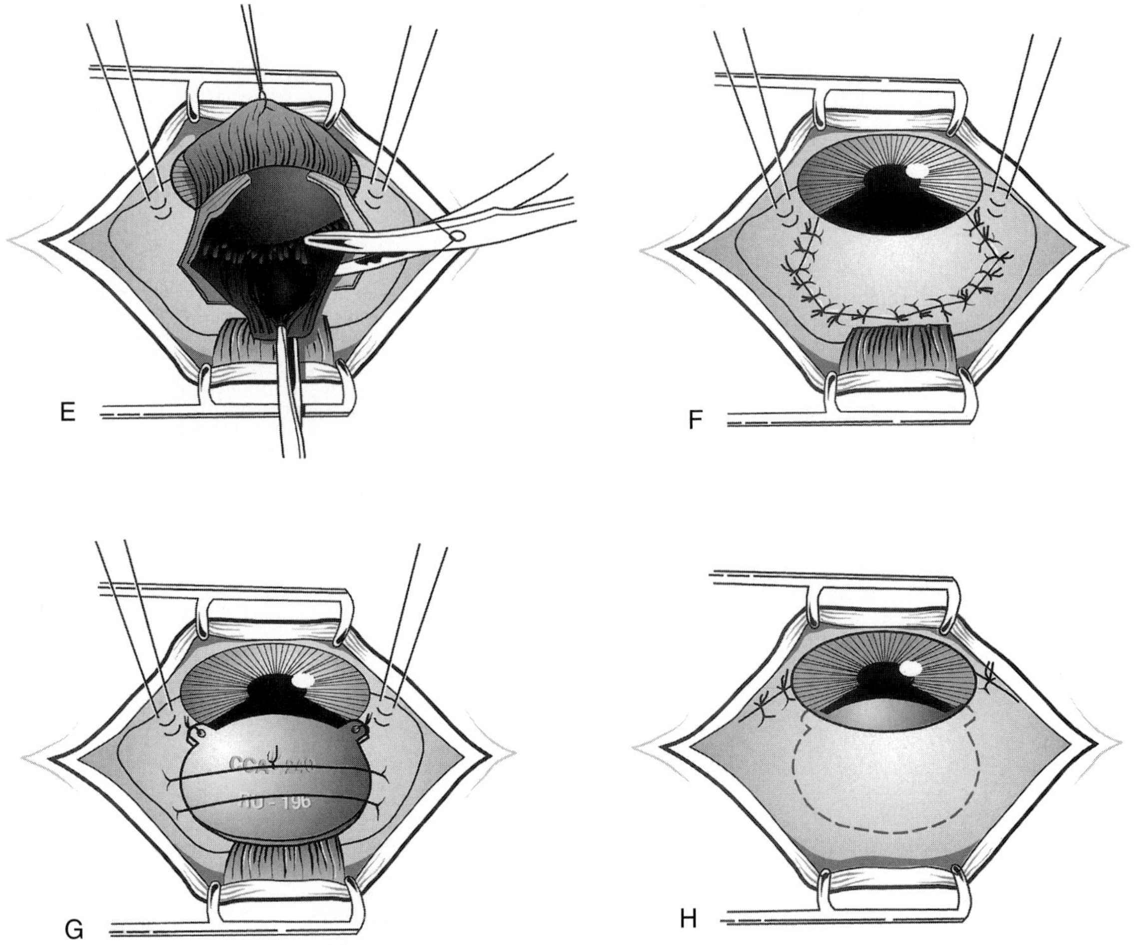

Figure 63–12 *Continued.* For legend see opposite page.

by vitrectomy through a separate sclerotomy. The superficial lamellar scleral flap is closed with interrupted, absorbable sutures. Some workers advocate full thickness corneoscleral excision over the tumor, performing a corneoscleral transplant at the end of the procedure.[62] An alternative precaution is to apply adjunctive plaque radiotherapy. This can cause severe hypotony, however, and is therefore best delayed a few weeks until the eye has healed from surgery.

Moderate hypotensive anesthesia helps to reduce hemorrhage, but is not essential, especially in elderly patients in whom there tends to be less bleeding.

Results

The chances of conserving the eye with good visual acuity are very good, unless extensive ciliary body excision is required.

Local tumor recurrence may occur if the tumor is incompletely excised, for example, if there is unrecognized tumor extension in the angle or ciliary body.

With excision of more than a third of ciliary body, there is a significant risk of hypotony and phthisis, as well as cystoid macular edema.

Despite conservation of the zonules, the lens may become subluxated anteriorly, to lie against cornea, causing keratopathy. The probability of cataract formation increases with the volume of ciliary body excised.

Preservation of an intact vitreous gel may reduce the chances of macular edema, but increases the risk of aqueous misdirection and malignant glaucoma.

Iridectomy and iridocyclectomy usually result in a large iris coloboma, to cause photophobia, refractive errors, and a cosmetic defect. Although these problems may be alleviated with a painted contact lens, not all patients can tolerate such a lens.

Contraindications

Iridocyclectomy is less likely to be successful if it is necessary to excise more than one third of the ciliary body. If the tumor extends posterior to ora serrata, then cyclochoroidectomy is necessary.

Endoresection

Indications

A very small number of surgeons have recently been performing trans-retinal resection of juxtapapillary tumors, to avoid optic neuropathy after radiotherapy and uncertainties regarding local tumor control after phototherapy.[63,64] Another indication is suspected tumor growth after radiotherapy or phototherapy.

Technique

This operation is highly controversial and will therefore be described only briefly. The procedure can be preceded by transpupillary thermotherapy (see below) or radiotherapy (N. Bornfeld) to destroy as much tumor as possible. A total vitrectomy is performed, in the standard fashion, with posterior vitreous detachment and removal of vitreous near the entry sites. The retina over the tumor is either folded away from the tumor, after making a peripheral circumferential incision, or removed with the vitrector. From a theoretical point of view, it would be ideal if before manipulation the tumor could be isolated from the general circulation, by incising or cauterizing the surrounding choroid, and if the tumor could also be destroyed, by laser treatment. The tumor is then resected piecemeal with a standard vitrector. Endo-diathermy is applied to any residual pigment as well as to any bleeding vessels. The retina is folded back and flattened with the help of fluid–air exchange. Endolaser is applied to create retinal adhesion. The eye is filled with silicone oil and closed. Cryotherapy is applied to the sclerotomies. If there is uncertainty regarding adequacy of tumor destruction then adjunctive plaque radiotherapy is given. The oil is removed after 12 weeks.

Results

Tumor recurrence can occur at the margins of the coloboma and in the scleral bed. Seeding to other parts of the eye has not been seen. Although the early results are encouraging, further follow-up is required to evaluate long-term local tumor control (Fig. 63–13).

Retinal detachment can occur as a result of entry site tears, inadequate retinopexy around the margins of any retinotomies, and inadequate vitrectomy, which causes retinal traction by vitreous bands. With experience, these complications should be preventable. Cataract eventually occurs in almost all cases from the use of silicone oil, but it is readily treatable. A proportion of patients develop a sudden and severe rise in intraocular pressure a few days or weeks after the operation, which is transient and responsive to medical therapy. Occasionally, the raised intraocular pressure persists until the silicone oil is removed. If trans-scleral cryotherapy is applied too close to the optic nerve, the patient may develop optic atrophy and poor vision.

Conservation of good vision is possible with endoresection, but it would be premature to recommend this form of treatment as a routine procedure.

Contraindications

Proponents of endoresection give the following contraindications (1) significant optic disc involvement, (2) diffuse melanoma, and (3) basal tumor diameter greater than 10 mm.

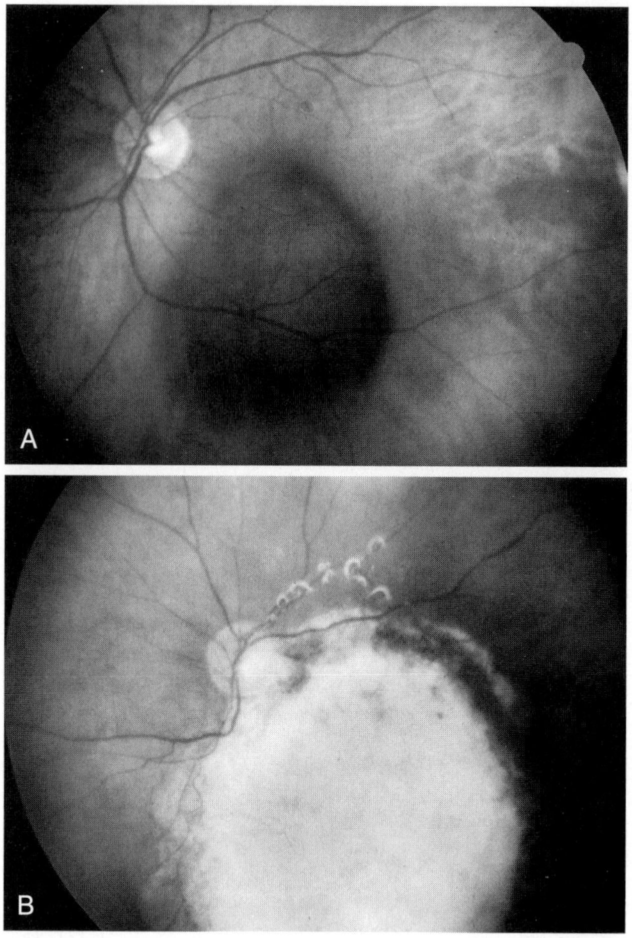

Figure 63–13. Fundus photograph of the left eye, *(A)* before endoresection, and *(B)* 21 months later (Courtesy of B. Damato, M.D.). The patient had no complications and died of a stroke several years later.

Phototherapy

Indications

The main indication for phototherapy is proximity of a small tumor to the optic disc, making optic neuropathy highly likely after plaque or proton beam radiotherapy. Phototherapy is also useful as an adjunct to radiotherapy and to salvage eyes with early tumor recurrence after local resection.

Technique

The initial form of phototherapy was flash photocoagulation with the xenon arc and then the argon laser.[65] The treatment was applied in two stages. First, the tumor was surrounded by a double row of heavy burns, to create a zone of choroidal atrophy, and next, the tumor was treated directly, at monthly intervals, until a flat grey scar remained ("gray mouse"). To increase the amount of tumor damage, at each treatment, the technique of low-energy, long-duration photocoagulation was developed, using the krypton laser.[66] This method is similar to techniques described previously, except that the tumor is treated with 500 micron burns, each lasting some 30 to 60 seconds. Another approach is photodynamic therapy, which uses light of an appropriate wavelength to activate a photosensitizer, such as a liposomal preparation of a benzoporphyrin derivative.[67]

A recent development is trans-pupillary thermotherapy (TTT) using the diode laser to raise the temperature of the tumor to between 45°C and 60°C for approximately 1 minute (Fig. 63–14).[68,69] The pupil is dilated with cyclopentolate and phenylephrine, and the eye is anesthetized by retrobulbar anesthesia. Using a panfunduscope lens or Mainster lens, infrared diode laser (810 nm) applications are placed over the entire tumor surface to include a 1.5 to 2.0 mm surround of clinically normal choroid. The beam width is usually 3.0 mm. Each exposure is approximately 1 minute long. The power is initially set at 300 mW and increased until the treated area develops blanching after 40 seconds of treatment, without closure of the retinal vasculature. A higher power is necessary if the tumor is amelanotic. Between two and four sessions are usually necessary and these are delivered at 3-monthly intervals. Oosterhuis, who originated the technique, recommends adjunctive plaque radiotherapy. Shields and co-workers use the same combination technique for medium-sized melanomas and have had success with small melanomas using thermotherapy alone.

Results

A single treatment of transpupillary thermotherapy is believed to cause tumor necrosis up to a depth of 3 to 4 mm[70] and therefore seems to be more effective than both flash photocoagulation and low-energy, long-duration laser photocoagulation, which it supersedes. The possible reasons for the greater tissue penetration include the longer wavelength of light, the wider beam diameter, the delayed loss of retinal transparency, and the long duration of each light application. It has also been suggested that tumor circulation remains patent, thereby transferring heat into the deeper parts of the tumor.

It is well recognized that tumor recurrence can occur several years after photocoagulation so that longer term follow-up is required to evaluate fully the efficacy of local tumor control with TTT.[70a]

The original intention of TTT was to destroy the choroidal tumor (and inevitably the overlying retinal receptors) while preserving the retinal nerve fibers and the major retinal vessels crossing the tumor surface. Whether such retinal preservation is possible depends on the amount of subretinal fluid present during each treatment. It seems that retinal damage is usually unavoidable. In addition, epiretinal membrane formation, retinal traction, and branch vein occlusion have been reported after this treatment. For these reasons, the final visual acuity depends on the tumor location and is likely to be best when the tumor is located away from the fovea.

Contraindications

The TTT procedure is contraindicated in the presence of (1) cataract and other media opacities preventing proper visualization of the tumor; (2) location in the far periphery, where access is difficult; (3) involvement of more than one third of the optic disc, because treatment would result in severe visual loss; and (4) tumor thickness more than 4 mm, because of an increased risk of inadequate tumor destruction. With small tumors, some workers would consider an additional contraindication to be uncertainty about the diagnosis of malignancy, although this is debatable.

Enucleation

Indications

Removal of the eye for an intraocular melanoma is indicated if the surgeon is not confident about achieving tumor control or conserving a useful eye by other means, or if the patient is not highly motivated to retain the eye or to attend for follow-up.

Technique

To prevent any possibility of enucleating the wrong eye, it is essential to visualize the tumor and to do this

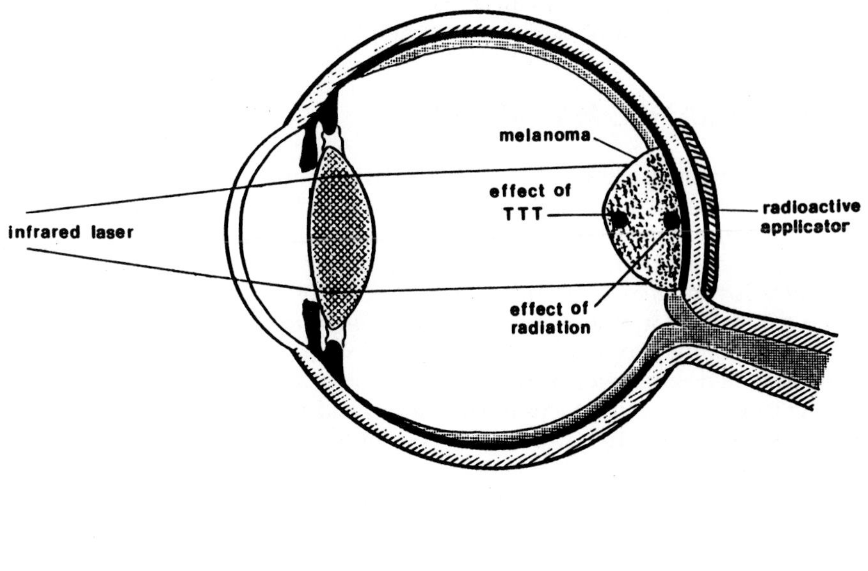

Figure 63–14. Principle of transpupillary thermotherapy with adjunctive plaque radiotherapy ("sandwich therapy") (Courtesy of Prof. Dr. J. A.Oosterhuis, Dr. H. G. Journée-de Korver, and Dr J.E.E. Keunen, Department of Ophthalmology, Leiden University Medical Center, The Netherlands.)

after draping the patient and covering the normal eye. The enucleation is performed as gently as possible, in case there is any truth in the Zimmerman's hypothesis that fatal tumor dissemination occurs as a result of physical trauma during surgery.[71] Some surgeons give a retrobulbar injection of long-acting anesthetic to prevent bradycardia from the oculocardiac reflex, and to control postoperative pain, in this case using a long-acting preparation. This may be administered after the conjunctiva is opened, to reduce the risk of perforating the globe. A variety of measures are advocated to minimize hemorrhage, and these include (1) adding epinephrine to the local anesthetic, (2) clamping the optic nerve for a few minutes, and (3) the use of a snare. The surgeon's preferred orbital implant can be used. A pressure bandage is applied for 1 or 2 days to prevent the formation of a peri-orbital hematoma.

Several groups have shown that pre-enucleation external beam radiotherapy is not useful in preventing metastatic disease.[72–74]

The management of patients with trans-scleral extension varies from center to center. Exenteration is no longer believed to improve the chances of survival, and removal of any visible tumor is considered adequate. Some workers advocate external beam radiotherapy to the orbit, delivering a total dose of approximately 45 Gy.[75] Others merely recommend observation. Factors that may influence the decision of whether to treat or observe patients with extraocular extension include the prognosis for survival, the size and integrity of the trans-scleral tumor extension, and the patient's attitudes toward cosmesis and risk of tumor recurrence.

Contraindications

Enucleation for intraocular melanoma is contraindicated if the patient has not been adequately informed of all possible forms of conservative therapy. If there is significant doubt about the diagnosis, it would be unwise to proceed to enucleation without first performing a biopsy or emphasizing to the patient that there is diagnostic uncertainty. The latter situation arises when an eye is blind and painful, with opaque media. Terminal metastatic disease is not necessarily a contraindication to enucleation, because without treatment the tumor may cause an acutely painful eye at a time when the patient is not well enough for enucleation.

POSTOPERATIVE MANAGEMENT

Protocols for the postoperative care of patients with uveal melanoma vary greatly. After conservative therapy, patients may be reviewed after 1 or 2 weeks, then every 2 to 6 months for the first year, then every 6 months for about 6 years, and, eventually, once a year if the risk of local tumor recurrence is considered to be small. Ophthalmoscopy and slit-lamp examination are supplemented with color drawings and photographs, echography, three-mirror lens examination, and other tests, as required. After enucleation, patients are reviewed to deal with any socket problems and, in selected patients with extraocular tumor extension, to screen for orbital recurrence.

The policy regarding the screening of metastatic disease varies from center to center. Some workers advocate no screening whatsoever, on the basis that treatment for metastatic disease is only palliative. Others recommend 6 or 12 monthly liver scans and serum biochemistry, in the hope of detecting any metastatic disease at a resectable stage, thereby prolonging life for a few months or even years in some patients.[76] Opinions differ as to how great the probability of metastasis should be before screening is recommended.

Treatment of hepatic metastases by systemic intravenous chemotherapy is disappointing, whereas direct intrahepatic perfusion is reported to induce a response rate of up to 40%, with such a response increasing the median survival from approximately 5 months to 13 months.[4,77]

A number of adjuvant systemic therapies have been recommended for patients with advanced cutaneous melanoma. At present, there is no form of adjuvant therapy that has been shown to be effective in improving survival in high-risk patients with uveal melanoma. It is hypothesized that because clinical metastatic disease responds so poorly to treatment, it is unlikely that similar treatment will be effective prophylactically.[78] Such a hypothesis, logical as it may seem, has yet to be proven. Ocular oncologists tend to remain in close collaboration with general oncologists and would offer high-risk patients the chance to take part in any randomized trials that may be in progress at the time.

At all stages of the management process, patients and their families should be offered psychological counseling.

NEVUS

INTRODUCTION

Choroidal nevi occur in more than 10% of the population, and are composed of spindle or polyhedral cells containing a variable amount of pigmentation. Nevi tend to be less than 2 mm thick and less than 10 mm in diameter. They may either have a featureless, gray surface or may cause degenerative changes in the retinal pigment epithelium, with drusen formation and secondary changes in retina. Serous retinal detachment and lipofuscin accumulation tend to be absent or minimal, and the presence of these changes increases the likelihood of malignancy.[79,80] In the iris, clinical features considered to be suggestive of malignancy include large size (i.e., > 3 mm), pigment scatter, and prominent vascularity.[81,82]

MANAGEMENT

Patients with suspicious choroidal and iris nevi are observed by comparing ophthalmoscopic and slit-lamp appearances with baseline photographs, using normal landmarks as reference points and taking into account variation in photographic magnification or exposure. It is also useful to measure tumor thickness by ultrasonography, at least at the first visit. Initially, patients are seen after 2 or 3 months and eventually after 6 to 12 monthly intervals.

MELANOCYTOMA

INTRODUCTION

Melanocytoma is a rare type of nevus,[83,84] which unlike melanoma is almost as common in non-Caucasians as in Caucasians. Most diagnosed melanocytomas arise within the optic nerve head, where they tend to be black, with feathery margins extending into retina. These tumors can arise anywhere in the uveal tract, including the ciliary body from where they may extend into the anterior chamber and into the episclera. It is likely that many melanocytomas away from optic disc are clinically mistaken for melanoma and are treated as such.[85] Some melanocytomas show minimal growth over several years. Optic disc tumors can cause acute visual loss as a result of venous occlusion or infarction and swelling of the tumor. Necrosis of a ciliary body melanocytoma may cause uveitis, pigment dispersion, and melanomalytic glaucoma.[86] Rarely, a patient diagnosed as having melanocytoma is eventually found to have a melanoma,[87] and there may be some debate concerning whether such a case represents a misdiagnosed melanoma or a melanocytoma that has undergone malignant transformation.

MANAGEMENT

Patients with melanocytoma are usually kept under observation, so that any malignancy is detected early. It is likely that some choroidal and ciliary body melanocytomas are misdiagnosed as melanoma and treated by brachytherapy. Ciliary body melanocytomas can be treated by local resection to prevent the complications mentioned above.

UVEAL METASTASIS

INTRODUCTION

Uveal metastases tend to arise from primary tumors in breast, lung, kidney, gastrointestinal tract, and pancreas.[88] The primary source is unknown in about 10% of females and 25% of males. Most metastases form in posterior choroid, growing rapidly to cause atrophy of the RPE, so that they appear as pale, white-yellow, smooth lesions with indistinct margins. Carcinoid tumors may have an orange or gold color, and metastatic cutaneous melanomas may be light brown or deeply pigmented. About 20% of all uveal metastases are multifocal and bilateral. There is usually an extensive serous retinal detachment, causing visual loss.

Rarely, metastases occur in the iris,[89] optic nerve head, or retina, where they tend to be irregular and friable.

INVESTIGATION

Patients with symptomatic uveal metastases usually present with a short ocular history. The ocular metastasis is often the first manifestation of the disease, except in patients with breast cancer, who usually give a history of previous treatment of their primary tumor. Most metastases can readily be recognized by their ophthalmoscopic appearance, and the diagnosis is facilitated in the minority of patients with multiple or bilateral tumors. Echography and MRI may demonstrate features characteristic of metastases, but neither test is pathognomonic. Documentation of rapid growth over a few weeks may aid differentiation from melanoma. A tissue diagnosis may be obtained by FNAB[90] or incisional biopsy, with the help of special immunohistochemistry.

If the site of the primary tumor is known, then investigations are guided by the need for staging. If there is no known primary disease, examination should focus on breast in women, and lung, kidney, gastrointestinal tract, and pancreas in both women and men. This would involve full history and physical examination, chest radiography or CT, sputum cytology, serum biochemistry, abdominal CT, fecal occult blood, urinalysis, and, in women, mammography. A tissue diagnosis is necessary, so that biopsy should be taken from the primary tumor, or an extraocular metastasis, or from the intraocular tumor, whichever is easiest. In all patients, it is important to perform a brain scan to identify intracranial metastases, which could be treated by radiotherapy at the same time as the intraocular tumor. Some workers also advocate radiological examination of weight-bearing bones, so that treatment of subclinical metastases might be given early to prevent pathological fractures and loss of mobility.

MANAGEMENT

Observation

If a metastatic tumor is small and asymptomatic, or if the patient is scheduled to receive systemic chemotherapy, it may be reasonable to keep the lesion under observation. After any treatment, patients need to be monitored periodically to detect possible local tumor relapse, which is especially likely after systemic chemotherapy.

External Beam Radiotherapy

Indications

External beam radiotherapy has long been the standard form of treatment for an intraocular metastasis and is indicated if vision is threatened.

Technique

Intraocular metastases in a patient with a poor prognosis for survival (e.g., lung carcinoma), are treated with 30 Gy delivered in ten fractions over 2 or 3 weeks. If the prognosis for survival is good, as in patients with breast carcinoma, or carcinoid, then a total dose of 45 Gy is delivered in 2 Gy fractions, that is, 5 days each week for 4½ weeks.

Results

The large majority of uveal metastases respond to external radiotherapy, with rapid regression within a few weeks, resolution of the retinal detachment, and improvement in vision. Most patients die before radiational complications have had time to develop, except for patients with breast carcinoma or carcinoid tumors, who have a better prognosis.

Contraindications

In patients with very extensive intraocular disease and an uncomfortable eye, enucleation may be the only way of relieving pain.

Plaque Radiotherapy

Indications

If the tumor is small, plaque radiotherapy may be as effective as and more convenient for the patient than external beam radiotherapy, being completed in a few days instead of several weeks. Such rapid treatment is especially beneficial if the patient is unwell or has a short life expectancy. Brachytherapy may also be useful as a secondary form of treatment, after failure of external beam radiotherapy, chemotherapy, or hormonal therapy.

Technique

The surgical techniques are similar to those described for uveal melanoma, except that the apex dose is smaller, usually being approximately 50–70 Gy. Wide safety margins are necessary, because metastases tend to have indistinct boundaries.

Results

In ideal cases, the results of plaque radiotherapy are good, most lesions showing rapid regression.[91] There is an increased likelihood of local tumor recurrence because small, posterior, amelanotic tumors may be difficult to localize accurately and because lateral tumor extensions may not be recognized.

Contraindications

The main contraindication is lack of confidence about delivering an adequate dose of radiation to the entire tumor, either because the tumor is thick or because it is poorly defined.

CHOROIDAL HEMANGIOMA

INTRODUCTION

Choroidal hemangiomas may be circumscribed or diffuse.[92] The circumscribed variety tends to present in adulthood as an indistinct tumor adjacent to the optic nerve or fovea. The diffuse type is usually diagnosed in childhood in association with the Sturge-Weber syndrome. Histologically, these hemangiomas are of the cavernous type, or the mixed, cavernous-capillary type. The circumscribed hemangiomas tend to cause a lacy-white fibrous proliferation over the tumor surface, occasionally with osseous metaplasia. Both varieties may remain asymptomatic or may progress, causing visual loss as a result of macular edema and serous retinal detachment. Ultimately the eye can become blind and painful as a result of neovascular glaucoma.

INVESTIGATION

Choroidal hemangiomas are diagnosed by their pink color, their posterior location, and their indistinct edges. Although they fill rapidly on fluorescein angiography, this is not a reliable diagnostic sign. Indocyanine green angiography is considered to be more helpful, showing rapid hyperfluorescence within a minute and "washout" of dye in the later frames.[18] High-intensity echoes are seen on echography, and Doppler scans may demonstrate pulsation, but these features are only suggestive and not diagnostic of hemangioma. Magnetic resonance imaging demonstrates features that are usually different from those of melanoma.[19] Computed tomography will demonstrate calcification within any osseous metaplasia.

MANAGEMENT

Photocoagulation

Indications

Treatment is indicated for symptomatic lesions. Photocoagulation aims to induce resorbtion of the subretinal fluid and to create extensive chorioretinal adhesions over the tumor (Fig. 63–15).[93,94] The entire tumor surface is covered with closely packed 0.2-second, 200- to 500-micron argon laser burns, which are just strong enough to produce a slight white reaction. A single treatment session may achieve resolution of the retinal detachment and improvement in vision, but many patients require repeat treatment.

Transpupillary Thermotherapy (TTT)

There are a few anecdotal reports of successful treatment of circumscribed choroidal hemangiomas using long-duration applications of diode laser phototherapy.[95,96]

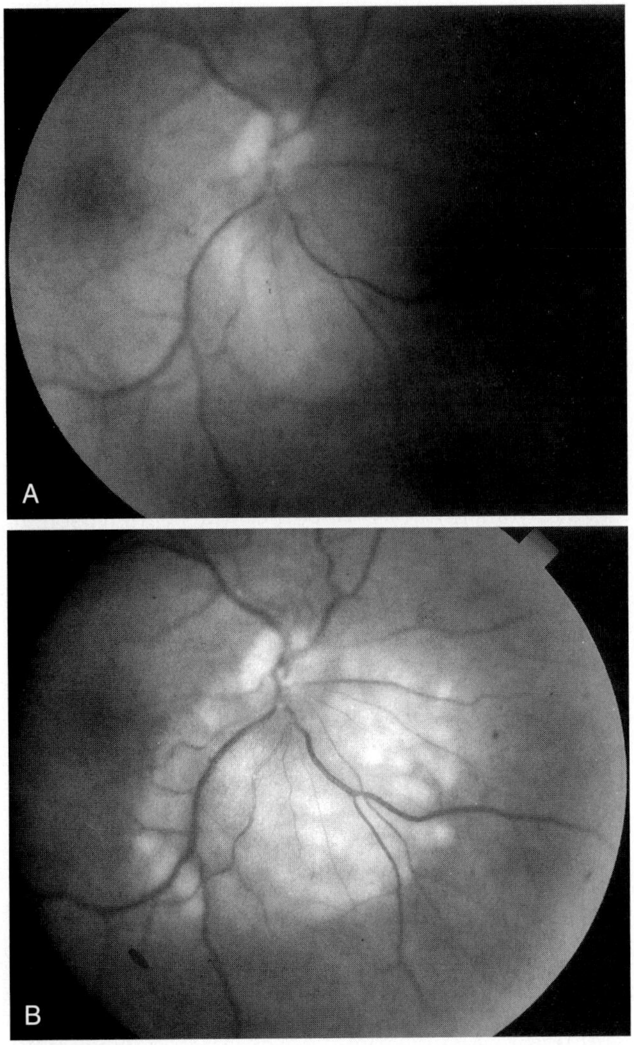

Figure 63–15. Choroidal hemangioma in the right eye before photocoagulation *(A)*, and immediately after treatment *(B)*. (Courtesy of Jerry A. Shields, M.D.)

PHOTODYNAMIC THERAPY (PDT)

A small number of circumscribed choroidal hemangiomas have been treated with photodynamic therapy using verteporfin, adopting the techniques used for choroidal neovascularization.[94a] Early results are very encouraging, with rapid resolution of the subretinal fluid, tumor flattening, and improvement in vision.

Radiotherapy

Indications

An alternative to phototherapy is radiotherapy, which has received much attention in recent years.[97,98] The treatment is aimed only at inducing resolution of the retinal detachment, and does not attempt to destroy the tumor itself.

Methods

External beam radiotherapy is delivered by giving a total dose of 12.5 to 20 Gy, in 6 to 10 divided fractions. A lateral field is used to prevent cataract. If the tumor does not extend close to the optic disc or fovea, then brachytherapy may be preferred, aiming to deliver a dose of 45 Gy to the tumor apex. Some workers prefer proton beam radiotherapy, which delivers smaller amounts of radiation to normal tissues.[99,100]

Results

The visual results are good if the tumor is both small and located away from the macula, and if the visual acuity is still good at the time of treatment. In patients with the Sturge-Weber syndrome, there may be other causes of visual loss, such as glaucoma, buphthalmos, amblyopia, and intracranial disease. Resolution of the retinal detachment may occur very slowly so that adjunctive photocoagulation may be useful. Prolonged exudative retinal detachment may cause a macular hole, which may rarely result in a rhegmatogenous retinal detachment.

Contraindications

Treatment is contraindicated if there are no symptoms. In very advanced cases, enucleation is the only treatment that can prevent pain.

RARE UVEAL TUMORS

Neurilemmomas, neurofibromas, and leiomyomas[101] are rare, benign tumors arising from ciliary nerves, fibrous tissue, and smooth muscle respectively.[94] They compress and displace normal tissues, causing lens damage and dilated episcleral vessels if located in ciliary body. Clinically, they usually resemble melanoma. If possible, they are treated by local resection, which also provides histological confirmation of the diagnosis.

EPITHELIAL TUMORS

MEDULLOEPITHELIOMA

Medulloepithelioma usually presents in childhood as a gray, white, or pink ciliary body mass, which may be polycystic and irregular, with a diffuse proliferation of tumor cells behind the lens, mimicking a cyclitic membrane.[102,103] The lens is sometimes cataractous and notched. Neovascular glaucoma is common. The tumor is usually malignant, but only rarely causes death, which is by intracranial spread or metastatic disease. Large tumors and those with diffuse spread are treated by enucleation. If the tumor is small and localized, then iridocyclectomy may be possible, although there is a high risk of local tumor recurrence.

ADENOMA AND ADENOCARCINOMA

Adenomas and adenocarcinomas usually arise in the ciliary epithelium, but may occur in the RPE.[104,105] In the ciliary body, they may be pigmented or amelanotic, depending on whether they arise in pigmented or nonpigmented epithelium.[106,107] They may be benign or malignant, in which case they tend to be only locally invasive, although rare deaths from intracranial spread or metastatic disease have been reported. Treatment is by local resection or enucleation, depending on tumor size.

CYSTS

Primary epithelial cysts posterior to the iris are deeply pigmented or transparent, according to the epithelium in which they arise.[94] They may be bilateral. Significant ocular morbidity is unusual.

Anterior chamber implantation cysts can enlarge to cause cataract, epithelial downgrowth, and glaucoma. They can be treated by iridocyclectomy, taking care not to rupture the cyst within the eye, using similar techniques described for iridocyclectomy (see above). If the cyst is adherent to cornea, then the internal corneal lamella or full-thickness cornea is excised *en bloc* with the cyst. If the excision is extensive, the patient may develop cataract and corneal decompensation, requiring lens extraction and corneal grafting at a later stage.

RETINAL TUMORS

RETINOBLASTOMA

INTRODUCTION

The division of each cell in the body is regulated by the RB1 suppressor gene, which is located at region 14 on the long arm of chromosome 13 (i.e., 13q14). Malignancy develops only when both the maternal and the paternal genes are inactivated (i.e., Knudson's two-hit hypothesis). In patients with germline RB1 mutations, all cells in the body have one defective gene, including the germ cells, which transmit the mutation to 50% of offspring. Neoplastic transformation occurs when the second gene mutates, resulting in multiple retinoblastomas and extraocular malignancies. In patients with the somatic form of the disease, both mutations take place in the same retinal cell, so that only a solitary retinoblastoma occurs without any increased risk of extraocular primary malignancies and no possibility of familial transmission. Sporadic retinoblastoma is due to somatic mutation in 75% of patients and germline mutation in the remainder.

Retinoblastoma cells have hyperchromatic nuclei and scanty cytoplasm. In well differentiated tumors, rosettes of columnar tumor cells may form around a membrane bound lumen or around a mass of neural fibres. Most tumors develop areas of necrosis, which give rise to calcification.

Retinoblastoma commences as a small, white or transparent intraretinal nodule, sometimes with visible flecks of calcification. The tumor can extend into the vitreous cavity to seed extensively, forming multiple preretinal tumors, vitreous opacities, nodules at the pupil margin, and a pseudo-hypopyon (endophytic growth). In other cases, white multilobulated masses form beneath a detached retina (exophytic growth). Most patients with retinoblastoma present with leukocoria and squint. Advanced retinoblastoma can cause a wide variety of complications, including rubeosis iridis, secondary glaucoma, corneal edema, vitreous hemorrhage, hyphema, uveitis, and severe periocular inflammation, mimicking orbital cellulitis. Retinoblastoma tends to invade the optic nerve to reach the subarachnoid space and disseminate throughout the central nervous system. Choroidal invasion can occur, with extraocular extension in advanced cases, resulting in proptosis, invasion of bone and sinuses, and metastasis to regional lymph nodes and other parts of the body. Rarely, a low-grade, diffuse retinoblastoma may infiltrate the retina without showing endophytic or exophytic growth, and this is more likely to develop in older children.

Patients with germinal retinoblastoma are at a high risk of developing multiple tumors in either eye, and these may be of the exophytic or endophytic variety. They also have an increased risk of developing nonocular primary tumors, especialy if they have received external beam radiotherapy in early life.[108,108a] There is debate as to whether the radiotherapy causes some of the nonocular tumors or whether it is a marker for other factors. The commonest second malignant neoplasms (SMNs) are osteosarcoma, leiomyosarcoma, and malignant fibrous histiocytoma. About 3% of patients with germline RB1 mutations develop a pinealoblastoma, also referred to as "primitive neural ectodermal tumor (PNET)" in the pineal gland or parasellar region, or "trilateral retinoblastoma" because it has similar histological features to retinoblastoma.[109–111] Clinical manifestations of this tumor include fever, vomiting, meningism, somnolence, convulsions, and headache.

Metastatic disease is now very rare in developed countries. It usually presents within 2 years and tends to involve regional lymph nodes, lung, brain, bones, and other organs. Prognostic factors for metastatic disease have been graded[112] and include tumor extension into optic nerve,[113,114] extensive uveal involvement,[113,115] tumor volume greater than 1 cm^3, molecular and genetic abnormalities,[114a] orbital invasion, and delayed treatment of orbital recurrence.

INVESTIGATION

Patients with retinoblastoma usually present with leukocoria, squint, or a positive family history. A thorough history is obtained from the parents, identifying any risk factors for conditions such as retinopathy of prematurity and toxocariasis, and enquiring whether any other family members had retinoblastoma or ocular malformations. In most cases, the diagnosis is straightforward and based on ophthalmoscopy. Once the main tumor is identified, a meticulous search for any other small tumor nodules is essential, and this requires complete mydriasis, 360-degree indentation, and usually examination under anesthesia. Full examination of the fellow eye may reveal bilateral disease. Examination is performed under the operating microscope or, if possible, with the slit lamp to identify any cataract, rubeosis, uveitis, or anterior chamber deposits, which may mimic inflammation and hypopyon. Detailed color drawings and color photographs using a wide-angle hand-held camera are invaluable (Retcam 120, Massie Research Laboratories Inc. Pleasanton, CA, USA).

Echography provides accurate measurements of the tumor dimensions and the tumor-to-disc distance. In addition, it may demonstrate calcification within retinoblastoma tissue. Such calcification is demonstrated more reliably, however, by computed tomography. The MRI features of retinoblastoma on pre- and post-contrast studies are shared by other solid intraocular tumors, such as medulloepithelioma and retinal hemangioma, so that MRI studies are most helpful in differentiating solid intraocular tumors from retinal detachment in conditions such as Coats' disease.[116] Magnetic resonance imaging with gadolinium enhancement and fat suppression may detect optic nerve invasion, perhaps also demonstrating the extent of such invasion. Both MRI and CT may demonstrate a pinealoblastoma in a patient with a germline RB1 mutation.

The diagnosis of retinoblastoma may be uncertain despite full examination in a small number of patients. Fine-needle aspiration biopsy and incisional or excisional biopsy are generally regarded as being absolutely contraindicated, except when there is a large tumor fungating out of the orbit. In very exceptional cases, some workers rarely perform FNAB and then only as a last resort. Because of the high risk of orbital seeding, the biopsy needle is passed through cornea and through the periphery of the iris.

Measurements of neuron-specific enolase and lactate dehydrogenase in the aqueous are no longer regarded as being of value.

The clinical findings are documented by color photography and by preparing annotated color drawings.

The Reese-Ellsworth Classification was developed for the prediction of ocular retention (not patient survival) after treatment.[117] It is still widely used for tumor classification, but newer systems are being designed.

With retinoblastoma, systemic examination may reveal dysmorphic features caused by the 13q deletion syndrome. In patients with pseudoretinoblastoma, systemic examination may identify conditions such as tuberous sclerosis and the rubella syndrome. In patients with germline mutations, pinealoblastoma and other systemic primary tumors should be excluded by a brain scan. If there is a high risk of metastatic disease, whole-body scans are indicated, together with bone marrow aspiration and lumbar puncture, which can be performed when the patient is anesthetized for treatment of the ocular disease.

TREATMENT

Photocoagulation

Indications

If a tumor is less than 2 disc diameters (DD) in size and less than 3 mm in thickness, and if it is post-equatorial but not close to the fovea, it may be treatable by photocoagulation.[1a,118]

Technique

The objective of photocoagulation is to deprive the tumor of its blood supply by placing a double row of heavy 0.5-second, 500-micron, argon burns around the tumor (Fig. 63–16). Special care is taken not to treat the tumor itself, as this may cause vitreous seeding and tumor dissemination in the eye. A visual field defect is inevitable and depends on the location of the tumor. Some tumors continue to grow even after repeated sessions so that other forms of treatment are required.

Contraindications

Photocoagulation is contraindicated when there is (1) optic disc involvement, (2) vitreous seeding, (3) tumor diameter greater than 3 DD, or (4) tumor thickness greater than 4 mm.

Transpupillary Thermotherapy

Indications

The indications of thermotherapy are similar to those of photocoagulation.[119] In addition, TTT is useful as consolidation therapy, to ensure that complete tumor destruction is achieved after another type of treatment is used. TTT can be combined with intravenous carboplatin for greater effect (i.e., chemotherapy).

Technique

An infrared beam is aimed at the tumor itself, using an appropriate contact lens. The power and duration of treatment is adjusted upwards in a stepwise fashion until a gray discoloration is achieved in the treated area without vascular spasm. The duration of each laser application varies between 5 and 20 minutes. Anterior tumors can be treated using a trans-scleral applicator.[120]

Cryotherapy

Indications

Treatment with cryotherapy is indicated for pre-equatorial tumors less than 3 mm thick and less than about 3 mm wide.[121] Cryotherapy is also useful for breaking the blood-ocular barrier and enhancing the penetration of systemic chemotherapeutic agents into the vitreous.

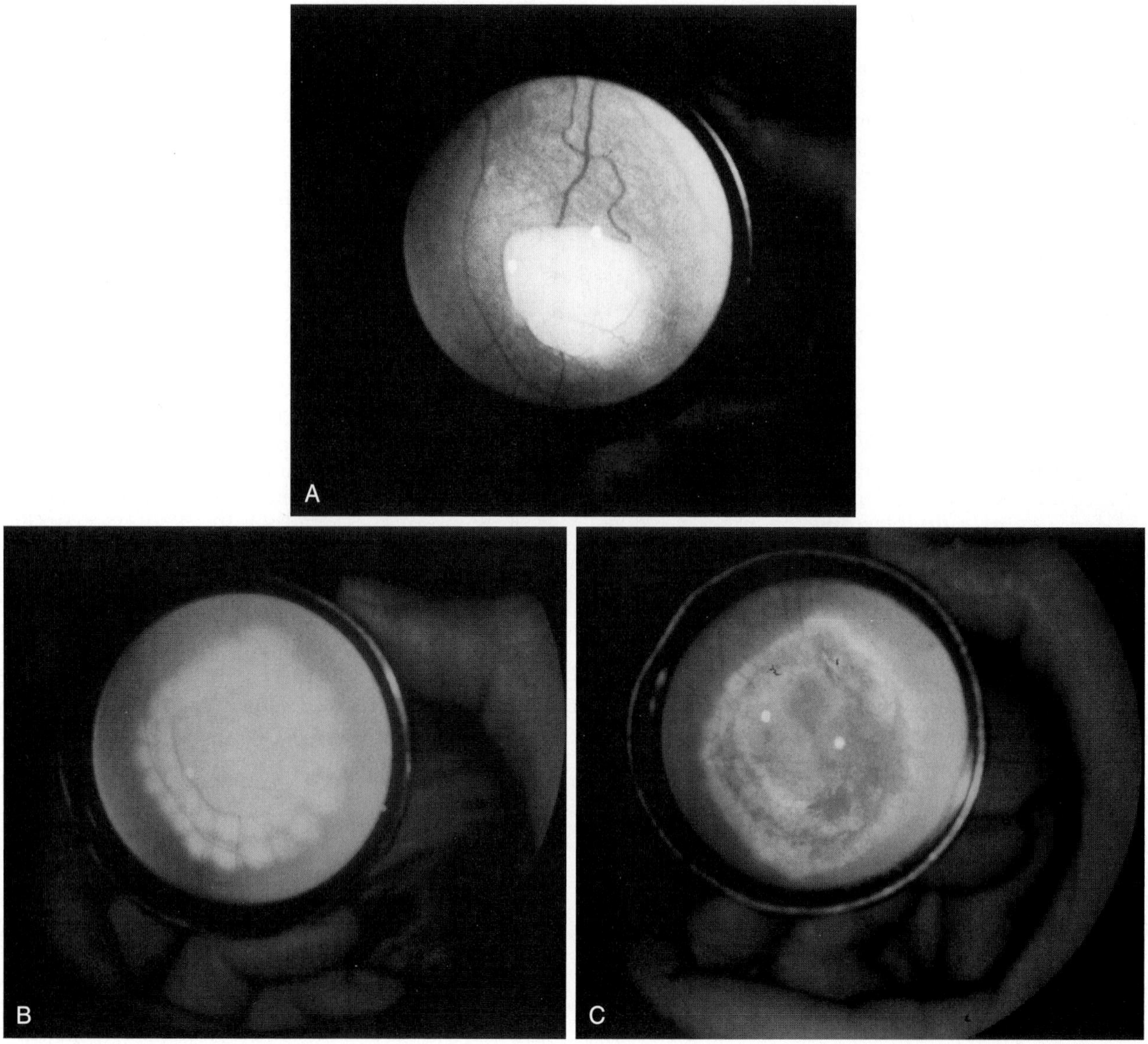

Figure 63–16. Fundus photograph showing a small retinoblastoma nodule before photocoagulation *(A)*, immediately afterwards *(B)*, and after resolution of the lesion *(C)*. (Courtesy of Jerry A. Shields, M.D.)

Technique

The triple freeze–thaw technique is used, ensuring that each ice-ball completely envelops the tumor.

Results

A single treatment is usually successful if the tumor is less than 1 mm thick. Larger tumors may require several sessions of cryotherapy.[122]

Contraindications

Cryotherapy is contraindicated if there is any vitreous seeding. Treatment of macular and juxtapapillary tumors with this method may cause visual loss as a result of a macular scar or optic atrophy.

Brachytherapy

Indications

Plaque radiotherapy is indicated for tumors up to 15 mm in diameter and 8 mm in thickness that do not extend close to optic disc or fovea, and that are too large for cryotherapy or photocoagulation (Fig. 63–17). Brachytherapy may also be useful in salvaging an eye when a tumor has not responded adequately to another form of treatment.[123]

Technique

The surgical techniques are similar to those described for melanoma, except that the usual apex dose is approximately 40 Gy.[123]

Contraindications

As a rule, brachytherapy is contraindicated if there is any vitreous seeding, unless there is minimal seeding very close to the tumor surface, which is likely to be included in the radiational field. Tumors greater than 15 mm in diameter or more than 8 mm thick are likely to recur, so chemoreduction may be performed beforehand.

Charged Particle Teletherapy

A very small number of patients with retinoblastoma have been treated with proton beam radiotherapy, but this technique is not widely accepted as a method of treatment for this tumor.

External Beam Radiotherapy

Indications

External beam radiotherapy is indicated when a tumor is not suitable for other forms of treatment, such as brachytherapy, phototherapy, or cryotherapy, because of large size or vitreous seeding.

In patients with hereditary retinoblastoma, external beam radiotherapy is used only when it offers the last hope of conserving some vision. This is because of the risk of inducing a second malignant neoplasm.

After enucleation, chemotherapy is employed if there is extension of tumor beyond the lamina cribrosa of the optic nerve or if there is macroscopic choroidal invasion. External beam radiotherapy to the orbit is added if there is tumor extension trans-sclerally or to the cut end of optic nerve, with the immediate fear of death from intracranial spread taking precedence over any concern about the future development of a second malignant neoplasm.

Technique

Retinoblastoma is usually treated with 45 to 50 Gy, delivered in 1.8 to 2.0 Gy fractions, with the total dose depending on the size of the tumor.[124]

If possible, a lateral field is used, to avoid cataract. If the tumor is post-equatorial, the anterior margin of the beam is generally aligned with the bony orbital rim, which corresponds to the equator of the eye. The beam is angled to avoid irradiating the contralateral eye unless there is bilateral disease.

If the tumor extends pre-equatorially, the lateral field can be combined with an anterior field, protecting the lens with a divergent block. The anterior extent of the lateral field can be placed as far anteriorly as the fleshy lateral canthus, which corresponds with the posterior pole of the lens. The amounts of radiation given by the lateral and anterior fields can be delivered in varying proportions, for example, 4:1 respectively. If possible, not more than 15 Gy is given through the anterior portal.

An anterior field irradiates the whole eye, to cause cataract. This complication can be avoided by placing a shield in front of the lens, but the dose of radiation directly behind the lens is reduced, increasing the risk of local tumor recurrence.

The Schipper technique uses a 6 to 8 MeV beam, which is highly collimated by means of a lead collimator. This is positioned by means of a rod resting on transparent corneal contact lenses (Fig. 63–18).[125] The beam can be aimed with an accuracy of 3 mm and has a penumbra of 1.5 mm. The field is D-shaped, and extends from a point 10 mm behind the globe, either to the posterior border of the lens, or, if a pre-equatorial tumor is present, to a point 3 mm more anteriorly. The fellow eye is avoided by rotating the table by 40 degrees. The head is immobilized using a transparent face mold and a vacuum pillow. Infants are treated under general anesthesia.

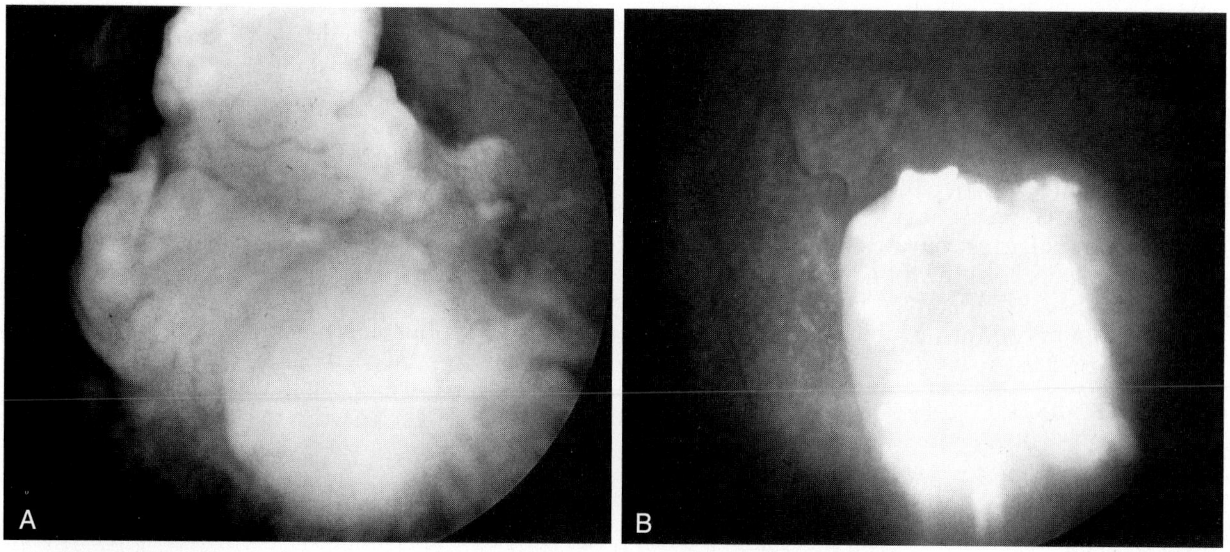

Figure 63–17. Fundus photograph showing a retinoblastoma nodule before plaque radiotherapy *(A)*, and after regression *(B)*. (Courtesy of Carol L. Shields, M.D.)

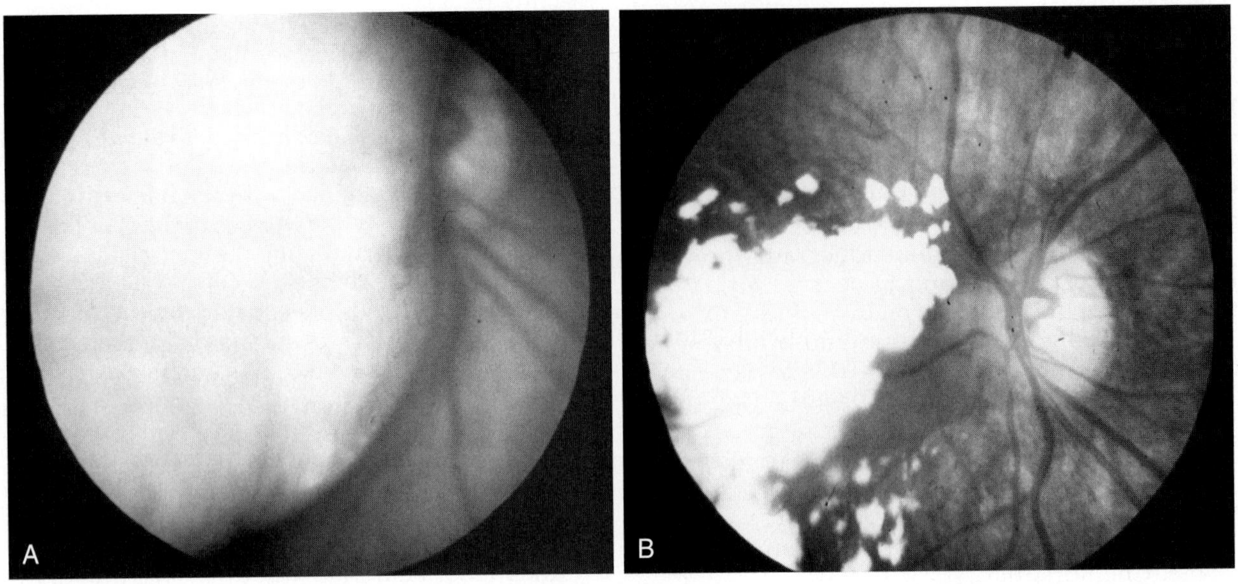

Figure 63–18. Fundus photograph of the left eye showing a large retinoblastoma before external beam radiotherapy *(A)* and after regression *(B)*. (Courtesy of Prof. Dr. N. Bornfeld.)

Results

With radiotherapy and appropriate salvage therapy in resistant cases, it is possible to conserve more than 90% of eyes classified in Reese-Ellsworth groups I–III, with the chances of success diminishing greatly in eyes with more extensive disease.[126,127]

Cataract is inevitable if the lens receives a sufficient dose of radiation. There may also be external eye complications as a result of lacrimal gland damage or conjunctival disease. In patients with hereditary retinoblastoma, radiotherapy increases the risk of a second malignant neoplasm approximately fivefold. Another problem is orbital bone growth arrest.[128] The chances of developing a second malignant neoplasm and orbital bone arrest diminish if radiotherapy is given after the first year of life. Radiation to the brain may cause pituitary insufficiency.

Contraindications

External beam radiotherapy should be avoided if at all possible in patients with hereditary retinoblastoma, to avoid a second malignant neoplasm, and in children less than 2 years old, to prevent orbital bone growth arrest. If more than 50% of the retina is involved by tumor the eye is usually enucleated because the chances of achieving tumor control are minimal, unless chemoreduction techniques are used.

Enucleation

Indications

Indications for enucleation include (1) no prospect of useful vision, (2) tumor filling more than 60% of the eye; (3) glaucoma, (4) diffuse infiltrating retinoblastoma, and (5) failed conservative treatment.

Technique

Enucleation is performed with special modifications. To ensure that the correct eye is removed, the forehead is marked on the side of the eye to be enucleated and, after draping the patient and covering the other eye, the tumor is visualized by indirect ophthalmoscopy. Scleral perforation is prevented by using a gentle technique, and by placing any traction sutures in the muscle stumps instead of the sclera, or avoiding sutures altogether and using artery forceps on long muscle stumps to hold the eye. An optic nerve stump of more than 10 mm is removed by using small, minimally curved enucleation scissors, which are pushed posteriorly along the medial wall of the orbit while the eye is pulled forward. It is important not to tilt the scissors laterally. Crushing of the nerve with clamps or snares may prejudice histological examination and is therefore avoided when tumor extension along the nerve is a possibility.

If the enucleated eye is opened fresh, for research or other purposes, artifactual spread of tumor tissue may complicate histological examination and subsequent management of the patient. Special precautions are therefore necessary to avoid these problems.

Complications

The most serious complications are (1) transection of tumor and orbital seeding when the optic nerve is cut too close too the globe and (2) inadvertent perforation of the globe, which carries the same risk.

Contraindications

As with childhood melanoma, enucleation is contraindicated if the parents have not been informed of any conservative forms of therapy having a reasonable chance of success.

Chemoreduction

Indications

Chemotherapy alone may completely destroy an intraocular retinoblastoma,[129,129a] but is usually administered to reduce tumor size prior to another form of treatment (i.e., chemoreduction) (Fig. 63–19). For example, with larger and more peripheral tumors, chemoreduction may allow plaque radiotherapy, phototherapy, or cryotherapy to be used instead of external beam radiotherapy, thereby reducing the risk of a second malignant neoplasm and orbital bone growth arrest.[130–132] In patients with advanced and bilateral disease, chemoreduction followed by external beam radiotherapy may allow conservation of some useful vision even in the presence of total retinal detachment.[133] A large fungating orbital tumor may be reduced to a size that can be treated surgically in a less mutilating fashion than would otherwise be possible. Chemoreduction for retinoblastoma may prevent intracranial neuroblastic malignancy (trilateral retinoblastoma).[133a]

Technique

Several protocols for administering chemotherapy have been developed, which generally use agents such as JM8 (carboplatin), VM-26 (teniposide) or Etoposide (VP-16). Focal treatment is administered when the tumor size has reduced sufficiently.

Complications

Recurrent tumor after chemoreduction is more likely in eyes with subretinal seeds at initial presentation.[137a] Such seeds are more common in patients with large tumors (i.e., diameter >15 mm) and young age at treatment (i.e., <1 year).

Systemic chemotherapy may be associated with a wide variety of monocular complications.[137b] Carboplatin can cause bone marrow suppression with immunosuppression and hemorrhage, nephropathy, and deafness. Etoposide has been rarely associated with leukemia.

Contraindications

In view of the uncertain long-term risk of second malignancy, chemotherapy for intraocular retinoblastoma tends to be avoided except as a means of preventing the use of external beam radiotherapy or if the tumor cannot be controlled satisfactorily with other means. Other exclusion criteria include iris neovascularization; tumor invasion into anterior chamber, optic nerve, choroid or extraocular tissue; and inadequate renal, hepatic or auditory function.

TREATMENT OF SYSTEMIC DISEASE

After enucleation, systemic chemotherapy is indicated if there is a high risk of metastatic disease from massive invasion of the choroid, orbit, or optic nerve.

Metastatic retinoblastoma is treated with high-dose chemotherapy, total body irradiation, intrathecal chemotherapy, and bone marrow rescue.[134–136] Some workers also use cyclosporine to inhibit multidrug resistance.[130]

Pinealoblastoma is treated with systemic and intrathecal chemotherapy combined with craniospinal irradiation.[137] Gamma knife radiotherapy seems promising for localized tumors.

FOLLOW-UP

After treatment, patients with retinoblastoma are observed for local tumor recurrence, late complications, and, in patients with a germline RB1 mutation, new tumor formation.

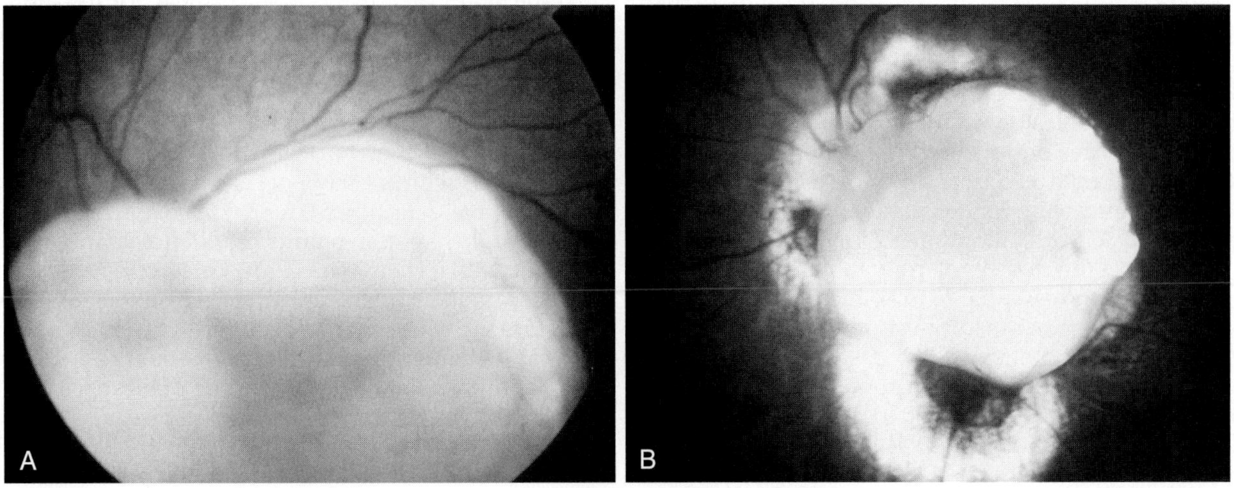

Figure 63–19. Fundus photograph of the left eye showing a juxtapapillary retinoblastoma before treatment *(A)*, and after chemoreduction and phototherapy *(B)*. (Courtesy of Carol L. Shields, M.D.)

After conservative therapy, patients are examined under anesthesia at 3 to 6 weeks and then every 2 or 3 months for the first year. After external beam radiotherapy, tumors may regress in several ways, with no visible change (type 0 regression); a "cottage-cheese" mass of calcification (type I regression), a 'fish-flesh' lesion (type II regression); or a mixture of these two types of regression (type III regression). Plaque radiotherapy tends to result in a flat scar (type IV regression).

The younger the child, the greater the risk of new tumors, which tend to develop more anteriorly in the eye. Patients with a germline RB1 mutation are observed for the development of new lesions and seen every 2 months until the age of 1 year, then every 3 months during the second year of life and every 4 to 6 months until the age of 4 to 6 years. There is no consensus as to whether examinations should be performed indefinitely (for example, once a year), or whether they can be stopped, and if so whether this should be when the child reaches the age of 8 or some other age. Because early diagnosis of pinealoblastoma improves the prognosis for survival, some workers (and certainly not all) advocate a contrast MRI brain scan for patients with a germline mutation, to be repeated every 6 months until the age 4 to 5 years.[109] Follow-up is not generally recommended for the screening of second malignant neoplasms, but patients are advised to seek a medical opinion if they develop any new symptoms lasting for more than a week.

After enucleation for advanced retinoblastoma, the risk of orbital recurrence diminishes after about 18 months.[138] Some workers advocate periodic scanning of the head and orbits in these patients.

FAMILY STUDIES AND GENETIC COUNSELING

In families with a germline RB1 mutation, it is possible to detect the mutation before birth, obtaining a chorionic villus biopsy sample by amniocentesis.

All patients with multifocal tumors and about 10% with a solitary lesion have a germline mutation. If a parent is known to have the mutation, then about 50% of all siblings will inherit the mutation. If there are multiple tumors and no parent has the disease, then about 2% of siblings will have the mutation. If the patient has a solitary retinoblastoma and the family history is negative the chances of having the mutation are approximately 1% in each sibling and 1% in each offspring.

Genetic counseling is offered after the acute crisis has passed and within 3 months of diagnosis, informing the parents of the chances of other family members being affected. It is essential to examine the eyes of both parents for retinocytoma. It is also necessary to examine all siblings and offspring (and, some would argue, even grandchildren) as soon as possible after birth, unless the mutation can be excluded in these individuals by molecular genetic techniques.[139] There seems to be agreement that the chances of developing retinoblastoma decline after the first 2 years of life, so that screening of relatives tends to be performed for about 4 or 5 years although there is no consensus about this.

RETINOCYTOMA

Retinocytoma is a rare, benign variant of retinoblastoma, which first grows a result of an RB1 gene mutation, and then undergoes spontaneous involution.[140,140a] Clinically, it resembles a retinoblastoma that has regressed after radiotherapy. Malignant transformation into a retinoblastoma can occur.[141]

ASTROCYTOMA

INTRODUCTION

Astrocytoma may occur in an otherwise healthy individual or as a manifestation of tuberous sclerosis or neurofibromatosis and is composed of fibrous or pleomorphic astrocytes.[142] It can occur as a flat, translucent, non-calcified, smooth lesion or as a white-yellow, multi-lobulated lesion (i.e. "mulberry tumor"), with yellow flecks of calcification. The tumor is usually located near or at the disc, but it may be peripheral. Multiple tumors may be present. Most tumors are asymptomatic but may rarely cause exudation or tractional retinal detachment. Vitreous hemorrhage may occur, especially if the lesion is disturbed surgically.

MANAGEMENT

The patient should be investigated for any systemic manifestations of tuberous sclerosis or neurofibromatosis. Molecular genetic studies are difficult because of the large size of the gene, the variety of mutations, and the high rate of mosaicism.[143]

RETINAL CAPILLARY HEMANGIOBLASTOMA

INTRODUCTION

Retinal capillary hemangioblastoma[144] is a hamartoma composed of capillaries surrounded by foamy interstitial cells. It commences as a tiny red nodule that grows into an orange mass with large feeder vessels. Fluid leakage results in circinate exudates, macular edema, and exudative retinal detachment. Fibrovascular proliferation into the vitreous with subsequent contraction can cause tractional retinal detachment, retinal tears, vitreous hemorrhage, and rhegmatogenous retinal detachment. Most retinal capillary angiomas are located peripherally, but some are juxtapapillary, showing either exophytic growth into the vitreous or diffuse endophytic growth in the retina. All patients with multiple retinal capillary angiomas and an unknown proportion of those with a solitary lesion have von Hippel-Lindau disease. This syndrome includes hemangioblastomas of the cerebellum and spinal cord, renal cell carcinoma, pheochromocytoma, and a variety of benign tumors.[144] The disease is inherited in an autosomal dominant fashion and follows Knudson's two-hit model similar to retinoblastoma.

INVESTIGATION

Retinal capillary angiomas are diagnosed by their characteristic ophthalmoscopic appearances. Multidisciplinary investigation is indicated for the detection of extraocular manifestations of von Hippel-Lindau disease. Patients and family members at risk require (1) annual retinal examination from the age of 5 years, (2) regular physical examination, (3) MRI brain scans for cerebellar and spinal hemangioblastomas, (4) abdominal CT or ultrasound scans for renal carcinoma and (5) urinary vanillyl mandelic acid (VMA) secretion measurements for pheochromocytoma.[145] Fluorescein angiography and fluoroscopy have been suggested as methods for facilitating the detection of early retinal lesions. If several members of the same family are affected, DNA studies may be possible, identifying which patients require regular screening.[146]

MANAGEMENT

Laser photocoagulation is still the first choice of treatment for small, retinal capillary angiomas, which should be ablated as soon as possible.

The surface of the angioma is treated with long-exposure, 500 micron, argon laser burns every week or two until the tumor is destroyed.[147] Treatment of the feeder vessels immediately prior to direct treatment of the angioma is controversial, as it may cause bleeding. If this is attempted, blood flow through the feeder vessels is stopped by pressing on the eye with the contact lens. If the tumor is not adequately destroyed, there may be increased exudation, with a risk of visual loss.

If a tumor is too large for photocoagulation (i.e. more than 2.5 DD) it may respond to cryotherapy, although this may need to be repeated after about 6 weeks (Fig. 63–20). Other methods include plaque radiotherapy,[148] and removal by vitrectomy.[149]

Juxtapapillary retinal capillary angiomas can sometimes be treated by photocoagulation without loss of vision.[150] An alternative approach is external beam radiotherapy,[151] although results are unpredictable (W. Friedrichs and associates, personal communication, International Symposium on Ocular Tumors, Israel, 1997).

CAVERNOUS RETINAL ANGIOMA

INTRODUCTION

A hamartoma, cavernous retinal angioma consists of a cluster of intra-retinal vascular aneurysms, which may

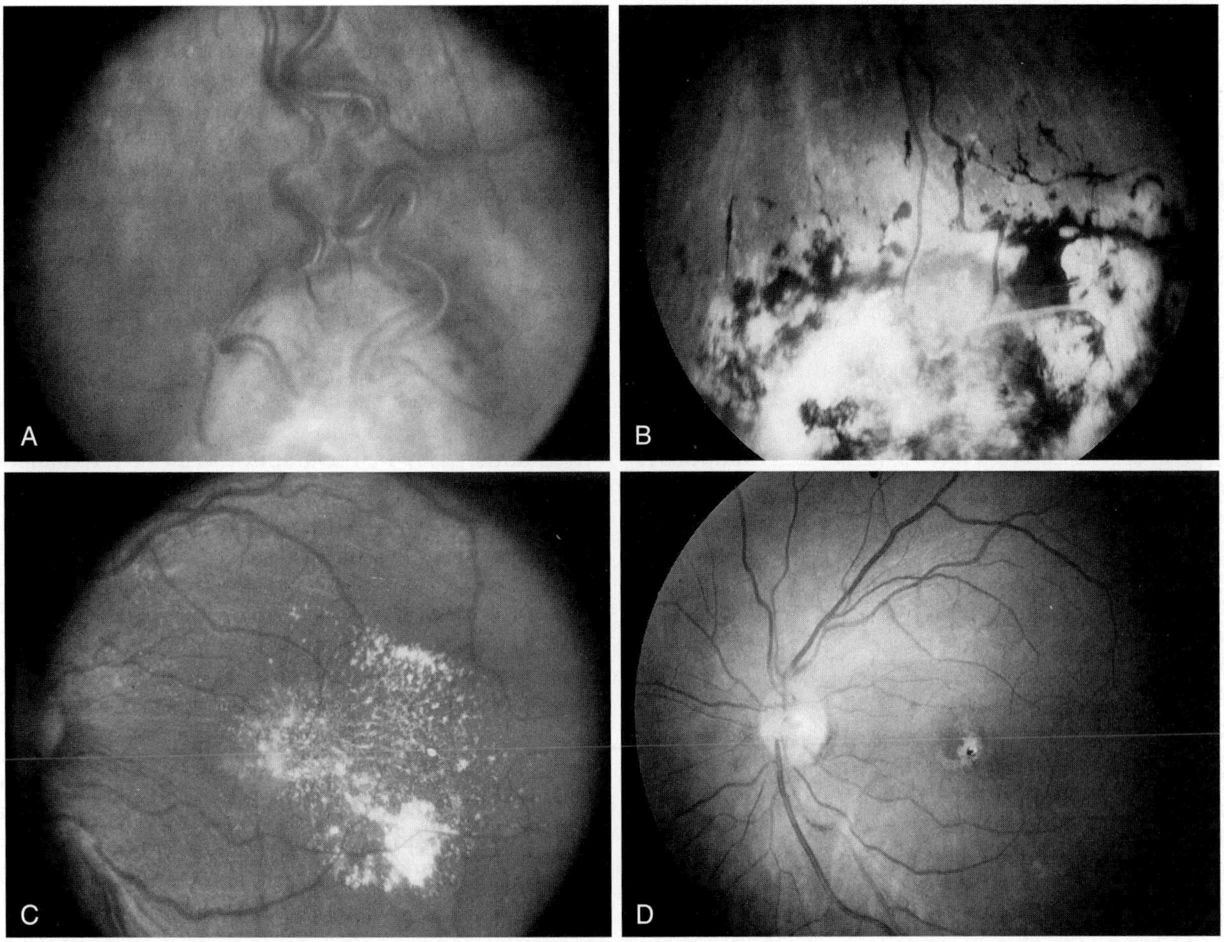

Figure 63–20. Fundus photograph of the left eye, showing an inferior retinal hemangioblastoma before cryotherapy *(A)*, and 17 years later *(B)*. Before treatment, there were extensive hard exudates at the macula *(C)*, which resolved with improvement of the visual acuity to 20/25 *(D)*. (Courtesy of Jerry A. Shields, M.D.)

cause visual loss as a result of epiretinal membrane formation or vitreous hemorrhage. It may be associated with cutaneous lesions and intracranial angiomas, which may cause intracranial hemorrhage. This syndrome may be inherited in an autosomal dominant fashion.

INVESTIGATION

An MRI brain scan is indicated to exclude intracranial disease. Family studies are also indicated in view of the inheritance of this condition.

MANAGEMENT

Treatment is not required unless there is recurrent vitreous hemorrhage, in which case it is suggested that cryotherapy may be preferable to photocoagulation (J. J. Augsburger, personal communication).

VASOPROLIFERATIVE TUMOR

This rare, non-neoplastic tumor is a raised, yellow, retinal or subretinal mass in the inferotemporal, preequatorial region, tending to form extensive retinal exudates that involve the fovea.[152,152a] Treatment is indicated when vision is threatened. A variety of techniques have been used, with mixed results.

INTRAOCULAR LYMPHOMA

INTRODUCTION

Intraocular lymphoma[153] (previously known as "reticulum cell sarcoma") usually develops after the age of 40 years, unless the patient is immunodeficient in which case it may occur earlier. The disease is a type of non-Hodgkin's lymphoma, composed of large, pleomorphic, B lymphocytes having large, indented nuclei and prominent nucleoli. Tumor cells form deposits between the RPE and Bruch's membrane and may infiltrate the retina, both diffusely and along the blood vessels, perhaps causing arteriolar occlusion. Other ocular manifestations include cells in the vitreous and anterior chamber, mimicking uveitis, as well as macular edema, exudative retinal detachment, and secondary glaucoma. Ocular involvement tends to be bilateral and asymmetric, presenting as blurred vision, floaters, photophobia, pain, and redness. Most patients with ocular lymphoma develop central nervous system disease within 2 years, dying about a year later. A minority of patients have infiltrates located predominantly in the choroid, and these are more likely to develop systemic, non-CNS disease. Rarely, patients with systemic lymphoma present with secondary ocular tumor, which usually involves the anterior uvea, perhaps mimicking a ring melanoma.

INVESTIGATION

Ocular lymphoma needs to be considered when a middle-aged, elderly, or immunocompromised patient presents with uveitis that is unresponsive to steroids. The diagnosis is confirmed by obtaining a vitreous sample, which may reveal cells with pathognomonic indented nuclei. Some workers advocate pars plana vitrectomy, whereas others report that better specimens are obtained using a 20-gauge needle attached to a syringe. The tumor cells are very fragile, and the diagnosis may be missed if the sample is not handled carefully. Steroid treatment should be stopped a few days beforehand as it may result in a false-negative biopsy. It is ideal to have a cytologist present in the operating room to receive and examine the specimen. Vitreous samples can also be analyzed for a raised interleukin-10 level[154] and for altered B- and T-gene rearrangements using the polymerase chain reaction.[155]

In view of the high risk of intracranial disease, the patient should have an MRI brain scan and a lumbar puncture. Bone marrow biopsies are also indicated.

TREATMENT

Ocular lymphoma is highly radiosensitive and responds to 40 to 50 Gy, delivered in 20 fractions over 4 weeks, to the whole eye. Recurrent disease can be treated with a course of intravitreal methotrexate.[156] The best visual results occur when vision is still good at the time of treatment. In view of the high incidence of CNS disease, all patients require regular assessment. Opinion is divided as to whether the CNS should be treated prophylactically.

REACTIVE LYMPHOID HYPERPLASIA

In this rare condition, follicular lymphocytic masses accumulate in the conjunctiva, ciliary body, and choroid, often simultaneously, to present as a white or pink tumor, which may be nodular or diffuse.[157] This condition can cause angle-closure glaucoma, exudative detachment, and features similar to uveitis. There may be a good response to systemic steroid therapy[158] or a small dose of external beam radiotherapy (i.e., 20 Gy).[153]

CONJUNCTIVAL TUMORS

NEVUS

Conjunctival nevi usually occur in the bulbar conjunctiva, and often contain numerous, small cysts. The likelihood of malignant transformation of histologically confirmed conjunctival nevi is presumed to be low.

Conjunctival nevi do not require treatment, but excision improves cosmesis, provides a diagnosis, and removes the threat of melanoma and is therefore advocated by some surgeons.

PRIMARY ACQUIRED MELANOSIS WITH ATYPIA

INTRODUCTION

Primary acquired melanosis with atypia is characterized by an increase in the number of conjunctival melanocytes, with loss of cellular differentiation and spread from the basal layer of the epithelium to other layers. It tends to arise in later life as an area of pigmentation in any part of the conjunctiva.[159] The risk of melanoma is negligible when there is no atypia, increasing to approximately 45% when atypical melanocytes are present. The presence of epithelioid cells and involvement of all layers of the epithelium increase the risk to 75% and 90%, respectively.[160]

INVESTIGATION

The degree of atypia in primary acquired melanosis is established by examining multiple biopsies, imprint cytology, or scrapings.

Microbiopsies are performed by grasping the conjunctiva with toothed micro-forceps and excising a 5-mm ellipse of tissue. Crush artifact is avoided by holding the specimen at only one place. The conjunctival specimen is gently placed flat on a small piece of paper; this is done without smearing or spreading the tissue on the paper, because this would cause crush artifact. Each specimen is placed in a separate pot of fixative with an indication of the anatomical location of the biopsy.

Imprint cytology is performed by blotting the conjunctiva with nitrocellulose paper, which is placed in fixative, carefully noting the anatomical location. Scrapings are obtained with a Bard-Parker knife and smeared onto a glass slide, which is air dried and then fixed with alcohol.

TREATMENT

Indications

Treatment is indicated when the melanosis is atypical enough to pose a significant risk of melanoma.

Technique

Either the patch of melanosis is excised, if the affected area is small enough, or the entire area is treated by cryotherapy. Both techniques may be used simultaneously. Cryotherapy is performed using a liquid nitrogen probe after infiltrating the subconjunctival space with local anesthetic[161] or air. The double freeze-thaw technique is used, reducing the temperature of the conjunctiva to −20°C to −40°C, using a thermocouple to measure the temperature. The iceball should be allowed to thaw spontaneously to enhance the effect of the cryotherapy. If the corneal epithelium is involved, this is removed by first wiping the cornea with an alcohol wipe and then performing debridement with a cotton bud. Care must be taken not to create any breaks in Bowman's membrane, as this serves as a natural barrier to invasion. If the entire conjunctiva is abnormal, the nasal and temporal conjunctiva are treated in two sessions.

Results

Cryotherapy rarely achieves total eradication of abnormal melanocytes, but it usually reduces the population of atypical cells so as to minimize the risk of melanoma. After each session of cryotherapy, there is significant conjunctival and lid edema, with little pain. This responds to topical antibiotics and steroids given for 1 or 2 weeks. Long-term complications of cryotherapy include conjunctival scarring, symblepharon, loss of eyelashes, and lax eyelids. If excessive treatment is given, there may also be intraocular complications, which include macular edema, cataract, and ocular hypotension.

Extensive primary acquired melanosis with atypia, which cannot be adequately controlled by cryotherapy, may respond to a course of topical mitomycin C.[162] This treatment is used only for flat intraepithelial disease and is not advocated for nodular tumor or when there is invasion of subepithelial tissues.

MELANOMA

INTRODUCTION

Conjunctival melanomas may arise from preexisting nevi, primary acquired melanosis, or *de novo*. Invasion can occur into lamina propria, along conjunctiva, down the nasolacrimal duct,[163] into eyelid skin,[164] and eventually into orbit and eye. Metastatic spread first tends to occur to preauricular and submandibular nodes, and then systemically. About 25% of patients with conjunctival melanoma ultimately die of metastatic disease. An increased risk is associated with tumor thickness greater than approximately 1.8 mm, as well as involvement of nonbulbar conjunctiva, and recurrence after treatment.[165–169]

TREATMENT

Conjunctival melanoma is treated by local excision of any nodules with cryotherapy to the bed and to the surrounding conjunctiva.[161,161a] An extensive conjunctival defect can be closed with an amniotic membrane allograft. Beta-irradiation using a ruthenium or strontium applicator may also be used to reduce the chances of recurrence. Alternatively, if there is extensive disease, for example at the caruncle, external beam radiotherapy may be applied to the entire area. Diffuse melanosis with atypia is treated with cryotherapy or mitomycin C, as described above, to reduce the chance of nodular recurrence, which is especially likely to occur in the fornices.

Previously, exenteration was advocated for extensive conjunctival melanoma and even for primary acquired melanosis with atypia, but such surgery is now performed only when there is extensive and aggressive melanoma that cannot be controlled by less mutilating treatment.

FOLLOW-UP

Patients are monitored periodically by slit-lamp examination, with biopsy in selected cases. The role of repeated and multiple conjunctival biopsies is controversial, with proponents having concerns about invisible, amelanotic disease, and opponents fearing subconjunctival tumor spread and conjunctival scarring.

CARCINOMA

INTRODUCTION

Conjunctival and corneal intraepithelial neoplasia (CCIN)[170] presents in later life and is characterized histologically by the loss of normal epithelial cell maturation so that the epithelium contains an increasing proportion of atypical cells. Clinically, there is a gelatinous area, usually at or near the limbus, with frosting of the corneal surface if there is extension across the limbus.

Squamous cell carcinomas may grow outward as a solid or papillary tumor, or inward, invading sclera and conjunctiva, in neglected cases eventually penetrating the eye and orbit. Metastasis to regional lymph nodes and systemically is rare.

MANAGEMENT

Nodules are resected with wide margins, after which histological assessment of clearance is performed, ideally examining frozen sections at the time of surgery.[170] Diffuse disease is treated with cryotherapy or radiotherapy. Encouraging results have been reported with mitomycin C[171] and topical 5-FU.[172] Orbital invasion requires exenteration, with radiotherapy if necessary.[173]

LYMPHOID TUMORS

Conjunctival lymphoid tumors tend to consist of reactive lymphoid hyperplasia or well differentiated B-cell lymphoma.[174,174a] They present as pink patches in the substantia propria of the conjunctiva, which can be moved over the eye. A poorly differentiated conjunctival lymphoid tumor should indicate the possibility of systemic disease.[174] Categorization according to the REAL classification is useful for determining prognosis.[174b]

Differentiation between benign and malignant lymphoid tumors relies on biopsy, with the help of immunohistochemistry. Systemic evaluation is essential and should include whole blood count, serum protein electrophoresis, body scans, and bone marrow biopsy. Conjunctival lymphoid tumors respond to 30 to 35 Gy of orthovoltage radiotherapy and to intralesional injections of interferon alfa-2b.[175,175a]

KAPOSI'S SARCOMA

Kaposi's sarcoma tends to occur in association with immunodeficiency and consists of fusiform endothelial cells and blood-filled vascular channels. Lesions may be left untreated if asymptomatic or if chemotherapy for systemic Kaposi's sarcoma is planned or in progress, as regression may occur. Small, bulbar lesions may be excised with wide clearance margins, perhaps using fluorescein angiography to delineate tumor margins. Small eyelid lesions can be treated with cryotherapy, resorting to external beam radiotherapy at a dose of 8 Gy if recurrence is a problem.[176,177]

CONCLUSIONS

The care of most patients suffering from an ocular tumor is usually a multidisciplinary process, involving not only ophthalmologists and anesthetists, but also pathologists, cytologists, radiologists, radiotherapists, oncologists, geneticists, and psychological counselors. Data on presenting features, treatment methods, and a wide variety of outcomes are computerized and analyzed routinely, so that data managers and statisticians are important members of the team. The quality of care is greatly enhanced when the general ophthalmologist and the family doctor in the patient's hometown continue to be involved in the patient's care. It is our hope that this text will help facilitate such collaboration.

REFERENCES

1a. Shields JA, Shields CL: Atlas of intraocular tumors. Philadelphia, Lippincott, Williams & Wilkins, 1999.

1b. Shields JA, Shields CL: Atlas of eyelid and conjunctival tumors. Philadelphia, Lippincott, Williams & Wilkins, 1999.

1c. Damato B: Ocular Tumors: Diagnosis and Treatment. Oxford, Butterworth Heinemann, 2000.

2. McLean IW, Foster WD, Zimmerman LE, Gamel JW: Modifications of Callender's classification of uveal melanoma at the Armed Forces Institute of Pathology. Am J Ophthalmol 1983; 96:502–509.

3. Shields CL, Shields JA, De Potter P, et al.: Diffuse choroidal melanoma. Clinical features predictive of metastasis. Arch Ophthalmol 1996;114:956–963.

4. Lorigan JG, Wallace S, Mavligit GM: The prevalence and location of metastases from ocular melanoma: Imaging study in 110 patients. AJR Am J Roentgenol 1991;157:1279–1281.

4a. Bedikian AY, Legha SS, Mavligit G, et al.: Treatment of uveal melanoma metastatic to the liver: A review of the M. D. Anderson Cancer Center experience and prognostic factors. Cancer 1995;76:1665–1670.

5. Seddon J, Moy CS: Choroidal Melanoma: Prognosis. In Ryan SJ, Schachat AP (eds), Retina, 3rd edition, St. Louis, CV Mosby, 2001; pp. 687–699.

6. Mäkitie T, Summanen P, Tarkkanen A, Kivelä T: Microvascular loops and networks as prognostic indicators in choroidal and ciliary body melanomas. J Natl Cancer Inst 1999;91:359–367.

7. Prescher G, Bornfeld N, Hirche H, et al.: Prognostic implications of monosomy 3 in uveal melanoma. Lancet 1996;347:1222–1225.

8. Gamel JW, McCurdy JB, McLean IW: A comparison of prognostic covariates for uveal melanoma. Invest Ophthalmol Vis Sci 1992;33:1919–1922.

9. Jensen OA: Malignant melanomas of the human uvea: A 25 year follow-up of cases in Denmark, 1943–1952. Acta Ophthalmol Copenh 1982;60:161–182.
10. Damato BE, Paul J, Foulds WS: Risk factors for metastatic uveal melanoma after trans-scleral local resection. Br J Ophthalmol 1996;80:109–116.
10a. Shields CL, Shields JA, Materin M, et al.: Iris melanoma: Risk factors for metastasis in 169 consecutive patients. Ophthalmology 2001;108:172–178.
11. McLean IW, Ainbinder DJ, Gamel JW, McCurdy JB: Choroidal-ciliary body melanoma. A multivariate survival analysis of tumor location. Ophthalmology 1995;102:1060–1064.
12. Zimmerman LE, McLean IW, Foster WD: Does enucleation of the eye containing a malignant melanoma prevent or accelerate the dissemination of tumour cells. Br J Ophthalmol 1978; 62:420–425.
13. Green RL, Frazier Byrne S: Diagnostic Ophthalmic Ultrasound. In Ryan SJ (ed), Retina. 3rd edition, St. Louis: CV Mosby, 2001; pp. 224–306.
14. Ossoinig KC: Standardized echography: Basic principles, clinical applications, and results. Int Ophthalmol Clin 1979;19: 127–210.
15. Coleman DJ, Silverman RH, Rondeau MJ, et al.: Ultrasonic tissue characterization of uveal melanoma and prediction of patient survival after enucleation and brachytherapy. Am J Ophthalmol 1991;112: 682–688.
16. Damato BE: Tumour fluorescence and tumour-associated fluorescence of choroidal melanomas. Eye 1992;6:587–593.
17. Sallet G, Amoaku WM, Lafaut BA, et al.: Indocyanine green angiography of choroidal tumors. Graefes Arch Clin Exp Ophthalmol 1995;233:677–689.
18. Shields CL, Shields JA, De Potter P: Patterns of indocyanine green videoangiography of choroidal tumours. Br J Ophthalmol 1995;79:237–245.
19. De Potter P, Shields J, Shields CL: MRI of the Eye and Orbit, Philadelphia, JB Lippincott, 1995.
20. Shields JA, Shields CL, Ehya H, et al.: Fine-needle aspiration biopsy of suspected intraocular tumors. The 1992 Urwick Lecture. Ophthalmology 1993;100:1677–1684.
20a. Bechrakis NE, Foerster MH, Bornfeld N: Biopsy in indeterminate intraocular tumors. Ophthalmology 2002;109:235–242.
21. Foulds WS: The uses and limitations of intraocular biopsy. Eye 1992;6:11–27.
22. Olsen KR, Curtin VT: Enucleation and plaque treatment. In Albert DM, Jakobiec FA (eds), Principles and Practice of Ophthalmology, 1st edition, Philadelphia, WB Saunders, 1994; p. 3226.
23. Shields JA: Counseling the patient with a posterior uveal melanoma. Am J Ophthalmol 1988;106:88–91.
24. Ah-Fat FG, Sharma MC, Damato BE: Taping outpatient consultations: A survey of attitudes and responses of adult patients with ocular malignancy. Eye 1998;12:789–791.
25. Morris J, Royle GT: Offering patients a choice of surgery for early breast cancer: A reduction in anxiety and depression in patients and their husbands. Soc Sci Med 1988;26:583–585.
26. Singh AD, Shields CL, De Potter P, Shields JA, Trock B, Cater J, et al.: Familial uveal melanoma. Clinical observations on 56 patients. Arch Ophthalmol 1996;114:392–399.
27. Augsburger JJ: Is observation really appropriate for small choroidal melanomas? Trans Am Ophthalmol Soc 1993;91: 147–168.
28. Shields CL, Shields JA, De Potter P, Singh AD, Hernandez C, Brady LW: Treatment of non-resectable malignant iris tumours with custom designed plaque radiotherapy. Br J Ophthalmol 1995;79:306–312.
28a. Finger PT: Plaque radiation therapy for malignant melanoma of the iris and ciliary body. Am J Ophthalmol 2001;132:328–335.
29. Bedford MA: The use and abuse of cobalt plaques in the treatment of choroidal malignant melanomata. Trans Ophthalmol Soc UK 1973;93:139–143.
30. Robertson DM, Earle JD, Kline RW: Brachytherapy for choroidal melanoma. In Ryan SJ (ed), Retina, 3rd edition, St. Louis, Mosby, 2001; pp. 739–752.
31. Lommatzsch PK: Treatment of choroidal melanomas with $^{106}Ru/^{106}Rh$ beta ray applicators. In Alberti WE, Sagerman RH (eds), Radiotherapy of Intraocular and Orbital Tumors, Berlin, Springer-Verlag, 1993; pp. 23–30.
32. Finger PT, Berson A: Szechter A: Palladium-103 plaque radiotherapy for choroidal melanoma: Results of a 7-year study. Ophthalmology 1999;106:606–613.
33. The Collaborative Ocular Melanoma Study Group: The COMS randomized trial of iodine 125 brachytherapy for choroidal melanoma, III: Initial mortality findings. COMS report no. 18. Arch Ophthalmol 2001;119:969–982.
34. Shields CL, Shields JA, Cater J, et al.: Plaque radiotherapy for uveal melanoma. Long-term visual outcome in 1106 consecutive patients. Arch Ophthalmol 2000;118:1219–1228.
35. Guthoff R, Frischmuth J, Jensen OA, Bjerrum K, Prause JU: Choroid melanoma. A retrospective randomized comparative study of ruthenium irradiation vs enucleation. Klin Monatsbl Augenheilkd 1992;200:257–261.
36. Collaborative Ocular Melanoma Study Group: Collaborative Ocular Melanoma Study (COMS) randomized trial of I-125 brachytherapy for medium choroidal melanoma: I. Visual acuity after 3 years, COMS report no. 16. Ophthalmology 2001;108: 348–366.
37. Summanen P, Immonen I, Kivelä T, et al.: Visual outcome of eyes with malignant melanoma of the uvea after ruthenium plaque radiotherapy. Ophthalmic Surg Lasers 1995;26:449–460.
38. Summanen P, Immonen I, Tommila P, et al.: Radiation related complications after ruthenium plaque radiotherapy of uveal melanoma. Br J Ophthalmol 1996;80:732–739.
39. Abramson DH, Servodidio CA, McCormick B, et al.: Changes in height of choroidal melanomas after plaque therapy. Br J Ophthalmol 1990;74:359–362.
40. Augsburger JJ, Gamel JW, Shields JA, et al.: Postirradiation regression of choroidal melanomas as a risk factor for death from metastatic disease. Ophthalmology 1987;94: 1173–1177.
41. Quivey JM, Augsburger J, Snelling L, Brady LW: ^{125}I plaque therapy for uveal melanoma. Analysis of the impact of time and dose factors on local control. Cancer 1996;77:2356–2362.
42. De Potter P, Shields CL, Shields JA, et al.: Plaque radiotherapy for juxtapapillary choroidal melanoma. Visual acuity and survival outcome. Arch Ophthalmol 1996;114: 1357–1365.
43. Vrabec TR, Augsburger JJ, Gamel JW, et al.: Impact of local tumor relapse on patient survival after cobalt 60 plaque radiotherapy. Ophthalmology 1991;98: 984–988.
44. Astrahan MA, Luxton G, Jozsef G, et al.: An interactive treatment planning system for ophthalmic plaque radiotherapy. Int J Radiat Oncol Biol Phys 1990;18:679–687.
45. Gragoudas ES, Char DH: Charged particle irradiation of uveal melanomas. In Albert DM, Jakobiec FA (eds), Principles and Practice of Ophthalmology, 1st edition, Philadelphia, WB Saunders, 1994; pp. 3233–3244.
46. Bercher L, Zografos L, Chamot L, et al.: Functional results of 450 cases of uveal melanoma treated with proton beam. In Bornfeld N, Gragoudas ES, Höpping W, et al. (eds), Tumors of the Eye, Amsterdam, Kugler, 1991; pp. 507–510.
47. Egan KM, Gragoudas ES, Seddon JM, et al.: The risk of enucleation after proton beam irradiation of uveal melanoma. Ophthalmology 1989;96:1377–1382.
48. Linstadt D, Castro J, Char D, et al.: Long-term results of helium ion irradiation of uveal melanoma. Int J Radiat Oncol Biol Phys 1990;19:613–618.
49. Munzenrider JE, Verhey LJ, Gragoudas ES, et al.: Conservative treatment of uveal melanoma: Local recurrence after proton beam therapy. Int J Radiat Oncol Biol Phys 1989;17:493–498.
50. Seddon JM, Gragoudas ES, Egan KM, et al.: Relative survival rates after alternative therapies for uveal melanoma. Ophthalmology 1990;97:769–777.
51. Egan KM, Ryan LM, Gragoudas ES: Survival implications of enucleation after definitive radiotherapy for choroidal melanoma: An example of regression on time-dependent covariates. Arch Ophthalmol 1998;116:366–370.
52. Seddon JM, Gragoudas ES, Egan KM, et al.: Uveal melanomas near the optic disc or fovea. Visual results after proton beam irradiation. Ophthalmology 1987;94:354–361.
53. Char DH, Castro JR, Kroll SM, et al.: Five-year follow-up of helium ion therapy for uveal melanoma. Arch Ophthalmol 1990;108:209–214.
54. Marchini G, Babighian S, Tomazzoli L, et al.: Stereotactic radiosurgery of uveal melanomas: Preliminary results with gamma knife treatment. Stereotact Funct Neurosurg 1995;64 Suppl 1:72–79.

55. Dieckmann K, Boyner J, Georg D, et al.: A linac-based stereotactic irradiation technique of uveal melanoma. Radiother Oncol 2001;61:49–56.
55a. Wilson DJ, Klein ML: Cryotherapy as a primary treatment for choroidal melanoma. Arch Ophthalmol 2002;120:400–403.
56. Damato BE, Foulds WS: Surgical resection of choroidal melanoma. In Ryan SJ (ed), Retina, 3rd edition, St. Louis: CV Mosby, 2001, pp. 762–772.
57. Peyman GA, Gremillion CM: Eye wall resection in the management of uveal neoplasms. Jpn J Ophthalmol 1989;33:458–471.
58. Shields JA, Shields CL, Shah P, Sivalingam V: Partial lamellar sclerouvectomy for ciliary body and choroidal tumors. Ophthalmology 1991;98:971–983.
59. Damato BE, Paul J, Foulds WS: Predictive factors of visual outcome after local resection of choroidal melanoma. Br J Ophthalmol 1993;77:616–623.
60. Damato BE, Paul J, Foulds WS: Risk factors for residual and recurrent uveal melanoma after trans-scleral local resection. Br J Ophthalmol 1996;80:102–108.
61. Foulds WS, Damato BE, Burton RL: Local resection versus enucleation in the management of choroidal melanoma. Eye 1987;1: 676–679.
62. Naumann GOH, Rummelt V: Block excision of tumors of the anterior uvea. Report on 68 consecutive patients. Ophthalmology 1996;103:2017–2028.
63. Damato B, Groenewald C, McGalliard J, Wong D: Endoresection of choroidal melanoma. Br J Ophthalmol 1998;82:213–218.
64. Lee KJ, Peyman GA, Raichand S: Internal eye wall resection for posterior uveal melanoma. Jpn J Ophthalmol 1993;37:287–292.
65. Bornfeld N: Laser treatment of choroidal melanoma. In Ryan SJ (ed), Retina, 3rd edition, St. Louis, CV Mosby, 2001; pp. 785–794.
66. Foulds WS, Damato BE: Low-energy long-exposure laser therapy in the management of choroidal melanoma. Graefes Arch Clin Exp Ophthalmol 1986;224:26–31.
67. Kim RY, Hu L-K, Foster BS, Gragoudas ES, Young LHY: Photodynamic therapy of pigmented choroidal melanomas of greater than 3-mm thickness. Ophthalmology 1996;103:2029–2036.
68. Oosterhuis JA, Journée-de Korver HG, Kakebeeke-Kemme HM, Bleeker JC: Transpupillary thermotherapy in choroidal melanomas. Arch Ophthalmol 1995;113:315–321.
69. Shields CL, Shields JA, De Potter P, Kheterpal S: Transpupillary thermotherapy in the management of choroidal melanoma. Ophthalmology 1996;103:1642–1650.
70. Journée-de Korver JG, Oosterhuis JA, de Wolff-Rouendaal D, Kakebeeke Kemme HM: Histopathological findings in human choroidal melanomas after transpupillary thermotherapy. Br J Ophthalmol 1997;81:234–239.
70a. Shields CL, Shields JA, Perez N, et al.: Primary transpupillary thermotherapy for small choroidal melanoma in 256 consecutive cases. Outcomes and limitations. Ophthalmology 2002; 109:225–234.
71. Zimmerman LE, McLean IW: An evaluation of enucleation in the management of uveal melanomas. Am J Ophthalmol 1979; 87: 741–760.
72. Augsburger JJ, Lauritzen K, Gamel JW, et al.: Matched group study of preenucleation radiotherapy versus enucleation alone for primary malignant melanoma of the choroid and ciliary body. Am J Clin Oncol 1990;13:382–387.
73. Char DH, Phillips TL, Andejeski Y, et al.: Failure of preenucleation radiation to decrease uveal melanoma mortality [see comments]. Am J Ophthalmol 1988;106:21–26.
74. Collaborative Ocular Melanoma Study Group: The Collaborative Ocular Melanoma Study (COMS) randomized trial of preenucleation radiation of large choroidal melanoma, II initial mortality findings. Am J Ophthalmol 1998;125:779–796.
75. Hykin PG, McCartney AC, Plowman PN, Hungerford JL: Postenucleation orbital radiotherapy for the treatment of malignant melanoma of the choroid with extrascleral extension. Br J Ophthalmol 1990;74:36–39.
76. Eskelin S, Pyrhonen S, Summanen P, et al.: Screening for metastatic malignant melanoma of the uvea revisited. Cancer 1999; 85:1151–1159.
77. Leyvraz S, Spataro V, Bauer J, et al.: Treatment of ocular melanoma metastatic to the liver by hepatic arterial chemotherapy. J Clin Oncol 1997;15:2589–2595.
78. Albert DM, Niffenegger AS, Willson JK: Treatment of metastatic uveal melanoma: Review and recommendations. Surv Ophthalmol 1992;36:429–438.
79. Augsburger JJ, Schroeder RP, Territo C, et al.: Clinical parameters predictive of enlargement of melanocytic choroidal lesions. Br J Ophthalmol 1989;73:911–917.
80. Shields CL, Cater J, Shields JA, et al.: Combination of clinical factors predictive of growth of small choroidal melanocytic tumors. Arch Ophthalmol 2000;118:360–364.
81. Char DH, Crawford JB, Kroll S: Iris melanomas. Diagnostic problems. Ophthalmology 1996;103:251–255.
82. Territo C, Shields CL, Shields JA, et al.: Natural course of melanocytic tumors of the iris. Ophthalmology 1988;95:1251–1255.
83. Joffe L, Shields JA, Osher RH, Gass JD: Clinical and follow-up studies of melanocytomas of the optic disc. Ophthalmology 1979;86:1067–1083.
84. Reidy JJ, Apple DJ, Steinmetz RL, et al.: Melanocytoma: Nomenclature, pathogenesis, natural history and treatment. Surv Ophthalmol 1985;29:319–327.
85. Char DH, Miller T: Accuracy of presumed uveal melanoma diagnosis before alternative therapy. Br J Ophthalmol 1995;79: 692–696.
86. Fineman MS, Eagle RC Jr, Shields JA, et al.: Melanocytomalytic glaucoma in eyes with necrotic iris melanocytoma. Ophthalmology 1998;105:492–496.
87. Shields JA, Shields CL, Eagle RC Jr, et al.: Malignant melanoma associated with melanocytoma of the optic disc. Ophthalmology 1990;97:225–230.
88. Shields CL, Shields JA, Gross NE, et al.: Survey of 520 eyes with uveal metastases. Ophthalmology 1997;104: 1265–1276.
89. Shields JA, Shields CL, Kiratli H, De Potter P: Metastatic tumors to the iris in 40 patients. Am J Ophthalmol 1995;119:422–430.
90. Augsburger JJ: Fine needle aspiration biopsy of suspected metastatic cancers to the posterior uvea. Trans Am Ophthalmol Soc 1988;86:499–560.
91. Shields CL, Shields JA, De Potter P, et al.: Plaque radiotherapy for the management of uveal metastasis. Arch Ophthalmol 1997;115:203–209.
92. Anand R, Augsburger JJ, Shields JA: Circumscribed choroidal hemangiomas. Arch Ophthalmol 1989;107:1338–1342.
93. Shields JA: The expanding role of laser photocoagulation for intraocular tumors. The 1993 H. Christian Zweng Memorial Lecture. Retina 1994;14:310–322.
94. Shields JA, Shields CL: Intraocular Tumors. A Text and Atlas, Philadelphia, WB Saunders, 1992.
94a. Madreperla SA: Choroidal hemangioma treated with photodynamic therapy using verteporfin. Arch Ophthalmol 2001; 119:1606–1610.
95. Othmane IS, Shields CL, Shields JA, et al.: Circumscribed choroidal hemangioma managed by transpupillary thermotherapy. Arch Ophthalmol 1999;117:136–137.
96. Rapizzi E, Grizzard WS, Capone A Jr: Transpupillary thermotherapy in the management of circumscribed choroidal hemangioma. Am J Ophthalmol 1999;127:481–482.
97. Schilling H, Sauerwein W, Lommatzsch A, et al.: Long term results after low dose ocular irradiation for choroidal haemangiomas. Br J Ophthalmol 1997; 81:267–273.
98. Zografos L, Bercher L, Chamot L, et al.: Cobalt-60 treatment of choroidal hemangiomas. Am J Ophthalmol 1996;121:190–199.
99. Hannouche D, Frau E, Desjardins L, et al.: Efficacy of proton therapy in circumscribed choroidal hemangiomas associated with serious retinal detachment. Ophthalmology 1997;104: 1780–1784.
100. Zografos L, Egger E, Bercher L, et al.: Proton beam irradiation of choroidal hemangiomas. Am J Ophthalmol 1998;126:261–268.
101. Shields JA, Shields CL, Eagle RC Jr, De Potter P: Observations on seven cases of intraocular leiomyoma. The 1993 Byron Demorest Lecture. Arch Ophthalmol 1994;112:521–528.
102. Broughton WL, Zimmerman LE: A clinicopathological study of 56 cases of intraocular medulloepitheliomas. Am J Ophthalmol 1978;85:407–418.
103. Shields JA, Eagle RC Jr, Shields CL, De Potter P: Congenital neoplasms of the nonpigmented ciliary epithelium (medulloep-

ithelioma). Ophthalmology 1996;103:1998–2006.
104. McLean IW, Burnier MN, Zimmerman LE, Jakobiec FA: Tumors of the uveal tract. In Rosai J, Sobin LH (eds), Tumors of the Eye and Ocular Adnexa. Washington, DC, Armed Forces Institute of Pathology, 1994; pp. 155–214.
105. Shields JA, Shields CL, Gunduz K, Eagle RC Jr: Neoplasms of the retinal pigment epithelium: The 1998 Albert Ruedemann, Sr, memorial lecture, Part 2. Arch Ophthalmol 1999;117:601–608.
106. Shields JA, Eagle RC Jr, Shields CL: Adenoma of nonpigmented ciliary epithelium with smooth muscle differentiation. Arch Ophthalmol 1999;117:117–119.
107. Shields JA, Shields CL, Mercado G, et al.: Adenoma of the iris pigment epithelium: A report of 20 cases: The 1998 Pan-American Lecture. Arch Ophthalmol 1999;117: 736–741.
108. Moll AC, Imhoff SM, Schouten-Van Meeteren AYN, et al.: Second primary tumors in hereditary retinoblastoma: A register-based study, 1945-1997. Is there an age effect on radiation-related risk? Ophthalmology 2001;108:1109–1114.
108a. Abramson DH, Melson MR, Dunkel IJ, Frank CM: Third (fourth and fifth) nonocular tumors in survivors of retinoblastoma. Ophthalmology 2001;108:1868–1876.
109. De Potter P, Shields CL, Shields JA: Clinical variations of trilateral retinoblastoma: A report of 13 cases. J Pediatr Ophthalmol Strabismus 1994;31:26–31.
110. Holladay DA, Holladay A, Montebello JF, Redmond KP: Clinical presentation, treatment and outcome of trilateral retinoblastoma. Cancer 1991;67:710–715.
111. Merriam GR: Retinoblastoma: Analysis of 17 autopsies. Arch Ophthalmol 1950;44:71–108.
112. Messmer EP, Heinrich T, Hoepping W, et al.: Risk factors for metastases in patients with retinoblastoma. Ophthalmology 1991;98:136–141.
113. Olver JM, McCartney ACE, Kingston J, Hungerford J: Histological indicators of the prognosis for survival following enucleation for retinoblastoma. In Bornfeld N, Gragoudas ES, Hoepping W, et al. (eds), Tumors of the Eye, Amsterdam, Kugler, 1991; pp. 59–67.
114. Shields CL, Shields JA, Baez K, et al.: Optic nerve invasion of retinoblastoma. Metastatic potential and clinical risk factors. Cancer 1994;73:692–698.
114a. Finger PT, Harbour JW, Karcioglu ZA: Risk factors for metastasis in retinoblastoma. Surv Ophthalmol 2002;47:1–16.
115. Shields CL, Shields JA, Baez A, et al.: Choroidal invasion of retinoblastoma. Metastatic potential and clinical risk factors. Br J Ophthalmol 1993;77:544–548.
116. Haik BG: Advanced Coats' disease. Trans Am Ophthalmol Soc 1991;89:371–476.
117. Reese AB, Ellsworth RM: The evaluation and current concept of retinoblastoma therapy. Trans Am Acad Ophthalmol Otolaryngol 1963;67:164–172.
118. Shields JA, Shields CL, Parsons H, Giblin ME: The role of photocoagulation in the management of retinoblastoma. Arch Ophthalmol 1990;108:205–208.
119. Shields CL, Santos MC, Diniz W, et al.: Thermotherapy for retinoblastoma. Arch Ophthalmol 1999;117:885–893.
120. Abramson DH, Servodidio CA, Nissen M: Treatment of retinoblastoma with the transscleral diode laser. Am J Ophthalmol 1998;126:733–735.
121. Shields JA, Parsons H, Shields CL, Giblin ME: The role of cryotherapy in the management of retinoblastoma. Am J Ophthalmol 1989;108:260–264.
122. Abramson DH, Ellsworth RM, Rozakis GW: Cryotherapy for retinoblastoma. Arch Ophthalmol 1982;100:1253–1256.
123. Shields CL, Shields JA, Cater J, et al.: Plaque radiotherapy for retinoblastoma. Long-term tumor control and treatment of complications in 208 tumors. Ophthalmology 2001;108:2116–2121.
124. Cassady JR: Radiation therapy for retinoblastoma. In Albert DM, Jakobiec FA (eds). Principles and Practice of Ophthalmology. Philadelphia, WB Saunders, 1994; 3285–3298.
125. Schipper J, Tan KEWP, van Peperzeel HA: Treatment of retinoblastoma by precision megavoltage radiation therapy. Radiother Oncol 1985;3:117–132.
126. Blach LE, McCormick B, Abramson DH: External beam radiation therapy and retinoblastoma: Long-term results in the comparison of two techniques. Int J Radiat Oncol Biol Phys 1996; 35:45–51.
127. Toma NM, Hungerford JL, Plowman PN, et al.: External beam radiotherapy for retinoblastoma: II. Lens sparing technique. Br J Ophthalmol 1995;79:112–117.
128. Imhoff SM, Mourits MP, Hofman P, et al.: Quantification of orbital and mid-facial growth retardation after megavoltage external beam irradiation in children with retinoblastoma. Ophthalmology 1996;103:263–268.
129. Greenwald MJ, Strauss LC: Treatment of intraocular retinoblastoma with carboplatin and etoposide chemotherapy. Ophthalmology 1996;103:1989–1997.
129a. Gombos DS, Kelly A, Coen PG, et al.: Retinoblastoma treated with primary chemotherapy alone: the significance of tumor size, location, and age. Br J Ophthalmol 2002;86:80–83.
130. Gallie BL, Budning A, DeBoer G, et al.: Chemotherapy with focal therapy can cure intraocular retinoblastoma without radiotherapy. Arch Ophthalmol 1996; 114:1321–1328.
131. Murphree AL, Villablanca JG, Deegan WF 3rd, et al.: Chemotherapy plus local treatment in the management of intraocular retinoblastoma. Arch Ophthalmol 1996;114:1348–1356.
132. Shields CL, De Potter P, Himelstein BP, et al.: Chemoreduction in the initial management of intraocular retinoblastoma. Arch Ophthalmol 1996;114:1330–1338.
133. Kingston JE, Hungerford JL, Madreperla SA, Plowman PN: Results of combined chemotherapy and radiotherapy for advanced intraocular retinoblastoma. Arch Ophthalmol 1996;114: 1339–1343.
133a. Shields CL, Meadows AT, Shields JA, et al.: Chemoreduction for retinoblastoma may prevent intracranial neuroblastic malignancy (trilateral retinoblastoma). Arch Ophthalmol 2001;119: 1269–1272.
134. Kingston JE, Hungerford JL, Plowman PN: Chemotherapy in metastatic retinoblastoma. Ophthalmic Paediatr Genet 1987; 8:69–72.
135. Saarinen UM, Sariola H, Hovi L: Recurrent disseminated retinoblastoma treated by high-dose chemotherapy, total body irradiation, and autologous bone marrow rescue. Am J Pediatr Hematol Oncol 1991;13:315–319.
136. White L: Chemotherapy in retinoblastoma: Current status and future directions. Am J Pediatr Hematol Oncol 1991;13:189–201.
137. Nelson SC, Friedman HS, Oakes WJ, et al.: Successful therapy for trilateral retinoblastoma [see comments]. Am J Ophthalmol 1992;114:23–29.
137a. Shields CL, Honaovar SG, Shields JA, et al.: Factors predictive of recurrence of retinal tumors, vitreous seeds, and subretinal seeds following chemoreduction for retinoblastoma. Arch Ophthalmol 2002;120:460–464.
137b. Benz MS, Scott IU, Murray TG, et al.: Complications of systemic chemotherapy as treatment of retinoblastoma. Arch Ophthalmol 2000;118:577–578.
138. Rubin CM, Robison LL, Cameron JD, et al.: Intraocular retinoblastoma group V—An analysis of prognostic factors. J Clin Oncol 1985;3:680–685.
139. Harbour JW: Overview of RB gene mutations in patients with retinoblastoma. Implications for clinical genetic screening. Ophthalmology 1998;105:1442–1447.
140. Gallie BL, Ellsworth RM, Abramson DH, Phillips RA: Retinoma: Spontaneous regression of retinoblastoma or benign manifestation of the mutation? Br J Cancer 1982;45:513–521.
140a. Singh AD, Santos MCM, Shields CL, et al.: Observations on 17 patients with retinocytoma. Arch Ophthalmol 2000;118:199–205.
141. Eagle RJ Jr, Shields JA, Donoso L, Milner RS: Malignant transformation of spontaneously regressed retinoblastoma, retinoma/retinocytoma variant. Ophthalmology 1989;96: 1389–1395.
142. Sharma S, Cruess AF: Tuberous sclerosis and the eye. In Ryan SJ (ed), Retina, 3rd edition, St. Louis, CV Mosby, 2001; pp. 585–595.
143. Verhoef S, Bakker L, Tempelaars AM, et al.: High rate of mosaicism in tuberous sclerosis complex. Am J Hum Genet 1999; 64:1632–1637.
144. Singh AD, Shields CL, Sheilds JA: von Hippel-Lindau disease. Surv Ophthalmol 2001;46:117–142.
145. Maher ER, Moore AT: Von-Hippel-Lindau disease. Br J Ophthalmol 1992;76:743–745.
146. Maher ER, Webster AR, Richards FM, et al.: Phenotypic expression in von Hippel-Lindau disease: Correlations with germline VHL gene mutations. J Med Genet 1996;33:328–332.
147. Lane CM, Turner G, Gregor ZJ, Bird AC: Laser treatment of reti-

nal angiomatosis. Eye 1989;3:33–38.
148. Kreusel KM, Bornfeld N, Lommatzsch A, et al.: Ruthenium-106 brachytherapy for peripheral retinal capillary hemangioma. Ophthalmology 1998;105:1386–1392.
149. McDonald HR, Schatz H, Johnson RN, et al.: Vitrectomy in eyes with peripheral retinal angioma associated with traction macular detachment. Ophthalmology 1996;103:329–335.
150. Johnston PB, Lotery AJ, Logan WC: Treatment and long-term follow up of a capillary angioma of the optic disc. Int Ophthalmol 1995;19:129–132.
151. Schlienger P, Desjardins L: [External electron irradiation in 2 cases of capillary hemangioma of the optic disk]. [Review] [French]. Bull Cancer Radiotherapie 1995;82:306–310.
152. Shields CL, Shields JA, Barrett J, De Potter P: Vasoproliferative tumors of the ocular fundus. Classification and clinical manifestations in 103 patients. Arch Ophthalmol 1995;113:615–623.
152a. Irvine F, O'Donnell N, Kemp E, Lee WR: Retinal vasoproliferative tumors. Surgical management and histological findings. Arch Ophthalmol 2000;118:563–569.
153. Akpek EK, Ahmed I, Hochberg FH, et al.: Intraocular-central nervous system lymphoma. Clinical features, diagnosis and outcomes. Ophthalmology 1999;106:1805–1810.
154. Buggage RR, Whitcup SM, Nussenblatt RB, Chan CC: Using interleukin 10 to interleukin 6 ratio to distinguish primary intraocular lymphoma and uveitis [letter]. Invest Ophthalmol Vis Sci 1999;40:2462–2463.
155. White VA, Gascoyne RD, Paton KE: Use of the polymerase chain reaction to detect B- and T-cell gene rearrangements in vitreous specimens from patients with intraocular lymphoma. Arch Ophthalmol 1999;117:761–765.
156. Fishburne BC, Wilson DJ, Rosenbaum JT, Neuwelt EA: Intravitreal methotrexate as an adjunctive treatment of intraocular lymphoma. Arch Ophthalmol 1997;115:1152–1156.
157. Ryan SJ, Zimmerman LE, King FM: Reactive lymphoid hyperplasia: An unusual form of intraocular pseudotumor. Trans Am Ophthalmol Soc 1972;76:652–671.
158. Desroches G, Abrams GW, Gass JDM: Reactive lymphoid hyperplasia of the uvea: A case with ultrasonographic and computer tomographic studies. Arch Ophthalmol 1983;101:725–728.
159. Folberg R, McLean IW: Primary acquired melanosis and melanoma of the conjunctiva: Terminology, classification, and biologic behavior. Hum Pathol 1986;17:652–654.
160. Folberg R, McLean IW, Zimmerman LE: Primary acquired melanosis of the conjunctiva. Hum Pathol 1985;16:129–135.
161. Jakobiec FA, Rini FJ, Fraunfelder FT, Brownstein S: Cryotherapy for conjunctival primary acquired melanosis and malignant melanoma. Experience with 62 cases. Ophthalmology 1988; 95:1058–1070.
161a. Shields CL, Shields JA, Armstrong T: Management of conjunctival and corneal melanoma with surgical excision, amniotic membrane allograft, and topical chemotherapy. Am J Ophthalmol 2001;132:576–578.
162. Frucht-Pery J, Pe'er J: Use of mitomycin C in the treatment of conjunctival primary acquired melanosis with atypia. Arch Ophthalmol 1996;114:1261–1264.
163. Robertson DM, Hungerford JL, McCartney A: Malignant melanomas of the conjunctiva, nasal cavity, and paranasal sinuses. Am J Ophthalmol 1989;108:440–442.
164. Robertson DM, Hungerford JL, McCartney A: Pigmentation of the eyelid margin accompanying conjunctival melanoma. Am J Ophthalmol 1989;108:435–439.
165. Shields CL, Shields JA, Gündüz K, et al.: Conjunctival melanoma. Risk factors for recurrence, exenteration, metastasis, and death in 150 consecutive patients. Arch Ophthalmol 2000;118: 1497–1507.
166. Folberg R, McLean IW, Zimmerman LE: Malignant melanoma of the conjunctiva. Hum Pathol 1985;16:136–143.
167. Jeffrey IJ, Lucas DR, McEwan C, Lee WR: Malignant melanoma of the conjunctiva. Histopathology 1986;10:363–378.
168. Lommatzsch PK, Lommatzsch RE, Kirsch I, Fuhrmann P: Therapeutic outcome of patients suffering from malignant melanomas of the conjunctiva. Br J Ophthalmol 1990;74:615–619.
169. Paridaens AD, Minassian DC, McCartney AC, Hungerford JL: Prognostic factors in primary malignant melanoma of the conjunctiva: A clinicopathological study of 256 cases. Br J Ophthalmol 1994;78:252–259.
170. Tunc M, Char DH, Crawford B, Miller T: Intraepithelial and invasive squamous cell carcinoma of the conjunctiva: Analysis of 60 cases. Br J Ophthalmol 1999;83:98–103.
171. Frucht-Pery J, Rozenman Y, Pe'er J: Topical mitomycin-C for partially excised conjunctival squamous cell carcinoma. Ophthalmology 2002;109:548–552.
172. Yeatts RP, Engelbrecht NE, Curry CD, et al.: 5-Fluorouracil for the treatment of intraepithelial neoplasia of the conjunctiva and cornea. Ophthalmology 2000;107:2190–2195.
173. Johnson TE, Tabbara KF, Weatherhead RG, et al.: Secondary squamous cell carcinoma of the orbit. Arch Ophthalmol 1997; 115:75–78.
174. Shields CL, Shields JA, Carvalho C, et al.: Conjunctival lymphoid tumors: clinical analysis of 117 cases and relationship to systemic lymphoma. Ophthalmology 2001;108:979–984.
174a. Coupland SE, Krause L, Delecluse H-J, et al.: Lymphoproliferative lesions of the ocular adnexa. Analysis of 112 cases. Ophthalmology 1998;105:1430–1441.
174b. Auw-Haedrich C, Coupland SE, Kapp A, et al.: Long term outcome of ocular adnexal lymphoma subtyped according to the REAL classification. Br J Ophthalmol 2001;85:63–69.
175. Dunbar SF, Linggood RM, Doppke KP, et al.: Conjunctival lymphoma, results and treatment with a single anterior electron field: A lens sparing approach. Int J Radiat Oncol Biol Phys 1990;19:249–257.
175a. Lachapelle KR, Rathee R, Kratky V, Dexter DF: Treatment of conjunctival mucosa-associated lymphoid tissue lymphoma with intralesional injection of interferon alfa-2b. Arch Ophthalmol 2000;118:284–285.
176. Dugel PU, Gill P, Frangieh GT, Rao NA: Treatment of ocular adnexal Kaposi's sarcoma in acquired immune deficiency syndrome. Ophthalmology 1992;99:1127–1132.
177. Ghabrial R, Quivey JM, Dunn JP Jr, Char DH: Radiation therapy of acquired immunodeficiency syndrome-related Kaposi's sarcoma of the eyelids and conjunctiva. Arch Ophthalmol 1992;110:1423–1426.

SECTION IX

Giora Treister, M.D.

Trauma

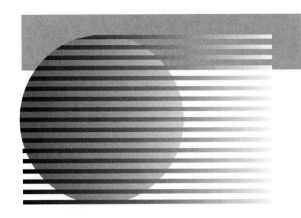

CHAPTER 64

Orbital and Adnexal Trauma

ROBERT ALAN GOLDBERG, M.D., JEFFREY L. JACOBS, M.D., GEORGE C. CHARONIS, M.D., and TINA G. LI, M.D.

INTRODUCTION

Injuries involving the eyelids, periorbita, and orbit are common after blunt or penetrating facial trauma. These injuries can vary from simple skin abrasions to more complex cases with extensive tissue loss and underlying fractures of the craniofacial skeleton. Complete assessment of the trauma patient to determine the extent of the underlying systemic damage is critical. Vital systems stabilization should be the first priority in the management of these patients. After successful stabilization of the patient's systemic condition has been achieved, attention can then be directed toward the specific ocular adnexal injuries. Restoration of structure and function with adherence to basic aesthetic principles should be the primary concern of the aesthetic reconstructive surgeon involved in the management of such injuries.

In this chapter general principles for the evaluation and management of orbital and adnexel trauma will be discussed. The most common types of adnexal injuries will be presented in a systematic approach. Ocular adnexal trauma can be very challenging and often tests the ingenuity of the aesthetic reconstructive surgeon. Several management principles and surgical techniques can minimize postoperative complications and improve aesthetic results and function. This can often have a dramatic impact on the patient's life, as secondary reconstructions can be very difficult or even impossible to correct in subsequent surgical attempts. These surgical principles also apply to periorbital and eyelid reconstruction following failed eyelid reconstruction.

PRINCIPLES OF EVALUATION AND MANAGEMENT

SYSTEMIC STABILIZATION

The evaluation of periorbital injuries begins after the traumatized patient has been stabilized and life-threatening injuries have been addressed. The role of the ophthalmologist in evaluation and management is very important. Good communication must be established between the trauma team and the ophthalmologist. Subjective symptoms related to the visual system or physical evidence of periorbital injuries demands the immediate attention of the ophthalmologist. The incidence of ocular injuries in craniofacial trauma is high, ranging between 15% and 60%.[1]

HISTORY

A complete history should be obtained to determine the time course and circumstances of the injury. For children, consideration must be given to the possibility of child abuse as the cause of ocular and periorbital injury. A history consistent with injuries from high-speed projectile particles may require appropriate imaging studies to determine the presence of intraocular or intraorbital foreign bodies. Animal and human bites deserve particular attention and are managed with the administration of appropriate antibiotics and tetanus prophylaxis. Chemical burn injuries should include identification of offending agent(s) and immediate thorough irrigation. The site of injury should be carefully inspected for any amputated tissue, and any tissue found at the site of injury should be preserved and placed on ice as soon as possible. In most cases such tissue can be sutured back to the proper anatomic location.

OPHTHALMOLOGIC EXAMINATION

Assessment of visual acuity is mandatory and should be done before any reconstructive efforts are undertaken. The pupils should be checked and the presence of a relative afferent pupillary defect noted. If such a defect is present, the surgeon should obtain neuroimaging studies. It may be necessary to discuss the potential of poor visual outcome despite best efforts at surgical repair. The extraocular muscles should be evaluated and any diplopia documented prior to surgery. The external examination should include a complete assessment of the craniofacial skeleton with particular emphasis on the periorbital region. Palpable step-offs, crepitus, or unstable bone needs radiologic evaluation. Baseline measurement of globe projection should be documented with Hertel exophthalmometry as enophthalmos is a common late sequelae of orbital trauma once swelling subsides. Eyelid position, orbicularis function, and any evidence of lagophthalmos should be documented thoroughly. Measurement of the intercanthal distance and evaluation of the integrity of canthal tendons is also necessary as traumatic tendon dehiscence and telecanthus are frequently associated with periorbital injuries. The integrity of the lacrimal system should be checked, maintaining a high index of suspicion for canalicular lacerations.

MEDICOLEGAL DOCUMENTATION

All injuries should be documented precisely and completely. This can be done with detailed drawings on the patient's charts and by photographic documentation. Bullets and other projectiles must be retained and marked so that there is no break in the chain of evidence. The medicolegal implications can be significant. Every effort should be made for complete preoperative documentation of every injury.

LABORATORY/RADIOGRAPHIC EVALUATION

Appropriate laboratory evaluation is usually performed by the emergency room team. A complete blood count and serum chemistry are often requirements for anesthetic purposes. Coagulation studies may be helpful in selected cases, and blood chemistry studies for alcohol and other toxic substances are necessary in others. When the clinical suspicion of orbital fractures is high, appropriate orbital imaging studies, mainly computed tomography (CT), should be ordered. Magnetic resonance imaging (MRI) and ultrasonic examination of the globe contents, extraocular muscles, optic nerve, and orbit can be important adjunctive studies.

INFECTION PROPHYLAXIS

The prevention of infection should be of primary concern. A complete tetanus immunization history should be obtained and the appropriate management followed if the patient is not up to date with immunizations. If an animal bite is known or suspected, all information regarding the site of injury, the owner of the animal, and any abnormal animal behavior must be obtained and the local animal care department contacted. The standard rabies protocol should be followed. (See the later section devoted to dog bites.)

Cat bites and even wounds caused by cat claws, carry a high risk for infection, mainly with *Pasteurella multocida* (see the later section of this chapter on dog bites). Appropriate prophylaxis includes penicillin VK 500 mg a day for 5 to 7 days. In allergic patients tetracycline may be given.[2]

Human bites have the potential for inoculating a large number of hearty bacteria and therefore require the administration of appropriate antibiotics, such as penicillin, amoxicillin, erythromycin, or dicloxacillin. Additional consideration for human immunodeficiency virus and hepatitis should also be given and appropriate testing administered.

After any type of bite injury copious irrigation of all injured tissues and removal of superficial foreign bodies lodged in the conjunctival fornices should be accomplished. Vigorous irrigation and removal of foreign bodies is sufficient to prevent wound infection from most bites.

TIMING OF INJURY REPAIR

The timing of the repair should be governed by several factors. Every effort should be made to reconstruct the injured tissues as soon as possible after the patient has been thoroughly evaluated and results of appropriate ancillary studies have been obtained. Waiting 24 to 48 hours in order to assemble the most efficient and experienced reconstructive team is a viable alternative unless the wound involves replacing amputated tissue. It should be emphasized that the best chances for restoration of structure, function, and cosmesis exist in the initial surgery. Trying to address secondary complications or a poor outcome can be difficult. Should a slight delay in treatment be deemed necessary, the wound should be kept moist with continuous application of saline-soaked gauze pads to prevent wound drying and desiccation. Adequate eye protection with copious lubrication or even a temporary tarsorrhaphy should be performed if the injury poses a significant threat for exposure keratopathy.

ANESTHESIA

The choice of anesthesia for the repair of adnexal injuries depends on several factors. Obviously, the patient's age is critical. Almost all children require general anesthesia in order to achieve the best reconstructive results. Large injuries with extensive soft tissue and bony involvement are best managed in a similar setting. However, even with general anesthesia, the addition of epinephrine is essential for hemostasis. Most adult injuries can be repaired with local infiltrative or regional anesthesia consisting of 1% to 2% xylocaine with 1:100,000 epinephrine. Infiltrative anesthesia can cause significant tissue distortion, which can be minimized with the use of hyaluronidase (Wydase), which facilitates the spreading of the anesthetic solution. Regional anesthesia of the infraorbital, supraorbital, infratrochlear, and supratrochlear nerves can be an effective adjunct to local infiltration.

MANAGEMENT OF COMMON INJURIES

DOG BITES

Of the 44,000 facial dog bites seen in emergency rooms each year, orbital and periorbital injuries occur in 4% to 8% of cases.[3,4] In a recent series in the ophthalmic literature, over half of such bites occurred in children under 5 years of age, and two thirds were in children under 10 years old.

It is essential to obtain information regarding the dog's health and rabies vaccination status. Immunocompromised patients, those who have undergone prior splenectomy, patients suffering from chronic obstructive pulmonary disease or alcoholism, and even healthy infants are at particular risk for development of fulminant septicemia 24 to 48 hours post-bite. *Pasteurella multocida* is identified in up to 50% of dog bite injury infections.[5] *P. multocida* infections commonly occur within 48 hours of inoculation and are characterized by prominent wound inflammation and drainage. The organism is a small, gram-negative coccobacillus that grows in both aerobic and anaerobic environments.[5] Septicemia, meningitis, and in rare cases, death have been reported from infection by a gram-negative, non-spore-forming rod, *Capnocytophaga canimorsus*. The organism was previously referred to as CDC group DF-2 (Dysgonic Fermenter-2), and can be cultured from the mouths of healthy dogs.[5–11]

Gonnering, in a study of periorbital dog bites, found no penetrating injuries of the globe and no tissue loss. Disruption of the lacrimal system was present in 14 of the 16 cases.[12] All dog bite wounds should be presumed contaminated and be decontaminated prior to surgical repair. While protecting the cornea with a scleral contact lens, forceful irrigation with at least 200 ml of normal saline using a 35-ml syringe and an 18-gauge irrigating cannula is recommended to limit infection.

Surgical repair should be carried out as in any other eyelid reconstruction with restoration of normal anatomic structure and function. Particular care should be taken in evaluating and repairing medial canthal tendon avulsions and lacrimal system injuries. Adjunct medical therapy includes tetanus prophylaxis and rabies prophylaxis if the rabies status of the dog is unknown or positive.

The need for prophylactic antibiotics in dog bites is controversial. Adequate wound decontamination is probably the single most important modality to prevent infection. Various studies have isolated multiple pathogens as the cause of post–dog bite infections. No single antimicrobial agent is optimal against these various pathogens, which include *Staphylococcus aureus, Pasteurella multocida, Pseudomonas aeruginosa, Streptococcus epidermidis, Capnocytophaga canimorsus,* as well as anaerobes.

Recommended choices of antibiotic prophylaxis include *penicillin, amoxicillin, cefuroxime,* and *cephalexin.*[14] Alternatives in the penicillin-allergic patient include erythromycin and tetracycline. Decisions regarding tetanus prophylaxis depend on the patient's immunization history and the character of the wound.

If rabies is suspected, health department officials should be contacted. The health department can assist in quarantine of the animal, as well as in offering current recommendations for rabies prophylaxis. The incubation period for rabies averages 30 to 50 days. Prophylactic treatment must be administered before the onset of clinical disease. Treatment consists of inactive rabies virus human diploid cell vaccine (HDCV) and rabies immune globulin (RIG). HDCV offers active immunity and RIG offers passive immunity.[5]

EYELID THERMAL AND CHEMICAL BURNS

Severe thermal burn injuries frequently involve the face, with the incidence of eyelid involvement reported as 20% to 30%.[15] Fortunately, Bell's phenomenon, the blink reflex, rapid reflex head movements, and shielding of the eyes with the arms and hands often prevent conjunctival and corneal injury.

Initial evaluation of an eyelid burn should include assessment of the depth of the burn wound. First- and second-degree burns are partial-thickness injuries, and third-degree burns are full-thickness injuries. First-degree burns involve only the epidermis. The mild swelling, erythema, and pain will generally resolve in 5 to 10 days without compromising eyelid function and structure as the damage is superficial.

Second-degree burns, at partial-thickness dermis depth, are characterized by erythema, formation of bullae, considerable edema, and pain. They often heal uneventfully in 7 to 14 days without sequelae. A deep second-degree burn can result in cicatricial eyelid deformity especially if superinfection occurs.

Third-degree burns are severe, full-thickness dermal injuries. The burned lids may have a dark, leathery appearance or appear translucent or waxy white. Such burns are not very painful because the terminal nerve endings have been destroyed. A thick black eschar will form and then separate in 2 to 3 weeks. Granulation tissue will then form and the myofibroblasts will lead to contracture wih ensuing eyelid retraction, cicatricial ectropion, and lagophthalmos.

Treatment

Acute treatment of all thermal eyelid burns requires frequent ocular lubrication with artificial tears and lubricating ointment at bedtime. If there is associated corneal and conjunctival injury, appropriate topical antibiotic ointment should be used as well. The topical antibiotic should be continued until the cornea has reepithelialized. Topical burn medications are placed on the periorbital skin in coordination with the burn team care.

Chemical burns should receive voluminous irrigation with saline or available nonirritating liquids, including water, at the initial site of the injury. It is critical to normalize the pH of the fornices and to debride any foreign materials, which may contain toxic substances. As a rule of thumb, acid burns are self-limited by the initial injury, causing coagulation of proteins and a barrier to further injury. Alkali burns can continue to damage tissues for an extended period. Important considerations at the time of evaluation are corneal clarity, extent of limbal ischemia, and presence of pain. The limbal blood supply is essential for healing, and pain indicates viable corneal innervation. In the intermediate phase (1–4 weeks) of eyelid burn healing, first-degree burns generally do not undergo significant cicatricial changes, and they often heal without sequelae. Second- and third-degree burns are accompanied by cicatrization and skin surface area shortage. This results in lagophthalmos secondary to lower and upper eyelid vertical and horizontal tissue inadequacy. Corneal exposure may lead to epithelial compromise and ensuing sterile or infectious corneal ulcers. In this intermediate period prior to full cicatrization, it is best to perform temporizing measures before the wounds are ready for skin grafting. If heavy ocular lubrication is not sufficient, surgical scar release with subsequent Frost suture eyelid splinting, or non-margin-injuring tarsorrhaphy can be performed.[16]

When burn wounds are completely healed, and the cicatricial phase of healing is over, definitive eyelid reconstruction may be undertaken. Full-thickness skin grafts are usually used for eyelid reconstruction. In less extensive situations, check mobilization with vertical transposition of anterior lamelle may be an aesthetic reconstructive alternative. Optimum donor sites for a full-thickness graft are the non-hair-bearing retroauricular skin, contralateral eyelid, and supraclavicular skin. In a severely burned patient, any available donor site may be used for full-thickness tissue, and split-thickness skin grafts may be used if necessary.

The technique of skin grafting in the burn patient is similar for both the upper and lower eyelids. The only exception is that the lower eyelid may require a horizontal eyelid shortening procedure in addition to the skin graft. The eyelid that is to receive the graft is placed on stretch (Fig. 64–1*A*). In the upper eyelid, the scar tissue is released with either an eyelid crease or supraciliary incision, and a subciliary incision is employed to release cicatricial scar tissue in the lower eyelid. After all scar tissue is released, the eyelid remains on stretch, and the skin graft is harvested and placed in the recipient bed. The graft is sutured into position with numerous interrupted 6-0 sutures leaving one arm of each suture long (Fig. 64–1*B*). A bolster is placed over the graft, and the sutures are tied over the bolster, compressing the graft down onto the host site (Fig. 64–1*C*). A pressure dressing is applied over the bolster with mild pressure, and in 5 to 6 days the dressing and the bolster are removed.[17]

The late phase of eyelid burn healing may also lead to scar formation and webbing of the lateral and medial canthi. Skin grafts and Z-plasty techniques can be employed to address this canthal webbing.[18]

In the treatment of the eyelid burn patient, critical emphasis should be placed on the protection of the cornea and conjunctiva. Skin deformities can often be repaired in the late postinjury period after temporizing measures to protect the cornea have been implemented.

EYELID RECONSTRUCTION

Most often, tissue can be conserved in trauma cases and the surgical repair involves aligning existing tarsal segments (posterior lamella) with care to accurately reconstruct the critical eyelid margin, then aligning successive layers of levator, orbicularis, and skin (anterior lamella). Small superficial eyelid lacerations that do not involve the eyelid margin and are parallel to the relaxed skin tension lines (RSTL) can be stabilized with skin tape or glue (Fig. 64–2*A*). Larger lacerations and those that are perpendicular to the RSTL require meticulous approximation and skin edge eversion (Fig. 64–2*B*). The orbicularis muscle contracts when severed and can markedly distort the wound, giving the false impression of tissue loss and the need for anterior lamellar augmentation with a skin graft or midface lift. Careful inspection and delicate manipulation of the laceration margins will more commonly demonstrate no actual tissue loss. Closure in several layers with interrupted 6-0 or 7-0 absorbable and nonabsorbable sutures often leaves little evidence of injury. Septal penetration with resultant levator injury must be ruled out in upper eyelid injuries.

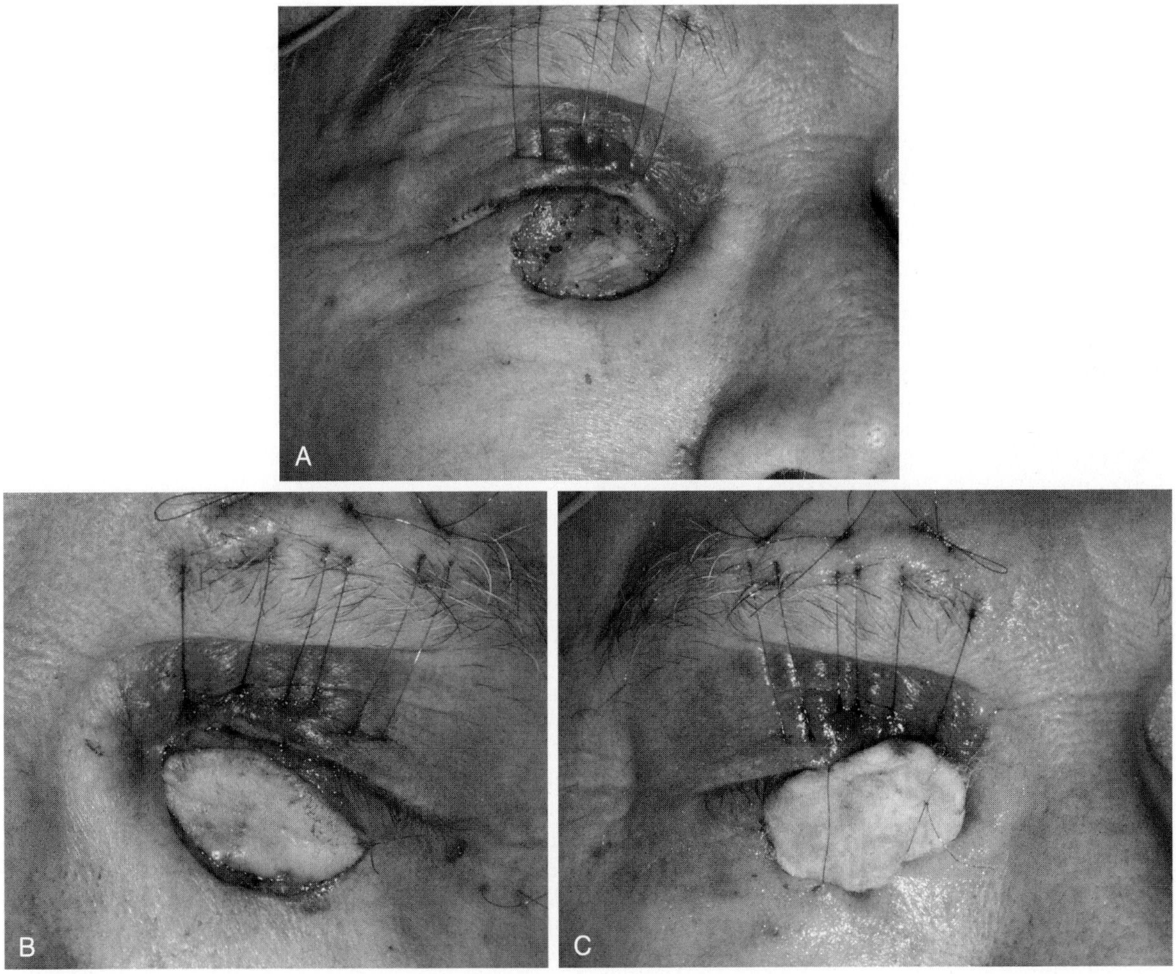

Figure 64–1. *A.* Eyelid with cicatricial shortening is placed on vertical traction to facilitate cicatrix dissection and graft placement. *B.* The graft is sutured into position with numerous interrupted 6-0 sutures, leaving one arm of each suture long. *C.* A bolster placed over graft to slightly compress the graft into the host bed is secured by sutures of appropriate length.

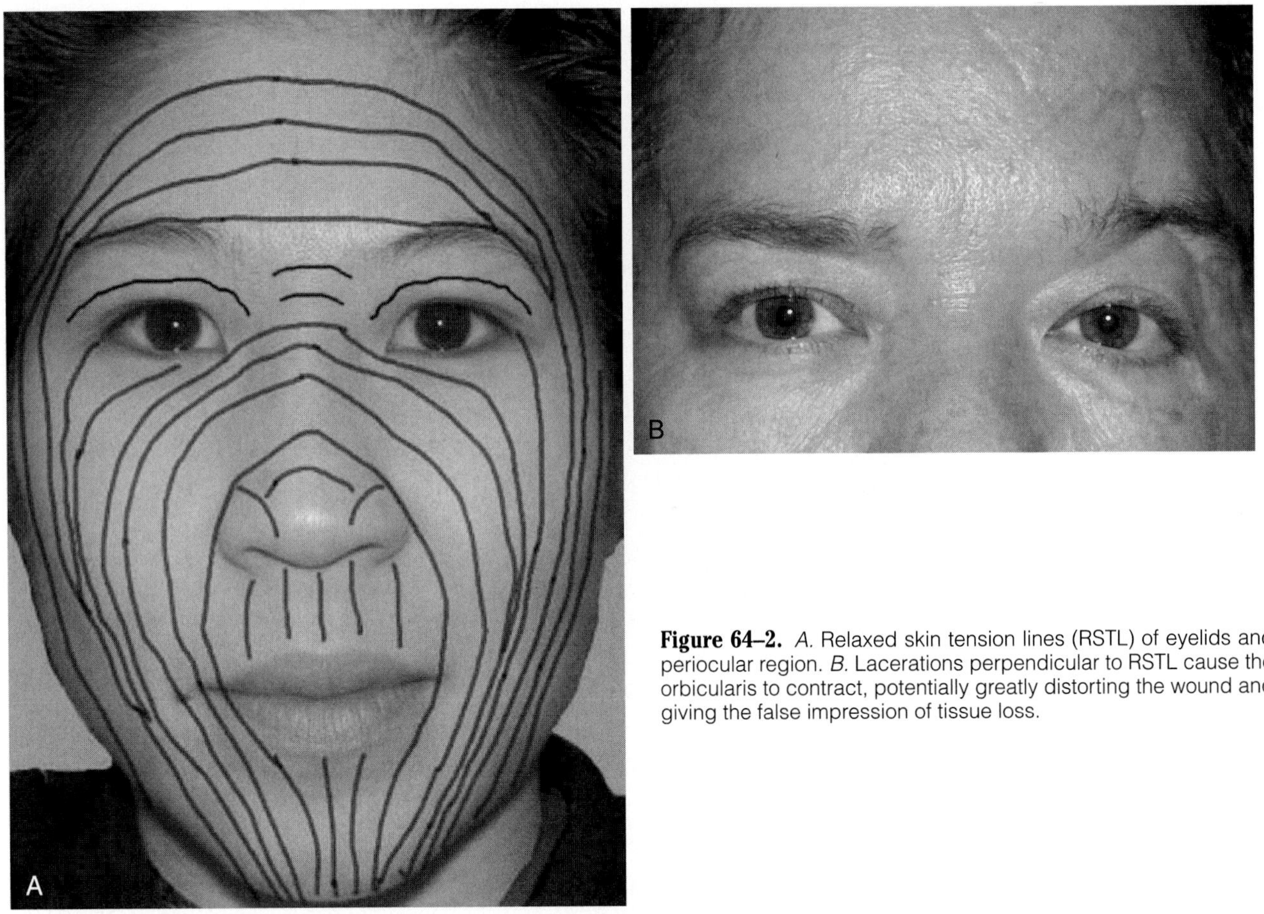

Figure 64–2. *A*. Relaxed skin tension lines (RSTL) of eyelids and periocular region. *B*. Lacerations perpendicular to RSTL cause the orbicularis to contract, potentially greatly distorting the wound and giving the false impression of tissue loss.

EYELID MARGIN LACERATIONS

Adnexal trauma to the eyelid margin requires the most meticulous eyelid approximation and must be precise to avoid eyelid notching and margin malposition. A good aesthetic result depends heavily on wound preparation. All tarsal irregularities at the wound edges should be trimmed to allow parallel tarsal-to-tarsal approximation of the repaired edges. This should be done from the eyelid margin to the peripheral tarsal border to prevent tarsal buckling, even though the primary laceration may only involve the nonmarginal tarsus. The repair begins with the placement of a 6-0 suture in the plane of the meibomian glands at the lid margin approximately 2 mm from the wound edges and 2 mm deep (Fig. 64–3*A*). Historically, these margin sutures are nonabsorbable. However, we have routinely used buried absorbable sutures (such as 6-0 Dexon, which comes with a convenient half-circle needle) without experiencing complications from premature suture absorption. This option is particularly useful in children.

The initial traction suture is pulled to determine whether satisfactory approximation of the margin edges has been accomplished. Eyelid margin eversion should be the goal. This suture is left long and untied to facilitate the repair of the tarsal segments. The anterior tarsus is next closed with fine interrupted partial-thickness sutures with 6-0 or 7-0 Dexon or Vicryl or 7-0 silk. The knots are tied on the anterior tarsal surface to avoid corneal irritation (Fig. 64–3*B*). Additional margin sutures are then placed, usually in the posterior eyelash line and in the gray line. These sutures are tied and left long. The anterior lamella of the eyelid is next closed with fine interrupted sutures. The margin sutures are tied through these sutures to prevent the suture ends from abrading the cornea (Fig. 64–3*C*). When nonabsorbable sutures are used, they are removed in 2 weeks.

CANALICULAR TRAUMA

The canalicular system is occasionally injured in lacerations or avulsions of the medial canthal region, and the anatomy of this area should be thoroughly studied so that the surgeon is comfortable evaluating injuries to the medial canthus and lacrimal outflow area. The canaliculus is farther posterior in the eyelid than many surgeons realize, running almost subconjunctivally. The lacrimal sac is also quite deep and is protected by bone. Lacerations of the sac itself are rare; it is more common to see the common canaliculus avulsed from the sac at the point of their junction.

All canalicular lacerations should be addressed surgically. Even though loss of one canaliculus does not al-

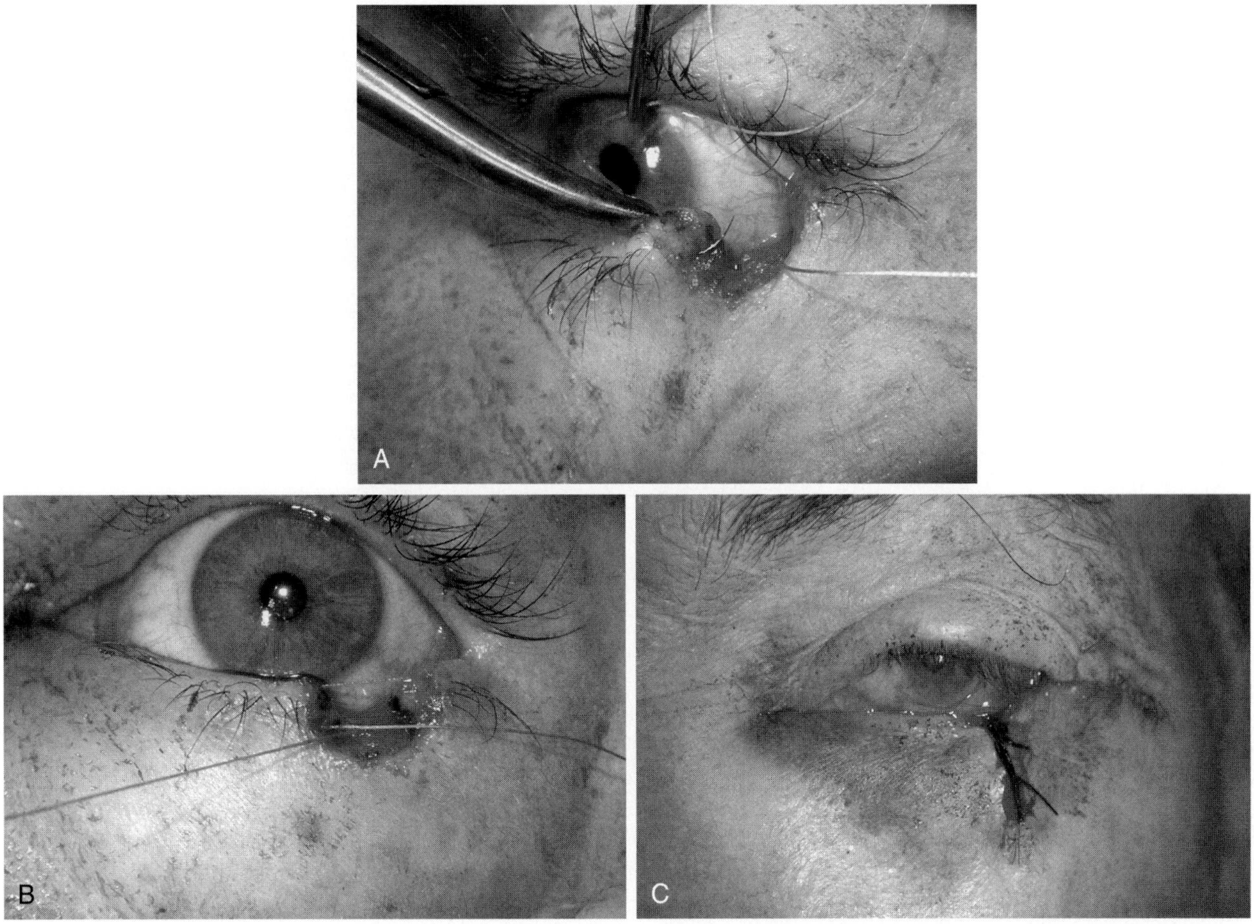

Figure 64–3. *A.* The suture is placed precisely in the plane of the meibomian glands at the eyelid margin approximately 2 mm from the wound edges and 2 mm deep. This placement should provide adequate margin eversion. *B.* Partial-thickness lamellar bites are placed on the tarsus and tied anteriorly to avoid corneal irritation. *C.* The two or three margin sutures are tied through the skin sutures to prevent corneal irritation from the suture ends.

ways lead to tearing, a percentage of patients will develop symptomatic epiphora if one canaliculus is blocked. Only superseding medical or ocular problems should prevent an attempt at canalicular reconstruction during the 72-hour window of primary repair. Silicone tubing is the preferred stenting material. The recent introduction of monocanalicular stenting hardware (FCI Monoka) is a great advancement in the treatment of such injuries. These stents, like their bicanalicular relatives, are left in place for as long as possible, up to 1 year if tolerated.

Repair Techniques

The more "tricks" one has to locate the cut medial canaliculus and perform bicanalicular silicone stenting, the better. For good reason, the pigtail probe has recently undergone something of a resurrection,[19-21] after a generation of ophthalmologists were frightened from its use.[22-23] There is no doubt that the pigtail probe can be pushed "around the corner" into the opposing eyelid even if it is not actually in the canalicular system. However, if used with a delicate touch, and if attempts at cerclage are immediately abandoned if it becomes apparent that the probe will not easily make the passage, the incidence of false passages should be minimal. Many oculoplastic surgeons favor the blunt-tipped (non-barbed) eyelet pigtail probe as their first approach to bicanalicular intubation in traumatic canalicular disorders. A nonabsorbable suture can be passed through the system using the eyelet on the tip of the pigtail probe (Fig. 64–4) and pulled back through the canalicular system. A 24-mm (in adults) length of hollow silicone tubing can be passed through the system over the suture. The suture is then tied and the knot is rotated into the common canaliculus, the end result being a cerclage of the upper lacrimal drainage system with a silicone stent.

If the pigtail probe will not pass easily, the surgeon must then identify the cut medial edge of the canaliculus in the wound. Adequate magnification, lighting, and retraction are critical. By focusing attention posteriorly in the medial eyelid stump near the caruncle, the cut edge can almost always be identified by its characteristic whitish color and rounded, rolled edges. The canaliculus is a white mucosal structure in a bed of red

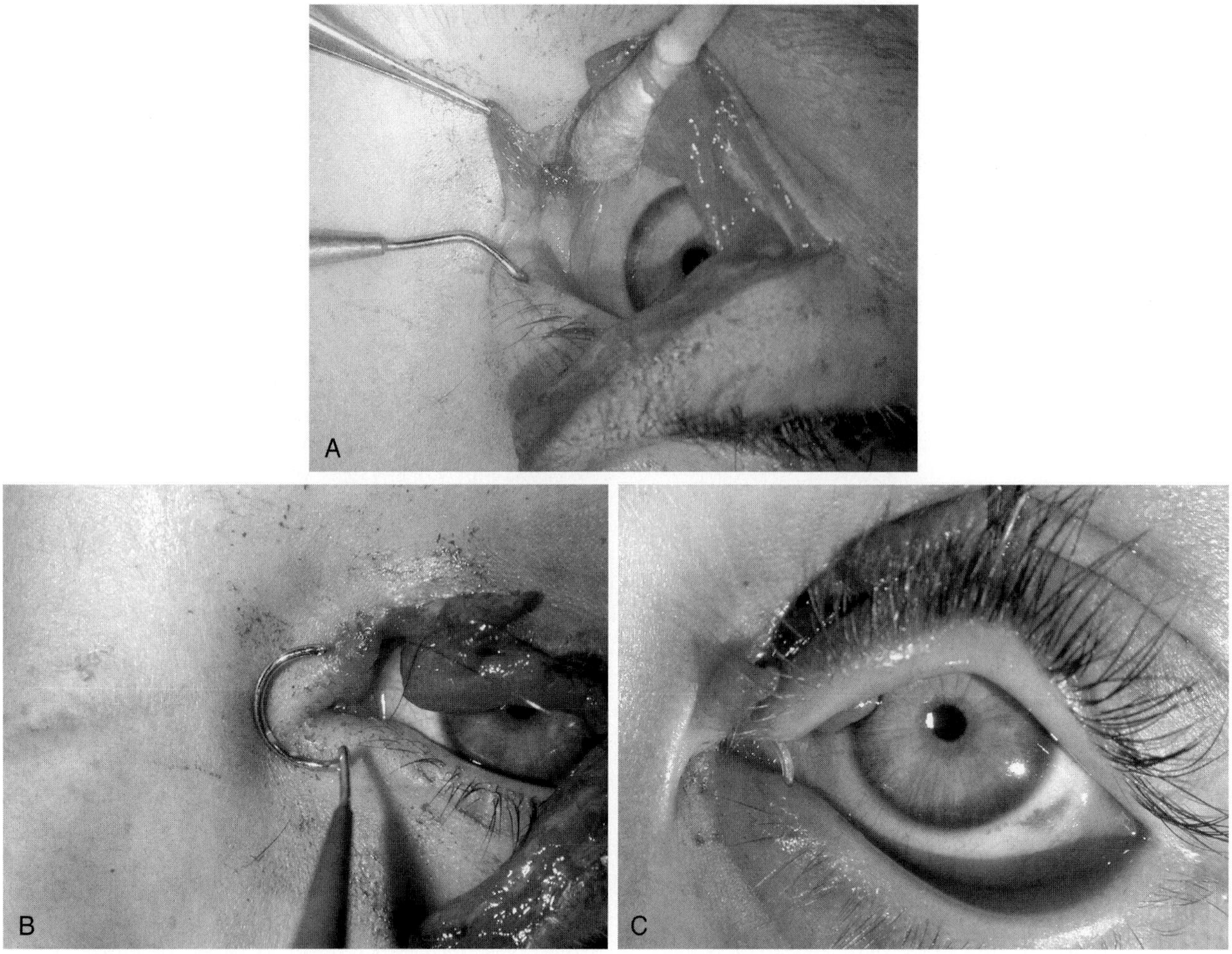

Figure 64–4. The pigtail probe is used to pass a silicone cerclage through the canalicular system to stent a canalicular laceration. *A.* The pigtail probe is inserted through the upper punctum and is delicately guided through the common canaliculus and inferior canaliculus, to exit through the cut edge of the inferior canaliculus into the wound. *B.* A 6-0 polypropylene suture is passed through the eyelet at the tip of the pigtail probe and is drawn back through the system. *C.* A 24-mm length of silicone tubing is threaded through the canalicular system over the preplaced 6-0 suture. The polypropylene suture is then tied under appropriate tension, and the knot is rotated to the internal common punctum so that only the smooth silicone tube with the suture resting inside is exposed between the upper and lower punctae in the medial palpebral fissure. The deep limb of the medial canthal tendon will next be reconstructed using absorbable sutures. Care is taken to accurately align the orbicularis muscle surrounding the cut canalicular edges.

muscle and connective tissue. As a last resort, air, dyed viscoelastic material, or identifiable fluids such as flourescein can be injected into the opposite canaliculus or even into the sac directly in hopes of identifying their exit through the cut canaliculus. If all else fails, the sac can be surgically opened, the internal common punctum exposed, and the canaliculus identified by retrograde probing. Once the cut edge of the canaliculus is identified, bicanalicular intubation into the inferior meatus of the nose can be performed. Adequate suturing of the deep orbicularis to allow appropriate union of the cut canalicular mucosal edges is a requirement; microscopic anastomosis of the mucosal surfaces with fine 8-0 or smaller sutures is advocated by some surgeons.[24] If the posterior limb of the medial canthal tendon is avulsed, it should be sutured to the periosteum of the posterior lacrimal crest to avoid anterior migration of the medial canthus. When the lateral canaliculus and punctum have been lost to tumor or trauma, the medial cut edge of canaliculus can be marsupialized into the conjunctival sac.

EVALUATION AND REPAIR OF ORBITAL FRACTURES

ORBITAL IMAGING

Computed tomography has revolutionized craniofacial fracture management. In many ways, the literature before CT scanning has become of historic interest only. The ability to accurately identify bony changes in three dimensions, to identify expansions in orbital volume, and to observe soft-tissue changes directly allows refined management of orbital fractures. Many of the controversies regarding fracture management that characterized the older literature have become irrelevant, because decisions are now based on the clinical examination and CT visualization of the precise bony and soft-tissue anatomic pathology of the fracture.

Computed tomography remains the "gold standard" for imaging of orbital and facial fractures because it is fast, provides excellent bony detail, and is relatively inexpensive compared to MRI. Plain films have very little role and except in unusual cases should be bypassed for immediate CT scanning in the axial plane and, if the patient can safely cooperate, the direct coronal plane.

When given the luxury of an additional orbital imaging study, MRI scanning can provide superb soft-tissue detail of the changes in the orbital fat and extraocular muscles that typically occur in orbital blow-out fractures. Tonami and collegues[25] have demonstrated the utility of MRI studies in detecting soft-tissue changes such as herniation and incarceration of muscle and fat. Because of the high soft-tissue resolution of MRI scanning, MRI is an ideal modality for this type of investigation. As more experience with MRI studies of orbital fractures is obtained, it should become possible to correlate the soft-tissue changes with motility outcome in the same way that Gilbard[26] was able to do with CT scanning.

With regard to entrapment of orbital soft tissues, however, orbital imaging studies must always go hand in hand with clinical correlation; cases that demonstrate no motility disturbance cannot be improved surgically, regardless of the findings on orbital imaging. Conversely, patients with blow-out fracture in which orbital imaging studies demonstrate no frank entrapment of the inferior rectus muscle may nevertheless go on to develop symptomatic cicatricial motility impairment. This finding was pointed out by Elsas and Anda,[27] who found in a series of blow-out fractures (treated based on CT findings and not on clinical examination with forced duction testing) that 2 of 6 patients with "hooked" but not "entrapped" inferior rectus muscles went on to develop restricted motility.

BLOW-OUT FRACTURE REPAIR: DECISION MAKING

The management of isolated orbital blow-out fractures is directed toward the two main treatable late complications of such injuries: change in globe position (enophthalmos and hypoglobus) and restrictive strabismus.[28–30] Management decisions must be based on the clinical examination and on orbital imaging studies. Decisions are also based on the acceptable amount of enophthalmos; our experience has been that patients have reached such a degree of sophistication that they will not accept 2 or 3 mm of enophthalmos as a post-traumatic result,[29] we are therefore aggressive in identifying and addressing expansions of orbital volume. If orbital imaging identifies significant expansion of the orbital volume (greater than 2 cc, typically in large floor fractures or fractures that involve the floor and medial wall), then immediate surgery is indicated to minimize the risk of late enophthalmos. Consequently, the surgeon must be careful to assure that the surgery restores the orbital volume, and this requires careful isolation of firm bony ledges on all sides of the fracture and adequate fixation of an appropriately sized alloplastic or autogenous implant.

These cases are easily surgically undercorrected, especially if a thin, nonrobust implant like Silastic is used for control of the orbital volume. In cases in which orbital imaging studies demonstrate a blow-out fracture but the orbital volume is not expanded significantly, there is no indication for immediate surgery. In these cases surgery is based on ocular motility considerations, with the goal of preventing or minimizing late restrictive strabismus. It is significantly more difficult in these cases to accurately identify surgical candidates and to achieve surgical success. Late orbital restriction is multifactorial,[31] and surgery that "reduces" a blow-out fracture by elevating the orbital connective tissues out of the maxillary sinus and plating across the defect may or may not alter the scarring of the septa of Koorneef[32–35] so as to improve the eventual orbital mobility. There are no absolute surgical indications and every case must be individualized. However, factors that tip the scales toward surgery include a restrictive motility pattern persisting beyond 2 weeks, positive forced ductions, and orbital imaging studies suggesting entrapment or incarceration of orbital connective tissues or extraocular muscle. A 1- to 2-week waiting period is recommended in these cases because the orbital edema that occurs immediately after the contusion injury can mimic a restrictive strabismus; steroid treatment may reduce this edema and clarify the clinical picture.[36]

Because these motility defects may clear completely with time, the surgeon is tempted to delay surgical therapy in cases of restricted orbital motility following blow-out fracture; however, the longer the wait the greater the chance of permanent restrictive scarring. If the surgical indications are present, orbital exploration should be performed within 2 weeks of the injury. Orbital surgery in these cases should involve careful repositioning of prolapsed orbital tissues and identification of the entire 360 degrees of bony fracture edge to be sure there are no residual scar bands from the orbital connective tissue to the fracture edges. Orbital fractures in children can cause significant muscle entrapment ("white-eyed blow-out fracture")[56] and in this case, urgent repair is indicated (Fig. 64–5).

Prophylactic antibiotics in orbital blow-out fractures are routinely given in many centers. Westfall and Shore[20] point to the rarity of orbital infection in uncomplicated blow-out fractures and the potential side effects of indiscriminate antibiotic therapy. They suggest a more tempered approach, with antibiotics used prophylactically only in potentially infected cases and then, used early on (preferably in the immediate preoperative period).

BLOW-OUT FRACTURE REPAIR: TECHNIQUE

Anesthesia for orbital fracture surgery can be general or monitored local. Kezerian and associates[38] report

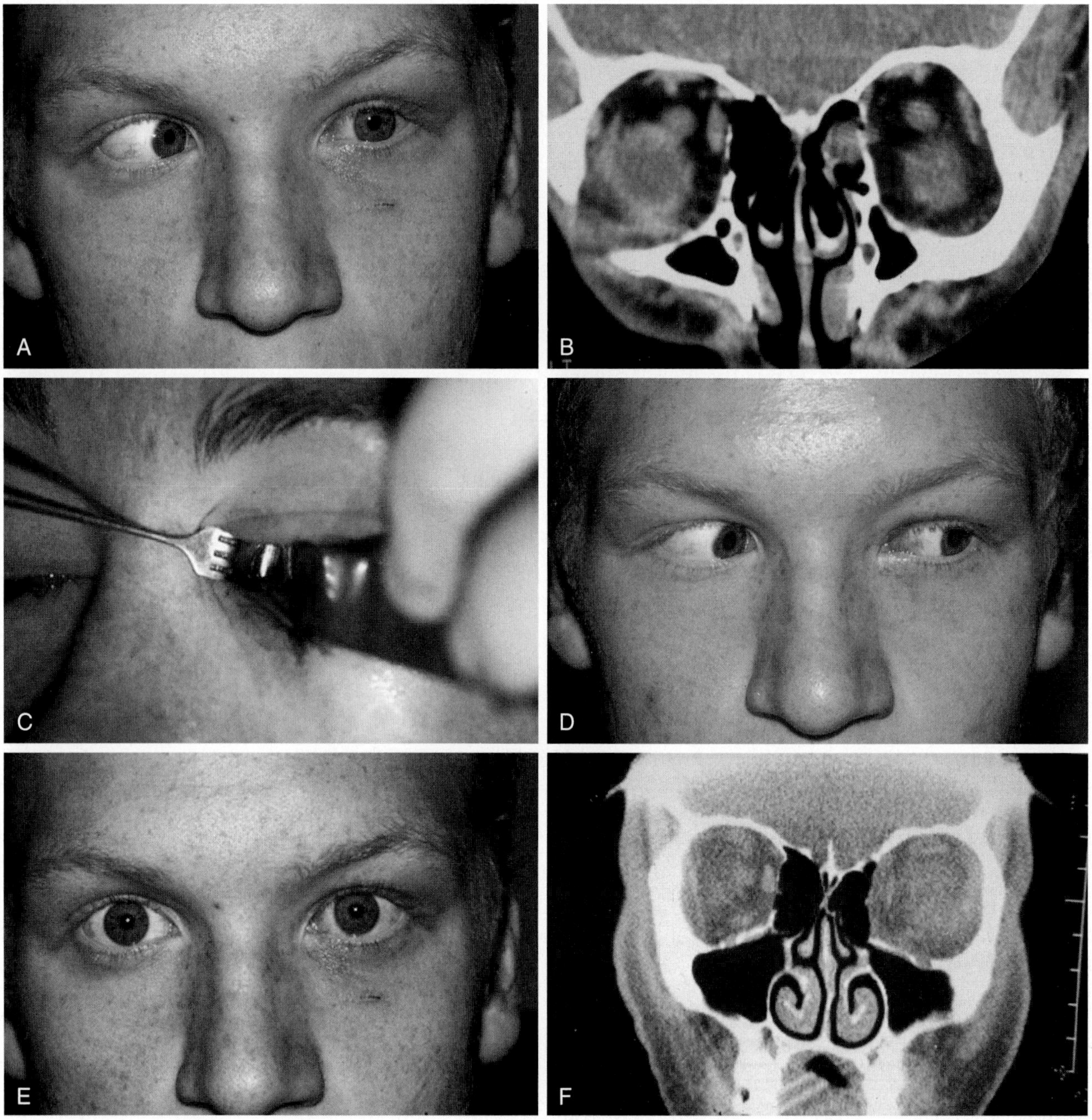

Figure 64–5. *A.* Preoperative photo of patient with medial wall fracture, enophthalmos, and entrapped globe. (© Figure copyright 1997: Regents UC, University of California, Los Angeles, reprinted with permission.) *B.* Preoperative CT scan demonstrating loss of the medial rectus muscle into the ethmoid sinus. *C.* Intraoperative photo. (© Figure copyright 1997: Regents UC, University of California, Los Angeles, reprinted with permission.) *D.* Postoperative result following transcaruncular placement of a Medpore implant bridging from the orbital roof to the lateral orbital floor. (© Figure copyright 1997: Regents UC, University of California, Los Angeles, reprinted with permission.) *E.* Invisible healed transcaruncular incision. (© Figure copyright 1997: Regents UC, University of California, Los Angeles, reprinted with permission.) *F.* Postoperative CT scan demonstrating adequate control of orbital volume and recreation of the medial wall contour. (© Figure copyright 1997: Regents UC, University of California, Los Angeles, reprinted with permission.)

four patients with isolated orbital floor fractures repaired under local anesthesia with peribulbar block, a technique that we have found useful in the office setting. We have not encountered complications related to the anesthesia in more than 24 patients seen over a 10-year period (Baylis and Shorr, personal communication). The transconjunctival approach to the orbital floor has considerable advantages over the cutaneous approach, including excellent exposure, rapid access, and minimal risk of causing lower eyelid retraction or ectropion.[39,40] The vast majority of the orbit, including the medial wall, floor, inferior orbital fissure, and lateral wall and superior orbital fissure can be accessed surgically through a conjunctival approach with cantholysis[41]; when additional superomedial exposure is required, we add a caruncular conjunctival or coronal incision. The medial orbit can be widely accessed through a caruncular incision, opening the medial conjunctiva at the lateral base of the caruncle and then dissecting medially along the posterior plane of Horner's muscle to the posterior lacrimal crest to expose at a subperiosteal level the roof, medial wall, and medial orbital floor. The caruncular approach is especially well-suited for large medial fractures that involve the superior lamina papyracea; in these cases the implant should rest on the stable fronal bone of the roof, and the caruncular conjunctival approach provides superb access to this area (Fig. 64–5).

The question of what material to place in the orbit to bridge the orbital fracture continues to engender significant controversy in meetings and in the literature.[30,40,42] The degree of controversy is out of proportion to the importance of the question. Far more critical are proper surgical technique, including appropriate surgical judgment in case selection as well as delicate handling, accurate dissection, and meticulous exposure of the orbital tissues and fracture edges. Properly placed and fixated, just about any well tolerated implant material will successfully bridge the fracture edges and accomplish the goals of surgery, which are to restore the orbital shape (and thus volume) and to normalize the orbital soft tissue relationships, thereby minimizing abnormal restrictive scarring within the orbital septa. Conversely, the newest, most sophisticated, exotic material implant will fail miserably if it is put in with crude surgical technique or in the wrong anatomic position. The size of the fracture can play a significant role in the decision regarding material choice: small fractures are well repaired with alloplastic sheet materials such as porous polyethylene (Medpor)[30] or absorbable materials such as lyophilized cartilage[40] or polydioxanone (PDS).[43] Recently available absorbable plating hardware (Lactosorb, Leibinger) confers the advantage of robust material that eventually absorbs with time, avoiding the risks inherent in leaving foreign material in the orbit. Current studies are under way to evaluate the effects for the long term of these promising implants on volume and motility. Larger fractures, particularly those with significant involvement of the medial wall, carry a much greater risk of undercontrol of orbital volume with late volume expansion and enophthalmos. These cases are best managed with rigid materials such as metal alloys, calvarial bone grafts, or thick porous polyethylene. The implant should be well stabilized in position; particularly in cases in which identification of 360 degrees of bony orbital ledge is difficult, the use of rigid fixation systems can be extremely useful in surgically controlling the orbital shape and volume (Fig. 64–6). A common mistake is to fail to realize that the posterior inferomedial orbit, rather than being concave away from the orbital contents, is actually convex toward the orbital contents. This postequatorial convexity must be recreated to avoid expansion of orbital volume into this space.

COMPLEX ORBITAL FRACTURES

Significant advances in craniofacial fracture repair technique have occurred over the past 15 years. Two technologic advances, computerized orbital imaging and improved osteosynthesis plating systems, have driven these advances. The ability to recognize and better stabilize and fix these fractures, together with appreciation for craniofacial principles of wide exposure and primary bony repair, have led to much more aggressive early management of orbital fractures. Ophthalmic orbital surgeons have always stressed the need for extensive knowledge of orbital anatomy and physiology in orbital fracture management. This knowledge and experience makes them especially well prepared to serve as the "captain" of the multidisciplinary team that typically manages patients with combined orbital and facial trauma.

Despite the widespread application of these principles, we still routinely see late cases of orbital trauma that are poorly managed, leading to late orbital dysfunction, which is much more difficult to address secondarily. Ophthalmologists, with their special knowledge and skills in orbital anatomy and physiology, should play an active role in the management of these patients; those with special interest and training in orbital surgery are ideally suited to act as primary surgeons in the management of these patients, and those ophthalmologists with a less active interest in orbital surgery should nevertheless stay abreast of conceptual and practical advances in orbital fracture management so that they can guide their patients through the diagnosis and management of their injuries in a way to avoid inappropriate therapy.

ORBITAL ROOF FRACTURES

Orbital roof fractures are seen in high-velocity facial injuries and may be harbingers of significant ocular, orbital apical, or intracranial injuries.[44,45] The diagnosis should be suspected in high-velocity facial injuries accompanied by exophthalmos, blepharoptosis, motility impairment, frontal nerve hypesthesia, or palpable step-off fracture of the superior rim. High-resolution CT is the diagnostic study of choice. These fractures typically have the configuration of "blow-in" fractures, with decreased orbital volume and exophthalmos re-

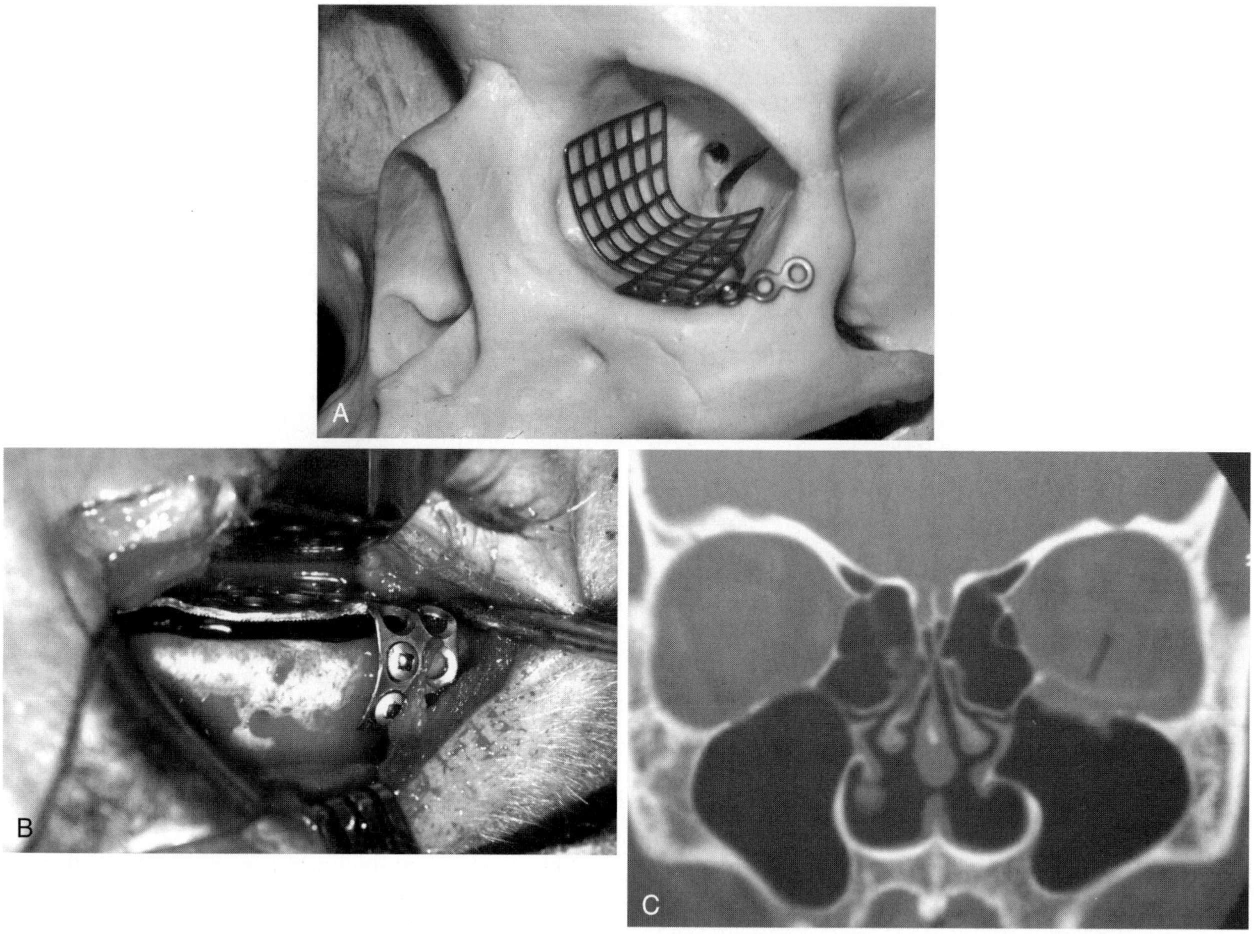

Figure 64–6. *A*. Titanium orbital floor plate is molded to fit the intact bony ledges in a large inferomedial orbital blow-out fracture; exposure is via transconjunctival incision. (© Figure copyright 1997: Regents UC, University of California, Los Angeles, reprinted with permission.) *B*. The plate has been inserted under direct visualization with care to recreate the normal orbital contour. The plate is rigidly fixated to the firm bone of the inferolateral rim and zygoma. (© Figure copyright 1997: Regents UC, University of California, Los Angeles, reprinted with permission.) *C*. Postoperative CT scan demonstrating adequate recreation of orbital shape and control of orbital volume. In this case, an outer table cranial bone graft was placed over the implant; the implants can be covered with porous polyethylene sheets or left bare. (© Figure copyright 1997: Regents UC, University of California, Los Angeles, reprinted with permission.)

lated to inferior displacement of the orbital roof. Minimally displaced fractures do not require surgical repair. In cases of significant bony displacement, open reduction of the fracture can be accomplished with a combined neurosurgical and orbital approach. When radiographic compression of the superior orbital fissure is noted in association with orbital apical neuropathies, most experts would recommend decompression of the fissure.

ORBITOZYGOMATIC AND NASO-ORBITAL-ETHMOIDAL FRACTURES

Ophthalmologists should be aware of the clinical setting, manifestations, and diagnosis and treatment of orbitozygomatic and naso-orbital-ethmoidal fractures.[30,40,42,46–50] In the setting of blunt trauma to the orbit, complex fractures of the midface can be masked by orbital and facial edema but may be suspected if canthal or orbital dystopia, zygomatic prominence asymmetry, or trismus, maxillary instability, or malocclusion of bite are present. The diagnosis is confirmed, and treatment decisions are largely determined, by high-resolution CT. The goals of surgery from an ophthalmic standpoint are to prevent late enophthalmos and orbital and canthal dystopia. Therefore, the indication for surgical repair is a significantly displaced fracture of the extended bony orbit including the maxilla, zygoma, and naso-ethmoidal complex. Early surgery (within 7 to 10 days) is far preferable to late repair; only overriding medical or ocular considerations should delay surgery beyond the period when primary repair can be performed. Surgical principles of repair include accurate repositioning and rigid fixation of key bony landmarks such as the medial canthal bony fragment[46,47,50,51] and the zygomatic tetrapod.[30,40,48] Rigid fixation systems[52,53] allow stable, accurate repositioning of bony fragments in three dimensions. The importance of detailed anatomic knowledge, accurate orbital imaging studies, and wide subperiosteal exposure of involved bony regions cannot be overemphasized.

LATE ENOPHTHALMOS

By far the best treatment for late enophthalmos after orbital fracture is prevention. Late enophthalmos is caused by unrecognized or poor control of expansion in orbital volume after orbital fractures (Fig. 64–7). The difficulty in treating late cases arises not only from the bony scarring with an expanded bony orbit, but also from soft-tissue changes that occur as the injured soft tissues both inside and outside the orbit heal abnormally over a distorted bony architecture.[51] Although many cases of late enophthalmos can be improved by decreasing the orbital volume with onlay grafts[54] or bony osteotomies,[55] in our experience there are some patients with severe late fibrosis of the orbital soft-tissue connective system and a positive "forced traction test," in which the globe cannot be grasped and tracted anteriorly in the orbit

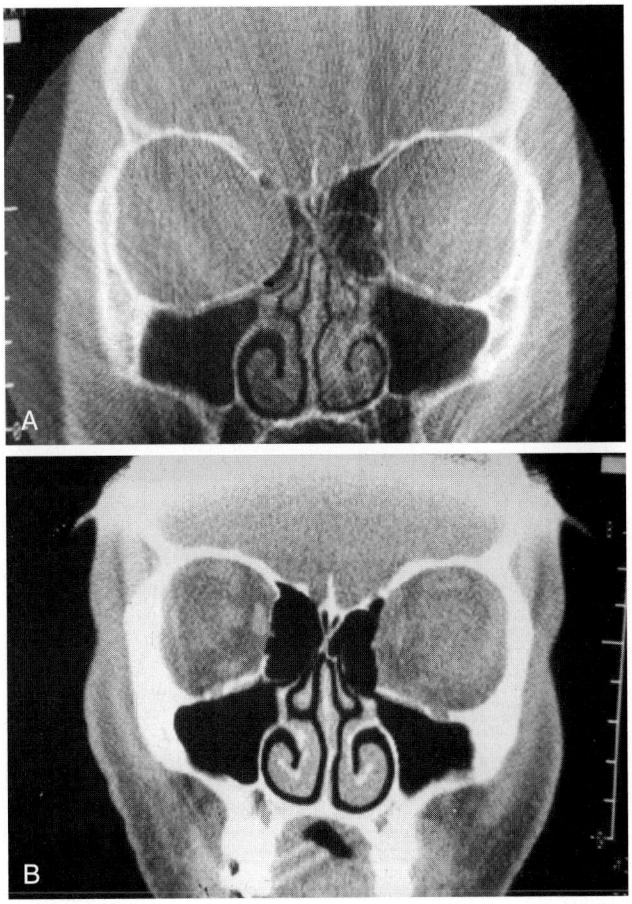

Figure 64–7. *A.* Coronal CT scan of patient with late enophthalmos after inferomedial orbital blow-out fracture. Orbital volume was poorly controlled at the time of initial surgery; the orbital shape has significantly expanded inferomedially. (© Figures copyright 1997: Regents UC, University of California, Los Angeles, reprinted with permission.) *B.* Postoperative CT scan demonstrating restoration of orbital volume. The implant rests on stable bone on the orbital roof and lateral orbital floor. (© Figures copyright 1997: Regents UC, University of California, Los Angeles, reprinted with permission.)

because of the tight leash of orbital cicatricial scar tissue. The defect may be surgically undercorrected in spite of extensive intraoperative attempts to lyse intraorbital scar tissue.

REFERENCES

1. Gossman MD, Roberts DM, Barr CC: Ophthalmic aspects of orbital injury: A comprehensive diagnostic and management approach. Clin Plast Surg 1992;19:71–85.
2. Walton RL, Matory Jr. WE: Wound care. In Ho MT, Saunders CE (eds): Current Emergency Diagnosis and Treatment, 3rd Edition. Norwalk, CT, Appleton and Lange, 1990;756–780.
3. Karlson TA: The incidence of facial injuries from dog bites. JAMA 1984;251:3265–3267.
4. Palmer J, Rees M: Dog bites of the face; a 15 year review. Br J Plast Surg 1983;36:315-318.
5. Herman DC, Bartley GB, Walker RC: The treatment of animal bite injuries of the eye and ocular adnexa. Ophthal Plast Reconstr Surg 1987;3:237–241.
6. Findling JW, Pohlmanss GP, Rose HD: Fulminant gram-negative bacillemia (DF-2) following a dog bite in an asplenic woman. Am J Med 1980;68:154–156.
7. Hicklin H, Verghese A, Alvarez S: Dysgonic fermenter 2 septicemia. Rev Infect Dis 1987;9:884–890.
8. Perez RE: Dysgonic fermenter-2 infections. West J Med 1988; 148:90–92.
9. Dankner WM, Davis CE, Thompson MA: DF-2 bacteremia following a dog bite in a 4 month old child. Pediatr Infect Dis J 1987;6:695–696.
10. Bailie WE, Stowe EC, Schmitt AM: Aerobic bacterial flora of oral and nasal fluids of canines with reference to bacteria associated with bites. J Clin Microbiol 1978;7:223–231.
11. Brenner DJ, Hollis DG, Fanning GR, et al.: *Capnocytophaga canimorsus* sp. Nov. (formerly CDC Group DF-2), a cause of septicemia following dog bite, and *C. cynodegnmi* sp. Nov., a cause of localized wound infection following dog bite. J Clin Microbiol 1989;27:231–235.
12. Gonnering RS: Ocular adnexal injury and complications in orbital dog bites. Ophthal Plast Reconstr Surg 1987;3:231–235.
13. Stevenson TR, Thacker JG, Rodeheaver GT, et al.: Cleansing the traumatic wound by high pressure syringe irrigation. J Am Coll Emerg Physicians 1976;5:17–21.
14. Gonnering RS: Orbital and periorbital dog bites. Adv Ophthal Plast Reconstr Surg 1987;7:171–180.
15. Glover AT: Eyelid burns. In Shingleton BJ, Hersh PS, Kenyon KR (eds): Eye Trauma, St. Louis, Mosby-Year Book, 1991;315–322.
16. Kulwin DR, Kersten RC: Management of eyelid burns. In Focal Points; Clinical Modules for Ophthalmologists. 1990; Vol 8, No. 2.
17. Hartford CE: Methods of reducing burn scar formation. In Stark RB (ed): Plastic Surgery of the Head and Neck, Vol 1, New York, Churchill Livingstone, 1987;282–285.
18. Waltman SR, Keates RH, Hoyt CS, et al.: Surgery of the Eye, New York, Churchill Livingstone, 1988.
19. Reifler DM: Management of canalicular laceration. Surv Ophthalmol 1991;36:113–132.
20. Jordan DR, Nerad JA, Tse DT: The pigtail probe, revisited. Ophthalmology 1990;97:512–519.
21. Baskin MA: Variations on pigtail probe technique [letter]. Ophthalmology 1990;97:1399–1400.
22. Saunders DH, Shannon GM, Flanagan JC: The effectiveness of the pigtail probe method of repairing canalicular lacerations. Ophthal Surg 1978;9:33–40.
23. Kennedy RH, May J, Dailey J, Flanagan JC: Canalicular laceration: an 11 year epidemiologic and clinical study. Ophthal Plast Reconstr Surg 1990;6:46–53.
24. Nelson CC: Management of eyelid trauma. Aust N Z J Ophthalmol 1991;19:357–363.
25. Tonami H, Yamamoto I, Matsuda M, et al.: Orbital fractures: Surface coil MR imaging. Radiology 1991;179:789–794.
26. Gilbard SM, Mafee MF, Lagouros PA, Langer BG: Orbital blowout fractures: The prognostic significance of computed tomography. Ophthalmology 1985;92:1523–1528.

27. Elsas T, Anda S: Orbital CT in the management of blow-out fractures of the orbital floor. Acta Ophthalmol (Copenh) 1990;68: 710–714.
28. Dutton JJ: Management of blowout fractures of the orbital floor [editorial]. Surv Ophthalmol 1991;35:279–280.
29. Putterman AM: Management of blow out fractures of the orbital floor: III. The conservative approach. Surv Ophthalmol 1991;35: 292–298.
30. Manson PN, Iliff N: Management of blow-out fractures of the orbital floor: II. Early repair for selected injuries. Surv Ophthalmol 1991;35:280–292.
31. Lipton JR, Page AB, Lee JP: Management of diplopia on downgaze following orbital trauma. Eye 1990;4:535–537.
32. Koorneef L: Current concepts on the management of orbital blowout fractures. Ann Plast Surg 1982;9:185–200.
33. Koorneef L: Orbital septa: Anatomy and function. Ophthalmology 1979;86:876–880.
34. Koorneef L: The architecture of the musculo-fibrous apparatus in the human orbit. Acta Morphol Neerl Scand 1977;15:35–64.
35. Koorneef L: New insights in the human orbital connective tissue: Result of a new anatomical approach. Arch Ophthalmol 1977; 95:1269–1273.
36. Millman AL, Della Rocca RC, Spector S, et al.: Steroids and orbital blowout fractures: A new systematic concept in medical management and surgical decision-making. Adv Ophthal Plast Reconstr Surg 1987;6:291–300.
37. Westfall CT, Shore JW: Isolated fractures of the orbital floor: Risk of infection and the role of antibiotic prophylaxis. Ophthal Surg 1991;22:409–411.
38. Kezirian GM, Hill FD, Hill FD: Peribulbar anesthesia for the repair of orbital floor fractures. Ophthal Surg 1991;22:601–605.
39. Westfall CT, Shore JW, Nunery WR, et al.: Operative complications of the transconjunctival inferior fornix approach. Ophthalmology 1991;98:1525–1528.
40. Zingg M, Chowdhury K, Ladrach K, et al.: Treatment of 813 zygoma-lateral orbital complex fractures: New aspects. Arch Otolaryngol Head Neck Surg 1991;117:611–620.
41. Shore JW: The fornix approach to the inferior orbit. Adv Ophthal Plast Reconstr Surg 1987;6:377–385.
42. Nguyen PN, Sullivan P: Advances in the management of orbital fractures. Clin Plast Surg 1992;19:87–98.
43. Ilzuka T, Mikkonen P, Paukku P, Lindqvist C: Reconstruction of orbital floor with polydioxanone plate. Int J Oral Maxillofac Surg 1991;20:83–87.
44. Sullivan WG: Displaced orbital roof fractures: Presentation and treatment. Plast Reconstr Surg 1991;87:657–661.
45. Karesh JW, Kelman SE, Chirico PA, Mirvis SE: Orbital roof "blow-in" fractures. Ophthal Plast Reconstr Surg 1991;7:77–83.
46. Leipziger LS, Manson PN: Nasoethmoid orbital fractures: Current concepts and management principles. Clin Plast Surg 1992;19: 167–193.
47. Markowitz BL, Manson PN, Sargent L, et al.: Management of the medial canthal tendon in nasoethmoid orbital fractures: The importance of the central fragment in classification and treatment. Plast Reconstr Surg 1991;87:843–853.
48. Rohrich RJ, Hollier LH, Watumull D: Optimizing the management of orbitozygomatic fractures. Clin Plast Surg 1992;19:149–165.
49. Dufresne CR: The use of immediate grafting in facial fracture management: Indications and clinical considerations. Clin Plast Surg 1992;19:207–217.
50. Markowitz BL, Manson PN, Yaremchuk M, et al.: High-energy orbital dislocations: The possibility of traumatic hypertelorbitism. Plast Reconstr Surg 1991;88:20–28.
51. Yaremchuk MJ: Changing concepts in the management of secondary orbital deformities. Clin Plast Surg 1992;19:113–124.
52. Ellis DS, Toth BA, Stewart WB: A micro system for rigid bony fixation in orbital surgery. Ophthal Plast Reconstr Surg 1991;7: 144–150.
53. Sargent LA, Fulks KD: Reconstruction of internal orbital fractures with Vitallium mesh. Plast Reconstr Surg 1991;88:31–38.
54. Geist CE, Stracher MA, Grove AS: Orbital augmentation by hydroxylapatite-based composites: A rabbit study and comparative analysis. Ophthal Plast Reconstr Surg 1991;7:8–22.
55. Pearl RM: Treatment of enophthalmos. Clin Plast Surg 1992; 19:99–111.
56. Jordan DR, Allen LH, White J, et al.: Intervention within days for some orbital floor fractures; the white-eyed blowout. Ophthal Plast Reconstr Surg 1988;14:379–390.

CHAPTER 65

Posterior Segment Trauma: Principles and Practice

GIORA TREISTER, M.D., TAMARA WYGNANSKI-JAFFE, M.D., and JOSEPH MOISSEIEV, M.D.

The management of ocular trauma is a challenge, and the outcome depends both on the nature of the injury and the ability of the ophthalmologist to cope with the variable and diverse nature of ocular trauma. In literature on the subject of ocular trauma there are abundant reports on series of patients that elaborate on prognostic factors and functional and anatomic outcomes.[1–10] The purpose of this chapter is to present a policy for the primary and definitive management of posterior segment trauma. Our approach to various aspects of posterior segment trauma is described, with special emphasis on the more severe types of penetrating trauma, with or without intraocular foreign bodies (IOFB). Key aspects in the decision–making process leading to treatment and the surgical procedures are described in detail, to familiarize ophthalmologists not routinely involved in the management of severe ocular trauma with this fascinating subject. Injuries from relatively minor blunt trauma are not discussed in detail.

TERMINOLOGY

Various classifications of ocular trauma have been used in the literature, making comparisons between studies difficult, and causing confusion with regard to the accurate definition of the terms in use. Recently, a standardized classification of ocular trauma that is simple and consistent was proposed,[11] and in our opinion it should be adopted by ophthalmologists for routine clinical use. The definitions of this classification are used throughout this chapter. The major definitions in this classification are:

1. *Rupture.* Full-thickness wound of the eye wall, caused by a blunt object. The impact results in a momentary increase in the intraocular pressure and an inside-out injury mechanism.
2. *Laceration.* Full-thickness wound of the eye wall, usually caused by a sharp object. The wound occurs at the impact site by an outside-in mechanism.

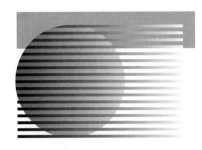

3. *Penetrating injury.* Single laceration of the eye wall, usually caused by a sharp object.
4. *Intraocular foreign body.* Retained foreign object(s) causing entrance laceration(s).
5. *Perforating injury.* Two full-thickness lacerations (entrance and exit) of the eye wall, usually caused by a sharp object or missile.

PRINCIPLES IN MANAGING PATIENTS WITH OCULAR TRAUMA

INITIAL EXAMINATION

History

A detailed history is of critical importance in the management of patients with ocular trauma. Information about the circumstances of the injury and the objects causing the injury should be obtained, as this information helps in evaluating the potential damage to the ocular tissues, and in indicating the potential presence of an IOFB and whether it is likely to be contaminated (Table 65–1).

Physical Examination

The examination of a patient with suspected penetrating injury to the eyeball must be carried out with great care. The eyelids should be opened carefully to avoid exerting unnecessary pressure on the globe, which could result in prolapse of ocular contents through a possible wound. When the eyelids are swollen they may be opened with blunt retractors under topical anesthesia, again taking care not to press on the globe. Young patients or agitated non-cooperating patients in significant pain should be examined under general anesthesia. In conscious cooperating patients the visual acuity should be determined, both for medico-legal reasons and because it is one of the strongest prognostic factors.[1,2,4,12,13] Uncertain or no light perception (NLP) in severely traumatized eyes is a poor prognostic factor, but it does not necessarily indicate that the eye is not salvageable, and occasionally a NLP eye will regain useful vision. If the patient can be examined at the slit lamp, the conjunctiva should be checked carefully to identify possible tears or hemorrhage, which could indicate a penetrating injury. The conjunctival sac and the cornea must be inspected for possible externally located foreign bodies. In eyes with a suspected IOFB, external foreign bodies should be kept for later determination of their composition, information that could be useful in determining the timing of surgery for removal of an internal IOFB. Eyes with small IOFBs consisting of inert material may be followed for some time, and occasionally not operated at all. The location and size of corneal or scleral wounds should be noted, as should the presence and extent of iris prolapse. If the corneal wound is small and the anterior chamber is deep, one should look for a possible defect in the iris, which might indicate the tract of a foreign body that penetrated to the posterior segment of the eye. The pupillary light reflex should be observed when possible, and the presence of traumatic mydriasis, relative pupillary afferent defect (Marcus-Gunn pupil), or inverse afferent defect should be noted. The iris must be carefully examined for possible foreign bodies, tears, or dialysis. In the absence of an open corneal or scleral wound, intraocular pressure should be measured. If the patient is unconscious or cannot be seated, all these steps may be done with the operating microscope. If possible, the pupil should be dilated to allow evaluation of the lens, including the presence of intralenticular foreign bodies, lens subluxation, anterior and/or posterior capsular tears, swelling and opacification of the lens material, and presence of lens material or vitreous in the anterior chamber. In severe blunt trauma vitreous may gain access to the anterior chamber through tears of the zonulae. In eyes with relatively clear media the vitreous and fundus can then be examined, both at the slit lamp if possible, and with the indirect ophthalmoscope. This examination is critical in assessing the severity of the injury to the posterior segment. Findings may include: vitreous hemorrhage, retinal edema, retinal tears and detachment, optic nerve head damage, and intraocular foreign bodies. When eye trauma is accompanied by head injury, consult a neurosurgeon before pharmacological dilatation of the pupils, because pupillary reaction may serve as the only indication of neurological deterioration in cerebral trauma. If incarceration of the iris into the wound is observed, it may be wise to delay dilatation of the pupil until the iris is surgically managed. This allows for better anatomical correction of the prolapsed tissues (Table 65–2).

TABLE 65–1. History to be Obtained in Posterior Segment Trauma

General	Date and Time of Injury
Location of injury	Household, job, sport, agricultural, etc.
Mechanism of trauma	High velocity, low velocity, blunt, penetrating, explosion, burns
Objects involved	Organic material, metal, glass, plastics, chemicals
Safety devices used	Safety glasses, safety mask
Former ocular status	Former visual acuity, amblyopia, other ocular diseases, former surgical procedures
General health	Assess systemic diseases such as clotting disorders, diabetes, hypertension, allergies to medications
Inquire	Time and content of last meal or beverage

TABLE 65–2 Ocular Examination in Posterior Segment Trauma

Visual acuity	Best corrected and pinhole acuity tested in both eyes
External examination	Ocular movements, proptosis (pulsatile/non pulsatile), murmurs Eyelids: hematomas, lacerations, ptosis, foreign bodies Nasolacrimal system, orbital bones, infraorbital sensation
Slit-lamp biomicroscopy	**Fornices:** burns, foreign bodies, hematomas **Conjunctiva:** hemorrhage, laceration **Sclera:** laceration **Cornea:** penetration, laceration, leakage (Seidel), erosion, foreign body, edema **Anterior chamber:** depth, reaction, hypopyon, hyphema, vitreous or lens material, foreign body **Iris:** prolapse, incarceration, hemorrhage, transillumination defects **Pupil:** equal, round, regular, direct and consensual response, pupillary afferent defect, inverse afferent defect
Tonometry	Applanation when possible Delay if globe is ruptured
Gonioscopy	Foreign body, bleeding, angle recess, cyclodialysis, angle closure Delay in cases of hyphema, perforation, or hypotony
Lens	Vossius ring, anterior and/or posterior capsular tear, opacity Dislocation/subluxation, foreign body
Ophthalmoscopy	**Vitreous:** reaction, PVD, hemorrhage, foreign body **Posterior pole:** optic nerve pallor/cupping **Macula:** edema, hemorrhage, hole **Retina:** hole, tear, detachment, incarceration, dialysis
Scleral depression	If no perforation

Special Testing

Imaging

Computerized tomography (CT) and ultrasound (US) examinations should usually be performed in patients with penetrating ocular injury, to eliminate the possibility of an IOFB. This can be done before the primary surgical procedure if the condition of the eye allows it, or later, after the lacerations are closed (Fig. 65–1*A*). Computerized tomography is increasingly helpful in assessing the location and size of the foreign body in the eye. However, some materials that make up foreign bodies may not be demonstrated by CT: plastics, wood, stone, glass, and metals such as zinc and aluminum.[14,15] Helical CT multiplaner imaging may offer several advantages over conventional CT assessment of metallic IOFBs. This includes shorter examination time, reduced motion artifact, less irradiation, and the ability to obtain coronal and sagittal reconstruction images without the need for additional scanning.[16] Ultrasound may be helpful in these cases, when the presence of an IOFB is suspected by history or by the findings on examination; however, it should not be performed on hypotonous eyes. When a metallic foreign body is large, it creates radial reflections in the CT scan and may interfere with determining the actual size and shape of the foreign body (Fig. 65–1*B*). In such cases, the size and shape of the foreign body can be better visualized by a routine x-ray. The US examination is also essential to exclude the possibility of retinal detachment,[17] again to be performed only after primary suturing of the globe has been performed. Ultrasound biomicroscopy may be helpful in detecting small nonmagnetic IOFBs that were missed by CT or US and to determine hidden locations of foreign bodies.[18,19] Ultrasound biomicroscopy in addition to imaging the anterior chamber may differentiate between hypotony caused by detachment of the ciliary body and that caused by an IOFB in the area of the ciliary body or parsplana. Magnetic resonance imaging (MRI) is traditionally contraindicated in cases in which one suspects an IOFB, because of the moving potential of magnetic metallic IOFBs during this examination. However, if ferromagnetic properties of the foreign body can be studied or excluded, and in the coil of the MRI the foreign body does not move, MRI may offer superior localization regarding soft tissue location. Nevertheless, MRI in the event of an IOFB should be reserved only for specific cases in which additional information is warranted.[20]

Electrophysiologic tests

If the retina is attached, a bright-flash electroretinogram (ERG) may be performed to evaluate the retinal function and the extent of damage to the retina from the trauma.[21] In some cases visual evoked potential (VEP) testing is also recommended, as it may be helpful in predicting the visual outcome following surgery[5] and reflects the integrity of the optic nerve and the visual pathways.

Other tests

In addition, it is necessary to assess the patient's ability to withstand general or topical anesthetic procedures. Note ocular and systemic conditions and diseases that may influence treatment such as clotting abnormalities, blood dyscrasias, sickle cell anemia, glaucoma, myopia,

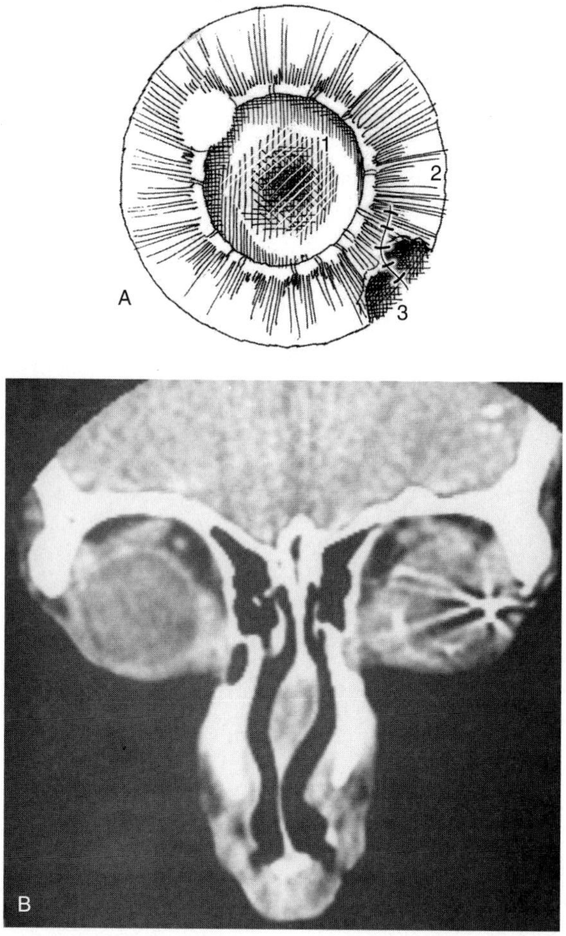

Figure 65–1. Primary management of penetrating injury with a suspected intraocular foreign body (IOFB). *A.* Suturing of the wound and restoration of ocular volume and pressure should be performed prior to any diagnostic procedures. View of the wound after closure: (1) traumatic cataract; (2) sutured corneal entry wound; (3) traumatic peripheral iridectomy. *B.* After closure of the wound computerized tomography is performed, revealing the presence and the location of the IOFB.

previous ocular injuries and surgical procedures, and mental well being. (For detection of ocular infection and typing of pathogens, see Chapter 3.) In addition extraocular injuries are to be carefully assessed.

Prognostic factors

The most significant factor in predicting good final visual outcome (20/40 and better) was initial visual acuity of 20/800 and better.[3–5,12,22] Other factors include the size of the wound. Wounds shorter than 10 mm were associated with a better prognosis. Wounds limited to the cornea and wounds located anterior to the horizontal muscle insertions have also been associated with better visual outcome.[4] Penetrating trauma in some reports was considered a better prognostic factor than blunt trauma. Others believe that presence of an afferent pupillary defect,[3] perforation of the globe and the finding of an IOFB are associated with poorer final visual acuity.[3,12]

MEDICOLEGAL CONSIDERATIONS

The patient or responsible individual should be informed of the nature of the trauma to the eye and recommended modes of treatment. The natural coarse of untreated traumatic eye injury should be explained. In addition the patient should be informed of details including hospitalization, anesthesia, surgery, postoperative care, and possible need for subsequent treatment both conservative and surgical. Anticipated visual recovery, side effects of treatment and risks of surgical procedures should be discussed and informed consent obtained.

TIMING OF SURGERY

Timing of the surgery is critical (Table 65–3). In the first 24 to 48 hours after trauma, other than primary wound closure as described elsewhere, a further posterior segment intervention is usually not recommended due to the risk of intraoperative bleeding, disturbed visibility, and the high rate of intraoperative complications.[23-25] Seven to ten days after the trauma, the tissues are much less edematous, the possibility of severe intraoperative bleeding is low, and posterior vitreous detachment may have occurred, making vitrectomy easier and safer. However, if surgery is delayed beyond 10 to 14 days the surgeon may encounter fibrous proliferation at the site of penetration[26] that is different from the type seen in proliferative vitreoretinopathy (PVR) and proliferative diabetic vitreoretinopathy (PDR). The proliferations take the form of thick and rigid fibrotic scars that include the sclera, choroid, and retina in one fibrotic mass. This can occur with or without retinal incarceration, and later results in severe traction retinal detachment (Fig. 65–2). The scar adheres so strongly to the eye wall that it may be very difficult to remove. It is therefore imperative that the eye is operated on before these scars form. Fibrous proliferation from a penetrating wound becomes significant usually within one week of the injury, so the best and safest time for definitive surgery is 7 to 10 days after the trauma.[24,27–29] Foreign bodies should be removed within the first 24 to 48 hours after the trauma if one of the following criteria exist: the foreign body contains organic material or is likely to be contaminated (as occurs in agricultural settings), risking the development of endophthalmitis[30–32]; there is an inflammatory response around the foreign body suggestive of toxicity; there are already signs suggestive of endophthalmitis, the foreign body is proven to be of pure copper (not alloy which is much less dangerous),[33] or if the foreign body is hidden by vitreous hemorrhage and its properties cannot be evaluated. It should be remembered that siderosis bulbi may occur even with small intralenticular foreign bodies.[34] The incidence of endophthalmitis in penetrating injuries in Israel, and perhaps in other developed countries, is lower than the 2% to 7% reported in the literature[32] and the 8% reported for war injuries.[35] It occurs in less than 2% of all cases, perhaps because most patients have easy access to major ophthalmic care centers and are seen promptly after injury. Therefore, in Israel we do not adopt the policy that every intraocular foreign body need be extracted immediately because of the danger of endophthalmitis, and we usually perform the surgery 3 to 4 days from the time of the injury.

CONTROL OF INFLAMMATION AND INFECTION

Traumatic endophthalmitis is a major concern in penetrating injuries, and occurs in 2% to 7% according to the literature.[32,35] Most cases are caused by agricultural accidents and mines, that is, from contaminated objects that were lying or buried in soil.

TABLE 65–3 Timing of Posterior Segment Surgery in the Setting of Acute Posterior Segment Trauma

General	During the first 24 to 48 hours after trauma perform primary wound closure When possible avoid posterior segment procedures due to: tissue congestion, risk of rebleeding, lack of posterior vitreous detachment and poor visibility
Timing of surgery	When possible 7 to 10 days following trauma
IOFB's to be removed within 24 to 48 hours	An IOFB containing contaminated material Inflammatory response around the IOFB Signs of endophthalmitis Pure copper IOFB IOFB hidden by vitreous hemorrhage
Avoid	Delaying surgery beyond 10-14 days, to reduce the likelihood of scar formation, membranes, and traction retinal detachment

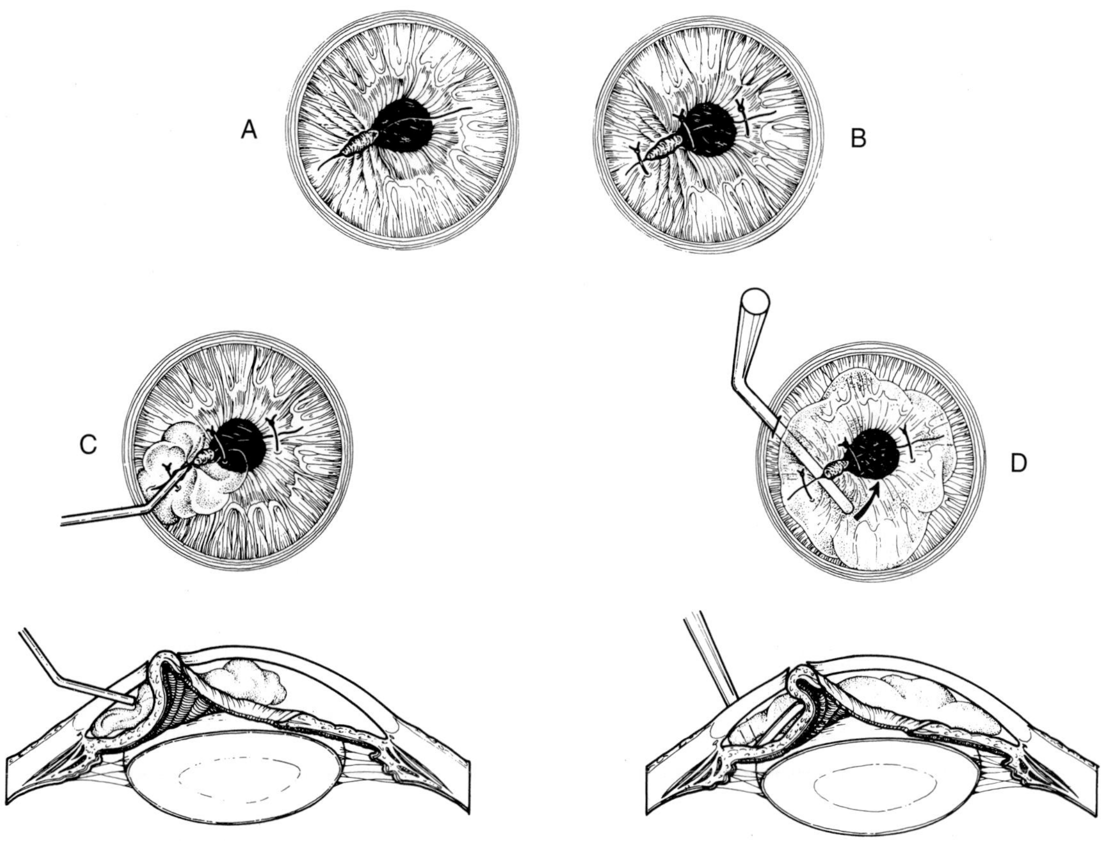

Figure 65–2. *A.* Initial appearance of a typical laceration with incarceration and prolapse of the iris through a portion of the wound. *B.* Before attempting to reposition the iris, the surgeon stabilizes the corneal laceration with several sutures to each side of the prolapsed iris. These sutures should not be excessively tight, constricting the iris, or inadvertently engage the incarcerated iris. *C.* A viscoelastic material is introduced adjacent to the prolapsed iris. The mass of the viscoelastic material gradually deepens the chamber and draws the prolapsed iris down and out of the wound. *D.* If the iris remains incarcerated, a cyclodialysis spatula sweeps the iris out of the wound, moving from the periphery toward the center. A viscoelastic material or a large air bubble is used to maintain the anterior chamber during this maneuver.

Diagnosis of Infection in Trauma

Endophthalmitis should always be suspected in cases of penetrating trauma and can be quite difficult to diagnose in such circumstances. Potential signs of endophthalmitis can actually result from the trauma itself. In many cases there is blood or inflammatory products in the anterior chamber or the vitreous space, the visual acuity is poor, and eye pain and swollen lids are present. Loss of the red reflex, a common sign of endophthalmitis in postoperative endophthalmitis, can also be due to the penetrating trauma and blood in the eye. Even a hypopyon, the typical sign of endophthalmitis, may not be easy to identify. Blood in the anterior chamber or a hyphema can mask a hypopyon, and the supine position of the patient may prevent formation of one. Fibrin visible in the anterior chamber or even a pupillary fibrinous membrane may be caused either by the trauma or by the endophthalmitis. The ophthalmologist must follow the development of the above signs and symptoms to detect whether they are increasing or diminishing in intensity. Specifically, the ophthalmologist should watch for pain that is increasing instead of being relieved and eyelids that are becoming increasingly swollen. A careful view of the anterior chamber may reveal two layers, the white layer of the hypopyon and the red layer of the hyphema (red cells). After several days the hyphema may turn white because of the breakdown of the blood products.

In summary, an increase in pain, increased swelling of the lids, and the beginning of a hypopyon are all probable indications of endophthalmitis. A culture should be taken from the conjunctiva and from the penetrating wound site. Any blood and tissue removed from the eye during surgery should be sent for culture. These cultures are often non-contributing because the treatment of a penetrating injury includes administration of systemic and topical antibiotics on admission to the hospital. It has been recently observed by the endophthalmitis research group that 62% of the vitreous cultures in posttraumatic endophthalmitis were positive. In these cultures 21% were polymicrobial, 46% were gram positive cocci, 17% gram positive bacilli, and 18% gram negative organisms. There still existed a comparably high percentage of *Actinomyces* organisms (5%) and 14% (a high percentage) were fungi.[36] When endophthalmitis is suspected, usually 1 to 2 days after admission, the chance of a positive culture is quite small. However, when growth of bacteria and fungi are obtained from an eye in the setting of penetrating trauma, organisms may grow without clinical signs of infection. Positive cultures should directly influence management in cases with clinically evident endophthalmitis. Nevertheless, routine intraoperative cultures failed to identify patients in whom endophthalmitis would develop, and they did not change the management regimen in eyes without clinical suspicion of endophthalmitis.[37] Prophylaxis and treatment of traumatic endophthalmitis are discussed in detail in Chapter 3.

SURGICAL PROCEDURES

POSTERIOR SEGMENT

Prophylactic Buckling

In most cases of penetrating posterior segment trauma, prophylactic encirclement is recommended to support the vitreous base and prevent traction in the vitreous base region, postoperative development of peripheral retinal tears, and late retinal detachment.[4,5,7,38–40] Therefore, in most cases of posterior segment involvement the definitive surgical procedure should begin with conjunctival peritomy, exploration of the sclera (for possible penetrating wounds), and suturing of an encircling element (e.g., silicone band style No. 41) even if the retina is attached (Fig. 65–3). In rare cases of minute scleral penetrating wounds with a small IOFB in the vitreous, the surgery may be performed without applying an encircling element.

Anterior Chamber and Lens Management in Patients With Posterior Segment Trauma

The following steps involve the management of the anterior chamber, to allow better visualization of the posterior segment. If there is a hyphema, it is evacuated using an anterior chamber maintainer to irrigate the anterior chamber with balanced salt solution. The blood is removed by a side-port 0.4-mm cannula inserted through another limbal paracentesis. A formed clot may be removed with intraocular forceps. In phakic eyes with a clear lens, attempts should be made to spare the lens. If residual red cells persist after irrigation and obscure the view of the posterior segment, the anterior chamber may be filled with viscoelastic material that will be removed only at the conclusion of the operation. If the lens is cataractous or if there is pathology in the region of the vitreous base that must be dealt with, the lens should be removed.

Removal of the lens can be performed in several ways depending on the age of the patient and the preferences of the surgeon. In young patients (until the age of 40 years), and at times even in older patients, the lens can be aspirated through the pars plana by the vitreous cutter or through a small limbal paracentesis with the 0.4 side-port cannula. When a less soft nucleus is present, either phacoemulsification or extracapsular cataract extraction (ECCE—particularly the Mini-Nuc technique),[41] could be adequate. Again, efforts should be made to preserve the posterior capsule if a posterior chamber intraocular lens (IOL) implantation is contemplated. Simultaneous IOL implantation with vitreoretinal surgery in well-selected cases allows for early vision rehabilitation. The lens can be implanted in the bag, sulcus, or sclerally fixated.[42,43] If ECCE is preferred, a scleral tunnel incision should be used, as it is watertight and may easily sustain the great pressures induced throughout posterior segment surgery. The

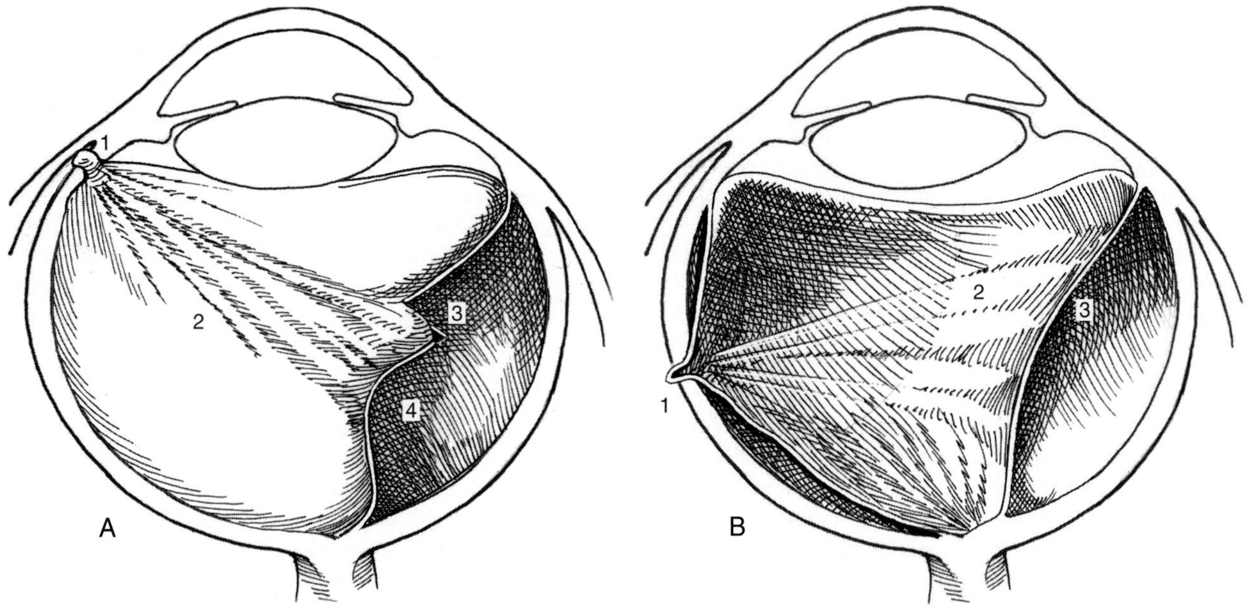

Figure 65–3. *A.* Late-onset traction-rhegmatogenous retinal detachment following an anterior scleral penetrating wound. There is vitreous incarceration (with or without fibrous proliferation at the entry site) (1), vitreous traction (2) on the retina on the opposite side, with resulting retinal break (3) and retinal detachment (4). *B.* Traction-rhegmatogenous retinal detachment resulting from posterior penetrating injury. The retina is incarcerated in the wound (1), with vitreous traction (2) on opposite side, and total retinal detachment (3).

scleral tunnel incision does not interfere with corneal clarity, and thus facilitates good visibility for posterior segment surgery.

Vitrectomy

In all cases where it has been decided to remove retained intraocular foreign bodies in the posterior segment, we recommend pars plana vitrectomy with removal of the IOFB only under direct visualization. Blind removal of a metallic IOFB with a magnet is contraindicated in our opinion. If the vitreous space is full of blood, a pars plana infusion cannula should not be inserted unless the cannula can be observed to be free in the vitreous cavity and is not covered by choroid or retina. If the eye is aphakic or pseudophakic a long infusion cannula (6.5 to 7 mm) can be inserted in the pars plana. The cannula is then illuminated by putting the fiber optic on the limbus at the opposite side or viewed with the indirect ophthalmoscope. Alternatively, the first steps of the posterior segment surgery can be done with an anterior chamber maintainer at the limbus, later to be replaced with a pars plana maintainer. In phakic eyes, the irrigating solution can be temporarily connected to a 20-gauge needle that will be held by the surgeon and inserted through the parsplana for volume replacement at the beginning of the vitrectomy. Because of its length, the needle can be clearly seen behind the lens, and vitrectomy can be performed safely (Fig. 65–4). After the opaque anterior vitreous is removed, the regular infusion cannula can be inserted in the usual location at the pars plana. These steps are necessary for prevention of iatrogenic choroidal or retinal detachment from inadvertent infusion of irrigation fluid under the choroid or retina, complications that may occur if the pars plana cannula is inserted blindly and its position cannot be ascertained. Ideally, the vitrectomy

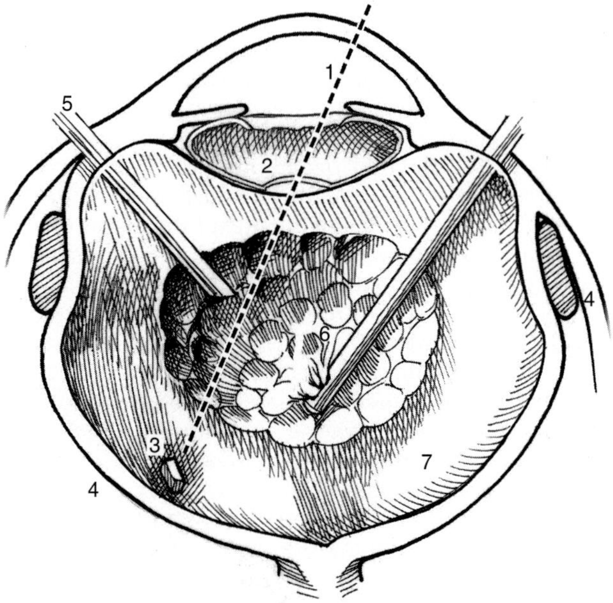

Figure 65–4. Prophylactic scleral buckle in penetrating posterior segment injury is important, even when there is no retinal detachment. (1) corneal penetration; (2) the lens was removed because of traumatic cataract, and the residual lens capsule was left in place; (3) there is a posteriorly located intraretinal foreign body; (4) a prophylactic scleral buckle was placed before the beginning of the vitrectomy; (5) fiberoptic probe; (6) vitrectomy probe; (7) vitreous hemorrhage without PVD.

is continued until most of the vitreous jelly is removed and the media becomes clear, then a thorough examination of the retina up to the vitreous base is possible. However, one of the gravest complications of vitreoretinal surgery in eyes filled with blood is iatrogenic retinectomy, particularly in the presence of retinal detachment. While removing a vitreous hemorrhage, it is important to determine whether there is a posterior vitreous detachment. This can often be determined by performing an ultrasound examination before the operation. In eyes with a posterior vitreous detachment, because of the patient's older age or the trauma itself, the vitreous can be removed safely and the retina can be nicely exposed. Removing the opaque posterior vitreous can be very difficult in young patients in whom a posterior vitreous detachment has not yet developed, and during the vitrectomy an inadvertent retinectomy may occur, causing retinal detachment or complicating the management of an existing retinal detachment. For this reason, attempts should be made to induce posterior vitreous detachment when a posterior vitreous hemorrhage is adherent to the retina, as described in the following section.

Removal of the Posterior Cortical Vitreous

Removal of the posterior cortical vitreous (PCV) is important not only for safe completion of the operation but also for improving the prognosis of the eye. The PCV may support the proliferative activity, and its presence may result in the development of a macular pucker and late retinal detachment. Posterior vitreous detachment (PVD) may occur after the trauma and before the definitive surgical procedure, facilitating the removal of vitreous hemorrhage and the repair of retinal detachment. In other eyes PVD does not occur and the surgeon faces the dilemma of whether to try to mechanically induce PVD to reduce the risk of late complications, or to leave the posterior hyaloid attached to the retina. It should be remembered that the attempt to create a PVD is sometimes time-consuming and may be associated with intraoperative and postoperative complications such as iatrogenic retinal breaks, retinal detachment, and visual field loss, as described in eyes following macular hole surgery.[44,45] Should the surgeon add these risks to the management of the traumatized posterior segment? A review of the literature reveals both direct and indirect evidence that removal of the posterior cortical vitreous in such eyes should be beneficial in the long term.

The importance of removing the posterior cortical vitreous in perforating injuries has been strongly emphasized by several authors[46–48] for prevention of the secondary complications. Failure to remove these structures may later be associated with contraction of the PCV and formation of traction folds in the retina. Depending on the location of the foreign body, these traction folds may involve the macula and significantly impair visual acuity. In more severe cases PCV can also cause traction retinal detachment and open previously existing breaks, particularly from perforating injury.

The major advances in techniques for creating PVD stem from the recent interest in macular hole injury. The main lesson from macular hole surgery was that the posterior cortical vitreous is a physical entity that has to be addressed separately, and that it may invisibly persist following vitrectomy in eyes without PVD. Several methods are used for obtaining this goal. Many surgeons use a flexible silicone-tipped cannula with active suction to engage the posterior hyaloid,[49] and induce detachment, usually around the optic nerve (Fig. 65–5*A*). The cortical vitreous is further detached to the equatorial zone and removed with the vitrectomy probe. Other techniques include use of several types of hyaloid lifters and cannulas to elevate the vitreous from the disc margin, creating an opening in the posterior hyaloid into which a 90-degree blunt membrane pick may be inserted.[50] In our opinion, active suction with the silicone-tipped cannulas is a safe technique, and probably is less likely to result in iatrogenic retinal breaks. We use this technique almost exclusively when performing vitrectomy in our trauma cases.

In cases with persistent posterior cortical vitreous with or without a vitreous hemorrhage, an attempt to create a PVD with a soft-tipped cannula and active suction may be dangerous, and we found the use of perfluorocarbon (PFC) liquids extremely helpful in such situations. We try to identify an area of partial PVD, and after creating a window in the vitreous face we inject PFC through the opening, and this separates the posterior hyaloid from the retina while flattening the detached retina (Fig. 65–5*B*), thus allowing a much safer and more complete vitrectomy. A similar approach was described by Desai et al.,[51] who report three cases in which they used perfluorophenanthrene in the management of traumatic vitreous hemorrhage and retinal detachment.

Sclerotomy for Removal of a Foreign Body

The sclerotomy through which an IOFB is to be removed must be large enough to permit as atraumatic a removal as possible. If the incision is too small, the foreign body can get caught inside the sclerotomy. Generally, the sclerotomy should be twice the size of the foreign body where it is to be grasped with a forceps. When removing uneven or irregular foreign bodies, we recommend adding a 1-mm posterior radial cut, converting the sclerotomy into an L-shaped opening (Fig. 65–6).

Another important point to consider while preparing the sclerotomy is that the opening in the parsplana should be as big as the opening in the sclera. If the parsplana opening is smaller, traction will be exerted on it during the passage of the IOFB, and this may result in a retinal tear, dialysis, or incarceration. Therefore the surgeon should always check the opening in the parsplana, and enlarge it to correspond to the scleral opening, using Vannas-like scissors, or other cutting instruments. After the sclerotomy is prepared, it is closed with temporary sutures to prevent collapse of the eyeball during extraction of the foreign body. When the surgeon grasps the foreign body with forceps or with a magnet, and

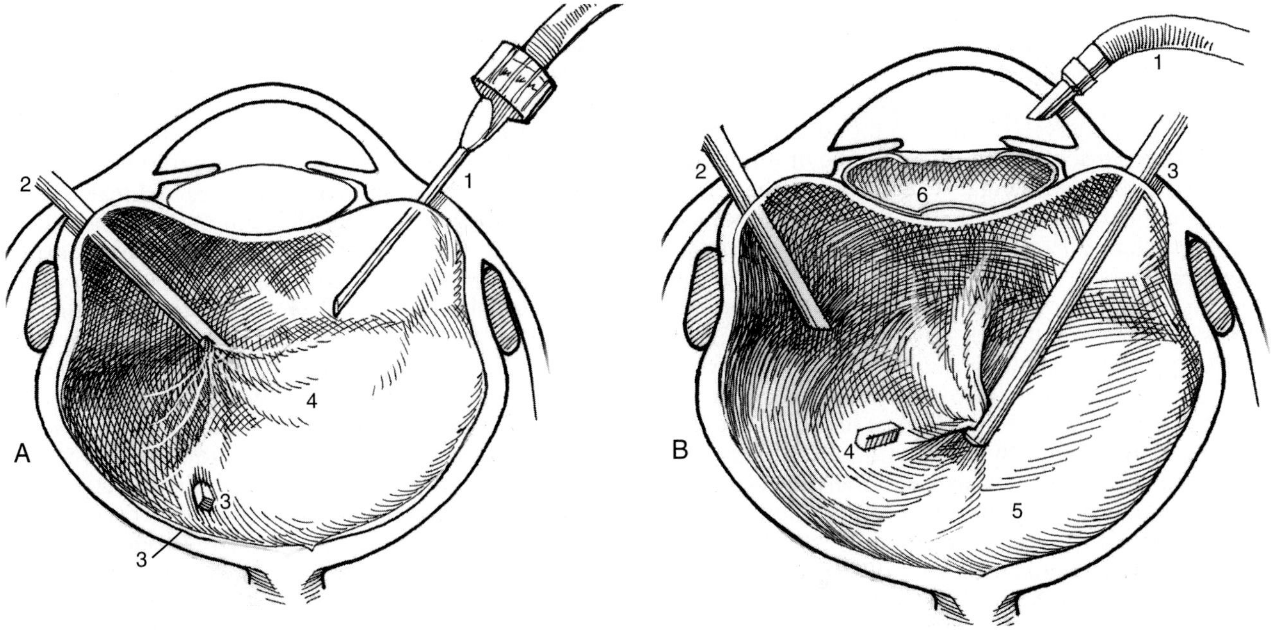

Figure 65–5. When there is a dense vitreous hemorrhage it may be difficult and dangerous to blindly insert the pars plana cannula. If the tip cannot be seen, it might be pushing the pars plana instead of penetrating through it. Opening the infusion valve may result in iatrogenic retinal or choroidal detachments that will further complicate the operation. *A.* In *phakic* eyes vitrectomy is first performed in the anterior vitreous with fluid replacement through a needle (e.g., 21-gauge) connected to the infusion bottle (1). Since the needle is long, it can easily be seen entering the anterior vitreous space. Caution should be exercised not to touch the crystalline lens. Later a pars plana cannula is inserted at the sclerotomy where the needle was, for completion of the vitrectomy; (2) vitrectomy probe; (3) intraocular foreign body; (4) dense vitreous hemorrhage. *B.* In *aphakic* or *pseudophakic* eyes, the first steps of the vitrectomy can be performed with an anterior chamber maintainer, and only after the anterior vitreous is clear, a pars plana cannula is inserted, preferrably a long one: (1) anterior chamber maintainer; (2) fiberoptic probe; (3) vitrectomy probe; (4) intraocular foreign body; (5) dense vitreous hemorrhage; (6) open capsule following traumatic cataract extraction.

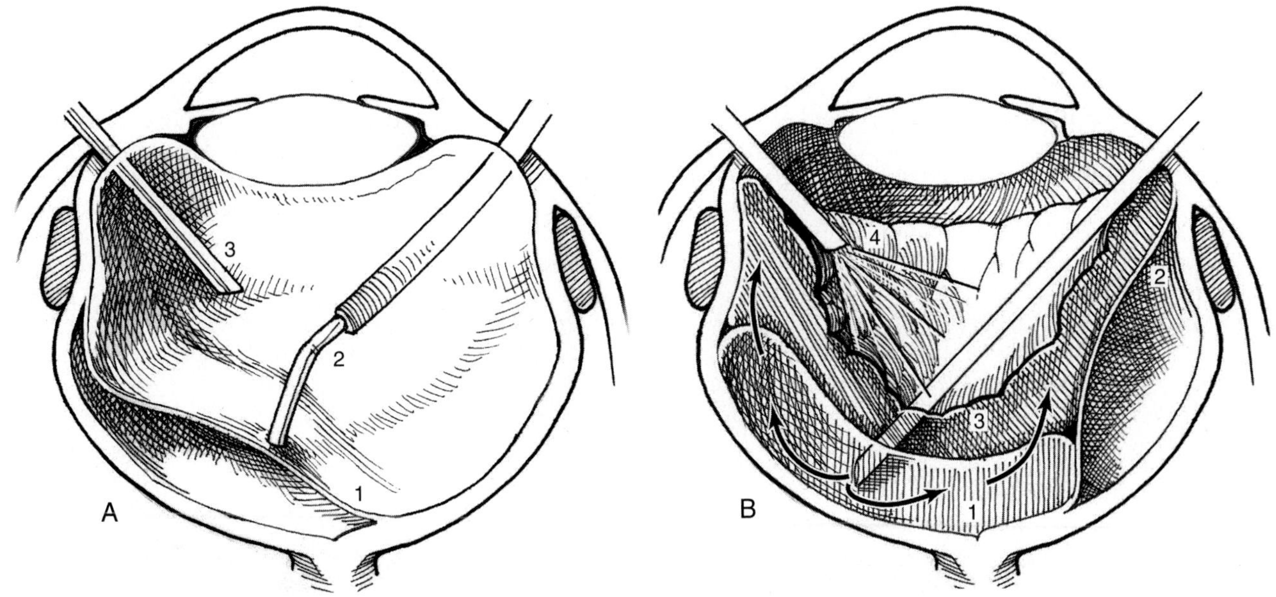

Figure 65–6. *A.* Mechanical posterior vitreous detachment in eyes with attached retina. The posterior cortical vitreous (1) is engaged with active suction through a silicone-tipped cannula (2), usually nasal to the optic disc. (3) fiberoptic probe. *B.* Separation of the posterior cortical vitreous with perfluorocarbon liquid in eyes with dense vitreous hemorrhage, retinal detachment, and no posterior vitreous detachment. An opening is created in the vitreous hemorrhage in one area, and the edges are gently released from the retina at that site. Perfluorocarbon liquid is then injected slowly through the opening, separating the vitreous from the detached retina, and flattening the retina at the same time (arrows): (1) bubble of perfluorocarbon liquid injected through a cannula; (2) detached retina; (3) dense vitreous hemorrhage; (4) fiberoptic probe.

brings it to the anterior vitreous space, the surgeon or the assistant can cut the sutures in the sclera.

Removal of an Intraretinal Foreign Body

Most retinal foreign bodies can be removed safely by a suitable intraocular forceps. The vitreous around the IOFB, whether encapsulated or not, should be cleaned, and if a reactive capsule exists its anterior surface should be opened. This can sometimes be done with a vitrectomy probe or with a sharp instrument (e.g., the MVR—microvitreoretinal blade), with the IOFB guarding against retinal damage from this maneuver. An attempt should then be made to grasp the IOFB with the forceps without pulling on adjacent tissues. This step should be done carefully, as intraretinal IOFBs often penetrate the choroid, and manipulations at the time of removal may cause significant choroidal hemorrhage, preventing safe conclusion of the operation, and increasing the risk of enlarging the existing retinal break. Choroidal injury and hemorrhage can also be caused by the arms of the intraocular forceps used for removing the IOFB. Therefore, when the foreign body lies directly on the retina or is intraretinal and also penetrates the choroid, a 90-degree intraocular forceps may be preferable to a straight one. If the foreign body is magnetic, an intraocular magnet is very helpful in pulling the foreign body from its bed, as it avoids the lateral movements inevitably made with the intraocular forceps, movements that increase the chance of choroidal hemorrhage (Fig. 65–7). The use of an intraocular magnet has another advantage in that the IOFB aligns itself along its longer axis at the tip of the magnet. This positioning assists in removing it through an opening tailored to its lesser width, through a smaller sclerotomy. Of course, this advantage is relevant to magnetic IOFBs located anywhere in the posterior segment, not only to intraretinal ones.

We prefer not to remove a foreign body by the transscleral posterior approach. This approach can lead to severe damage to the eyeball, including choroidal hemorrhage and incarceration of the vitreous and retina, which may in turn lead to rhegmatogenous or traction retinal detachment. At the present state of vitreoretinal surgery, the intraocular approach is much safer for IOFB removal, because removal of the foreign body is not the final surgical procedure. As described in a previous section of this chapter it is important to remove the posterior cortical vitreous, if there was no PVD, as well as the reactive capsule that often forms around the IOFB. This is particularly true for intraretinal IOFBs.

Although several publications have indicated that once the PCV is removed there is no need to treat retinal tears with endophotocoagulation[41,47] we treat all retinal breaks with the endolaser during the operation unless they are adjacent to the fovea. For this we use argon green endolaser during the operation to obtain moderately white burns, usually with an intensity of 0.3 to 0.7 watts.

Incarcerated Retina

Incarceration of the vitreous and the retina can occur in penetrating and perforating wounds of the eye. More frequently it occurs in perforating injuries, as previously described.

In double perforating injuries there is also an exit

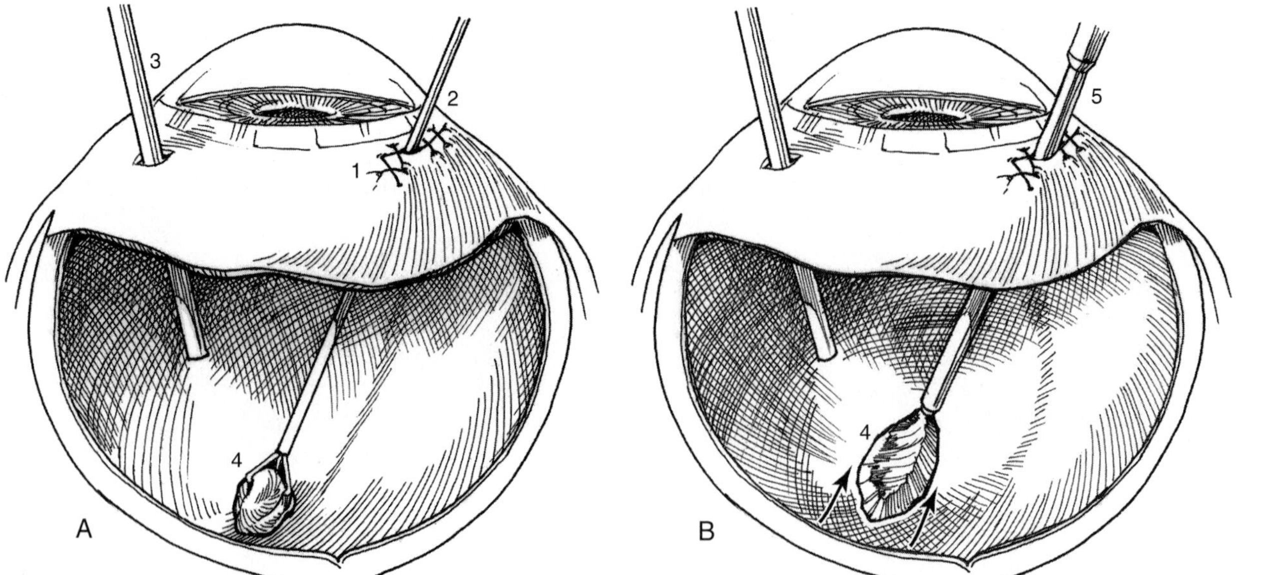

Figure 65–7. *A.* Preparation of an L-shaped sclerotomy for removal of larger IOFBs. The size of the sclerotomy is determined by the estimated size and shape of the IOFB, and should be large enough to allow its passage easily. It is important to ascertain that the incision in the pars plana corresponds in size to the scleral incision. The sclerotomy is sutured temporarily to maintain closed system conditions until the IOFB is brought to the opening: (1) L-shaped sclerotomy with temporary sutures; (2) intraocular forceps; (3) fiberoptic probe; (4) intraocular foreign body. *B.* An intraocular rare earth magnet (5) is often very useful in removing intraretinal foreign bodies, as it allows them to be removed without direct manipulations at the level of the retina.

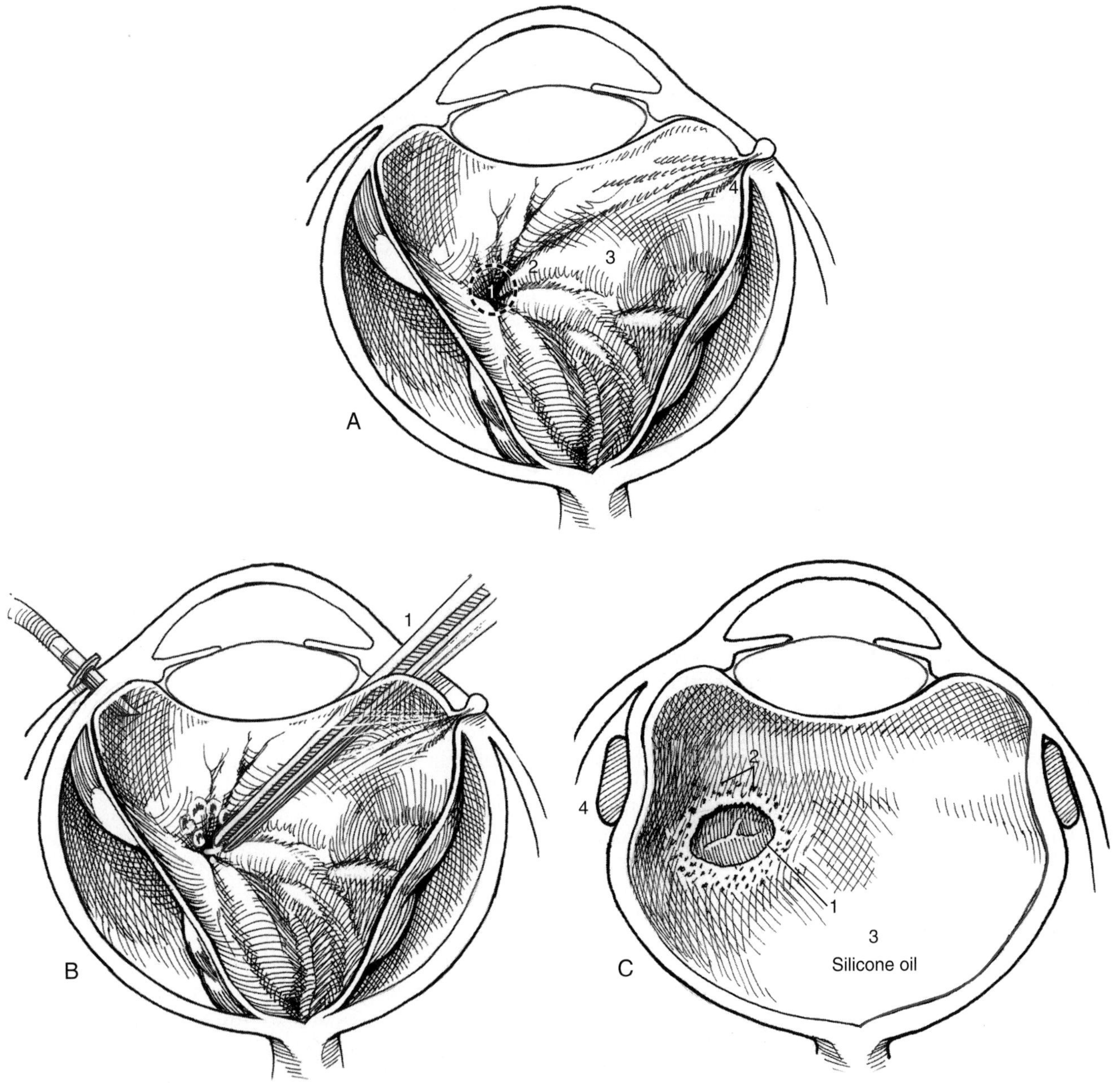

Figure 65–8. The management of perforating injury ("double perforation") with retinal incarceration at the exit wound. *A*. The retina is incarcerated in the exit wound (1) with retinal folds and total retinal detachment. The circle (2) centered on the incarceration marks the perimeter of the planned retinotomy. There is vitreous hemorrhage (3) and vitreous incarceration in the entry wound. *B*. Multiple diathermy (1) burns are carefully placed on the center of the retinal incarceration. The resulting retinal coagulation necrosis enables the surgeon to release the retina from the incarceration site with intraocular forceps. This maneuver reduces retinal tissue loss, and results in a much smaller retinectomy then that created with intraocular scissors. In addition, the diathermy prevents bleeding from torn retinal vessels. *C*. After the retinectomy the retina is flattened. The retinectomy usually results in a much larger than anticipated retinal opening (1). Several rows of laser burns are placed around it (2). In such cases silicone oil injection (3) may be preferable to gas. Usually, a scleral buckle is also placed (4).

wound, and the vitreous and the retina may become incarcerated in the exit wound (Fig. 65–8*A*). The incarcerated retina must be released in order to flatten the retina and prevent severe traction detachment. This can usually be done only by cutting the retina around the incarceration site, thus creating a large retinectomy. Sometimes it is possible to decrease the size of the retinectomy by performing intraocular diathermy as close as possible to the center of the funnel of the incarceration. The incarcerated retina becomes very friable, and can be released from the incarceration with intraocular forceps, usually with less loss of retinal tissue, and a smaller retinectomy (Fig. 65–8*B*). In most cases releasing the retina from the wound creates a very large retinectomy or a giant tear. Since the advent of perfluorocarbon fluids, the difficult management of these giant tears has become much simpler.[52] After the retina is reattached with the PFC, the borders of the tear are photocoagulated with the endolaser; then, depending on the condition of the retina, PFC–gas or PFC–silicone exchange is performed (Fig. 65–8C).

Treatment of Traumatic Giant Retinal Tears

Giant retinal tears may occur in a penetrating injury as well as in blunt trauma. Basically, treatment of a traumatic giant tear is the same as treatment of a nontraumatic giant tear.[52–54]

Silicone Oil in Posterior Segment Injuries

Silicone oil can be used to fill the vitreous cavity at the end of the surgery.[55] If the lens was removed and the surgeon plans to use silicone oil, it is recommended to remove the entire lens capsule. A residual lens capsule may be incorporated later in the anterior PVR complex with organization and formation of a thick fibrous ring. This structure may either pull on the ciliary processes and ciliary body, resulting in hypotony, or pull on the pars plana and peripheral retina, resulting in traction retinal detachment. After removal of the nucleus and cortex, by means of either ECCE or phacoemulsification, the remaining capsular sac is removed with intraocular forceps via a pars plana sclerotomy, or through a limbal paracentesis.[56,57] The same technique is used in pseudophakic cases in which the intraocular lens is removed in order to facilitate dissection of the vitreous base area in cases of anterior PVR. The use of chymotrypsin is optional, and the capsule can often be removed without pharmacological zonulolysis.[57] Silicone oil may be indicated instead of intraocular gas when the surgeon suspects that not all the retinal breaks were identified during surgery, and particularly when a large and/or inferior retinotomy is performed. It may also be used in cases in which the eye is so severely damaged by the injury that there are large lacerations of the retina (above 4 disc diameters), a large primary retinal detachment (larger than two quadrants), or persistent hemorrhage during surgery.[58] Silicone oil provides a long-term tamponade for the unidentified retinal tears, prevents retinal detachment, and allows for much easier follow-up and laser treatment after surgery, because there is better visibility than in a gas-filled eye.

The use of silicone oil is associated with many complications, among them band keratopathy, cataract, glaucoma, and toxic retinopathy. Therefore, these eyes should be followed carefully.[59,60] Emulsification of the oil is a major determinant for the development of complications, particularly glaucoma. The time to emulsification is very variable; it depends on the viscosity and purity of the oil and on some ocular factors as well.[61,62] In one study[63] it was found that residual blood remaining in the eye after surgery is the primary cause of oil emulsification. Therefore at the end of surgery an effort must be made to remove any remaining blood from the vitreous space and the retinal surface. In most cases, after a relatively short period of follow-up (usually 2 to 3 months), when the condition of the eye is stabilized, the retina is attached, all retinal breaks are treated, and no new retinal holes or traction are observed, the silicone oil can be removed from the eye before the development of complications. To decrease the possibility of re-detachment of the retina after removing the silicone oil, it is advisable to treat the retinal periphery and buckle with 360-degree laser photocoagulation.

COMBINED SEVERE ANTERIOR AND POSTERIOR SEGMENT INJURIES

In cases of severe corneal opacities, posterior segment surgery can be performed only with a temporary keratoprosthesis (Eckhardt or Landers lenses).[64] This is required when the cornea becomes opaque from the trauma (e.g., large irregular lacerations, staining from blood), and posterior segment surgery cannot be performed because of poor visibility. After removal of a button of the opaque cornea, the anterior chamber can be reconstructed in an "open-sky" technique, which involves removing the whole lens or lens material, fibrin, blood, iris remnants and adhesions, and then performing an anterior vitrectomy.

At the beginning of the procedure the keratoprosthesis is placed and secured with sutures. Vitrectomy is then performed, vitreous hemorrhage is removed and the retina is exposed and treated, in accordance with the findings. The older types of keratoprosthesis (e.g., Landers-Foulks lens) offer a limited field of view. To obtain a wider field it is recommended that they be used in conjunction with a wide field system. Methylcellulose or another viscoelastic material is placed on the keratoprosthetic lens, and a wide-field contact lens is placed on top. We have found that the combination of these two lenses provides the surgeon with a wide visual field including the fundus periphery and the vitreous base area. This is important because when using this type of keratoprosthetic lens it is difficult to indent the fundus periphery from the outside to allow the surgeon to work on the vitreous base area.

POSTOPERATIVE CONSIDERATIONS

FOLLOW-UP OF BLUNT OCULAR TRAUMA

Any blunt trauma to the eyeball must be carefully assessed for at least 2 months after the trauma, because retinal holes and tears may develop during this period.[65,66] Contusions of the eye can cause both anterior and posterior retinal edema, including macular edema macular hole, retinal breaks, and retinal dialysis.[67,68] The retinal breaks may be hidden by retinal or vitreous hemorrhages. In young patients who have a healthy vitreous and no PVD, traumatic retinal tears usually do not cause an immediate retinal detachment. On follow-up examinations of the periphery, however, newly developed retinal tears may be identified and they can be effectively treated by laser. Failure to detect retinal tears may result in late retinal detachment. In more severe contusions, examination of the periphery of the retina may reveal retinal dialysis or a giant tear.[69] The difference between retinal dialysis and giant tears is that in giant tears the vitreous base adheres to the anterior border of the tear and pulls it anteriorly, while the posterior border of the tear is free and may roll due to the elasticity of the retina (or PVR in neglected cases). In dialysis, the vitreous is adherent to the posterior border of the dialysis and pulls toward the center of the eye. If the dialysis is small, without surrounding retinal detachment, it can be effectively treated with laser. When there is vitreous traction, a scleral buckle might be considered.[70] Dialysis of more than 90 degrees usually has to be treated with vitrectomy, intraocular gas, and endolaser.[71] Dialysis can be present in the eye for a relatively long time without producing retinal detachment. The ophthalmologist needs to conduct a thorough examination of the peripheral retina in order to rule out a dialysis that can be present in the absence of symptoms. A detailed description of the management of retinal breaks, retinal detachment, and giant retinal tears is given in other chapters.

FOLLOW-UP OF RETAINED INTRAOCULAR FOREIGN BODIES

In the modern era, many of the intraocular foreign bodies are made of inert materials. In this respect certain patients with a retained IOFB present a diagnostic and treatment challenge to the ophthalmologist. In cases with a relatively small foreign body in the vitreous, a self-sealing penetrating wound, good visual acuity, and no retinal involvement, it is possible to observe the eye for some time before making the decision to operate (see the earlier section on sclerotomy and removal of IOFB). If the IOFB has a bright appearance without any inflammatory reaction in the vitreous, the patient could be followed closely without the need for immediate surgery. The risk associated with retained metallic foreign bodies is that they may contain iron and copper that will cause toxic changes to the ocular tissues (chalcosis and siderosis).[33] Therefore, besides clinical examination, the classic approach was to perform repeated ERGs and look for reduction in the response.[72] However, changes in the ERG may occur only after significant toxic damage has already occurred. We recommend prompt removal of IOFBs in the following settings:

1. Pure iron or copper IOFBs because the risk of siderosis and chalcosis
2. All non-inert IOFBs that cause a toxic inflammatory response to the surrounding tissues
3. All IOFBs penetrating the retina and choroid
4. All IOFBs that cannot be observed directly because of vitreous hemorrhage or any other opacity

Foreign bodies that are believed to be of inert material, that cause no reaction in the tissue around them, and that are directly observable can be followed closely (Fig. 65–9).

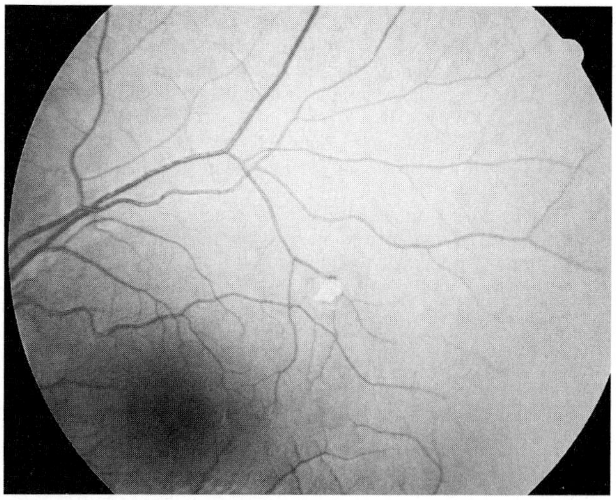

Figure 65–9. A retained intraocular foreign body, 12 years after the injury. There is no evidence of retinal toxicity or encapsulation. The visual acuity was 20/25.

POSTTRAUMATIC OCULAR HYPOTONY

Ocular hypotony is one of the most difficult complications to manage in eyes with severe penetrating injury following vitreoretinal surgery. The management of hypotony involves extensive dissection in the vitreous base area, with release of traction on the ciliary body.[73,74] In injured eyes suffering from hypotony as a late stage complication, the ciliary body and the ciliary processes are covered with relatively thick fibrotic membranes that in our experience are different from those observed in eyes with anterior PVR.[73] In most of these cases in addition to detachment of the ciliary body, the ciliary processes are intermingled within and strangulated by the fibrotic tissue, and it may be very difficult, if not impossible to find cleavage planes for dissection. Removing the membranes is associated with avulsion of the ciliary processes along with the membranes, thereby contributing to the continuation of hypotony. Immediate intervention at the onset of hypotony allows removal of the membranes before they become integrated with the ciliary body and processes, and the surgical results may be improved. In certain cases filling the eyeball with silicone oil may prevent hypotony and restore intraocular pressure.

REFERENCES

1. Sternberg P, de Juan E, Michels RG: Multivariate analysis of prognostic factors in penetrating ocular injuries. Am J Ophthalmol 1984;98:467–472.
2. Gilbert CM, Soong HK, Hirst LW: A two year prospective study of penetrating ocular trauma at the Wilmer Ophthalmological Institute. Ann Ophthalmol 1987;19:104–106.
3. de Juan E, Sternberg P, Michels RG: Penetrating injuries: types of injuries and visual results. Ophthalmology 1983;90:1318–1322.
4. Esmaeli B, Elner SG, Schork MA, Elner VM: Visual outcome and ocular survival after penetrating trauma. A clinicopathological study. Ophthalmology 1995;102:393–400.

5. Hutton WL, Fuller DG: Factors influencing the final visual results in severely injured eyes. Am J Ophthalmol 1984;97:715–722.
6. de Juan E, Sternberg P, Michels RG: Evaluation of vitrectomy in penetrating ocular trauma: a case control study. Arch Ophthalmol 1984;102:1160–1163.
7. Ahmadieh H, Soheilian M, Sajjadi H, et al.: Vitrectomy in ocular trauma. Factors influencing final visual outcome. Retina 1993;13: 107–113.
8. Koval R, Teller J, Belkin M, et al.: The Israeli ocular injury study. A nationwide collaborative study. Arch Ophthalmol 1988;106:776–780.
9. Martin DF, Meredith TA, Topping TM, et al.: Perforating (through and through) injuries of the globe. Surgical results with vitrectomy. Arch Ophthalmol 1991;109:951–956.
10. Brinton GS, Aaberg TM, Reeser FH, et al.: Surgical results in ocular trauma involving the posterior segment. Am J Ophthalmol 1982;94:271–278.
11. Kuhn F, Morris R, Witherspoon CD, et al.: A standardized classification of ocular trauma. Ophthalmology 1996;103:240–243.
12. Williams DF, Mieler WF, Abrams GW, Lewis H: Results and prognostic factors in penetrating ocular injuries with retained intraocular foreign bodies. Ophthalmology 1988; 95:911-916.
13. Heier JS, Enzenauer RW, Wintermeyer SF, et al.: Ocular injuries and diseases at a combat hospital in support of operations Desert Shield and Desert Storm. Arch Ophthalmol 1993;111:795–798.
14. Topilow HW, Ackerman AL, Zimmerman RD: Limitations of computerized tomography in the localization of intraocular foreign bodies. Ophthalmology 1984;91:1086–1091.
15. Zinreich SJ, Miller NR, Aguyao JB, et al.: Computed tomographic three-dimensional localization and compositional evaluation of intraocular and intraorbital foreign bodies. Arch Ophthalmol 1986;104:1477–1482.
16. Lakits A, Prokesch R, Scholda C, et al.: Multiplanar imaging in the preoperative assessment of metallic intraocular foreign bodies. Helical computed tomography versus conventional computed tomography. Ophthalmology 1998;105:1679–1685.
17. McNichols MMJ, Brophy DP, Power WJ, Griffin JF: Ocular trauma: evaluation with ultrasound. Radiology 1995;195:423–427.
18. Deramo VA, Shah GK, Baumal CR, et al.: Ultrasound biomicroscopy as a tool for detecting and localizing occult foreign bodies after ocular trauma. Ophthalmology 1999;106:301–305.
19. Barash D, Goldenberg-Cohen N, Tzadok D, et al.: Ultrasound biomicroscopic detection of anterior ocular segment foreign body after trauma. Am J Ophthalmol 1998;126:197–202.
20. Lanzl IM, Hess U, Harms J: MRI for metallic foreign bodies? Ophthalmology 1999;106:1232–1234.
21. Fuller DG, Knighton RW, Machemer R: Bright flash electroretinography for evaluation of eyes with opaque vitreous. Am J Ophthalmol 1975;80:214–223.
22. Pieramici DJ, MacCumber MW, Humayum MU, et al.: Open globe injury update on type of injuries visual results. Ophthalmology 1996;103:1798–1803.
23. Benson F, Machemer R: Severe perforating injuries treated with pars plana vitrectomy. Am J Ophthalmol 1976;81:728–732.
24. Ryan SJ, Allen AW: Pars plana vitrectomy in ocular trauma. Am J Ophthalmol 1979;88:483–491.
25. Coleman DJ: Early vitrectomy in the management of the severely traumatized eye. Am J Ophthalmol 1982;92:543–551.
26. Faulborn J, Topping TM: Proliferations in the vitreous cavity after perforating injuries: a histopathological study. Graefes Arch Klin Exp Ophthalmol 1978;205:157–166.
27. Conway BP, Michels RG: Vitrectomy techniques in the management of selected penetrating ocular injuries. Ophthalmology 1978;85:560–583.
28. Meredith TA, Gordon PA: Pars plana vitrectomy for severe penetrating injury with posterior segment involvement. Am J Ophthalmol 1987;103:549–554.
29. de Juan E, Sternberg P, Michels RG: Timing of vitrectomy after penetrating ocular injury. Ophthalmology 1984;91:1072–1074.
30. Boldt HC, Pulido JS, Blodi CF, et al.: Rural endophthalmitis. Ophthalmology 1989;96:1722–1726.
31. Parish CM, O'Day DM: Traumatic endophthalmitis. Int Ophthalmol Clin 1987;27:112–119.
32. Brinton GS, Topping TM, Hyndiuk RA, et al.: Post traumatic endophthalmitis. Arch Ophthalmol 1984;102:547–550.
33. Neubauer H: Ocular metallosis. Trans Ophthalmol Soc UK 1979;99:502–510.
34. O'Duffy D, Salmon JF: Siderosis bulbi resulting from intralenticular foreign body. Am J Ophthalmol 1999;127:218–219.
35. Anderson WD: Prophylactic antibiotics and endophthalmitis in Vietnam. Am J Ophthalmol 1973;75:581–585.
36. Endophthalmitis Research Group: Microbiologic spectrum and susceptability of isolates: part II. Posttraumatic endophthalmitis. Am J Ophthalmol 1999;128:242–244.
37. Rubsamen PE, Cousins SW, Martinez JA: Impact of cultures on management decisions following surgical repair of penetrating ocular trauma. Ophthalmic Surg Lasers 1997;28:43–49.
38. Charles S: Vitreous microsurgery, 2nd Edition. Baltimore, Williams & Wilkins, 1987:190–191.
39. Moisseiev J, Belkin M, Bartov E, Treister G: Severe combat eye injuries in the Lebanon war. Isr J Med Sci 1984;20:339–344.
40. Rosner M, Bartov E, Treister G, Belkin M: Prophylactic scleral buckling in perforating ocular injuries involving the posterior segment. Ann Ophthalmol 1988;20:146–149.
41. Blumenthal M: Manual ECCE, the present state of the art. Klin Monatsbl Augenheilkd 1994;205:266–270.
42. Chaudhry NA, Belfort A, Flynn HW, et al.: Combined lensectomy, vitrectomy and scleral fixation of intraocular lens implant after closed-globe injury. Ophthalmic Surg Lasers 1999;30: 375–381.
43. Tyagi AK, Kheterpal S, Callear AB, et al.: Simultaneous posterior chamber intraocular lens implant combined with vitreoretinal surgery for intraocular foreign body injuries. Eye 1998;12:230–233.
44. Sjaarda RN, Glaser BM, Thompson JT, et al.: Distribution of iatrogenic retinal breaks in macular hole surgery. Ophthalmology 1995;102:1387–1392.
45. Kerrison JB, Haller JA, Elman M, Miller NM: Visual field loss following vitreous surgery. Arch Ophthalmol 1996;114:564–569.
46. Gregor Z, Ryan SJ: Complete and core vitrectomy in the treatment of experimental posterior penetrating eye injury in the rhesus monkey. I. Clinical features. Arch Ophthalmol 1983;101:441–445.
47. Gregor Z, Ryan SJ: Complete and core vitrectomy in the treatment of experimental posterior penetrating eye injury in the rhesus monkey. II. Histologic features. Arch Ophthalmol 1983;101: 446–450.
48. Sternberg P: Trauma: principles and techniques of treatment. In Ryan SJ (ed.), Retina, 2nd Edition, Vol III. St. Louis: CV Mosby, 1994:2351–2378.
49. Kelly NE, Wendel RT: Vitreous surgery for idiopathic macular holes: results of a pilot study. Arch Ophthalmol 1991;109:654–659.
50. Han PD, Abrams GW, Aaberg TM: Surgical excision of the attached posterior hyaloid. Arch Ophthalmol 1988;106:998–1000.
51. Desai UR, Peyman GA, Harper CA: Perfluorocarbon liquid in traumatic vitreous hemorrhage and retinal detachment. Ophthalmic Surg 1993;24:537–541.
52. Chang S, Lincoff H, Zimmerman NJ, Fuchs W: Giant retinal tears: surgical techniques and results using perfluorocarbon liquids. Arch Ophthalmol 1989;107:761–766.
53. Glaser BM, Carter JB, Kuppermann BD, Michels RG: Perfluorooctane in the treatment of giant retinal tears with proliferative retinopathy. Ophthalmology 1991;98:1613–1621.
54. Hirose T, Schepens CL, Lopansri C: Subtotal open sky vitrectomy for severe retinal detachment occurring as a late complication of ocular trauma. Ophthalmology 1981;88:1–9.
55. Azen SP, Scott IU, Flynn HW, et al.: Silicone oil in the repair of complex retinal detachments. A prospective observational multicenter study. Ophthalmology 1998;105:1587–1597.
56. Lewis H, Aaberg TM, Abrams GW, et al.: Management of the lens capsule during pars plana lensectomy. Am J Ophthalmol 1987; 103:109–110.
57. Moisseiev J, Bartov E, Cahane M, et al.: Cataract extraction in eyes filled with silicone oil. Arch Ophthalmol 1992;110:1649–1651.
58. Spiegel D, Nasemann J, Nawrocki J, Gabel VP: Severe ocular trauma managed with primary pars plana vitrectomy and silicone oil. Retina 1997;14:275–285.
59. Silicone Study Group: Vitrectomy with silicone oil or sulphor hexafluoride gas in eyes with severe proliferative vitreoretinopathy: results of a randomized clinical trial. Silicone Study Report 1. Arch Ophthalmol 1992;110:779–791.
60. Silicone Study Group: Vitrectomy with silicone oil or perfluoropropane gas in eyes with severe proliferative vitreoretinopathy: results of a randomized clinical trial. Silicone Study Report 2. Arch Ophthalmol 1992;110:792-805.

61. Crisp A, de Juan E, Tiedema J: Effect of silicone oil viscosity on emulsification. Arch Ophthalmol 1987;105:546–550.
62. Savion N, Alhalel A, Treister G, et al.: Role of blood components in ocular silicone oil emulsification. Invest Ophthalmol Vis Sci 1996;37:2694–2699.
63. Bartov E, Pennarola F, Savion N, et al.: A quantitative in vitro model for silicone oil emulsification. Role of blood constituents. Retina 1992;12(Suppl 3):S23–S27.
64. Soheilian M, Ahmedieh H, Sajjadi H, et al.: Temporary keratoprosthesis for surgical management of complicated combined anterior and posterior segment injuries to the eye: combat versus noncombat injury cases. Ophthalmic Surg 1994;25:452–457.
65. Johnston PB: Traumatic retinal detachment. Br J Ophthalmol 1991;75:18–21.
66. Cox MS: Retinal breaks caused by blunt nonperforating trauma at the point of impact. Trans Am Ophthalmol Soc 1980;78:414–466.
67. Avila MP, Jalkh AE, Murakami K, et al.: Biomicroscopic study of the vitreous in macular breaks. Ophthalmology 1983;90:1277–1283.
68. Menezo JL, Suarez-Reinolds R, Frances J, Villa E: Shape, number and localization of retinal tears in myopic over 8D, aphakic and traumatic cases of retinal detachment. Ophthalmologica 1977; 175:10–18.
69. Archer DB, Canavan YM: Contusional eye injuries: retinal and choroidal lesions. Aust J Ophthalmol 1983;11:251–264.
70. Tasman W: Peripheral retinal changes following blunt trauma. Trans Am Ophthalmol Soc 1972;70:190–198.
71. Freeman HM: Current management of giant retinal breaks and fellow eyes. In Ryan SJ (ed.), Retina, 2nd Edition, Vol III. St. Louis: CV Mosby, 1994:2313–2333.
72. Knave B: Electroretinography in eyes with retained intraocular foreign bodies—a clinical study. Acta Ophthalmol 1969;100 (suppl):1–63.
73. Lewis H, Aaberg TM: Causes of failure after repeat vitreoretinal surgery for recurrent proliferative vitreoretinopathy. Am J Ophthalmol 1991;111:15–19.
74. Zarbin MA, Michels RG, Green WR: Dissection of epiciliary tissue to treat chronic hypotony after surgery for retinal detachment with proliferative vitreoretinopathy. Retina 1991;11:208–213.

CHAPTER 66

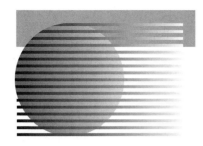

Management of Endophthalmitis Associated with Trauma

TRAVIS A. MEREDITH, M.D.

Posttraumatic endophthalmitis is perhaps the most significant complication after penetrating ocular trauma. Posttraumatic endophthalmitis occurs in 2.4% to 16.5% of traumatized eyes, depending on the series,[1–4] and approximately 25% of endophthalmitis cases are related to nonsurgical trauma.[2,5,6] Infection after trauma is very different from infection after planned intraocular surgery. Posttraumatic endophthalmitis occurs approximately 100 times more frequently than after planned surgery, and the infecting organisms are often more virulent. After treatment the outcome of therapy is often much worse for posttraumatic cases than after treatment for postoperative cases.

A broad spectrum of infecting pathogens is encountered in traumatic endophthalmitis (Table 66–1). Contaminated material introduced into the eye at the time of surgery is often the source of infection, and the patient's own periocular flora may also contribute in some cases. The type of trauma and the setting of the injury thus are important determinants in posttraumatic endophthalmitis (Table 66–2). Young men are most often the victims of intraocular infections, and most injuries occur at home or at work. In urban areas rates of infection are reported to be from 2% to 10%,[3,7] whereas injuries in rural settings may become infected in up to 30% of cases, perhaps because of more contact with soil contamination.[1] The specific organisms are different from postoperative cases although gram-positive organisms still predominate. *Bacillus* species and *Streptococcus* organisms are more common in posttraumatic endophthalmitis than postoperative endophthalmitis, and multiple organisms are frequently cultured from the infections.[8,9]

Intraocular foreign bodies (IOFB) are more likely to produce infection than other types of penetrating ocular trauma. The rate of infection has been reported to be between 6.9% and 13% of cases, and there is no difference in risk from different types of IOFB.[2,10,11] In a large national survey of IOFB, infection was four times greater when surgery was undertaken to remove the foreign body longer than 24 hours after injury as compared to removal within in the first 24 hours (3.5% vs. 13.4%).[10] When removal of the IOFB was delayed, older patients appeared to be at higher risk. Eyes suffering lacerations are at higher risk than those ruptured by blunt trauma, and disruption of the crystalline lens has been found to be associated with an increased incidence of endophthalmitis.[7]

The treatment results are often disappointing and the range of postoperative vision is worse than after postoperative cases. More eyes are lost entirely and enucleated after traumatic endophthalmitis. Prevention of infection is important, but there is no known definitive regimen or strategy that is universally successful in avoiding these infections.

TABLE 66–1. Organisms Causing Traumatic Endophthalmitis

Streptococcus epidermidis	21%
Bacillus species	20%
Multiple organisms	18%
Streptococcus species	10%
Gram-negative	10.5%
Fungi	8.5%
Staphylococcus aureus	7%
Other	5%

TABLE 66–2. Risk Factors for Traumatic Endophthalmitis

Rural setting
Intraocular foreign bodies
Delayed removal of intraocular foreign body
Rupture of crystalline lens

CLINICAL PRESENTATIONS AND DIAGNOSIS

Most patients present after suffering a penetrating injury which is repaired and then develops an infection within the first few days. Self-sealing corneal and scleral wounds are also at risk for infection. Inflammation and pain from the original injury may mask the signs and symptoms of infection, making early diagnosis difficult. Increasing inflammation, particularly the development of vitritis, causes concern about the possibility of infection. The appearance of a hypopyon makes it highly likely that the eye is infected. Scleral abscesses and local ulcerations of the cornea may be part of the presenting picture. *Bacillus* infections present in a particularly explosive pattern, with a dramatic increase in pain and inflammation within a 24-hour period. Fever, proptosis, leukocytosis, and a ring infiltrate of the cornea (ring abscess) may be features of these infections.[13–15]

In some cases endophthalmitis may be the presenting syndrome after occult trauma. A patient may have suffered what appeared to be a minor injury that in reality left an unsuspected IOFB or occult ocular penetration. Decreased vision and pain lead patients to consultation, at which time the infection and injury may be diagnosed.

Fungi produce an entirely different pattern, in which signs of infection may occur weeks to months after the initial injury. There may be gradually increasing inflammatory signs in the vitreous cavity and anterior chamber with a long, slow onset. Focal opacities of the vitreous ("fluff balls") and more diffuse vitreous inflammation may develop. In rare cases bacterial infections have been noted years after the initial trauma.[8]

Traumatic filtering blebs remain at risk for infection throughout the life of the patient.

MICROBIOLOGICAL CONSIDERATIONS

A single gram-positive agent was responsible for 62.5% of cases in a summary of several clinical studies in the pathogens causing postoperative endophthalmitis. *Staphylococcus epidermidis* (21%), *Bacillus* species (20%), and *Streptococcus* species (10%) were the major gram-positive pathogens (Table 67–1).[8] In a review of pediatric postoperative endophthalmitis, streptococci were responsible for 50%.[12] In the combined series gram-negative pathogens (10.5%), fungi (8.5%), and mixed infections with multiple organisms (8.5%) were responsible for the remaining cases. As compared to postoperative endophthalmitis, *Staphylococcus aureus* was relatively infrequently encountered in traumatic endophthalmitis (7%). Gram-positive coagulase-negative micrococci were responsible for 70% of the postoperative infections in the Endophthalmitis Vitrectomy Study (EVS); cases of fungal infection were excluded.[16,17]

The pathogen creating the infection plays a determinate role in the final visual acuity as demonstrated by EVS outcome data.[17] Final visual acuity of 20/100 or better was achieved at the following rates: gram-positive, coagulase-negative micrococci, 84%; gram-negative organisms, 56%; *S. aureus*, 50%; streptococci, 30%; enterococci, 14%. The organisms demonstrated associated with poor outcomes are much more common in posttraumatic cases than in acute postoperative cases.

Bacillus infections create the most devastating outcomes and are far more common in posttraumatic endophthalmitis than in postoperative cases. Intraocular foreign bodies are associated with most *Bacillus* infections,[1,2,15] and *Bacillus* species were the sole isolate in 36% of a large series of cases of endophthalmitis related to retained IOFB. In rural settings *Bacillus* species were identified in 46% of infections.[1] *Bacillus* species are spore-forming, gram-positive, aerobic bacilli. *Bacillus cereus* is the most common pathogen isolated from traumatic endophthalmitis, but there are at least 33 other species. *Bacillus* are common in farm environments where they are ubiquitous and may live in soil, dust, and water. Toxin production from *Bacillus* creates severe inflammation and tissue necrosis, and inoculation of toxins alone has been demonstrated to produce a marked tissue reaction.[14] *Bacillus* infections may produce severe clinical signs within 12 to 24 hours and may cause fever and leukocytosis as well. Although a small number of patient eyes have been salvaged after *Bacillus* infections, most of these unfortunate cases result in loss of the eye.[15]

After penetrating trauma, many types of fungi have been isolated in the eye. *Fusarium* was the most common isolate from the combined series,[8] but many other varieties of fungi have been reported. The average onset of symptoms of fungal endophthalmitis after trauma was 57 days in one report.[4]

TREATMENT

The selection of treatment strategy depends on the nature of the injury and on the clinical presentation of the infection. The rapidity of onset, severity of inflammation, setting of trauma, and ocular structures involved may lead the clinician to suspect more or less virulent organisms. The clinical problem of traumatic endophthalmitis differs so significantly from postoperative cases that the recommendations of the EVS do not apply to traumatic endophthalmitis.[18]

ACUTE POSTTRAUMATIC ENDOPHTHALMITIS

In the most common presentations there is either a rapid onset of infection after surgical intervention, or the patient may present with the infection already established. Most authorities recommend vitrectomy as the mainstay of initial management of these presentations.[2,4] Virulent pathogens are often found in these eyes. Actual killing of bacteria may be more difficult in some of these cases; vitrectomy and antibiotic injection have been demonstrated to be more effective in bacterial eradication than intraocular antibiotic injection alone.[19–21] Toxin release may also be a factor in virulence, and early removal of the vitreous and its bacterial load may reduce toxin damage in some cases.[14]

Surgery may also allow repair of intraocular damage produced by the injury itself. Vitreous blood may be removed, lens fragments or swollen lens may be extracted, and the view of the posterior segment may be improved so that retinal tears and detachment may be identified and treated. Foreign body removal may be combined with treatment of infection in some cases.

DELAYED INFECTION

Occasionally, presentation may be 10 days to 2 weeks after injury with a slow crescendo of presenting symptoms, possibly implying infection with less virulent organisms. In some cases the anterior chamber alone may be involved when there is an intact lens. Corneal infection is often part of this presentation. Cultures of the anterior chamber and treatment with topical, subconjunctival, and intravenous antibiotics may be appropriate because higher levels of aqueous antimicrobial may be achieved with intravenous administration than those levels achieved in the vitreous. A reasonable anterior chamber concentration of some antibiotics may be achieved with hourly topical antibiotics.[22–25] Specially prepared antibiotics may be made up with significantly higher concentrations of antimicrobial than the commercially available preparations.

Subconjunctival antibiotics may also provide significant antibiotic concentrations to the cornea and anterior chamber. The dosages recommended for intraocular concentration are calculated for the vitreous cavity and should not be injected directly into the anterior chamber because the smaller volume creates a much greater potential for corneal toxicity. If there appears to be spread of the infection into the vitreous cavity, intravitreal injections may also be considered.

In the evaluation stage, a thorough ocular examination should be carried out, although pain and periocular tissue swelling may limit the assessment of ocular structures. If there is no large laceration or gross distortion of the globe, ultrasound may be helpful in determining the extent of intraocular damage. For surgical planning, the presence of choroidal hemorrhage, retinal detachment, and displacement of the lens are important to determine. Occasionally a computed tomography (CT) scan is used to assess the degree of distortion of the globe, often in conjunction with assessment of periocular trauma. The CT scan is probably the "gold standard" for evaluation of the presence and location of intraocular foreign bodies.

In the preoperative period, povidone-iodine instillation in the conjunctival sac is appropriate only if there is no possibility that the antiseptic will gain access to the interior ocular structures. The same is true for administration of topical antibiotics. Undue pressure on the globe during preparation for surgery must be avoided, even if there has been a prior repair of the laceration. Lid sutures are sometimes better than a lid speculum if there is significant periocular swelling.

If there has been a previous surgical repair of a penetrating injury, the adequacy of closure must be assessed and additional corneal and scleral sutures added if necessary. It is desirable to place the infusion cannula 3.5 to 4 mm posterior to the limbus early in the operation when the eye is still firm. The inferior temporal quadrant is usually chosen if this area is not compromised by choroidal detachment, scleral wound, or elevated retinal detachment. The position of the cannula in the vitreous cavity must be verified prior to turning on the infusion to avoid infusion under the retina or into the uvea. On many occasions a separate infusion must be given through a more superior incision until the media can be cleared sufficiently to visualize the infusion cannula.

If there is apparent infected material withdrawn from the anterior chamber, it must be submitted for culture and gram stain. The initial vitreous is also removed without infusion of intraocular fluid so as to obtain the most concentrated specimen possible. Manual suction may be applied by a small syringe attached to the vitreous cutter by a short segment of tubing. In some cases the entire syringe is submitted for processing to the microbiology laboratory. The next stage is to carefully remove the central vitreous, taking care to evaluate for the presence of retinal detachment or choroidal detachment. Thorough removal of vitreous is desirable, but poor visibility often limits the amount of vitreous that can be safely removed. Often there is white material on the surface of the retina which cannot be differentiated from underlying tissue necrosis. For this reason, attempts to strip the vitreous away from the retina are usually ill-advised.

Once the media has been cleared, the retina should be examined carefully for breaks or detachment and treated when necessary with cryotherapy or laser photocoagulation. If there are breaks for which vitreous cannot be easily removed, support by a scleral buckle is advisable when possible. In some instances a prophylactic encircling band should be considered, as it is for penetrating trauma without concomitant infection.

If a gas bubble must be used in the eye, it compromises the ability to inject a full dose of intraocular antibiotic. Detachments from peripheral breaks may be treated externally to avoid an intraocular gas bubble, but if there are posterior breaks an internal drainage and fluid–gas exchange may be necessary. Favorable outcomes have been reported in recent years in repair of detachment in posttraumatic endophthalmitis.[27,28]

After adjustment of the buckle height, one anterior sclerotomy is closed and a suture for closure of the second sclerotomy is preplaced. Approximately 0.2 cc of fluid is withdrawn from the vitreous cavity and appropriate intraocular antibiotics are injected, closing the sclerotomy by drawing the suture tight around the needle as it is removed. Current choices for prophylaxis are vancomycin 1 mg, and ceftazidime 2.25 mg.

When an air bubble has been placed in the eye at the closure of surgery, an injection of the usual dose of antibiotic will reach concentrations in residual fluid higher than desired and may result in toxicity. Several strategies may be adopted for this problem. Prior to the fluid–gas exchange the standard concentration of antibiotic may be injected and a short period of time allowed for diffusion. The air–fluid exchange will then leave the correct concentration in the residual fluid. Another approach is to leave smaller bubbles (perhaps 50%) in the vitreous cavity and inject a proportionately smaller amount of antibiotic. Antibiotic may also be used in the infusion fluid during the procedure, thus assuring intraocular antibiotic concentrations during the procedure and leaving some antibiotic in the residual fluid at the end of the fluid–gas exchange.

After conjunctival closure, subconjunctival antibiotics are usually injected and the eye is dressed with antibiotic dilating drops, a sterile pad, and a Fox shield.

POSTOPERATIVE CARE

Frequent topical antibiotics in the postoperative period are probably unnecessary unless there is external infection because intraocular concentrations remain high for 24 to 48 hours after intraocular injection. Intravenous antibiotics should be considered for 5 to 10 days because vancomycin, ciprofloxacin, cefazolin, and ceftazidime will penetrate into the vitreous cavity.[29–34] Aminoglycosides do not have sufficient penetration to recommend them for intravenous administration. Systemic corticosteroids should be considered, and frequent topical corticosteroids are also beneficial in many cases. Intraocular corticosteroids have not been proven to be superior to systemic administration,[21,35] although they have been advocated by some authors.[36] Their half-life is short in inflamed eyes.[37] Topical cycloplegic drops are useful unless the iris has been lost to the trauma. The eye should be re-evaluated carefully for the first several days after surgery. Forty-eight hours after the procedure is a critical moment. Effective concentrations of intravitreal antibiotics are nearly at an end, but by this time culture results should be known. A judgment may be made about the clinical progress of the eye. If there is improvement, no further intervention may be necessary. An unfavorable clinical course suggests the possibility of continued infection. A repeat tap of the vitreous cavity for culture and a second round of injections may be considered. If an initial vitrectomy has not been performed, it should be considered at this juncture.

TREATMENT OF DELAYED-ONSET ENDOPHTHALMITIS

In most cases of delayed-onset endophthalmitis there is less inflammation and an indolent course, making it less necessary to undertake immediate therapy. When the rare case of sudden-onset endophthalmitis presents months to years after trauma, the management is similar to that outlined above. More often, a fungal etiology is suspected and a standard vitrectomy may be undertaken on a more elective basis. Because fungal infections are difficult to eradicate, as much vitreous as possible should be removed. Vitreous specimens may be sent for fungal stains during the procedure; a positive result will guide the choice of intravitreal antimicrobial injection. If the stain is positive for fungus, 5 μg of amphotericin is usually administered. If the stain is negative, the surgeon may inject an antimicrobial, antifungal agents, or wait for culture results before choosing an intraocular injection. Because of the slow growth of fungus on culture media, a report may be delayed for weeks, allowing the infection to go untreated.

Systemic antifungal agents are used postoperatively, but the precise choices have not been a subject of systematic study. Systemic amphotericin is sometimes used, but it may have highly significant side effects. Oral fluconazole and itraconazole have also been administered. Repeat injections of intraocular amphotericin are considered if the infection persists for several months. Unusual cases have been reported to be resistant to amphotericin B (e.g., *Paecilomyces lilacinous*)[38] and require intravitreal miconazole, 0.025 mg, and systemic fluconazole.[39]

OUTCOMES

Most series of posttraumatic endophthalmitis demonstrate that the majority of eyes have final vision of less than 20/400. A significant number are phthisical or enucleated. This contrasts sharply to the EVS, in which 53% of the eyes regained 20/50 vision or better and only 26% were 20/200 or less.[39] It is likely that these poor results of treatment reflect both the types of pathogens creating the infection and the severity of initial injuries. By contrast, in most series of posttraumatic infection most eyes have final vision of less than 20/400, and a significant number are enucleated or are phthisical.[8]

REFERENCES

1. Boldt HC, Pulido JS, Blodi CS, et al.: Rural endophthalmitis. Ophthalmology 1989;96:1722–6.
2. Brinton GS, Topping TM, Hyndiuk RA, et al.: Posttraumatic endophthalmitis. Arch Ophthalmol 1984;102:547–50.
3. Gilbert CM, Soong HK, Hirst LW: A two-year prospective study of penetrating ocular trauma at the Wilmer Ophthalmological Institute. Ann Ophthalmol 1987;19:104–6.
4. Affeldt JC, Flynn HW Jr, Forster RK, et al.: Microbial endophthalmitis resulting from ocular trauma. Ophthalmology 1987; 94:407–13.
5. Bohigian GM, Olk RJ: Factors associated with a poor visual result in endophthalmitis. Am J Ophthalmol 1986;101:332–41.
6. Puliafito CA, Baker AS, Haaf J, et al.: Infectious endophthalmitis: a review of 36 cases. Ophthalmology 1982;89:921–9.
7. Thompson WS, Rubsamen PE, Flynn HWJ, et al.: Endophthalmitis following penetrating trauma: risk factors and visual acuity outcomes. Ophthalmology 1995;102:1696–701.
8. Alfaro DV, Roth D, Liggett PE: Posttraumatic endophthalmitis: causative organisms, treatment, and prevention. Retina 1994; 14:206–11.
9. Parrish CM, O'Day DM. Traumatic endophthalmitis. Int Ophthalmol Clin 1987;27:112–9.
10. Thompson JT, Parver LM, Enger CL, et al.: Infectious endophthalmitis after penetrating injuries with retained intraocular foreign bodies. Ophthalmology 1993;100:1468–74.
11. Williams DF, Mieler WF, Abrams GW, et al.: Results and prognostic factors in penetrating ocular injuries with retained intraocular foreign bodies. Ophthalmology 1988;95:911–6.
12. Alfaro DV, Roth DB, Laughlin RM, et al.: Paediatric post-traumatic endophthalmitis. Br J Ophthalmol 1995;79:888–91.
13. Davey RT, Tauber WB: Posttraumatic endophthalmitis: the emerging role of *Bacillus cereus* infection. Rev Infect Dis 1987;9:110–23.
14. Beecher DJ, Pulido JS, Barney NP, et al.: Extracellular virulence factors in *Bacillus cereus* endophthalmitis: methods and implication of involvement of hemolysin BL. Infect Immun 1995;63: 632–9.
15. Foster RE, Martinez JA, Murray TG, et al.: Useful visual outcomes after treatment of *Bacillus cereus* endophthalmitis. Ophthalmology 1996;103:390–7.
16. Han DP, Wisniewski SR, Wilson LA, et al.: Spectrum and susceptibilities of microbiologic isolates in the endophthalmitis vitrectomy study. Am J Ophthalmol 1996;122:1–17.
17. Endophthalmitis Vitrectomy Study Group: Microbiologic factors and visual outcome in the endophthalmitis vitrectomy group. Am J Ophthalmol 1996;122:830–46.
18. Meredith TA: Post-traumatic endophthalmitis (editorial). Arch Ophthalmol 1999;117:520–1.
19. Cottingham AJ Jr, Forster RK: Vitrectomy in endophthalmitis: results of study using vitrectomy, intraocular antibiotics, or a combination of both. Arch Ophthalmol 1976;94:2078–81.
20. Aguilar HE, Meredith TA, Drews C, et al.: Comparative treatment of experimental *Staphylococcus aureus* endophthalmitis. Am J Ophthalmol 1996;121:310–7.
21. Meredith TA, Aguilar HE, Trabelsi A, et al.: Comparative treatment of experimental *Staphylococcus epidermidis* endophthalmitis. Arch Ophthalmol 1990;108:857–60.
22. Barza M: Antibacterial agents in the treatment of ocular infections. Infect Clin North Am 1989;3:533–51.
23. Barza M, Lynch E, Baum JL: Pharmacokinetics of newer cephalosporins after subconjunctival and intravitreal injection in rabbits. Arch Ophthalmol 1993;111:121–5.
24. Barza M, Kane A, Baum JL: Intraocular levels of cefamandole compared with cefazolin after subconjunctival injection in rabbits. Invest Ophthalmol Vis Sci 1979;18:250–5.
25. Barza M, Kane A, Baum J: Ocular penetration of subconjunctival oxacillin, methicillin, and cefazolin in rabbits with staphylococcal endophthalmitis. J Infect Dis 1982;145:899–903.
26. Yoshizumi MO, Leinwand MJ, Kim J: Topical and intravenous gentamicin in traumatically lacerated eyes. Graefes Arch Clin Exp Ophthalmol 1992;230:175–7.
27. Mieler WF, Glazer LC, Bennett SR, et al.: Favorable outcome of traumatic endophthalmitis with associated retinal breaks or detachment. Can J Ophthalmol 1992;27:348–52.
28. Foster RE, Rubsamen PE, Joondeph BC, et al.: Concurrent endophthalmitis and retinal detachment. Ophthalmology 1994; 101:490–8.
29. Alfaro DV, Liggett PE: Intravenous cefazolin in penetrating eye injuries. Effects of trauma and multiple doses on intraocular delivery. Graefes Arch Clin Exp Ophthalmol 1994;232:238–41.
30. Alfaro DV, Runyan T, Kirkman E, et al.: Intravenous cefazolin in penetrating eye injuries II. Treatment of experimental posttraumatic endophthalmitis. Retina 1993;13:331–4.
31. Nossov PC, Alfaro DV, Michaud ME, et al.: Intravenous cefazolin in penetrating eye injuries. Retina 1996;16:246–9.
32. Alfaro DV, Davis J, Kim S, et al.: Experimental *Bacillus cereus* posttraumatic endophthalmitis and treatment with ciprofloxacin. Br J Ophthalmol 1996;80:755–8.
33. Aguilar HE, Meredith TA, Shaarawy A, et al.: Vitreous cavity penetration of ceftazidime after intravenous administration. Retina 1995;15:154–9.
34. Meredith TA: Antimicrobial pharmacokinetics in endophthalmitis treatment; studies of ceftazidime. Trans Am Ophth Soc 1993;91:653–99.
35. Meredith TA, Aguilar HE, Sawant A, et al.: Intraocular dexamethasone produces a harmful effect on treatment of experimental Staphylococcus Aureus endophthalmitis. Tr Am Ophthalmol Soc 1996;94:241–52.
36. Schulman JA, Peyman GA: Intravitreal corticosteroids as an adjunct in the treatment of bacterial and fungal endophthalmitis. A review. Retina 1992;12:336–40.
37. Kwak HW, D'Amico DJ: Evaluation of the retinal toxicity and pharmacokinetics of dexamethasone after intravitreal injection. Arch Ophthalmol 1992;110:259–66.
38. Pflugfelder SC, Flynn HWJ, Zwickey TA, et al.: Exogenous fungal endophthalmitis. Ophthalmology. 1988;95:19–30.
39. O'Day DM, Head WS, Robinson RD, et al.: Intraocular penetration of systemically administered antifungal agents. Curr Eye Res 1985;4:131–4.
40. Endophthalmitis Vitrectomy Study Group: Results of the Endophthalmitis Vitrectomy Study: a randomized trial of immediate vitrectomy and of intravenous antibiotics for the treatment of postoperative bacterial endophthalmitis. Arch Ophthalmol 1995;113:1479–96.

Index

NOTE: Page numbers followed by f refer to illustrations; page numbers followed by t refer to tables.

D

E

H

I

J

K

L

M

N

O

T